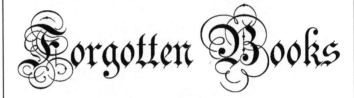
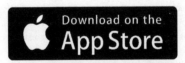
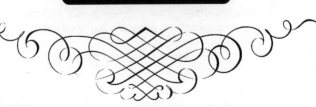

ISBN 978-0-282-95436-9
PIBN 10859003

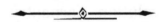

AN EPITOME

OF

BRAITHWAITE'S RETROSPECT

OF

PRACTICAL MEDICINE AND SURGERY;

CONTAINING

A CONDENSED SUMMARY OF THE MOST IMPORTANT CASES; THEIR TREATMENT, AND ALL
THE REMEDIES AND OTHER USEFUL MATTERS EMBRACED IN THE FORTY VOLUMES—THE
WHOLE BEING ALPHABETICALLY CLASSIFIED, AND SUPPLIED WITH AN ADDENDA,
COMPRISING A TABLE OF FRENCH WEIGHTS AND MEASURES, REDUCED TO ENGLISH
STANDARD—A LIST OF INCOMPATIBLES—EXPLANATION OF THE PRINCIPAL
ABBREVIATIONS OCCURRING IN PHARMACEUTICAL FORMULÆ—A VOCA-
BULARY OF LATIN WORDS MOST FREQUENTLY USED IN PRESCRIP-
TIONS, AND A COPIOUS INDEX.

BY WALTER S. WELLS, M.D.

VOL. II.

NEW YORK:
DICK & FITZGERALD, PUBLISHERS,
18 ANN STREET.

AN EPITOME

OF

BRAITHWAITE'S RETROSPECT.

HYSTERIA.

Essential Oil of Valerian a Remedy in Nervous and Hysterical Affections.—[Mr. Gore relates the case of a lady, and accompanies his remarks with the following practical observations:]

I viewed her case as one arising from a lesion of innervation of an adynamic character, out of which the other morbid phenomena arose—the diminution in the animal temperature, the absence of the pulse, and the general tremor, as the results of the circulation forsaking the periphery, for an impeded action in internal organs; and the result of the treatment entirely confirmed this view.

A jar of warm water was applied to her feet, warm flannel to the surface, and a teaspoonful of the following mixture in a wineglass of water every hour, until relief followed:

Mist. camphoræ; spt. ammon. aromat, aa. ʒij.; ol. ess. valer., gtt., xxv. M.

She got a little warm wine whey occasionally. A restless feeling of languor continuing, she got:

Some warm leaf tea, and at nine o'clock a pill containing the eighth of a grain of morphine, one drop of oil of valerian, with some extract of hyoscyamus.

She slept well, and when I called in the morning, I found her quite enlivened at the idea of being so much sooner well of this attack than of former ones, though she considered it more severe.

[Speaking of another case, he says:]

Soon after this time, I was called to the country to see a lady of wealth and importance, who labored under many distressing nervous symptoms—disturbed rest, irregular bowels, impaired digestion, headaches, a partial palsy of the left arm, with nervous twitchings in the left side of the face, colicky pains across the abdomen, with much inflation of the bowels. Throughout the continuance of her illness the catamenia continued undisturbed. She was of a spare habit of body, and every indication of plethora absent. The dyspeptic symptoms were those which first called for attention, out of which I conceived, the nervous disturbance arose; but long after her bowels became regular, the evacuations healthy, and the appetite good, *her nervous symptoms remaining unaltered.* she was subjected to the influence of electricity, and of the following mixture she took a small teaspoonful in half a tumbler of porter twice a day:

Rhubarb root, sliced, ʒiij.; chirayeta, ʒij.; coriander seeds, bruised, ʒiiss.; Bradishes' alkaline solution, ʒviij.

This was allowed to stand for ten days, and on being filtered, sixteen drops of oil of valerian were added, which made a very good antacid, anti-spasmodic, tonic, aperient mixture, and from the use of which she derived much signal benefit.

[It will be observed that in this case Mr. Gore used the *chirayeta*, and as this remedy is not generally known, we would just remind the profession that in many cases of indigestion, and especially when accompanied with an unpleasant giddiness after eating, this will be found a valuable remedy. The following is a good way of preparing and taking the infusion of chirayeta: Add half an ounce of chirayeta to one pint of boiling water; let it stand closely covered for twelve hours, and then strain it through a fine sieve, and pour it into a wine bottle in which has been put half an ounce of the subcarbonate of soda; this to be well shaken together. A wineglassful of the infusion to be taken three times a day, one hour before each meal. A larger quantity of the above, not to be made at once, as it does not keep good for many days. Mr. Gore ends his observations as follows:]

In the abdominal pains, and in that pain of the side peculiar to many young females, a combination of aloes, assafœtida, and oil of valerian, proves exceedingly advantageous.

I had one case of chorea, which, after a little attention to the bowels, derived inestimable benefit from a single drop of the oil, in a lump of sugar, three times a day. After about three weeks this young woman was quite restored. It occurs to me that this would be a very suitable remedy to drop into a carious tooth accompanied with pain, where inflammation of the fang was absent, but having no opportunities to test this since the idea occurred to me, I can only give it as a suggestion.

Part ii., *p.* 54.

Efficacy of Opium Injections in Cases of Nervous Excitement.—It seems that both tobacco and opium, when administered in the form of an injection, take even a more powerful effect than when taken into the stomach. Dupuytren explains this fact with respect to opium, by supposing that in the stomach its effects become modified by the process of digestion, whereas, when administered by the rectum it becomes absorbed, unaltered, into the system. This is well illustrated in a case of nervous excitement, published by Dr. Maddock, in which the opium injection was used with remarkably good effects; and no doubt, in many cases of nervous excitement, produced either by disease or by operations, this remedy would be found valuable.

Part iv., *p.* 44.

Tobacco in Hysteria.—In a case of hysteria, related by Dr. J. H. Thomson, where all the usual remedies seemed comparatively useless, tobacco leaves, soaked a few moments in hot water, and then spread over the epigastric region of the patient, succeeded in arresting three consecutive attacks.

Part vi., *p.* 82.

Ioduret of Silver—Suggested in various painful hysterical affections, in doses of from one-eighth of a grain to one or two grains, two or three times a day, in the form of a pill. *Part* vii., *p.* 82.

Ergot of Rye.—Mr. Nardo has found the internal administration of ergot of rye, followed by the rapid removal of the disease, depending on atony of the nervous and genital systems.

His practice consisted in administering about a scruple of the ergot, with sugar, in divided doses, each day, intermitting the dose every third or fourth day. *Part* vii., *p.* 90.

Local Hysteria.—Dr. R. B. Todd, after alluding to the power of the mind to create pain, or to perpetuate it after it had been excited by some physical cause, observes: I do not profess to give an account of *all* the forms that local hysteria may assume, so many and so various are they. I shall, however, briefly refer to the principal varieties that are likely to be met with in practice.

Pain in the Side.—Among the most common forms of local hysteria are those pains in the right or left side; of these I believe the most frequent is that on the left side; the pain is referred to a spot immediately beneath the left mamma, corresponding very nearly to the situation of the apex of the heart. In most cases the pain is increased on pressure; sometimes, however, firm and steady pressure gives ease, and I have sometimes observed patients to make pressure themselves, in order to obtain some relief. It is quite extraordinary what a common symptom this pain is, or that on the right side. It is very frequently (that on the left side especially) accompanied with leucorrhœa or some form of uterine derangement, so much so, that now, after I have learned that a young woman of hysterical appearance complains of this pain, my next question invariably refers to the existence of leucorrhœa. In some instances this pain is always increased on inspiration, and is attended with a short but frequent cough, without expectoration. If there be any emaciation, or if there has been phthisis in the family, the fears of the patient's friends become excited, lest this cough and pain should be the forerunners of consumption. And it is not always easy to assure oneself that the irritation of nascent tubercles may not have some share in the production of the phenomena.

Irritable Spine.—The irritable spine is another form of local hysteria, which, if treated on erroneous principles, or if its real nature be not detected, may lead to very serious consequences. This affection has been deemed of sufficient importance by some practitioners, to merit its being designated by the special name of *spinal irritation.* But this term is highly objectionable. Many who have written upon this subject have striven, on very insufficient evidence, to show that the spinal cord itself is at fault. The truth, however, is that the spinal irritation is but a symptom of a general state, a local malady, depending on a constitutional cause. These cases are often mistaken for actual disease of the vertebræ, and patients have been confined to the recumbent posture for its cure, a mode of treatment admirably calculated to perpetuate the real complaint. It often happens that the patient has difficulty in walking, and this is regarded as the consequence of the spinal affection. She at first finds herself easily fatigued; the pain in her back is increased by walking or standing; she gradually becomes disinclined to move, and gets accustomed to the horizontal position, and, therefore, readily yields to any suggestions in favor of quiet, or reluctantly obeys the advice which recommends an opposite plan. The most acute pain is felt over a particular spot on the back. Slight pressure will produce it, when the patient's attention is alive to it; and firm pressure will often fail to create it when her attention has been diverted from it. But there is always a good deal of tenderness in the whole course of the spine and in other parts also. You will derive great assistance in your attempts to distinguish the real nature of this affection, by attending to the nature of the pain; it is always of that *exaggerated* kind which is characteristic of hysterical pain. It is much more acute than the pain which attends diseased vertebræ; it is more superficial, so as often to appear, as I believe it is, seated in the skin that covers the spinous processes.

Local Pulsation.—We had lately a case in which this form of local hysteria was very well marked; and it was accompanied with another symptom not uncommon in hysterical persons. This was a strong pulsation of the aorta in the epigastric region, simulating aneurism. For some time the pulsation appeared so strong, and was so circumscribed, that had I not known the decidedly hysterical character of the patient's constitution, I should have felt considerable apprehension on her account. However, as her strength improved, and her catamenia became regular, these symptoms disappeared.

Hysterical Affection of Joints.—The profession is much indebted to Sir Benjamin Brodie for having directed attention to the frequency with which local hysteria manifests itself, especially among the higher classes, in the form of affections of the large joints, simulating those diseases with so much accuracy that practitioners have frequently been misled by it. Sir Benjamin states the remarkable fact, which no one is so well able to ascertain as a surgeon of his great experience, that four-fifths of the supposed cases of joint-disease which occur among the higher classes are hysterical. This statement ought to impress us strongly with the importance of being well acquainted with the peculiar features of these hysterical affections of the joints.

You will, of course, expect to find in these cases indications of the hysterical constitution; globus; perhaps, occasional hysterical paroxysms; general irritability; enfeebled nutrition; pain easily excited on pressure at various parts of the body; irregular catamenia, or some uterine disturbance. The joints which are most frequently affected are the hip and knee. The patient keeps the painful joint quite at rest, being fearful of the least disturbance. When the joint is moved, she will call out with much more expression of pain than if there were actual ulceration of the cartilages. "There is always exceeding tenderness," Sir Benjamin Brodie remarks, "connected with which, however, we may observe the remarkable circumstance, that gently touching or pinching the integuments in such a way as that the pressure cannot affect the deep-seated parts, will often be productive of much more pain than the handling of the limb in a more rude and careless way." As, however, in most hysterical affections, if you can succeed in engaging your patient's attention about some other object, and thus directing her thoughts from her own sufferings, you will find that the joint can be moved with comparatively little or with no pain.

Irritable Breast.—Another very serious form of painful hysterical affection is the irritable breast. It is not generally attended with swelling or enlargement. The irritability is excessive, and the patient shrinks quite as much from superficial as from deep-seated pressure, and even before she has been actually touched at all. These characters, along with the evidence of hysterical constitution, are sufficient to enable the attentive practitioner to distinguish the real nature of the affection.

Paralysis of the Bladder.—Hysterical paralysis of the bladder is also common, and much mischief may arise from neglect of constitutional treatment, and too close attention to the local affection. Sir Benjamin Brodie lays down the rule, that in these cases the catheter should not be had recourse to; and the only exceptions to it are in those extreme cases in which actual paralysis has taken place, and the bladder is likely to become diseased, if not artificially relieved. A similar want of power over the rectum may occur in hysterical women. I have known women complain that they were unable to expel the contents of the rectum, although they were conscious of fæces having passed into it. With respect to many of these cases of hysterical paralysis, there is much truth in Sir B. Brodie's remark, "that it is not that the muscles are incapable of obeying the act of volition, but that the function of volition is suspended."

Spasmodic Affections.—Among the various forms of local hysteria, we may class some singular spasmodic affections, which often prove exceedingly troublesome; for example:

Laryngeal Affection.—In the woman Collier, whose case I have had occasion to refer to as an instance of paraplegia, we had an example of a spasmodic affection of the muscles of the larynx, very much resembling the spasmodic croup, or laryngismus stridulus, which occurs in children. This attack was always preceded by depression of spirits and hysterical crying; the breathing became difficult, and both inspiration and expiration were attended with a stridulous noise; there was also a loud barking cough, which could be heard at a considerable distance. The attack passed off as the temporary excitement disappeared.

Hysterical Sobbing.—One of the most singular cases I ever saw was that of a girl named Howe, aged 19, who was admitted in consequence of a peculiar spasmodic affection of the diaphragm, of a most severe kind, and which, while it lasted, was most troublesome and painful.

At her admission, she stated that for the last three months she had been very subject to leucorrhœa. In other respects, she was in good health. Her face has the aspect of hysteria; the full upper lip is very well marked. Four days before her admission, in taking down a bedstead, she fell and struck the right side of her abdomen. In half an hour she was seized with a catching of her breath, and with pain in the right side of the abdomen. This continued for two or three hours, so as to interrupt her work, and then went off. Her bowels were open at the time, but she is of costive habit. In the evening, the catching of her breath and the pain returned; it now continued some time, so that she scarcely lay down during the night. Next morning there was great epigastric tenderness, and she was unable to bear the pressure of her stays.

At our first visit, we found her affected with this catching of the breath, It exactly resembled a violent fit of sobbing, unattended with flow of tears. There is a jerking movement of the neck from side to side with each sob, but the limbs are motionless. Any excitement increases the sobbing. It was much increased by our visit, and subsided after we left. The upper extremities are now thrown into jerking movements, resembling those of chorea, shortly after the sobbing begins.

Her treatment consisted in free purging for the first few days, lest there should be any lodgment in the intestinal canal, and subsequently tonics. Her attacks ceased, and as she remained quite free up to the 5th of April, and her health was much improved, she was discharged. She was, however, readmitted on the 10th, with a recurrence of the paroxysms, without any apparent cause. They are accompanied with jerking movements of the upper limbs and tremblings of the lower ones, which give her an unsteady gait in walking. Pressure excites or increases the sobbing, particularly when applied on the right side; and if the pressure be continued, the sobbing becomes excessively violent, and the whole body is thrown into convulsive movements.

She had followed a tonic treatment for a considerable time without any benefit to these paroxysms. I determined now to try a succession of blisters to the epigastrium. The first excited a very severe paroxysm; however, by perseverance in the use of them, she has not only become able to bear them, but the paroxysms have considerably diminished in frequency and severity, so that now she can bear a good deal of pressure without inducing the sobbing.

Sir B. Brodie has recorded a case very similar to this.

Hysterical Sneezing.—Women are sometimes attacked with violent fits of sneezing, coming on at particular periods and lasting for a considerable time. Of my own knowledge, I am aware of but one instance of this, in a newly married lady, in whom the fits of sneezing used to come on early in the morning. There was, I had reason to believe in this case, great disappointment that the signs of pregnancy did not appear about the usual time; and it was curious that these attacks should have come on chiefly when the morning sickness would have shown itself in the early stage of pregnancy.   *Part* viii., *p.* 59.

Treatment.—The following formula is very highly lauded by Dr. Debreyne:

R P. camphoræ, ℥ss.; P. assafœtida, ℥ss.; extr. belladonnæ, Ʒiv.; extr. aquos. opii, Ʒj.

Mix and divide into 120 pills; commence with two at first *per diem*, and gradually increase the dose to six in the 24 hours; they should always be taken before food. Occasionally a wineglassful of the infusion of valerian or orange leaves may be given with much advantage along with each dose of the pills.

Dr. D. is in the habit of administering them also for the cure of general or partial nervous trembling, and of *chorea*. Sometimes he exhibits, in the latter disease, the belladonna by itself; and, he says, very generally with success. When it fails, he has recourse to cold bathing.

Part x., *p.* 25.

Hysteria treated by the application of Cold to the Region of the Uterus.—M. Butignot mentions the case of a young woman, eighteen years of age, attacked for the first time with hysteria, which lasted seven days. She was quite blind during this period, but remained perfectly sensible. There was permanent contraction of the muscles of the trunk and extremities, with occasional convulsive movements. She could only swallow a few drops of liquid at a time, and speak a few words in a low voice. Treatment was of no avail, soothing and antispasmodic remedies did no good, but M. B. remarked on the fifth day that the paroxysm became aggravated about noon; he immediately gave quinine, under which treatment the symptoms gradually subsided. The following year she was again attacked as before, and from pain in the hypogastric region, with suppressed catamenia, he was led to infer the existence of over-excitement in the uterus. He ceased all treatment, and applied cold compresses to the lower part of the abdomen and upper part of the thighs. In half an hour the patient was relieved, and had no return of her symptoms.

Part xiii., *p.* 68.

Hysteria.—M. Gendrin gives opium, in large doses, commencing with gr. v. daily, and increasing to gr. x. or gr. xij.: 'The appearance of an hypnotic effect is a sign that the disease, and the tolerance of opium induced by it, are on the decline, and the dose must then be lessened.

Part xv., *p.* 72.

Treatment of Hysteria.—Occurring in a patient of *plethoric habit*, and accompanied by *cerebral symptoms:* leech the head, or cup between the shoulders; if this is ineffectual, give two grains of digitalis twice a day, and put a blister on the nape; for the convulsions of the voluntary muscles, give half a grain of extract of belladonna, every eight or twelve hours.

Produced by Accumulation in the Colon.—Clear out the bowels by the repeated exhibition of pills composed of extract of jalap, compound extract of colocynth, and compound rhubarb pill.

Combined with Pyrosis.—Give trisnitrate of bismuth, with a bitter infusion.

From Anæmia.—Give chalybeates.

Hysterical spasms may be subdued by the inhalation of ether vapor, or chloroform.

Part xvi., *p.* 90.

Observations on Hysteria.—Referring to cases in which females have become outrageously excited, Mr. Corfe says:

Now, all attempts to pacify such persons by ordinary means, as by argument, by medicine, or by reasoning, are fruitless; they are like eels for wriggling, and like bulls for fierceness and strength; our only alternative is to fix them on the stretcher, and strap them there, mount a chair placed on each side of the head, and keep up a constant stream of cold water on the face; and the more they scream the more cold water they are obliged to gulp down their throat, until the globus is conquered, the head cooled, the passions subdued, and, when they really find that we give them more in proportion to the screaming, they become calm and sue for pity.

Part xvii., *p.* 58.

Belladonna in Hysteria.—Marked benefit is derived from belladonna, given as follows: Take of camphor, 12 grammes (about ʒiij. and gr. v.); assafœtida, 12 grammes; extract of belladonna, 4 grammes (about ʒj.); aqueous extract of opium, 1 gramme (about gr. xvss.); sirup of gum, enough to make 120 pills. Give one pill the first day, two on the second, and gradually increase the dose to six pills daily. *Part* xxi., *p.* 77.

Treatment of Cerebral Hysteria.—Employ as a prophylactic and curative agent in this affection, the persevering and systematic application of electro-galvanism to the abdominal and pelvic regions, in combination with other means. Amongst the adjuvants that should be administered concurrently with its use, Dr. Laycock mentions tar in small doses, the introduction of which we owe to Professor Simpson, and which is in itself an excellent remedy for habitual constipation, without the aid of electro-galvanism.   *Part* xxii., *p.* 82.

Colchicum in Hysteria and Chorea.—Thirty drops of the tincture of colchicum, taken every eight hours, was followed by complete relief. In *chorea*, also, the same remedy has proved valuable.   *Part* xxv., *p.* 300.

Hysteric Hemiplegia.—This may be known from hemiplegia depending on disease of the thalamus opticus and corpus striatum by its occurring generally in young subjects, by the muscles of the face not being affected, and by loss of sensation preponderating over loss of motion. The best treatment is steel and valerian. (Prof. Gull.)   *Part* xxxiv., *p.* 28

—•♦•—

INDIAN HEMP.

Indian Hemp.—There are few medicines which have excited more interest than Indian Hemp, and few medicines of known medicinal powers have so often and so signally failed to fulfill the hopes respecting it. The reason of this seems to be that the preparations which have been used by different experimenters have not been alike. One man has used the simple tincture of the *seed*, another the tincture of the *resin*, and another the resin itself. Again, one preparation may be very useful in India, but the same, when brought to this country, may be so deteriorated as to be useless. Dr. O'Shaughnessy may have found the resin of the plant powerful in India, while it is necessary, when used in this country, to make a tincture of the resin, prepared in India from hemp, collected at the proper season. Mr. Donovan, from numerous experiments on his own person, and on others, especially recommends the *tincture of the resin* as superior to all the other preparations of this drug. The resin itself seems to be totally insoluble in watery liquids, and it should therefore be made into a tincture. The pilular form will often pass undissolved through the alimentary canal. This is corroborated by the fact that Mr. R. O'Shaughnessy found that one drachm of the tincture, which contains three grains of the resin, had a much more powerful effect than five grains of the latter. Mr. Donovan prepares his tincture of the resin by mixing two grains of the resin with one drachm of rectified spirit; and of this he gives at first from eight to fifteen minims in a very small quantity of proof-spirit. If the draught be mixed with water, the resin will be rapidly precipitated and adhere to the vessel, and will thus escape being swallowed.
                                                Part xi., *p.* 16.

Indian Hemp as an Oxytocic.—This seems to be a valuable oxytocic remedy. Several cases are given by Dr. Christison illustrative of its powerful effects. The extract may be given in the form of pill, but in this form the hemp is rather uncertain. Another form recommended is the emulsion, made by rubbing a scruple of the extract in a warm mortar in a drachm of olive oil, to which may be added half an ounce of mucilage, and seven and a half ounces of distilled water. The tincture is perhaps the best form, of the strength of three grains of the extract to a drachm of rectified spirit. The dose of the extract is from one to six grains, of the tincture ten to thirty drops. To promote uterine contraction, less than thirty drops is of little service. In tetanus one or two drachms must be given. *Part* xxiv., *p.* 320.

INFANTS.

Nursery Treatment of.—No other kind of milk to be given to an infant in addition to the milk of the mother or wet-nurse. The less rocking the better. When asleep, to be laid upon its *right* side. The best food is "Lemann's biscuit-powder," soaked for twelve hours in cold spring water, then *boiled* for half an hour, not simmered, or it will turn sour. Very little sugar to be added to the food, and then only at the time *when given*.

Sweets, of every kind, are most injurious, producing acidity, flatulency, and indigestion, sores in the mouth, and disordered secretions. An infant will take medicine the more readily if made lukewarm in a cup placed in hot water, adding a very little sugar *when given*. The warm bath (at ninety-four degrees of heat, *not less*, for *ten* minutes, every other night) is a valuable remedy in many cases of habitual sickness or constipation.

"Soothing-sirup," sedatives, and anodynes, of every kind, are most prejudicial. They stop the secretions. A very small dose of laudanum given to an infant may produce coma and death. When an infant is weaned, which is generally advisable at the age of nine months, it is of the utmost importance that it be fed with the milk of *one cow*, and *one only* (a milch cow), mixed with "Lemann's biscuit-powder" (prepared as before directed), and *very little sugar.*

Solid meat is not generally required until an infant is fifteen months of age, and then to be given sparingly, and cut very fine. Roasted mutton, or broiled mutton-chop (without fat), is the best meat; next to that, tender *lean* beef or lamb; then fowl, which is better than chicken; no pork or veal; no pastry; no cheese; *the less butter the better.* An infant should not be put upon its feet soon, especially while *teething*, or *indisposed*. *Avoid over-feeding* at all times, more particularly during *teething*. It is very likely to produce indigestion and disordered secretions, the usual *primary causes* of convulsions, various eruptive complaints, and inflammatory affections of the head, throat, and chest. *Part* vii., *p.* 90.

Hint on the Feeding of Children.—Nurses in general, who have the charge of young infants brought up by the hand, have an invincible objection to thin food, as the object is to make the child look as fat and hearty as possible, and we have to struggle against this prejudice sometimes in cases even of imminent danger.

In most of these cases we find the alvine dejections to consist of a thick, pasty mass, without a proper admixture of bile, constipation being a fre-. quent accompaniment; and it is not till the secretions become less consistent, and of a better color, that we observe decided signs of amelioration as to the spasmodic attacks. The generality of authors who have written on this subject allude to this state of bowels. Dr. Underwood mentions, that he has known some of the largest and finest infants he had ever seen, die suddenly *within the month*, immediately after the nurse had boasted of their having taken "three boatfuls of victuals." There are numerous cases, also, of general convulsions occurring soon after being fed with thick food. In a family in which twelve children were successively subject to this disease, they were all fed by hand, principally owing to the mother having sore nipples. *Part* xvi., *p.* 293.

Diet of Infants.—We have had a considerable experience in directing and observing minutely the rearing of infants upon a substitute for mother's milk. We never allow a healthy infant, for the first two months, to have any other food as a substitute for its mother's milk than cow's milk diluted with two-thirds of water, and well sweetened with fine sugar. Of this fare we sanction *an unlimited supply*, at intervals of from one and a half to two hours during the day, and three or four hours at night, provided it be sucked from a teat. Upon this simple fare, we have seen children grow up in the plenitude of health and strength. If the food be as thin as we have described, no evil can arise from over-feeding; and by allowing an interval to elapse between the times of feeding, digestion goes on better, and fretfulness is averted. To weak or scrofulous infants, the addition of a little mutton suet is good, or the same benefit may be obtained by giving two teaspoonfuls of cod-liver oil daily. Oatmeal, and all farinaceous foods, are unsuitable and unnatural for the first two months, and are certain to induce fits of feverishness and griping pains. After the second month, rusk, melted down in the sweetened milk and water, is useful; but the food must still be thin, and sucked from a teat by the infant. The exertion of sucking is, for many reasons, very salutary.
Part xxviii., *p.* 291.

Prolonged Retention of Life by Infants who have not Breathed.— The long period during which life may, under certain circumstances, be retained by the infant who has never breathed, is a fact full of interest to the physiologist, the medical jurist, and the accoucheur. The experiments of Legallois show that, in the mammalia, the fœtus which has not breathed can resist death from submersion much longer than the fœtus in which respiration has been carried on. Puppies and kittens, immediately after birth, may be kept under water for twenty-eight minutes with impunity; when five days old, they perish after sixteen minutes' submersion; and, when fifteen days old, they die as rapidly as other warm-blooded animals of any age, from deprivation of air. The human still-born fœtus can probably live longer without respiration than any other mammalian fœtus. The following cases are collected in the "Gazette Hebdomadaire" for December 1st, 1824, from different sources. They are very striking, and very suggestive to the practical accoucheur.

A woman aged 25, who had tried to conceal her pregnancy, was delivered when seated on a tub. The infant, born without any signs of life, was buried in a sand-pit, and, after remaining there for half an hour, was removed, and lived. This case is described by Dr. Weese in 1845, in "Badisch. Ann. f. Staatsarz," x. 2.

In 1850, a young woman was tried by the tribunals of Berlin, who had buried her new-born male infant, believing it to be dead. After an hour, the infant was disinterred, and recalled to life.

T. P., a servant, aged 23, was delivered in a stable, when leaning against the wall, alone, and in a state of unconsciousness, about half-past four, A. M. When she came to herself, she found the infant on the ground, having a spade lying upon it, with its cutting edge turned to the body. She took the infant, which was perfectly cold, believing it to be dead, and, with the placenta attached, wrapped it up in her apron, and buried it in the garden. Suspicions arose that she had been confined: she confessed; and at half past nine the infant was dug up from a depth of thirty *centimètres*. It was found lying on its face, with the placenta under the abdomen. Though cold, apparently dead, and pulseless, the cord was tied. For two hours, P., a surgeon, used means to reanimate it, when at last it began to breathe feebly, gradual signs of life became more evident, and it cried. Some slight wounds were observed on its body: wounds in the neck, which did not bleed at first, bled when the infant was restored. It took the breast greedily. On the 17th and 18th, the wounds suppurated; and on the 19th, it died of convulsions. The physicians intrusted with the judicial autopsy, reported that it had been inhumed before it breathed; and that it had not breathed till after it was exhumed; and that the statement of the mother was possibly true. She was therefore acquitted of the charge of infanticide, but was found guilty of concealment of pregnancy. *Part* xxxi., *p.* 213.

Defective Assimilation in Infants.—This disease, which is the most frequent and fatal of all infantile disorders, is almost always the result of want of breast-milk, and the use of injudicious food. Fatty acids, and already artificially digested animal and occasionally vegetable substances, and especially breast-milk, must be supplied. It is a very good plan to mix human and cow's milk. Simple juice of meat is very useful. The remedies of use are phosphate of soda, producing an emulsion with fats, thus allowing of their assimilation; chloride of potassium to dissolve carbonate of lime; phosphate of lime, to enable the blood to take up more carbonic acid, and thus hold in solution more carbonate of lime (these substances severally strengthening muscular and bony tissue). Nitrate of silver and sulphate of copper are the best remedies for the diarrhœa. Wine is also required even in large quantities. Dr. Routh. *Part* xl., *p.* 57.

INFLAMMATION.

Hints on the Treatment of Inflammation.—Dr. Watson enters into the treatment of inflammation, and places his chief reliance on blood-letting, copiously used at the commencement of the disease. Respecting venesection from the external jugular vein, he says:

There is a distinct and peculiar danger attending the incision of this vein, that, namely, of admitting *air* into it. You perhaps are aware that if air enters a large vein near the heart, and passes on to that organ, it kills outright.

[When on the subject of mercury in the treatment of inflammatory diseases, he offers the following valuable hints:]

Patients who are kept under the influence of mercury grow pale as well as thin: and Dr. Farre, who has paid great attention to the effects of this drug, remedial and injurious, holds that it rapidly destroys red blood: as effectually as it may be destroyed by venesection.

But the great *remedial* property of mercury is that of stopping, controlling, or altogether preventing the effusion of coagulable lymph ; of *bridling adhesive inflammation.*

In common adhesive inflammation, whether of serous or the cellular tissues ; whenever, in fact, you have reason to suppose that coagulable lymph is effused, or about to be effused, and mischief is likely to result from its presence, then you may expect much benefit from the proper administration of mercury ; as an auxiliary, however, to blood-letting, not as a substitute for it.

[Speaking of antimony, Dr. Watson says:]

Antimony, as far as my own observation goes, is admirably suited to cases of active inflammation, in which mercury would either be not so useful, or could not be brought to bear. It is in inflammation of the mucous membrane of the air passages that antimony is so signally beneficial.

On the other hand, antimony does not appear to be nearly so valuable a remedy as mercury, when serous membranes are inflamed.

As to the form in which the antimony should be exhibited, I apprehend that we shall all come at last to freshly dissolved tartar emetic.

Part iii., *p.* 32.

Blood-letting in Inflammation.—In commenting on the practice of bleeding in the erect posture in inflammation, and then giving a large dose of opium to prevent reaction, Dr. Craigie believes it will often be found to give rise to a great fallacy ; the faintness thus produced being often merely mental, and always too temporary and too trifling to facilitate the removal of the congested blood from the vessels of an important organ or membrane in a state of intense inflammation ; except, perhaps, when the disease is in the head, eyes, or upper parts of the body, in which case, the erect position must certainly be the most proper, and during venesection, must cause the greatest drain of blood from the parts. *Part* iii., *p.* 39.

Use of Poultices in Inflammations of the Great Cavities.—Nothing is more remarkable in the practice of physic in France, than the constant use of cataplasms in the treatment of inflammations of the great cavities. The moment inflammation is supposed to exist in the chest or abdomen, the first order given is to apply cataplasms.

In the bronchial irritation attendant upon the exanthematous fevers, poultices to the chest are universally employed ; and where any want of energy appears to exist in the system, preventing the coming out of eruption, cataplasms, consisting of the usual linseed meal, with the addition of a very small quantity, say a twelfth or fifteenth part of mustard meal (not flour), are applied to the feet, and maintained for days together ; thus keeping up both the temperature of the extremities, and gently stimulating the skin. The same mixture is also, when necessary, applied to the calves of the legs and thighs.

Pleurodynia, diaphragmitis, and many other affections of a painful nature, are likewise treated by poultices ; and it is certain, that their effects are often, in such cases, very satisfactory. *Part* iii., *p.* 42.

Opium in Acute Internal Inflammations.—Recommended by Dr. R. Christison, particularly in inflammations of the mucous membranes.

Part iii., *p.* 45.

Hemostasis.—A substitute for blood-letting in cases of inflammation. *Vide* Art. " Congestive Fever."

Nitrate of Potash.—In large doses, suggested in inflammatory affections.
Part ix., *p.* 19.

Treatment of Chronic Inflammation.—[Chronic inflammation generally indicates a scrofulous diathesis, and we must direct our treatment to the constitution, and employ alteratives if any medicines are used; but improved diet, change of air, and removal to the sea-side, will often be sufficient. Mr. Cooper observes:]

In chronic inflammation of the joints, glands, and in the formation of indolent tumors, and even those of a specific character, as fungus and scirrhus—which go on increasing insidiously and almost without pain—too active means prove highly injurious, and small doses of bichloride of mercury, with sarsaparilla, or Plummer's pill with hyoscyamus at night, seem to be the best remedies, assisted by generous diet and free air. Our London hospitals are the worst possible places for such patients to be sent to. Mercury in these cases is not given with the same view as in syphilis, to act specifically, but merely to act gently upon the chylopoietic viscera, and is given in very small doses; and so soon, therefore, as the secretions are restored, the mercury should be withheld and iodine prescribed. The formula which I usually order it in is as follows:

℞ Iodini, gr. ss.; potass. iodidi, ℨss.; sirup. papav., ℥ss.; infus. gent. co., ℥viij. M. Capt. cochl. larga ij. bis quotidie, with tepid applications to the chronic swellings, either warm water dressings or the following lotions, if the warmth does not prove agreeable to the patient's feelings: ℞ Ammon. hydrochlor., ℨj.; sp. vini rect., liq. ammon. acetat. aa. ℨij.; aquæ destillat., ℥iv. M. ft. lotio.

Friction, steaming and bandaging, will, each of them, in certain cases, prove advantageous, as well as a variety of stimulating applications; as, for instance, equal parts of camphor and soap liniments, with a small quantity of tincture of opium, often prove of great service.
Part xvi., *p.* 307.

————•••————

INFLUENZA.

Opium.—Dr. Christison finds opium of the most use in inflammations of the mucous membranes, especially coryza, catarrh, influenza and dysentery. He would cure coryza at once by causing the patient to avoid all meals after dinner, to use liquid sparingly, and by giving a full dose of muriate of morphia or Battley's solution at bedtime; and breakfast before getting up the next morning. It seems necessary, however, that the remedy should be administered early in the attack. "Febrile catarrh too may be checked abruptly in the same way, if patient and physician are lucky enough to meet during the first or second day at farthest."

Dr. Christison has repeatedly seen epidemic *influenza* thus checked at the outset—the local inflammation vanishing, while the strange lassitude, listlessness and ennui, so characteristic of this disorder, went on as usual for some days during convalescence. *Part* iii., *p.* 45.

Ipecacuan—Suggested in influenza. Proportion, one or two scruples of ipecacuan to five or seven ounces of water. Dose—Half an ounce every two or three hours. *Part* viii., *p.* 22.

Eupatorium Perfoliatum in Influenza—Manner of Administration.— In the severest cases, where it was determined to treat the disease with the herb alone, the patient, after being covered in bed, was induced to swallow a wineglassful of the infusion, prepared by infusing an ounce of the dried leaves in a pint of boiling water, warm, every half hour. After the fourth or fifth dose, considerable nausea, sometimes vomiting, with free diaphoresis, ensued, and there was an immediate amelioration of all the symptoms. Along with the nausea, free expectoration commenced; and after the former symptom had subsided, the patient was freed from every annoyance, and remained in every respect comfortable. Sufficient to keep up the impression on the system, the infusion was now given only every third or fourth hour in the same dose. The bowels were generally opened in about six hours after the commencement of the treatment, and afterward continued in a lax condition. Toward the evening of the second day, and particularly if the patient had been guilty of imprudent exposure, the symptoms frequently returned, and it was necessary to repeat the course adopted at first. But generally the medicine, continued as directed, kept the symptoms completely in check, and the patient was out on the fourth day. In cases where the treatment was commenced with calomel, etc., the infusion, to secure its diaphoretic and expectorant effects, was introduced on the second day in wineglassful doses every second hour. To correct the debilitating effects of the disease, frequently remaining after all its acute and more violent symptoms had subsided, a wineglassful of the cold infusion was directed three times a day.

The treatment of the disease in old persons, or in other cases where there was a marked tendency to prostration, was commenced in the same manner. As soon as the effects already mentioned as occurring were induced, the cold substituted for the warm infusion was directed in the same dose every second hour, to be continued, gradually lessening the period throughout the disease, unless the violent symptoms returned, when it was to be discontinued until the same course was repeated with the warm infusion, and then resumed. (Dr. Peebles.) *Part x., p. 33.*

———•♦•———

INSANITY.

Seclusion, as employed at Hanwell, in the Treatment of the Insane.—In the management of the insane, seclusion of the patient is advised during the period of the paroxysm, or fit of passion. To acquire the confidence of the patient, by kind and soothing treatment, is considered indispensable, and nothing will so much oppose its acquisition as brutal, or even impatient usage during the paroxysm. *Part iii., p. 63.*

Non-restraint System in the Management of the Insane.—The appearance and general state of the patients in the wards of Hanwell, the order, activity and cheerfulness, which pervade the asylum, and the rapid subsidence of the wildness of new patients, are all alleged by Dr. Conolly as proofs of the superiority of the gentle plan of treatment. It occasionally happens that patients are brought into the asylum in severe restraints. They are immediately set free; nor is the restraint ever put on again; yet the patient remains quiet. *Part vii., p. 87.*

Injurious Influence of Tobacco in Insanity.—Vide Art. "Tobacco."

Insanity produced by the use of Chloroform during Labor.—[At a meeting of the Westminster Medical Society, a few months ago,]

Dr. Webster related the following case, communicated to him by a professional friend, in consequence of perusing in "The Lancet" a report of the three similar instances he had mentioned at a previous meeting of the Society. Only one drachm of chloroform, sprinkled upon a handkerchief, was used; but the effect it produced was so sudden and violent, that the patient, after inhaling, remained quite insensible, which greatly alarmed the attendants; with the insensibility there was likewise deadly paleness of the countenance; however, she slowly rallied, but had a painful and protracted labor. During several days subsequently, the lady continued in a very nervous condition, although not then actually incoherent; but she soon became so furiously maniacal as to require coercion by a strait-waistcoat. After being insane during many months, the patient gradually recovered her reason, and ultimately got convalescent.

Part xxi., *p.* 361.

Medical Jurisprudence of Insanity.—A careful distinction, says Dr. Jameson, must be made between *diseases having mental symptoms,* and diseases of the mind; betwixt madness and such affections as hypochondriasis and hysteria. Hypochondriasis consists of illusions and hallucinations regarding one's bodily sensations, and is, therefore, not insanity until these become deep-seated and permanent delusions, compelling to irrational conduct. Hysteria, hypochondriasis, and various other affections, which often precede, cause, and accompany insanity, are not diseases of the mind, but, more strictly speaking, diseases having mental symptoms, until by generating delusions they pass into insanity, and afterward continue as complications of the disorder which they have created. Thus, we have hysterical mania, which is not hysteria merely, but hysteria and mania combined; so also there is hypochondriacal monomania, which is not hypochondriasis alone, but hypochondriasis and insanity together.

Simple defect of intellectual power, *intellectual dullness,* must not be confounded with the imbecility which constitutes a variety of insanity, which is not merely a feeble intensity of mind, but a positive deficiency of faculties. Wherever there is a feeble exercise of attention, or defective memory, there will be imperfect comparison and resulting inaccuracy of judgment; but not from these, or similar causes, any necessary tendency to be governed by delusions. In all cases of imbecility included in the term unsoundness of mind, there are both emotional and intellectual deficiency, a loss of control over conduct, and from the antecedence of judgment being in some part defective or diseased, a liability to confound the actual with the unreal. Delusion is not a prominent characteristic, however, for in such cases feebleness is the type of all the mental manifestations, whether healthy or disordered.

Eccentricity has also to be distinguished from insanity. All the insane are eccentric in their ideas, their language, or their conduct; but the merely eccentric have but a voluntary resemblance to the insane. Eccentricities differ from lunacies, in not arising from a loss, but from an undue exercise of, the faculty of judgment; very often from a vanity or self-respect in the individual, that leads him to prefer his own judgment to all other judgment, experience and authority. They offend against custom

and experience more than against reason. The eccentric, if he cannot give
a satisfactory reason for his *outre* conduct, can at least assign an intelligible motive: the lunatic has no explanation to afford that does not involve
an absurdity. A certain individual behaves in all respects like other men,
unless that he constantly walks about without a hat, or any other artificial
covering for his head. When questioned upon this point of disagreement
with the custom of his neighbors, he says that nature did not intend the
head to have any other protection than what she herself had afforded, that
a bare head is more becoming, that he feels himself in every way more
comfortable as he is, and that he is certain that he will live longer in consequence of acting in this rational way. In two instances in which lunatics
adopted the same habit, the causes assigned by them were of a very different description. One did not have his head covered, because it had
grown so large that he could not get a cap to fit it; and the other was so
annoyed by certain mischievous tormentors of an invisible kind drumming
upon the crown of his hat, that in general he preferred to carry it in his
hand. The eccentric man had a rule of conduct, the result of his own
narrow judgment; the two lunatics were impelled by fancies upon which
their judgment was entirely inoperative. Lord Monboddo, insisting that
the human family were originally adorned with tails, showed himself an
eccentric theorist; had he asserted that they actually retained them, he
would have had an insane delusion, instead of a philosophic crotchet. He
would have had a false perception on which his judgment was inoperative,
whereas he was guided *by his judgment* to a strange conclusion.

  Eccentricities no more constitute insanity, than idiosyncrasies constitute
disease; and as these are competent with a sound state of body, so are
those with even a vigorous judgment. For example: There was an old
man well known in London in the last century, who was of an ungainly
appearance, and subject to occasional attacks of hereditary melancholy.
So inconsistent was he in his habits, that sometimes he practised great ab-
stemiousness, and at other times devoured huge meals, with brutish
slovenliness and voracity: sometimes he would persist in drinking nothing
stronger than water, but occasionally he drank wine by tumblerfuls. His
income was far from large, and not of a certain amount, yet he kept a set
of old men and women about his house, whose bickerings and disagree-
ments now and then drove him out of doors. He was in general very
loquacious, but had been known to sit in company and drink a dozen cups
of tea without speaking a syllable. When not engaged discoursing, it was
his custom to keep muttering to himself. In walking he performed
strange gesticulations with his limbs, and would not go in at a door, unless he could effect his entry in a certain preconceived number of steps,
and so as to introduce himself on a particular foot, turning back, and re-
commencing, until he succeeded as he desired. There was a row of posts
near his house, which he would not pass without touching singly, and if
he found that he had omitted one in the series, he retraced his steps to
remedy the neglect. He hoarded up orange skins for some mysterious
purpose which he would never divulge. He suffered remorse of conscience
for once having taken milk with his coffee on Good Friday. He believed
in ghosts, and went ghost-hunting in Cock-lane; and he maintained
that he had heard his mother calling upon him by name from the other
world. Yet Dr. Johnson was so far from insane, that his judgment commanded respect and admiration everywhere, and by the common consent

of eminent contemporaries he was the most vigorous thinker and the greatest sage of his time.

There are, however, instances of eccentric conduct resulting from *abuse of the imagination*, which verge closely upon madness, and occasionally pass into it. The distinction is, that the individual's voluntary power over his thoughts is capable of bringing the comparing faculty into efficient operation, when he chooses duly to exert his will. Thomas Hood speaks of one who, in consequence of exciting his fancy by German tales of diablerie, used to fly upstairs at his utmost speed from the street door to the attics, because a sort of wager with the devil came into his head, that he would gain the top before counting a certain number, or forfeit eternal happiness. Every one possibly experiences moods which differ in no respect from insanity, than that they are neither permanent nor independent of the will. These may be common in imaginative minds, but instead of being indulged, they should be guarded against and restrained, for, though they exist at first by sufferance of the will, they sometimes gain a strength that defies control, and triumphs over the reason. Hoffman, a master in fantastic fiction, suffered so much from intemperate abuse of the imaginative faculty, that solitude became terrible to him. He was never quit of a mysterious sense of danger; things the most cheerful became incongruously associated with thoughts the most dreadful, while monsters and spectres, which he himself had created, tyrannized over his reason. To appease his terrors, he had frequently to summon his wife from bed to sit by him as he studied at night. He was constantly on the verge of insanity, and died of spinal disease, his mind being tortured by his fancy to the last hour of his existence.

Often it is not an easy matter to draw a distinction between insanity and *moral depravity*. In every case of mental alienation there is disorder of moral as well as of intellectual manifestations. The moral disturbance is usually the earliest developed feature of the malady, frequently it is the most prominent, and occasionally no other is distinguished; so that the bad have been liable to pass as mad, and the mad for bad, according to the philosophy and fashion of the time. There is no problem in law, medicine, and ethics, of greater social importance, or of more difficult solution, than the discrimination of insanity and vice. A wicked deed may be the result of an undeveloped moral sense, as for example in a child or an idiot; it may be the consequence of such extremity of passion as impels to instinctive, instead of deliberative action; and it may be the indication of a conscience enfeebled by voluntary neglect, and the habitual gratification of evil desires. Any of these states may be simulated by disease; but it is with the last two only that the jurist will have difficulty; for in all cases of insanity in which the moral sense is non-existent, the powers of the understanding are also either undeveloped or destroyed. No hideousness of depravity can amount to proof of insanity, unsupported by evidence of a judgment incapacitated, or a will fettered, by disease. In those cases of mental disorder in which the emotions are perverted, and where there is no clear proof of deranged intellect, cases which do from time to time occur, the presumption of insanity, in regard to a criminal action, has to be upheld by evidence of suspension of the will. The actions of an individual in such a state ought to be impulsive, involuntary, and irreconcilable with the idea of a healthy state of the emotional faculties.

Part xxii., *p.* 358.

Medical Treatment of Insanity.—[The following is a brief outline of
Dr. Winslow's views on the pathology and medical treatment of insanity :]

It is necessary that we should, before being able to appreciate the effect
of medical treatment, entertain just and enlightened views as to the *cura-
bility of insanity.* I now speak from a somewhat enlarged experience,
from much consideration of the matter, and I have no hesitation in affirming that, if brought within the sphere of medical treatment in the earlier
stages, or even within a few months of the attack, insanity, unless the result of severe physical injury to the head, or connected with a peculiar
conformation of chest and cranium, and a hereditary liathesis, *is as
easily curable as any other form of bodily disease for the treatment of
which we apply the resources of our art.* It is a lamentable error to suppose, and a dangerous, a false, and unhappy doctrine to promulgate, that
the disordered affections of the mind are not amenable to the recognized
principles of medical science. The vast amount of incurable cases of
insanity which crowd the wards of our national and private asylums,
is pregnant with important truths. In the history of these unhappy persons—those lost and ruined minds—we read recorded the sad,
melancholy, and lamentable results of either a total neglect of all efficient
curative treatment at a period when it might have arrested the onward
advance of the cerebral mischief, and maintained reason upon her seat; or
of the use of injudicious and unjustifiable measures under the mistaken
notions of the nature and pathology of the disease. In no class of affections is it so imperatively necessary to inculcate the importance of early
and prompt treatment, as in the disorders of the brain affecting the mani
festations of the mind. I do not maintain that our curative agents are of
no avail when the disease has passed beyond what is designated the " curable stage." My experience irresistibly leads to the conclusion that we
have often in our power the means of curing insanity, even after it has
been of some years' duration, if we obtain a thorough appreciation of the
physical and mental aspects of the case, and perseveringly and continually
apply remedial measures for its removal ; but I cannot dwell too strongly
upon the vital necessity of the early and prompt exhibition of curative
means in the incipient stage of mental derangement.

I believe insanity (I am now referring to persistent insanity, not to those
transient and evanescent forms of disturbed mind occasionally witnessed)
to be the result of a *specific morbid action of the hemispherical ganglia,
ranging from irritation, passive and active congestion, up to positive and
unmistakable inflammatory action.* This state of the brain may be con·
fined to one or two of the six layers composing the hemispherical ganglia ;
but all the layers are generally more or less implicated, in conjunction
with the tubular fibres passing from the hemispheres through the vesicular
neurine. This specific inflammation, from its incipient to the more advanced stage, is often associated with great vital and nervous depression.
It is, like analogous inflammation of other structures, not often accompa·
nied by much constitutional or febrile disturbance, unless it loses its
specific features, and approximates in its character to the inflammation of
active cerebritis or meningitis. This state of the hemispherical ganglia is
frequently conjoined with active sanguineous circulation and congestion,
both of the substance of the brain and its investing membranes. The
morbid cerebral pathological phenomena—viz., the opacity of the arach·

noid, the thickening of the dura mater, its adhesions to the cranium, the depositions so often observed upon the convoluted surface of the hemispheres, and on the meninges, the hypertrophy, scirrhus, the cancerous affections, the induration, the depositions of bony matter in the cerebral vessels and on the dura mater, the serous fluids in and the ulcerations upon the surface of the ventricles, the alterations in the size, consistence, color, and chemical composition of the vesicular neurine and fibrous portion of the brain—are all, in my opinion, the results, the sequelæ, more or less, of that specific inflammatory condition of the hemispherical ganglia to which I have referred. It does not necessarily follow that the *fons et origo mali* of insanity is invariably to be traced to the brain. The preliminary morbid action and irritation are often situated in the heart, the stomach, the liver, the bowels, the lungs, or the kidneys, the brain being secondarily affected; nevertheless, in all cases inducing actual insanity, the hemispherical ganglia are involved in the morbid action. The most recent pathological doctrine propounded to explain the phenomena of insanity—I refer to the views of a recent writer—that derangement of mind is the effect of "*loss of nervous tone*," and that this loss of nervous tone is "*caused by a premature and abnormal exhaustibility of the vital powers of the sensorium*"—conveys to my mind no clear, definite, or precise pathological idea. It is true that we often have, in these affections of the brain and disorders of the mind, "loss of nervous tone," and "exhaustion of vital power;" but, to my conception, these are but the *effects* of *a prior morbid condition of the encephalon*, the *sequelæ* of specific inflammation of the hemispherical ganglia. To argue that insanity is invariably and exclusively the result of "loss of nervous tone," is to confound cause and effect, the *post hoc* with the *propter hoc ;* and would, as regards therapeutical measures, act as an *ignis fatuus*, alluring us as pathologists from the right and legitimate path. I feel anxious that my views upon this important subject should be clearly enunciated, and not open to misconception. I think much mischief has arisen from a belief in the existence of active ordinary cerebral inflammation in cases of insanity, for it has led to the adoption of treatment most destructive to life, and has seriously interfered with the permanent restoration of the reasoning powers. Nevertheless, insanity is occasionally complicated with acute cerebral symptoms sufficient to justify us in the cautious use of somewhat active measures for its removal. We must avoid the fatal error of a too rapid process of generalization, and be careful of not looking to symptoms instead of to the disease itself, and of permitting ingenious and well constructed *à priori* theories of the nature of insanity to dazzle our imaginations and abstract the mind from the steady and patient investigation of pathological science and individual cases of disease. If we allow our judgment to be warped by the inflammatory theory on the one side (I am now speaking of *ordinary*, not of *specific* inflammation), and conclude that the excitement of mania is to be subdued by copious depletion or the administration of antiphlogistic measures—or if, on the other hand, we adopt the speculative opinions of those who believe that, in every case of insanity, irrespectively of its origin, its progress, or its character, there exists "mere loss of nervous tone," caused by "a premature abnormal exhaustibility of the vital powers of the sensorium"—how lamentably shall we be misled as to the real character of insanity, and in the application of our therapeutic agents? These circumscribed and partial views of the pathology of insanity often

lead to serious solecisms in practice. In ninety per cent. of the cases of
acute mania there is found in the brain and its meninges a state of sangui
neous congestion, particularly of the hemispherical ganglia, combined
with alterations in the grey nervous matter. In forming an opinion of the
actual pathological condition of the cerebral substance, we should remember that, particularly in public asylums, it is a rare occurrence for recent
cases to be admitted; that the acute and sub-acute active cerebral conditions have subsided, and the disease has assumed a chronic form, before
the patient is examined and placed under treatment; consequently many
deductions recorded by pathologists have been based upon the study of
chronic, and not of acute mania. A large percentage of the cases, before
admission into our national asylums, have passed through the primary and
acute stages, and have probably been subjected to medical treatment.
This fact must never be lost sight of in forming our opinion, not only of
the nature of the disease itself, but of the medical treatment necessary for
its cure. In private practice the acute forms of insanity are often met
with; but even with the advantages which the physician can command, of
investigating the earlier stages of deranged mind, he often discovers that
the mental affection has been allowed to exist and slowly progress for a
considerable period, no treatment, either medical or moral, having been
adopted for its removal. In the incipient form of insanity, particularly
when it manifests itself in plethoric constitutions, has been sudden in its
development, is the result of physical causes, and is connected with the
retrocession of gout, or is rheumatic in its character, there can be no doubt
the nature of the changes induced in the brain is more allied to that of
inflammation than that of nervous exhaustion. The attacks from the slow
and insidious operation of moral causes are less likely to be accompanied
by active symptoms. In many instances the maniacal excitement is
asthenic or *atonic* in its character, resembling the delirium of the last
stages of typhus fever.

The most simple classification of insanity, the one best adapted for useful
and practical purposes, is its division into the *acute* and *chronic* forms; the
insanity ushered in by *excitement* or by *depression* into *mania* and *melancholia—amentia* and *dementia*. The minute divisions and subdivisions,
the complicated and confused classification to be found in books, may serve
the ostentatious purposes of those desirous of making pompous display of
scientific lore, but I think they have tended to bewilder and obscure the
understanding of the student, and lead the man in search of practical truth
from the investigation of the disease itself to the mere study of its symptoms, and to the consideration of unessential points and shades of difference. Adhering to this division of the subject, each form should be viewed
in relation to its *complications*, as well as to its *associated diseases*. Among
the former are epilepsy, suicide, homicide, paraplegia, hemiplegia, and
general paralysis. The associated disease implicate the lungs, heart, liver,
stomach, bowels, kidney, bladder, and skin.

Before speaking of the preliminary examination of the patient supposed
to be insane, and the prognosis in cases of insanity, I would premise that
those inexperienced in the examination of this class of cases would often
arrive at false and inaccurate conclusions, if they were not cognizant of the
fact, that the insane often describe sensations which they have never experienced, and call attention to important symptoms which have no exis
tence except in their own morbid imaginations. A patient will tell you

that he has a racking headache, or great pain and tenderness in the epigastric region, both symptoms being the fanciful creations of his diseased mind. This is particularly the case in the hysterical forms of insanity, in which there always exists a disposition to pervert the truth, and exaggerate the symptoms. Again, serious bodily disease may be present, the patient not being sufficiently conscious to comprehend the nature of the questions asked, or able to give intelligible replies to the anxious interrogatories of the physician. Insanity often masks, effectually obscures, other organic affections, the greater malady overpowering the lesser disease. When Lear, Kent, and the Fool are standing alone upon the wild heath, exposed to the merciless pelting of the tempest, Kent feelingly implores the king to seek shelter from the "tyranny of the open night" in an adjoining hovel; it is then that Lear gives expression to the psychological truth just referred to:

> " Thou think'st 'tis much that this contentious storm
> Invades us to the skin; so 'tis to thee;
> But *where the greater malady is fixed,*
> *The lesser is scarce felt;*
> . . . . The tempest *in my mind*
> Doth from my senses take *all feeling else*
> *Save what beats there.*"

Disease of the brain may destroy all apparent consciousness of pain, and keep in abeyance the outward and appreciable manifestations of other important indications of organic mischief. Extensive diseases of the stomach, lungs, kidneys, bowels, uterus and heart have been known to have progressed to a fearful extent without any obvious recognizable indication of the existence of such affections. Insanity appears occasionally to modify the physiognomy and symptomatology of ordinary diseases, and to give them peculiar and specific characteristic features.

Again, it is necessary for the physician to watch the operation of medicine in masking important diseases. The different forms of narcotics, if given in heroic doses, often mislead us in our estimate of the nature of bodily diseases not directly connected with the mental affection. The most essential preliminary matters of inquiry have relation to the age, temperament, and previous occupation, and condition in life of the patient. It will be necessary to ascertain the character and duration of the attack; to ascertain whether it has resulted from moral or physical causes; if of sudden, insidious, or of slow growth; whether it has a hereditary origin, or is the effect of a mental shock, or of mechanical injury; whether it is the first attack; and if not, in what features it differs from previous paroxysms. It will also be our duty to inquire whether it is complicated with epilepsy, paraplegia, or hemiplegia, suicidal or homicidal impulses. If any prior treatment has been adopted, we must ascertain its nature; whether the patient has suffered from gout, heart disease, rheumatism, cutaneous affection, or syphilis. It is important in cases of females to obtain accurate information in relation to the condition of the uterine functions, and to ascertain the state of the moral affections. We should also inquire whether the patient has been suspected of habits of self-abuse. Having obtained accurate information upon these essential points, our own personal observation will aid us in ascertaining the character of the mental disturbance; the configuration of the head, chest, and abdomen; the gait of the patient, the

degree of sensibility and volitional power manifested; the state of the retina, the pulse, the urine, and temperature of the scalp and body generally; the condition of the skin and chylopoietic viscera; the action of the
heart, lungs, and nature of any existing disease of the uterus. If a patient
complains of any local mischief, however imaginary it may appear to be at
the time, it is essentially necessary that we should clearly satisfy our minds
upon the point before dismissing it as not entitled to serious investigation. A patient once bitterly complained of retention of urine; upon examination the bladder was found to be distended, and the man had passed
no urine for twenty-four hours. I was about to introduce a catheter, when
the patient burst into a fit of laughter, and immediately emptied his bladder. Esquirol relates a case of a merchant, who, whilst suffering from
melancholia, declared that some foreign body was sticking in his throat.
No notice was taken of this supposed fanciful idea. The patient died, and
an ulcer was discovered at the upper third of the œsophagus. A patient
complained of devils being in his stomach and bowels, and declared that
they were acted upon by electric or magnetic agencies. After death he was
found to have scirrhus of the stomach, and chronic inflammation of the
bowels. A patient refused to eat; he said he could not swallow his food
without great pain. As he had exhibited other symptoms of a disposition
to suicide, it was thought by myself and others, that his obstinate refusal
of food was associated with ideas of self-destruction. He died, and at the
post-mortem examination a stricture in the pylorus was discovered. These
illustrations, and they could easily be extended, will prove the importance of paying minute attention to particular delusions, with the view
of ascertaining whether they have not a particular and *actual* physical
origin.

The *prognosis* in cases of insanity will mainly depend upon the duration
of the attack, its character and origin, and the diathesis of the patient.
The prognosis is generally unfavorable if the disease is hereditary—if the
symptoms are similar in character to those exhibited by other members of
the family when insane. Insanity, accompanied by acute excitement, is,
cæteris paribus, more easy of cure than when it has been of slow and gradual growth, and is marked by great mental depression. The prognosis is
favorable in cases of puerperal mania; it is unfavorable when there exists
a want of symmetry between the two sides of the head, with small anterior, and large posterior cerebral development. Any great inequality in
the cranial conformation would be a suspicious indication. The existence
of any malformation in the development of the chest is also an unfavorable sign, and would induce us to give a guarded prognosis. Dr. Darwin
says, when a person becomes insane, who has a small family of children to
absorb his attention, his prospect of recovery is but small, as it establishes
that the maniacal hallucination is more powerful than those ideas which
usually interest us most. The prognosis is unfavorable when patients are
under the morbid delusion that they are poisoned, and are constantly suffering internally from peculiar sensations. Religious delusions are more
difficult to eradicate than other morbid impressions. The age of the patient will materially guide us in forming a correct prognosis. Hippocra-
tes says the insane are not curable after the fortieth year; Esquirol maintains the greater portion recover between the ages of twenty and thirty;
Haslam, between the ages of ten and twenty. As a principle, we may

conclude that the probability of recovery in any given case is in proportion to the early age, physical condition, and duration of the attack. When a patient has youth and a good constitution to aid him, and is advantageously placed, having at command remedial measures, and is excluded from all irritating circumstances, the prognosis may be favorable. I have seen patients after the advanced age of sixty and seventy recover; and cases of cure are upon record where insanity has existed for ten, fifteen, and twenty years. In forming our prognosis, it is important to ascertain the educational training of the patient. Has he been in the habit of exercising great self-control? Has his mind been well disciplined? Has he kept in abeyance the passions, or have the motions and impulses of his nature obtained the mastery over him? He who has been taught to practise self-denial and self-control in early life, is, *cœteris paribus*, in a more favorable position for recovery than he who has permitted himself to be the willing and obedient slave of every passion and caprice. Insanity, accompanied with criminal propensities, is said to be incurable; because, as Ideler urges, such patients " cannot bear the torments of their consciences, and relapse into the stupefaction of insanity to flee from the consciousness of their guilt." The prognosis is unfavorable when the insanity is complicated with organic disease of the heart and lungs, with deafness, and paralysis in any of its forms. Lesions of the motor power are very unfavorable indications. Great impairment of mind, accompanied with delusions of an exalted character, and associated with paralysis, is generally incurable. Esquirol says, epilepsy, if associated with insanity, places the patient beyond all prospect of cure. I should be loth to adopt this sweeping condemnation. I have seen cases of epilepsy, combined with mental derangement, recover; although, I admit, they constitute a difficult class of cases to manage.

[As it would be impossible to describe in detail the particular class of remedial agents adapted to each class of deranged minds, in the succeeding lecture the subject has been generalized, the most prominent kinds of insanity, and the difficulties of their management, only being discussed.]

In regard to the treatment of acute mania, the important and much-litigated question at issue among practitioners of all countries, is that relating to the propriety of depletion. Whilst some practitioners of great repute and enlarged experience fearlessly recommend copious general depletion for the treatment of insanity, and refer to cases in which this practice has been attended with the happiest results, others, equally eminent, and as much entitled to our respect, denounce the lancet as a most fatally dangerous weapon, and shudder at the suggestion of abstracting, even locally, the smallest quantity of blood. In avoiding Scylla, we must be cautious of being impelled into Charybdis. The error consists in a vain effort to discover a uniform rule of treatment, and attempting to propound some specific mode of procedure adapted to all cases. He who maintains that blood-letting is never to be adopted in the treatment of mania, without reference to its character, its origin, the peculiar constitution of the patient, and the existence of local physical morbid conditions, which may be materially modifying the disease, and giving active development to delusive impressions, is not a safe practitioner. Neither would I confide in the judgment of the physician who would, in every case of violent maniacal excitement, attempt to tranquillize the patient by either general or local depletion.

In attacks of insanity, when the symptoms are acute, the patient, young and plethoric, the habitual secretions suppressed, the head hot and painful, the eyes intolerant of light, the conjunctivæ injected, the pupils contracted, the pulse rapid and hard, and the paroxysm sudden in its development, *one* general bleeding will often arrest the progress of the cerebral mischief, greatly facilitate the application of other remedies, and ultimately promote recovery. In proportion as the symptoms of ordinary insanity approach those of phrenitis, shall we be justified in the use of general depletion. Although it is only occasionally, in instances presenting peculiar characteristic features—cases occurring in the higher ranks of life, where the patient has been in the habit of living *above par*, and is of a sanguineous temperament—that we are justified in having recourse to the lancet, there is a large class of recent cases presenting themselves in the asylums for the insane, both public and private, in the treatment of which we should be guilty of culpable and cruel negligence, if we were to omit to relieve the cerebral symptoms by means of the local abstraction of blood. It is the fashion and caprice of the day to recklessly decry the application of cupping-glasses or of leeches in the treatment of insanity, in consequence, I think, of the slavish deference shown to the opinion of a few French pathologists of eminence, who have, by their indiscriminate denunciation of *all depletion*, frightened us into submission, and compelled us to do violence to our own judgment. The local abstraction of blood is, in the hands of the discreet and judicious practitioner, a powerful curative agent; and yet it is the practice of some men, and men, too, of position, to discard altogether the remedy.

I will briefly refer to the kind of case in which the local abstraction of blood will be found most beneficial, if proper regard be had to the temperament, constitutional condition, and the local circumstances modifying the character of the attack. In insanity, when the exacerbations occur at the menstrual period, *cæteris paribus*, leeches to the vulva and thighs, with the use of foot-bath, and the exhibition of aloetic purgatives, will be attended by the most favorable results. In irregular and obstructed menstruation, the local abstraction of blood will be very serviceable. In suppressed hemorrhoids, leeches to the neighborhood of the sphincter ani will greatly benefit in unloading the hemorrhoidal vessels, and relieve the brain of undue excitement. In cases of nymphomania, leeches to the vulva are indicated, and have been known to greatly benefit. In cases of intermittent insanity. the paroxysm may often be cut short by relieving the overloaded state of the vessels of the head by means of cupping or the application of leeches. In some instances I have tried Dr. Wigan's plan, and have applied leeches to the Schneiderian membrane, particularly for the treatment of insanity of early life, and connected with conduct evidently the effect of cerebral irritation. I have seen this mode of procedure of essential benefit in persons of plethoric constitution and of sanguineous temperament. Occasionally the insanity is found to be associated with active visceral disease, or with hypertrophy and other affections of the heart. Under these circumstances, when there exists great tenderness over the region of any of the visceral organs, and we are satisfied, by a careful stethoscopic examination, that hypertrophy of the heart is present, leeches applied over the seat of the local mischief, conjoined with other appropriate treatment, will materially aid us in subduing the maniacal affection. In cases of illusions of hearing, or of vision, it will often be necessary to apply leeches behind the ears, or over the superciliary ridges. I have known this practice entirely remove the morbid illusions which had been embittering the person's life.

But apart entirely from the local affections to which I have referred, for the treatment of idiopathic insanity, apparently without any complications, or modified by any of the associated diseases, the careful and temperate local abstraction of blood, when general depletion is inadmissible, will often materially shorten the duration of an attack of insanity, and restore the mind to a healthy condition. I am anxious to record my favorable opinion of this mode of treatment, because I have witnessed so many sad results from an opposite timid and reprehensible neglect of the means placed within our power for the treatment of the varied forms and degrees of mental derangement. Sad consequences have undoubtedly followed the indiscriminate use of depletory measures; the presence of violent mental excitement has occasionally led the practitioner to the conclusion that the disease was of an active character; and in the attempt to allay the undue cerebral excitement by means of antiphlogistic measures, the patient has sunk into incurable and hopeless dementia. But recognizing an *anæmic* class of cases, where great excitement is often associated with loss of nervous and vital power, we must be cautious in permitting serious disease to be creeping stealthily on in the brain, no effort being made to relieve the congested cerebral vessels or inflamed tissue, until serious disorganization has taken place in the delicate structure of the vesicular matter, and the patient is forever lost. In the treatment of acute mania, the remedy next in importance to cautious depletion is that of *prolonged hot baths.* To Dr. Brierre de Boismont, of Paris, at whose excellent institution I first witnessed the application of this remedial agent, the profession is indebted for reviving a practice which had long fallen into disrepute. In treatment of acute mania, the prolonged hot baths will be found of the most essential service. Dr. Brierre de Boismont has recorded the history of sixty-one of seventy-two cases that were subjected to this mode of treatment. Three-fourths of this number were cured in a week, and the remainder in a fortnight. The patients remain from eight to ten and fifteen hours in warm baths, whilst a current of cold water is continually poured over the head; the temperature of these baths is from 82° to 86° Fahr.; the affusions 60° Fahr. Among the therapeutic effects of these baths, Dr. B. de Boismont reckons a diminution of the circulation and respiration, relaxation of the skin, alleviation of thirst, the introduction of a considerable quantity of water into the economy, an abundant discharge of limpid urine, a tendency to sleep, a state of repose This mode of treatment is said to be ineffectual in cases of periodic intermittent mania, in mania beginning with great mental impairment, or associated with epilepsy or general paralysis. . The result of my own experience of this plan of treatment has produced a very favorable impression upon my mind, and I think it is entitled to a fair trial in all our public asylums where they admit acute and recent cases.

In some forms of acute mania it is desirable, as a substitute for depletion, to diminish the activity of the circulation by the exhibition of nauseating doses of the tartrate of antimony; it may be serviceably combined with the tinctures of digitalis and hyoscyamus. This remedy, however, requires careful watching, as it often has been known to suddenly reduce the vital powers to a low ebb, and extinguish life. It will be found beneficial in proportion to the recent character of the ease, and the positive activity of the cerebral circulation. The tincture of digitalis was formerly in great repute as an anti-maniacal remedy; the experience of late years has not encouraged us in administering it in the doses prescribed by some of the old writers; nevertheless, it is a useful agent, and occasionally proves a valuable auxiliary in the hand of the practitioner who carefully watches its operation.

For the cure of the acute forms of insanity, the douche bath has been much lauded; but this remedy is now rarely used in British asylums. I have occasionally seen benefit derived from its exhibition, but it requires great caution in its use. A patient has been subjected, whilst in a paroxysm of acute delirium, to the douche bath, and has sunk almost immediately into incurable idiocy! The physical shock has occasionally been known to produce a good moral impression. For illustration: a patient imagined himself emperor of the world, and would not allow any one to address him by any other title. The immediate application of the douche bath destroyed his idea of royal dignity, and he was willing to admit that he had never been, nor was at any time a regal personage. A few hours subsequently, the delusive impression returned in all its original force; the douche bath was again had recourse to, and a second time the morbid impression vanished; by a series of baths he was restored to sanity, and after his complete recovery, when the particulars of his case were placed before him, he observed, "Why did you not whip me, and beat this nonsense out of my head? I wonder how you could have borne with my folly, or I have been guilty of such contemptible arrogance and obstinacy." As a substitute for the douche, the shower-bath is often used with great benefit, particularly in certain forms of melancholia, associated with nervous depression and general debility. In cases of melancholia, or other kinds of chronic insanity connected with a congested state of the liver, the nitro-muriatic bath will occasionally do much good. In a few instances I have noticed marked benefit from Bertolini's sedative bath, composed of henbane, two pounds, and equal parts of hemlock, and cherry laurel leaves, well infused in a sufficient quantity of hot water. But the simple hot-bath in certain conditions of the nervous system, particularly in some forms of suicidal mania, is of the utmost benefit. A warm bath a short period before retiring to rest, bathing the head at the same time with cold water, particularly if the scalp be unnaturally hot, will often insure a quiet and composed night when no description of sedative, however potent its character and dose, would influence the system.

In the early stages of insanity, and throughout its whole course, the bowels are often in an obstinately constipated condition. The concentration of nervous energy in the brain appears to interfere with that supply which should proceed to other structures; consequently there appears to be a want of healthy sensibility in the mucous membrane of the bowels, and an interruption to the peristaltic action of the intestinal canal. There is no class of agents which act so certainly and effectually in relieving the mind when under the influence of depressing emotion, as cathartics. The ancients considered hellebore as a specific in certain forms of melancholia. In the hands of modern practitioners, it has not been found to merit the high encomiums which have been passed upon it. It is important in every case of insanity, but particularly in the acute stages of mental derange-ment, to act powerfully upon the bowels by means of a succession of brisk cathartics. The bowels are often found gorged with fecal matter, and immediate relief often follows the administration of two or three doses of calomel and colocynth, or of croton-oil. It will often be necessary to assist the operation of the cathartics by means of enemata. In hysterical and some other forms of insanity, there is always a disposition on the part of the patient resolutely to resist the calls of nature, and, knowing this peculiarity, we must carefully watch the condition of the bowels, otherwise serious mechanical obstructions may ensue, followed by intractable diseases of the rectum. Insanity is often associated with gastric and intestinal dis-ease, with an irritable condition of the mucous membrane of the alimentary canal; and, in such cases, although it is important to relieve the bowels and prevent them from being constipated, we must bear in mind that the injudicious exhibition of irritating drastic cathartics may aggravate the mental disease, by increasing the gastric and intestinal irritation, and thus do permanent and irremediable mischief. Much injury may arise from the indiscriminate and injudicious administration of cathartics. In insanity associated with menstrual obstructions, it will be necessary to exhibit the class of purgatives known to act specifically upon the lower bowel; consequently aloetic cathartics, such as the compound decoction of aloes, are found of most service in these cases. In plethoric habits, when there is a marked determination of blood to the head, no medicine will relieve so speedily as active doses of the compound powder of jalap.

In the treatment of insanity, the class of medicines termed *sedative* play an important part. If exhibited with judgment, the most gratifying results often follow *their continuous and persevering administration.* The sedative treatment of insanity is a subject of itself, and I quite despair of touching even upon the confines of many interesting and important points involved in the consideration of this division of my lecture. In insanity unassociated with active cerebral circulation, congestion, or paralysis, or after the head symptoms have been relieved by the local abstraction of blood and the administration of appropriate medicine, the exhibition of sedatives will be followed by the most beneficial results. In recent cases they are generally inadmissible, except in delirium tremens and puerperal insanity, and other forms of derangement analogous in their pathological character and symptoms to these affections. In chronic insanity, in melan-cholia unconnected with abdominal repletion, or visceral disease, the per-severing use of sedatives in various combinations will often reëstablish sanity, when no other course of treatment is likely to be successful in dis-pelling the illusive impressions, or raising the drooping and desponding spirits. Battley's solution, the tincture of opium, the meconite, acetate, and hydrochlorate of morphia, the preparations of hyoscyamus, conium, stramonium, camphor, hops, aconite, ether, chloroform, hydrocyanic acid, Indian hemp, are all of great and essential service if administered with judgment and sagacity. In suicidal insanity, when local cerebral conges-tion is absent, and the general health and secretions are in good condition, the meconite and hydrochlorate of morphia often act like a charm, *uninterruptedly and perseveringly given* until the nervous system is com-pletely under its influence. I have witnessed the most distressing attacks of suicidal mania yield to this treatment, when every other system has failed. I could cite the particulars of numerous cases of this form of

insanity radically cured by the occasional local abstraction of blood from
the head, the administration of alteratives, the warm bath, and sedatives.
In the use of this powerful curative agent, our success will often depend
upon a *ready adaptation of the kind of sedative to the description of case
in which it may be deemed admissible, and a judicious combination of
various kinds of sedatives.* I do not think we pay sufficient attention to
such combinations. I have often seen an apparently incurable and un
manageable case yield to several kinds of sedatives combined, when it
resisted the operation of any one or two. The extract of conium is often
of service in cases of insanity combined with epilepsy; conjoined with
mineral tonics, conium is occasionally of benefit, particularly in melancholia
connected with chronic diseases of the digestive organs and with neuralgia.
In cases of uterine irritation, I have seen great good result from the com
bination of hops, camphor, and hyoscyamus. In illusions of vision, belladonna, commencing with quarter-grain doses, will be found a useful remedy.
In insanity complicated with dysmenorrhœa, the combination of camphor
with hyoscyamus, opium, or conium, may be given with great advantage.
The hydrochlorate of morphia, in union with dilute hydrochloric acid, is
said to be useful in cases where the sedative treatment is desirable. I am
often in the habit of exhibiting sedatives and tonics in a state of combination, particularly conium with iron, opium with quinine, or with the infusion or compound decoction of cinchona. In debility, with irritability of
the nervous system, accompanied by restlessness, Battley's solution, with
the preparations of cinchona, will often prove of great benefit. The tincture of sumbul I have occasionally administered, and I think with advantage, in paroxysmal or convulsive forms of insanity. I have given to the
extent of one or two drachms for a dose. In hysterical derangement, the
tincture of Indian hemp will occasionally allay the excitement, and produce
sleep more rapidly than any other form of sedative. The valerianate of
zinc has not answered the expectations of those who have spoken so highly
of its medicinal virtues. Tincture of opium with camphor, and the tartrate
of antimony, is an excellent combination in cases of doubtful cerebral congestion. Tincture of hops in doses of from one to four drachms, it will be
necessary to give when no other formulæ are admissible. As a mild form
of sedative, compound ipecacuanha powder is occasionally recommended;
but a good substitute for Dover's powder is a pill composed of opium,
ipecacuanha, and soap.

In treating the more chronic forms of insanity, particularly melancholia,
it will be essential to bear in mind that they are difficult of cure, because,
owing to the slow, obscure, and insidious character of the disease, the
mental affection has been of some duration before the attention of the
practitioner has been directed to its existence. As this form of derangement generally exhibits itself in trifling perversions of the affections and
propensities leading to little acts of extravagance and irregularity of
conduct, associated with great depression, we often find the attack has
existed some years before a necessity is felt for any medical advice or
treatment—perhaps a suicidal propensity has manifested itself, this being
the first apparent overt act of the insanity.

It is necessary, before suggesting any course of treatment in melancholia, to ascertain whether any latent visceral disease be present. Occasionally the local irritation will be found either in the liver, or the
stomach and bowels, and in women the uterine functions are frequently

disordered. In the religious and other forms of melancholia in females, the delusive ideas are often associated with uterine irritation; and under such circumstances, if actual physical derangement of an active character exists in this organ, the best treatment will be, the application of leeches to the neighborhood of uterus, combined with warm hip-baths, sedatives, and mineral tonics. In cases of melancholia, the digestive functions are often much vitiated, the circulation languid, the skin cold and flaccid; and these symptoms being conjoined with a general loss of physical tone, such patients require generous diet, good air, gentle exercise, and occasional stimuli. When dyspeptic symptoms are combined with an inactive state of the bowels, I have often administered the compound tincture of guaiacum with great benefit. It is important to watch the particular features in these cases, and to improve the general health by the exhibition of mild alteratives and vegetable tonics, with alkalies. I have occasionally administered, with success, in this form of insanity, apparently associated with an abnormal condition of the nutrition of the brain, cod-liver oil, with preparations of iron.

My time will not admit of my submitting for your approval the treatment best adapted for those forms of mental disease associated with an atrophied or softened condition of the nervous matter. I think more is to be done for the cure of these cases than the writings of medical men would lead the student to suppose, particularly if the disease be seen and subjected to treatment in the early stages. I have recorded the details of several instances of cerebral disease, exhibiting all the legitimate features of ramollissement, and yielding to the persevering administration of the preparations of iron, phosphorus, zinc, and strychnia, combined with generous living, and the occasional application of a leech behind the ear, should indications of cerebral congestion be present. I have also derived benefit in these cases from the use of the milder forms of mercury, associated with cinchona. In cases of impairment of the mind, loss of memory, defective power of attention, occasional paroxysm of *mental* paralysis, unconnected with lesions of the *motor* power, I have found a solution of the acetate of strychnine, and a solution of the phosphate of strychnine, of great advantage.

In some chronic forms of insanity, in dementia, and persistent monomania, connected, as it was supposed, with morbid thickening of the dura mater, and with interstitial infiltration of the membranes, as well as with exudations upon its surface, I have occasionally had the head shaved, and have perseveringly rubbed over the scalp a strong ointment of the iodide of potassium combined with strychnine. In other instances I have kept the head painted with the mixture of iodine. I have seen marked benefit from this mode of treatment. In several cases where the mental symptoms were supposed to be associated with effusions of serum, I have ordered the iodine to be applied externally, at the same time exhibiting minute doses of calomel, or mercury with chalk, to slightly affect the system: this, conjoined with occasional tonics, diuretics, and stimuli to support the vital powers and enable the patient to undergo this treatment, is occasionally productive of considerable benefit, in cases apparently placed quite beyond the reach of improvement in cure.

I have only briefly spoken of two distressing, and often unmanageable forms of insanity—viz., of suicidal mania, and of those cases where the patient obstinately refuses to take either food or medicine. In insanity associated with suicidal tendencies, it will be important to ascertain whether any cerebral congestion exist, as such is often the case. A few leeches applied to the head, followed by an active cathartic, will relieve the local irritation, and often dissipate the idea of self-destruction. In the absence of any positive active cerebral symptoms, the prolonged hot bath, and the persevering exhibition of some form of sedative, is the best treatment to be adopted. I have seen the suicidal impulse removed after the administration of a few doses of belladonna; but the meconite and hydrochlorate of morphia, if given for a sufficient length of time, will, in the great majority of cases, distinct from actual incurable visceral or cerebral disease, effect a cure. Occasionally the shower-bath, and counter-irritation in the vicinity of the head, will aid us in reëstablishing health. Cases sometimes present themselves where the patient determinedly refuses to take either food or medicine. This character of case gives those who have the care of the insane much anxiety. The refusal of food may be connected with determination to destroy life, or it may be associated with delusive impressions. I am inclined to believe that in the majority of these cases the symptom is the result of some local mischief remote from the brain, and sympathetically affecting the organ of thought. Upon examination we often find, in these cases, great gastric derangement, obstinate constipation, considerable tenderness upon pressure in the epigastric region, hepatic disease, the tongue foul, breath offensive, and other symptoms of derangement of the chylopoietic viscera. The determination to resist nourishment arises, under such circumstances, from a *positive loathing of food—a want of all inclination for it.* I have seen cases of this description, where it has been deemed necessary, in order to prolong life, to introduce food forcibly into the stomach, speedily cured by the adoption of means for improving the state of the general health and digestive organs. Mild alteratives, vegetable tonics, blisters over the region of the stomach, if the patient complain of pain in that region upon pressure, the warm and shower-bath—is the most successful treatment to adopt in cases connected with obvious visceral derangement. Instances sometimes occur, where the refusal of food is clearly traceable to a delusive impression—a hallucination of taste, which makes everything appear to the patient bitter, disgusting, and poisonous. The unhappy patient imagines that he is commanded, either by good or evil spirits, not to eat. These unhappy persons must be treated upon general principles, and the remedies be adapted to the peculiar character of each individual case. Under such hallucinations of taste, patients often swallow the most extraordinary articles. The case of a lunatic is recorded, who imagined that his stomach required to be strengthened with iron. He was seized with inflammation of the œsophagus, of which he nearly died. He then confessed that he had swallowed the blade of a knife. After his death, there were found in his stomach seven oxidated lath nails, each two inches and a half long; thirty-three nails, two inches long; forty-nine smaller iron nails and rivets; three pieces of wound-up iron wire; an iron screw, an inch long; a brass image of a saint; part of the blade of a knife; and other articles; amounting in number to 100, and weighing about twenty ounces. It will be necessary, in cases like those to which I have been referring, to ascertain whether the determination not to eat is the effect of such perversions or hallucinations of taste.

The time will only admit of my alluding generally to the importance, as a principle of treatment, of the administration of tonic remedies, active exercise in the open air, and to good and generous living. It is rarely necessary, in the treatment of insanity, to deprive the patient of animal food. Individual cases occasionally come under our notice, in which it is necessary, for a time, to enforce a farinaceous diet; but such is not often our duty. Among paupers, insanity is frequently cured by the free use of good animal food, and a generous supply of porter. Even when we are satisfied of the necessity of local depletion, it will often be necessary to give wine, and allow the patient a generous diet. *Part* xxvii., *p.* 313.

INTESTINAL AFFECTIONS.

Treatment of Injured Intestine from a Blow upon a Hernial Sac.— Accidents of this kind usually occur either by a direct blow, or by the person being forced against some hard body. Mr. Key says:

The extent of injury which the intestine sustains will vary according to the violence of the blow. The contusion may be insufficient to burst the bowel, or to occasion such a lesion of tissue as shall end in gangrene, its effects being only inflammation of the coats of the intestine: or the violence may be such as at once to rupture the intestine: or, failing to rupture the bowel, the contusion may be so severe as to be followed by sloughing and escape of fæces. These three states require distinct consideration, as the treatment required for each necessarily varies.

The mildest form of injury which a blow inflicts on a hernia is analogous to the contusion of other soft parts. Such contusions, it is probable, are not followed by any serious consequences.

Collapse, vomiting, and abdominal tension, are wanting to give a charter of severity to the injury.

The two first indications that immediately force themselves on the surgeon's attention, are, the necessity of returning the contents of the hernial sac, and obtaining free evacuations from the bowels. To the former of these proceedings there can be no objection, as the vitality of the bowel is scarcely endangered: and if it were left in the sac, adhesion might form between the injured bowel and peritoneum, that would afterward interfere with its return into the abdomen. The administration of purgatives ought to be wholly abstained from, notwithstanding the confined state of bowels usually consequent upon an accident of this nature. A bruised bowel is placed by nature in a state of rest: the exhaustion of the nervous energy of the part diminishes in the muscular tissue the disposition to contract. Such inactivity of the bowel should be encouraged, and not thwarted by irritating purgatives. The safety of the bowels depends on the non-occurrence of inflammation; but if, by undue interference, the bruised structure is hurried into a state of inflammation, sloughing or ulceration will probably be the result. Beyond an occasional enema, to unload the larger intestines, nothing need be done. Opium may be required, if pain come on, indicating peritonitis; and if joined with calomel, care should be taken that the action of the former should preponderate, in order to prevent the probability of stimulating the bowel. Food should also be given in the smallest quantity, and in a fluid form, that little or no feculent residue may remain to oppress the part. In this respect nature is our guide : vomiting which usually ensues immediately after the accident, empties the upper part of the canal ; and the little desire that the patient feels for food, prevents, if nature be allowed her own way, any chance of repletion.   Thus the part is placed in a state of repose ; and the circulation soon regaining its healthy condition, the functions of the intestines are restored.

The necessity for repose in an injured state of bowel it would be well to bear in mind, after the operation of strangulated hernia.   The bowel is gorged by the strangulation, bruised by the taxis as it is too often practised, or inflamed by long incarceration in the sac.   An intestine in such a condition cannot but be injured by an early administration of purgatives, which irritate and inflame the bowel, or exhaust what little remains of vital energy.

If the contusion be so severe as to destroy the vitality of the bowel without rupturing it, the condition of the patient, both immediately after the accident and for several days subsequently, sufficiently attests the severity of the lesion which the part has sustained.   The hernial sac is usually found filled with the injured bowel ; but the absence of distention serves to distinguish it from a state of strangulation.   The integuments appear to be bruised, though sometimes but slightly.   The part is very tender when handled, but feels soft and pliant ; and very moderate pressure is sufficient to reduce the contents of the sac.

The shock which the nervous system receives, is followed by a feebleness of the circulation, a corresponding pallor of the whole surface, and a sense of syncope.   This condition is, however, only transient : re-action almost immediately ensues : the patient passing from the state of collapse, and gradually rising into a state of inflammatory excitement, as the injured bowel becomes the seat of more or less inflammation.

The speedy recovery of the patient from a state of collapse, quickly dissipates the suspicion of a rupture of the intestine ; and the surgeon usually endeavors to replace the contents of the hernial sac as soon as reaction takes place.   To this proceeding there is no objection, if it be done with gentleness.   The danger of abdominal extravasation will not be increased by replacing the injured bowel at the neck of the sac ; for should sloughing of its coats ensue, the slough may be walled in by adhesion of the surrounding peritoneum, and fecal extravasation be prevented ; or, should this salutary process of adhesion fail to insulate the slough, the sac will receive the fecal matter, and quickly give intelligence of the impending mischief, by the tumefaction that will ensue within the scrotum.

The symptoms that arise in this state of things, in some points resemble those of a strangulated bowel.

It does not appear that persons are always aware of being the subjects of hernial protrusion.   Their ignorance of the fact is not to be taken as evidence of a rupture not having existed previously to the blow ; and it is of no little importance to establish the existence of a hernia, as without it, a rupture of a bowel is in the highest degree improbable, by a blow received upon the pelvis, or scrotum, or even upon the inguinal canal.

When the blow or injury has been so severe as to cause the rupture of the bowel, or the violence of the symptoms are such as to apprehend sloughing of the injured intestine, and the escape of the fæces into the peritoneal cavity, the most judicious practice, according to Mr. Key, is to open the sac, and if fæces are present to liberate them; and if not, to wait, in order to see if the bowel should slough. In either case, the opening of the sac will allow a free exit to any fæces which are, or which may be present. In one case, the patient experienced no relief for three days from the opening of the sac, when a copious discharge of fæces took place and completely relieved him. ◄In another case, the blow was so severe, and followed by such severe symptoms, that the bowel was supposed to be ruptured. On opening the sac, however, no fæces escaped for four days; at the end of which time, the fæces appeared and escaped freely. On the 7th day, the fæces escaped by the rectum, although they continued to pass through the wound for five or six weeks, when ultimately the part healed. These facts will recall to the minds of most practical men cases of such contusion, which have been left to themselves and have proved fatal by extravasation of the fæces into the cavity of the peritoneum, when an opening into the sac would have prevented such an occurrence; for although such an opening ought not to be undertaken except from the strongest suspicions that rupture or sloughing has been caused, yet, when we remember how often the sac is opened in cases of supposed strangulated hernia, without any danger resulting, we need not risk the life of a patient by an unnecessary delay in such a procedure. *Part* v., *p.* 104.

Wounds of the Intestines.—M. Boutard recommends a method of obtaining direct union in wounds of the intestines; in longitudinal wounds, by approximating the edges of the wound by means of suture; in transverse wounds, either by the same method or by invagination. To effect this, the author excises the projecting lip or ring of mucous membrane at the level to which the mucous and serous coats have retracted; the everted mucous membrane, with its epithelium, which prevents all union, being thus removed, on bringing the lips of 'the wound together, serous membrane is in contact with serous membrane, muscle with muscle, and bleeding mucous membrane with the same structure. If invagination is to be practised, the mucous membrane is scarified and excised to the extent of four or five millimetres in the portion of the intestine which is to be the recipient; and thus the serous surface of the invaginated intestine is placed in contact with a mucous surface reduced to a condition favorable to union. *Part* ix., *p.* 189.

Chronic Intestinal Eruption—Therapeutic Action of the Salts of Cerium.—The salts of few metals were at present in our pharmacopœia, and Prof. Simpson saw no reason why many more might not be added to their number. He had recently drawn the attention of the profession to the salts of nickel, which, as far as his observation went, presented much similarity in action to those of iron and quinine, and seemed to be of use in cases of sick headache. He now proposed to read to the society some very imperfect observations on the therapeutic action of some other metals: and first, as to cerium, which, given in the form of nitrate, and in one-grain doses twice or thrice a day, appeared to act as a sedative tonic of considerable value, strongly resembling bismuth, and the salts of silver. He had employed it, in the first instance, in cases of general chronic intestinal eruption—a peculiar and intractable form of disease, for which arsenic and nitrate of silver were generally prescribed; and where these remedies had failed, cerium had been tried with marked advantage. In irritable dyspepsia, with gastrodynia and pyrosis, and in chronic vomiting, its exhibition was attended with satisfactory results; and in the vomiting which occurs during pregnancy prompt relief was afforded. It was a good tonic, and a useful substitute for the salts of silver, bismuth and hydrocyanic acid. Dr. S. had not employed it much in convulsive diseases, as chorea and epilepsy, in which nitrate of silver was used, but the exhibition of the salts of cerium was certainly attended with this advantage, that it could be persevered in without any fear of discoloration of the skin. As far as his experiments with cadmium went, it bore much resemblance to the preparations of antimony, and excited diaphoresis and vomiting. Tellurium, besides its expense, was precluded from being used in practice by its disagreeable effects. Dr. S. mentioned a case where a dose had been inadvertently given to a student of divinity, and had been followed by the evolution of such a persistent odor, that for the remainder of the session the patient had to sit apart from his fellow-students.　*Part* xxxi., *p.* 222.

———•◦•———

INTESTINAL OBSTRUCTION.

Intestinal Obstruction from Stricture of the Sigmoid Flexure of the Colon.—The operation of M. Callisen, of Copenhagen, to produce an artificial anus in the lumbar region, over that portion of the intestine, not covered by the peritoneum, has been revived by M. Amussat with great success. In all the old operations for this purpose in the iliac region, by MM. Littre and Pillore, the peritoneum was wounded, which seems to have been the chief cause of death in numerous cases. In his operation in the lumbar region, Callisen " proposed to make a vertical incision extending from the edge of the false ribs parallel to the anterior border of the quadratus lumborum muscle. He thus hoped to reach the colon between the layers of its short and imperfect mesentery." This operation, however, was attended with some difficulties, till modified by Amussat, who " has shown that the failure of the operation on the dead subject was owing to the intestine being empty, and that in such cases as require the formation of an artificial anus, the colon is greatly distended; in which condition the layers of the peritoneum, forming its imperfect mesentery, are so far separated as to allow the intestine being reached without opening the peritoneum." Amussat has, moreover, adopted the transverse instead of the vertical incision. This important operation has not only been performed on the adult, but also in an infant of forty-eight hours old.
Part v., *p.* 107.

Treatment of Volvulus.—Mr. Pilcher has recorded a case of volvulus occurring in a child, in which all the remedies commonly employed for the removal of the disease had been unavailingly employed, when he was induced by the recollection of a former case to order thin gruel to be injected by the rectum until the lower intestines had become completely distended, regurgitation being prevented by pressure around the anus. The effect was almost immediate, the obstruction giving way and the patient completely recovering.　*Part* viii., *p.* 73.

Internal Strangulation of the Intestines.—[Mr. Mackenzie remarks that, considering the great fatality of this disease, if left to itself, it is strange that operative interference is not more frequently resorted to.

An operation cannot make matters worse than, in the majority of cases, they are; while it is not unlikely to be successful if a correct diagnosis can be made. There is one class of cases which Mr. Mackenzie thinks can be diagnosed with almost certainty—cases of "*dislocation of the sigmoid flexure of the colon.*" Mr. M. says:]

I use the term dislocation, as being more applicable, inasmuch as it implies the operation of some active force, considering that condition necessary before a sudden displacement can take place. That the intestine is torn from its attachment by a sudden force, I am fully convinced, from having discovered the mesocolon lying in loose shreds amongst the intestines, saturated with extravasated blood: a circumstance which could not in any other manner be accounted for.

What renders this sigmoid flexure so peculiarly liable to dislocation, I am at a loss to determine. In those cases which have come under my observation, the imprudent use of raw indigestible substances, as cranberries, turnips, cabbage, etc., was suspected as the cause of the disease. Possibly violent distention of the tortuous gut, by flatus, may force it, on physical principles, to assume a straight position, and thereby a strain being necessarily made on its attachments, contribute to its separation. In whatever manner the displacement is effected, the result is remarkably uniform: the intestine is thrown from its natural situation toward the centre of the abdomen, and receives a twist at its termination in the rectum, which causes complete obstruction of the passage; the small intestines get coiled round it in such a manner as to strangulate the gut by the free margin of the mesentery. In these cases, while all the symptoms of strangulation and obstruction of the bowels are present, there is one symptom never absent, which, respect being had to the history of the case, leads to a correct diagnosis, namely, that it is impossible to throw up injection per rectum in any quantity, for as soon as the gut is filled as far as the twist or volvulus, which is always low down, the water or fluid injected flows out as fast as it is thrown up, independent of any action of the rectum itself. Besides, the introduction of the long tube is impracticable, being always arrested at the obstruction.

It is evident that no method of treatment, save by operation, can possibly do any good in this class of cases. The administration of purgatives in these as well as in every other case where there is mechanical obstruction, cannot be too severely reprobated, inasmuch as they invariably accelerate the fatal result, and add to the sufferings of the patient. ·

Part xvii., *p.* 162.

Ileus, or Volvulus.—The abdominal cavity should certainly be only opened as a last resource. When an exploration is determined on, it should be performed in the linea alba, except the obstruction is in the large intestine, when an artificial anus must be formed in the lumbar region.

Part xviii., *p.* 185.

Ileus.—In cases of intestinal obstruction, when the constipation is complete, and there is fecal vomiting, and these symptoms are not relieved by the use of ordinary means, for three or four days, it is justifiable to resort to operation. If there are satisfactory indications of the seat of the obstruction, make the incision at or near that point, but if there is much doubt, make it in the median line. If the cause of the obstruction cannot be removed, or it is deemed imprudent to make an extended search for it, make an artificial anus as near as may be to the seat of obstruction.

Part xix., *p.* 169.

Treatment of Obstruction of the Bowels.—[Let us suppose an instance of this kind. We are called to a patient who has had no proper evacuation from the bowels for the last seven or eight days, though he has taken repeated doses of powerful aperient medicines, none of which have operated effectually. On examination you find some degree of distention about the umbilicus, with a varying degree of tenderness on pressure. In severe cases you may find permanent sickness, mucus or bile being rejected from the stomach. The tenderness on pressure is not so great as we might expect. Flatus is felt to rumble in the intestines, and proceeds, as it were, downward to a certain point, and then stops. With all this the tongue is moist and often clean; the pulse is not perhaps accelerated, generally weak; the urine, provided the obstruction is not high up in the bowels, is not necessarily affected, though generally high colored.]

Under these circumstances, and especially in the milder cases, the first thing that perhaps you do is to order a large enema to be thrown up. It is found to traverse the large intestine easily; the patient assures you that he feels it go as far as the ilio-cæcal valve, and after a short time it returns without any tinge of fecal matter. The obstruction is not in any part of the colon, but somewhere in the small intestine.

We must not forget that the most simple case of obstruction is liable to run on into a fatal form, if, with the view of obtaining an action of the bowels, we are incautious in the prolonged use of irritating medicines. Concerning treatment, Dr. E. Wells continues:

Endeavor, in the first place, to compose and soothe the mind of the patient. A slight faintness, produced by blood-letting, has often acted beneficially in this state. After these measures, the safest plan is to give repeated doses of calomel and opium, the latter in half to one grain doses every four hours. Wait now until the bowels begin to act, which they generally will do, and when they do, then a small dose of castor oil will do good. Gruel may be taken now, as it prevents the sense of sinking, and probably acts mechanically in propelling the contents of the intestinal tube.

In those severer cases, where there is frequent sickness, with pain in the bowels, and a rumbling of flatus, abstain from giving any food by the mouth for some days. The support should be entirely trusted to beef-tea injections, these not exceeding a quarter of a pint, and administered every four hours. If there is difficulty of retention, add to them a few drops of laudanum.

It is proved that these are sufficient to maintain the strength for some time—at any rate, for a period sufficient to allay the irritating symptoms, which forbid the exhibition of food by the mouth. This part of the treatment I am inclined to consider as of the highest importance: for as long as food continues to be administered by the mouth, and is rejected by vomiting, there will be little chance of arresting the inversion of the peristaltic action of the intestinal tube.

Part xxiii., *p.* 119.

INTESTINES.

Intus-susception—Recovery from, by Sloughing of the Intestines.—
[At a meeting of the Royal Medical and Chirurgical Society, Mr. Jeaffreson read an account of a case of intus-susception of the bowel, which he had attended, and recovery by sloughing of a portion had occurred. The patient was a young man, 17 years of age. He was laboring under general febrile symptoms; the countenance was anxious, the abdomen becoming tympanitic: nothing would stay on the stomach: the matters vomited had a grass-green color. Calomel and opium, and purgatives, were given for three days, and clysters used, when decided symptoms of inflammation of the peritoneum and bowels appeared.]

Leeches, fomentations, etc., were used in addition to the other means, but no evacuations took place till the 31st, when there were very copious and offensive discharges from the bowels, and the vomiting ceased. From this date the patient gradually recovered. Copious evacuations took place, charged with gelatinous-looking mucus, and on one occasion a small quantity of blood. On the 8th of June, there was discharged from the bowels what the author supposed to be either a portion of the small intestine, or a cast of it (of coagulable lymph): it was about $2\frac{1}{2}$ or 3 inches in length, and of a tubular form; smelt horribly putrid, and one or two minute points presented the appearance of sphacelus. After this, with some slight interruption, the patient recovered. The substance voided was examined under the microscope by Mr. Toynbee, who stated that he found cellular tissue, traces of blood-vessels and nerves, and epithelium.

[Dr. Williams could not agree that such cases were remarkably uncommon, though they might rarely be met with by any one individual.]

In tropical climates it was by no means uncommon for even a foot or more of intestine to come away in severe cases of dysentery. It would seem almost as if this were the mode established by nature to effect a cure.

[Mr. Fitzmaurice had practised many years in Ceylon, where severe sloughing dysentery was very common among the natives.]

It was no uncommon occurrence for six, eight, or even eighteen inches of intestine to slough away, and yet recovery take place. In the Museum at Woolwich are many preparations illustrative of this fact.

Part xii., *p.* 199.

Wounds of the Intestines.—[When after a wound of the abdomen, we find symptoms of wounded intestine, without there being protrusion, we must keep the patient perfectly quiet, administer stimuli if needed, but insist upon total abstinence from food for some time.] B. Cooper says:

When the wounded intestine protrudes, its contents may be perceived issuing from the wound, although the opening itself appears to be closed by the protrusion of the internal mucous membrane. The size of this opening and its direction, as to whether it be longitudinal, or transverse, must now regulate the treatment to be adopted. If the wound be very small, its edges may be pinched up by a pair of forceps, and a thin silk tied round so as to include the whole of the wound; the intestine is then to be returned into the cavity of the abdomen, but must be kept as close as possible to the external wound. The ligature produces a sloughing of all the included tissues, and adhesive inflammation of the peritoneum being set up, an external wall of plastic matter is formed around the dead part, which ulcerates off into the intestines, and is carried away with the fæces. Sir Astley Cooper successfully employed this method of treatment in one or two cases in which the intestine had been inadvertently wounded in the operation for strangulated hernia.

When the opening in the bowel is large, different kinds of stitches are used to keep the edges of the wound in apposition. The uninterrupted suture, however, or glover's stitch, is, I believe, the best, but the finest procurable needle and silk must be employed; and after the bowel has been returned into its natural cavity, the same precaution as I have already mentioned to keep it in proximity to the external wound, should be adopted. When the intestine has been completely divided by a transverse wound, various plans have been recommended for reëstablishing its continuity. For this purpose, some animal substance of a cylindrical form, such as the trachea of a sheep, has been introduced. This serves as a sort of mold and enables the surgeon to keep the edges of the severed bowel in juxtaposition during the application of the suture, the foreign substance easily passing away afterward with the stools. Some have recommended that the upper extremity of the intestine should be passed into the lower, and that a ligature be then applied around the whole. This produces contact of the peritoneal coat of the intestine, above and below the ligature, and, as adhesive inflammation is set up, an effusion of plastic matter soon covers the ligature, and reëstablishes the continuity of the external part of the canal, the ligature itself, and the constricted portion, ultimately sloughing off internally, and being conveyed away with the excretions.

It has been objected to this operation, that, in bringing the severed ends of the intestines together, a serous is presented to a mucous surface, and that these two structures are ill fitted for union; but it is not intended in this operation that they shall unite; the union is caused by the effusion of the plastic matter from the external surface above and below the ligature, and from serous to serous membrane, the whole of the intestine included in the ligature being destroyed and sloughing away. M. Jobert has proposed, as an improvement in the above operation, to invert the inferior extremity before the superior is introduced. In that case, two serous membranes are brought in contact, and the union may take place at once between them; but, under these circumstances, the invaginated portion would not be included in a ligature, but retained in position by suture.

After all, however, from the result of the experiments, it remains questionable whether, in complete division of an intestine by a transverse wound, it is not better to establish an artificial anus and leave nature to her own efforts for the ultimate restoration of the patient; and this does not indeed appear to be so difficult a process as may be supposed, particularly if nature be judiciously assisted by the art of the surgeon.

Almost immediately after the divided intestine has been replaced in the cavity of the abdomen, an adhesive inflammation shuts out the open extremities of the intestine from the peritoneal cavity, so that after a few hours have elapsed the stitch employed to secure the wounded intestine near the external wound in the abdomen may be removed, and as soon as the feculent matter passes partly through the latter the patient may be considered safe, as far as refers to the danger of extravasation of the fæces mto the abdomen.   But as the formation of an artificial anus renders the patient loathsome to himself, and unfitted for a social state, subsequent means must be adopted to reëstablish the integrity of the intestinal canal.

With this view, one of the first steps is to diminish as much as possible a tendency which the upper portion of the bowel has to prolapsus or eversion of its mucous membrane; and this object may be attained by keeping the fæces in a semi-fluid state, and by maintaining slight pressure upon the extremity of the protruded part.   The lower portion of the intestine is liable to contract at its extremity, so that the ready passage of the contents of the upper portion is prevented from passing into the lower; this may be in some measure obviated by the use of enemata, which stimulate the natural action of the bowel and prevent it from falling into the abnormal condition always produced by disuse.   The strictest attention to cleanliness of the external wound should constantly be observed, otherwise the presence of the feculent matter will interfere very materially with the progress of the healing process.   As the wound goes on uniting it gradually contracts into a narrow fistula: this contraction is still further promoted by gentle pressure; and after a while, as the fæces meet with some resistance in the direction of the wound, they acquire a tendency to pass on through the natural passage—a change which is first indicated by the escape of flatus and mucus per anum; upon which enemata, should be freely employed to reëstablish the natural function of the rectum and anus.

By such treatment, a recent artificial anus may very generally be .cured, but if neglected, the lower part becomes so much retracted, and at the same time contracted, as to render the cure almost impossible.

In gun-shot wounds where the ball has penetrated the parietes of the abdomen and wounded a viscus, nature has sometimes effected the reparation of the part—the ball passing away with the fæces.   A musket ball has also been known to penetrate and lodge in the urinary bladder, from which it has afterward been removed incrusted with calcareous matter, the patient ultimately recovering. ·   *Part* xviii., *p.* 175.

Peculiar Affection of the Intestinal Mucous Membrane.—Treatment by Electro-Galvanism.—[Dr. Cumming gives a detailed account of a disease, which, he says, is not described in systematic works, but which is, nevertheless, very common, and is productive of serious discomfort to the patient.   Dr. C. says:]

We are often consulted by patients who, at the first glance, convey the impression that they are imperfectly nourished: they have an emaciated appearance.   In detailing their symptoms, they lay great stress on a feeling of emptiness, or rather faintness, at the epigastrium: they complain of exhaustion there.   They generally next direct our attention to a more or less fixed pain either in the left hypochondriac or iliac region, sometimes both, more frequently the latter—a pain from which they are rarely exempt, and which is sometimes very severe and acute, though oftener annoying and irritating.   If they have ever been induced to apply a mustard blister to the seat of pain, they dwell on the relief, great, though temporary, they have experienced from it.   The stomach, in most of the cases I have seen, has not been irritable;·it commonly retains and 'digests the food; ·but pain is frequently felt in the course of the colon, in a period varying from an hour to two hours thereafter. · The bowels are at one time constipated, at another lax, in the same person. Some are uniformly costive, others more frequently loose ; but in all (*and this is the characteristic mark of the disease*), a peculiar membranous, fibrinous matter is discharged. In some cases it is stringy, in others tape-like in its form ; in others again, in small masses, resembling fat ; while in the milder cases it is more diffluent and gelatinous. That the disease has, from want of proper examination of the intestinal evacuations, frequently eluded observation, I know too well from my own experience, and that it has consequently been maltreated does not admit of doubt.

To take the report of the appearances from the patient is, in too many instances, the surest way to deceive both you and himself. In addition to this, there is not unfrequently a considerable discharge of blood from the bowels, and that, too, where no hemorrhoids can be detected. Almost uniformly there is great pain during evacuation, and always a feeling of exhaustion for some time after. In most of the patients there is a peculiar expression of countenance. It is an expression of anxiety, quite different, however, from that which usually marks organic disease. You do not conclude, as is too often the case with the latter, that your patient is laboring under an incurable malady.

Scarcely less characteristic of the disease than any of the preceding symptoms is the state of the mind. In all there is more or less nervousness, greatly increased toward night, inducing sleeplessness : and when, toward morning, sleep does come on, nightmare is frequent—dreams (generally of an unpleasant nature) invariable.

When the affection has been of long duration (and too frequently this is the case before we are consulted) the mental irritability is very great.

It is vastly more common in the female than in the male sex, though by no means uncommon in the latter ; and in the former it is very often accompanied by dysmenorrhœa, and occasionally by the membranous form of that affection.

In the treatment, the primary, and, I believe, indispensable point is total, or almost total, abstinence from aperient medicine ; and secondly, external counter-irritation.

Circumstances, which I need not at present detail, led me to surmise that electro-galvanism would accomplish both these indications of treatment. The results of its use in a considerable number of cases of this disease, warrant me, I think, in affirming that it is competent of itself to the cure of almost every ease, and that, aided by the internal exhibition of tar, it will cure both certainly and speedily. In the first place, it acts as an aperient—seemingly by its action on the muscular coat, as well as the mucous membrane of the bowels. *In every case* in which I have used it this has been the effect ; and if it had no other consequence than this, the advantage would be prodigious ; for, as in a multitude of instances, the disease has been traced to the use or abuse of laxative medicines as a cause, and as during the treatment even the mildest aperients irritate the membrane, and so far aggravate (temporarily) the disease, the evacuation of the bowels, by any means that do not irritate, is obviously of great consequence. It supersedes counter-irritation. The pain in the side, for the removal of which the counter-irritant was employed, is relieved by an application of the galvanism for at least twenty-four hours ; in many cases for a much longer period ; but as the agent is applied once a day, where no contra-indicating cause exists, till the disease is removed, the pain may be said to be abolished.

Galvanism, therefore, might of itself effect a cure; but I have generally combined it with the administration of tar, suggested first, I believe, by Dr. Simpson, and have found it of all internal means by far the most effectual. It relieves the feeling of exhaustion at the epigastrium, imparts an agreeable warmth, and promotes appetite and digestion. The plan I have hitherto adopted has been, to give the tar, in the form of pill or capsule, thrice a day; the electro-galvanism (Kemp's, of Edinburgh, machine is the one I have used), is applied for a quarter of an hour daily, the intensity being increased from time to time. Steady perseverance is requisite. With this, the case must be obdurate indeed that will resist a cure.

One remarkable fact connected with the treatment by galvanism is, that it *determines* the portions of the bowels where the greatest amount of irritation exists—a knowledge which manual pressure fails to convey; for it is a singular truth, that when the instrument is in action, extreme tenderness is complained of in more than one well-defined spot or tract, of which the patients were not previously aware. And it is extremely interesting to observe how this tenderness, after a time and the continued use of galvanism, diminishes till a mere point is fixed on as its seat, and how this also is removed. *Part* xxi., *p.* 150.

Intestines—Stricture of.—If the stricture is low in the colon, the vomiting does not come on until some time afterward; if it is in the small intestines, the vomiting comes on early. If the vomiting is not stercoraceous, it is not likely to be an obstruction of the small intestines. When it is in the larger intestines, it takes a longer time to produce stercoraceous vomiting than when it is in the small. When the seat of obstruction is below that point, Amussat's operation of an artificial opening is the most preferable in the left colon. When this, from the circumstances of the case, cannot be effected, then the opening should be made in the right colon.
Part xxv., *p.* 204.

Wounds of the Intestines.—Mr. Guthrie gives the following: When an incised wound in the intestine is not supposed to exceed a third of an inch in length, no interference should take place; for the nature and extent of the injury cannot always be ascertained without the committal of a greater mischief than the injury itself. When the wound in the external parts has been made by an instrument not larger than one-third, or from that to half an inch in width, no attempt to probe or to meddle with the wound, for the purpose of examining the intestine, should be permitted. When the external wound has been made by a somewhat broader and longer instrument, it does not necessarily follow that the intestine should be wounded to an equal extent; unless it protrude, or the contents of the bowel be discharged through the wound, the surgeon will not be warranted in enlarging the wound, in the first instance, to see what mischief has been done. It may be argued that a wound four inches long has been proved to be oftentimes as little dangerous as a wound one inch in length; yet most people would prefer having the smaller wound, unless it could be believed that the intestine was injured to a considerable extent. Few surgeons even then would like to enlarge the wound to ascertain the fact, unless some considerable bleeding, or a discharge of fecal matter, pointed out the necessity for such an operation.

If the first two or three hours have passed away, and the pain, and firm but not tympanitic swelling in the belly, as well as the discharge from the wound, indicate the commencement of effusion from the bowel, or an extravasation of blood, an enlargement of the opening alone can save the life of the patient. The external wound should be enlarged, the effused matter sponged up with a soft, moist sponge, and the bowel or artery secured by suture. When a penetrating wound, which may have injured the intestine, has been closed by suture and does not do well, increasing symptoms of the inflammation of the abdominal cavity being accompanied by general tenderness of that part, with a decided swelling underneath the wound, indicating effusion beneath, the best chance for life will be given by re-opening the wound. It is a point in surgery which a surgeon should contemplate in all its bearings. The proceeding is simple, little dangerous, and under such circumstances can do no harm.

When the wounded bowel protrudes, or the external opening is sufficiently large to enable the surgeon to see or feel the injury by the introduction of his finger, there should be no difficulty as to the mode of proceeding. A puncture or cut, which is filled up by the mucous coat so as to be apparently impervious to air, does not demand a ligature.

An opening which does not appear to be so well filled up as to prevent air and fluids from passing through it, as such wound cannot usually be less than two lines in length, should be treated by suture. When the opening is small, a tenaculum may be pushed through both the cut edges, and a small silk ligature passed around, below the tenaculum, so as to include the opening in a circle, a mode of proceeding I have adopted with success in wounds of the internal jugular vein, without impairing its continuity; or the opening may be closed by one, two, or more continuous stitches, made with a very fine needle and silk thread, cut off in both methods close to the bowel, the removal of which from the immediate vicinity of the external wound is little to be apprehended under favorable circumstances. The threads or suture will be carried into the cavity of the bowel, as has been already stated, if the person survive; and the external part of the wounded bowel will either adhere to the abdominal peritoneum, or to one or other of the neighboring parts.

When the intestine is more largely injured, in a longitudinal or transverse direction, or is completely divided as far as, or beyond the mesentery, the continuous suture is absolutely necessary.

When the abdomen is penetrated and considerable bleeding takes place, it is necessary to look for the wounded vessel. When the hemorrhage comes from one of the mesenteric arteries, or from the epigastric, the wound is to be enlarged until the bleeding artery is exposed, when ligatures are to be placed on its divided ends, if they both bleed. I have seen the epigastric artery tied several times with success.

A Portuguese caçador, on picquet, was wounded at the second siege of Badajos, in a sally made by some French cavalry. He had three or four trifling cuts on the head and shoulders, and one across the lower part of the belly, on the right side. He bled profusely, and when brought to me had lost a considerable quantity of blood, which came through a small wound made by the point of a sabre. This wound I enlarged until the wounded but undivided artery became visible; upon this two ligatures were placed, and the external wound was sewed up. The peritoneum was opened to a small extent, but the bowel did not protrude, and the patient (not being an Englishman, and not, therefore, so liable to inflammation), recovered.

The recollection of other nearly similar cases, causes me to say, that when hemorrhage takes place from within the abdomen, the wound should be enlarged; and that if an artery in the mesentery, or in any other place which can be got at, should be found bleeding, a very fine silk ligature should be placed, if possible, on each side of its divided extremities, and cut off close to the knot, the external wound being afterward accurately closed. This is a point of practice to which future attention is directed.

When a musket-ball penetrates the cavity of the belly, it may pass across in any direction without injuring the intestines or solid viscera. It usually does injure one or the other, and it has been known to lodge without doing much mischief. The symptoms are generally indicated by the parts injured, although in all, the general depression and anxiety are remarkable; their continuance marks the extent, if not the nature, of the mischief. *Part* xxviii., *p.* 190.

Intestinal Catarrh.—In those cases of intestinal catarrh in children in which the mucous membrane becomes ulcerated around the anus, give an enema containing about a drachm of borax. *Part* xxxvi., *p.* 300.

———•••———

INTOXICATION.

Results of Drinking.—Of all diseases of the internal organs produced by drinking, the granular liver seems to have attracted most attention; perhaps justly; but there is no doubt, that of all organic diseases, the two most to be feared in intemperate persons with recent surgical injuries, are the granular kidney, and slight but general emphysema, with a dilated, but not always much diseased heart; and in persons past the middle of life, dying rapidly in hospitals after operations and surgical injuries, combined with much loss of blood, these two affections of the urinary and respiratory organs are very far from uncommon. The three chief affections destroying patients after operations and injuries — namely, the general habit produced by drinking; secondly, organic disease of the lungs and kidneys, especially emphysema in the former, and granular disease in the latter; and, thirdly, tubercle—act very differently and at different periods. During the early period, and often for weeks after operations, patients laboring under tubercular disease do well; and it is often only at the absolute return to health, rather than during the recovery of the patient from the operation itself, that the effects of tubercle begin to show themselves. Organic disease produced by drunkenness, and habitual drunkenness, act differently; the organic disease presses heavily at every period, and may destroy life early or late; but the mere habits of the drunkard show themselves chiefly at a very early period. The patient who nearly sinks from his unsound organs within the first few days, often lags on for weeks and months in danger; but the man who has simple delirium tremens is taken ill directly, and often dies; but if he recovers from his delirium, he generally gets well from the operation, and sometimes quickly. *Part* xiv., *p.* 324.

Intoxication.—It is sometimes puzzling to distinguish intoxication from cerebral disease.

Mr. Corfe says: A patient is brought into the hospital, perhaps on a policeman's stretcher, or he is carried in by friends, who state that he was picked up in the streets, senseless. His pupils are dilated, immovable; his breathing is deep, and low, and heavy, the expiration being short and abrupt, whilst the inspiration is a prolonged deep sigh, with more or less stertor; pulse is full and strong. The suspicion arises that the man has sanguineous effusion into one or both ventricles of the brain. But it must be again acknowledged that, of all the perplexing, deceitful, and varying symptoms which diseases occasionally put on, those of cerebral lesions or mere cerebral disturbance are, of all others, the most difficult to decide upon. We have admitted cases into the hospital in the dead of the night, brought here by policemen, who have found the patient senseless, or he has been seen to fall senseless on the pavement; we have bled, blistered, leeched, and purged; shaved the head, and given turpentine enemas, but all to no purpose; insensibility has remained; when, to our surprise, in twelve hours afterward we have gone to visit our patient, we have found him perfectly sensible and tolerably well, not more surprised at the loss of a head of hair than we have been at the sudden revival of our supposed case of apoplexy. Whilst, on the other hand, I have admitted a case as one of "dead drunk," perfectly inanimate, and have, for the sake of precaution, sent him into the ward to bed, and yet have found it to prove an instance of apoplexy. I have, however, learned a valuable lesson by even these difficulties: for in every instance of late years when a case of complete insensibility is admitted, I have requested the house surgeon to empty, and then wash out, the stomach by means of the pump; and if it has been from drunkenness, the "sot" has shown his character up before we have finished this operation; and if it has been one of apoplexy, it has done no harm, and it has proved that it was more than intoxication, as no alcoholic fetor has been detected in the contents of the stomach.

In all cases of intoxication the mental faculties become roused before the operation of thoroughly washing out the stomach by the pump is concluded; whilst, on the other hand, it may be said, the reverse is ordinarily the case in cerebral lesions, or in mere concussions of the brain. Before we allow the tube to be withdrawn from the stomach, in cases of inebriety, we usually inject three ounces of the diluted acetate of ammonia draught, which has an extraordinary effect—sometimes in "sobering" the head, and calming the stomach too.

I am aware that it is much easier to recommend the employment of the stomach-pump than to administer it to persons who are sometimes in the highest state of excitement bordering on maniacal fury. I am anxious, therefore, to describe the mode in which we employ this remedial agent in such cases:

The patient is seated in a strong wooden chair, another chair is placed behind him, and an attendant is ordered to sit in it, and taking the arms of the patient, he pinions them by holding the wrists firmly against the back of the chair. This method serves to fasten the trunk securely in the chair; the legs are then swung in a round towel, which is passed round the ankles by a noose, and, a second chair being placed, so that the back of it shall be toward the legs of the patient, another attendant is placed in it; he carries the towel over the back of the chair, and sits upon it, and thus the legs are at right angles with the trunk, and consequently they are almost powerless. If, however, the man offers to flex the knees, the ankles are instantly raised higher, and the power of the flexors of the thigh is thereby overcome in an instant. By this position, it will be observed, that the patient is deprived of all muscular power, and the only fixed point on which his body rests is the ischiatic tubera. I am satisfied that the stomach-tube may not only be introduced with comparative ease, but that the operation of the pump is perfectly harmless, when judiciously administered, upon a refractory patient thus immovably fixed. *Part* xvii., *p.* 49.

Action of Alcohol.—From an elaborate series of experiments, the following conclusions are arrived at by Dr. Duchek : 1. Alcohol in the organism is subservient to an increased combustion, the intermediate products of which are found in the blood. 2. Intoxication is dependent upon the existence of aldehyde in the blood at the time. 3. The effect of aldehyde upon the blood is that of rapid consumption of oxygen ; and, finally, 4. Hereby the combustion of other substances is interrupted, or rather diminished.

[In these short remarks the reader will at once perceive the most powerful inducements to abstain from alcohol. It runs away with that oxygen which he is always inspiring for the oxidation which is required in almost every process of the animal economy. We live, as it were, to oxidize. Almost all the changes in the body are the results of oxidation, and yet the spirit drinker continually checks this process of nature.] *Part* xxx., *p.* 298.

Chronic Alcoholic Poisoning.—From the long-continued use of alcoholic drinks, even long after their discontinuance, various nervous symptoms sometimes arises, as hallucination and loss of sleep. Oxide of zinc in two grain doses, twice a day, an hour after each meal, is the best medicinal treatment that can be adopted, this dose may be gradually increased till the patient takes six or eight grains twice a day. Of course it is necessary for the patient to cease drinking. By the use of the above remedy, sleep was induced, and the trembling of the body and limbs along with other nervous symptoms, rapidly disappeared. *Part* xxxix., *p.* 56.

IODIC PREPARATIONS.

Hints for the Administration of Iodine.—Dr. Mojsisovitz, of Vienna, has contributed an elaborate paper to the Medicinische Jahrbucher, on the administration of iodine and its various preparations, in which he has pointed out certain precautions which are probably not generally known, and the ignorance of which may account for the unsatisfactory results so often derived from their use.

As the feculent matters decompose the preparations of iodine, we find this substance in the state of ioduret of starch, in the stools of those who eat bread, potatoes, rice, gruel, and vegetables, while taking the medicine. It is therefore necessary to interdict the use of every sort of food containing fecula to patients to whom iodine is given. It is probably owing to a decomposition of this kind having taken place, that we are to explain the inert effects of those enormous doses of the medicine which have been exhibited by some physicians, as Dr. Elliotson, Dr. Buchanan of Glasgow and Professor Forget of Strasbourg.

According to the experience of our author, the use of saline baths greatly promotes the action of iodine on the system. He has also reason to believe that the activity of its operation is a good deal influenced by the condition of the weather at the time. When the air is clear and dry, it seemed to have most effect, and more especially when there was a tendency to inflammatory complaints : whereas, on the other hand, its action seemed to be almost null during the endemic prevalence of small-pox, puerperal fever, and diarrhœa.

The crises, which iodine has a tendency to provoke, are salivation, and a cutaneous eruption like scarlatina or miliaria ; the secretion of the urine is usually the more abundant in proportion as the diet of the patient is kept low and restricted.

Dr. M. prefers the hydriodate of potash, and the proto and deuto-iodurets of mercury, to either pure iodine or to any other of its preparations. He regards the tincture of iodine as one of the very worst formulæ that can be used ; it is more likely, he says, to cause a wasting of the testicles or mammæ, hemoptysis, palpitations of the heart, etc., than any of its salts.

The dose of the hydriodate which he recommends for adults is about fifteen grains dissolved in distilled water, in the course of the day.

If there be any open ulcers, they should be kept wetted with a solution of the hydriodate ; but if the local affection be a tumor, then he recommends that it should be well rubbed with the ointment composed of two parts of the proto-ioduret of mercury and twenty-four of lard.

The disease in which Dr. M. has used iodine with advantage are, œzena, ulceration of the tongue, palate, etc., various forms of obstinate cutaneous disease, and of secondary syphilis, white swelling, and other maladies of the joints, periostitis, tumefaction of the lymphatic glands, scrofulous induration of the subcutaneous cellular tissue, and many of the other kinds of strumous disease.   *Part* iv., *p.* 58.

Iodide of Potassium—Therapeutical Action of.—Dr. Lisfranc obtains great success from the administration of this substance, in white swellings, necrosis, ulcers of the legs, engorgement of the breasts and testicles, chronic syphilis, and some diseases of the skin. When a patient is about to be submitted to this mode of treatment, certain precautions are necessary, since some persons may take ʒj., without experiencing any inconvenience, whereas others cannot take gr. iv., and even grs. ij., without offering untoward accidents. Formerly Dr. L. added from Ɵss. to Ɵj. of iodine to the iodide, but, having remarked that it gave rise to intestinal irritations, he omitted it, and now employs the following formula : ℞ Aq. destill. tiliæ Europ. ℨv., sirup. aurant. ℨj., iodid. potas. Ɵj. M. Ft. mist. cuj. cochl. mag. mane nocteque sumend. ex aqua, decoct sapon offic. vel infus humul lup. This quantity is usually taken in the space of a week, and, on renewing the draught, the dose of iodide is raised to Ɵiss., and an equal quantity is added to each succeeding one, until the patient takes ʒiiss., ʒiij., ℨss., and even ʒv., which last Dr. L. very seldom surpasses. The advantages resulting from the administration of this substance are : amelioration of the general health, especially in lymphatic patients affected with necrosis, and abundant suppuration, or marasmus, caused by an old white swelling. The inconveniences are: an astringent, metallic taste in the mouth, with some patients very disagreeable, every morning on waking; this may be remedied by the use of the tooth-brush, or gargles, with water alone, or water to which, for every half tumbler, a tablespoonful of the spirit. cochlear. is added; a cutaneous eruption, similar to urticaria, and when the remedy is continued, resembling eczema, or prurigo; when the face is the seat, the subcutaneous cellular tissue is swollen, and forms small tumors, like tubercles. These accidents ought not to prevent the administration of the remedy, when the disease is very serious; but when it is slight, the medication must be ceased for a time, and then recommenced. As to the iodic salivation, observed by Mr. Wallace, Dr. Lisfranc, in upward of one hundred patients, never witnessed it once. The disease in which Dr. L. has advantageously had recourse to it, are: tertiary syphilis, and that in spite of irregularities in regimen and excess of drink; this was especially manifested in one of the lesions produced by the affection, which is seated in the rectum, and resembles cancer; so much so, that he always commences by administering the iodide, and it is only when that substance, aided by compression, etc., has failed, that he decides upon operating. In necrosis of the bones of the extremities, and for which amputation seemed to be the only means of obtaining a cure; the parts thus affected, were the femur, the tibia, the phalanges, after whitlow. White swellings; ulcers of the legs; for instance, in those of atonic nature, or in wounds which, on individuals of a lymphatic temperament, from want of attention and cleanliness, or from friction, have become covered with vegetations, bleeding with the greatest facility, and, in every respect, analogous to a cancerous ulcer. The cicatrix thus obtained, is, from its very formation, white, firm, resistant, and allows the patient to move about at a very early period. Cancer of the uterus, and of the breast; in the pain caused by these affections, opium is administered in some cases; at first it soothes, but very soon becomes inefficacious; nor does it ever prevent the disease progressing; their cure may then be attained with the iodide of potassium. In engorgements of various organs, chronic orchitis, tumors of the breast, etc.

It sometimes happens that, when this substance has been given a few days, the accidents above described appear; in such cases we must cease to administer it for eight or ten days, and then recommence it, to be ceased again should the accidents reappear; and it is very rare that, after having prescribed it thus, it is not tolerated on the third or fourth trial. Again, in diseases which require it to be taken for a very long time, certain peculiarities may be observed; for instance, when the iodide is administered to a patient affected with white swelling, at first a notable amelioration manifests itself, but very soon after the disease becomes stationary, and anorexia and insomnia declare themselves. Such a state is what Dr. L. calls iodic saturation; here, the continuation of the remedy is not only useless, but even hurtful; it must therefore be discontinued for a time, the patient be ordered to amuse himself, to take a nourishing diet, some tonics, etc., and to go into the country, if possible. Finally, when the system has thrown off the iodide, it may be prescribed anew, and with the same success as at first.   *Part* xi., *p.* 103.

Iodide of Potassium.—The iodide of potassium was shown by the late Dr. Robert Williams to be of great certainty in rupia and hard periosteal node; that its power is much less in roseola, purpura, and ecthyma, but still it is better than mercury; while, in lichen, lepra, psoriasis, and iritis, mercury is more beneficial than the iodide. If suppuration has commenced in the node, then sarsaparilla is the remedy, the iodide being useless. In soft node and prurigo, he showed the true power of sarsaparilla; and in syphilitic angina and rupia, the invariable good effects of combining local mercurial applications with the internal administration of the iodide of potassium.   *Part* xxiv., *p.* 268.

Iodine rendered Soluble by Sirup of Orange-peel and Tannin.—M. Debauque has found means of keeping iodine in a state of solution, when added to mixtures in the form of tincture. The author uses, for that purpose, sirup of orange-peel, which answers the purpose perfectly. It was suspected that *tannin* was mainly instrumental in this result; and this was rendered evident by putting a few grains of tannin into a quantity of water to which tincture of iodine had been added, and in which the iodine had of course been precipitated. The addition of the tannin caused the iodine to be immediately re-dissolved. Thus will the sirup of orange-peel be advantageously added to mixtures containing tincture of iodine, and tannin to injections composed of water and the same tincture.
                                                Part xxv., *p.* 306.

Topical Application of.—The topical application of this remedy is very general. The following is the formula : ℞ Iodini, ʒj.; sp. vini rect., ʒj.; ft. solutio. It is better to keep this some time before using. It should be applied in glandular affections beyond and around the enlarged parts, so that the absorbed fluid may be carried through the gland by the lymphatic vessels. It is used topically, 1st, in *pleuritic and neuralgic stitches;* 2d, to the throat in cases of *aphonia* or hoarseness; 3d, to the mucous lining of the throat itself in cases of congestion and of *enlargement of the tonsils;* 4th, around the external parts of the eye, in cases of *strumous inflammation;* 5th, in all forms of *periostitis,* whether syphilitic or strumous; 6th, in *glandular affections* as above mentioned; 7th, as injections into cysts and cavities of *abscesses,* provoking adhesive, but not suppurative inflammation, as in hydrocele.   *Part* xxix., *p.* 326.

Iodide of Potassium with Ammonia.—It is said that this medicine is more valuable when combined with ammonia, gently stimulating the stomach, diffusing the blood, and with it the medicine through the system, and, by chemical decomposition, liberating the free iodine, and thus sending it on its salutary message.
The proportions usually prescribed are, two to three grains of the iodide with four to five of the ammonia.   *Part* xxx., *p.* 300.

Iodine Adhesive Paint.—The following is the formula for an iodine paint, made adhesive by the addition of mastic, which is used at the Moorfields Ophthalmic Hospital:
℞ Spirit. vin. rect., ʒij.; sp. æth. nitr., ʒiv.; mastic., ʒss.; iodini, ad saturat.
This is very useful where iodine is required about the eyes, as it does not run on the skin.   *Part* xxxiii., *p.* 292.

Effects of the Tincture of Iodine applied locally on the Mucous and Serous Membranes, in relation to Pain.—Dr. Boinet remarks that the contact of tincture of iodine with the mucous membranes is not at all painful'; and that it is possible to paint, almost without the consciousness of the patient, the pharyngeal and buccal mucous membranes, the tonsils, the neck of the uterus, the vagina, etc., without causing any pain; on condition, however, of not allowing the tincture to touch the orifices of the mucous cavities—namely, the points where the mucous membrane terminates and the skin commences; for the pain is very severe, and is prolonged for a considerable time, whether the tincture is applied to the lips, the anal orifice, or the female external parts of generation. In these cases the patients experience a pain as intense as when the tincture of iodine is applied to the skin denuded of its epithelium, or to a recent wound. There is the same pain when the ocular or palpebral conjunctiva is touched for the treatment of certain inflammations of the eye, the removal of granulations, etc. If several successive paintings take place, the same change ensues on the mucous membrane as on the skin—namely, that desquamation having taken place, the pain becomes then very severe after the subsequent application. As to the serous membranes, the tincture of iodine always produces in them very severe and cutting pains, and in an instantaneous manner. But this pain is much less severe upon the articular membranes than on the peritoneum. The acute pain produced by the contact of the tincture of iodine with the peritoneum is, in fact, a certain sign which indicates that an ascites has been mistaken for an ovarian dropsy; inasmuch as, in the latter affection, the iodine injection is never painful. This pain is also a proof, when it arises with less intensity in injecting an ovarian cyst, that a certain quantity has penetrated into the peritoneum.   *Part* xxxv., *p.* 281.

Iodide of Lime.—This preparation, made with one part of iodine and seven of lime, is recommended by Dr. Pidduck as superior to the iodide of potassium—in the comparative smallness of its dose; in its ready combination with the blood and tissues, manifested by its alterative effects; in not passing so quickly through the kidneys; in not producing gastro-enteric and vesical irritation: and in being nearly tasteless. Dr. Pidduck uses a solution of one drachm (containing eight and a half grains of iodine) in a pint of boiling water, which, when cold and filtered, is colorless and transparent. The iodine is found to exist in the solution in the form of iodide of calcium and iodate of lime.   *Part* xxxvii., *p.* 251.

IPECACUANHA.

Practical Remarks upon Ipecacuanha.—The value and efficacy of ipecacuanha, as an emetic or expectorant in many affections of the respiratory organs, more particularly of children, are too generally conceded and acted upon to require an extended notice.

In dysentery, ipecacuanha has been, and continues to be, much used. By Mosely, who held it in high repute, ipecacuanha was given in doses of half a drachm to two scruples; and by the late Professor B. S. Barton, it was regarded as almost a specific, particularly in cases of a typhoid character. In chronic diarrhœa, small doses of the powder, repeated several times a day, either alone, or preferably in conjunction with opium or Dover's powder, will be found of great value, and frequently, with strict attention to a proper regimen, will succeed in curing many most unpromising cases. In these last cases, when dependent upon, or connected with, derangement of the biliary secretion, additional power will be given to the above doses, by uniting with them two or three grains of blue mass, to be repeated every night as long as requisite.

In hemorrhage from the lungs or uterus, small doses of ipecacuanha, combined with sugar of lead and opium, are used with decided benefit. In hemorrhage from the stomach, large doses of ipecacuanha have been strongly recommended, particularly by Dr. Condie.

In the early stages of the bowel affections of children, no less than in adults, an emetic of ipecacuanha will often succeed in arresting the progress of the disease, and rarely fail to prove beneficial.

By combining from one-fourth to half a grain of ipecacuanha with a minute portion of opium, and two or three grains of blue mass, the alterative properties of this last are materially enhanced. This method will be found of great benefit in most mild cases of biliary and bowel derangement.

Formula for the Sirup.—Finding the process for the sirup, recommended in the United States Dispensatory, attended with unnecessary trouble, and uncertain as to uniformity, I adopted, after many trials, the following formula: ℞ Ipecacuan. rad. contus., ʒiv.; aquæ Oij.; sp. vin. rect., ʒx.; sacch. alb. lbs., iiij. Macerate the bruised ipecacuanha in one pint of boiling water for twelve hours, then add the remainder of the water and alcohol, and continue the maceration for five or six days. Place the whole in a small displacement apparatus, returning the fluid that passes until it becomes perfectly clear, and then continue to pour a small quantity of water occasionally upon the surface, until two pints and ten ounces by measure shall have passed. Now add the sugar, and with a gentle heat, evaporate until the syrup shall be of a proper consistence, readily ascertained by occasionally taking out a small portion and allowing it to cool. When of a proper consistence, pass it through a small quantity of fine tow placed in the tube of a funnel, to render the sirup clear and transparent. Three pints and ten ounces of sirup is the quantity obtained. It is, in strength, nearly double of that prepared by the usual formula; and this I consider an additional recommendation. *Part* xxiii., *p.* 299.

Saccharized Alcoholic Extract of Ipecacuanha.—Mr. A. G. Dunn recommends the employment of a saccharated extract of ipecacuanha in preference to the usual preparation of the drug, such as the wine and sirup, which he considers liable to vary in strength; and the powder is, he thinks, objectionable, from its insolubility. The following is the formula for preparing the extract:

Rad. ipecac., ʒiv.; bruise to a coarse powder, and macerate for thirty days in f. ʒxvj. of diluted alcohol, shaking it occasionally, then filter and express. Evaporate the tincture thus formed to ʒij. with which mix powdered white sugar, ʒviij., and triturate them in a mortar until they become dry.

The extract thus prepared has the peculiar odor and taste of ipecacuan; it is of a brownish-yellow color, and soluble in water, ether, alcohol, mucilage of acacia, and, in fact, in all the solutions with which this remedy is usually combined. The dose required to be exhibited is the same (twice as much) as the genuine powdered root. From its agreeable taste and perfect solubility in fluids, it is much preferred to the other preparations of the drug, by those who have employed it; more especially in prescribing for children, for whom its sweet taste renders it an excellent form for combining with other remedies.   *Part* xxx., *p.* 300.

———•••———

IRON.

Bisulphate of Iron and Alumina.—When ten parts of well washed alumina, three of soft iron filings, and five of carbonate of soda or potass, are compressed by fixed air for a considerable time in distilled water, a clear carbonated solution is obtained. But when the pressure is removed and the consolidation of the carbonic acid ceases, the solution no longer remains clear or permanent. When the fluid, however, is treated with sulphuric acid in excess, a *bi-sulphate* results in the crystals of which the iron is permanently safe from rusting or peroxidating in the air, or even when dissolved, as is the case with other salts, or preparations of that metal. When used as an *internal tonic* or *astringent*, the iron of this salt does not irritate; when applied as a lotion, it does not rust or stain the linen. Sir James Murray continues:

Great care must be taken not to confound this new saline remedy with a salt called by writers " *iron alum.*"

This new salt is also entirely different from a " *sulphate of alumina and iron,*" mentioned in some chemical works.

The new salt is very soluble in any cordial or aromatic water. I give it in doses of five or ten grains every two or three hours, till its effects succeed. In order to stay the bowels, in wasting looseness during cholera, it might be repeated much oftener. The iron is not a stimulant in this salt, but rather calms whilst it sustains. The aluminous quality abates tormina and soothes the mucous membranes. Even alum itself diminishes pain, and does not increase or induce paralysis of the intestines, as salts of lead are sure to do when long continued.   *Part* xix., *p.* 312.

Preparations of Iron: Ammonio-Acetas Ferri.—Dissolve one drachm of iron wire in half an ounce of hydrochloric acid, mixed with an equal quantity of water (by measure); then add half a gallon of water, and precipitate with an ounce of liquor potassæ; set aside for twenty-four hours; draw off the supernatant liquor with a syphon; fill again with water, and repeat the process a third time. Lastly, collect the precipitate on a linen filter; dissolve the oxide thus prepared in two ounces of strong acetic acid, and make up the measure to ten ounces with distilled water; set aside for twenty-four hours, and filter. To every twenty ounces of the filtered liquor add half a drachm of strong liquor ammoniæ. Dose ten minims to half a drachm.

Sirupus Ferri Acetatis.—Dissolve two pounds of sugar in ten ounces of water, in a water bath; to the sirup, whilst hot, add eleven ounces of the acetate of iron prepared as above (without the ammonia); when cold, filter through paper. Dose, twenty minims to one drachm.
          Part xxiii., *p.* 301.

Phosphate of.—Two specimens, one solid the other fluid, have been introduced, of phosphate of iron dissolved in the metabasic acid in a boiling state, and allowed to cool. If exposed to the air for a day it hardens, but can be made at once into pills, by means of liquorice powder or flour. It is stated to be superior to the other preparations of iron. Dose, one to two grains, three times a day.   *Part* xxiii., *p.* 303.

Administration of Iron in Food.—M. Martens read an essay before the Belgian Academy of Medicine, on Ferruginous Medicines. Among his conclusions, we find the following :

" Wheaten bread may be rendered much more nutritive " for chlorotic patients, " by adding a small quantity of sulphate of iron. In this way, alone, it can be capable of forming a substitute for meat."

In the discussion, it was suggested that the same method of medication would be beneficial to patients recovering from acute diseases, especially when the system was not yet able to bear animal diet. This idea is good ; and would be easy of application.   *Part* xxiii., *p.* 304.

Pyrophosphate of Iron.—There is no tonic which acts so promptly and favorably as the pyrophosphate of iron and soda, prepared in a liquid form ; it is easy to administer, rapidly absorbed, and does not produce fatigue to the digestive organs.   *Part* xxxvi., *p.* 254.

Sirup of Protocarbonate of Iron.—The facility with which protocarbonate of iron dissolves in organic acids, and its perfect harmlessness in irritable subjects, render it one of the most valuable agents in therapeutics ; accordingly, all the new preparations into which sugar has been introduced, for the purpose of giving stability to this saline compound, have been adopted in practice.

M. Dannecy, a distinguished pharmacien in Bordeaux, having ascertained that the precipitate of protocarbonate of iron obtained by mixing sweetened and boiled solutions of carbonate of soda and of protosulphate of iron possesses the singular property of dissolving in simple sirup without becoming colored, conceived the idea of thus preparing a new ferruginous sirup.

This preparation being permanent, will be employed in cases in which the form of sirup is preferable to that of pills ; for example, in the treatment of children.   *Part* xxxvii., *p.* 250.

—————•♦•—————

IRRIGATION.

Improved Method of Continuous Irrigation.—The instrument consists of a zinc reservoir, with a vulcanized India-rubber tube opening from it at its side, close to the bottom. The entrance of water into the tube is regulated by a stop-cock ; at the other end of the tube is affixed a broad zinc head, resembling a compressed or flattened rose of a watering-pot, a linear series of perforations being cut through its lower or convex edge. Equidistant from each other, and about half an inch apart, threads of worsted were passed through these holes from within, and made to project about three-quarters of an inch below the metal. This end was suspended over the part to be irrigated ; the reservoir charged with water placed upon the usual little shelf situated at the head of the bed, and the stop-cock being turned, allowed the water to escape into the tube. The extent and rapidity of the irrigation were, by the aid of the stop-cock, perfectly regulated.

A small sheet of oil-skin was placed under the arm and separated from the bed, the oil-skin being so arranged as to conduct the water which had passed over the limb into a basin or upon the floor of the ward. It is obvious that water of any temperature, or medicated in a prescribed manner, may be made, by this simple and cheap apparatus, to distribute itself over any part, however small or extensive it may be.

By enlarging or diminishing, by elongating or shortening, the head, or varying its form, the drops may be carried simultaneously over a larger or smaller, or any irregularly-formed surface.   *Part* xxvii., *p.* 257.

———•••———

ISSUES.

Mode of Inserting.—Dr. Geoghegan recommends the application of kali to the surface of the true skin, denuded of its cuticle by the application of a blister. The blister should be of precisely the same size as the issue to be inserted, and having been applied for the usual time, the cuticle should be gently but completely removed, and the superfluous moisture absorbed by a piece of lint (the surface of the skin not being rendered altogether dry). The stick of potass should be then passed once lightly over the entire surface, no friction whatever being necessary. The operation is now complete, save the removal of superfluous potass by the press-ure of a piece of lint applied after the lapse of about half a minute—a procedure which is, however, unnecessary, where due care has been observed in its application.

The caustic at once extends its influence into the substance throughout its entire depth, and the pain, which is of an active burning kind for some moments, rapidly subsides, and, in a great measure, disappears in from 15 to 30 minutes, in the generality of cases. By the mode of procedure just described, the more prolonged pain and apprehension attendant on rubbing in the caustic, is avoided; and from the simplicity and facility of the operation, the latter may be administered in the guise of a stimulant application to the blistered surface without inflicting on the sufferer the formalities of an issue, or the horrors of expectation. The destruction of the skin to an unlooked-for and undesirable extent, which is so frequent by the ordinary methods, is entirely avoided by the proposed modification.

Part xii., *p.* 251.

Issues—May be made by applying to the part, slightly excoriated or denuded of cuticle, a smooth zinc plate of proper size, having a silver wire soldered to its back; to the other end of the wire is soldered a smooth silver plate of the same diameter as the zinc, and this is closely applied to an abraded surface, *lower* down in the body than the zinc plate. In a few days an eschar will form beneath the zinc plate.

Part xviii., *p.* 340.

Issues—May be thus conveniently made by means of galvanism. Get a piece of perforated zinc fastened or riveted to a sixpence, shilling, or half-crown. Place this on the spot where the issue is to be made, with the zinc surface next to the skin, and cover it with a piece of spongio-piline moistened with salt and water. Moisten the spongio-piline with salt and water every twelve hours. An eschar will be thus formed in about twelve days, or, if the cuticle is removed before applying the little battery, the slough will be formed in from four to six days, but more irritation is created than by the former method.   *Part* xx., *p.* 272.

Issue-making.—Cut a hole the size of the issue required in a piece of leather plaster, and apply it to the part, then introduce into this hole powdered potassa cum calce, just sufficient to cover the skin, drop upon this two or three drops of spirits of wine, and cover the whole over with a large piece of plaster. In twenty-four hours the plasters may be removed.
     Part xxxv., *p.* 308.

—•••—

JAUNDICE.

Inspissated Ox-gall in Jaundice.—Dr. Johnson states that he has, in some very bad cases of jaundice, administered inspissated ox-gall in doses of five grains, gradually increased to ten grains, three times a day, with the best effect.   *Part* iii., *p.* 31.

Treatment of Jaundice.—[Dr. Budd recommends the following treatment in cases of jaundice arising from suppressed secretion :]

From ʒss. to ʒj. of sulphate of magnesia, in conjunction with gr. xv. of carb. of magnesia, and ʒss. of aromatic spirits of ammonia three times a day—the sulphate of magnesia to keep up free action of the bowels; the carbonate of magnesia to neutralize any excess of acid in the stomach or bowels ; and the aromatic spirits of ammonia to support the nervous system, and to keep up the action of the skin.   *Part* xxvi., *p.* 95.

Use of Turpentine in Jaundice, etc.—Turpentine has long been used in purpura hemorrhagica, and cases where the blood seems to become more diffluent than natural. Its efficacy in yellow fever has latterly been well shown by Dr. Laird, who considers the pathology of yellow fever as primarily connected with a morbid alteration of the blood, and that the turpentine, besides its general properties as a sedative, styptic, and antiseptic, possesses also peculiar power of action on the skin and kidneys. I can bear ample testimony to its success in another form of jaundice, which we meet with much more frequently in fever, and arising from a totally distinct cause ; I allude to jaundice from excessive secretion of bile. In the year 1845, Dr. Corrigan treated, with turpentine, a case of this kind ("considerable discharges of blood, mixed with bile, from the intestines") which occurred in the Hardwicke Hospital, and which recovered, even after the brain began to be affected. I have had in my wards several cases of this kind within the last three months, all of which recovered under the use of turpentine. The usual dose ordered is a drachm every two or three hours. It is frequently given with nitrous spirit of ether, to promote perspiration and avoid strangury. Dr. L. continues:

There is a form of jaundice occasionally met with in fever, and which is of great practical importance to be acquainted with. A patient in continued fever, without any appearance of jaundice or hepatic symptoms on the previous day, suddenly becomes quite yellow about the fourteenth or fifteenth day of fever, and all the tissues become impregnated with bile ; besides giving the usual tint to the skin and conjunctiva, the bile passes off by the bowels most copiously, and the urine is loaded with it. In one case I observed that the posterior part of the dorsum of the tongue, the soft palate, and fauces, had assumed the yellow hue, and that not merely the saliva, but the expectoration, was deeply tinged with it.

These cases are purely critical, and differ from other forms of crisis only in the organ in which the critical action takes place. Instead of occurring in any of the usual modes, such as perspiration or diarrhœa, etc., it occurs by a profuse secretion of bile, which endeavors to pass rapidly away through all the outlets of the body. Such cases require but little treatment; the rapidity with which all the icteric symptoms pass off is most surprising. There are two facts, however, to be noticed regarding it; one is, that the premonitory symptoms of this form of crisis are more severe than I have ever seen in any other; the other important feature in this mode of crisis, is the excessive debility which follows it.

I have also very frequently seen jaundice arise in the course of fever, as a symptom of pneumonia. *Part* xxx., *p.* 68.

Properties of Carbazotic Acid.—It is formed by the action of nitric acid on indigo, aloes, silk, and other organic substances. It forms yellow shining scales, soluble in water, to which it gives an intense yellow color and bitter taste. The process recommended by Liebig for preparing it consists in boiling ten parts of diluted nitric acid in one of indigo, and adding to the liquid, when cold, a quantity of potassa. The potassa combines with the carbazotic acid, and forms carbazotate of potass; which, in its turn, is decomposed by the addition of another acid, by which the carbazotic is set at liberty, and is deposited in brilliant yellow crystals. It is soluble in alcohol and ether. Dr. T. Moffat says:

I have prescribed carbazotic acid and the carbazotates of potass, ammonia, iron, and zinc, in eight cases, and in four of these the skin and conjunctiva became yellow during the administration of the remedies. They were completely jaundiced; and I believe that the yellowness was owing to the coloring matter of the remedies having tinged the serum of the blood. The coloration may have been owing to some change produced in the biliary system by the remedies; but I am inclined to the former opinion. The tinge of the skin and conjunctiva so perfectly resembles jaundice, that the keenest observer would be deceived.

Part xxxii., *p.* 41.

Jaundice.—The first principle to be borne steadily in mind in all cases, whatever their cause, is to promote in every way the functions of those organs compensatory by which elimination of bile is effected, using warm and vapor baths, saline purgatives, and the various kinds of diuretics. In employing blisters, cantharides is inapplicable, from its action on the kidneys.

In jaundice from acute congestion of the liver, leeches, cupping fomentations, etc., over the region of the liver, and saline purgatives to unload the engorged portal system, are the curative measures most likely to be followed by relief. When the congestion is primary, due to spirit-drinking, and such as may go on to inflammation of the adhesive character, mercury pushed to slight specific action is indicated; but in cases of closure of the ducts, mercury can do no good, here we can only carry out the principle of elimination by other channels. *Part* xl., *p.* 67.

JOINTS.

The Excision of Diseased Joints.—The removal of diseased articulating surfaces may certainly be ranked amongst the greatest triumphs of modern surgery. Instead of leaving the disease to wear out the constitution of the patient, or amputating the limb, and thereby crippling him for life, the joint is boldly laid open, the diseased portions excised, and the wound allowed to heal by granulation; taking care to place the limb in the most suitable position for its after use, after anchylosis has taken place.

Mr. Cooper says: Now, as to the *rationale* of the operation, I cannot help believing that those who have recommended the excision of joints, have dwelt too strenuously upon its advantages, as to the quantity of diseased structures which, by mechanical means, they remove. In my opinion, the great benefit which is derived is from exposing and perfectly laying open all the affected tissues, so that nature is not herself obliged to produce sinuses and ulcerations through the soft parts. It is not the quantity of bone you cut away, but, by exposing a large surface, you allow the diseased tissues to readily come away, instead of burrowing through the soft parts. No more should be removed than is evidently already destroyed by disease, and we find that this is generally confined to the articulating surfaces alone of the bones implicated. If you remove beyond this, you do no good, but, on the contrary, detach muscles which would otherwise have been of the greatest service to the new joint, and thereby render it far less capable of natural and useful motion. *Part* ii., *p.* 122.

Removal of Foreign Bodies in Joints by means of Subcutaneous Incisions.—The proceeding recommended by the author, Dr. Goyraud, of Aix, consists in pushing the loose body (if in the knee joint) into the synovial pouch above and to the outer side of the patella, beneath the vastus externus muscle, and while an assistant holds it fixed there, passing a narrow knife through the skin at some distance above the joint, and through all the intermediate tissue down to the foreign body. Without enlarging the opening in the skin, the synovial membrane and adjacent tissues over the loose substance are now to be freely divided, till, by the pressure on the latter, it slips out of the joint through the wound and lodges itself in the subcutaneous cellular tissue, or in some of the other tissues between the skin and the joint. After this the patient must remain at rest for several days (the small external aperture being merely covered by sticking-plaster), till all chance of inflammation occurring has passed away. The foreign body dislodged from the interior of the joint will form a cyst for itself, and remain in its new position without producing any annoyance; but if it should be deemed necessary, it may easily be removed by a single incision through the skin over it, which will no longer be likely to excite any inflammation of the joint itself. *Part* iii., *p.* 95.

Treatment of Cartilaginous Bodies in Joints.—Mr. Liston, in his lectures on the "Diseases of the Joints," says he has, in several cases, pursued the plan recommended by Dr. Goyraud, of Aix, with excellent success. *Part* ix., *p.* 185.

Use of Issues in Diseases of the Joints.—Dr. Brownless condemns the indiscriminate employment of issues in chronic diseases of the joints, believing that the continual and profuse discharge sometimes kept up by them is very injurious, by weakening the powers of life in diseases where so much depends upon the state of the general health.

If issues are used, make one of moderate size, and when it is nearly healed, make another at a different part of the joint; and do this again and again. If an issue is kept open (which is not advisable), it must not be with peas, but by occasionally retouching with caustic.

Part xv., *p.* 169.

Joints—Scrofulous Disease of.—Secure rest of the joint by plasters, leather or gutta percha splints, and bandages; but confine the patient to the house no more than is absolutely necessary, or the health will be injured, and the local disease thereby aggravated. Apply tincture or ointment of iodine, night and morning, so as just slightly to irritate the skin; and alternate its use with other stimulating liniments, blisters, or, in slight cases, the cold douche. When abscesses form, allow them to burst spontaneously. *Part* xxi., *p.* 25.

Chronic Disease of.—In chronic diseases of the joints, connected with gout and rheumatic gout, much may be done to prevent its progress at its very commencement. Place the patient on a careful system of diet, partaking very moderately of animal food, avoiding fruit, acids, etc., and taking little or no fermented or spirituous liquors. Perspiration should be induced by exercise or by the hot-air bath, once in a week or fortnight. Acetic extract of colchicum, in alterative doses, combined with mercurial pill, and occasional purgatives, should be given from time to time. Moderate doses of potash and magnesia (always avoiding soda) may be given three or four hours after the principal meals, to neutralize any superabundant acid in the stomach. If the patient is depressed by the colchicum, give Dr. Gregory's powder. Little is to be done locally. If pain is severe in the part, leeches may be applied, and, if need be, a bandage for the purpose of limiting motion. When the disease is fully established, these remedies may be still used to mitigate the symptoms, but we must then give the iodide of potash in two or three grain doses twice daily, and continue it for weeks, if it agrees with the patient. No general rule can be laid down. In one case, great benefit was found from the use of cod-liver oil locally, and from its administration internally. *Part* xxii., *p.* 192.

Iodine Injections in Hydrarthrosis.—M. Velpeau says, in his opinion, there is not more danger in injecting a joint than in injecting the tunica vaginalis, and that he has done it with complete success, the smallest possible trocar being employed. Neither does the question of injecting the abdomen in ascites with iodine seem to him one of mere hypothesis. Many French surgeons have related numerous cases followed by complete success, where the practice has been employed, while others consider the conclusions drawn to be somewhat hasty. *Part* xxii., *p.* 198.

Inflammation of the Synovial Membranes of Joints.—[As to the constitutional origin of these affections, Sir Benj. Brodie remarks:]

Inflammation of a synovial membrane may arise as a local affection, the consequence of a sprain, a contusion, or other mechanical injury. In other cases, various joints being affected, either simultaneously or in succession, it is manifestly the effect of a disordered state of the general system.

I must confess that, in proportion as I have acquired a more extended experience in my profession, I have found more and more reason to believe that local diseases, in the strict sense of the term, are comparatively rare. Local causes may operate so as to render one organ more liable to disease than another; but everything tends to prove that, in the great majority of cases, there is a morbid condition, either of the circulating fluid or of the nervous system, antecedent to the manifestation of disease in any particular structure.

[Sir Benjamin insists in the treatment " on the necessity of regarding them as constitutional and not local affections." When the joint is greatly and distressingly distended with serum, it is recommended to make a few minute punctures, and apply an exhausted cupping-glass; and as soon as pu is known to have been secreted, to make a free incision into the joint. He then says :]

" If it be a question whether the collection of fluid in a joint be purulent or otherwise, it is prudent, in the first instance, to make a puncture with a grooved needle. If it prove to be purulent, a free opening should then at once be made with a lancet, in a depending situation. It is important that this operation should not be long delayed, lest the matter should make its way out of the joint in other directions, and form irregular and circuitous sinuses among the neighboring tendons and muscles. It is equally important that the opening should be sufficiently large to allow the matter to flow spontaneously, without it being necessary to have recourse to pressure on the joint. If afterward there be reason to believe that there is still a lodgment of matter in any part of the joint or among the neighboring soft parts, the original opening should be dilated, or the surgeon should avail himself of the first opportunity which occurs of making another opening in a convenient situation; and it will often happen that several such openings will be required before the cure is completed."   *Part* xxiii., *p.* 271.

Joints—Diseased.—That as the separation of diseased cartilages from the extremity of the bone is commonly by a process of "shedding;" that as the portions so exfoliated tend to keep up a constant irritation within the joint; that as the natural outlets for these portions, the sinuses, are inadequate for that purpose; that as for their removal they have to be dissolved in the discharges of the joint, which is necessarily a very slow process; but as, whenever they are removed, an immediate process of reparation commences, Mr. Gay recommends that free and deep incisions should be made along the side of the joint, so as to lay open its cavity freely, and to allow of no discharges being retained by any possibility within it. The incisions should be made in the long axis of the limb. They should extend into the abscesses of the soft parts so as to lay them open, and the incisions should pass through sinuses, unless out of the way of the incision. If either of the bones be carious or necrosed, the incision should be made deep into them, to allow the free escape of diseased portions. Important vessels should be avoided. The wounds should be kept open by pledgets of lint, and free suppuration encouraged.   *Part* xxv., *p.* 179.

Scrofulous and Rheumatic Inflammation of Joints.—Mr. Stanley remarks upon the difference in the frequency with which certain joints are attacked by disease, and how exempt others seem to be from the like affections. An example of the former fact may be taken in the hip and knee joints, and of the latter in the lower jaw, the sterno-clavicular articulation, or the heads of the ribs with the vertebræ. Some explain this by their greater or less exposure to external influences; but this cannot be the case, else why should the hip be more frequently attacked than the ankle joint? Others say that joints are more susceptible from the activity of their functions; but few joints are more exercised than the lower jaw, and yet few are more free from disease.

I now come to the consideration of strumous inflammation of joints, and before proceeding to investigate its phenomena, the following questions demand attention: 1st. What are the circumstances which would lead us to regard the disease as strumous, when brought to the bedside of a patient? 2d. In what condition should we expect to find the structures, viz.: the bones, cartilages, and synovial membranes of a joint, provided the disease be strumous? With reference to the first question, I am unacquainted with any local symptom, any precise condition in the affected joint itself, which would enable us at once to decide on its strumous nature. We must look elsewhere. The age and aspect of the patient, the past or present existence of scrofulous disease in other parts, such as enlargement and suppuration of the cervical absorbent glands, strumous ophthalmia, tubercle in the lungs and other organs—any of these, especially if actually coëxistent, would justify us in regarding the disease as scrofulous. Often, indeed, these cases are obscure, and sometimes we are led to a wrong conclusion. The aspect of the patient is delusive, and should not be too much relied upon. Many instances occur in which the patient's appearance seems indicative of the existence of scrofula, whose subsequent progress and favorable recovery prove that such evidence is fallacious.

We have now to answer the second question. What is the state of a joint invaded by strumous disease? The morbid specimen I now exhibit shows the condition of the articular extremity of a bone in an extreme attack of this nature. The end of the bone is softened from absorption of its earthy matter, and its cancelli are filled with tuberculous deposit. It is, however, according to my experience, rare to meet with so complete an example of strumous disease as this specimen furnishes. In the majority of cases, I believe that no tubercular matter is found deposited, and when found, it is only in the last stages of the affection. Such a condition of bone, when it does exist, is, in my opinion, irreparable; and, when the surgeon is summoned to a case exemplifying the disease in this its latest stage, he can do nothing to restore the bone to its natural state, nothing to accomplish a cure. There is, however, an earlier stage in these affections, which you will often have to treat in private, although it is seldom seen in hospital practice—a stage amenable to treatment, a stage in which, generally speaking, the morbid impairment of the bone may be arrested, and its integrity restored. It is characterized by increased heat, and enlargement of the bone, immediately above the joint. There is, indeed, increased vascularity, and low inflammation of the bone, which is quickly followed by expansion of the cancellous texture, and absorption of earthy matter. Ultimately in bone thus degenerated, tubercle is sometimes deposited. Such, then, is the state of the bone in a joint affected with struma. The other structures—the cartilages, synovial membrane, etc., are in a state of low inflammation, inflammation which has commenced either in the bone or the synovial membrane itself, and which, if suffered to advance, is followed by its usual consequences—exudation, thickening of tissues, and sometimes suppuration. Now, the appropriate treatment for an attack of this sort is, perfect rest for the limb, and removal of all weight and pressure from the inflamed joint, so as to insure, as far as possible, its complete tranquillity. If inflammation exists in any activity, the judicious application of leeches will be beneficial; but it should be borne in mind that leeches must not be lavishly employed, as strumous patients cannot stand depletion. The remainder of the treatment is constitutional, and should be directed to the restoration of the general health, if that has failed; to its maintenance if it has not. To this end country air, or, where it is practicable, a resort to the sea-side should be recommended; a light, nutritious diet enjoined, and the state of the stomach and bowels be carefully attended to.

Not unfrequently disease in the soft tissues around a joint, inflammation, and abscess, are mistaken for disease inside the joint; and, in some instances, eminent surgeons have amputated limbs under the impression that an irremediable articular affection existed, while in reality, the exterior tissues alone were involved, the joint itself being sound.

Joints are liable to another form of inflammation, differing from that we have just reviewed—"rheumatic inflammation." The diagnosis of articular rheumatism is not usually difficult. When rheumatic fever is present, it is, of course, obvious; but, when it is not, the implication of other joints, the cause and symptoms of the attack, and the history of prior rheumatism, will generally guide us to a right decision; the implication of other joints, because it is extremely rare to find rheumatism affecting one joint only; it attacks two or three simultaneously, or flies about from one to another: the cause and symptoms of the attack—because we shall almost invariably find that the patient has been exposed to cold or. dampness, and because muscular pains are generally precursory to the articular inflammation. Rheumatic disease thus induced, is commonly marked by pain in one particular spot; the patient does not complain of general pain in the joint, but points to one especial locality, and describes it as the seat of all his sufferings.

Articular rheumatism is, moreover, intractable, leaving one joint and assailing another, or departing and recurring in the same joint. Joints are attacked by rheumatic inflammation in two ways; either their fibrous structures, their ligaments, suffer, or their synovial membranes. Now, the consequences of rheumatic inflammation of the ligaments may be serious, such, indeed, as may terminate in dislocation of the bones of a joint. For, under its influence, the ligaments become soft and elongated, so as to permit the bone to slip out of the cavity in which it is naturally fixed. In this way the head of the femur may be displaced upward on the dorsum ilii without rupture or ulceration of either the capsula or the ligamentum teres.

Rheumatic synovitis commonly ends in effusion. Ulceration of the articular cartilages may, however, supervene; and I have witnessed a case in which this condition was set up within nine weeks from the commencement of the attack, so that it was found necessary to amputate the limb. More usually, however, rheumatic synovitis gives rise to anchylosis, such anchylosis as may result from the adhesion of opposite synovial surfaces by effusion of fibrin, and which is called spurious, in contradistinction to true or osseous anchylosis.

Gonorrhœal rheumatism is a form of the disease occurring in conjunction with gonorrhœa, brought on by exposure to the vicissitudes of weather, and to the development of which, a certain unhealthy constitu-

:ional state appears necessary. Unlike ordinary rheumatism, it confines itself to one or two joints, and, unshifting, clings to them with remarkable tenacity. It is, in truth, an affection that has long baffled the powers of medical surgery. In many instances the patients appear to recover, but the complaint returns on the slightest exposure, and no permanent cure is effected. There is now under my care a Pole suffering from gonorrhœal rheumatism of the wrist-joint. In him the disease has yielded for the present to three grain doses of the iodide of potassium, given three times daily; and I am informed that the gonorrhœal discharge, which had become scanty, has reappeared since the mitigation of the articular disease. The best possible termination in these cases, a termination which has ensued in the instance I have mentioned, is serous effusion into the joint; for when the fluid is absorbed, it is not unlikely a useful joint may remain. Some time back, a young man, aged twenty-one, was my patient in the hospital, in consequence of a most acute attack of rheumatism in the shoulder-joint, following gonorrhœa. Though he was in a reduced state, I ordered him to be bled from the arm; mercury was administered; in fact, very active treatment was adopted. Serous effusion in the joint resulted, and within five weeks I had the gratification of seeing him leave the hospital with the functions of the joint in a great measure restored.

We occasionally meet with examples of rheumatic synovitis occurring after parturition, which may originate anchylosis. The affection differs in no shape from ordinary rheumatic synovitis; but it requires gentle treatment, as the patients attacked by it are generally much debilitated, and frequently suffering from some uterine complication.

Part xxvi., *p.* 118.

Joints, Diseased.—M. Tessier, of Lyons, has shown that prolonged rest alone, even where little or no disease previously existed—a rest for five or six months—is sufficient to cause absorption or ulceration of the cartilages of joints. This prolonged rest also aggravates existing disease.

In the early stage of inflammation of joints, apply plenty of leeches, except in scrofulous subjects. To relieve pain, use the following: moisten a bit of lint with twenty or forty drops of chlorinated hydrochloric ether, and apply it to the joint. After bleeding bring the patient rapidly under the influence of calomel, or 'give tartar emetic. The limb should have absolute rest in the most favorable position, for five or six weeks, but not longer, for fear of stiffness, etc. The joint may be splintered with leather in the following way: Get some thick leather, soften it in warm water, and mold it, when pliable, to the joint, and when hard, remove it and line it with wash leather. This forms an admirable splint. One may be made for each side of the joint. Evacuate any pus that may be formed, in good time. Promote the absorption of such materials as the inflammation may have deposited, by counter-irritation, by means of blisters, croton oil, discutient plasters, composed of equal parts of galbanum and mercurial plaster, pressure, friction, the cold douche.

Ulceration of Articular Cartilages of.—Acute inflammation is marked by rapid effusion within the joint, and uniform swelling; in disease of cartilage, the swelling is slower, and outside the joint, not coming on till some time after the first sensations or uneasiness. In chronic degeneration of synovial membrane, the swelling, although indolent, is more rapid than when the cartilage is diseased. The swelling is sloughy, elastic, and superficial. Scrofulous disease of the heads of the bones is most likely to be confounded with disease of cartilage; but ulceration of cartilage chiefly belongs to the middle and after periods of life, and to dyspeptics. In scrofulous disease, the pain generally comes on *after* the formation of pus. In ulceration of cartilage, the pain comes on earlier, and may con tinue a long time without pus forming at all. Perfect repose, accomplished by *splinting* the joint, either by Mr. Scott's method, or by leather or gutta percha splints *molded* to the joint. Give mercury early, when not contra-indicated, colchicum, with alkaline aperients. By and by apply counter-irritation.

Scrofulous Disease of.—In the early stage of the disease, Sir B. Brodie says, "All kinds of counter-irritation, such as blisters, issues, setons, and tartarized antimonial ointment, are not only not useful, but actually mischievous." The only exception is in cases of hip-joint disease of a painful character. These counter-irritants certainly excite absorption of fluid which may exist in the joint, but do not act on the diseased structure. Perfect repose of the parts in the horizontal position, with leather or gutta percha, or other kinds of splints lightly applied, is, no doubt, the best local treatment; at the same time, allowing the patient as much outdoor amusement as possible. *Part* xxx., *p.* 93.

Veratrine Ointment as a Local Application in Scrofulous Affections of the Joints.—To promote absorption in these cases, use the following ointment: veratrine, grains five to ten, dissolved in spirits of wine, and add to one ounce of axunge. This is not to be used in acute affections, but in chronic. Rub about the size of a small bean upon the joint for a quarter of an hour daily. If violent itching be produced, use a little glycerine and water. *Part* xxx., *p.* 123.

Articular Disease illustrating the Advantages of the Actual Cautery. —[The following case commenced after cold and fatigue, about four months before admission into the Edinburgh Royal Infirmary. The pain in the shoulder was at first intense.]

On admission she complained of constant gnawing pain in the left shoulder, and extending down the limb as far as the elbow, and sometimes to the fingers; when in the sitting posture she held the affected limb with the other hand, to ease the pain: the arm was also affected with a feeling of numbness and weakness; and although the shoulder was not very tender on pressure, and very gentle passive motion of the arm could be performed through a considerable angle without pain, yet any attempts on her own part to move it produced great aggravation of her sufferings. As a result, no doubt, of habitual disease, the muscles about the shoulder were much atrophied, and this caused a remarkable apparent prominence of the bony points, viz., the spine of the scapula, the acromion, the anterior border of the outer part of the clavicle, and the head of the humerus. The shoulder had an appearance that suggested at first sight the idea of dislocation.

The patient being under the influence of chloroform, Mr. Syme cauterized thoroughly the skin over the anterior and posterior aspects of the joint, rubbing a red hot cautery iron freely backward and forward four or five times over each part. It had the effect of raising and rubbing off the cuticle, but did not char the skin. An hour afterward the patient was suffering but little pain. Said she slept well that night, the first time for four months, and feels now no pain save that of the burns.

A poultice was applied yesterday; the pain of the burn is now gone, and she feels *no pain at all.* Says that she has not only lost all pain, but also that the feeling of numbness is gone from the limb, and that she seems to have more power in it. The burned parts present a white sloughy appearance.

The poultice was continued till the sloughs separated, when simple cerate was substituted for it with a view of retarding, rather than promoting cicatrization.

In time, this case fully recovered. Other cases are given showing in an equally striking manner the beneficial effects of the actual cautery in certain forms of articular disease. It will be observed that it is by no means so painful a remedy as is generally supposed, and also that its good effects are more than can be attributed to the mere discharge of pus from the sore which it produces, seeing that a great improvement commonly occurs within a few hours of its application, and long before suppuration is established. *Part* xxx., *p.* 120.

Incisions into Joints.—According to Mr. Gay, these may be made with advantage: 1st. In cases of chronic inflammation, with effusion and pain, if these have resisted ordinary remedies and health is declining; 2nd. In cases of acute or subacute synovitis, when the symptoms are unusually severe, and the external coverings show a tendency to ulceration, or when there is reason to believe that there is pus within the joint; 3rd. When the joint is occupied by bony or cartilaginous debris, which cannot find exit; and 4th. In cases of carious disease of the bones.

Mr. Hancock thinks that these can only be beneficial when, from the long duration of the disease, the actual structure of the joints have become so changed as to diminish the danger of opening into their cavity. When the disease is recent and progressing, opening the joint is attended with an aggravation of the symptoms. *Part* xxxv., *p.* 71.

Affections of the Joints following Operations on the Genito-Urinary Organs.—Mr. Coulson, Surgeon to St. Mary's Hospital, in his lecture, remarked as follows:

It is known that certain affections of the genito-urinary organs are occasionally followed by severe disease of the joints.

The injuries and diseases of the genito-urinary organs with which they may be connected are various. They may follow lithotomy and operations on the urethra. They may follow lithotrity; the introduction of instruments into the bladder; irritation of the urethra from the passage of foreign bodies, and gonorrhœal abcess, with ulceration of the urethra. In fact, any injury or disease which gives rise to primary suppuration in or about the genito-urinary organs of the male, may be followed by secondary articular disease. Besides these, there are joint affections, which appear to be excited by mere irritation of the same parts without suppuration.

The articular affections are sometimes purulent, sometimes non-purulent; and this distinction is well marked, the two varieties being seldom mixed in the same case. The attack of the joint sets in very soon after the appearance of constitutional symptoms. Thus it frequently happens that the joints begin to swell on the first or second day after the rigors and fever. The secondary deposits are often confined to the joints and muscles, and do not extend to the principal viscera. Notwithstanding the apparent limitation of the general disease, death ensues rapidly after the first appearance of the constitutional symptoms—on the fourth, sixth, tenth, and twelfth days.

On the other hand, many of these cases, though extremely severe, terminate by recovery of the patient; yet the joints have been extensively injured, as is shown by the anchylosis which ensues.

The purulent affection of the joints generally sets in under the following circumstances; a slight injury has been inflicted on the genito-urinary organs, or the patient may have irritated the urethra by attempting to pass a catheter himself. Severe rigors, followed by fever of a nervous kind, ensue; and in one or two days the joints are attacked by pain and swelling. The tumefaction may increase to a considerable size in a few hours the joint becoming red and hot. The knee, shoulder, ankles, and elbow are the joints most commonly affected. Some of these cases terminate fatally in a fortnight; others again are chronic; even in these the joint disease may commence as early as the second day.

The morbid changes in these cases are various. They are usually inflammatory. The synovial membrane is injected, and sometimes lined with false membrane, and the joint contains pus; but ulceration of the cartilages is not common. In other cases the lesions are confined to the periarticular tissues, which are infiltrated with pus; or the purulent inflammation may occupy the interior as well as the exterior of the joint, although the capsular ligament has nowhere given way. In a few cases the joint has been the seat of simple inflammation, and does not contain any pus; and matter may be discoved in joints which did not seem during life to be attacked. It is very rare to find pus in a joint which appeared healthy up to the time of death; but this has occurred in one case.

In chronic cases the periarticular swelling often contains pus, and the cartilages are softened or eroded. Indeed, we may infer that the cartilages and even ligaments have been extensively diseased from the anchylosis which ensues.

In the milder form of the disease, the joints become painful and swollen; but these symptoms are not severe, and the skin is not red. In a few days the affection may subside, and pass to another joint; hence this form is often mistaken for rheumatism. The effused fluid is sometimes purulent; in the majority of cases, we may infer that the effusion is serous from the manner in which it disappears. I should observe that many of the acute and some of the chronic cases are accompanied by intermuscular abcesses in the limbs.

The nature of the articular affections just described is not well understood. M. Velpeau attributes them to poisoning by urine. M. Civiale confesses that he is unable to explain how they are produced. For my own part I am inclined to attribute the severe cases accompanied by constitutional symptoms, and followed by purulent deposits, to the influence of pus poisoning.

I have found small abcesses along the urethra, produced by the frequent passage of instruments for stricture. I have also found inflammation of the prostatic veins. In other cases, small primary abcesses have been found in the prostate or wall of the bladder, or suppurative inflammation in the cellular tissue of the scrotum. All these are sufficient causes.

Part xxxvii., *p.* 120.

Hysterical Joint Affections—Mr. F. C. Skey says, that in three-fourths of diseases of the knee joint occurring in young women from fifteen to twenty-five, you will find more or less palpably the traces of hysteria ; for even the presence of real disease of the joint is no guaranty or safeguard against the existence of some symptoms really attributable to hysteria.

Part xxxix., *p.* 133.

ANKLE JOINT.

Amputation at the.—One reason, Mr. Fergusson says, why surgeons refuse to perform amputation at the ankle joint, is, that the integuments are often swollen and ulcerated. But this is no objection to the proceeding, the disease being produced entirely by, and kept up by, the irritation of the carious bone, a principle of the greatest importance to be remembered. Sloughing of the lower flap has been often observed, and in order to obviate this, Mr. Syme has recommended a shorter flap to be made ; and Mr. Fergusson states that he has even made a shorter one than that recommended by that gentleman. It is desirable to make the flap no longer than is absolutely necessary. *Part* xxiv., *p.* 185.

Caries of the Ankle Joint.—Amputation of the leg, below the knee, used to be the common operation for caries of the ankle joint and bones of the tarsus ; but when the disease does not extend above the articulating extremities of the tibia and fibula, the foot may be removed, and the thick integuments about the heel preserved to form a cushion for supporting the weight of the body. Besides this, there is much less fatality about this operation than in that of amputation of the leg.

Part xxvii., *p.* 352.

Amputation at the Ankle Joint.—Take care to make as much use as you can of the sole of the foot for the flap. It will have to bear all the pressure afterward, and is skin ready formed for such purpose. Preserve not only the skin but the whole of the fibrous and fatty granular structure of the sole. Keep the knife free from the posterior tibial artery, which is best done by cutting quite behind the flexor tendons, close to, or even shaving the periosteum. Instead of using adhesive strips and bandages afterward, make use of sufficient sutures, and then apply straps of linen about a foot long and an inch wide, soaked in warm water, to the stump between the sutures. Keep the parts warm generally, with warm water on lint covered with oil-silk, and keep up gentle pressure on the flap.

Part xxix., *p.* 184.

Astragalus—Non-Excision of.—This is a modification of Syme's operation ; but Mr. Simon believes the stump to be better than Syme's, because of its greater breath, its mobility in the joint, and the saved inch and a half of leg. The operation is performed similar to that of amputation at the ankle joint, the knife running between the astragalus and os calcis. The flap is taken in the same manner as in amputation at the ankle joint. *Part* xxix., *p.* 186.

Ankle Joint—Exarticulation of.—Peregoff, of St. Petersburg, modifies Mr. Syme's operation at this joint. He preserves the posterior portion of the os calcis, which is thus left to fill up the heel flap. The operation is conducted in the same way as Mr. Syme's, except that, after the exarticulation of the astragalus, the os calcis is divided by the saw behind the posterior extremity of the astragalus, and the heel is thus preserved, instead of being peeled out. The saw is then applied to separate the malleoli, and a thin slice of the articular surface of the tibia. The cut surface of the tibia is then brought into apposition with the cut surface of the os calcis, and the skin flaps accurately united by sutures. *Part* xxix., *p.* 322.

Lines of Incision Suitable for Operations at the Ankle Joint.—In operations at the ankle joint, arrange your incisions so that you can gain access to the tarsal bones, and if the disease be more extensive than anticipated, that you can even remove the entire foot at the joint, if you wish. Make "a transverse incision across the sole of the foot, commencing about three-quarters of an inch in front of one malleolus, and ending at a similar point in front of the other malleolus: a second incision is then made in the median line, beginning over the tendo-Achillis on a level with the ankle joint, and joining the former at right angles in the sole of the foot. The two lateral flaps thus marked out being next dissected upward, close to the bones, the calcaneum and astragalus are freely exposed. By division of their ligamentous and tendinous connections, one or both of these bones may be easily removed;" and other parts may be easily reached by extending the median incision a little forward. If, from the great extent of disease, it is found necessary to remove the entire foot, it may be done by uniting the two extremities of the transverse incision by a curved incision across the dorsum of the foot. *Part* xxx., *p.* 117.

Tarsus—Excision of the.—When the calcaneum and astragalus are not diseased, Chopart's operation is the best; if these two bones are very much diseased, then Syme's; if the calcaneum be sound, then Peregoff's; or the calcaneum, astragalus, scaphoid, and cuboid, may any or all of them be removed, if the disease is confined to the tarsus, and the foot saved, by Mr. Teale's operation. In Peregoff's operation, the calcaneum has to be cut through with a saw. The chain-saw has been generally used, but Mr. Simon thinks the "Dublin saw" much preferable, and does away with the objections usually urged against the chain-saw. In Peregoff's operation, as performed by Mr. Simon, first make the usual transverse incision across the sole of the foot, from the external malleolus to the opposite point on the inner malleolus; next cut rapidly across the instep meeting the ends of the former incision; then disarticulate the astragalus, and cut through the end of the calcaneum. *Part* xxxii., *p.* 111.

Ankle Joint—Excision of the Os Calcis.—[William S., aged thirty-four years, states that three years ago he had a fall and injured his ankle; in a few months an abcess formed on the dorsum of the foot, which, after some time, healed, but broke out and healed again repeatedly. He has not been able to move excepting with crutches since the accident, and has repeatedly been advised by different medical men to have the foot removed. On examination, the soft tissues about the heel were found very much swollen. There were the openings of two sinuses, one under the the outer ankle, and the other near the tendo-Achillis, which both led to dead bone in the os calcis. The ankle joint was free from any serious lesion. Removal of the calcaneum was recommended, and was submitted to on August 22d, 1854. On September 17th he was discharged cured; in twelve weeks he could walk with only the aid of an ordinary walking-stick; and in eighteen months after the operation, he could walk ten miles a day without any inconvenience.] Dr. R. W. Coe observes: •

The first incision must be begun where the calcaneum, astralagus, scaphoid, and cuboid bones meet, and carried in the direction of the calcaneo-cuboid articulation outward across the dorsum of the foot, a finger's breadth behind the projection of the fifth metatarsal bone, and directly inward across the sole of the foot, as far as a line drawn from the fourth toe. A second incision must be commenced where the first terminated, nearly at right angles to it, and carried backward so as to terminate on the inner side of the tendo-Achillis, an inch above its insertion. This flap must be turned back, keeping the knife close to the bone, excepting where crossed by the peroneal tendons. The tendo-Achillis must now be divided, and the knife carried through the articulation of the calcaneum with the astragalus, then the calcaneo-cuboid joint must be laid open, and the bone will be found pretty movable, but it must not be torn away, neither must other parts be used as a fulcrum to pry it out; the connections must be cut. The greatest difficulty is in separating its deep connections, which cannot be seen, and scarcely felt, the bone being in the way. You must take care to keep the knife close to the bone, so as to avoid wounding the posterior tibial artery and nerve.

Part xxxiv., *p.* 128.

Amputation at the Ankle Joint—Peregoff's Operation.—The essential point in this operation for removal of the foot is to leave the posterior part of the os calcis so as to fill up the heel flap; by this means the limb is lengthened by an inch and a half or two inches more than by other operations, and the posterior flap has not the bag shape of Syme's, and so does not form a receptacle for a collection of pus. The os calcis is sawn through immediately behind the disarticulated astragalus, the remnant of the os calcis uniting by its divided surface with the inferior extremities of the tibia and fibula. The tendo-Achillis is not divided.

Part xxxvii., *p.* 116.

Excision of the Os Calcis by a New Method.—In the removal of this bone, the incisions, one transverse and one longitudinal, are usually made *across* the sole of the foot, but here there is a great disadvantage, namely, that cicatrices are left along the line of most pressure. A better plan is to carry a horse-shoe incision from a little in front of the calcaneo-cuboid articulation round and behind the heel to a corresponding point on the opposite side of the foot; dissect up the semi-circular flap thus formed by carrying the bistoury close to the os calcis, the under-surface of which is exposed. Then make a perpendicular incision about two inches in length, over the middle of the tendo-Achillis, falling into the horizontal one. Detach the tendon and dissect the flaps up close to the bone, carry the blade over the upper and posterior part of the os calcis, open the articulation with the astragalus, divide the ligaments, and turn the bone out. Thus there is no cicatrix over the parts most exposed to pressure.

Part xxxvii., *p.* 119.

Resection of the Ankle Joint.—Syme's and Peregoff's operations or modifications of them, are frequently performed in diseases of the ankle-joint, when, by resection of the joint the otherwise healthy foot might be saved. These former operations should never be performed unless there is so large an amount of disease as to preclude all hope of preserving a good and useful foot. Mr. Hancock, at the Charing Cross Hospital, has now performed this operation four times, three times successfully, and once unsuccessfully, owing to pulmonary affection. The success of the operation depends upon leaving the anterior and posterior tibial arteries intact, and not opening the sheaths of the tendons; the only parts cut through are, the external and internal lateral ligaments, and the bones. Neither the extensor nor flexor tendons, the anterior nor posterior tibial arteries are injured, consequently, there are no vessels to tie; when successful, the patients are able to walk and run about with scarcely any perceptible limp.   *Part* xl., *p*. 81.

ELBOW JOINT.

Excision of.—M. Robert presented a woman, aged 26 years, on whom he had practised the operation of excision of the elbow joint. The disease rendering the operation necessary was caries of the humero-cubital articulation, following a fall on the elbow. There were several fistulous openings about the olecranon. In the fold of the arm were two deep sinuses penetrating into the joint. The soft parts around were moderately engorged. The operation was effected by dividing and reflecting the integuments over the olecranon. The humerus was sawn through immediately above the condyles, the ulna below the coronary process, and the radius just below its articular extremity. The limb was placed in the apparatus of M. Guizot. But little reaction ensued, and the fever and sleeplessness which had previously harassed the patient ceased immediately. The patient recovered sufficient use of her arm to resume her occupation as sempstress.   *Part* vi., *p.* 148.

Operation for the Removal of Loose Cartilages in the Elbow Joint.— [Mr. Solly's patient was left, after a severe attack of rheumatism, with pain and swelling of the elbow joint. This was treated by rest, counter-irritation, iodine, and mercurials; and on the subsidence of the general swelling, there was found a small circumscribed swelling, which appeared to be a sac containing several hard and movable bodies, situated above and behind the inner condyle. It was determined to remove these bodies by operation. Mr. Solly says :]

I made an incision about one inch in length over the swelling above the inner condyle, dividing the skin, fascia, and synovial membrane, till I exposed the loose cartilages, for such they proved to be. They were easily pressed out of the opening. I introduced my little finger into the sac, and felt the articulating surfaces or the humerus and radius, and I thought I felt an irregular surface on the ridge between the radius and ulna, like an attached portion of a false cartilage, but there were no more loose bodies in the joint. Those removed were eight in number. I brought the edges of the wound into close apposition, put one suture in through the skin, and the isinglass plaster over it. I placed a pasteboard splint on the back of the joint, fixing it to the upper and fore-arm, so as to prevent the slightest motion in the joint. The wound was quite healed in forty-eight hours, but I kept the joint at rest for a week: after this he was able to move it without the slightest pain—he did not suffer in any way after the operation, except for the confinement occasioned by the splint. I have seen him repeatedly since he left the hospital, and he has remained quite well and resumed his occupation on the river.   *Part* xix., *p.* 130.

Disease of the Elbow Joint.—Amputation of the whole limb, excision of the articulating surfaces, and the bringing about of anchylosis are the three modes which have been hitherto resorted to, not to cure diseased joints, but to prevent the constitution from sinking under the drain of a disease but too often found incurable, and to render the portion saved in some degree useful to the individual.

It is almost needless to say, that in a vast many instances all ordinary means of curing these diseases fail. Rest, splints, bandages, tonics, change of air and diet, mercurials, iodine, all fail to stay the progress of the disease, until it no longer becomes a question as to whether we shall have recourse to the knife or not, but how soon, and in what way it is most advisable.

Mr. Gay has for some time past been in the habit of treating cases of diseased joints by a plan which has so far been found to be at one and the same time simple, rapid, and effectual. It is nothing more or less than to make one or more incisions right down to the diseased joint, with a view of letting out the debris of the diseased articulation, the remnants of the cartilages, etc., which seem to him one of the principal obstacles to the procuring of anchylosis; a healthy inflammation is by these means set up in the cavity, which speedily results in firm and complete anchylosis. The constant success which has attended this plan seems calculated to bring about a complete revolution in the treatment of these complaints.

J. T., a laborer, entered the Royal Free Hospital, under Mr. Gay, with disease of the elbow joint. Of its origin and cause he knew nothing, and only remembers that it began about seven years ago, and since then it has run its course unchecked by any means. On admission, the state of the limb was as follows : The arm was straightened and the elbow joint almost immovable, even the slightest attempt to procure motion being followed by excessive pain. The joint itself was very much enlarged, but the remaining part of the limb was wasted to a considerable extent. There were six sinuses leading to the joint, two on either side, one in front, and another on the inner side of the olecranon. Around their orifices the skin was livid and unhealthy-looking, and they all conducted direct to the joint, so that the probe passed immediately into it. A quantity of thin, ichorous fluid was consequently poured out from them. The man's health was much impaired.

Although the state of the joint seemed to hold out scarcely the remotest hope of success, Mr. Gay made an incision on either side, carrying it along the course of the lateral sinuses, and fairly down to the joint. These incisions were each four inches long, and left behind great gaping wounds, laying open to view the interior of the joint. The ends of the bones were found completely bereft of cartilage, and so soft that portions were as readily torn away by means of a steel director as if they had been so much cork. But little bleeding followed the operation, which was concluded by filling up the cavities with lint, and confining the joint with a bandage. The first thing that ensued was a most profuse discharge, which continued unabated until about nine days after, when it gradually began to lessen, owing to the evident healing of the wounds, which now appeared strongly disposed to close. The patient was seized with simple fever, but eventually recovered, with complete anchylosis. *Part* xxiv., *p.* 171.

Excision of the Elbow Joint.—Always remember that in caries of the joint, little more than the articular surface is engaged in the disease. It is the ignorance or neglect of this point which has made many cases unsuccessful. The incisions originally practised by Moreau are the best, viz., a transverse one across the back of the articulation, immediately above the olecranon, from the ulnar nerve to the external condyle, and two longitudinal through the extremities of the transverse, so that the incision altogether has the form of the letter H. When the flaps have been raised, free access is gained to the articulation; and when the operation is completed the edges of the transverse incision, if brought accurately together, generally adhere by first intention. Having dissected up the flaps, do not attempt to remove all the articulation at once, as otherwise there will be a risk of cutting the ulnar nerve; but having exposed the olecranon, cut it off in the first instance, so as to get free access to the joint; then divide the external lateral ligament, and having pushed the ulnar nerve over the inner condyle, free the end of the humerus and saw it off on a line with the tuberosities; and lastly, remove, in succession the ends of the radius and ulna on a line with the base of the coronoid process. More than the extent thus defined would be unnecessary and injurious, while less would hardly remove the disease, and even if it did, would incur the risk of anchylosis.

Part xxxi., *p.* 106.

Excision of the Elbow Joint.—When this joint has been anchylosed in a wrong position, so as to be useless, a certain degree of motion may be secured by the following operation : cut out a large portion of the end of the ulna, radius, and humerus, making, in fact, a resection of the anchylosed joint. *Part* xxxi., *p.* 108.

Wounds of.—To excise the elbow joint, because a compound fracture of the olecranon had been sustained, would, of course not be warrantable, as it may heal and unite without the occurrence of inflammation ; but if articular inflammation do take place, the question does admit of serious consideration whether it would not be best to excise the ends of the bones with the hopes of saving the patient's constitution, and of gaining a mobile joint. *Part* xxxiv., *p.* 122.

Elbow Joint—Severe Injuries of.—Primary amputation ought never to be thought of in compound fracture of the elbow, excepting the artery be torn through, or the soft parts both before and behind hopelessly damaged. The ill consequences to be feared are in inverse proportion to the amount of external laceration inflicted. In cases sufficiently severe to warrant it, it is far better surgery to freely enlarge the wound behind the joint, and excise the projecting ends of the bones, than to be content with a simple reduction.

Much less of suppuration and of constitutional disturbance appears to follow cases so treated, and the chance of good motion being obtained after an excision is infinitely greater than it is when the ends of the injured bones remain. It may be worth a question whether, even in certain cases not usually deemed sufficiently severe to warrant it, for the reasons above mentioned, it might not be well to enlarge the wound and excise the joint. Crushed elbows with but small external wound, undoubtedly, as a rule, do badly. The excision of joints during the acute or commencing stages of inflammation, would seem hitherto to have been regarded with suspicion, though probably with no very definite reason. In cases of slight injuries, in which at the time it had been thought best to do nothing, but which have subsequently gone wrong, it might, perhaps, be good practice to do *secondary* excision, say within the first week or two. The immediate relief afforded by free incisions under such circumstances is well known, and it would probably be increased by the removal of the bones and their ulcerating cartilages.

In treating these cases poultices and warm fomentations should be utterly eschewed.

W,hen it has been decided to preserve the arm, it is the surgeon's duty (excepting, perhaps, in a case of sloughing), to persevere, in spite of discouraging circumstances, afterward. *Part* xxxiv., *p.* 127.

Elbow-Joint—Resection of.—The last improvement in this operation is that of Langenbeck, who makes only one long incision on the inner edge of the ulna. The ends of the bones may be readily turned into the wound and sawn away with a key-hole saw, cutting from before backward. In certain cases, where there is great swelling and the ligaments are sound, this plan will be more difficult, and a cross incision will be necessary.
Part xxxv., *p.* 69.

Excision of the Elbow Joint.—There are two objects to be attained by this operation, viz.: First, to remove all the diseased bone, and second, to do this in such a way that a useful and movable joint may result. It is always far better to remove the whole of the articular surfaces of the joint than to remove the diseased portion only, for the disease often extends afterward to the other bones; and there is often more suffering and fever than when the whole is removed. *Part* xxxvi., *p.* 148.

Excision of the Elbow—Heath's Splint.—The great object in this operation is to obtain a movable joint; to this end always remove not a mere slice from the edge of the bones, but a full inch or so; there is then less tendeney to anchylosis. Employ a splint invented by Mr. Heath, late house-surgeon to King's College Hospital, consisting of four iron plates, well padded, concave on their front surface, to fit the limb, convex behind; these are intended to be placed opposite to one another, one pair above and the other below the joint, projecting portions perforated with a female screw spring from the convex back of each plate. Two iron rods with hinges in their centres, and a small screw at either end, cut in opposite directions, to fit in the female screws of the iron plates, connect the plates above the joint with those below. The plates are now attached firmly by means of straps and buckles, and, if necessary, additional strips of plaster. By turning round the rods the extremities of the bones are separated to the required distance, while by means of the hinges in the centres of the rods motion can be made with the greatest facility. *Part* xxxvii., *p.* 108.

HIP JOINT.

Treatment of Disease of.—Dr. Evans believes that *mercury* may be regarded as a *specific remedy* in hip disease.

That we may apply it with equal *certainty* and *benefit* in *scrofulous* and non-scrofulous subjects.

That it is better to bring the system at once and fully under its action than to give a *long* and *lingering* alterative course of mercury.

That in the majority of cases, mercury alone, when pushed to salivation, will effect a cure. That the application of leeches are occasionally, though not always required, and when any little pain remains at the groin, a small blister will then be of benefit.

That rest, the horizontal posture, and attention to regimen, etc., must be strictly enjoined.

That hip-joint disease, if not in all, certainly in nearly all cases, is caused *not* by *primary ulceration* of the *cartilages*, but by *scrofulous inflammation* of the *synovial membrane*—this morbid state being the first link in the chain of pathological actions.

Lastly. That the diseased limb is *really elongated* during the second stage of coxalgia, and that this appears to be in a great measure effected not by curvature of the spine, etc., but by the pushing out of the head of the femur; this is caused by the inflammation within the joint, aided by the organic relaxation of the surrounding muscles.   *Part* vi., *p.* 152.

Hip-joint Disease.—[Affections of the hip joint are too seldom seen at the commencement, when properly applied remedies might restore the joint. In the second stage, we have no longer a simple case of erythema of the synovial membrane, but an active form of inflammation extending to the more dense parts of the capsule and cartilage, attended with severe pain in rotation and abduction of the limb.]

Often in the earliest part of the second stage, the limb will not admit of perfect extension, and by careful examination of the joint it may be discovered that the thigh is permanently flexed on the pelvis. It is this state of the limb to which Mr. Key directs attention, as fraught with the worst consequences to the patient. This state of flexion of the femur on the pelvis usually takes place slowly and imperceptibly, but sometimes it is rapidly induced by a sudden attack of inflammation in a joint that has previously exhibited signs of disease in its mildest form. This is the worst form of the disease, so far as the deformity of the joint is concerned; for the intense pain which the patient experiences on the slightest movement of the limb induces her to seek for ease in positions that add greatly to the distortion of the limb by the obliquity given to the pelvis. The patient is seen lying usually on her sound side, with the affected limb drawn up to nearly a right angle with the pelvis. As the patient lies on her side the affected limb appears to be three or four inches shorter than the other. When she is placed on her back, which position she assumes with difficulty, and the bearings of the two patellæ, and the spinous processes of the ilia noticed, the former are seen to differ as much as from two to three inches, while only a difference of an inch is perceptible in the level of the iliac spinous processes. This would seem to show that the limb was actually shortened; such, however, is not the case, and by examination of the pelvis it will be seen that the twist of the pelvis on the lumbar vertebræ, by carrying the affected joint backward, is the cause of the great shortening of the limb.

During the stage of inflammation it is impossible to use any means of counteracting this distorted position of the pelvis, and by the time that the patient is able to bear extension so as to restore the pelvis to its natural bearing, and to diminish the angle which the femur makes with the pelvis, the parts have become so fixed in their new position as to render it difficult to alter their position, and impossible in the majority of cases to restore them to their natural bearings. The consequence is, that when the patient is convalescent with a somewhat stiffened joint, the foot cannot be brought down to the ground, and a shoe with a sole of two inches is required to enable her to walk with the foot flat on the ground. How is this state of things to be prevented? The only remedy for the evil is in every case of disease of the hip joint to maintain the straight position, as soon as the nature of the affection is ascertained. It is a position applicable in all stages of the disease.

In the early stage characterized only by a slight limping in the gait, or by an occasional slight pain in the knee or thigh, it possesses the advantage of maintaining the joint in a state of complete repose. The articulation being at rest, the muscles do not act, but remain in a passive state. On the contrary, when the limb is kept bent with a pillow placed under the knee, a position usually resorted to in the early stage, the pelvis and thigh in a child are continually in motion; little or no pain is felt by the little patient, and injunctions to preserve rest are made in vain. In the bent position, therefore, rest, one of the most important elements in treating a diseased joint, is not maintained, and the disease, therefore, fails often to be arrested. By a long splint applied along the outer side of the limb, and made to extend from the toe to the axilla, entire rest is given to the joint, and absolute inaction of the muscles preserved.

The arrest of the disease is greatly expedited by the entire tranquillity obtained by the straight position in conjunction with the mercurial treatment. The principal advantage of preserving the limb in a straight position is seen in the second stage of the disease, when under the united effects of inflammation and ulceration of the cartilage of the joint, the tendency of the flexor muscles to contract, induces such a degree of deformity in the lumbar vertebræ, pelvis, and hip-joint, as when once allowed to take place, can never afterward be wholly remedied.

The course which abscess takes when suppuration takes place in the joint seems to be in some degree modified by the straight position. When the limb is allowed to bend upon the pelvis, matter is usually formed at the back part of the joint under the glutæi muscles, or at the side of the joint on the anterior margin of the glutæus medius. But when the straight position is observed, the suppurative action is inclined to the fore part of the joint, and the collection of fluid is formed on the outer edge of the iliacus muscle, by the side of the tensor vaginæ femoris. This course of the matter may be accidental; but in two cases now in the hospital, suppuration has taken this course, one having burst and discharged itself; and in the other case the abscess is making its way toward the surface in the same direction.

But there is an advantage gained in the advanced stage of the disease too important to be passed over; namely, the prevention of dislocation of the head of the bone on the dorsum ilii—an occurrence, though by no means frequent, yet found sometimes to take place, and greatly adding to the deformity and shortening of the limb. It can only occur in the flexed position of the limb, which thrusts the head of the bone backward against the capsular ligament and posterior part of the acetabulum; and these structures, together with the head of the bone, being partly destroyed by the ulcerative process, the femur gradually escapes from the cotyloid cavity, and becomes lodged upon the dorsum of the ilium.

The state of anchylosis in which this disease usually leaves the joint requires a concluding observation in reply to any objection that might be raised to the utility of a limb anchylosed in a straight line with the body. The only inconvenience arising from it occurs in the sitting position, in which the patient being unable to flex the limb sufficiently to sit on a chair in the usual manner, is compelled to drop the affected limb in a nearly perpendicular posture, and to sit with the pelvis resting on the side of the chair. This is the only evil attending the straight position, and is more than counterbalanced by the uniform length of the two limbs, and the absence of almost all lameness in the act of progression. Care, however, should be taken to prevent the patient bearing too early upon the unsound imb during convalescence, when the straight position has been observed in the treatment of the case; for a sense of weakness, as in the first stage of the disease, induces him to raise the pelvis on that side in order to prevent much weight being thrown upon the weak limb. The effect of this elevation of the ilium is to curve the lumbar vertebræ in a lateral direction; and this distortion becomes permanent. *Part* xii., *p.* 241.

Formation of an Artificial Joint.—This method, for which we are indebted to the ingenuity of Dr. John Rhea Barton, has been applied as yet but to the anchylosis of a single articulation—that of the hip joint. It has, however, been suggested by this surgeon, that it might likewise be found applicable to similar affections of the lower jaw, knee, elbow, fingers, and toes, when the muscles of these respective articulations remain uninjured. The method consists in the uncovering of the bone at or near the diseased point, dividing it across with the saw, and subsequently moving the lower portion from time to time upon the upper, to prevent a solid reunion of the divided parts. By this mode of proceeding, there is the same disposition on the parts for the formation of a false joint, as we often find producing that result in fractures where the bones are not kept sufficiently at rest. Under such circumstances, the two opposing surfaces of bone may be expected to unite by flexible ligamentous matter, or become smooth and polished by the friction; the lower fragment, in the latter case, rounding itself into the form of a head; and the other hollowing itself more or less into the shape of a cup, in which the former plays; the periosteum and surrounding cellular tissue becoming condensed and thickened, so as to perform the office of a fibrous capsule, and the muscles modified to a certain extent, to accommodate themselves to the new articulation. *Part* xii., *p.* 243.

Inflammation of the Hip Joint.—[The test proposed by Dr. O'Ferrall, as a means of diagnosing between hip-joint disease and other affections resembling it, we made use of, and it was found that when adduction and abduction of the affected limb was made, the entire pelvis moved, forming an angular lever, whose fulcrum was the acetabulum of the opposite side. On disease in this locality, Dr. O'Ferrall remarks :]

When a hip joint case is brought under our notice, it is of great practical importance to determine its probable duration, before the period at which we are consulted; for the success of the mercurial treatment will depend much on this question. In T.'s case, the nates of the affected side drooped, as in cases of some standing; but when he was laid on his face and the muscles of both nates were equally at rest, there was no remarkable loss of bulk in the muscles themselves. The measurement of the thigh of the affected side, showed also a circumference equal to that of the sound one. There could be no doubt, then, that the case was comparatively recent, for the characteristic wasting which belongs to disuse, had not yet been established. It might be thought that the history of the case would be sufficient to determine this point. Nothing could be more fallacious.

[In another case, a young gentleman, whilst hunting, in crossing a hedge, his left foot was caught in a bramble, and forcibly everted; he experienced great pain in the hip, groin, and knee, and there was perceptible shortening of the limb of one inch.]

The diagnosis arrived at was—recent sprain of the hip joint, previously in the state of morbus coxæ. This diagnosis, most startling and unpalatable to himself and friends, was grounded, 1st, on the constitution of an angular level by the pelvis and thigh bone, when the latter was moved; 2ndly, on the obliquity of the pelvis, which was certainly not of sudden occurrence; and 3dly, the fact of a remarkable wasting of the muscles of the entire limb.

In the one, the absence of wasting, marked the case as one of recent occurrence, and promising a recovery from antiphlogistic treatment. In the other the presence of wasting, with obliquity of the pelvis enabled him to distinguish an actual case of morbus coxæ, when presented to him as an instance of recent accident only. The value of the mercurial treatment introduced by Dr. O'Beirne, is lessened by employing it in unsuitable cases. The diagnosis of stages, in joint diseases, is, therefore, of the utmost importance in practice. *Part* xiii., *p.* 194.

Hip Disease.—[After alluding to the severe measures formerly adopted in the treatment of hip disease, Mr. Syme says:]

The great object now held in view is to prevent motion of the joint, and this is effected by means of mechanical support, in addition to the horizontal posture. The splint employed should not be limited to the neighborhood of the hip, but be made to extend over the whole length of the limb and a portion of the trunk; or, in more precise terms, from the sole of the foot to the false ribs, since it is only by preventing motion of the knee, and ankle also, that the hip joint can be maintained in a state of perfect rest. Together with this local treatment, due attention is of course requisite in regard to the diet and state of the digestive organs. Cod-liver oil, which so remarkably corrects the condition of system that predisposes to derangement of the scrofulous kind, should, at the same time, be freely administered.

Under this simple and gentle mode of treatment, steadily pursued, a large proportion of cases terminate favorably, without any alteration of the limb in regard to form, mobility, or strength. On some comparatively rare occasions, the pain continues without abatement, or increases in severity, and then counter-irritation becomes requisite. For this purpose the actual cautery affords by far the most efficient means, and if employed during the influence of chloroform, is divested of the only objection that can be alleged against its use. The sore established should not exceed three inches in length and one in breadth.

In the event of suppuration taking place, the abscess should not be opened until it has nearly approached the surface, when an aperture of adequate size, and so situated as to afford a free drain from the discharge becomes proper. Water-dressing is preferable to ointments and the long splint; or if the limb has been allowed to get into a position which prevents the employment of this, a piece of leather, fashioned to the shape of the hip and thigh, should be still carefully applied, to prevent the irritation attending movement of the joint, great attention being at the same time paid to the maintenance of the patient's general health and strength. The result depends chiefly upon the state of the bones composing the joint. If they are carious, he *must* die; if they are not, he *may* recover. The risk of caries being induced, is proportioned inversely to the age of the patient; so that the prognosis becomes less and less favorable from childhood to maturity.

Some operations have been lately performed in London, with the view of remedying caries of the hip joint, by cutting out the head of the thigh bone; but this proceeding must have originated and been conducted in forgetfulness of the well-established pathological fact, that when caries attacks the surface of a joint, it is never limited to one of the bones which compose the articulation. If the articulating surface of the head of the thigh bone be carious, it follows, as a matter of absolute certainty, that the acetabulum must be in a similar condition. But as the acetabulum does not admit of removal in the living body, with any prospect of safety or advantage, no benefit can be derived from taking away a part of the articulation, and, therefore, excision of the head of the thigh bone for caries of the joint should be regarded as no less erroneous in theory than objectionable in practice.

In an old volume of "The Lancet," it is stated that Mr. Syme cut out the head of the humerus for disease of the shoulder joint, leaving the glenoid cavity to "shift for itself"—the fact really being that the patient labored under necrosis of the upper end of the bone, so that the head was expanded into a thin shell containing an exfoliation, which was removed with the effect of preventing amputation at the shoulder joint, previously deemed requisite, and enabling the subject of the case, then a boy, to grow up into a strong healthy man. This statement, like others, having no foundation except in the depraved imagination of their authors, was treated with the silence that it deserved, and would not be noticed now unless there seemed a risk of its being stumbled on by some one in search of authorities for bad practice. It is true that Mr. Syme did once cut out the head of the humerus for caries, but in that case the disease, instead of affecting the surface of the bone, which was perfectly sound, had hollowed out the interior substance into a cavity, so that the circumstance of the patient recovering the use of her arm, and enjoying good health for ten years after the operation, in no wise invalidates the rule, that caries of an articulating surface is never limited to one of the bones which compose the joint.

In the London operations the hip joints must have been either carious or not; and the proceeding, therefore, either useless or unnecessary. That it is possible for patients laboring under disease of the hip joint to recover, after excision of the head of the thigh bone, could hardly be doubted by any who has remarked the shrunk and distorted limbs which result from morbus coxarius, terminating in anchylosis, or examined the preparations illustrative of this condition obtained after death. The scars of old sinuses, and the histories of persons who have regained good health after suffering from hip disease in their youth, frequently afford evidence that the joint must have suppurated; that the articular structure must have been seriously deranged; that the respective surfaces of the bones must have been more or less extensively denuded of their cartilaginous covering; and that there must have been great displacement before consolidation was accomplished by anchylosis. It is very probable that in some of these persons the head of the thigh bone might have been cut out during the suppurative stage, without preventing recovery, especially if the most careful attention had been subsequently bestowed upon the maintenance of the patient's strength. But in what respect they would have derived benefit from the operation it is not so easy to see. *Part* xix., *p.* 119.

Scrdfulous Disease of the Hip Joint.—An opening having been made freely with an abscess lancet, the limb may be wrapped up in a flannel, wrung out of hot water, and this may be continued until the first flow of matter has ceased, a poultice or water-dressing being applied afterward. The opening should be free, so that the abscess should heal from the bottom; and also that no pressure need be used to cause it to escape. All rough manipulation is to be carefully avoided. The treatment of a sinus which is left after the opening of an abscess may be comprised in a few words. If the orifice be disposed to heal prematurely, it may be prevented by the occasional application of the caustic potash, care being taken that the caustic does not enter the sinus itself; otherwise, some simple ointment or water-dressing is all that is required. The old practice of probing a sinus yields us no accurate information, nor is it useful; and the same remark applies, but with greater force, to the use of stimulating injections.

The determination of the question of amputation in instances of this species of articular disease, Sir Benjamin Brodie makes to depend upon the point, whether or not there be indications of other tubercular disease in any of the internal organs. It too frequently happens, that when one diseased joint is removed by amputation, another becomes the seat of the same malady, or tubercular deposits in the lungs, the bronchial glands, or in the mesentery, finally destroy the patient. When there is any reason to apprehend such results, amputation, of course, is worse than useless. *Part* xxii., *p.* 189.

Hip Joint Disease treated by Cod-liver Oil.—Several cases of this disease have been successfully treated at St. Thomas's Hospital by the use of cod-liver oil. It changes the abnormal molecular condition of the blood, so well known to exist in these cases, and so often connected with scrofula and other constitutional disorders. *Part* xxii., *p.* 195.

Hip Joint—Hysterical Affections of.—[Mr. Coulson was consulted in the case of a young lady, nineteen years of age, highly nervous and excitable in temperament, with an affection of the hip joint. Leeches had been applied, the recumbent position enforced, and counter-irritation in every available form employed—but all of no avail. The pain was diffused and complained of as insupportable. The joint under examination seemed natural, and her general health had not suffered in proportion to the duration of the disease; indeed, there seemed as much pain excited if the integuments alone were examined. No persuasion could prevail upon her to make use of the limb. Steel and quinine were prescribed, but with no success. At length, by the death of her father, the means of living became much reduced, and the different members of the family were obliged to exert themselves to meet the calamity.]

This young lady, upon being made acquainted with the particulars—for misfortune it was none to her—one day suddenly rose from her couch and walked. She exerted herself much, both mentally and bodily, for the good of those around her, seemed to forget her long illness, and has ever since remained well.

It has been calculated, that at least four-fifths of the females among the higher classes of society supposed to be suffering from diseases of joints, are, in truth, affected with hysteria, and with nothing else.

In hysterical affections of the hip joint, the patient from the first complains of pain in the part, and not in the knee, as is frequently the case when organic changes are commencing in the joint itself. The pain which the patient describes as most severe is not limited to one spot, but extends over the buttock to the lumbar region, and down the thigh. It is this general diffusion of pain which constitutes one of our most useful distinctions between this affection and disease of the hip joint. From the commencement, the patient complains of such aggravation of pain by pressure and motion, that she confines herself to one position of the limb ; and yet upon occasions, when the mind is otherwise occupied, or during sleep, she will move it without complaint. The sensibility of the limb to the touch is frequently so great that the slightest pressure on any part of the hip or thigh will cause the patient to scream ; she shrinks involuntarily from the mere approach of the hand ; but, nevertheless, upon a careful examination, these morbid conditions will be found to exist more in the skin than in the deep-seated parts. As Sir Benjamin Brodie, who first directed attention to these important affections, observes : " If you pinch the skin, lifting it at the same time off the subjacent parts, the patient complains more than when you forcibly squeeze the head of the thigh bone into the socket of the acetabulum." The more the patient's attention is directed to the part, the more the pain is increased ; but if her attention be directed otherwise, she will hardly complain, and the pain does not interfere with her rest. In disease involving the structures of the joint, there is nothing of which the patient complains so much as the inability to sleep at night—a sudden start, or pain, or cramp, banishes sleep, and the patient dreads again to close her eyes. In hysterical affections, on the contrary, the sleep is calm and refreshing ; and this, perhaps, is a great reason why the general health so slightly suffers, even in long-protracted cases.

Treatment.—The vegetable tonics seem to be more efficacious than the metallic. But when the appetite is tolerably good, the tongue clean, the bowels regular, then the metallic tonics may be employed with good effect. In most neuralgic affections the preparations of iron are valuable, none more so than the carbonate. To relieve pain, no remedy is preferable to valerian. Dr. Copland says the remedy he has found most useful is the spirit of turpentine, prescribed in various modes, internally and externally, and administered in enemata ; the preparations of iodine alone, or with narcotics and camphor. By being compelled to move the limb and enter into society, patients have been known to recover, after the complaint had resisted every other kind of treatment.　　　　　*Part* xxiv., *p.* 167.

Treatment of Hip Joint Disease.—The mode of treatment pursued by Professor Carnochan in morbus coxarius has been very successful. He relies principally on constitutional treatment, abandons the use and motion of the affected side, and allows the abscess to open spontaneously. The number of cases now in progress, of convalescence, the general improvement in the physical appearance of the patients, and the absence of the distressing hectic, indicate the soundness of the principle upon which he proceeds. . . . . The number of victims of Pott's disease, of all ages, is by no means the least interesting feature of practice to be seen here. With these also the principal attention is given to constitutional treatment, rest and counter-irritation of a mild character being the adjuvant means employed. *Part* xxix., *p.* 168.

Sinuses of the Hip depending upon Exfoliations from the Pelvis.— Mr. Syme remarks as follows :

It is necessary that you should recollect the distinction between necrosis and caries. In the former disease a portion of bone dies, and separates from the living substance, so that no obstacle to recovery exists after the exfoliation or detached piece escapes from the position where it is situated; but in the latter the bone retains its vitality, and obstinately remains in a diseased condition, without any natural limit of duration, except the life of the patient or conversion of the caries into necrosis. It must further be recollected that the dense osseous substance which composes the shafts of bones is chiefly liable to necrosis, and that the spongy or cancellated texture is almost exclusively the seat of caries. Now, sinuses about the pelvis are unhappily met with very frequently as the attendants or consequences of disease in the hip joint, vertebræ, or sacrum, where the disease, being of an incurable kind, and the part concerned not admitting of removal, any sort of treatment can produce no better effect than a very imperfect degree of palliation, and it has hence been usual to regard such cases as of a very hopeless character. But nearly thirty years ago there happened to fall under my notice a case which showed that such a judgment should not be passed as a matter of course, or without more caution and discrimination than had been supposed requisite. The patient was a young man, aged 28, who for the preceding seven years had suffered from sinuses about the hip and upper part of the thigh, which being regarded as proceeding from fistula in ano, had been treated by the late Mr. George Bell and other surgeons, without obtaining the relief desired. He had then applied to quacks with no better success, and finally abandoning all hope of recovery, had allowed the disease to pursue its course. It was a considerable time after this resolution that my assistance was asked. I found him extremely emaciated, and so weak that he could hardly leave his bed, with a large abscess of the thigh, and several sinuses about the hip, discharging matter profusely. Having opened the abscess, I examined the sinuses, and found that one, which opened in the fold between the buttock and thigh, led to the tuberosity of the ischium, in which there was a cavity containing an exfoliation of bone. I therefore dilated this sinus by incision, introduced my finger, and having found an opening between the origins of the extensor muscles, enlarged it by the bistoury, so as to obtain access to the interior, whence I removed a small bit of dead bone. The patient then quickly recovered, and ever afterward enjoyed good health.

I am inclined to think that violent muscular contraction may have been the exciting cause of inflammation and death of the bone. The subject is curious, and worthy of investigation, but of little importance when compared with the practical benefit which may result from a knowledge of the fact that sinuses of the pelvis sometimes depend upon loose exfoliations, which will not find their way out unassisted, but which may be readily removed artificially, with the effect of a speedy and permanent recovery. *Part* xxxi., *p.* 117

Hysterical Affection of the Hip Joint.—The pain is more severe than in chronic inflammation. Pressure produces greater pain when slight than when firm, and is more general than when there is inflammation. It is most relieved by a belladonna plaster round the joint, and general tonics, such as quinine, iron combined with hyoscyamus, or valerian and camphor.

Part xxxii., *p.* 121.

Hip Joint—Excision of.—Great advantage will be obtained by the use of Mr. Butcher's saw: the blade is pressed behind the bone, and then being turned in a horizontal direction by a screw, the head and trochanters are readily removed.   *Part* xxxv., *p.* 70.

Excision of the Hip Joint.—After the performance of this operation, a swing should be used, sufficiently strong to suspend the entire body. The wound should be left uncovered, except by the dressings, in order to secure a depending escape for the discharge. By this means there is no necessity to disturb the patient to allow of the evacuation of the bowels, and the accumulation of the discharge from the wound is prevented.

Part xxxvi., *p.* 137.

KNEE JOINT.

White Swelling of the Joints.—[Lisfranc distinguishes white swellings into those in which a sub-inflammation exists, and those in which no trace of this is present. He thinks that:]

It is not always an easy matter to distinguish the *engorgement* of the soft parts from an enlarged condition of the bone itself, but that in time the induration often becomes movable upon the bony parts, these last remaining nearly or quite healthy; in this case the disease spreads from without inward.

In cases of white swelling, it is very important to be assured of the condition of the thoracic and abdominal viscera; for, where diseases of any of these exist, they have sometimes been found to make progress in proportion as the affection of the joint becomes amended—even requiring that irritation should be reproduced in the latter. When the visceral affection is incurable, but stationary, we do not treat the white-swelling actively, unless it becomes dangerous.

Unfortunately the thoracic and abdominal affections are often *latent*, and resist our means of investigation—so that death may speedily follow the cure of the disease of the joint, in consequence of some unsuspected organic affection.

Abscesses, formed *around* the white-swelling, should be opened as promptly as possible, while, when formed *within* the substance of the engorgement, exit must be given to the pus as late as possible—providing the inflammation be not acute, and there be no danger of the pus penetrating the joint. It is very easy to be deceived as to the existence of pus—while the sojourn of this fluid in contact with the indurations proves to be one of their most powerful solvents. The most experienced surgeons often have great difficulty in deciding whether a collection of fluid or pus be situated within, or external to the joint. The alternative of amputation decides the surgeon in determining to open the collection, and, if symptoms follow which denote that the cavity of the joint is exposed also, he proceeds at once to amputate.

M. Lisfranc considers that, in general, much too little importance is attached to *regimen*, in *chronic surgical disease*. The ordinary, and sometimes an excessive diet is permitted, and the great aid in dissipating engorgements, derived frcm allowing patients, in some degree, to what he calls "live upon their own substance" (*i. e.* a starvation regimen), is lost sight of. He has repeatedly known these tumors, which have resisted every other means, to become dispersed after diminishing the diet one-third or a half. Exceptions will occur to this, when the patient is excessively feeble or scrofulous, and when the digestive organs suffer from the change.

If the patient be strong, and any acute inflammation exist about the joint, one or more bleedings from the arm, and afterward leeches, will be required. But the periods of employing these must not succeed each other too rapidly—for chronic diseases, by their duration, frequently induce great debility.

Local emollient and anodyne baths, continued for two hours at a time, are useful. Although, by appropriate means, the inflammatory element may disappear in a month, it may persist in other cases for three, six, or nine months, and, to such cases, which may also have resisted mercury and barytes, we must oppose time, and the continued application of small relays of leeches. Eventually the moxa may be employed. It is rare, indeed, to find one of these swellings dissipated by antiphlogistics alone. A slight diminution of volume only results from the subsidence of inflammatory action. After the employment of antiphlogistics, an interval must be allowed prior to commencing the use of stimulants—but the presence of occasional pain, or pain which has resisted depletion, must not deter us. *Leeches* may be applied for other than the ordinary reasons. From three to six, or eight, placed around the base of the tumefaction, will cause a degree of heat and excitement in the swelling, when torpid, and favor absorption.

[The leeches may be repeated in this way several times, taking care that the bites do not bleed for more than a quarter of an hour, for fear of the debilitating effects. Cupping may be substituted, and acts as an antiphlogistic or stimulant, according to the quantity of blood drawn.]

Compression is useful by preventing the too free access of blood to the tumor, and causing a slight degree of excitement at its surface. It is most advantageously applied so that it may extend an inch beyond the circumference of the tumor. If employed in improper cases, it may occasion inflammation or gangrene, and, in all, requires regulation in its various degrees, according to the stages and peculiarities of each. Thus the mere application of diachylon, the use of bandages and agaric, and the application of leaden plates to the part, excite different degrees of compression. The compression may be readjusted every twenty-four hours, and its employment does not exclude the use of iodine ointments, and the various internal remedies. Even after the tumor has disappeared, especially when of a scirrhus consistence, compression must be continued for several weeks longer.

It is to be rejected—1. When considerable inflammation exists. 2. When the tumor, though small, is very hard, unequal, knotted, adherent to the skin, and especially if this latter be red or discolored. When, however, the scirrhous mass has been removed, we may employ pressure. 3. When the tumor is in some parts indurated, and in others pultaceous.

The author believes Dr. O'Beirne's conclusions concerning the utility of *salivation* in these cases, are too general, and too premature.

Mercurial inunction, carried to salivation, is equally useful as the calo-mel. When no inflammation of the part exists, the mercurial ointment, applied by topical friction, is an excellent solvent, but, when inflammation does exist, it must be applied in thick layers, to remain in contact with the part, as recommended by M. Serres, when it acts as an antiphlogistic, and not, as in the case of friction, as a stimulant to absorption.

Lisfranc recommends applying the *ioduret of lead*, if properly watched that no injurious excitement be produced ; and he finds that in scrofulous subjects, the internal use of iodine, and especially the iodide of potassium, is very useful. The iodide of lead is certainly a valuable agent in many cases, and especially when the cervical or axillary, and perhaps also when the mesenteric glands are enlarged; but it ought to be given in-ternally as well as applied externally. The usual dose internally is from four to ten grains.

Blistering must not be employed when even sub-inflammation is present, being, as it is, essentially stimulant.

When the blister occasions an injurious degree of inflammation, we must meet this with leeches, etc. We must judge of the ultimate effects they are likely to produce by the degree of irritation that results.

The application of the *moxa* follows the same rules as the use of blister-ing. When a repetition is likely to be required, the moxa must be of only a small size, somewhat less than a shilling.

The *seton* is the most exciting of all exutories, and must not be em-ployed until the inflammatory action has subsided. It should not be passed through the substance of the engorgement, but on one side of it. It is only to be employed when all other excitants have failed.

There are cases of white swelling, which, after proceeding well on to-ward a cure, remain, at length, quite stationary, treat them how we will. In these we must abandon all active measures, contenting ourselves with hygienic precautions, and sometimes in a few weeks we may find the swell-ing much dissipated, and, even if still persistent, the various therapeutical agents will usually be resumed with much greater advantage after such an interval.

M. Lisfranc states that, under his hands, the *muriate of barytes*, given in large doses, has been found very successful, the patient being also during its use confined to a vegetable diet and water drink, upon which, however, he often gains both flesh and strength. He begins with six grains, and reaches, in some cases, as high as forty-eight grains per diem, while, at Marseilles, and in Italy, two drachms have been given in the same period.

When the white swelling dates from a *rheumatic* origin, it has been re-commended to place an irritant, such as a blister, upon the joint itself. This practice is attended with the danger of fixing the locality of the in-flammatory action; and M. Lisfranc prefers, in the case of the knee joint, *e. g.*, placing the blister at the upper and outer part of the thigh; and in following this practice he has met with great success. In some of these cases the pain, which is so distressing, has disappeared under salivation as if by enchantment.

After a cure, the joint is not at once enabled to resume its functions. The patient has remained at rest during a long space of time, and pain attends his first movements.

Relapses were formerly very frequent, but M. Lisfranc has found them to be rare, since he has given his patients a padded knee-cap to wear. This limits the movements of the joint, and supports it during their performance, prevents any stagnation of the fluids, and aids the resorption of any effusion that may occur. Atrophy of the joint sometimes follows, which may be persistent, or may disappear, as the general health improves.

Part vii., *p.* 158.

Various Diseases of the Knee Joint—Inflammation of Synovial Membrane.—When the disease has been of long duration, says Sir B. Brodie, a change takes place in the condition of the synovial membrane, quite different from what is ever observed in the serous membranes. It becomes thickened, of a soft pulpy consistence; the inner surface is no longer smooth and uniform, but processes of soft vascular substance project from it, in the manner of fringes, into the cavity of the joint. In the commencement of this disease the morbid changes are, of course, confined to the synovial membrane; in a more advanced stage these changes extend to the other textures. That portion of the membrane which covers the cartilages, though it resists the disease in the first instance, becomes affected afterward. The cartilages themselves adhere less closely to the bone than under ordinary circumstances, and by and by they begin to ulcerate; generally on the patella in the first instance, on the femur and tibia afterward.

The fluid found in the cavity of the joint, when the synovial membrane is inflamed, is serous. In cases of a slight degree of inflammation, it is slightly turbid; in severer cases it is very turbid, with flakes of coagulated lymph floating in it. Under certain circumstances the synovial membrane will secrete, not mere serum, but actual pus. In like manner, serous membranes occasionally secrete pus, though under ordinary circumstances they merely secrete serum. The cavity of the knee joint is then converted into one large abscess; the abscess being bounded in some parts by inflamed synovial membrane, and in others by the bones of the joint. I say by the bones of the joint; for the cartilages whenever they come in contact with the purulent secretion, become absorbed. Now let us suppose that there has been inflammation of the synovial membrane, and that it has subsided. In what condition is the joint afterward? Sometimes the membrane is left thickened, of a gristly texture, and that may happen even where the cartilages and bones have altogether escaped the invasion of the disease. In other cases, the cartilages being absorbed, the cavity of the joint is completely filled up by the thickened synovial membrane, and the coagulated lymph effused from its surface. The parts all adhere the one to the other, and anchylosis by soft substance, in the first instance, and by bony substance ultimately, is the consequence. However, complete anchylosis does not occur except the cartilages have been completely absorbed. Where the cartilages have been only partially absorbed, a healing process is established. A kind of membrane is formed upon the surface of the bone in the place of the cartilage, and the joint retains its complete mobility.

With regard to treatment in all cases of inflammation, and, I may add, of other diseases of a joint, the first and most important thing is to keep the joint in a state of quietude.

The best contrivance for keeping the joint quiet is splints, made of thick and stiff leather, macerated in warm water, and allowed to dry on the part. They should be pretty broad splints, one being applied to each side of the joint, nicely adjusted to it, and kept on by a bandage. These splints, when dry, become as hard as a board, but they are easy to be worn, because they exactly fit. When the cure is nearly completed, the patient should wear an elastic bandage, so as to allow of a little motion, within certain limits, and the heel of his shoe should be raised a little, to keep the knee slightly bent.

In cases of acute inflammation, general antiphlogistic measures may be required as well as the local abstraction of blood.

After giving a brisk purgative, then give twelve minims of vin. colchici in a saline draught three times a day; in two or three days stop its exhibition, and after an interval of a day or two give it again; it is most useful when there is a gouty diathesis, with lithates in the urine; an occasional purgative is necessary during the administration of the colchicum, and also small doses of blue pill to keep up the secretion of bile which colchicum diminishes. Give mercury so as to affect the system; this may be done not only in the gouty diathesis, but also where there is rheumatic inflammation, and combine it with opium, as in iritis.

In chronic inflammation the same measures as in the acute, only not quite so active: leeches; blisters; apply them in succession, or keep one open with savine cerate; give colchicum as an alterative, two grains of the extract with as much blue pill, every night, and an aperient every third or fourth morning: or give the acetous extract, with calomel and comp. ext. of coloc. every second or third night. Give, also, iodide of potassium in small doses, combined with alkaline remedies. In slight cases, use lini ments to the joints, lin. vol. camph., and sp. terebinth.; or olei olivæ ʒiss.; acid. sulph., ʒj., and sp. terebinth. ʒss.; or paint the knee with a solution of iodine.

I said that mercury was useful in another and more advanced stage of the disease, when the altered character of the pain, attended with starting of the limb at night, indicates that ulceration is going on in the cartilages. Here the only remedy is mercury, and the effect of it is remarkable. Make the gums sore, and the patient who was suffering tortures, will, in a few days, be quite relieved. If it be administered at a sufficiently early period, it will save the limb, but will not prevent anchylosis. Mercury should be given here in the same manner as in cases of iritis, or chronic inflammation of the testicle. Calomel and opium may be administered two or three times a day till the gums are sore, mere alterative doses being insufficient.

Treatment of Abscess of the Knee Joint.—[In these cases the suppuration often involves the whole joint, which is one large abscess. The treatment is comparatively simple.]

Make an opening as soon as you can, and let out the matter. But what kind of opening? Not a small or valvular one.

All large abscesses, and those of joints especially, should be opened by a very free incision, so that the pus may flow out without squeezing, or any kind of rough manipulation.

There should not be the pressure even of a finger on the abscess, with a view to force out its contents. Make a free opening, let the matter flow of its own accord, at the same time keeping the joint in a state of absolute and complete repose by means of leathern splints, or by supporting it with pillows and cusions, and it will scarely ever happen that any mischief follows. If the first opening be made in a depending part, it may be all that is wanted. It may be, however, that one or two openings will be required in other situations afterward. In these cases the disease has its origin in the soft parts. The bones are in the first instance in a healthy state, and the progress of the disease is so rapid, that, although deprived of their cartilages, there is not time for the bones to become materially diseased afterward.

The articular cartilages will have become absorbed, and recovery by anchylosis is the result: the joint during recovery must be supported with leathern splints: or if the leg be bent on the thigh, use the screw instrument, with splints at the posterior part of the leg and thigh. In using the screw, however, you should observe that it is better to leave the leg a very little bent on the thigh rather than quite straight. The former position of the leg is more convenient for walking than the latter, especially if the patient has the heel of his foot or shoe a little raised.

Gouty Inflammation of the Synovial Membrane of the Knee-Joint.— This disease is met with in those who lead an indolent life, and indulge too freely in wine and animal food; some of the smaller joints are generally affected first, and it has this peculiarity that there is seldom much effusion within the joint; the synovial membrane becomes thickened, and then absorbed, and the cartilages are not unfrequently removed by a continuation of the disease of their structure.

In the course of time, that is, after the lapse of some years, the cartilages, and even the bones, become absorbed; the fingers being actually shortened and twisted in a variety of ways. Not unfrequently, in cases of long standing, the bones of the knee, examined in dissection, present a singular appearance, as if they had actually been worn away by friction.

In some instances there is a deposit of lithate of soda, or chalk-stone, in the joint itself, and in its neighborhood. This, like the last, is a very troublesome form of the disease, and is very little under the dominion of remedies.

Give a grain of acet. ext. of colchicum, a grain of blue pill, and three grains of ext. of hop, every night, with a gentle aperient every third or fourth morning; after giving these pills for a fortnight, stop them for two months, and then give them a fortnight again, and so on: give also a grain and a half or two grains of iodide of potassium, with ten or twelve grains of bicarbonate of potash twice a day, for six or eight weeks at a time. This system must be continued, with occasional intermissions, for one or two years, or even longer. This chronic gouty affection is not in itself dangerous, but it shows a bad constitution, and the person thus affected is liable to other diseases.

Scrofulous Disease of the Knee Joint.— Never abstract blood, nor make use of counter-irritation. Here, as in all diseases of joints, a state of perfect repose is necessary; use the leathern splints. As soon as the digestive organs are brought into a proper state, give tonics, particularly chalybeate tonics. To children give the vinum ferri of the old Pharmacopœia, for three weeks, and then omit it for ten days, and so on for several years, so as to improve the weak constitution. If fever be produced, decrease the dose, or omit it altogether for a while; or give the tinct. ferri mur.; or the sirup of iodide of iron; or the latter and the vin. ferri alternately. When you have a patient with whom no form of iron will agree, then give quinine, bark, or alkaline solution of sarsaparilla; the latter is very useful to delicate children. Change of air is highly beneficial, the sea-side; when the joint has become stiff, do not use force to straighten it; it should be done gradually by means of a screw apparatus; if an abscess forms in the joint, continue the use of the splints, but have them lined with oil-silk. If the disease have been neglected, or it has been found impossible to save the joint, amputate as soon as possible. If, by examination with a probe it is found that there be a piece of dead bone within the joint, so that it cannot exfoliate, the sooner the limb is amputated the better. Bony anchylosis takes years for its completion, so that if the limb be bent there will be plenty of time to get it into its proper place.

Primary Ulceration of the Cartilages of the Knee. — [This disease apparently may originate either in the cartilage itself, or in the orifice of the adjacent bone; but in what Sir Benjamin considers primary ulceration, it invariably begins in the surface next to the articular cavity. He says:]

On examining the joint in an early stage of the disease, the cartilage is found to be absorbed at one point, and the surface of the bone exposed and carious. Probably there is no effusion of any kind in the joint, neither serum nor pus; but the exposed surface of bone is more vascular than under ordinary circumstances. As the disease advances, the ulceration of the cartilage becomes more extensive, and when it has attained a certain point, pus is formed in the joint. As in some cases there is suppuration without ulceration, so in these there is ulceration without suppuration. As I have observed in a former lecture, the two processes are generally combined, but there is no necessary connection between them. The cartilages at last become destroyed throughout the knee—on the femur, the patella, and the tibia. Sometimes when abscess forms, it is limited by adhesion to one part of the joint, and then perhaps suppuration takes place in another part of it. In other cases the abscess is not so limited; the whole joint is distended with matter, so as to form one large abscess; and in this stage of the disease, the bones in the neighborhood of the joint become inflamed and dark-colored; the matter lodging in the cancelli becomes putrid, probably a portion of the bone loses its vitality and exfoliates into the articular cavity, while the abscess finds its way out in various directions, making numerous sinuses under the fascia, and among the tendons, before it presents itself externally.

While these changes take place in the affected joint, they are indicated by the following symptoms. Generally there are rheumatic pains in other joints in the first instance; by and by the pains are, as it were, concentrated in the knee. The pain is very severe, and yet the joint is scarcely at all swollen, or rather I should say there is no swelling in the first instance. After a time there is a slight general enlargement of the joint, the consequence of a deposit of lymph, or serum, outside of the synovial membrane. The swelling assumes the shape of the articulating ends of bones, and appears greater than it really is; because the muscles of the thigh are wasted above, as those of the leg are below. The pain is aggravated by motion, and there is a painful starting of the limb at night. The pain is especially aggravated by pressure on the patella, and whenever, in this or any other case of disease of the knee, this symptom exists, you may suspect that the cartilages of the joint are beginning to ulcerate. The disease may go on not only for weeks but for many months, the patient's health suffering all the time, from disturbed rest at night and constant pain in the day, and yet without suppuration taking place. By and by matter forms, and then there is an aggravation of all the symptoms. The matter, as in all other cases of abscesses connected with the knee joint, burrows in various directions among the muscles and tendons, making numerous and circuitous sinuses.

Keep the joint perfectly at rest, and use setons, issues, blisters, and counter-irritants. The great remedy is mercury ; two grains of calomel and one-third of a grain of opium, three times a day, until the gums are affected. Where mercury cannot be borne, give sarsaparilla and iodide of potassium ; sarsaparilla should also be given after the course of mercury. Ung. hydrarg. may be rubbed into the thighs where it cannot be borne internally. A caustic issue inserted on each side the patella will very often stop the pain and the starting of the limb at night, when other means have failed.

Morbid Alteration of Structure of the Synovial Membrane.—There is a curious condition of the synovial membrane in which it seems to have undergone a peculiar morbid alteration of structure. It is thickened in various degrees, sometimes to the extent of an inch and a half, having assumed a sort of pulpy structure intersected by white membranous bands. In some instances there is a preternatural vascularity, and vessels injected with blood are seen ramifying in it to a considerable extent. In other cases no increased vascularity is perceptible. There is little doubt that in some cases this is the result of long-continued chronic inflammation ; but in others I am glad to believe that it takes place independently of the inflammatory action.

[The disease may progress for some time, even years, without any other symptoms.]

As it has advanced to the layer of the synovial membrane, which is reflected over the cartilage, the latter has begun to ulcerate, the ulceration being marked as on other occasions, by aggravation of pain and startings of the limb at night. At this stage of the disease small abscesses form in the substance of the diseased synovial membrane. These gradually make their way to the surface, one coming in one place, and another in another, discharging a very small quantity of matter.

When the cartilages are thus ulcerated, the matter is formed in the joint, and perhaps in the substance of the synovial membrane also, the patient's health begins to be affected, as in other cases of articular abscesses, and at this period nothing can be done for him but to amputate the limb. Can any remedial means be employed with success in the early stage of the disease ?

Apply pressure by means of several alternate layers of diachylon plaster and bandage ; and afterward by leathern splints, and a firm bandage ; attend also to the general health.

Sir B. Brodie considers the affection to be of rare occurrence : he then speaks of

Loose Cartilages in the Knee.— Remove them by operation ; get the cartilage fixed over the outer or inner condyle, and while it is retained in that situation, divide slowly, the skin, cellular membrane, fascia, ligaments, and synovial membrane : hold the knife with a loose hand, or the cartilage will be pressed into the joint ; lay hold of it with a tenaculum, but should it recede within the joint, never grope for it, but bring the edges of the wound together, and perform the operation at some other time. A valvular operation has been proposed.   •   *Part* xiii., *p.* 185.

Case of Scrofulous Disease of the Knee, treated by Sulphur and Electro-Galvanism.—This was a case of scrofulous enlargement of the knee joint, occurring in a young woman, the swelling being of three months' duration. The general treatment consisted in the administration of small quantities of the purest *sulphur*, combined with carbonate of iron, nutritious diet, and such open-air exercise as the case would admit of. And the local applications were first hot poultices to relieve the pain, next compression by means of strips of iodine plaster and a bandage, and then the hot water douche. When she had been about sixteen weeks under treatment, Mr. Bulley began to use electro-galvanism. He says:]

After the electro-galvanism had been applied every other day for a fortnight or three weeks, I could observe a very perceptible alteration in the shape of the affected joint, the more than natural quantity of synovial fluid which remained in its cavity up to the time she left the hospital having become absorbed; and I could plainly perceive that the rounded appearance occasioned by the more solid deposit in the ligamentous tissues was gradually becoming less and less apparent, until at the end of about five weeks from her leaving the hospital, it had almost completely disappeared, and she could walk about upon the limb without any particular pain or stiffness in the joint, which, by admeasurement, did not exceed to any appreciable extent the size of the other knee; it was, in fact, evident that the morbid deposit which I could have no doubt was of the same solid character as usually accompanies the more advanced forms of scrofulous exudation, had been absorbed and taken away by the processes employed.

Part xviii., *p.* 152.

Joints Diseased—Issues.—The best kind of counter-irritation is that exerted by the issue made with caustic potash. In synovial disease of the knee the issue is particularly useful.   *Part* xix., *p.* 122.

Removal of Loose Cartilages from Joints.—In his description of the subcutaneous or valvular mode of removing loose cartilages, Professor Miller remarks:]

" In the first place, the patient is to be prepared for the operation. For a day or two, the limb is to be disused, so that previous excitement may have thoroughly subsided. Low diet is enjoined, the primæ viæ are gently yet efficiently cleared, and general secretion is seen to be in a satisfactory state, so that there may be no predisposition to inflammation. Then the foreign body, having been made superficial, is gently pushed to the extreme verge of the synovial pouch; either on the inside or on the outside of the patella, as may be most convenient. The internal position is usually the most preferable; and there it is retained fixedly, by the fingers of an attentive and steady assistant. A tenotomy needle, or thin and narrow bistoury, of fine edge, is passed in an oblique direction; and an incision a little larger than the outline of the cartilage, is made through the tense synovial membrane. The instrument is then withdrawn slowly and cautiously, the finger gently yet firmly following and consolidating its track. A few drops of blood escape, but not a particle of synovia; and no air has obtained admission, even to the areolar tissue. The integumental wound is immediately and carefully occluded, by plaster or collodion.

" The foreign body is then gently pressed through the aperture in the synovial capsule, which aperture, as has just been stated, is made sufficiently free to admit of this being accomplished without force or difficulty.

When exterior to the capsule it is coaxed through the areolar tissue—sufficiently lax readily to admit of this—by gentle pressure of the fingers; not in the track of the puncture, but in a different direction, probably at nearly a right angle to it. When about an inch and a half, or two inches, from the synovial wound, it is there permitted to remain. Not permanently, however, as has been proposed. Otherwise, acting still more as a foreign body in its recent and raw site, inflammatory action is excited, suppuration is all but inevitable, and extension to the synovial membrane becomes extremely probable; the very result to the avoidance of which all our pains had been directed. For two days, or three at the utmost, it is suffered to remain in its new locality, undisturbed; the most careful prophylactic treatment being meanwhile employed, both generally and locally, so as to avert undue excitement. By that time the synovial wound will have closed by adhesion; and both tracks—that of puncture as well as that of extrusion—will have been consolidated. Then, the substance having been fixed as before, a direct incision is made upon it; not more than is sufficient for its ready removal. After it has been lifted out, the superficial and slight wound is brought together by strap: and, in all probability, it unites by adhesion." *Part* xxiii., *p.* 273.

Knee Joint—Excision of.—The following description of the operation of excision of the knee joint as performed by Mr. Jones, of Jersey, in a case under his care, will show the formidable nature of the operation.

The case was one of extensive ulceration of the cartilages. It is gratifying to know that the result was completely successful. It was performed as follows: A longitudinal incision was made on each side of the knee joint, midway between the vasti and flexors of the leg, full five inches in extent; rather more than half the length was over the femur, and rather less than half over the tibia. These two cuts were down to the bones; they were connected by a transverse one just over the prominence of the tubercle of the tibia, care being taken to avoid cutting the ligamentum patellæ by this incision; the flap thus defined was reflected upward, the patella, its ligament, and the joint thereby exposed. The synovial capsule was cut through as far as it could be seen; the patella and its ligament were now drawn over the internal condyle, while the joint was kept extended. It was next forcibly flexed, the crucial ligaments, almost breaking in the act, only required a slight touch of the knife to divide them completely; the articular surfaces of both bones were thus completely brought to view, and nearly two inches of the femur and half an inch of the tibia were sawn off, the soft parts being drawn aside by assistants. The external condyle of the femur was found hollowed out by a large abscess, and it was necessary to saw off a portion of the carious bone, and to gouge the remainder, until healthy cancellous tissue was reached. The entire synovial membrane was in a state of pulpy degeneration, and was carefully dissected off. The hemorrhage had been rather great, but had now almost ceased, and no vessel required deligation. The blood was sponged out of the wound, the patella (after the diseased portion had been gouged out) and its ligament were replaced as nearly as possible, in their natural state, the bones brought in apposition, the flap brought down and held by sutures, the limb bandaged on a slight undersplint and laid in a box, the wound covered with moist lint, and the boy put to bed yet asleep. The operation occupied full twenty minutes, and was performed while the patient was under the influence of chloro-form.

Preserving the patella, and not dividing its ligament, makes the operation more tedious and difficult ; but this is a very secondary consideration, where it results in obtaining a more favorable issue. That it proved so in this instance is abundantly established by the fact that, in less than seven weeks after the operation, this patient is able to raise his foot without any assistance ; while a young man who occupies the next bed, and in whose case everything has gone on favorably, was only able to do so in as many months.   *Part* xxviii., *p.* 155.

Knock-knees.—An operation is described by Dr. Mayer, of Wurzburg, whereby this deformity was remedied. The front and inner side of the head of the tibia having been deprived of integument and periosteum, a wedge was cut from this portion nearly of the thickness of the bone. By straightening the limb the bony surfaces were brought in contact, and the limb acquired its natural shape. In a month the parts were completely healed and the weight could be borne upon the leg. Soon afterward the other leg was operated upon with the like success. *Part* xxviiii., *p.* 164.

Excision of Joints.—There is one important view always to be observed with respect to this operation on the knee and the elbow. In the knee joint endeavor to promote *firm anchylosis.* In the elbow joint endeavor to insure *mobility.*   *Part* xxix., *p.* 183.

Incision into the Knee Joint.—[The following case by Dr. Jordison, shows the extent to which injury of this large joint may be carried, with ultimate safety, and even without anchylosis.]—G. G., aged 20 years, an agricultural laborer, of strumous habit, whilst in the act of mowing, came in contact with the scythe of his fellow-laborer producing an incised wound of about five inches in length, extending transversely across the anterior part of the thigh immediately above the superior edge of the patella. The hemorrhage, which had been considerable, had in a great measure subsided. On introducing my finger into the wound to ascertain its course, I could readily pass it into the cavity of the joint, the aperture into which was to the extent of about an inch. I lost no time in closing the wound, which I did by a number of sutures, covering the entire wound with numerous strips of adhesive plaster, and incasing the whole in oil-skin, so as to exclude the air as much as possible. I then placed the leg and thigh upon a long, straight splint, and had him conveyed home. In the course of two hours reaction commenced, and for about six hours he suffered excruciating pain, which I successfully combated with large doses of opium, combined with small doses of calomel. I allowed the dressings to remain undisturbed for several days, and for a fortnight there was not the least constitutional disturbance, but at the expiration of that time (he being still under the most rigid antiphlogistic discipline), the pulse suddenly rose to 135, the tongue became loaded, and the countenance anxious ; the knee was very much enlarged, exquisitely tender, and discharged large quantities of synovia. I ordered two dozen leeches to be applied, hot fomentations, and to take calomel and opium every four hours. In the course of a few days the constitutional disturbance gradually subsided, but the size of the knee remained unaltered ; the integuments now sloughed to a considerable extent, and the discharge of synovia still continued very profuse.

It was upward of two months, before the wound commenced for the first time to wear a more healthy aspect, and the tenderness to subside. In fifteen weeks from the infliction of the injury it was cicatrized. The motion of the joint was at first very limited, but as time wore on it obtained greater mobility, and I have now the satisfaction of seeing him industriously employed in his wonted avocation, with his once afflicted knee as strong, as flexible, and of as much service to him as it was prior to the accident. *Part* xxix., *p.* 183.

Knee Joint—Amputation at the.—First make a small anterior flap, drawing the knife across the front of the joint, and then inserting the point of the blade behind the femur, thrust it through to the other side, close to the condyles; then carrying it downward cut the posterior flap from the calf of the leg. The saw is then applied a little above the condyles, and the flaps brought together as in an ordinary amputation. Mr. Potter, of Newcastle, saws through the bone before making the posterior flap. Take the full length of the calf for the posterior flap, as the soft parts at the back of the thigh contract very much in the course of time. *Part* xxx., *p* 110.

Knee Joint.—In operations for diseases of the knee joint, *save the patella, if possible*, with its ligament. *Part* xxxi., *p.* 105.

Excision of the Knee Joint.—Take care to clear away from the face of the flap the whole of the synovial membrane. Be careful of the direction of the saw as you saw through the femur and tibia—take care that you cut through these bones *parallel to each other*, else their surfaces will not meet properly. The line of section in the femur should be close to the edge of the articulating cartilage of the inner condyle, which will remove all the articular surface likely to be implicated in disease, and still leave a breadth of bony surface about equal to the cut surface of the tibia. The patella must be left. It is indispensable. *Part* xxxi., *p.* 108.

Excision of the Knee Joint.—Having turned back the flap containing the patella, apply the saw carefully, and divide the required amount from the femur and tibia, without disturbing the soft parts by the needless introduction of a spatula; remove both ends together, first raising the separated extremity of the femur, and dissecting from above downward. By thus keeping the articular extremities in connection, their dissection from the popliteal vessels is rendered safe and easier, time is saved, and the operator can have the upper soft parts depressed by an assistant when the continuity of the vessels is unimportant, whilst he is enabled himself to raise the back part of the joint from the more perilous vicinity of the vessels inferiorly. *Part* xxxii., *p.* 109.

Knee Joint—Diseases of.—In obstinate cases, which defy the usual forms of treatment, local depletion by means of leeches or cupping is injurious. You will find the most benefit from the inunction of mercurial ointment, with one-third its quantity of fluid extract of opium, followed by perfect rest in the recumbent position, and firm application of a flannel roller. *Part* xxxiii., *p.* 137.

Contractions of the Knee.—When from nervous irritation, as a symptom of general hysteria, there will be no evidence of disease within the joint; in these cases put the patient under the influence of chloroform, and the limb will almost of its own accord fall into a straight position, in which it must be retained by means of a long splint. When depending on spasmodic contraction of the ham-strings from irritation of the nerves at some distance, as by the pressure of fæces, etc., give powerful cathartics to clear out the bowels. When from subacute inflammation within the joint, it will generally yield without the necessity of extending force, by the application of leeches, blisters, and other remedies to reduce the inflammatory action, as small doses of mercury and morphia, etc. When from consolidation of ligamentous structures in and around the joint, you will generally succeed by gradual and forcible extension. Never mind the snaps and cracks which may be heard; there is no fear, if you only take care that there is no inflammatory action going on in the joint at the time.

Part xxxiii., *p.* 137–160.

Anchylosed Knee Joint.—During the acute inflammatory stage, keep up counter-irritation by a *repetition* of caustic issues made with potassa fusa; this method is preferable to keeping an issue open by peas, as there is greater advantage to be gained by the primary burning than the subsequent suppuration. If the joint be obliterated, and the disease entirely subdued, you may strengthen the limb by forcibly breaking through the anchylosing bands; this may be accompanied by a loud crack, but there is no danger; they generally do very well. *Part* xxxiii., *p.* 144.

Excision of the Knee Joint.—The following two suggestions may be worthy the attention of practical surgeons in the management of these cases. The first is the *division of the hamstring tendons*, so as to prevent the displacement of the bones, which is so troublesome in the after-treatment. The second is the *making of an opening into the popliteal space*, for the direct escape of pus, to prevent it bagging and burrowing.

Part xxxiii., *p.* 145.

Excision of the Knee Joint.—Dr. Vitalis suggests that after the operation the limb be put up in one of Ester's swinging fracture apparatus, having an opening at the posterior part through which pus may escape, and the wound be dressed without disturbing the limb.

Part xxxiii., *p.* 307.

Excision of the Knee Joint.—An error in diagnosis as to the suitableness of a case for excision by no means debars the patient from the likelihood of cure by amputation. If the patient be under the influence of chloroform the shock is not greater, and if the bones are found extensively diseased, amputation should be performed at once. *Part* xxxv., *p.* 67.

Resection of the Knee Joint.—There is a great practical distinction between strumous diseases of the knee joint, commencing within the cavity of the articulation, and those originating in the cancellous structure of the heads of the bones entering into the formation of the joint; for every diseased joint, with the exception of that form of diffuse strumous infiltration of the head of the two bones, is, in general, well suited for the adoption of resection in preference to amputation. The surgeon should not always decide which operation he will perform, till he has obtained a clear view of the state of the joint. *Part* xxxvi., *p.* 140.

Dropsy of the Knee Joint.—Provided that the case be one of simple uncomplicated chronic dropsy, Dr. Macdonnell's plan of injection with iodine will probably prove successful. The puncture should be made at the part most remote from the joint. If the sac is very large the injection should not be used directly after the first tapping, but time should be allowed for the sac to collapse somewhat. When the injection is going to be used, apply a wet bandage from below the knee upward to a level with the upper edge of the patella, so as to push the remainder of the fluid above the joint into the pouch of synovial membrane. When the fluid is drawn off, inject about two drachms of the strongest tincture of iodine, with an equal quantity of lukewarm water. Allow this to remain, moving the joint a little, that the fluid may be diffused. The wet bandage must now be carried further up the limb, the aperture being first closed with adhesive plaster. A long padded splint should be afterward applied.

Part xxxvi., *p.* 143.

Removal of the Patella from an Excised Knee Joint.—Mr. Fergusson is an advocate for the removal of the patella even when healthy, unless it is bound to the condyles of the femur by osseous material. It is liable to give subsequent annoyance.

   *   *   *   *   *   *

After-Management of Excisions of the Knee Joint.—It is not only " meddlesome midwifery " which is bad, but meddlesome surgery. There is no one cause so productive of ill effects after the above operation as changing the splints too soon, and constantly examining to see if consolidation has commenced. After the operation the limb should be placed on a straight back splint very carefully padded, that there may not be any unequal pressure, especially about the heel and the malleoli, where it is especially liable to take place. The two side splints should be movable, that the wound may be readily dressed. The pads should be secured from soiling by being covered with oil silk. *Part* xxxvii., *p.* 115.

Anchylosis of the Knee.—In the treatment of this affection there has not hitherto been shown, generally speaking, sufficient patience on the part of the surgeon. In infants of six years of age the joints have been excised, that is, just at that period of life when successful treatment by extension is most to be hoped for. Even where from strumous disease, the tibia is dislocated backward, by *gradual* efforts the bones may be restored to their places, and the disease subdued. (Cases related.) As the result of rheumatic disease, bony anchylosis is not uncommon, and requires much more energetic, or rather forcible treatment than strumous disease. In the straightening of contracted joints extension is wanted, not forcible rupture of contracted tendons and uniting bands, though subcutaneous tenotomy may be practised if necessary. If the slightest amount of motion be attainable on manipulating the joint, a favorable prognosis should be given. *Part* xxxviii., *p.* 130.

Suppuration of the Knee Joint—Free Incision.—When suppuration has taken place in the knee joint, it is absolutely necessary that an incision should be made. You will commit a fatal error to leave a patient unrelieved of abcess in the interior of the joint, under the impression that you are likely to add to the mischief already existing by opening so large a joint as that of the knee. The incision must be free, and the cyst allowed by its inherent faculty of contraction to force out its own contents. It is desirable to leave the opening patent, and not to bring the edges of the wound together by strapping and bandaging, although this practice may sometimes succeed. *Part* xl., *p.* 92.

SHOULDER JOINT.

Arthropathia of the.—A peculiar form of chronic arthritis sometimes affects this joint, leading to atrophy both of the soft parts and the bones. The treatment of these cases will vary according to the stage of the disease. During the early and inflammatory period, use repeated leechings and small cuppings, mercurial and belladonna ointment, and emollient and resolvent poultices. During the second stage, that of muscular atrophy, apply large blisters, moxas, or the cautery before and behind the joints, and use baths, with local stimulants and tonic douches, of plain, sulphureous or aromatic waters. Lastly, when the bones become affected, lay aside antiphlogistic and derivative treatment, and employ friction, especially with oil of turpentine; use also passive motion, taking care, however, not to excite fresh inflammation by doing this too soon, and not to run the risk of anchylosis, by delaying it too long.

Part xx., *p.* 107.

Peculiar Affection of the Shoulder Joint.—[Sir Benj. Brodie describes a most tedious and annoying affection of this joint, seeming to depend in many instances on a chronic inflammation of the substance of the deltoid muscle, or of the bursa under the deltoid and to be greatly benefited by the employment of counter-irritation and the iodide of potassium.]

"The cases here referred to occur more frequently in private than in hospital practice: and (whether it be accidentally or not I do not know) it certainly has happened that I have met with it more frequently in the female than in the male sex. The patient complains of pain, which, however, is referred not so much to the joint itself as to the arm a little below it, near the insertion of the deltoid muscle. At first the pain is trifling, but it soon becomes severe and constant. The patient describes it as a *wearing* pain, of which she is constantly reminded. It is aggravated by every motion of the limb, and by pressing the articulating surfaces against each other. Not only is there no perceptible enlargement of the shoulder, but after some time, in consequence of the want of use and wasting of the deltoid muscle, it seems to be actually reduced in size. It is not long before the mobility of the joint is impaired, becoming gradually more and more limited. When the patient attempts to raise the elbow from her side, it is observed that the scapula is elevated at the same time with the humerus. She is unable to raise her hand to her face, nor can she rotate the limb so as to place it behind her. When the progress of the disease is stopped at an early period, the mobility of the joint may be restored; but otherwise, although the pain and all other symptoms of the disease have subsided, the joint remains stiff, and to all appearance completely anchylosed. Whatever motion the arm is capable of, under these circumstances, depends not on the humerus, but on the scapula.

"It certainly is seldom that this disease terminates in abscess of the joint, when proper attention has been paid to the treatment of it.

"Whether it be from this, or from any other disease, that the joint of the shoulder is brought to such an extreme state of disorganization, one result is, that it is liable to dislocation, or, more properly, to sub-luxation in the direction forward. In one case in which I had the opportunity of examining the parts after death, I found the anterior margin of the glenoid cavity of the scapula destroyed by ulceration, the head of the humerus permanently resting on the ulcerated surface. In another case, in the living person, I found the dislocation to be only occasional, the head of the bone slipping forward so as to make a visible projection in certain motions of the arm, and in certain other motions returning to its natural situation.

"I may take this opportunity of noticing another circumstance, which, though not of much interest in pathology, is of some importance in practice. An abscess originating in the shoulder joint sometimes presents a peculiar appearance, when it is making its way to the surface. A dissection, which I once had the opportunity of making, will explain at once the nature and the cause of this peculiarity. The abscess, taking the course of the tendon of the long head of the *biceps flexor cubiti* muscle, had suddenly emerged from the joint at the lower end of the bicipital groove of the humerus: then, having taken a direction forward, on the anterior edge of the deltoid muscle, had presented itself under the integuments, having a spherical form, so that it might have been mistaken for an encysted tumor. I met with one case, in which this mistake respecting an abscess of this kind, was actually made by a surgeon of considerable experience, who proposed the removal of the tumor by the knife.

Part xxiii., *p.* 272.

Shoulder Joint, Disease of.—In a case which required excision of the head of the humerus, Mr. Syme enlarged an opening existing on the inner side of the shoulder; he then, by means of a probe-pointed bistoury, guided on his finger, detached the connections of the spinati muscles, and pushing the arm upward, protruded the head of the bone, which was then removed. We may remark that ball and socket joints are most liable to chronic inflammation, suppuration, and caries; while the hinge joints are more subject to ulceration of the cartilages, and gelatinous degeneration of the synovial membranes. But the shoulder joint is apt to suffer from disease entirely peculiar to itself; one is, removal of the osseous substance by absorption, so that a cavity is left in place of the round extremity, from inflammation affecting the head of the humerus, independently of the scapula. Again, excessive action of the biceps will produce an injurious effect upon its osseous attachments, leading to exfoliation of the coracoid process, and disease of the humerus, along which the long head of the muscle passes. *Part* xxxiii., *p.* 134.

Shoulder Joint—Resection of.—Resections of the shoulder, unlike those of the knee, generally necessitate the removal of but one of the articular extremities entering into the joint; it is very seldom that more than the head of the humerus need be removed, either from disease or injury, and this, from the very nature of the affections of the joint, which, while they seriously damage or even destroy the head of the humerus, rarely attack the glenoid cavity of the scapula. Again, the exposed position of the humerus, which renders this bone so peculiarly liable to injury from gun-shot wounds, forms a protection for the scapula. Fortunately, the full benefit of resection may be secured by the removal of one articular extremity, as it is not our object to obtain bony anchylosis.

This operation is applicable to compound dislocations, to cases where a bullet may have lodged in the head of the bone, and to all wounds of the shoulder joint complicated with crushing or fracture of one or both bones entering into the articulation, unless, of course, the severity of the injury, by division of the great vessels, or by extensive laceration of the soft parts, necessitates ex-articulation of the limb. Nor need the extension of the injury to the shaft of the humerus deter the surgeon from attempting the operation.

In disease, either one or both articular extremities of the joint may be removed for caries, or, indeed, for any other incurable affection of the articulation, which renders it not merely useless as a joint, but by its presence either destroys the utility of the whole extremity, or seriously affects the general health of the patient. Lastly, this operation may be substituted for ex-articulation, in cases where tumors affecting the head of the humerus do not by their extension to the shaft necessitate the removal of the entire limb. We apprehend that resection of the joint is by no means justifiable for mere anchylosis, provided that this is the only inconvenience the patient suffers from.

The operation is contra-indicated where, together with compound fracture, there is any excessive destruction of the soft parts, or injury to the great vessels or nerves. Neither should cases of necrosis or caries be submitted to operation, unless the disease be confined to the articular extremity of the bone, or at any rate be within reach of removal.

It appears, from the history of former operations on this articulation, that, previous to its performance by Professor Langenbeck, the long tendon of the biceps had always been divided. He it was who first practised an operation which had for its object the preservation of this tendon. Langenbeck's method consists in an incision commencing at the acromion, and extending downward on the anterior aspect of the joint for three or four inches; this should fall just over the bicipital groove, which is then opened, and the tendon drawn inward; the muscles inserted into the tuberosities are now divided, and the head of the bone thrust out of the wound and removed by an ordinary saw. The operation is sufficiently easy of execution when the head of the bone retains its connection with the shaft, and the soft parts are not tense or swollen. On the other hand, it is difficult by this incision to remove the disconnected head of the humerus, and especially when the integuments are swollen and oedematous. To remedy this, and to provide a more dependent aperture for the escape of the secretions from the wound, Stromeyer made use of a semicircular incision, commencing at the posterior edge of the acromion, and extending downward and outward for three inches, having its concavity forward; the joint is thus freely opened from above and behind, the tendon of the biceps can be preserved, and a free and dependent aperture is left for pus. Stromeyer states that patients recover from this operation much more quickly than from Langenbeck's, owing to the much greater facility it affords for cleansing the wound. That perfect recovery may take place after division of the tendon of the biceps is well known, and, indeed, Esmarch relates three cases of resection in which it had been torn across by a ball, and yet in each case the patients recovered, with good use of their arms. It may also be gathered from similar evidence that transverse division of the fibres of the deltoid but little affect the ultimate success of the case Whatever mode of incision be adopted, the deltoid, with few exceptions, becomes much atrophied after the operation; perhaps, this is caused by the division of its nerve, which, with the posterior circumflex artery, are the only nerve and vessel of importance that are liable to injury.

The after-treatment of these cases is far more simple and more easy of execution than that of excision of some other joints. Absolute rest, cleanliness, and appropriate constitutional support constitute the principal measures to be adopted; but we will refer to the plan pursued during the Schleswig-Holstein war. Absolute quiet was maintained by bandaging the arm to the side. Ice was freely applied to the parts, and maintained there until suppuration was fully established. Bleeding, both constitutionally and locally, was unsparingly employed during the stage of reaction, and upon this Stromeyer strongly insists. The wound was never, if possible, disturbed, all cleansing was effected by allowing water to flow over the wound. Matter, if it formed, was let out by incisions, and not squeezed out. Cicatrization was promoted by dressings of nitrate of silver lotions; flannel bandaging was employed to consolidate the parts; passive motion was commenced as soon as the cicatrix had formed, and was continued at the discretion of the surgeon, and as the patient could bear it, until considerable voluntary motion of the extremity had been regained. *Part* xxxvi., *p.* 129.

WRIST JOINT.

Endermic use of Morphia in Articular Contractions.—[Dr. Haygarth published an account of an arthritic affection, which he termed "Nodosity of the Joints." He described it as almost peculiar to women, as occurring at the period of cessation of the menses, principally affecting the fingers, and considered it an affection of the whole of the tissues composing the wrist, and near akin to gout. The joints were painful at night, often tender to the touch, swollen, and, in old cases sometimes actually dislocated. Dr. Thompson has met with an affection much resembling this, which he has successfully treated by the endermic application of some of the salts of morphia. Cases of real nodosity he has also found much benefited by the same treatment.]

The disease which is the subject of this communication does not display itself at any particular period of life; nor is it confined to either sex.

Dr. T. has never seen it in persons under the age of puberty. It appears, in every instance, to be the sequel of repeated severe attacks of acute rheumatism; and has great affinity to inflammation of the synovial membranes, as described by Sir Benjamin Brodie.

[A number of cases are given, from which the following conclusions may be drawn.]

1. That in painful, swollen, and contracted joints, depending on rheumatism, or other causes the topical application of hydrochlorate, or acetate of morphia, to a blistered surface, on the affected joint, is capable of reducing the swelling, abating pain, and restoring the motion to the joints. 2. That these salts seem to produce these beneficial effects, by reducing the sensibility of the nerves of the joint, and favoring absorption by their counter-irritant influence. 3. That they do not act as general narcotics, until the joints are relieved. 4. That they frequently excite a pustular eruption over the body; but this disappears spontaneously, soon after the use of the topical application is discontinued. *Part* xii., *p.* 252.

Wrist Joint, Excision of.—Mr. Erichsen and Mr. Fergusson have removed the bones of the wrist by lateral incisions. Mr. Simon has removed them by making two long incisions in the anterior and posterior aspects of the joint, reaching from about two inches above the wrist, back and front, to the centre of the palm and dorsum of the hand, the incision being so managed as to run between the tendons coursing down to their destination on the metacarpal bones and fingers.

Part xxix., *p.* 195.

Carpal Bones, Excision of.—In cases of partial disease of the wrist joint, in place of amputation of the forearm, excision of the diseased bones is sometimes preferable, as by this means the disease is equally removed, and a very useful hand preserved. It should be conjoined with the use of cod-liver oil and tonics, etc., especially in strumous cases.

Part xxxiii., *p.* 145.

KIDNEY AFFECTIONS.

Treatment of Renal Disease.—Dr. Bright gives the following outline of his treatment of renal disease:

In the first steps, and the more acute forms of disease, bleeding may be considered the most important remedy; but this is, of itself, wholly inadequate to cure unless we purge freely, and at the same time call upon the skin to do its duty. Of all the measures for effecting this latter purpose, the strictest confinement to bed is the most effectual; and without that, I do not believe that in this climate we have a chance of cure. That preliminary, however, being adopted, antimonials are probably the best diaphoretics; but the liquor ammoniæ acetatis is likewise very useful; and a simple saline draught of citrate of potash or soda is, I believe, when diligently persisted in, of much avail, and the warm bath, in its various forms, may in many cases be brought to act most beneficially.

Amongst the purgatives, I shall only mention that elaterium and jalap, with the bitartrate of potash, appear to be the most effectual. When the disease has made further progress, and has become chronic, perhaps organic, I should still recommend the greatest attention to the full effects of purgation, and to the state of the skin, and to protection from atmospheric changes. A voyage to the West Indies, and a residence in one of the more healthy islands, often produce a great change in the constitution, acting chiefly upon the pores of the skin. We have, at least, the negative experience that confirmed cases rarely recover in this country, whatever treatment be adopted.

There are certain remedies whose actions in this disease are less obvious than those to which I have referred; but many of them probably act by affording a degree of stimulant or astringent action to the kidney; of these I may mention the mineral acids as applicable in the declining stages of more acute attacks; the uva ursi, in its different preparations, in the chronic disease; the pyrola umbellata, and the diosma crenata where great irritability of the urinary organs exists—a remedy which I have been led to adopt, in many cases, from the very favorable reports of Sir Benjamin Brodie; nor have I been disappointed of some good effect, though I should perhaps employ with greater confidence a long-continued course of soda, conium, and uva ursi.

Dr. Barlow one of the editors of " Guy's Hospital Reports," strongly recommends tartarized antimony in this formidable disease : with respect to which he says :

"I have never found it necessary to give more than half a grain at a dose to an adult; neither have I attempted to push it to the greatest extent possible; the object not being to give heroic doses of the remedy, but, if possible, to cure the patient." *Part* i., *p.* 55.

Ischuria Renalis.—Dr. Theophilus Thompson has recorded an unusual example of complete interruption of the renal secretion, unattended with the urgent symptoms which protracted anuria usually induces. Death will generally ensue within three days of such an event : Dr. Prout thinks that five days will often elapse before coma takes place. In this case of Dr. Thompson's, no urine was secreted for about 120 hours, and during the next 48 hours, only half an ounce was passed, and the natural quantity was not restored for a month, and yet no urgent cerebral symptoms at any time occurred. Dr. T. attaches some importance in the treatment of the case to the application of nitrate of silver. The final result of the case does not seem to invalidate the value of this opinion. The case was that of a lady aged 45, who had for five years suffered in the region of the colon from frequent and severe attacks of pain. January 28th, the secretion of urine was suddenly suspended, so that only half a drachm was obtained on introducing the catheter. Nine ounces of blood were removed from the loins by cupping, and small doses of tincture of cantharides were administered. In the evening, two drachms of turbid urine were passed. The loins were cupped again, and blistered: prussic acid, creasote, etc., were given, but still, on the 3d February, *i. e.*, seven days after the first suppression, little or no urine had been voided. The nitrate of silver was now freely applied to an old issue on the loins which had lately been dried up, with the view of restoring it : in the evening, a drachm of urine was discharged, and during the night $3\frac{1}{2}$ ounces. The secretion became gradually restored. *Part* ix., *p.* 67.

Injuries of the Kidneys.—The kidney may be injured in a variety of ways, giving rise to very different symptoms. 1. It may be lacerated and cause death by hemorrhage into the cavity of the peritoneum, with the addition likewise of urine escaping into the same cavity. 2. It may be lacerated, with its capsule, and both blood and urine may escape into the cellular tissue around it, without the serous membrane being torn ; and the fatter the person is, the more distant the peritoneum will of course be from the gland. In these cases it has happened that death has ensued from secondary hemorrhage into the parts around the kidney, behind the peritoneum, many days (in one case as late as the 10th day) after the accident, and when the patient appeared to be doing well. 3. There may be no laceration of the capsule of the kidney, but an injury may extend into the infundibula and pelvis of the gland, so that the effused blood escapes into the interior, and hence there is *hematuria.* A great quantity of blood may be lost in this way ; as much as three pints at once. 4. Another consequence of injury of the kidney is *suppuration* within the organ. 5. And another effect is illustrated by two examples published by Mr. Stanley, in which, besides suppuration, there were formed fluctuating tumors or cysts, containing a clear, yellow fluid, resembling urine. With respect to the treatment of some of these cases, Mr. Hawkins says:

"In the first place, with regard to the hematuria, it is seldom that its amount causes any alarm; but if the blood comes away in great quantities, you have the same resources as in other internal bleedings, to which alone you can look for checking hemorrhage from the kidney which does not pass down with the urine. You can cause syncope by bleeding, and you can give styptics, which I have seen do much good in some cases of hematuria. Of these, the best is lead; so that you can give three grains of the acetate with a quarter of a grain of opium every three or four hours for a time. In some cases, in which the lead failed, or alternately with it, I have seen the powdered galls stop the bleeding.

"This medicine is, however, rather nauseous, and sometimes irritating to the stomach. You can also give a dessertspoonful of Ruspini's styptic every three or four hours. You might reasonably expect that, if these medicines have power in any case of hemorrhage, they would be of especial service in hemorrhage from the kidney, to which organ so large a quantity of blood is constantly passing. Another styptic—turpentine— which is useful in passive bleeding from the kidney, does not seem to be applicable to cases of injury in which inflammation is present. The presence of blood in the bladder does not usually occasion much trouble; it did so in the patient from whom this blood passed, and I was obliged to wash out the bladder to free it from coagula and enable the urine to escape, not after an accident, indeed, but for fungus hematodes of the kidney. With a double catheter and warm water, there is no difficulty in doing this, if you are obliged; at all events, there can be no occasion to perform the high operation, as for lithotomy, which was done in one case by Mr. Copland Hutchinson, where blood lodged in the bladder. In most cases, however, you may disregard the amount of hemorrhage, and treat the case as you would another in which there was no bleeding, and you will find it cease gradually in two or three days. I need not say that rest is necessary, and with this you must employ antiphlogistic remedies. You see that our patient now in the house has been cupped once, and has had leeches also once, and fomentations to the painful side; and such means are usually enough. In the case, however, which I read to you, of recent suppuration, I was obliged to bleed as often as five times; cupping, however, is generally sufficient. Then you saw that I gave calomel and saline purgatives; and if you have occasion for purgatives in these cases, and particularly when the lithates abound, as they did here, the salts you select should be the vegetable ones, the potassio-tartrate of soda, or the tartrate of potash, so that the alkalies may at once pass to the kidney and neutralize the excess of acid. Then, again, you may give saline draughts, and add to this sometimes some colchicum if the inflammation does not easily yield.

"After the first symptoms have subsided, you must next look carefully for remaining pain and weakness in the loins, and use counter-irritants; apply blisters, taking the precaution of using some muslin or tissue-paper under them, in order that the cantharides may not be absorbed and pass to the injured or inflamed kidney; and finally, if such pain and weakness continue long, you should insert a seton or an issue over the affected part, which you will do with the view of preventing the formation of abscess or other chronic disease of the kidney, and also to obviate another future mischief, which has been pointed out by Mr. Earle, in a paper in the 'Medico-Chirurgical Transactions,' namely, the formation of calculi in the kidney; though it does not seem very probable that these bodies would be deposited unless the patient's urinary secretion was otherwise disordered."   *Part* x., *p.* 135.

Granular Disease of the Kidney—Bright's Disease, or Albuminuria— Treatment.—Enjoin a general tonic regimen; avoid as articles of food, fat and other highly carbonized materials; attend to the functions of the skin and bowels; relieve congestion of the gland, and, if necessary, use small bleedings. (Dr. Johnson.) Make use of cautious small blood-lettings in the early stages, particularly if acute; give hydragogue cathartics, and improve the general health: do not deplete where the disease is chronic. (Dr. Williams.) In the very early stages change the mode of life and habits of the patient, enjoin pure air and careful attention to diet and exercise; in this stage, application for relief is seldom made. In the second and third stages, relieve congestion; promote the flow of urine and the action of the skin, and prevent the deposition of fatty matters by a diet which contains neither fat, nor butter, nor any of those non-azotized substances nearly allied to it, as starch, sugar, potatoes, etc. (Dr. Todd.)

In the *acute* form, remove congestion of the kidneys by blood-letting, regulated according to the intensity of the disease and the patient's strength; restore the function of the skin, by keeping the patient in a warm atmosphere, giving mild diaphoretics, and the use of the warm or vapor bath. Dr. Barlow gives tartar emetic. Next, remove the dropsy, by diuretics and purgatives, nitrate of potash, in doses of two scruples or more, with digitalis and cream of tartar; the nitrate should be largely diluted.

In the *chronic* form, first attend to the function of the skin by warm clothing, diaphoretics, and the warm bath. Give tincture of cantharides in doses of from four to twelve drops, in some emulsion (Dr. Bright); Dr. Wells and M. Monneret advise thirty to sixty drops in twenty-four hours; or give ioduret of iron (M. Gutbrod); or hydriodate of potash, and use iodine ointment (M. Alken); or give chalybeate tonics, saline purgatives, and nutritious diet (Dr. Rees); or equal parts of tinct. of cantharides and tinct. of sesquichloride of iron (Dr. Copland).

Treat the *dropsy* with cream of tartar and digitalis (Dr. Christison), give from a drachm to a drachm and a half of the former three times a day, and at the same time a pill containing one or two grains of powdered digitalis, or twenty drops of the tincture in cinnamon water: give a blue pill (grs. 5) every night for four or five nights. Diuresis may often be established by an emetic of ipecac., and tartar emetic, or by a hydragogue cathartic; should these fail, give squills, broom, spirit of nitric ether, or Hollands and water, or carbonate, nitrate, or acetate of potash; or decoction of horse radish (Rayer). Diuretics do not cure the disease; they can only relieve the dropsy.

Try seidlitz or Pullna water; cream of tartar in half ounce doses (Rayer); give five, seven, or nine grains of gamboge, once every two days, triturated with bitartrate of potash, to prevent griping. Combat the concomitant affections of the digestive organs with creasoté (Dr. Christison); give it as a pill, one drop of creasote, two grains of rhubarb, and one grain of extract of gentian, for the mass; or with the sedative solution of opium; or with extract of opium and nitrate of silver, half a

grain of each in a pill. Apply sinapisms, turpentine epithems, or a cantharides blister, externally; sprinkle the blistered surface with muriate of
morphia; check diarrhœa by chalk, astringents, and opiates; or give
acetate of lead with opium, or strychnine with opium (Dr. Wood).

Part xiii., *p.* 108.

Case of Excessive Secretion of Earthy Phosphates by the Kidneys,
with long-continued Irritability of the Stomach.—[This case, recorded
by Dr. Bird, is an excellent illustration of the relation existing between
the function of the stomach and kidneys. The patient, in 1841, was
attacked with vomiting, after dinner, with severe pain at the pit of the
stomach. This vomiting occurred after every meal for six months, being
always preceded by intense pain, which was relieved as soon as the
stomach was emptied. The next eight months the vomiting became less
frequent, only recurring after dinner. He was admitted into Guy's Hospital on the 9th of April, 1845. The following was his condition at
the time:]

On admission into Guy's Hospital, the lad's complexion was pale and
bloodless, with a slightly icteric tint; he was emaciated to an extreme
degree, his bones being barely covered; and his face bore no small resemblance to a fleshless skull, over which a skin of parchment had been
tightly drawn. His general appearance was that of a person worn out by
malignant disease. He chiefly complained of a burning, gnawing pain, at
the scrobiculus cordis, and of a heavy pain across the loins. Tongue
clean and red; pulse quick and sharp; skin dry and imperspirable. He
vomits shortly after each meal, bringing up his food slightly changed, and
according to his own account, has never passed a single day, during four
years, without vomiting once, and more frequently several times. He
complains of great thirst. The bowels act daily. Flatulent eructations
frequent, and possessing the odor of stale fish. Urine copious, pale, loaded
with crystals of the triple phosphate, not albuminous, alkaline; specific
gravity 1.020, and evolving a disgusting fishy odor. The abdomen is distended with flatus; there is some tenderness at the scrobiculus cordis,
where no tumor is perceptible. He had, shortly after his admission,
vomited nearly four pints of thin, acid, yeast-like matter.

Misturæ magnesiæ, ʒj. ter in die. Milk diet.

April 11th.—Has vomited daily after dinner, the vomited matter presenting the same yeast-like appearance. Urine has an ammoniacal odor,
and deposited crystals of phosphates.

R Strychniæ, gr. j.; acidi nitrici dil. ʒj.; aquæ, ʒxij; solve et sumat
æger, ft. ʒj ter in die.

He was strictly confined to milk diet, consisting of eighteen ounces of
bread, an ounce of butter, and two pints of milk daily, and ordered to
take the medicine fifteen minutes before each meal.

[On the 16th, a liniment of croton oil was applied to the scrob. cord.,
after which he ceased to vomit; the pain also ceased, the urine became
neutral, and contained but few phosphatic crystals. On the 22d, the urine
was free from deposit, and the skin acted freely. Dr Bird adds:]

From the date of this report the same treatment was continued, and
the patient steadily improved; the vomiting ceased, the urine became
acid, he recovered his flesh—indeed became decidedly fat; it was scarcely
possible to recognize in him the wretched skeleton admitted but a month

before. On May 19th, he suffered a slight relapse both of pain and vomiting, following a severe paroxysm of pains in the region of the left kidney, and relieved by a copious discharge of urine loaded with triple phosphate, and rapidly becoming alkaline and fetid. He appeared to recover from this in a few hours, and left the hospital strong enough to attend to his work, and apparently well; having continued the strychnia during six weeks, and taken altogether about eleven grains of that alkaloid.

I am not aware of attention having been previously directed to the connection of this condition of urine, and attending diuresis, with intense irritability of stomach, or, at all events, of their standing to each other in the relation of cause and effect. I may venture to express my own conviction of the etiology of the case in a few words. A lad of delicate frame is engaged in laborious occupations, often far beyond his strength for years, during that part of life which is most susceptible to marked influences; functional derangement of the spinal marrow ensues, marked by the pain across the loins, and altered state of the urine. The stomach thus rendered irritable scarcely retains food, emaciation results, the patient is unable to obtain a sufficient supply through the medium of the stomach for the sustenance and reparation, much less for the increase of tissue. The necessary result is, his stunted growth, extreme emaciation, and the excretion of an unhealthy fluid from the kidneys, the necessary result of the impaired condition of the vital chemistry of these organs, itself an almost constant, although often transitory, result of the slightest mechanical injury to the spine.

The strychnia was administered in consequence of its well-known influence upon the functions of the spinal marrow, and believing that where alkaline urine is really secreted as such by the kidneys, independently, of course, of the character of the ingesta, there is always some lesions of that important structure. Its effects were certainly most satisfactory; for, after years of almost incessant vomiting, the patient soon acquired the power of retaining his food, the urine slowly losing its alkaline character. I would, indeed, venture to press this important remedy upon the notice of surgeons, to whose province cases of alkaline urine following injury to the spine more immediately belong. Nor can I avoid here taking the opportunity of alluding to the value of the drug in the distressing vomiting so frequent in uterine affections, especially in the irritable stomach of hysteria, in which it is almost always successful as an important palliative.

Part xiv., *p.* 98.

Bright's Disease.—The diet must be free from fat, and from those non-azotized substances which are easily converted into fat; as starch and sugar. Enjoin a removal to pure air, regular exercise, attention to cleanliness, and temperature of the skin; and give tonics and other chalybeates. The congestion of the kidney will be relieved by attention to skin and bowels, but local bleeding may sometimes be cautiously employed.

Part xv., *p.* 126.

Depuration of the Blood.—It is found that the kidneys can depurate the blood, not only of matters generally regarded as proper to their function, but of substances usually separated by other emunctories; in fact, they remove all soluble noxious matter. When, therefore, disease is excited or aggravated by noxious or lethal effete matter in the blood, we should endeavor to procure the decomposition and elimination of this matter, by stimulating the depurating functions of the kidneys. And this may be accomplished by the exhibition of the alkalies, and their carbonates, citrates, acetates, and tartrates, which not only stimulate the kidneys, as do the vegetable diuretics, but also increase the metamorphosis of tissue going on in the capillary system. (Bird.) *Pt.* xviii., *p.* 57.

Case of Injury to the Kidneys.—In consequence of death in general so speedily following the suspension of the excretion of urea by the kidneys, owing to its consequent quick absorption into the blood, and poisonous influence on the brain and nervous system, it rarely happens that time is given for a practitioner to determine decidedly, both chemically and pathologically, that the comatose symptoms depend altogether on the non-elimination of urea by the kidneys. The following case, by Dr. Shearman, from the attending circumstances, elucidates this point fully:

Edward C——, aged eight years, in perfect health, while at play was run over across the loins by a heavy truck. In two hours after the accident I saw him. He was then in a state of collapse, and my impression was, that some internal hemorrhage was then going on, for he was blanched, cold, and pulseless. He complained of acute pain in the left lumbar region, which was very tender to the touch, spreading to both the inguinal and the pubic region. I gave him stimulants, and kept him warm, by which means, in the course of thirty-six hours, he gradually improved; and he then passed a large quantity of blood with his urine, not having previously voided any urine since the accident. This was repeated several times during the next twenty-four hours.

I examined this urine and blood most carefully, but failed to detect the least particle of urea or urates in it. My little patient became restless; fever set in, with a pulse at 130; and the pain in the region of the kidneys increased, notwithstanding the application of leeches, etc. But these symptoms, in the course of two days, were succeeded by coma; he could not be kept awake.

I now bled him in the arm, and reapplied leeches to the tender part. On examining this blood, urea was most distinctly detected in it, and in considerable quantity. The urine, at the same time, contained not a particle of urea, urates, uric acid, or albumen, and its specific gravity was only 1.005.

I got him under the influence of mercury as quickly as possible; as soon as its specific effect was apparent, urea gradually reappeared in the urine, and its specific gravity increased. By degrees the comatose symptoms subsided, and in the course of five weeks the usual health was reëstablished. He continues quite well.

The mode of detecting urea in the blood, which I adopted, was the one recommeded by Dr. G. O. Rees ("On the Analyses of Blood and Urine, in Health and Disease," second edition, page 40). *Part* xviii., *p.* 135.

Diagnosis of Renal Disease.—An observation of great importance in the diagnosis of renal disease has been recently made by Dr. Johnson, viz., that disease of the kidney, of a recent acute nature, is indicated chiefly by the presence of fibrinous matter entangling "entire epithelial cells " with albumen, and very commonly blood; while, on the other hand, "granular particles of disintegrated epithelium" indicate a disease of a chronic character. *Part* xxiii., *p.* 136.

Bright's Disease.—Ascertain whether the coagulability of the urine present depends on albumen, by the aid of heat first, and then by the addition of nitric acid. All intercurrent diseases are more unmanageable, and more apt to prove fatal, in consequence of the renal disorder. The most mortal of all signs are, a very scanty urine of very low density, an extremely impoverished condition of the blood corpuscles, and stupor gradually verging toward coma. The treatment of Bright's disease is two-fold; to remove the fundamental disease, and to cure the secondary diseases. The main remedies for the former object are general and topical depletion, local counter-irritation, diaphoretics, diuretics, and astringents. The best diuretics are digitalis, squill, and bitartrate of potash, but when all these have failed, diuresis has been established by Hollands. The cathartic plan should not be adopted for the dropsy; it is apt to excite a permanent diarrhœa, and mercury should be shunned as inducing in this disease excessive action. The best remedy for the diarrhœa is the Edinburgh lead and opium pill, in a dose of five or ten grains, twice or three times a day, to which may be added, in severe cases, a fatty suppository of morphia. Vomiting may be removed sometimes by bismuth, more frequently by morphia, hydrocyanic acid, creasote, chloroform, or little fragments of ice; when these fail, by a blister applied over the epigastrium.

Part xxiv., *p.* 142.

Bright's Disease.—Dr. Jones looks upon the fibrinous cylinders which are found in the urine in this disease to be produced by congestion, causing effusion of liquor sanguinis, and thus fibrin and albumen being effused together, the fibrin coagulating in the ducts producing the cylinders, and the granular matter within them. When these appear in the urine, Dr. Jones always suspects the presence of granular disease of the kidney. Dr. George Johnson was the first who attempted the solution of the problem between this deposit and granular degeneration. Dr. Johnson subsequently extended his views, and distinguished four conditions of the kidney: 1. Acute desquamative nephritis. 2. Chronic desquamative nephritis. 3. Simple fatty degeneration. 4. Fatty degeneration with desquamative nephritis. He imagined that the microscope would enable us to distinguish the sediments peculiar to each of these several diseases, but the sediment unfortunately in the same case varies exceedingly at different periods. Sometimes even microscopic examination fails altogether when the chemical evidence has been decided enough.

[With regard to the treatment.]

The intense action of mercury in Bright's disease has so frequently and so forcibly been presented to my notice, that I have formed a general rule never to give mercury in cases of albuminous urine. I have seen the most violent salivation from single doses even of grey powder, and on this account, even in serous inflammation consequent on Bright's disease, I advise you not to give mercury. Why mercury should act so energetically in this disease is probably explained by the altered state of the kidney. In health, most probably, mercury no sooner passes into the system than it begins to pass out again by the kidney, like hydriodate of potash or the salts of iron. For example, if a single grain of hydriodate of potash is taken in an ounce of distilled water, in twelve minutes it can be detected passing off in the urine; but if the kidney is diseased, then most probably this rapid excretion does not so easily take place, and the intensity of the action of this and other medicines may thus be greatly increased.

In the treatment of urinary poisoning, I know no single remedy which has produced an effect at all equal to that of a blister on the back of the neck. This appears to me to indicate that there is some local congestion of the brain, as well as some poison in the blood. I have as yet had no good opportunity for trying what the free administration of vegetable and mineral acids can do when head symptoms are present; in one case, large quantities of lemon-juice appeared to have a beneficial effect. The theory of Dr. Frerichs indicates the acid treatment, and it is worthy of a fair trial.

Dr. Watson is, without doubt, right in saying that these head symptoms may arise from insufficient supply of blood. Just, as in children, symptoms resembling hydrocephalus may arise from anæmia, when, instead of depletion, counter-irritation and stimulants are required. On this theory, no poison is considered to be present in the blood. The truth probably is, that too little blood, too much blood, and poisoned blood— each of these states, in different cases, is the cause of the head symptoms in Bright's disease.

As I cannot make any separation of Bright's disease into different diseases, so I am unable, from observation, to find that different kinds of treatment are desirable. The indications are, first, to relieve the congested kidney; and, secondly, to improve the general health. Gentle but decided action on the skin and bowels appear to me best to fulfill the first indication; cupping, vapor-bath, and elaterium, are the three most energetic remedies; cream of tartar, compound jalap powder, and abstinence from stimulants, are the milder agents. To improve the health, proper air, exercise, food, and small doses of iron, are essential.

Specific treatment by gallic and nitric acid has not benefited my patients in St. George's Hospital. In so-called chylous urine, I know well the use of gallic acid, in doses of two drachms daily; but, in Bright's disease, when ten-grain doses were given, I have more than once known bad symptoms to occur. In one case, violent convulsions made their appearance soon after the gallic acid was taken. In no case have I found that it stopped the albumen from passing away. I may here mention, that tannic acid appears to affect the stomach much more than gallic acid does.

With regard to the treatment by nitric acid, which has been extensively tried in Germany, I have not found any good result, even when dilute nitric acid has been taken daily for many weeks.

As to the result of treatment, omitting the cases which follow scarlet fever, which constantly recover perfectly, temporary relief is generally all that is obtained. Life may be prolonged for years. Even with ascites, I have known a patient in and out of St. George's Hospital for ten years. Usually, although every complication may be removed, the albumen continues in the urine. The patient resumes his work, and considers that he is recovered; but heat and nitric acid show that this is not the case; and it is only by great care that the tendency to a return of the former symptoms, or to gout, can be prevented.   *Part* xxv., *p.* 126.

Bright's Disease.—Urea in this disease accumulating in the blood, is best eliminated by the administration of colchicum.   *Part* xxv., *p.* 142.

Renal Disease—Acute.—Dr. Johnson correctly remarks, how very frequently acute renal diseases, with dropsy and albuminous urine, are preceded by chills upon the surface, produced often by working or standing in wet clothes. The same in cases occurring after scarlatina: hence it is, that the chief means of preventing consequences ensuing after scarlet fever, are protection from cold until the period of desquamation has passed by. The circumstances under which these attacks of acute renal disease occur, and of the appearances observable in the urine and in the kidneys, warrants the inference, that the renal changes are the result of an effort to eliminate some abnormal products, which have been conveyed to the kidneys by the blood. In cases of scarlatina, for instance, it is probable that exposure to cold has the effect of checking the process by which the fever-poisou, or ferment, or the product of fermentation, is eliminated from the skin, and that the morbid materials are then transferred to the kidney, in accordance with the well-known tendency to vicarious action of the skin and kidneys. An instructive illustration of this principle is afforded by the fact of several medicines, such as, for instance, the acetate or citrate of ammonia, acting either as diaphoretics or diuretics, according as the tendency is imparted to them by the skin being kept warm, or the contrary. These facts may assist our comprehension of what probably happens when a patient is exposed to cold too early after the onset of scarlatiua. The work of elimination is then transferred from the skin to the kidney; and, as a result of this, there is, in some instances, a free desquamation of the renal epithelium, analogous, as it appears, to the cutaneous desquamation which follows the eruption of scarlatina.

Where we have albuminous urine and dropsy, the greatest possible care should be taken to guard against cold, because it is the chief cause in the production of renal disease, and therefore must tend to perpetuate it, if it already exist. In cold weather the patient must be absolutely compelled to keep in bed, both on account of insuring the horizontal positiou, and also the equable warmth of the skin. The diet should be scanty, and, unless specially indicated, alcoholic stimulants should not be given. The next thing is to obtain free action of the skin and bowels; the first by the hot-air bath and diaphoretic medicines, the latter by saline aperients, and the pulv. jalapæ comp.

The free action of these great excretory surfaces is a very efficient means by which to lessen the injurious over-work of the kidneys. It scarcely need be said, that however scanty may be the urine, no stimulant diuretic is to be given; indeed, the more scanty the secretion, the more injurious 'would be the effect of any irritating drug.

During the convalescence, the urine is usually twice as abundant as in health, in consequence, probably, of the naturally diuretic influence of the urea and other urinary products which, having accumulated in the blood during the acute stage of the disease, find a free outlet when that stage is passed. A practitioner who has been perseveringly giving diuretics, and who is ignorant of this pathological fact, will be likely to attribute to the influence of his drugs this abundant flow of urine, which is, in fact, only a natural and a spontaneous diuresis.

It will be understood that, in deprecating the use of diuretics, it is only with reference to cases of *acute* renal disease. When the disease has become chronic, and when an excessive dropsical accumulation constitutes the most distressing and dangerous symptom, we must endeavor to remove the dropsical accumulation by means of diuretics, whether these accelerate the progress of the disease in the kidney or not.

After the acute stage of nephritis has passed, Dr. Johnson recommends that the patient, especially in winter, be kept in-doors, until no albumen can be detected in the urine. If he rebels, he will very probably bring on a relapse, of which he should be warned. If, after every precaution has been taken, and the period of confinement prolonged, still the urine contains albumen, though natural in other respects, gallic acid may be given; and if after this the quantity of albumen continues, Dr. Johnson advises that he should be removed to the sea-side, and allowed to take a daily airing. If the malady still persists, and assumes a chronic form, the patient must be urged to take a sea voyage as early as possible. As to the treatment of cerebral symptoms, consequent on acute inflammation of the kidneys, as after scarlatina, or exposure to cold, we must relieve the congested state by cupping over the region of the kidneys, and abstracting a moderate quantity of blood, and by exciting free action in the mucous membrane of the bowels, by means of elaterium or pulv. jalap. co., with a few grains of calomel sometimes added.

If we can excite copious discharges from the mucous membrane of the bowels, we shall by that means eliminate some of the excreta which are poisoning the blood, for urea has been detected in the watery stools produced by elaterium.

If the patient's appearance be not decidedly anæmic, we may venture to abstract a small quantity of blood; but we shall do this with much caution, if we bear in mind Dr. Watson's suggestion—sanctioned, too, by the high authority of Dr. Todd—that an impoverished condition of the blood may favor the tendency to coma and the poisonous action of urea. Cold lotions may be applied to the head when the scalp is hot, and blisters when the skin is cool. Since, in any case, it is a more hopeful task to prevent drowsiness from passing into coma, than to bring a patient out of a comatose condition when once he has fallen into it, it is important to keep a watchful eye upon the premonitory symptoms. In some cases, it appears that the most successful mode of keeping them in check is to give a nutritious but unstimulating diet, with moderate doses of steel, and, at the same time, to keep up a free action of the bowels.

Can the kidney perfectly recover from an acute inflammatory attack? Dr. Johnson answers, yes, if the case has come early under treatment, and yielded to it in moderate time. No harm will result, except the spoiling of a few of the tubes and wasting of the parts, unless the disease has been so long prolonged as to destroy the epithelial lining of the tubes and render them liable to be converted into cysts.   *Part* xxviii., *p.* 134.

Passive Hemorrhage from the Kidneys.—[It is not always easy, when we are quite certain that the urine contains blood, to be able to state definitely from what part of the urinary apparatus it proceeds. Dr. Crooke is of opinion that it often precedes that condition in which albumen is present in the urine, viz., " *chronic albuminous nephritis;*" and that it often insidiously follows " *acute desquamative nephritis,*" which is supposed to have yielded to treatment.]

Symptoms.—Passive renal hemorrhage offers to our notice two classes of symptoms—the general and the local. The general are those of anemia, the result of a continual draining away of that vital fluid, the blood; the local refer chiefly to the bladder. The general symptoms are, a pallid complexion, of a dirty-white or muddy color; with dilated pupils; occasional headache and singing in the ears; the tongue is large, flabby and furred, the edges thereof indented by the teeth; the bowels are open and loose; there is much flatulence and nausea, with irregular appetite; palpitation is frequent; the surface of the body is cool; the skin soft and relaxed, but dry; the pulse full, soft and bounding, or small and soft, putting on the former condition upon change of posture; there is gradual but progressive emaciation, irritability and gloominess of temper, with great disinclination to any exertion, bodily or mental. These symptoms vary in degree according to the longer or shorter duration of the disease.

2d. The local symptoms are in some cases an aching pain in the loins, but this is, perhaps, rather an exception than the rule. They, the loins, are rather the seat of an uneasiness and feeling of weakness, which is increased upon pressure; the calls to micturate are frequent and urgent, attended with pain, sometimes referable to the penis, sometimes to the inside of the thighs and to the perineum; the urine is not much, if at all, increased in quantity when compared with the amount of fluids imbibed.

Treatment.—The therapeutical indications are three in number. First, to check the hemorrhage by relieving the congestion; secondly, to restore the general health; thirdly, to guard against relapse, and this is an important point, as there is a great tendency thereto upon the application of any exciting cause. The first indication may be effected by rest, daily use of the warm bath, with friction to the bodily surface, local depletion, abstinence from diuretic drinks, bland farinaceous diet, and the use of astringent remedies. To relieve the gastro-hepatic derangement, a small quantity of blue pill, with a sedative saline draught, will be found useful at intervals during the exhibition of astringent remedies, the best of which is gallic acid. It has been given in the following form: Gallic acid, a drachm; dilute hydrochloric acid, two drachms; solution of hydrochlorate of morphia (E. P.), one drachm; distilled water, five ounces and a half, as a mixture; a tablespoonful to be taken every fourth hour. The therapeutical effects of gallic acid are well described by Dr. Golding Bird: "Gallic acid acts as a direct astringent, reaching the renal capillaries, and finding its way into the urine, which becomes strongly charged with it," etc. To relieve the irritability of the bladder, five grains of soap-and-opium pill should be used every night as a suppository. These medicines should be continued until the hemorrhage ceases, and the vesical irritability which remains for some time after the cessation of the hemorrhage is relieved by tincture of cantharides, in doses of from ten to twenty drops, combined with an anodyne. When the urine is free from blood discs, the general hygienic rules for restoring tone to the system should be enforced; animal diet, with a few glasses of sherry daily, may be allowed, and quinine with iron prescribed. As preventive measures, the warm bath with friction should be daily persisted in; flannel should be worn next the skin, and all exposure to exciting causes studiously avoided. *Part* xxix., *p.* 147.

Kidney—Irritation and Inflammation of, from a Calculus.—Prevent the increase of the concretion by correcting the unhealthy state of the urine according as acid, alkali, or oxalate of lime, predominate. Avoid severe exercise. Allay pain by the hottest hip-bath, at a temperature of 110° or 112° Fahr.; by chloroform internally and externally; by opium and the injection of warm water into the rectum. Guard against inflammation, by general or local bleeding; by aperients and sudorifics.

The complaints which may be mistaken for a nephritic attack are lumbago and colic. The absence of vomiting in lumbago, and the seat of pain in colic, may lead you to a correct opinion; but the presence of blood-globules when the urine is examined with the microscope, is the sure indication that the attack is caused by the descent of a renal calculus, and the affection of the testicle may be generally found confirmatory of this opinion. Do not think that in every case in which blood is found by the microscope in the urine a calculus necessarily exists in the kidney. Blood globules may appear in the urine from simple congestion of the kidney in many diseases—from Bright's disease, from inflammation of the mucous membrane alone, from congestion or disease of the prostate, from scrofulous disease, or malignant disease; and in some of these diseases the difficulty of distinguishing between them and renal calculus is by no means easy. (Jones.)
Part xxx., *p.* 85.

Malignant and Scrofulous Renal Disease.—Renal diseases are often very difficult of diagnosis. We ask ourselves first, perhaps, whether it be Bright's disease; next, whether any concretion be present, or whether inflammatory action exist; and, lastly, we ask whether the case be one of malignant or scrofulous disease. Neither malignant nor scrofulous disease admits of easy relief, and, therefore, the medical attendant should be careful in giving his prognosis.

Sometimes, says Dr. H. B. Jones, no urinary symptoms whatever are observed, the malignant disease existing in another more vital part, causing the renal disease to be entirely overlooked.

Sometimes another urinary disease exists at the same time, and thus the symptoms are made obscure. Thus granular disease of the kidney may exist with encephaloid disease, and the secondary symptoms produced by the former may alone force themselves on the attention.

As far as I have hitherto observed, the microscope has not enabled me certainly to predict the presence of malignant disease of the kidney. I must say the same of incipient malignant disease of the bladder. The symptoms of this disease are more distressing than when the kidney is affected; but even when I have felt confident of my diagnosis, I have sometimes been unable to confirm it by the microscopic discovery of malignant cells, in consequence of the highly alkaline urine acting on the cells. In other cases, in which small masses of malignant matter were passed, the microscope has confirmed the diagnosis which the general symptoms had made most probable. Nor has the microscope as yet enabled me to speak certainly regarding the commencement of scrofulous disease. The means of distinguishing between scrofulous disease and calculus of the bladder or kidneys, are very insufficient; but by careful attention to the progress of the symptoms, more certainty may be attained than by help of the microscope.

In conclusion, then, as no certain microscopic or chemical test exists for the early stage of scrofulous and malignant disease, it will be best, in doubtful cases, to refuse to give a positive opinion. Suspend your diagnosis until, by carefully watching the progress of the case, you find sufficient evidence of the nature of the disease.
Part xxx., *p.* 87.

Morbus Brightii.—According to Dr. Handfield Jones, this is not an inflammatory affection, but purely a disease of depraved nutrition; therefore, you must endeavor to improve the general vigor and power of the system, and therewith its nutrition, in every possible way. After the dropsy is removed, you must still continue your treatment until the urine is restored to its healthy condition, the blood improved, and the system reinvigorated. The following is very useful in these cases: R Acid. nitrici, miij.; tinct. cinchon., ʒj.; inf. gent. co., ʒj. Ter die. R Tinct. ferri mur., mx.; aquæ, ʒj. Ter die c. cibo. *Part xxxii., p.* 100.

Iodide of Potassium in Dropsy, with Bright's Disease of the Kidney. —In the sub-acute or chronic form, give five grains of iodine and five grains of bicarbonate of potass in one ounce of water three times a day. It has been very successful in reducing the general anasarca and improving the condition of the health. *Part xxxii., p.* 103.

Supra-Renal Capsules—Disease of.—The combination of the bronzed state of the skin with great systemic debility may be held indicative of disease of the supra-renal capsules; and the more marked these conditions are, the more positively may the opinion be formed. A differential diagnosis may sometimes be requisite, however, as regards the following diseases: 1. *Jaundice.* In some states of chronic jaundice, the skin may be brown rather than yellow, and great vital depression may exist. Here, however, the conjunctiva and the matrices of the nails would, by their discolored state, prevent the possibility of deception. The tint in jaundice is also a diffused one, and does not occur in patches, as in true bronzing. 2. *Browning from exposure to the sun,* etc. In these, the examination of parts protected by the clothes would generally be sufficient to prevent error. 3. *Pityriasis versicolor.* The patches of pityriasis versicolor sometimes remarkably resemble those of the bronzed skin. Their limitation to the abdomen and chest, their defined outline, their furfuraceous surface, the slight itching which attends them, their contagious character, and above all, the microscopic examination of the cuticle, furnish, however, abundant means by which to distinguish between the two. 4. *The diffused brown muddiness of some other cachexiæ.* The dark areola round the eye, so often seen in states of disordered menstruation, is in rarer cases found coincident with a loss of healthy tint in the skin generally, which assumes a dirty, sallow brownish appearance. This, in exaggerated instances, might be mistaken for bronzing.

It should be borne in mind that in all cases, in which bronzing is to be held as positively indicative of diseased capsules, there ought to be traces of patching and mottling in some parts, and that in proportion as the tint is equally diffused over the whole body is the diagnosis doubtful.

We can never give any other than an unfavorable prognosis—no recovery from true bronzing of the skin has ever been recorded; but as we believe that the changes which the supra-renal bodies undergo, are allied to inflammation, we should expect the most benefit from mercury, in very small doses, or the use of iodide of potassium—the patient's strength being meanwhile supported by a nutritious, but non-stimulating diet.

Part xxxiii., p. 129.

Bright's Disease.—Liquor ammoniæ acetatis, by acting on the skin and relieving the congested condition of the kidneys, is the best of all remedies for this disease; diuretics at the same time being strictly avoided, but not mercurials. (Dr. Addison.) *Part xxxiii., p.* 237.

Frequent Micturition.—Dr. G. Owen Rees, gives the following:

Among the causes of frequent micturition is rena. calculus. In this distressing affection little or nothing can be done. To the patient's own feelings the bladder is often the seat of the disease, and even by medical men these cases have been mistaken for irritation of the neck of the bladder caused by stricture, and the most lamentable results brought about by the violent measures resorted to for relief. A correct diagnosis may however generally be formed.

Frequent micturition, with small quantities of pus in the urine, loin pain and lassitude, if we have an early history of hematuria, should guide us to diagnose renal calculus; and even if frequent micturition and a small quantity of pus be the only symptoms, we shall generally be right in giving the above opinion, even if history fail to afford us evidence of hematuria. The presence of a small quantity of pus in the urine would appear easily explained in its relations to renal calculus.

The hollowing out of the nephritic structure, which we find occurring in order to make room for calculi about to become encysted in the kidneys, must have been effected by a gradual process of disintegration, and this we know is preceded by inflammation. The purulent discharge would thus seem to attend the formation of a convenient cavity for the lodgment of the calculus. So long as this action is going on, the patient will pass pus in the urine, and it may be some years before matters are adjusted. The constitution has much to go through. A scrofulous taint leads to abscess in the kidney, and death. The more fortunately constituted generally do well, provided they can be induced to avoid the catheter and the sound.

In speaking of the condition of the urine in this calculous affection of the kidney, I have made use of a somewhat indefinite expression, viz., " a small quantity of pus." By this I would wish my readers to understand a urine depositing a yellowish-white sediment, but not in such quantity that the patient's attention need be attracted by it. It renders the urine but slightly turbid as it is passed, or when the deposit is shaken up in it.

This is the general state of things when nephritic calculus is encysting, or when it fails to find its way down the ureter, provided constitutional causes do not interfere to produce suppurative disease, which may appear in the form of pyelitis or of general abscess of the kidney. This purulent impregnation is constant, and, if it fail to show itself so as to be evident to the unassisted eye, the microscope rarely fails to demonstrate the presence of pus so long as the bladder is irritable.

There is a cause for frequent micturition so nearly connected in its symptoms with that last noticed, that it naturally suggests itself in this place. It consists in a state of kidney known as strumous kidney, or phthisical kidney, as some authors have designated it. If calculous disease develop itself in a strumous subject, we find very early that abscess results; but in all subjects some amount of pus may be expected during the time of encysting. In phthisis of the kidney, however, the bladder becomes irritable without any evidence of a calculous disposition; and we find that pus can be clearly proved in the urine. The symptoms are generally at first considered to depend on calculus, and it too often happens that the disease has made great progress before the real state of the case becomes evident. The symptoms are at first nearly identical with those of nephritic calculus. The same degree of sharp lumbar pain, however, is not present, and there is no history of hematuria; but the symptoms presenting themselves at the time of examination bear a striking similarity; and if the previous history be not ascertained, a diagnosis is next to impossible. It is both for the advantage of the practitioner and of the patient that this distinction should be early made; for if calculus be the exciting cause, of course our prognosis will be more favorable.

The two points for consideration are—1st. The diathesis of the patient. 2nd. The history as to hematuria. If frequent micturition and purulent urine, such as I have described, be present in a strumous person, and we have no history of hematuria, we may diagnose phthisis of the kidney. If frequent micturition and purulent urine coëxist with a history of hematuria, then, in all probability, there is calculus. We must not conclude, however, that because calculus is present we have no fear of the worst results, for if the patient be of strumous habit, abscess may result as a consequence. In all cases, however, the history of hematuria is an advantage, inasmuch as even should the patient be strumous, the calculus may be voided, and, the exciting cause of mischief being thus removed, the kidney may recover itself, and the patient do well.

Amongst causes for frequent micturition, we find diabetes enumerated. The quantity passed on each occasion is, however, so large, compared with that characterizing most of the other states I have described, that the patient's attention is attracted by the large discharge, as well as by the frequent call, and the former is related as the more prominent symptom. This should lead at once to the examination of the urine for sugar, and if that be *not* found, we may perhaps determine the presence of insipid diabetes by the low specific gravity, the increased flow, great thirst, and other characteristic symptoms. It does, however, now and then happen in diabetes that frequent call to pass urine has been the symptom most noticed by the patient, and then, if due care be not taken, the practitioner is a long time led astray. Cases such as these by no means infrequently occur. They are sometimes treated as dependent on the gouty diathesis, a uric acid deposit having attracted the attention of the medical attendant. Treatment is then persevered in until all the more aggravated symptoms of diabetes appear. The early detection of this disease, which is so important for its relief, is thus prevented.

I now have to speak of two forms of cancerous affection which may produce frequent micturition, viz., malignant disease of the kidney and of the bladder. These two states are characterized by hematuria. It sometimes happens that the irritability of the bladder is so great, when the kidney alone is involved, that this sympathetic affection may be mistaken for the primary disease, and the nephritic mischief entirely overlooked. What I would wish to enforce is, that these two symptoms, hematuria and frequent micturition, taken together, should be regarded (the prostate being excluded) as indicating calculus or malignant disease, and that either the kidney or the bladder may be in fault. The indications of cystitis, shown by the urine when calculus exists, have been already dwelt upon; but when malignant disease is present, there may be none of these. The urine may be clear, or may only contain such a small quantity of blood that very careful examination is requisite in order to detect it by the naked eye. Here the kidney might be considered in fault, and the diagnosis is not always to be made.

If we have a tumor of the abdomen over the region of the kidney, then we may safely diagnose that organ involved; but this indication is not always afforded us, and then we should examine the bladder very carefully. If, on sounding, hemorrhage occur to an extent exceeding that usually produced by exploration, there is most likely a growth on the mucous surface of the bladder.

Before leaving this part of my subject, I must say a word or two respecting the seat of tumor in these forms of disease. First, with regard to the kidney. It is necessary to guard against being led astray by the tumor appearing in a position somewhat removed from that in which it ordinarily exists. Nephritic enlargement sometimes occurs at the upper portion of a kidney, and in abscess of the organ especially, there is often considerable bulging upward. This may occur to such an extent that the tumor eventually may be felt in that part of the abdomen usually occupied by the liver, and in malignant affections also, if the right kidney be involved, the tumor may exist over nearly the whole of the right hypochondriac region. An able paper will be found in the "Guy's Hospital Reports," in which Dr. Bright has given sketches illustrative of this fact.

As regards the production of frequent micturition by malignant disease of the bladder, the tumor must be situated near the neck of the organ in order to cause the symptom. I have had two cases within the last few years especially illustrative of this point. In the one, so little inconvenience was felt that had it not been for the microscopical indications of the urine, I should have inevitably mistaken the disease. There was no increased desire to pass urine, and no pain; and hematuria was only an occasional symptom. Post-mortem examination showed the advantage to be derived from microscopic research, the diagnosis being verified by the presence of a large mass of villous growth on the fundus of the bladder. The situation of the tumor, far removed from the neck of the organ, explained the absence of the symptom of frequent micturition. In the other case, a tumor of the same kind existed near the neck of the bladder, and the irritation was most torturing. The symptoms otherwise exactly resembled those of the former case. There was the same hemorrhage after sounding, and hematuria was of very frequent occurrence. I have spoken of certain microscopical appearances which determined my diagnosis: these were merely such as I have detailed in former lectures, consisting in the presence of those corpuscles or cells which are found in the villous growths from mucous membranes, and which, when they can be satisfactorily determined to exist in the urine, are always most significant.

Before leaving the analytical symptomatology of frequent micturition, I would speak of the influence of habit and of nervousness in continuing the symptom, even after the obvious causes producing it are removed. With regard to habit, it is in some cases of the greatest importance to inform the patient of his position, and to instruct him to restrain himself as much as possible. If he will do this, his malady becomes of necessity of shorter duration. We often find the subjects of this symptom acquainted with every corner suitable for the relief of their wants. They are reminded of their malady on approaching their wonted haunts. An effort is required to pass them, and it is well to instruct such patients to make a point of doing so if they possibly can. The nervous feeling which arises in sufferers from this infirmity when they find themselves in company is very distressing. They are certain to feel the inclination when there is the greatest difficulty in gratifying it. They consequently refuse to go into society. They are, perhaps, urged to do so; they suffer great misery, and their complaint becomes aggravated. This should never be allowed. Let them avoid company, and as their complaint improves they get more courage; and there is no fear of a return of this nervousness, except they again become the subjects of those physical ailments which originated the disease. *Part* xxxv., *p.* 310.

Movable Kidneys.—A knowledge of the fact that the kidneys may, in a healthy person, be in abnormal position in the abdomen, and detectible by external manipulation, is important, lest any errors in diagnosis should be caused from suspecting the presence of some malignant or otherwise dangerous tumor. In these cases the mass is smooth, hard, and resisting, rounded in outline, can be moved upward and slightly downward.
Part xxxvii., *p.* 84.

Bright's Disease.—Our diagnosis as to the state of advancement of this disease will be materially assisted by observing the size of the waxy casts, which increases in diameter as the disease progresses, owing to the tubes becoming denuded of their epithelial lining.

The larger casts, which have the full diameter of the uriniferous tubes, and a remarkably sharp outline, having been formed in tubes which have lost their epithelial lining, and with it their proper secretory function. These large casts then indicate a more serious degeneration of the tubular structure than the small ones. They are often combined in the urine of the same patient, but the existence of a large proportion of the full-sized wax-like casts in the urinary sediment is usually a sign of serious import, and indicates an advanced form of disease. *Part* xxxvii., *p.* 89.

Employment of Sugar in the Dyscrasia attending Bronzed Skin.—Dr. Todd, in a case of bronzing of the skin under his treatment in King's College Hospital, ordered the free dietetic employment of sugar. The patient, a woman, is believed to have derived considerable benefit from it in relief to the malaise and debility from which she suffered. The theory of the treatment is, we believe, based on the belief, founded on analyses of the blood, that the sugar-making function of the liver is interfered with by the disease. *Part* xxxvii., *p.* 104.

Addison's Disease—Case of Diseased Super-renal Capsules, with Asthenia.—A young man died lately at Guy's Hospital, who was affected with the asthenia or debility to which Dr. Addison has drawn attention in his curious monograph—an affection now pretty generally known in practice as "Addison's Disease." The duskiness or blotching of the skin was peculiarly well marked, for a period extending over two years, and of a deeper tinge at the navel, nipples, and scrotum. He had dizziness and failure of vision on attempting to walk, and no appetite. He was laboring, in fact, under what is called at Guy's, by some, as "Asthenia Addisonii."

We believe the term "Melasma" gives a very absurd idea of the disease; and the word "bronzing" Dr. Addison has, over and over again, repudiated, as not occurring in any of his writings on the disease.

Post-mortem Appearance.—The color of the darker portions of the skin was very deep, something between the tinge of the quadroon, and the greenish brown of some bodies long kept in the dead-house; the axilla, umbilicus, and genital organs, were particularly dark or blotched; the margin of the lips also were dark; the hair darkish; eyes grey; the mueles were red and of good size; the contents of the chest presented nothing abnormal; the brain was healthy; the lungs—with the exception of the apex of the right lung—were healthy; the heart was small, but firm, red, and healthy; the veins full of blood; the mucous membrane of the stomach was very much injected, and the surface covered with tenacious mucus, as if a low form of gastritis existed; intestines healthy; mesenteric and other glands healthy, as were the liver, spleen, and pancreas.   Coming to the suprarenal capsules, they were found to be entirely destroyed, by a deposit of an albuminous cretaceous deposit; there appeared, also, signs of inflammation of their investing capsules, as the latter were firmly adherent to surrounding parts; the right capsule was thus united to the liver and top of the kidney, and the surrounding fat could not be removed in the ordinary way; the right capsule was about the size of the healthy organ, but the left was puckered into a roundish mass about the size of a walnut; both, in fact, seemed filled with a cretaceous matter, or white amorphous substance like tubercle; the right capsule was softened in its middle, containing a fluid like pus. In rough terms we would say the capsules, as is usual while they are diseased, in this affection, were full of a chalky, tuberculous matter that injured the nervous tissues around them. The most suggestive feature in the case, in fact, was the condition of the semilunar ganglion, the nerve branches of which ran quite into the diseased capsules, and were lost in them.

We need only say the pigmentary matter in the skin presented nothing of importance, being found in the *rete mucosum*, where it was probably deposited in a passive manner; the destruction of the semilunar ganglia prevented its normal assimilation or absorption.

This disease is not so much due to any vital action which the supra-renal capsules perform in the economy, as to the pressure or injury exerted by the enlarged organs on the semi-lunar ganglia and solar plexus, with both of which the capsules are intimately associated. Dr. Habershon adopting this view, first proposed by Dr. Copland, treated this case by the use of electricity, together with bark and iodide of potassium. Considerable relief was afforded.   *Part* xxxviii., *p.* 114.

————•◦•————

LABIUM.

Case of Encysted Tumor of the Labium.—Dr. Macdonnell was consulted by a lady on account of a tumor in the labium, of three years' duration, which presented some of the characters of hernia. It differed, however, from that disease in so many respects as to justify, in Dr. Macdonnell's opinion, exploration. The following is the account he gives of the treatment:

March 20th. An exploratory puncture was made, and water of a dark olive color, devoid of odor, escaped. The opening was enlarged, and a tumblerful of thick fluid flowed out, which was of a creamy consistence, and on microscopic examination was found to be composed of decomposed pus-globules, with a large quantity of what appeared to be epithelial scales intermixed. The sac of the tumor was freely cauterized with nitrate of silver conveyed on a probe, and the orifice kept open by means of a plug of lint.

· 27th. The sac of the tumor has been filled up with solid secretion, and has undergone great diminution in size; no general disturbance.

April 1st. Scarcely any trace of the tumor to be detected, except some thickening of the labium, giving to it a greater fullness and prominence than the other. Ordered to apply mercurial ointment.

10th. Perfectly recovered; no traces of the disease left.

Four plans of treatment have been recommended for the cure of these tumors: 1st. Complete dissection out of the whole cyst—a plan which must be extremely difficult in most cases, in all extremely painful, and in such a case as mine quite impracticable. 2d. Laying open the cyst, and filling it with charpie. 3d. Seton. 4th. Removal of the fluid, and then compression, so as to bring the walls of the cyst into close apposition. The plan of treatment which I have employed for some years past has been to cauterize with nitrate of silver the lining membrane of the cyst, so as to cause adhesive inflammation, and this process I have found to be so readily excited by the caustic, that I have never been obliged to repeat it a second time. *Part* xix., *p.* 271.

Fibrous Tumor of the Labium.—In a case of this nature, in Guy's Hospital, Mr. Massey made an incision in a longitudinal direction from one extremity of the labium to the other, to the inner side of the large venous trunk, and just within the mucous surface. A finger was then introduced between the integuments and tumor, and its loose connections with the surrounding tissues forcibly torn through, and the mass completely enucleated. It is of some practical importance to remember that these tumors are closely coated with cellular tissue of a dense character, and it is necessary to cut through this in order to turn out the growth. It is quite easy for the operator to mistake the capsule for the surface of the tumor, and to be trying to separate the integument from it, which would be a long process; and to prevent this it is better to cut slightly into the tumor itself, when the edge of the capsular covering is at once indicated, from whence the enucleation is readily completed. *Part* xxv., *p.* 290.

LABOR.

Case of Complete Detachment of the Os Uteri during Labor.—[In this extraordinary case the os uteri remained obstinately closed for a considerable period, and notwithstanding the regular action of the womb, aided by the gentle use of ergot, it remained but little dilated to the last. Mr. Carmichael proceeds to say:]

The os uteri did not yield, but the head was propelled fully into the pelvis, pushing the cervix before it. In the course of the evening of the second day the patient's condition grew worse, she became delirious, the pulse quick and irregular; and, in a word, she must have quickly sunk if interference had not been resorted to. To apply the forceps, I can only say, the circumstances of the case were such as decidedly to preclude it. The perforator was resorted to, and the cranium evacuated of its contents; the crotchet was then introduced, and traction, of a very gentle nature, made on one of the parietal bones. During this, however, a strong contraction of the uterus succeeded, when the head was at once expelled, carrying before it the os uteri and a part of the cervix of the womb, the diameter of which measured about three inches and a half.

The placenta came away in the usual manner; there was, however, considerable hemorrhage, and such difficulty in getting the womb to contract, that the cold affusion became necessary. Two hours after the delivery I became much alarmed for my patient; jactitation, restlessness, difficulty of breathing, etc. I gave her a full anodyne, and having procured tranquillity and given all the necessary instructions to a competent person as to the state of the uterus, which was padded, and other parts to be attended to, left her for the night. On my visit the next morning, to my surprise, she was sitting up in bed, eating her breakfast, expressing how comfortable her condition was compared with that of the preceding day. *Part* ii., *p.* 148.

Use of the Perforator and Crotchet.—The following series of aphorisms from the researches of Dr. Churchill, will be found useful to be known at the bed-side.

It may be asked, when the responsibility is so serious, what evidence will be sufficient to satisfy a conscientious practitioner that he may not be committing a crime in his anxious endeavors to afford relief? To this it may be answered:

1. That the continuance of strong labor pains for a certain time, without any advance of the head of the child, is so far evidence of a fixed obstacle to the passage of the child.

2. The failure of a cautious attempt to introduce the forceps will, to a certain extent, demonstrate the amount of the disproportion between the head and the pelvis; and the failure of a careful, yet firm attempt at extraction by the forceps (when the application has been effected), will prove that the disproportion cannot be remedied by compression.

3. A well educated finger will enable us in most cases to ascertain whether the diameters of the pelvis are such as will allow of the passage of a living child. And even though this mode be uncertain, we have a means of correcting our estimate, by comparison with the child's head in apposition with the pelvis. If the natural efforts after several hours, or the forceps with a proper and safe amount of compression and force, cannot bring the widest part of the head of the child through the narrow part of the pelvis, we may fairly conclude that the only resource is craniotomy.

4. The general condition of the mother will also aid our decision. If she be much exhausted, if fever be present, the uterus powerless, the life of the child doubtful, and the success of the forceps dubious, we may shrink from inflicting the double shock of an unsuccessful application of the forceps and subsequent delivery by the crotchet. But these cases are very rare: they only happen when the patient has been mismanaged, and it requires experience and judgment to decide upon the propriety of terminating them by embryotomy.

The *cases* in which the operation is demanded are:

1. When the child is dead, and the labor tedious. But we must be quite sure that the child *be* dead, before this is made the ground of interference.

2. In distortion of the pelvis, when the antero-posterior diameter of the brim is less than three inches, we have no chance of delivery by the natural efforts, or by the forceps; so that to save the mother we must destroy the child.

3. When the transverse diameter of the lower outlet is diminished to the

same extent by the approximation of the tubera ischii, if the forceps, applied antero-posteriorly, are insufficient to move the head, we must have recourse to craniotomy.

4. When the calibre of the pelvis is diminished to a certain degree by a fixed obstacle—as, for example, a fibrous tumor, or an exostosis growing from the bone or periosteum, it may not be possible for the natural efforts alone, or aided by the forceps, to expel the child. In such a case, it will be necessary to lessen the head, and apply the crotchet.

In these three latter classes of cases, the passage through the pelvis may be so much diminished as to render it necessary to break up the skull, or to eviscerate the child.

5. In some cases of ovarian disease, where the tumor has formed adhesion within the pelvis, so as to prevent its being pushed above the brim, it has been found necessary to lessen the head before the child could be extracted. We are not, however, to decide upon this measure until the natural powers have had a fair trial, as it sometimes happens, that in the progress of labor, the tumor is so much displaced as to allow of the passage of the child. Further, it will be worth while, before sacrificing the infant, to ascertain whether the contents of the tumor may not be drawn off, by passing a long trocar into it. If a small quantity of fluid escape, it may allow of the application of the forceps, and so enable us to save the child. If, however, the tumor prove to be solid and immovable, we must, as a "*dernier ressort*," have recourse to the perforator and crotchet.

6. When a child is hydrocephalic to such an extent as to prevent its entering or passing through the pelvis, whether distorted or of the natural size, there can be no question as to the propriety of opening the head.

7. In some cases of convulsions, rupture of the uterus, etc., where immediate delivery is necessary, *and where the forceps cannot be applied*, craniotomy must be performed.

8. If an arm descend along with the head, the diameters of which correspond closely to those of the pelvis (whether the latter be of the usual size or not), it may be necessary to terminate the labor by opening the head.

9. I have already alluded to a class of cases, where, from mismanagement the patient has been allowed to continue too long without help, and in consequence is greatly exhausted with fever, quick pulse, delirium, etc. In such cases the patient will die if she be not assisted; and from the unfavorable state in which she is, she cannot bear a prolonged or very painful operation. Now, if there be sufficient space for the forceps, they ought to be preferred, and it would be very wrong to use the perforator; but if this be doubtful, and the probabilities against our succeeding with that instrument, then the consideration of the patient's inability to bear a severe operation may in some cases decide us in favor of embryotomy. These cases, however, are but few, and they must be well marked, to justify our adopting at once such extreme measures.

10. In footling or breech cases, when the head (separated or not from the body) cannot be extracted, we must evacuate its contents.

The next question to be decided, is the *period of labor* at which the operation should be performed.

1. In all cases where the diminution of the pelvic diameters is so great as to render it impossible that a living child can be born naturally or extracted, there can be no hesitation in recommending that the head

should be opened at an early period of the labor, say as soon as the os uteri is dilated, or fully dilatable.

2. When the distortion is less, we cannot be sure as to the result of the natural efforts, and we must wait until it is evident that they are inadequate; then an endeavor should be made to use the forceps, and if this fail, there should be no delay in the performance of embryotomy.

3. These observations will apply equally to the case of morbid growths, ovarian disease, etc., obstructing the passages.

4. In cases of convulsions, ruptured uterus, etc., the time for the operation is determined by circumstances connected with those accidents, and which will be found laid down in the works on the subject.

5. In the mismanaged cases to which I have alluded, the condition of the woman, which determines the necessity for the operation, will also point out the importance of promptitude. If the case be so bad that we dare not risk a failure with the forceps, it is clear that we cannot afford to delay embryotomy.

After the head is extracted, the body generally follows without much difficulty; but should this not be the case, we must have recourse to evisceration. The scissors must be plunged into the chest and the contents broken up; the crotchet hooked upon the ribs, and traction exerted. The contents of the abdominal cavity may be evacuated in a similar way, and after this we shall generally be able to extricate the child.

Part iii., *p.* 121.

Parturition without Consciousness.—Mr. Rawson was called to this case immediately on the waters being discharged. No pain was present, and she was asleep on his arrival.

On examination, I found the os uteri dilated, and the head presenting. The child was slowly and *unintermittingly*, but forcibly, expelled. She betrayed no symptoms of uneasiness whatever, and though I watched her countenance, she did not exhibit the least consciousness of the child's expulsion, but expressed her surprise on seeing it. The child was strong and lively, and, with the mother, did well. The mother was about two-and-twenty, short, plethoric, and *healthy*.

I conceive the above case is interesting in a medico-legal point of view. Dr. Montgomery doubts the possibility of such an occurrence, " excepting under peculiar circumstances, *certainly not in a first delivery*."—(Dr. M.'s "Exposition of the Signs and Symptoms of Pregnancy.") In Beck's " Medical Jurisprudence," it is said that " the possibility of a woman being delivered without being conscious of it, is disbelieved, *excepting some extraordinary and striking cause intervene*." But if such a circumstance *can happen* with a *first child*, it must have its full weight in cases of infantieide. *Part* iv., *p.* 135.

Advantages of keeping the Umbilical Cord whole for some short time after Birth.—In all cases where the infant is born weakly or in a state of asphyxia, M. Baudelocque recommends not to cut the umbilical cord for some time at least after birth. He relates that since he has followed the opinions of Smellie, Levret, Chaussier, etc., on this subject, he has not lost a single case, although when born the child might be in a state of pretty complete asphyxia or apoplexy. He states that, though a child be born in an apoplectic or asphyxiated state, the circulation still continues through the umbilical vein, even though the umbilical arteries should have ceased to beat, and that premature section of the umbilical cord takes away one of the chief aids to its revival. *Part* iv., *p.* 135.

Remarkable Birth of Twins.—Dr. Schroder gives the following case: On the 16th of November, I was sent for, to a robust healthy woman, who, *three days before* had been delivered of a first child about 29 weeks old, in order to remove the after-birth. I very soon discovered that there was a second child in utero. The woman appeared to be vigorous; there had been no pain since the birth of the first child; there was no hemorrhage; the bladder was not distended; the situation of the child was not high, the head presenting: and I saw no reason for forcing delivery. I visited the woman several times, to ascertain the progress. *At last on the sixth day the second child was born*, and immediately afterward the after-birth came away, without any assistance. Both children are living.

Part v., *p.* 160.

Alternate Warmth and Cold as an Excitement to Uterine Action.—Mr. C. Simpson writes as follows:

Some little time ago I had under my care a case of puerperal convulsions which terminated well. The patient became conscious, but was obstinate. With great difficulty I forced some liquid into the mouth, but she would not swallow; I therefore dashed cold water in the face, and the contents of the mouth were instantly gulped down. This novel mode of making patients swallow was repeated, I should say, a dozen times, and with the same invariable effect. During the convulsions the labor stopped. There was, as it were, a metastasis of muscular action, from the apparatus of parturition, distributed over the whole system. Every resource in this state of things which was employed to produce uterine pains did but aggravate the general convulsions without acting on the uterus itself. After the lapse of many hours, however, the labor was resumed, and now the cold water, applied suddenly to the abdomen, was most effective in producing uterine contractions. After a little while, however, this lost its utility. The abdominal surface becoming *cold* from the repeated application, the water no longer acted as an *excitant*. Accordingly warm flannels were applied to restore the temperature, and then cold water was again applied with decided effect. This alternate application of cold and heat is of great value in cases of hemorrhage from the uterus.

Part vii., *p.* 182.

Tartar Emetic in Tardy Labor.—Ramsbotham, speaking of *rigidity of the os uteri*, says that antimony, in doses sufficient to keep up a feeling of nausea, has been exhibited in these cases with marked effect. Dr. Gilbert also highly recommends the same in doses sufficient to induce and maintain emesis, retching, etc., in cases of tedious labor consequent upon insufficiency of uterine contractions, and rigidity of the os tineæ. These cases are most frequently found to occur in patients of tense fibre and robust constitutions. *Part* ix., *p.* 203.

Injection of the Uterus as a means of Expediting Delivery.—The editor of the "Medical Gazette" mentions a singular process which was adopted near Edinburgh, at the suggestion of Mr. Dick, the veterinary surgeon, to expedite the delivery of a cow. The animal had been in labor a considerable time, and was nearly exhausted; six or eight quarts of tepid water were now injected into the uterus, which in five minutes caused such vigorous pain that the animal was speedily released. This plan has since been adopted in the human subject, by a surgeon, in a case where nothing but the long forceps could have effected delivery. He injected about a quart of tepid water, with similar success.

Part x., p. 195.

Obstructed Labor—Division of the Symphysis Pubis in certain Cases of.—Dr. Smith says that division of the symphysis pubis is a much less formidable operation than either cæsarean section or craniotomy, and advocates its adoption in certain cases. The operation was founded on the opinion that the ligaments of the pelvis relaxed during labor, a fact well known to occur in many of the lower animals, and which authors of the highest respectability, as Ruysch, Harvey, and Denman, affirm to be not uncommon in the human female; Dr. Denman also mentions a case where it existed in a woman who died three or four days after delivery. Dr. Churchill mentions three cases in which the operation was performed, and all the patients recovered, after having the ossa pubis separated for three inches, two inches and a half, and two and a sixth respectively. Dr. Menzies and Dr. Smith made a number of examinations on *recently dead females*, and found that an inch and a sixth was the greatest extent to which the pubic bones could be separated without injuring the sacro-iliac ligaments. But experiments on the recent subject are far from satisfactory, since in the one case the ligaments seem possessed of an unusual degree of elasticity, while in the other they have the rigidity of dead animal fibre. They satisfied themselves also that the antero-posterior was the diameter least increased by it; that the distance to which the bone could be separated was greatly influenced by the position of the trunk and limbs; that the force required to separate them, such as drawing down a fœtus into and through the pelvis, was much greater than could be justifiably applied to the structure of the living female, and lastly, that, with care, neither bladder, peritoneum, nor urethra, need be injured. The fatal result of many of those cases in which this operation was performed on the continent, show that these structures had been injured.

[The gist of this paper rests on the assumption, that in the human race the maternal passages and fœtal head are so adapted, that a slight deviation from their relative normal proportions becomes a cause of obstructed labor, and Professor Simpson has shown that the slight difference between the head of the male and female child is quite sufficient to account for many of the difficulties and dangers of parturition.]

The conclusions may be summed up as follows:

1. Craniotomy is, in all cases of obstructed labor, justifiable when the entire fœtus cannot be extracted through the pelvis, from deformity at the brim, from osseous and certain other tumors, and from great contraction of the outlet by the near approach of the tuberosities of the ischia to each other—the obstruction being more than can be overcome by the forceps, *or other means*, yet not so much but that a mutilated fœtus may pass. 2. The cæsarian section must be resorted to whenever the deformity is so great that a mutilated fœtus cannot be extracted through the natural openings; and for which operation symphysotomy can never be substituted. 3. Symphysotomy is only applicable to cases in which the de-

lıvery cannot be accomplished by the forceps, and would require that craniotomy should be performed—the obstruction being dependent on the
funnel-shaped form of the pelvis, and satisfactorily ascertained to be such
that a slight increase to the contracted diameter would permit an entire
child to pass; but in no instance would it be justifiable to resort to this
operation if any uncertainty existed either as to the degree of deformity
of the pelvis, or the vitality of the child. *Part* xi., *p.* 205.

Turning.—[Many writers on midwifery recommend that in the operation of turning, both feet should, if possible, be grasped and pulled
down. We entirely agree with Professor Simpson in the following very
judicious remarks.]

In most cases I hold this method to be improper and unjustifiable, because it is almost always more difficult to seize both extremities than to
seize one; because one is quite sufficient for our purpose, and more safe for
the life of the mother; and because by pulling at one extremity (when
pulling does happen to be required after the version is accomplished) we
more perfectly imitate the natural oblique position and passage of the
breech of the infant, than when we drag it down more directly and more
upon the same plane, by grasping and dragging at both limbs equally.
The infant also assuredly incurs less risk of impaction of the head, and
above all, less chance of fatal compression of the umbilical cord, when the
os uteri and maternal canals have been dilated by the previous passage of
the breech, increased in size by one of the lower extremities being doubled
up on the abdomen, than when both extremities being seized and extended, these same passages are more imperfectly opened up by the lesser-
sized wedge of the breech alone. Notwithstanding, however, the great
difficulties, and consequently the greater dangers attendant on the operation, when we search for and grasp both lower extremities, instead of one,
it is still so dogmatically laid down as a rule by most obstetric authorities,
that many practitioners seem to deem it a duty, not to attempt to turn
the child without having previously secured both feet.

In few or no cases of turning is it proper or requisite to bring down both
extremities, unless in the complication of turning under rupture of the
uterus. In that case, but in that only, ought we to follow at once this
procedure—and here we follow it because, if we left the other extremity
loose in the uterus or abdomen it would be apt to increase the lesion in
the walls of the organ, if it happened to get involved in the aperture, or
impacted against its edges. In some very rare instances in which, after
version by one leg has been effected, and immediate delivery is necessary,
the cervix and os interum occasionally contract so forcibly and strongly
upon ·the protruded limb, whenever we drag upon it, as not to allow a
sufficient amount of traction being applied to this extremity without
fear of lacerating its structures. In such cases it may be well to attempt
to repass the hand to secure the other extremity, for then by pulling at
both extremities together, we incur less chance of injuring them than
if we applied the same required amount of force to either of them singly.

I believe the seizure of the knee to be preferable, in most, if not in all
cases, to the seizure of the foot, or, rather, as it should be more correctly
stated, to the seizure of the ankle of the child. I speak, you will recollect,
of turning in cases of shoulder or arm presentation, in which the liquor
amnii has been for some time evacuated, and the uterus by its tonic con-

traction, has clasped itself around the body and head of the child. Under such circumstances, it is an object of importance not to be obliged to introduce our hand further than is absolutely necessary, into the cavity of the uterus, because the contraction of the organ, in many cases, opposes its introduction, and the forced introduction of it is apt to produce laceration. It is an object also of equal moment to attempt to turn by a part which produces as little change as possible in the figure and form of the infant ; because, if we thrust any of the angulated parts of the child against the interior of the contracted uterus, we should also thus be still more liable to produce rupture of that organ. Now, holding those points in view, it appears to me, that the turning of the child, by seizure of the knee, presents several decided advantages over turning of the child by seizure of the foot.   For, 1st. The knee is more easily reached. As we slip our hand along the anterior surface of the protruding arm, and along the anterior surface of the thorax of the child, we always, if the attitude of the child has not been altered by improper attempts at version, or very irregular uterine action, find the knees near the region of the umbilicus of the infant—the lower extremities, as you are aware, being folded up *in utero* so that the knees are brought up to that part, and the legs flexed upon the thighs in such a manner that the heels and feet lie nearly in apposition with the breech of the child. To seize a foot, therefore, we should require to pass our hand about three inches (or in fact, the whole length of the leg) *further* than we require to do in order to seize a knee. 2nd. The knee affords the hand of the operator a much better hold than the foot. By inserting one or two fingers into the ham or the flexure of the knee, we have a kind of hooked hold which is not liable to betray us. Every one, on the other hand, who has turned by the foot or feet, knows how very apt the fingers are to slip during the required traction, and how much in this way the difficulties of the operation are sometimes increased. 3rd. We produce, I believe, the necessary version of the body of the child more easily by our purchase upon the knee—because thus we act more directly on the pelvic extremity of the infant's spine, than when we have hold of a foot. 4th. Turning by the foot appears to me to endanger greatly more the laceration of the uterus than turning by the knee. The reason of this is sufficiently evident. When we turn by the foot, we have to flex the leg round upon the thigh, and thus at *one* stage of the operation and during one part of the flexion of the leg, we are obliged to have the leg bent to a right angle with the thigh, and the foot of the infant thus projected and crushed against the interior of the uterus.

It is needless to say how much all this danger is increased, when, after having brought down one foot, we pass again our hand, and attempt to bring down a second foot (as is recommended by some authors), for thus we only double the danger of the laceration of the uterus, from the forced and obstructed passage along its interior, of this other extremity.

One point remains for our consideration. Granting that it is proper to seize a knee, I think it matter of the very first moment to know which knee should be seized.   On this point you will find no directions in any of our modern obstetric works, British or foreign, as far I know them ; and yet I believe the secret of turning with facility and safety in a case with the waters evacuated and the uterus contracted—depends upon the knowledge of which of the two lower extremities of the infant should be seized. If we turn with one of the extremities—and whether the foot or the knee—it should be the foot or knee of the limb on the *opposite side of the body* to that which is presenting. Thus, if the right shoulder or arm presents, we should take hold of the left knee or foot; and if the left arm or shoulder presents we should take hold of the right knee or foot.

When we do this, by carrying the knee diagonally across, if I may so speak, the abdomen of the child to the os uteri, we both *flex and rotate* at the same time the trunk of the infant, and in doing so, the semi-rotation of the trunk inevitably carries up the presenting arm, in proportion as the knee which is laid hold of is pulled down by the operator.

I have insisted upon the advantages of taking hold of the knee that is highest and furthest from you, and believe this to be a matter of the very first moment. Both knees of the child, as the infant lies folded up in utero, are generally in juxtaposition, and lying upon the abdomen of the infant, near the umbilicus. If, therefore, in passing your hand into the uterus, you insinuate it as you ought to do, along the anterior surface of the thorax and abdomen of the child, you come in contact with both knees at the same time. And the rule which I would give you is this, that instead of hooking your finger or fingers into the flexure of the lower or nearer knee, you hook them instead into the flexure of the upper, more distant, or opposite one. Both are so far, in general, equally near, or equally distant, and you seize the one or the other according as you take care to turn your finger so as to hook it into the flexure of the lower or the flexure of the upper. *Part* xi., *p.* 213.

Protracted Labor from Insuperable Rigidity of the Os Uteri—Operation.—Dr. Lever makes the following observations respecting the propriety of incising the rigid ring-like edge of the os uteri in cases of protracted labor arising therefrom: The operation itself is exceedingly simple and painless; and, if performed in the way I shall recommend, unattended with hemorrhage. The patient should be on her left side, in the usual obstetric position, and brought to the edge of the bed; the forefinger of the left hand should, in the absence of that part of the os uteri intended to be incised, and, if possible, its point should be slipped within; then, directing a probe-pointed bistoury or hernia-knife along the finger, we should wait for the occurrence of pain, when the incision may be made by passing the cutting edge of the instrument against the indurated margin of the os. The immediate effects of the incision will be the discharge of a small quantity of thin watery blood; especially in those cases where œdema of the cervix is present. In the case under consideration, the external tissues of the uterus contracted more than the internal, so that the wound seemed longer without than within. I selected the sides of the mouth for the situation of the incision, for several reasons: firstly, at the sides of the womb, the rigidity was the greatest; secondly, it is at the sides of the womb we usually find lacerations, when they take place spontaneously, as is frequently seen in protracted labors. Where the waters pass off early, and when the os uteri is thin and tense, such a lesion is by no means unusual.

Again, in making the incision at the sides there is no danger of wounding the bladder in front, or the rectum behind; and, lastly, as in most cases there will be found an elongation, swelling, and congestion of the anterior lip, serious hemorrhage might result if this part of the womb were divided. Some writers have recommended a crucial incision; but, in my opinion, such will be found unnecessary. A further tearing of the parts may take place during the passage of the head; but it is usually slight, and confined to the vagina. Before the operation a careful examination of the os uteri should be made; for we sometimes find this part of the womb communicating to the finger a strong pulsation, from the presence of a large vessel coursing along the rim; and in the truth of this observation I am confirmed by the experience of Mr. Power. After the incision the pains may moderate, or may subside for a time; but on their renewal the obstruction will give way; and, if there exist no pelvic deformity, they will suffice to terminate the delivery. Not unfrequently a slight and temporary degree of faintness follows the operation, during which uterine contraction is lulled.

[Dr. L. concludes his paper by a few remarks on artificial dilatation, which are well worthy of attentive perusal. He affirms that, when attempted in cases like the foregoing, it is almost certain to produce laceration with irritation, inflammation, gangrene, or even death. At a post-mortem on a female at which he was present, who died within forty-eight hours after her delivery, in which this practice was used, extensive peritonitis with effusion of lymph, and lacerated os uteri in several places were found. This affords strong confirmation of the above opinion. At the same time it is needful to warn the young and enthusiastic practitioner that none of the gentler modes of producing relaxation, such as tartar emetic, the warm bath, etc., should be neglected; nor should the use of the knife be delayed until symptoms indicative of an approaching state of collapse appear. The following propositions are submitted as the result of experience on this subject :]

1. That insuperable rigidity of the os uteri occasionally occurs, over which the usual remedies exercise no influence. 2. That such insuperable rigidity may lead to a partial or complete separation of the cervix. 3. That to prevent such a serious lesion, two methods of treatment have been recommended: the one consisting in artificial dilatation; the other, in incising the rigid and contracted os uteri. 4. That artificial dilatation, in most cases, is unjustifiable, from the serious injuries it occasions, and the consequent irritation and inflammation. 5. That, under such circumstances, an incision of the os uteri, in one or more places, should be performed. 6. That the operation is unattended with danger, unaccompanied by pain, and, if rightly performed, free from copious or dangerous hemorrhage. 7. But the operation, to be successful, must be performed before there are symptoms of approaching collapse.

Part xii., p. 290.

Use of the Forceps—How to Apply.—Having ascertained the exact position of the head, introduce the hand well smeared with lard, within the os uteri; search for, and pass the fingers over the ear, so as to guide the blade over that organ, whatever may be its position. When the instrument is locked, do not tie the handles with tape, as it keeps up a degree of pressure on the child's head not consistent with its safety. In acting with the forceps, always bear in mind the different axes of the pelvis, viz., of its brim, cavity, and outlet; therefore, keep the handles of the instrument back to the perineum, till some part of the occipital bone has cleared the arch of the pubis, and when this occurs, gradually bring the handles toward the pubis, when the chin will pass over the perineum. The three powers of the forceps are brought into operation, viz., compression, traction, and leverage; but compression ought never to be made beyond diminishing the child's head to three inches, indeed, instruments are seldom constructed to admit of more.

Part xiii., *p.* 349.

Inversion of the Uterus from Short Funis.—[Mr. Smith's patient was enduring very severe labor-pains, which suddenly subsided as soon as the child's head rested upon the perineum, and the most violent rigor set in. She became deadly pale, and covered with a cold clammy perspiration. Mr. Smith suspected rupture of the uterus to have taken place; he gave a stimulant, and afterward an opiate. The rigor soon ceased, but as soon as it had done so, she gave a most terrific scream, and the child's head and shoulders were born. The bystanders, apparently suspecting, by their looks, that there was some mismanagement, could scarcely be persuaded to stay to give assistance. The patient still endured agonizing pain, and begged for the child to be taken away. Mr. S. extracted the arms, and on turning down the bed-clothes, the following appearances presented themselves:]

The infant, a boy, was lying on his back, apparently lifeless, his legs and part of the thighs retained in the vagina, and the funis so much on the stretch, that the skin of the abdomen was dragged out about an inch and a half. Having used smart friction over the region of the heart, he gave a slight scream, and having lifted him up toward the body of the mother so as to relax the cord, the extremities passed out with a little assistance. The child was immediately separated, and handed to an assistant; but the mother still continued to complain of the most acute pain. On making an examination, I found the placenta so near the os externum, that I thought I had nothing to do but to lift it out; but such was not the case, for I found it attached to the uterus. I immediately nibbled away the attachments with my finger and thumb with the greatest caution, and on removing the placenta, the pain still continuing with great severity, I immediately examined again and found the *uterus* (fully three fourths, according to the feel of it) *inverted*, the os girding it round like a cord, and of course I lost no time in reducing it; this was done with the greatest ease; and in order to insure permanent contraction, I thrust my hand into the cavity, which gave no pain, and having kept my doubled fist there for about half a minute, it gradually closed upon it, and thrust it out, precisely as if it had been another placenta. The mother was immediately bound up firmly, the pains having entirely ceased, and in the evening she was sitting up in bed, suckling her baby as if nothing had happened.

The patient lost very little blood, and complained of no pain whatever after the uterus was reduced. The funis was not more than six inches long, perhaps about eight when on the stretch. The placenta was remarkably small; the child was of full size. *Part* xiii., *p.* 350.

Inversion of the Uterus.—Syncope without hemorrhage may depend, according to Dr. Mitchell, upon the following causes:

1st. The labor may have been tedious and the patient faint from mere exhaustion. 2nd. From rupture of the uterus or bladder. 3rd. From internal uterine hemorrhage; or 4th. From inversion of the uterus. How necessary, therefore, that the practitioner should at once be aware of the cause of syncope. In the three first to which I have alluded, the uterus may be felt over the the pubes; in the last it cannot. As a general rule, it will be well in every case of doubt, at once to make a vaginal examination, as it has ere this occurred that the accident has not been detected until after the woman's death, or where it has not proved fatal until all chance of reduction has passed by. In cases of this description, the accoucheur should be certain that there is no escape of blood externally, to ascertain which, he ought not to be content with merely examining posteriorly, but in every instance he ought to look if any has escaped in front, as I have several times found the bed soaked with blood in consequence of a constant stream running over the woman's thigh, although none appeared to come from between the vulva.

Inversion of the womb may be mistaken for polypus, prolapsus uteri, or vaginæ. It has also been ignorantly removed by the crotchet, supposing it to be the head of a child. It may be distinguished from polypus by being rough externally, and very sensitive to the touch. Polypi are smooth and glistening, and the mouth of the uterus can be felt by encircling their necks. From prolapse of the uterus it may be known by the absence of the os uteri, and from that of the vagina (which rarely assumes so large a size), by our being able to discover a second opening above the tumor—the true os. I may mention, however, that many first-rate practitioners have mistaken polypus for inversion—accounts of which will be found in the different periodicals.

The treatment of inversion of the uterus will greatly depend upon the fact, whether the placenta be attached to the inverted organ, or if it has been expelled. In the former case—viz., where the placenta is attached, there is less danger to the patient from flooding, as the uterine sinuses are closed by the adherent placenta. In either case, as soon as the accident is discovered, reduction should be accomplished as soon as possible; but a very important practical question remains to be decided. In the event of the placenta being adherent to the displaced uterus, ought we first to detach it, and then reduce the uterus; or, on the other hand, should we attempt the reduction, the placenta being still adherent? Now, in answering this question, I should state that there is considerable difference of opinion amongst the highest authorities.

I think the practitioner can have no difficulty in making up his mind as to the proper plan of treatment, which appears to be in every case to attempt the reduction of the displaced organ without detaching the placenta, but if that be impracticable, he should then detach it and proceed with the greatest promptitude to reduce it.

There can be no doubt that in all cases of inversion, whether attended with hemorrhage or not, the presence of syncope renders the reduction much easier than it would be without it. Sir C. M. Clark says that he has been called by other practitioners to cases of inverted uterus, where the patient has expired from hemorrhage before the accident was discovered, and that in every instance the displaced uterus was reduced with very little trouble, all difficulty being removed by the depressed condition of the woman prior to death. Upon the same principle we find that Dewees recommends bleeding to syncope in cases of inversion unattended with hemorrhage.

Now as to the termination of this difficulty we have seen that it may prove fatal in a few hours from flooding. In some instances the hemorrhage has been followed by inflammation terminating in gangrene, induced by a kind of strangulation of the uterus in its cervix. There are several cases mentioned by Rousset, in which recovery took place after the spontaneous separation of the mortified organ. It may become chronic, and either prove fatal by exhausting discharges, or as in some rare instances be spontaneously cured. It has been fully proved that the inverted organ may be removed with impunity by ligature or excision; successful cases are given by Granville, Gooch, Newnham, etc. *Part* xiv., *p.* 276.

Hemorrhage during Labor.—When the patient is sinking from loss of blood, administer ether vapor as a *stimulant ;* and after the labor, even if the uterus has contracted well, give a dose of secale cornutum.

Part xvi., *p.* 251.

Treatment of Post-Partum Hemorrhage—Dr. Torbock proposes to arrest flooding by the injection of stimulants into the uterine cavity. He gives two cases in support of the proposed practice.

The first was the subject of recto-vaginal fistula; the head was delayed at the mouth of the womb by bands of adhesion, the results of violence used in a previous labor, but after these were divided, the uterine efforts were inefficient to effect delivery, which was therefore accomplished by the aid of the forceps.

It was at this moment, from the atonic state of the uterus, frightful hemorrhage followed. The ordinary means were used to produce uterine contraction, as pressure, grasping the uterus, secale, and the introduction of the hand into the uterus. At this critical moment was suggested the introduction of a piece of rag, saturated with brandy, diluted one-third with water, into the uterine cavity, which was very promptly done; when on a second application it was grasped by the contracting uterus, all hemorrhage ceased; the patient progressed favorably. The stimulant used in the second case was rum. *Part* xvi., *p.* 273.

Rigidity of the Os Uteri.—When there is a hot skin, and a quick, full pulse, we may bleed, and nauseate with tartar emetic, give a turpentine or emollient enema to clear out the bowels, and then a full opiate, and smear the os and cervix freely with extract of belladonna. If these means fail, incise the os uteri on each side with a probe-pointed bistoury.

Part xvii., *p.* 241.

Turning as an Alternative for Craniotomy and the Long Forceps, in Deformity of the Brim of the Pelvis.—It is proposed to turn the child, and extract by the feet, instead of performing embryotomy, or applying the long forceps. By this operation, the narrowest portion of the cone formed by the fœtal head is first engaged in the contracted brim, and the skull will usually become so indented and compressed in its biparietal diameter, as to allow of its extraction by such force as may be safely applied to the child's neck. Thus the best chance of life is afforded to the child, while, from the early period of labor at which the operation is performed, the mother is spared all the evils which result from protracted pain and long-continued pressure on the soft parts.

  *   *   *   *   *   *

When the head is prevented from entering the brim of the pelvis by reason of the diminished diameter of the latter, turning should be had recourse to, in preference to embryotomy or the long forceps; and should be performed early—the earlier the better. But it should not be under-

taken when labor has been long continued—when the strength is exhausted
—the uterine energy gone, or the uterus painfully and permanently
contracted; nor is it recommended when the child is dead, the pelvis *very*
much contracted, or when the accoucheur is not familiar with the operation.   *Part* xvii., *p.* 242.

Deformity of the Brim.—When the use of the long forceps comes into
competition with the employment of craniotomy, the former is generally
to be preferred. Now, when the pelvis is contracted in its conjugate or
antero-posterior diameter, the long or fronto-occipital diameter of the
child's head occupies the transverse diameter of the brim. The blades
of the long forceps should, therefore, be placed obliquely upon the child's
head; one, the posterior, over the side of the occiput; and the other, or
anterior, over the side of the brow or temple; or, in other words, they
should be applied in the oblique diameter of the brim, for in this situation
there is the most room for them.   *Part* xviii., *p.* 276.

Unusual Cases of Utero-Gestation.—On the 16th of Nov., 1822, a
woman in the parish of Farnham, Surrey, after having had irregular
uterine action for two days, was delivered by a midwife of a dead fœtus,
of a little more than thirteen inches long, and having the appearance of a
seven months' fœtus. The placenta was shortly afterward expelled, and
it was then found that there was a second fœtus, living and active, in
utero: but as there were no pains and no hemorrhage, it was determined
to wait the event. The woman recovered favorably: and on the 14th of
January, 1823, or fifty-nine days from her premature accouchment, she
was again taken in labor, and delivered of a fine healthy child. She had
been regularly unwell on the last week of March, and expected her confinement to take place about Christmas.

　　*　　　*　　　*　　　*　　　*　　　*　　　*　　　*

In the "London and Edinburgh Monthly Journal of Medical Science,"
Dec., 1842, a case is related by Dr. Jameson of a blighted twin being
retained, with its placenta and membranes, for seven weeks after the birth
of its fellow twin alive, and which was presumed to have arrived at the
full period of utero-gestation. This is very remarkable! We can easily
conceive the uterus to be endowed with the power of ridding itself of a
blighted or dead fœtus before the period of utero-gestation is accomplished,
even allowing the second fœtus to be retained to the full period; but to
throw off the healthy, and retain the blighted one, and that beyond the
usual period of pregnancy, is an anomaly proving that the laws of nature,
in many cases, are extremely difficult of explanation. In the "Lancet,"
Jan., 1843, a Mr. Vale recites the case of a woman, being pregnant with
twins, giving birth to the first alive, at the seventh month; and the second
also alive, two months afterward, being the completion of the proper
period of utero-gestation. Drs. M'Clintock and Hardy, in their work,
entitled, "Practical Observations on Midwifery," 1848, record the case of
a female at her sixth pregnancy producing twins, both children being
girls, the first of which was strong and healthy, and apparently at full
time—the second much smaller, dead, copper-colored, and in a state of
putrefaction. In this case there was but one placenta, and that part of it
which was inclosed by the membranes of the dead child was slightly
darker and more consolidated than the rest. We (the Ed.) have in our
practice experienced three cases in which the births of twin children were

separated by a space of time; in two cases an interval of three weeks occurred, and in the other fourteen days. In all three cases the first-born fœtus was dead. Such examples go far to prove that in cases of plural births each fœtus possesses its independent involucra. We do not detect any of the characteristics of super-fœtation in these cases; in fact, we experience considerable doubts respecting the majority of cases published under that title.—*Ed. Brit. Record.* *Part* xviii., *p.* 284.

Hysterocele.—[Hernia of the uterus, whether inguinal, femoral, or ventral, is a very rare occurrence, but Mr. Bell has met with two cases.] I attended Mrs. M——, at her fourth confinement. At five o'clock, A.M., after a tolerably severe labor of sixteen hours' duration, a fine female child was born. As soon as the cord was separated, and the child handed to the nurse, in accordance with my usual practice, I applied my hand to the abdomen, when, to my astonishment, I found the anterior-superior part of the uterus protruded through a rent in the linea alba, which was completely torn through from the ensiform cartilage to pubis. The uterus felt so large and firm, that little doubt existed of its containing another child.

On making a vaginal examination, a second set of membranes was detected, on rupturing which the child was ascertained to present with nates to mother's abdomen. The uterus was pressed back into the abdominal cavity, and firmly maintained in this position with both hands until the child (a male) was born; this occurred half an hour after the first birth. The conjoined placenta came away immediately—the uterus contracted firmly, and descended into the hypogastrium. A compress was placed on each side of the rent along its whole extent, and a bandage firmly applied. A smart attack of peritonitis occurred, but it was fortunately subdued by the ordinary treatment. Three months after delivery I carefully examined the abdomen, and could detect no trace of the rupture.

The great distention to which the abdominal parietes were subjected from the uterus containing two very large children, must have stretched the fibres of the linea alba to the utmost extent, the contraction of the abdominal muscles during labor producing the complete separation of the tissues. *Part* xviii., *p.* 301.

Treatment of Rigidity of the Os Uteri.—Dr. Scanzoni, who has carefully examined the conditions of the os and cervix, in the latter months of pregnancy, believes that the constriction, which sometimes declares itself in the first stage of labor, is due to rigidity of the upper orifice of the uterine neck, and not the lower, which is generally sufficiently dilatable. Instead of the treatment usually recommended, viz., bleeding, antimony, belladonna, frictions, etc., he advises a continuous douche of warm water upon the os and cervix, directed by means of an appropriate instrument. *Part* xix., *p.* 225.

Excision of Malignant Tumor of the Os Uteri during Labor.—When the disease involves only a portion of the os uteri, and proves an impediment to the dilatation of the latter during labor, it may be excised with safety and advantage. *Part* xix., *p.* 226.

Use of Ice in Promoting Uterine Contraction.—Dr. Mackall, in a communication to the committee of the American Medical Association, states, that for several years past he has been in the habit of employing pounded ice in cases of suspended or protracted labor. That when this had been swallowed freely, the pains had immediately returned, the uterus had contracted strongly, and the labor been speedily completed.

In cases where labor pains had been suspended for twelve or twenty-four hours, they have been renewed promptly and efficiently. In cases of inevitable abortion, where the uterine contractions are feeble and inefficient, and where hemorrhage is considerable; in retention of the placenta from imperfect contraction of the uterus, and in cases of alarming hemorrhage after delivery and expulsion of the after-birth, it is equally applicable—in short, whenever the firm contraction of the uterus is desirable, that object will most certainly be attained by the administration of ice.

*　　*　　*　　*　　*　　*　　*　　*

Decoction of the Roots of Cotton Plant.—Dr. Blackburn of Barnesville, states that he has used a strong decoction of the roots of the cotton plant in two cases of labor with successful issue, to promote uterine contraction where ergot failed.　　　　　　　　　　*Part* xix., *p.* 233.

Treatment of After-Pains.—Consists in the removal of coagula from the vagina and os uteri, the avoidance of all the extra-uterine causes of uterine contraction, and the administration of opiates. Gentle friction with the linimentum opii over the abdomen is often very useful; but I have found still greater benefit from the application of this liniment to the mammæ. By a reflex action, it allays the excessive sensibility of the uterus, when thus applied.

In excessive after-pains, without hemorrhage, without the presence of coagula, and in the absence of other signs and consequences of inertia, the infant should never be applied to the breast for some hours after delivery; not, in fact, until the uterus has become calmed from its state of morbid excitability. Early and constant stimulation of the breasts by the child is a common cause of irritable uterus for many days after delivery. This agent, so salutary in all cases of impending inertia, is often made, unnecessarily, a cause of suffering, at a time when the patient is little able to endure it, and without any counterbalancing good, if the uterus has contracted healthily. I repeat, we want no more than safe contraction; every after-pain beyond this point is both unnecessary and mischievous.

　　　　　　　　　　Part xix., *p.* 258.

Breech Presentations.—The child dies from hemorrhage into the placenta, caused by compression of the umbilical vein. To obviate this, tie the cord early, before the complete birth of the child; and endeavor to get respiration carried on while the head is still in the vagina.

　　　　　　　　　　Part xix., *p.* 275.

Impropriety of Frequent Operative Interference in Midwifery.—Never be anxious to promote hasty delivery, and use all operative measures as seldom as it is possible. The late Dr. J. Clarke, of Dublin, who used the forceps only once in 3,847 labors, was singularly successful in saving the lives of both mothers and children.　　　　　*Part* xx., *p.* 193.

Hemorrhage—Post-Partum.—In extreme cases, pass one hand into the uterus; introduce the pipe of an enema apparatus by the side of the arm a little way into the vagina, and inject suddenly ice-cold water, which will pass up into the uterus. By the ordinary plan of injecting the vagina, we are not sure that the injection enters the uterus; but by having one hand introduced into this organ, we learn whether it is really injected, and we ascertain also the effects of the injection. This method is very much better than that of introducing a bladder into the uterus and then distending the former, as it is the influence of the cold, and not the pressure, that we want to employ. *Part* xx., *p.* 194.

Labor—Use of Chloroform in.—The careful inhalation of chloroform is quite innocuous. It may therefore be given in *natural labor*, simply for the purpose of allaying pain, *if the patient requests it.* And it ought to be given when the regularity and efficiency of the pains are interfered with by emotion, nervous excitement, or cerebral congestion. In all such cases the inhalation must only be carried to the extent of allaying pain—not to make the patient unconscious. In *operative* midwifery, chloroform should be given in difficult cases of turning, and of retained placenta; and the full surgical effect, of unconsciousness and muscular relaxation, should be produced. In forceps and craniotomy cases, chloroform should not be used. *Part* xxi., *p.* 315.

Prolapsus of the Pregnant Uterus.—Mrs. P., a delicate woman, had already two children. After the birth of the second, she was much troubled with a sensation of bearing down, and sometimes of a slight protrusion of the uterus, which she endeavored, very ineffectually, to remedy, by wearing some kind of bandage. The protrusion became greater when she next became pregnant, but diminished, and was at length wholly removed, as the uterus enlarged from gestation. When, however, the labor drew near, she was again sensible of much weakness and bearing down; and at length when the pains actually came on, she was much alarmed by finding that a large fleshy mass had passed through the os externum with a good deal of fluid discharge. She sent for Mr. Gristock, who found that not only a considerable portion of the vagina was protruded, but that the os uteri was to be felt considerably without the os externum. He ordered her to bed, had the parts freely fomented, and requested a friend to visit the patient with him. They found her much alarmed, but presenting no symptoms indicative of danger. It was, therefore, determined not at present to employ any active interference. The pains at first were not strong, but as they increased in strength, it was *thought advisable to expand the hand over the protruded part, so as to make the ends of the fingers afford five points of support to the prolapsed vagina.* By degrees it appeared to recede during the pains, and, at last, during a very strong pain, the whole mass slipped up into the pelvic cavity; the infant was speedily born, the placenta came away, and the uterus contracted firmly, remaining in its proper situation. This woman got quite well, and in less than two years became pregnant again; she then came under the care of Dr. Hugh Ley. The same procedentia again took place, and was managed in the same way, with the same happy result.

Part xxii., *p.* 274.

Entrance of Air by the Open Mouths of the Uterine Veins After Parturition.—Dr. Cormack arrives at the following conclusions. He says:

1. The entrance of air into the veins does not necessarily give rise to

exactly the same symptoms; the intensity of the effects depending upon the degree in which the action of the right side of the heart is arrested or impeded by its over distention, and upon the degree of asphyxia induced by the impediment to the passage of the blood through the lungs.

2. The indications of treatment are three-fold; *first*, to relieve the distended right auricle; *secondly*, to treat the impending or actually present asphyxia; and *lastly*, to prolong life by every possible means, in the hope that the air may be all absorbed, and the passage of the blood through the small vessels of the lungs again be made easy.

3. In the most rapid class of cases, in which death is suddenly threatened from paralysis of the heart from over-distention, we must first strive to relieve the organ from that condition; when the phenomena are chiefly those of asphyxia from more gradually increasing obstruction of the lungs, the various means for treating asphyxia must be resorted to, and among these, in many cases, I believe the alternate use of the hot and cold douches will be found to be very valuable, especially if combined with stimulants judiciously varied and skillfully administered externally and internally. In many cases, repose, dashing cold water in the face, keeping the surface warm, and TIME may be the only means which ought to be used.

From the facts already stated, it is plain that the treatment, both preventive and curative, is to obtain natural and permanent contraction of the uterus after delivery. As it is extremely probable that loss of blood, and the entrance of air, in many cases conjointly cause death, it is satisfactory to feel assured that the proper treatment for the one is the best also for the other, so far as the one thing primarily essential is to strive to get the uterus to contract. Plugging will also be specially proper when there is convulsive contraction and expansion of the uterus, with or without much hemorrhage; for then there exists the greatest aptitude for the atmospheric air to enter, or be forced into the uterine veins.

If a large quantity of air have entered the circulation, unequivocal evidence of this will be found by listening to the heart, when the churning sound will be heard.   *Part* xxii., *p.* 309.

Indian Hemp as an Oxytoxic.—The administration of the Indian hemp seems markedly and directly to increase parturient action, and Dr. Churchill states that it possesses powers similar to those of the ergot of rye in arresting hemorrhage, when dependent upon congested states of the impregnated uterus.   *Part* xxii., *p.* 316.

Ergot of Rye in Labor.—Dr. Meigs, of Philadelphia, only uses ergot of rye at the moment or just before the birth of a child; in order to secure, if possible, a permanent and good contraction of the womb after labor, in women who are known in their preceding labor to have been subject to an alarming hemorrhage.   *Part* xxiii., *p.* 257.

Head Presentation—Turning in.—On this subject, Dr. Ramsbotham says, the following are the circumstances only under which he would resort to this operation: If the clear available space in the conjugate diameter were about $3\frac{1}{4}$ inches, or from that to $3\frac{1}{2}$—if the woman's children had all previously been born dead—if the membranes were still whole, or the liquor amnii having been evacuated, the uterus had not contracted closely round the child's body, the head being perfectly free above the pelvic brim, not having as yet descended into the pelvic cavity;

and if the attendant, by being in the habit of performing obstetrical operations, had acquired a certain dexterity in regard to them, and had perfect confidence in himself. *Part* xxv., *p.* 276.

Galvanism in Obstetric Practice.—Do not employ the apparatus in which two currents are produced, but simply the single current machine, for a direct current tends to produce contraction, an inverse current, paralysis. In using the single current machine, place the positive conductor over the lumbo-sacral region, and carry the other over the abdominal surface, with a gentle friction. In this way powerful uterine contractions may be easily excited. *Part* xxv., *p.* 278.

Treatment of unavoidable Hemorrhage.—In treating *unavoiduble hemorrhage*, attended with exhaustion, Dr. Murphy very much prefers having resource to Dr. Simpson's plan of artificial separation of the placenta, to turning ; and thinks this last operation is quite unjustifiable, on Smellie's plea that the woman must not die undelivered—the very attempt to prevent her doing so being, in fact, sometimes the cause of her death. His rules are thus summed up. (1.) In cases where no exhaustion has taken place, or where this is only commencing, the child should be turned and delivered the moment the os is sufficiently dilated or dilatable. When this is not so, the placenta should be compressed by the plug and by the discharge of the liquor amnii, and other means employed to prevent exhaustion, until delivery is practicable. (2.) In extreme exhaustion, turning should not be performed, but the placenta should be separated, and the child left undisturbed until decided reaction takes place. (3.) When the os is rigid, means should be employed to compress the placenta and increase the action of the uterus, so as to give time for dilatation and turning. Should exhausting hemorrhage, however, come on in the meantime, the placenta should be removed, rather than the hand be forced into the uterus. *Part* xxvi., *p.* 312.

Hemorrhage after Delivery accompanied by severe After-pains.—In several cases which Dr. Ramsbotham has met with, there have been most severe after-pains, with great hemorrhage, though the uterus was still firm and comparatively small. His explanation is, that a clot having filled the cavity of the uterus, the womb is unable to expel the offending mass. The more fluid parts are squeezed out, and the firmer remain behind, clinging with such tenacity to the uterine walls as to be almost as difficult of removal as a piece of adherent placenta. The treatment of such cases is to introduce the hand, remove the clot from the cavity of the uterus, and immediately the after-pains and the hemorrhage dependent thereon will cease.

Dr. R. gives the following, among other cases :

My assistance was sought by a medical practitioner, for Mrs. C. H., who had been delivered of her first child three hours. The placenta had been retained by irregular contraction, and removed from the uterus by the hand ; previously to which she had lost about two pounds of blood. When I arrived, she was faint, cold, and pale ; the pulse was very small ; the uterus was excessively hard, and rather larger than natural ; there was an uninterrupted draining going on, and she was suffering excruciating pains at intervals, evidently proceeding from uterine contractions. She had taken three drachms of laudadum without relief. I passed my hand into the cavity with considerable ease, notwithstanding the strength of the uterine contractions, and removed a quantity of tough, fibrinous coagula, considerably larger than an orange. She felt immediate freedom from pain, and the discharge ceased almost as suddenly. She became a little faint, but soon rallied; at four she was sleeping comfortably; and her recovery was uninterrupted. *Part* xxvii., *p.* 180.

Peculiar Accidental Uterine Hemorrhage.—Sudden syncope or faintness, with great distention and pain of the abdomen, supervening in cases of advanced pregnancy, should lead you to suspect internal uterine hemorrhage. Mr. Harrinson asks:

What would stop the bleeding most effectually for the time till the patient could rally? The coagulum at the mouths of the vessels supported in its position as it would be by the foetus, membranes, etc. Withdraw this plug, and the hemorrhage would almost certainly return. Therefore the practice would naturally be to keep the plug there till we saw a fit occasion to allow it to come away. Bringing the child away, and emptying the womb by artificial means, would insure the separation of this plug at a time perhaps when the woman was not fit for such a process. We should say, therefore, in such a case:

1. Give stimulants in moderation and keep the woman horizontal.

2. If syncope continued, rupture the membranes, give a dose of ergot of rye, and keep up the patient as well as you can by stimulants and food, but don't bring away the child yourself—let the womb expel it, and be ready the moment the child is born to compress the fundus uteri with a cold hand or cold wet towel, so as to compel it to contract rapidly and to expel placenta and coagula. If you save the woman from the first gush of blood, you will probably save her altogether. *Part* xxvii., *p.* 183.

Galvanism in Obstetric cases.—A continual current is by no means so effectual as repeated shocks; these rarely fail to excite muscular contractions, for this stimulus acts directly on muscular fibre. The discs of the apparatus may be covered with thin flannel, and applied on either side of the uterus, the flannel being moistened with water. This plan is equally effectual as the application of the discs to the spine of the cervix uteri.

In cases of hemorrhage before the birth of the child, apply the poles of the galvanic battery to the side of the uterus. *Part* xxix., *p.* 259.

Galvanism as an Obstetric Agent.—[Dr. Radford was first led to the use of galvanism in midwifery from observing its value in a case of atony of the bladder. He has used it]

1st. In cases of tedious labor arising from uterine inertia.

2d. In cases of accidental hemorrhage, either before or after the rupture of the membranes, and especially when exhaustion from loss of blood exists.

3d. In cases of "placenta prævia," in which the practice of detaching the placenta is adopted, and the vital powers are greatly depressed.

4th. In cases of internal flooding before or during labor.

5th. In cases of post-partum floodings.

6th. In cases of hour-glass or irregular contraction of the uterus.

7th. To originate, *de novo*, uterine action, or in cases in which it is desired to induce premature labor.

8th. In cases of abortion, when the indications show the necessity, or justify the expulsion of the ovum.

9th. In cases of asphyxia in infants.

Galvanism is especially advantageous as a general stimulant in all those cases in which the vital powers are extremely depressed from loss of blood. •Its beneficial effects are to be observed in the change of the countenance, restoring an animated expression; in its influence on the heart and arteries; in changing the character of respiration; and its warming influence on the general surface. *Part* xxix., *p.* 268.

Uterine Douches in Tedious Labor.—The tepid douche, used in the way adopted to induce premature labor, may sometimes stimulate the uterus when inactive. You may use the douche for ten minutes or a quarter of an hour at a time. The same means may assist in dilating a rigid os uteri. *Part* xxxi., *p.* 207.

Flooding after Delivery.—Inject cold water into the womb. Use a Weiss's syringe, and introduce the nozzle of the tube an inch or two fairly into the os uteri. *Part* xxxi., *p.* 208.

Hemorrhage after Delivery.—Generally the more powerfully the uterus contracts after delivery, the less the danger of flooding; not so, however, in all cases; if a portion of the placenta, a fold of the fœtal membranes, or a quantity of coagulated blood, be retained in its cavity, it may be adherent to the internal surface, so that no efforts of the uterus can dislodge it; the more fluid parts may be squeezed away, but the tougher particles remain, and bleeding still go on so as to endanger the life of the patient. By the introduction of the hand, and the withdrawal of the coagula, the agonizing pains and the further loss of blood are at once put a stop to, and instantaneous ease and immediate safety secured. *Part* xxxii., *p.* 221.

Uterine Hemorrhage.—When threatened abortion is from a debilitated condition of the uterus, which, in its relaxed condition, opens the os, small doses of ergot act as a tonic, and close the bleeding orifices of the vessels. If the patient be near the full time, and delivery cannot be prevented, whether a case of placenta previa, or not, rupture the membranes at one side, and give a good dose of ergot, so as to force the presenting part of the child firmly down upon the bleeding surface, and thus to dam up the stream; if this be not successful, deliver, if you can pass the hand; but if you cannot without much force, plug, until such time as you can deliver.

In women peculiarly liable to flooding, as soon as the child is born, be careful not to interfere unnecessarily during delivery. *Imitate nature,* or rather *let nature alone.* When the head is expelled, don't seize upon it and pull for your life, like a madman, but wait patiently, not only until nature has expelled the shoulders, but the hips also, for the body and legs of the child will stimulate the uterus to action as effectually as the hand of the accoucheur, and thus prevent flooding. But some may say, supposing the head is expelled and the pains cease, would you not employ traction then? No! certainly not! you must not lend so much as the strength of a finger toward completing the delivery, but "*compel the uterus to do its own work.*" Besides being careful not to interfere in these cases, as soon as the head presses upon the perineum, give a full dose of ergot as a precaution against flooding, and repeat if necessary.

In cases of abortion, if the flow of blood be great, give large and repeated doses of ergot, so that the presenting part may be forced down, to act as an internal plug. In addition to this, it may be advisable to employ the plug, by pushing a piece of alum into the vagina before the plug.

After the child is delivered, the first aim is to secure uterine contrac-' tions; it is worse than useless to deliver the placenta if this is not effected; it must be excited by ergot, firmly grasping the uterus, abdominal frictions, ice, the cold and hot douche alternately; if these means are not sufficient, introduce the hand and remove the placenta. In cases of abortion where the placenta is retained, the general treatment is to trust to time; if there is hemorrhage, plug and give ergot; but there is a great deal of uncertainty about this. The placenta should be removed if possible; some recommend hooking it down with one finger, but this cannot always be done; in such cases, perhaps, a pair of polypus forceps would be best to seize the placenta, twist it round and round again so as to detach it and bring it away. After the placenta is expelled, there may be hemorrhage from irregular contraction, loss of power and nervous energy, or from some mechanical impediment to contraction, as a clot of blood. In all these cases you must introduce the hand, and when it is contracted, keep it so, by external pressure and ergot.

In cases of severe flooding, don't apply the bandage; it is in the way, and prevents more certain manipulations; after all danger has passed, it may be applied for support to the abdomen. *Part* xxxii., *p.* 222.

Labor—Induction of.—The uterine douche possesses many advantages over ergot—1st. It will excite contractions; 2d. It does not endanger' either the mother or the child; 3d. Its action can be better regulated according to the effect required; and, 4th. It may be employed at the commencement of labor, and in all degrees of dilatation of the neck.

Part xxxiii., *p.* 262.

Turning—Use of Forceps.—In all cases where the head is detained after the delivery of the body, the use of the forceps is greatly preferable to pulling by the body or neck of the child. They may be applied easier than in vertex presentation, because you have the head fixed and know its exact position. The extracting force is certainly safer.

Part xxxiii., *p.* 263.

Tartar Emetic, in Obstetric Practice.—In the early stages of primiparæ, where the os uteri is hard, undilatable, and fails to yield to time and the ordinary remedies, one grain of tartar emetic with six ounces of soapwater may be given by the rectum with very beneficial and relaxing effects. It is particularly applicable for the robust and plethoric.

Part xxxiii., *p.* 273.

Post-Partum Hemorrhage.—In cases where women have suffered from flooding in several previous labors, you should give one or two doses of ergot during the last pains which expel the child. Immediately after delivery, in suspicious cases, the hand should be placed on the abdomen, and pressure made until efficient contraction is felt to take place. The uterus should be grasped and held firmly by the hands. The application of cold to the vulva and abdomen, by douching with a wet towel, or dashing the water on, is very effectual in rousing the uterus to contraction. If these means fail, the hand should be washed and introduced into the uterus. In addition to this, if the uterus appear paralyzed, cold water may be injected in a full stream into its cavity, or galvanism may be tried if there be time and convenience. Cold and heat applied alternately are much more efficacious than cold applied alone to excite reflex action. When one reflex surface is exhausted you may appeal to another, dashing cold water on the face, swallowing a gulp of cold water, an enema to the rectum, etc. Whenever coagula collect in the uterus or vagina, they produce irritation, keep up the hemorrhage, and must be turned out with the hand. If the placenta be only partly separated, or remain in the uterus, it must be immediately removed; if the patient is very much reduced, do not wait, pour some brandy down her throat, and proceed at once.

Part xxxiv., *p.* 233.

Elm Tents for Dilating the Cervix Uteri.—Elm bark possesses many advantages over sponge for dilating the cervix uteri. It is less expansible, and so dilates more gradually; it is not decomposed, and furnishes an abundant mucilage, which protects irritated or diseased surfaces.

Part xxxiv., *p.* 247.

Metastatic After-pains.—Among the different cases noted by Dr. Power, we find a marked instance of uterine metastasis upon the bladder: Mrs. P., at the beginning of the labor, had genuine uterine contractions, which dilated the os uteri with sufficient rapidity, when we remarked that the pains became suddenly more distressing, though they had no longer their former influence upon the mouth of the uterus. Placing our hand upon the fundus uteri during a pain, we could not perceive any contractions at all, but the woman complained of a very painful sensation just above the symphysis pubis, which ceased after some time, and came back in regular intervals. Mrs. P. had not evacuated her bladder for a considerable time, and was prevented from doing so by the pressure of the head against the symphysis pubis. We considered this a case of metastatic pains in the bladder, produced by an irritation of this organ, arising from its being overloaded with urine, and the vain attempts to empty itself. We therefore introduced the catheter, and drew off a considerable quantity of water. This being performed, regular uterine contractions set in, and labor was soon ended in the most satisfactory manner. Prof. Stein gives, among other cases, one of metastasis to a part of the nervous system, which is quite removed from the sphere of the uterine nerves. He says: "In this case a great quantity of liquor amnii was present, and, in consequence, the pains were very irregular. Suddenly, all uterine action ceased, and the woman was taken with a violent facial neuralgia. This affection lasted for one hour, when it gave entirely away, and another succession of labor pains set in; these, after some time, ceased, and the prosopalgia commenced, which was exchanged once more for activity of the womb, and so on by turns. At length the membranes were ruptured; after which, regular uterine action began and continued till the child was born."

Another very singular case was observed by the same author. A woman, when at the full term of her confinement, was taken with general convulsions, which ceased suddenly, but continued in the musculus orbicularis of both eyes, so that she could not open them for two days. Now the womb began its work, and with the first contraction her sight was re-established.

Pilger observed that, during a confinement the pains gave way, and the patient was suddenly taken with an alarming dyspnœa, which ceased as soon as another contraction of the uterus commenced. Others witnessed . that the abdominal muscles were the seat of metastatic labor.

This kind of dystochia is of rare occurrence. But there is another very severe and most tormenting affection occurring after confinement, namely, those very painful affections of the lower extremities, which commence a few hours after the child is born, and last sometimes for two or even eight days. The authors who treat of the said affection, call it " *the crural neuralgia of women in childbed*," and believe it to be the result of pressure of the fœtal head, or the forceps, or of an inflammatory exudation upon the crural nerves as they pass through the pelvis. This is the case in a few instances. But when these pains follow after an *easy* confinement, where neither a large-sized head, nor a forceps operation, nor an inflammation of the bowels, can be referred to as explaining this symptom, then we have to seek for another explanation.

[Dr. Nœggerath has had several cases under his observation which have exhibited this curious phenomenon. In one remarkable case, the pains began to come on about nine hours after delivery of a living, full-grown child.]

This morning, at about seven o'clock, the right thigh was suddenly seized with a pain, which soon increased to such violence, nay, fury, that the patient was afraid to move the leg the slightest degree from its position. The lower part of the thigh was the seat of the greatest pain, and especially its external surface extending over the dorsum pedis. The least pressure could not be endured. After the child was born, the woman had not the slightest perception of after-pains. She felt as if her *abdomen was empty*, or rather *not existing*. The uterus was enormously distended, its limit or outlines being scarcely distinguishable, texture remarkably soft and relaxed. Considering this to be a case of metastatic after-pains, I thought the chief indication would be to bring on uterine activity, after which the pain in the thigh should disappear. The result of my treatment proved that I was right.

Shortly after ten o'clock I gave her a large teaspoonful of powdered ergot of rye (secale cornutum). Ten minutes after, the patient remarked a discharge of blood from the vagina, the first after her delivery; a quarter of an hour after the administration of this remedy, the woman became more quiet, she ceased to cry, except occasionally, and a painful expression was noticed in her features. Twenty minutes past ten o'clock she said that the former kind of pain had left her thigh and yielded to a very bearable sensation of smarting. At half-past ten o'clock she took the same quantity of ergot, and fifteen minutes later I had the pleasure to see that the patient moved to lie upon her right side; she could bend her knee, and move her leg up and down; she even told me now that she *had not the least pain*. When I left her (before eleven o'clock), I could ascertain that the uterus was well contracted, lessened in size, and considerably harder than when I made the first examination. The woman had no relapse afterward.

In explanation of these singular pathological occurrences, we must bear in mind, that there is always present a limited amount of nervous power in the central organs. Therefore, if one part of the body receives a nervous impulse in excess, other organs must be more or less deprived of it; or, when there is prepared in the nervous centres a certain amount of material for the purpose of setting one department of nerves into action, and this department being in itself not properly disposed to receive it, then, another portion of the nerves must attract this amount, and show a greater activity. The same result must happen, when some other part of the system is in such an unnatural condition, that it attracts more nervous force from the centres than is due to it. In this case another organ must lose part of its activity.

These principles applied to the uterine system, we are able to explain the pathology of metastatic pains. When labor begins, the sympathetic nerves and the spinal cord secondarily are called to a physiological energy, which is seen in no other instance of life. Their activity is provoked by the uterus, and in ordinary circumstances directed to the uterus. But in order to perform their duties properly, the womb must be sufficiently disposed to attract the nervous fluid to its own sphere. In case of its being in a state of weakness, other organs receive the effect of the overloaded centres, and thus exhibit the phenomenon of metastatic pains. Therefore, this complaint is most commonly observed in connection with atonic labor-pains. But if some part or other of the system was previously, or during parturition, in an unhealthy condition, it would be liable to attract to itself the nervous energy originally due to the uterus, even if the latter was in a state of health. Therefore, we see that, in very many instances of metastasis, the affected organs stood under some morbid influence before or during confinement. *Part* xxxvi., *p.* 230.

Tedious Labor.—In cases where labor is arrested, not from any obstacle, but from simple atony and want of pains, where in fact the polarity of the cord is exhausted, try the effect of strychnia; in doses of one-sixteenth of a grain to commence with, repeated and gradually increased as necessary. It induces uterine contractions in a very remarkable manner, each dose being distinctly followed by this effect; it does not cause violent or continued action of the womb. In not one of nine cases in which it was administered, did any bad effects follow, and in all the labor was accomplished within an hour and a half after commencing the use of this drug.

Dr. Vernon prepares a solution of strychnine in very dilute hydrochloric acid, of the strength of one grain to the fluid ounce, and administers in divided doses, repeated upon each subsidence of uterine contractions. He says:

In the "Lancet," of June 14, 1856, I published a short letter in which I incidentally referred to the use of strychnia as an oxytoxic. Curiously enough, a letter from Dr. Matthew Corner appeared in juxtaposition with my own, detailing a case of poisoning by strychnia. The patient swallowed two grains of strychnia by mistake. She was pregnant, and aborted in the course of the action of the poison. The case terminated favorably. I have since become acquainted with the case of a lady who aborted five times consecutively whilst under the influence of nux vomica given as a tonic.

Part xxxvii., *p.* 234.

Galvanism in Obstetric Practice.—Individual shocks applied to the uterus produce no appreciable effects upon it; and a current directed transversely through the organ produces only a partial contraction of it in the direction of the current; but a sustained current of electricity directed longitudinally through the uterus, from the upper portion of the spinal cord, excites the action of the uterus. and singularly enough also accelerates the dilatation of the os uteri. A case of placenta prævia is mentioned, in which several alarming hemorrhages had occurred before labor had commenced. A sustained current of electricity applied in the manner stated for six hours, not only prevented further hemorrhage, but so accelerated the dilatation of the os uteri, that the hand was readily introduced and delivery completed with safety to the patient, although the child, from the extensive separation of the placenta, was still-born. In another case this mode of treatment speedily induced the expulsion of an organized membrane remaining after an early abortion, the ovum having been previously expelled. The patient was much exhausted by repeated floodings.

Part xxxvii., *p.* 271.

Chloroform in Natural Labor.—The great rule in administering chloroform in natural labor, is to give it so as to allay pain, without destroying consciousness. You may thus, without danger, give chloroform for any length of time. *Part* xxxviii., *p.* 206.

Uva Ursi in Labor.—In ordinary delayed labor, fifteen grains given in infusion every hour is as efficacious and far more innocent in its operation than secale cornutum. When rapid effects are desired, as in metrorrhagia, a decoction of 4 drachms to a quart of water should be employed, and given in frequent and divided doses. *Part* xxxviii., *p.* 206.

Dilatation of the Os Uteri.—The natural sickness of labor always has a beneficial influence in inducing relaxation, unaccompanied by a subsequent evil; and for the same reason artificial nausea has a powerful influence in subduing rigidity of the os uteri or vagina, and is so safe in the administration that it is a well-known fact that puerperal or peritoneal inflammations are rarely seen where tartar emetic as a nauseant has been judiciously given; there seems an almost perfect immunity of system from these diseases afterward. An emetic dose should be given at first, and the nausea continued by diminished doses. It must always be first ascertained that there do not exist certain unhealthy conditions of system, as organic disease of the heart or lungs, etc., in which case continued nausea might be productive of serious mischief.

[Dr. Gilmour has omitted what we consider the most important and safest medicines to accomplish dilatation of the os uteri, viz., chloroform and ipecacuanha. We have been highly pleased lately with the effects of chloroform. Early in labor, when the pains are regular and the os uteri rigid and small, by slightly influencing the patient with chloroform during almost every pain, the parts become much more rapidly softened and dilated. We have simply dropped a little chloroform on the pillow, near the nose of the patient, and told her to inspire it pretty freely each time, or just before the pain comes on. Instead of waiting six or eight hours for the dilatation of the os, we have thus accomplished it in less than two hours. One grain or two grains of ipecacuanha every half hour, will have also a good effect; but in a less pleasing way, and not so certainly.—Ed. "Retrospect."] *Part* xxxviii., *p.* 322.

Passage of the Fœtal Head.—The diameter of the different parts of the pelvis are so managed that the fœtal head undergoes a screw-like twist in its transit. It behooves the accoucheur to be mindful of this in applying the forceps. *Part* xxxix., *p.* 279.

PLACENTAL COMPLICATIONS.

Treatment of Placental Presentations.—The practice of removing the placenta, in cases of placental presentation, seems to have been well known and practised in Manchester for years, and originated in the practice of the late Mr. Kinder Wood. Mr. Wood says:]

If we find so much exhaustion as to make us fear the effects of further hemorrhage, during artificial delivery, the first step after passing the hand must be to detach the whole of the placenta; by this the hemorrhage will be completely suppressed, for the effect of passing the hand through the os uteri, and throwing off the placenta, will always be to produce so much contraction as to arrest the bleeding from the small decidual or uterine mouths. It is satisfactory to know that the child is rarely living in these cases of exhaustion, its blood being poured out through branches of the placental structure, along with that of the mother; and when brought down, its appearance, like that of the mother, is bleached and exsanguined. The time required to separate the placenta is very short, and the loss of blood during the attempt exceedingly trifling. I know from experience, that when the placenta is wholly detached, the hemorrhage will cease.

In some cases I have been called to attend, when the ordinary method of delivery has been adopted, the patient died, and this led me to modify the practice, by detaching the placenta, rupturing the membranes, and then delivering the child; but after due consideration I was again induced to vary my plan, and in those cases where we can have no hope in saving the patient if we proceed to delivery, however well the operation be conducted, I have no hesitation in recommending that the placenta be separated completely, and the membranes ruptured, and that the hand be withdrawn immediately upon this being effected, leaving the child and placenta behind. By this practice the patient will be placed precisely in the situation which occurs in the most favorable cases of recovery by the natural efforts. I conceive no fact in midwifery rests upon a more solid foundation, than that this hemorrhage will cease upon separating the placenta, and by this practice the patient is placed in as favorable a situation as is possible for recovery. Time will be gained to support her by proper means, and which can be used with greater freedom, as the hemorrhage is infallibly suppressed by this operation. *Part* xi., *p.* 195.

Placental Presentation—Extraction of the Placenta before the Child in Cases of.—All obstetric authors agree that no complication in midwifery occasions more anxiety to the practitioner, or danger to the patient, than hemorrhage from placental presentation, and the results of practice fully support this opinion. Of 174 cases which Dr. Churchill has collected, 48, or nearly one-third of the mothers died. Dr. Simpson has attempted a still more extensive analysis, and finds that of 399 cases recorded, in 115 the result was fatal to the mother, a mortality as great as that of malignant cholera in 1832–33, and twice as great as the average in cases of lithotomy. Looking at the results, any attempt to diminish such fearful mortality is entitled to the most careful notice of the profession. Hitherto two great principles of treatment, which some have supposed to be applicable to the two different stages of the complication, have been pursued, viz.: 1st, the evacuation of the liquor amnii; an 2d, delivery of the child by turning.

[Some accoucheurs, as Drs. Burns and Hamilton, Baudelocque, Capuron, and others, think this the *only* mode of treatment advisable under any circumstances in these cases. Drs. Merriman, Conquest, Dewes and Denman, are unanimous in the opinion that turning must be resorted to.]

Cases of placenta prævia, says Dr. S., frequently occur in practice in which neither of the two preceding plans can be successfully adopted—where the artificial evacuation of the liquor amnii is insufficient to moderate the hemorrhage to a safe degree, and where forced delivery by turning is inapplicable or extremely dangerous if adopted. In these and other cases, I would beg to submit to my obstetric brethren an additional principle of treatment, viz.: The complete separation, and, if necessary, extraction of the placenta before the child. Obstetric pathologists seem unanimous in the opinion that all the more formidable varieties of hemorrhage, which occur from the uterus in the latter months of utero-gestation, or the earlier periods of labor, are attributable to the separation of the vascular connections between the placenta and the interior of the uterus, and the escape of blood from the vessels which are laid open in consequence of this separation. Paradoxical as it may appear, there are sufficient grounds and facts for believing, that when the placenta is separated slightly and partially, the chance of fatal hemorrhage to the mother is greater than when the disunion of the organ is more entire and complete. Various authors have detailed cases in which the death of the mother speedily took place though the portion of the placenta separated from the uterus was exceedingly small.

Dr. S. has collected notes of 141 cases in which the placenta was expelled before the child, which he throws into a tabular form, and divides into—1st, Cases in which a considerable interval elapsed between these two occurrences; 2d, Cases in which the interval was less than ten minutes; 3d, Cases in which the child was born immediately after the placenta, or along with it; and 4th, Cases in which the period is not mentioned. I believe, says Dr. S., that the data which I have collected are amply sufficient to establish, as a great physiological and practical fact, that, when the placenta, in cases of unavoidable hemorrhage, is once completely detached from its connections with the interior of the uterus, the accompanying flooding in general entirely ceases, or become quite moderate and inconsiderable in quantity.

Summary of Results.—1. The total separation and expulsion of the placenta before the child, in cases of unavoidable hemorrhage, is not so rare an occurrence as accoucheurs appear generally to believe. 2. It is not by any means so serious and dangerous a complication as might *a priori* be supposed. 3. In nineteen out of twenty cases in which it has happened, the attendant hemorrhage has either been at once altogether arrested, or it has become so much diminished as not to be afterward alarming. 4. The presence or absence of flooding after the complete separation of the placenta, does not seem in any degree to be regulated by the duration of time intervening between the detachment of the placenta and the birth of the child. 5. In ten out of one hundred and forty-one cases, or in one out of fourteen, the mother died after the complete expulsion or extraction of the placenta before the child. 6. In seven or eight out of these ten casualties, the death of the mother seemed to have no connection with the complete detachment of the placenta, or with results arising directly from it, and if we do admit the three remaining cases (which are doubtful), as leading by this complication to a fatal termination, they would still only constitute a mortality from this complication of three in one hundred and forty-one, or about one in forty-seven cases. 7. On the other hand, under the present established rules of practice, one hundred and thirty-four mothers died in three hundred and ninety-nine placental presentations, or about one in three. *Part* xi., *p.* 203.

Placenta Prævia—Partial.—Rupture the membranes as soon as possible, and excite uterine action by friction, the application of a binder, ergot of rye, or galvanism.

Complete.—If the os is undilated and rigid, *plug* with a sponge dipped in vinegar and water; when the os is sufficiently dilated, seize a foot and deliver cautiously. In head presentation with a dead child, use craniotomy; and in both this case and that of foot presentation, rupture the membranes early through the placenta, by a silver catheter. (Dr. Tyler.)

* * * * * * *

When the vital powers are much depressed, and the placenta partially detached, plugging is dangerous. So are the administration of secale cornutum, and delivery of the child, because they lower still more the powers of the system. Detach completely the placenta, and employ galvanism, which both rouses the uterus, and stimulates generally.—(Dr. Radford.)

* * * * * * *

Turn as soon as possible, extract the placenta, and get the uterus to contract: taking care to keep up the pulse. If the strength is too much exhausted for this, or if the os uteri will not admit the hand, separate the placenta if possible; rupture the membranes with the nail, and *plug the vagina completely*, then give ergot of rye, and apply cold, or galvanism. When the pulse rallies withdraw the plug, and if possible turn; if this cannot be done, plug again and wait. It is plain that if we cannot deliver, we must directly stop the bleeding; and plugging in the case supposed, where the placenta is low down, is quite effectual.

Dr. Simpson advises when the hemorrhage and exhaustion are very great, and when turning, etc., are impracticable, on account of the undilated state of the os and cervix, especially in primiparæ, or the contracted state of the uterus itself, or the narrowness of the pelvis; or when turning is dangerous on account of the exhaustion of the mother, or not required for the safety of the child, on account of its death or prematurity, to *detach the placenta*, and leave the expulsion of the child to nature, if the hemorrhage, as is usually the case, ceases, and no particular complication arises. *Part* xv., *p.* 274–279.

Retained Placenta.—Empty the umbilical vein, and forcibly inject cold water slightly acidulated with acetic acid; or if there is much hemorrhage, cold decoction of ergot, or solution of tannic acid. *Part* xv., *p.* 280.

Placental Presentations.—The practice recommended by Dr. Simpson, of entirely detaching the placenta, and leaving it, is likely to be of use in very many instances; as where there is such an unyielding condition of the soft parts as to prevent speedy delivery, or where the flooding has been going on for a considerable time, and the practitioner, on his arrival, finds the bleeding still continuing, and the woman so much exhausted that the sudden emptying of the womb would be dangerous. But this plan by no means supersedes delivery by turning, which, if adopted in a prompt and energetic manner, is a safe and proper method of treatment.

    *   *   *   *   *   *   *

The practice of detaching the placenta is inapplicable in the most formidable cases—is as difficult to accomplish as turning, and does as much violence to the uterus—is almost certainly fatal to the child, and affords no increased chance of safety to the mother. If the cause of hemorrhage is ascertained to be placenta prævia, rupture the membranes, introduce the hand, and turn and deliver the child—provided that the os is sufficiently dilated, or easily dilatable; if it is not, wait, and act upon general principles, till sufficient relaxation has taken place.—(Mr. Newnham.)

    *   *   *   *   *   *   *

When copious and repeated hemorrhage occurs in the eighth or ninth month of pregnancy, and signs of labor do not appear, evacuate the liquor amnii, pass a conical plug into the os uteri, fill up the vagina behind it, and then give one or more doses of secale. The plug occasions the formation of a large coagulum within the uterus, the presence of which, combined with the irritation caused by the plug, excites uterine contraction. By the expulsion of the clot, the os is dilated, and we are then able to introduce the hand and turn with more facillty. (Dr. Reid.) *Pt.* xvii., *pp.* 225-237.

Placenta Prævia.—The chief methods of treatment are: 1. The plug. 2. Puncturing the membranes. 3. Turning the child. Plugging is adapted to those cases which occur at the sixth or seventh month, when a continuous drain is going on after the first loss. The best method of plugging is to introduce strips of lint, pieces of sponge, or a silk handkerchief dipped in vinegar and water. Do not plug too tightly, or uterine contraction may be excited, and further separation take place. Puncturing membranes is adapted to those cases, not very severe, where the os uteri is only dilated to a slight extent, and turning is impracticable; it arrests the hemorrhage by lessening the vascular supply, and bringing down the presenting part of the child to act as a plug to the placental site. Turning is the grand remedy in placenta prævia; if performed at the proper time, it affords the greatest chance of safety to both mother and child.

    *   *   *   *   *   *   *

The most prompt and efficient method in almost all cases is to introduce the hand, dilate the os uteri, separate the intermediate portion of placenta, rupture the membranes, seize one foot, turn, and deliver. In selecting the time when to do this, the great thing is to distinguish the dilatable character of the os uteri; if this be present, the extent of dilatation is of no importance comparatively. It requires great care that the dilating force be steadily applied and evenly distributed, so as to guard the cervix from laceration, which might prove fatal from hemorrhage. Version is sometimes prohibited by the immediate exhaustion of hemorrhage, or from rigidity of the os uteri, in spite of hemorrhage; in the former case plug and give stimulants freely, as a temporary resource. In the latter case, separate the entire connection of the placenta, rupture the membranes, and excite uterine action. (Dr. Tyler Smith.)   *Part* xxxiv., *p.* 226.

Encysted Placenta.—That is, where the placenta is retained by the contraction of the os uteri after parturition, must be removed by gently dilating the os first by the placenta itself, if possible, or if this do not succeed, by the fingers, drawing gently at the cord, and at the same time having firm pressure made on the abdomen. *Part* xxxiv., *p.* 227.

Placenta Prœvia.—In those terrible cases where the os is rigid and unyielding, and the flooding profuse, do not delay, but introduce one or two fingers through the os, and detach all that part of the placenta which adheres within the cervical zone, or region of dangerous placental seat. The contraction of the womb present in such a case as this, is the very element which will secure the success of this operation, as it constricts the mouths of the bleeding vessels. If contraction is not present, it must be induced by ergot of rye or galvanism. By the performance of this operation, moreover, the os and cervix are released from a mechanical impediment to dilatation. If necessary, the hemostatic process may also be assisted by the use of the plug. By these means the hemorrhage will have been arrested in the great majority of cases, but, if not, time will have been gained, and forced delivery rendered more easy. *Part* xxxvi., *p.* 221.

Placenta Prœvia.—A case is related in which, the os being dilated to the size of a small teacup, the separation (as advised by Dr. Barnes) of the whole circumference of the placenta which was presenting, sufficed at once to check the hemorrhage. By further separating the posterior portion of the placenta the membranes were reached, and the presentation discovered to be a footling. The child was delivered in a short time alive, and the mother did well. *Part* xxxix., *p.* 292.

Placenta Prœvia—Air Pessary.—An interesting case is related by Mr. Jardine Murray, of Brighton, in which the os uteri being dilated sufficiently to admit two fingers, and syncope impending from hemorrhage, a flattened caoutchouc air-pessary was introduced between the wall of the uterus and the presenting surface of the placenta. The pessary being then inflated by means of the attached syringe, it acted admirably as a direct plug and dilator of the os uteri. Whenever, from time to time, the trickling of blood recurred, it was effectually checked by further dilatation of the pessary, by a few strokes of the syringe. In two hours the os was sufficiently dilated to admit the hand, and though turning was necessary, as the shoulder presented, the case was soon brought to a favorable conclusion. *Part* xl., *p.* 196.

PREMATURE LABOR.

Mode of Inducing.—Dr. Meissner's mode of operating, which is a modification of that by puncture of the membranes was the following: A very slender canula is provided of about 13 to 14 inches in length, and bent regularly in the form of a segment of a circle. It has a ring soldered on the convex side of its lower extremity, in order to give a more secure hold, and allow of the point of the instrument being accurately guided. This canula is provided with two trocars, one with a blunt point and the other with a sharp-cutting point. When the instrument is to be used, the blunt pointed trocar is introduced into the canula, and projects beyond its orifice so far as to prevent the edge of the tube injuring the parts. The patient then stands before the practitioner, who kneels before her, the usual manner in which vaginal examinations are made on the continent, or she may sit on the very edge of a chair, or of the bed. The forefinger of the left hand is then introduced into the vagina, and the canula guided along it to the orifice of the uterus, making the convexity of the instrument correspond to the curve of the sacrum. The point of the instrument is then pushed slowly backward and upward, so as to make its rounded point slide between the uterus and the back of the membranes. When the point is once past the neck of the uterus, it advances easily, care only must be taken to detach the membranes as little as possible. When the point of the instrument is about 10 or 11 inches within the *os uteri*, the blunt-pointed trocar is withdrawn, and the handle of the instrument is pressed against the perineum, to detect, if possible, against what the point of the canula is pressing. If it be felt to be a hard body, the point is made to move to one side or other till an elastic fluctuating spot be reached, which shows it is opposite the membranes alone ; the sharp-pointed trocar is then introduced and perforation of the membranes is made. The trocar is then withdrawn, and about a tablespoonful of the *liquor amnii* is allowed to escape; after this the canula also is removed, and the woman is allowed to walk, sit, or lie down at her own pleasure. *Part* iii., *p.* 124.

The Use of the Plug to produce Premature Labor.—Two modes of producing premature labor are resorted to at the present day. Either the membranes are punctured, or a tent of sponge is introduced into the os uteri, as recommended by Professor Kluge. The former method is liable to the objection of causing the too rapid escape of the liquor amnii, and thus endangering the life of the child when labor pains are tardy in their occurrence. The second is often extremely difficult to accomplish, or even impossible when the os uteri is directed very much backward, or when the patient has never before been pregnant.

Dr. Scholler was led to try the plug, from having observed that when used to suppress hemorrhage, in cases of placental presentation or of threatening abortion, it had a considerable influence in exciting uterine action. He had observed, also, one case where its employment to restrain hemorrhage was followed by premature labor, which it seemed to have occasioned. He recommends filling the upper part of the vagina with balls of charpie, which, for the sake of cleanliness, should be renewed every twenty-four hours. The action of the uterus is usually very speedily excited, and, when fully established, the plug may be withdrawn and secale cornutum administered to prevent the diminution of labor pains. The finger may likewise be used to aid the dilatation of the os uteri, but great care must be taken to leave the membranes uninjured.

The average length of time which elapsed between the application of the plug and the birth of the child was five days and fourteen hours.

Part v., *p.* 162.

Induction of Premature Labor.—M. Dubois confines himself to those cases where the safety of the mother is in question, not regarding in any respect whether the child is viable or not. This absolute abandonment of the interests of the infant, when the life of the mother is seriously endangered, although not admitted by many accoucheurs, now finds less and less opposition every day.

The first mechanical condition requiring the operation, is *excessive dilatation of the uterus by superabundance of the liquor amnii.*

The second set of cases sometimes demanding the operation are those where, in addition to the pregnant uterus, *the abdomen contains a large tumor.* Thirdly, cases where, from *malconformation of the pelvis and trunk*, there is not sufficient space for the uterus to develop itself. We may remark, however, that in these last sets of cases, premature labor generally comes on spontaneously.

Fourthly, cases of *retroversion of the uterus*, in which it becomes impacted in the small pelvis.

Fifthly, those cases of *uterine hemorrhage* where nothing but the evacuation of the ovum, and the contraction of the uterus, will stop the bleeding. We now come to another series of cases demanding the operation ; and, firstly, we mention those nervous diseases which may demand it when they exist to an excessive and dangerous degree, as *chorea, convulsions*, etc. But M. Dubois inculcates extreme caution in such cases, as also in cases of *obstinate vomiting* during pregnancy. Two cases are mentioned in which *cholera* supervened upon pregnancy ; in one labor was induced, in the other it came on spontaneously ; both women recovered.

There is another series of cases sometimes demanding the operation, namely, where there exists chronic disease, very much agravated by the mechanical distention of the uterus, *as disease of the heart, of the aorta, asthma, etc.*

Again, it is proprosed to bring on labor in cases where the child has been previously found to *die at some regular time*, before the completion of the ninth month. But this ought to be done only when the infant is alive and viable, and even then it should be resorted to with reserve, as there may be hope that the disease which caused the death of the child in a former pregnancy may have now disappeared.   *Part* xix., *p.* 234.

Premature Labor.—The following method, proposed by Kirnsch and Cohen, has been successful in inducing premature labor : Pass the nozzle of a large syringe, containing 11 or 12 oz. of water, at 92° F., half an inch within the cervix, and inject the water with some degree of force for a number of times (*e. g.* eight or ten, up to seventeen times) ; and repeat this process twice a day until labor is induced.   *Part* xxi., *p.* 308.

Premature Labor—Induction of.—Dr. Simpson recommends the dilatation of the os uteri by sponge tents, gradually increasing them in size. The membranes are also separated to a certain extent. This he had never found to fail, although he had employed it in numerous cases. In this manner the first stage of the labor is almost entirely accomplished before labor begins, and consequently, the child is saved from the pressure, etc., incidental to the earlier and protracted part of the first stage.

Part xxiv., *p.* 348.

Premature Labor—Induction of.—The following is the method of Professor Kiwisch : A piece of India-rubber tubing, about eleven feet long and half an inch in diameter, is connected with a straight tube from an injecting apparatus five or six inches in length, the latter forming the extremity of the siphon. A vessel containing about two gallons of water of about 110° Fahr., is placed nine or ten feet from the ground, the patient being placed in an empty hip-bath. The proper end of the tube is to be passed into the vagina, and directed toward the os uteri, where it is to be held steadily. After exhausting the tube, the other end is to be placed in the warm water. The stream flows with considerable force against the os uteri, and continues until the whole contents of the vessel are discharged. Two gallons of cold water are then to be placed in the vessel, and disd irged in the same way. The douche may be repeated if necessary on the next day.

*   *   *   *   *   *

In another case the plan adopted was somewhat different. The common elastic bottle-syringe, manufactured by Roberston, of Dublin, was used. To this was attached a flexible tube, with a bone pipe at the end. This was introduced into the vagina, and directed against the os uteri. Tepid water was then forced, by means of the syringe, along the tube, from some convenient vessel, another smaller one being placed to catch the water as it poured from the vagina. The process had to be continued about five minutes. A second and third application was made on successive days; and on the third, labor came on at half-past three o'clock P. M., and terminated at half-past ten at night.   *Part* xxvii., *p.* 170.

Premature Labor.—There is a great and undoubted sympathy between the breasts and other parts of the sexual apparatus. It was supposed that irritation of the mammary nerves might induce uterine action. This was tried. Sucking pumps, made of caoutchouc, were applied for two hours seven times during three days: after the third application the cervix uteri was shortened, after the sixth severe labor pains came on, and after the seventh the child was born.   *Part* xxviii., *p.* 263.

Premature Labor—Induction of.—To give the child the best chance of surviving, instead of rupturing the membranes, you must separate them from their connection in the vicinity of the os. Various plans have been devised for this purpose; but perhaps Dr. Weir's instrument, which combines the uterine introduction of a female catheter, with the injection of tepid water, is the best. It consists of a large flattened female catheter, to which can be attached a common injecting syringe. In using it, the tube is first cautiously introduced within the os for about three inches, and then by means of the syringe a quart of tepid water is injected so as to act by slowly separating the membranes. A sponge tent should now be introduced within the os, and the injection may be repeated, at inter vals of two or three hours, until successful.   *Part* xxxii., *p.* 229.

Premature Labor—Induction of.—In the early months, while the cervix uteri is as yet undeveloped, and the ovum is contained in the cavity of the fundus uteri, the douche cannot be relied upon, and the better plan will be to introduce the uterine sound and turn it round once or twice; this will never fail to produce expulsion. When th: life of the child is no object, as before the seventh month, the stilette m.r · be used, but before the fifth month this is a dangerous instrument.   *Part* xxxv., *p.* 208

———•◆•———

LACTATION.

Use of the Bofareira, Ricinus Communis, or Palma Christi.—In cases of child-birth where the appearance of milk is delayed, a decoction is made by boiling well a handful of the white Bofareira (Ricinis Communis or botanists) in six or eight pints of spring water. The breasts are bathed with this decoction for fifteen or twenty minutes. Part of the boiled leaves are then spread thinly over the breasts, and allowed to remain until all moisture has been removed from them by evaporation, and probably, in some measure, by absorption. This operation is repeated at short intervals, until the milk flows upon suction by the child, which it usually does in the course of a few hours. If the milk is required to be produced in the breasts of women who have not given birth to or suckled a child for years, the mode of treatment is as follows: A similar decoction is made, and it is poured, while yet boiling, into a large vessel, over which the woman sits so as to receive the vapor over her thighs and generative organs, cloths being carefully tucked around her, so as to prevent the escape of the steam. In this position she remains for ten or twelve minutes, or until the decoction cooling a little, she is enabled to bathe the parts with it, which she does for fifteen or twenty minutes more. The breasts are then similarly bathed and gently rubbed with the hands, and the leaves are afterward applied to them in the manner described. These operations are repeated three times during the first day, on the second the process is repeated as to the breasts three or four times; on the third day the whole process is repeated. A child is now put to the nipple, and, in the majority of instances, it finds an abundant supply of milk. In the event of success not following, the treatment is continued for another day; and if there be still want of success, the case is abandoned.

Part xxii., *p.* 316.

Case of Lactation in a Male.—Dr. Horner gives a case of lactation occurring in an adult male, aged 22 years. The patient's attention was first drawn to his left breast, which appeared to be enlarging, and continued to increase in size for three weeks, when he came to Philadelphia. After being in this city for three weeks, he became quite anxious in regard to his condition; for, although he suffered very little pain, the mamma had become quite as large as that of a female nursing.

He was induced to apply at the Clinic of the Jefferson Medical College to consult the faculty of that Institution. His case came up before Prof. Mütter, who, upon examination, found the mammary gland largely developed, and filled with lacteal secretion, which differed in no wise from that of a mother. He could assign no cause for this freak of nature: his health was very good, and the other breast natural. A soap plaster was prescribed, and compression ordered to be kept up, which he persisted in for full six weeks, when the gland returned to its usual size.

Part xxiii., *p.* 258.

Suckling—Impairment of Vision during.—This affection arises from the drain there is upon the system; therefore, if severe, the child should be immediately weaned; if slight, it should not be put to the breast more than twice in the twenty-four hours. The anæmic condition of the patient naturally indicates the employment of a stimulating plan of treatment. You must give iron in some form, combined with ammonia, which is the most generally useful of all stimulating medicines; quinine also may be necessary. If the patient does not improve, try mercury, but you must give it very cautiously in these cases. Leeches or blisters should never be applied; you must increase the quantity and improve the quality of the blood.

[Whatever reduces the powers of the system, and impairs the quality of the blood, such as diarrhœa, leucorrhœa, or excessive natural secretions, so as to act as a drain on the system, may be followed by impairment or

loss of vision, which, when detected early, is very amenable to treatment, whereas, when neglected, it not unfrequently terminates in total blindness.]
Part xxxii., *p.* 237.

Effects of Belladonna in arresting the Secretion of Milk.—Dr. Burrows of Liverpool cites the following striking case : The child was dead owing to the nature of the labor, and the resuscitative measures adopted did not prove successful. On the fourth day the breasts assumed their maternal functions ; on the seventh day they were full, tense, painful, and knotty, with a slight inflammatory blush, though spirit lotion had been applied.

I directed the areola, and a circle extending half an inch beyond it, of each breast, to be painted thickly over with the extract of belladonna, reduced to the consistence of thick paste by the addition of the acacia mixture. As the late Mr. C. T. Haden recommended the use of colchicum for the purpose of controlling arterial action in inflammation of the breast and nipples, with the same intention I gave the following mixture :

℞ Infusi rosæ comp. ℨvj.; magnesiæ sulphatis ℨj.; vini colchici ℨiij.; aquæ menthæ piperitæ ℨxv. M.   Fiat mistura cujus sumatur ℨj. 4tâ quâque hora. The result was most satisfactory. In thirty-six hours after the application of the extract, the mammæ were cool, pale and flaccid ; and the knots softened and reduced in size. I advised the repainting of the areolæ ; and in two days after—*i. e.* three and a half days from the first application— they were so reduced in size that they were smaller than during the latter period of pregnancy, and the knots could scarcely be felt.
Part xxxv., *p.* 234.

Suppression of Milk.—If from any cause the lacteal secretion should become suppressed, and it is desirable to again renew it, it may be accomplished by the application of electricity.   *Part* xxxvi., *p.* 236.

Abortive Treatment of Milk Abscess.—Dr. Goolden has found this mode of treatment eminently successful.— *Case.*—M. S——, confined of her first child. According to her reckoning and the appearance of the infant at its birth, the labor was premature. On the third day the breasts were swollen, hard, tender, throbbing, and red ; the superficial veins enlarged, with feeling of great distention. The nipples were retracted and cracked, and the child was too feeble to suck, even if the nipples had been more prominent. The milk partially oozed away, and a little was drawn by means of a breast pump, but not enough to produce any sensible diminution of their bulk ; besides which, the abortive efforts were attended with the greatest suffering. There was fever, anxiety of countenance, and depression of mind ; as she had a great dread of a " bad breast." This was evidently one of those cases that must inevitably result in abscess, unless something more than the ordinary remedies were resorted to. I gave directions to paint the areolæ and nipples with extract of belladonna, and to take a saline mixture with half-drachm doses of colchicum every six hours. Upon visiting her on the following day I was as much gratified as surprised at the result of the treatment. The fever had entirely disappeared ; the breasts were quite soft ; the *milk had flowed away in great abundance* into a bread and water poultice ; a cheerful expression of countenance was exchanged for the former one of anxiety and dread ; and all apprehension of evil had disappeared. I ordered the mixture to be omitted, but to continue the local application. The case required no further treatment, and she was " about " in the course of a few days.

In the cases related by Dr. Goolden, the belladonna, with the internal administration of colchicum, appeared to have had the effect of arresting the secretion of the milk. In the case above detailed it is seen that the milk *flowed away abundantly*; and that the mother was enabled to continue lactation shortly after the application.

The long-recognized power which this drug is known to possess of relaxing muscular contraction, at once suggests the *modus operandi* in these cases.

Doubtless, any of the active forms of belladonna would answer the purpose equally well with the extract; such as a solution of its active principle, atropine.

The latter is undoubtedly more elegant, and I dare say would be more speedy in its effect; but the extract, from its being a messy and unsightly application, is much more likely to be carefully washed off, so as not to be injurious to the infant when replaced at the breast. *Part* xxxvi., *p.* 237.

Dispersion of the Milk.—Iodide of potassium given in doses of from six to eight grains per diem, has the effect of suspending, and in less doses, of moderating, the secretion of milk. This property may be made of the greatest use in arresting impending inflammation and abscess; the pain and fever will often disappear next day. After the cure the milk returns again two or three days after the suspension of the iodide.

[Probably this treatment might be advantageously combined with the external application of belladonna, first recommended by Dr. Goolden, and since found so eminently successful by other practitioners.]

Part xxxviii., *p.* 221.

Defective Lactation—Dietetic Treatment.—Experience proves that much may be effected by proper diet; the food should be "analogous." First among the grains are lentil powder, or the so-called revalenta: but pea-soup and bean-soup have also a marked effect in improving the flow and richness of milk. The lentil and bean, however, are preferable to peas, when they are as easily procurable. Shell-fish, as oysters, are peculiar in containing much phosphorus. If, on trial, they do not produce urticaria or roseola in the child, they will on the above account be advantageous, as the phosphates are beneficial to both mother and child. *Part* xl., *p.* 310.

LARYNGEAL AFFECTIONS.

Transverse Divisions of the Larynx and Trachea.—In cases of divisions of the trachea, or larynx, we would strongly recommend surgeons to bear in mind the advice given by Mr. Stanley, viz., not to be satisfied to bring the outward parts together by means of ligatures, etc., trusting afterward to position to complete the cure, but to introduce a ligature or two through the windpipe itself, or through the fibrous tissue connecting the cartilages, so as to prevent the lower portion retracting. In a case of cut throat, however, the surgeon must not apply his sutures immediately, as he might very naturally feel inclined to do, but wait a little to see wha blood has escaped into the windpipe, and allow it to make its escape befor closing up the aperture.

Rust, of Berlin, observes, that "in wounds dividing only partially th trachea or larynx, a suitably inclined position of the head and neck is generally all that is required to effect a speedy union; but where the larynx or trachea is completely cut across, it becomes expedient to have recourse to sutures. The tendency of the lower portion to sink down from the upper is often so great, that we must not limit our sutures to the cellular tissue, but pass them through the substance of the trachea itself, and even through the cartilages of the larynx." He relates a case of cut throat which occurred in Charité Hospital at Berlin, where the thyroid cartilage was divided, and adds, "that in this patient, the tendency of the lower end of the divided larynx to sink down from the upper, was such as to occasion the necessity of a suture through the substance of each portion of the cartilage (thyroid), that sutures passed simply through the soft tex tures repeatedly gave way, and that the healing in this case was perfect.

Mr. Stanley remarks that in such cases when a liquid is swallowed, it often passes down the trachea, and comes out at the wound, giving rise to a suspicion that the œsophagus is also wounded, but this is owing to a loss of irritability of the glottis, which thus allows the liquid to pass.

Part x., *p.* 136.

Coin removed from the Larynx by Inversion of the Body.—Dr. Duncan relates a case of this accident which occurred to a man who was amusing himself with tossing up a shilling, and catching it in his mouth, when it slipped into the larynx. At first, violent coughing with great dyspnœa were produced, but these after some time subsided. From the favorable result of Sir B. Brodie's case, it was determined to try inversion of the body, which plan had also occurred to the patient himself. Instruments were, however, kept ready in case the shilling should change its position so as to produce suffocation. The mode in which the experiment was performed, though rough, was quite effectual.

The man was placed with his shoulders against the raised end of a pretty high sofa, and then being seized by three of the most powerful of those present by the loins and thighs, he was rapidly inverted, so as to bring the head into the dependent position, and, after a shake or two, Dr. Simpson at the same time moving the larynx rapidly from side to side, the shilling passed into the mouth and fell upon the floor. Not the slightest cough or dyspnœa was produced, and the patient immediately started up, delighted with the result. He was now perfectly free from uneasiness, and there was a marked change in the character of the voice. He had not the slightest subsequent bad symptoms. *Part* xi., *p.* 173.

Cynanche Laryngœa.—Dr. Budd believes that this disease is really erysipelas, and that its not being recognized as such, is owing to its so frequently proving fatal, before it has had time to spread. In support of this, he relates in his paper read to the Medico-Chirurgical Society, five cases which have recently occurred in the London hospitals.

These cases, the author observes, were clearly examples of the same disease; but they did not all begin exactly in the same manner. In three, the inflammation commenced in the fauces; in one, it commenced in the parotid gland; and in one, the first appearance of it was an erysipelatous blush at the angle of the lower jaw. In all the cases the inflammation soon spread to the glottis, and produced there the same effects—namely, redness and great thickness of the epiglottis, and of the lips of the glottis, with effusion of sero-purulent fluid in the submucous cellular tissue—to such a degree as, in three of the cases, to produce almost sudden closure of the glottis, and consequent suffocation.

The occasional connection of laryngitis with erysipelas was noticed by Dr. Cheyne in his article on laryngitis in the "Cyclopædia of Practical Medicine:"

The author cites the facts related by Mr. Ryland, and observes that they prove conclusively that inflammation of the larynx, causing great swelling of the lips of the glottis, and infiltration of the fluid in the submucous cellular tissue, and thus leading to speedy suffocation, occasionally results from the poison of erysipelas. He considers the following circumstances favor the opinion he has expressed as to the nature of the disease. That the inflammation spreads in the same mode as in erysipelas of the skin, presenting the deep redness and swelling, and infiltration of a serous or sero-purulent fluid, which occur in that disease; that it is more fatal than ordinary laryngitis; and that it occurs most frequently among the inmates of hospitals in which erysipelas prevails, and among such of them as are peculiarly liable to erysipelas, viz., convalescents from continued fever or eruptive fevers, and those laboring under secondary syphilitic ulcers.

Mr. Arnott, to show the erysipelatous nature of the disease under discussion, related the following cases: A gentleman was seized with a pain in the back of the throat, attended by difficulty of swallowing. Nothing could be seen. Leeches were applied, and blood afterward taken from the arm. The blood was buffed and cupped. He appeared better; but a few hours after was suddenly seized with dyspnœa and died. The only disease found was inflammation of the glottis, one of the margins of which had sloughed. Four days after, his wife, who had attended him, was seized with an affection of the throat; the tonsils were enlarged. Erysipelas of the head and neck shortly afterward developed itself. The daughter, who came from the country to see her mother, suffered from inflammation of the larynx and pharynx, and afterward from erysipelas of the head and face. When there was infiltration of purulent matter, he believed that in these cases the operation was always fatal. He did not know what to do after the operation in these cases. *Part* xv., *p.* 93.

Syphilitic Laryngitis.—Dr. Watts relates the case of a man who, when suffocating with syphilitic inflammation of the larynx, was saved by tracheotomy.

Dr. W. saw him for the first time Sept. 29th, after he had been given up for death by three medical gentlemen; the patient was then so breathless as to be scarce able to make the effort to whisper single words at intervals; his voice was nearly extinct, and the inspirations were accompanied with a loud hissing noise in the larynx. The friends stated he had not slept for twelve days, owing to the intensity of the orthopœna. After a careful examination of the chest and air passages, and having obtained a perfect history of the circumstances, syphilitic laryngitis was diagnosticated; the iodides of mercury and potassium, with other appropriate treatment were prescribed, and the case was viewed as being favorable for the performance of tracheotomy. In consultation with Dr. Dumville, the plan of operation was agreed upon; but it was determined to wait until the last extremity before having recourse to it, and in the meantime the patient was carefully watched. In the evening of Oct. 1st, the powers of life seemed fast failing, and it appearing impossible for him to continue the

-struggle for breath longer with safety, the operation was undertaken at his own instance, and most happily perfor ned by Mr. Dumville. The fit of spasmodic coughing usually attendant on the introduction of the tube having subsided, the man fell into a sound sleep even before the dressings were completed: so signal was the relief from suffering, so completely was he worn out by anxiety and fatigue, and deprivation of rest. The case progressed favorably; the patient continuing to take the medicines, was soon under mercurial influence, and gradually improved in health. On the 30th Oct., precisely thirty days after the operation, the use of the tube was finally dispensed with; the wound closed up within a week, but required other seven days before the skin healed perfectly. The iodide of potassium was administered for a few months longer, to insure the thorough eradication of the lues; but from the period of the removal of the tube he continued steadily improving, until he regained more perfect health than he had enjoyed for many years.

Dr. Watts remarked, that notwithstanding the case had been treated by others as asthma, the circumstance of the syphilitic constitution, the chronic cough without pulmonary disease, the apparent origin of the cough in the larynx, the periodical relapses of the laryngeal affection, and the peculiar aching in the bones, appeared to him as sufficiently indicative of syphilitic laryngitis—an opinion which was further strengthened by the radically curative effect of the remedies employed. As promoting the success of the operation, he dwelt on the importance of the patient's room being made very warm before operating, as also on the propriety of maintaining a high temperature afterward. He had known death follow, as if by shock or spasm, the sudden inhalation of the chilly atmosphere of the operating theatre in winter when this precaution had been neglected.

Part xv., *p.* 201.

Follicular Disease of the Throat and Larynx.—Dr. Green advocates the use of nitrate of silver as a local application in chronic laryngitis, " clergyman's sore throat," and similar affections, some of which not unfrequently simulate, or complicate phthisis. The mucous membrane lining the fauces pharynx, and larynx, is abundantly studded with muciparous follicles. At the back of the tongue they open into the foramen cæcum and the lenticular papillæ; in the uvula and pharynx they are large; and the tonsils seem to be entirely composed of them; in the œsophagus they are like Brunner's glands, and are imbedded in the submucous tissue. In the upper part of the larynx these follicles are numerous, and still more so in the trachea: they secrete a fluid to lubricate the passages, which in the healthy state is bland, transparent, and not abundant in quantity, but is increased and vitiated by disease.

Apply solution of *crystallized* nitrate of silver, of from one to four scruples to the ounce of distilled water. Use a piece of whalebone, ten inches long and curved at the extremity, having a small round piece of fine sponge securely attached to it. The mouth being opened wide and the tongue depressed by a spatula of a peculiar form, carry the sponge, dipped in the solution, over the top of the epiglottis, and while the patient breathes gently out, press it downward and forward through the aperture of the glottis into the laryngeal cavity. Apply this every other day or oftener, for two or three weeks, and then twice a-week till the surface assumes a healthy appearance. If there are extensive ulcera s on the epiglottis, and about the month of the larynx, apply for once or twice a solution of double the strength of that above mentioned For a few days before cauterizing the interior of the larynx, *educate* the arts by applying the solution to the more external parts. Give iodide of potassium internally; or sesqui-oxide of iron; with sedatives, such as belladonna, conium, hyoscyamus, morphia; and expectorants. *Part* xvi., *p.* 119.

Ulceration of the Epiglottis, and Opening of the Larynx.—In a case of ulceration of the epiglottis, and opening of the larynx in a child, consequent upon swallowing sulphuric acid, Dr. Green used the solution ot crystallized nitrate of silver with the greatest success. *Part* xvi., *p.* 126.

Spasm of the Windpipe in Infants.—During the paroxysm dash cold water in the face, and expose it to the fresh air. Lance the gums if there is the least fullness or tenderness; and unload the bowels by a dose of calomel, followed by castor oil, and a warm water injection. Afterward give small doses of calomel or grey powder, and the following mixture; Fetid spirits of ammonia, half a drachm; dilute hydrocyanic acid, five minims; tincture of henbane, seven minims; spirit of aniseed, one drachm; sirup of orange peel, four drachms; water an ounce and a half. A teaspoonful twice or thrice daily. And rub a little liniment upon the chest and spine occasionally; as a drachm of tincture of cantharides, a drachm of laudanum, and an ounce of soap-liniment. Or give assafœtida enemeta. Depletion is rarely required. Take the child into the country, and keep it as quiet as possible. *Part* xvi., *p.* 131.

Laryngismus Stridulus.—*Inhalation of Ether* recommended, by means of a sponge saturated with ether and held to the nose and mouth of the patient upon the first indication of an accession of the spasm.

Part xvi., *p.* 132.

Laryngitis—Acute.—Besides the ordinary treatment by leeches and tartar emetic, if there is œdema of the epiglottis (indicated by there being difficulty in swallowing, and a sensation of a swelling in the throat, without affection of the tonsils) blow powdered alum into the throat, through a quill. *Part* xvii., *p.* 71.

Application of Nitrate of Silver to the Fauces and Larynx.—[A variety of methods have been adopted to apply nitrate of silver, either solid or in solution to the fauces and larynx. We have seen several methods of applying the solution to the larynx; but we would warn the practitioner to be very cautious how he adopts this method, for fear of suffocation. There is no doubt, however, that if nitrate of silver could be safely and easily applied to the laryngeal and bronchial surfaces, it would have a wonderfully beneficial action, as it has upon all mucous surfaces.]

Mr. Coxeter's Laryngeal Shower Syringe, is by far the most convenient form in which a syringe can be used for these applications to the interior of the throat and the posterior nares. It consists of a seamless tube, composed of silver—not unlike that of a medium-sized catheter. It is curved in a form suitable to its intended uses. The distal extremity is somewhat flattened from side to side, and is perforated by fine openings, which admit of the emission of the contained fluid in the form of a delicate shower. The proximal extremity is fitted with an elastic suction-bottle, which, by its own action, charges the instrument with the fluid, which is then emitted by simply compressing the bottle with the thumb. Rings are attached for holding the little instrument, and an ingenióus arrange-ment is made, by which the quantity of fluid ejected can be accurately re-gulated. The inventor says that his shower syringe possesses the advan-tage of applying gently, and without friction, to an irritable surface, the remedial agent intended to be employed. It does this more generally and uniformly than the sponge, and is entirely free from the risk to which the latter, in becoming detached from the whalebone, is liable.

Part xxvii., *p.* 74.

Laryngotomy.—Place the patient on his back, and completely expose the crico-thyroid membrane by dissection before opening the larynx. This is necessary, as an artery (the inferior laryngeal) is often passing this space, and requires a ligature. Then make a vertical incision into the larynx, through the crico-thyroid space, and insert a full sized trachea tube. It is sufficient, in dyspnœa arising from causes in the larynx *of the adult*, to make the opening in the crico-thyroid space, but not so *in the child.* In the adult, any inflammatory effusion, or thickening, arising from acute affections of the larynx, takes place in the submucous tissue, and is more local. In the child, it takes place more on the free surface of the mucous membrane, and spreads downward, thus becoming tracheal as well as laryngeal. Laryngotomy, therefore, is not so applicable to the child as to the adult. *Part* xxx., *p.* 132.

—•◆•—

LARYNX.

Larnyx—Inflammation of.—In the first stage of an inflammatory attack of the larynx or trachea, when the mucous membrane is dry, an emetic will restore the moisture. Cauterization should be used locally at the same time that the emetic treatment is adopted internally. In treating these inflammations by the application of the nitrate of silver, it is important to bear in mind that *the more intense the degree of inflammation of the lining of the larynx is, the weaker ought to be the solution of the nitrate applied to it.* The first effect of the application is to coagulate the albuminous film upon the surface of the membrane which has been stripped of its epithelium, and thus to cover and protect it. As the good effects of the application are worn off in a few hours, the touching of the larynx must be repeated frequently for some days, until all the symptoms of laryngitis have completely disappeared; as in most severe cases, especially in adults, a chronic thickening is liable to be left, it is a good precaution to give a little mercury toward the end of the acute attack. In true exudative croup, where the inflammation is of a much more intense and fibrinous character, and where it is almost of a purely local nature, seizing at once on the larynx or trachea, the treatment by the application of caustic is unsuitable, the symptoms being increased rather than diminished, by its use. *Part* xxvi., *p.* 63.

Topical Medication of the Larynx.—Instead of thrusting a piece of sponge into the larynx, in applying the solution of nitrate of silver, Dr. Cotton, by means of a pair of forceps made by Mr. Coxeter, squeezes the sponge saturated with the solution over the larynx, so that it passes into its interior. This plan is stated to be much less irritating than the one commonly employed. *Part* xxvi., *p.* 70.

LEAD.

Acetate of Lead.—[It is important that the prejudice of the poisonous nature of the acetate of lead should be exploded, and its value as a medicament established.]

Several interesting cases wherein acetate of lead has been administered in large quantities without destroying life, are recorded by Dr. Christison and Professor Taylor.

A woman was admitted into Guy's Hospital in May, 1846, having swallowed *an ounce and a half* of sugar of lead dissolved in water, from which she recovered, and left the hospital in five days.

Mr. Gorringe reported two cases in which two girls swallowed by mistake *one ounce* of the acetate, and another in which a girl swallowed one drachm, and all recovered.

Dr. Hirding gives a case in which a girl swallowed *three drachms ;* she, too, recovered.

Dr. Iliff records *four* cases in which individuals swallowed each *an ounce ;* and Dr. Evans one, in which *three drachms* were swallowed, and all in a very short time recovered. These cases, with the "observations and experiments of Orfila, prove that the belief that sugar of lead is an active poison, is erroneous."

Dr. Sweeting suspects that where acetate of lead, internally administered, has occasioned dangerous symptoms, the preparation has not been free from oxidation—it is the *oxide* which is injurious.

The same obtains in *painter's* colic ; these people mix considerable quantities of litharge and red lead, technically called driers, with their oils, and neglecting careful ablution before taking their meals, imperceptibly swallow a material of a very dangerous character. *Part* xxiv., *p.* 114.

Use of Acetate of Lead.—The only point on which I presume to differ, says Dr. Burridge, from Mr. Sweeting, is this—that of combination. In accordance with the practice of Dr. Christison, and the rule laid down by the late Dr. A. T. Thomson, of University College, I always give acetate of lead in a fluid form ; *never* without acetic acid, and very rarely indeed without Battley's liq. opii sedativ. *Part* xxiv., *p.* 116.

Saturnine Poisoning.—Neither sulphuric acid nor sulphates can serve as antidotes to slow poisoning by the salts or compounds of lead, the sulphate of lead being itself a slow but sure poison, capable of killing vigorous dogs in twenty or thirty days. *Part* xxvii., *p.* 240.

———•♦•———

LEECHES.

How to make Leeches bite.—The leech which it is intended to apply, is thrown into a saucer containing fresh beer, and is to be left there till it begins to be quite lively. When it has moved about in the vessel for a few moments, it is to be quickly taken out and applied. This method will rarely disappoint the expectation, and even dull leeches, and those which have been used not long before, will do their duty. It will be seen with astonishment how quickly they bite. *Part* viii., *p.* 157.

Leeches—Mode of applying.—Place the leeches on the skin and slightl
exhaust the air around them by means of a cupping glass placed ove
them, after the air is rarefied in it in the ordinary manner.

Part xxvi., *p.* 327

Leeches—Revival of.—As soon as the leeches come off, they should
submerged in a mixture consisting of one part of vinegar and eight o
water; they immediately begin to disgorge, and must then be pressed
gently toward the mouth between the thumb and finger. After disgorge
ment the leech must be washed twice in common water, and then placed
in an earthen vessel with plenty of water, and kept at a uniform temperature. The water must be changed every morning, and the dead leeches
cast out. In four or five days the leeches will bite and draw as much as
before.   *Part* xxxiv., *p.* 283

———•◦•———

LEECH BITES.

Hemorrhage from Leech Bites—Modes of Arresting.—Wipe the orific
with a bit of lint or fine linen, and when nearly dry, seize a small portio
of integument around the bite with the thumb and finger, and make mo
derate pressure, until the hemorrhage is completely suppressed, which will
be from five to fifteen minutes.

Or, take a small pinch of down from a beaver hat, and pile it upon the
orifice; then put over the down a piece of thin muslin, and draw it tightly.
If blood oozes through both, dry it, until the hemorrhage ceases, and in
short time the down and muslin will have become matted with coagulum.
All superfluous down may be cut off, and in two days the orifice will have
healed, and the matted matter will fall off.

Or, apply a piece of lint dipped in a strong solution of alum, or apply to
the place, tobacco, such as is used for smoking.   *Part* xiv., *p.* 194.

Leech Bites—Bleeding from.—Roll a very small piece of lint into a hard
knot, smaller than a pea, and wiping the orifice clean, place this little pad
upon it, and draw a long strap of adhesive plaster over it. The elasticity
of the skin, pulling upon the plaster, supplies the requisite pressure.

Part xvii., *p.* 291.

To Arrest the Bleeding from Leech Bites.—Dr. Tucker states that he
has arrested bleeding from leech bites by dipping some of the flocculent
portion of lint in collodion, and pressing it on the orifice; and then applying
collodion freely over the whole surface with a camel-hair pencil Mr. E.
Wilson advises that the compress of lint should be covered by a little disc
of thin paper as soon as applied, so as to prevent it sticking to the finger
or the instrument (a pencil or pencil-case), by which pressure is applied.

Part xix., *p.* 144.

Hemorrhage from Leech Bites.—This may be arrested by the application of caustic. To apply this properly, crush a small piece of lunar caustic
to powder, heat the point of a silver probe in a candle, and dip it into the
powder; it thus becomes crusted over with the nitrate, and forms a fine
button of caustic, which will easily reach the bottom of any such wound.

Part xxii., *p.* 347.

Tincture of Mastic as a Hemostatic.—It is stated in "Schmidt's Jahrbucher," that Dr. Frankl has found the tincture of mastic an excellent hemostatic. He employs it in epistaxis, and in troublesome bleeding from leech bites. It is applied to the points whence the blood issues, by means of a camel's-hair pencil. Terzer, a dentist of Vienna, is also reported to have used it successfully in hemorrhage following the extraction of teeth.

Part xxvii., *p.* 132.

Styptics.—*Vide* "Matico," "Oil of Ergot of Rye," "Creasote," etc.

———•••———

LEUCORRHŒA.

Decoction of Elm Bark.—Four ounces of the fresh bark, bruised, and boiled in four pints of water, form a thick decoction. Dose, four ounces three times a day; may also be used locally as a wash in almost every stage of cutaneous disease, and in that disordered state of the functions of the skin induced by dram-drinking, attended with redness of the skin.

Part i., *p.* 61.

Tincture of Muriate of Iron.—Recommended in leucorrhœa as follows : ℞ Tinct. of muriate of iron, one drachm ; tinct. of opium, half a drachm ; infusion of Iceland moss, infusion of gentian, of each four ounces. M. Dose, an ounce every three or four hours. A wash of sulphate of zinc may be used locally at the same time. *Part* iii., *p.* 30.

Secale Cornutum.—Suggested in cases of leucorrhœa entirely devoid of inflammation. *Part* iv., *p.* 15.

Ioduret of Silver.—Suggested in cases of leucorrhœa of long standing, in doses varying from one-eighth of a grain to one or two grains, in the form of pills, two or three times a day. Alum lotion, locally.

Part vii., *p.* 82.

Creasote in Leucorrhœa.—Dr. Allnatt says : The following is the formula I generally adopt for adults : ,

℞ Creasote, minims xx. ; solution of potash, ℨij. ; white sugar, ℨij.

Rub together in a mortar ; afterward add, by degrees, eight ounces of water. Mix. Make an injection, to be used three times a day.

In obstinate cases of gleet, occurring in flabby leucophlegmatic *males*, I propose this remedy to the notice of the practitioner with great confidence.

Part vii., *p.* 86.

Use of Astringents—Tannin.—Mr. Druit says :

In obstinate leucorrhœa, I have used it as a vaginal suppository, ten grains being made into a mass with tragacanth, and introduced and allowed to dissolve. But in this disorder I believe alum and the other mineral astringents to be of more service ; and that in many cases such treatment as will reduce a swelled and congested uterus is of more consequence than any mere local application. *Part* x., *p.* 139.

Treatment of Leucorrhœa by Iodine.—M. Van Steenkiste has made use of a dilute tincture of iodine with great success in cases of obstinate chronic leucorrhœa.

R Iodine, **gram. iv.**; alcohol, gram. lx.; solve; et aquæ destil., grammes cxxv.; about 30 fluid grammes (or f.℥xv.) are to be thrown into the vagina as an injection, and repeated every day, or every other day, according to the excitement it occasions. *Part* x., *p.* 195.

Leucorrhœa.—There are two species of *uterine* leucorrhœa; in one the disease is in the cervix, and the secretion is alkaline; and in the other, the secretion is acid, and the disease in the fundus. Introduce the speculum and pass a gum tube containing a stilet armed with litmus paper, for about an inch into the cervix: protrude the stilet and let it remain till moistened. Thus we find the nature of the secretion; if it is alkaline, again introduce the tube without the stilet, and inject by means of a gum-elastic bottle, a solution of sulphuric acid, half a drachm of acid to an ounce of water, or of acetate of lead of the same strength. If the lips of the os are abraded, touch with arg. nit. before passing the instrument. If the mucous glands of the cervix are enlarged, pass the tube; and having wiped it clean from mucus, smear the end with ointment of arg. nit., gr. x.; to ung. cetac., ℥j., and again pass it. (Dr. Mitchell.) *Pt.* xv., *p.* 320.

New Remedy for Leucorrhœa.—Dr. Braman states that for nine years he has been in the habit of using preparations of helonias diœca (unicorn plant) as a remedial agent. "In leucorrhœa," he says, "I consider it invaluable. I use it with a confidence I *attach to no other medicine.* Under its influence the patient, whose life has been almost a burden, soon revives. Her uncomfortable sensations vanish, and ultimately, an entire recovery of health and strength is established." It may be given in the form of powder, tincture, or sirup; but the latter is the most eligible. The doses which Dr. Braman recommends are of the powder, one drachm and a half; of the tincture, one fluid drachm; of the sirup, three fluid drachms. These doses are to be taken thrice a day, half an hour before the ordinary meals; and according to the urgency of the case, the quantity administered may be increased, if the patient bears it well. In irritable stomachs, nausea is sometimes produced; and when this occurs, the dose must be diminished. *Part* xx., *p.* 229.

Vide Selections from Favorite Prescriptions, Art. "Medicines."

Iodide of Potassium in Leucorrhœa.—Dr. Payne recommends the iodide of potassium as an injection in leucorrhœa. It is to be used (℥iss. to a pint of water) three or four times daily. *Part* xxxvii., *p.* 211.

Bichromate of Potash as an Astringent.—To remove the fetor from sloughing wounds, syphilitic sores, ulcers, etc., and where an astringent is useful, a lotion of bichromate of potash, five grains to the ounce, and increased, is very serviceable. In a case of chronic leucorrhœa, where the lips of the os uteri were swollen and spongy, it effected a complete cure after many other remedies had wholly failed. *Part* xxxvii., *p.* 268.

———•◆•———

LIGATURES.

Use of Ligatures formed of Animal Substances.—The substance which Mr. Wragg prefers is the fibrous tissue of the deer, dried, then twisted so as to form a small round thread, smooth and regular on the surface, non-elastic, sufficiently strong to resist the traction made on it by the surgeon in tying the knot. The mode of preparing these ligatures appears to the author to be a matter of great importance, and one capable of insuring or compromising the success of the operation: These tendinous slips ought to be dried slowly, and not used until all the moisture has disappeared; the author prefers those which have been dried for some years. During the ten years he has employed these ligatures, he has never used any others; and during this period he has tied arteries in fingers, hand, forearm, arm, leg, and thigh, and has never seen any symptoms to show that the absorption of the knot had not taken place. Some cases, chosen from a large number, will confirm the truth of these.propositions: In 1836, Mr. Wragg amputated the leg of a woman above sixty years of age for a malignant ulcer; the ligatures made of the fibrous tissue of the deer were cut close to the knot, and the wound brought together; the stump was healed at the end of three weeks. No part of the ligature could be seen; no abscess, no ulceration, indicative of the threads having been on the tissues as foreign bodies.

In the case of a young man, one of the cutaneous branches of the posterior tibial artery was cut by a blow from a hatchet. Mr. Wragg tied it with one of these ligatures, which he cut close to the knot; he then brought the wound together by four points of the interrupted suture made of a thread of the same substance. Nothing further was seen of the knot of the ligature; as to the threads used for the suture, they became softened, and, from the time suppuration commenced, had a macerated appearance, their volume diminished by degrees, so that at the end of a certain time he saw, by the effect of a gradual eating away, a segment of the circumference of the thread disappear, and at last the knot gave way just as if it had been divided by scissors. *Part* xix., *p.* 141.

LIGAMENTS.

Diagnosis of Inflamed Ligaments.—According to Prof. Cooper, if inflammation of ligament be primary, it may generally be diagnosed by the slight degree of swelling which occurs at the joint, and by the absence of acute pain while the patient is standing on the diseased limb in the erect posture. The least attempt at motion is, however, productive of severe suffering, and this constitutes an important distinction between disease of ligament and that of synovial membrane or cartilage; as in the latter case, the most painful position is when standing upright, with the weight of the body pressing on the affected articulation.

Part xvii., *p.* 130.

LINIMENT.

Exanthemic Liniment.—The following liniment is particularly recommended by Dr. Morris, when desirous of keeping up a mild rash upon the skin: R Ol. crot., mxx.; antim. tart., Ðj.; liq. potassæ, ℥j.; aq. puræ, ℥vij. M., while Dr. Hannay, of Glasgow, considers ipecacuanha one of the most manageable and efficient applications. His formula is pulv.

ipecac. ol. olivæ, aa. 3ij.; adipis suill 3ss. M.   It requires to be rubbed in for fifteen to .twenty minutes, and is, he thinks, peculiarly adapted to cases of cerebral irritation in children, dependent on receded eruption.

Part xii., *p.* 254.

———•♦•———

LINT.

Preparation of— With Nitric Acid.—Dr. Rivallie lately communicated to " L'Union Médicale," his mode of cauterizing cancerous tumors with *solidified* nitric acid.   He proceeds as follows: Some lint is placed in an earthen vessel, and a certain quantity of nitric acid, in its highest degree of concentration, is gradually dropped upon it.   A gelatinous paste is the result, and to this, a shape in keeping with the tissues to be cauterized, is to be given.   The caustic mass is then seized with long forceps, and placed upon the part.   After a quarter of an hour, or twenty minutes, it is carefully to be taken off, and an eschar, four or five lines in thickness, is thus obtained.   There are cases, however, where the caustic may be left for twenty-four hours, when the surgeon wishes to destroy a large encephaloid cancer.   The pain is trifling except the skin intervene; and when the caustic is left a long time, there is no pain after the first three or four hours.   With large diseased masses the cauterization should be repeated every day after the eschar has been carefully removed.   When the caustic is applied for a few minutes only, the part should, on its removal, be dressed with lint dipped in a solution of alum.   *Part* xxi., *p.* 24.

———•♦•———

LIP.

Case of Enlargement of the Labial Glands.—[This was a curious case of enlargement of the upper lip.   The lip had been increasing in size for two years; its progress had been unattended with pain, but he had had some irritation from exposure of the mucous membrane to the air.   He had no scrofulous or venereal taint.   Mr. Wilde says :]

Upon examination, I found the lower lip totally unaffected, as well as the extreme angles of the upper ; but all the rest of the red border of this lip was immensely thickened, and so much enlarged that, when the mouth was closed, it formed a large, projecting, red mass, not unlike a pair of ripe strawberries, the division between them being caused by the natural central sulcus of the lip.   If these projections were allowed to remain unwiped for some time, a number of globules of a clear fluid formed upon the surface of the mucous membrane.   The membrane itself was rather more vascular than usual; where the drops exuded, it was particularly smooth and polished, but toward the edge of the lip it had become thickened, covered over with adhesive crusts, and cracked in several places.   The external surface of the lip was natural.

As the young man was very anxious to be relieved of this deformity, I removed it in the following manner.   Assistants having commanded the coronary circulation, by holding the angles of the lip, as in the operation for the removal of cancer of this part, I made an incision, with a small, sharp scalpel, through the mucous membrane, parallel with and about three-eighths of an inch from the edge of the lip, and about two inches and a half in length. By another incision, through the membrane, upon the dental surface of the lip, which was everted for the purpose, I completely included and dissected out the diseased mass, which, during the progress of the operation, I found to consist of a congeries of small globular bodies, nearly transparent, and about the size of advanced trout-spawn. There was scarcely any hemorrhage during the operation, and any granules of the disease which were cut across, or adhered to the surface of the wound, having been completely removed, the edges of the incision were accurately adjusted, and sewed together by a fine silk ligature, after the manner of the continued suture. Upon shutting the mouth, the deformity was found to have been completely removed, and the edges of the lips met as before the supervention of the disease. A few hours after, a smart hemorrhage occurred from the surface of the wound, but it was checked by the use of tincture of matico, and occasional pressure, which the patient was able to effect for himself. *Part* xvi., *p.* 184.

Hydatids of the Lower Lip.—Dr. Heller, of Stuttgard, has seen five cases in which acephalocysts were developed in the lower lip, and always on its inside. This affection appears first as a small and hard lump, which rapidly increases, so that in one month it may attain the size of a cherry; it gives rise to pain, deformity, and difficulty in moving the lip. The hydatids are seated immediately beneath the mucous membrane, and are transparent. If they can be removed without opening their cavity, they are found to be made up of a rounded vesicle, full of fluid, transparent as water, and with a diaphanous and tender wall. The only cure consists in extirpating the cyst, which must be total, or it will reappear; hence nitrate of silver may be applied after the operation.

In a case which came under our own notice about six months ago, in a young, delicate lady, seventeen years of age, the hydatid, situated on the internal part of the lower lip, had, in the space of three months, acquired the size of a small hazel-nut. We touched it with tincture of iodine once, twice, or thrice a-day, as the patient could bear it, and in three weeks the transparent sac entirely disappeared, leaving a small ulcer with a hardened base; to this we applied occasionally nitrate of silver, which healed the wound. Gentle external friction twice a-day, with a little iodine ointment, eventually removed every vestige of hardness. *Part* xvi., *p.* 229.

Malignant Tumefaction of the Under Lip, rapidly following the Appearance on its Surface of a Papula near the angle of the Mouth.— (The following was communicated by Dr. Samuel B. Wells, of Middleburgh, N. Y.)

As some benefit might accrue from the communication of a few cases of an anomalous character, which have occurred during a somewhat extensive practice in the Valley of the Schoharie, I herewith transmit a short account of them which you are at liberty to make public for the use of the profession.

In the summer of 1842 I was called to see a case of disease of the under lip, then in charge of Dr. P. S. Swart, in the village of Schoharie. The patient was a man about 25 years of age, and had enjoyed good health up to the time of the attack, although his habits had been somewhat intemperate. Three days before I saw him, a small pimple appeared on the surface of the under lip, toward the left angle of the mouth. It com-

menced with swelling and redness, which soon assumed a purple hue, and
increased rapidly. At first there was not much constitutional disturbance,
very little pain, fever, or acceleration of the pulse. In less than thirty-six
hours the lip had attained four times its normal size, and had assumed a
gangrenous aspect, the swelling extending downward as far as the clavicle, involving the areolar tissue, together with the integuments of the parts
concerned, occasioning great difficulty of respiration, from pressure of
the larynx. During the incipient stage of the disease, the patient had
been freely evacuated, and an antiphlogistic regimen adopted. Externally,
discutients, such as solution of muriate of ammonia and acet. plumb., had
been applied. But as soon as the septic tendency of the disease became
manifest, cataplasms of yeast and Peruvian bark were substituted, and a
corresponding change was also made in the use of internal remedies—the
infusion of serpentaria, quinine, wine and ammonia being substituted.
Notwithstanding, the patient grew worse every moment—the engorgement of the lip and the adjacent parts continued to increase until mortification ensued, when, on the following day, he died.

An interval of ten years elapsed, when I was called to see a second case
of the kind: Mrs. B——, a lady of robust constitution, and who, up to
this time, had enjoyed excellent health. She had been taken ill the preceding day. A small pimple occupied the surface of the lower lip, as in the
foregoing case. This was accompanied with pain, redness and swelling.
There was also considerable increased excitement of the system, together
with much cerebral disturbance. This patient was bled freely, and general antiphlogistic measures speedily adopted. Notwithstanding, the
violence of the symptoms continued unabated. During the night, the lip
became greatly enlarged, and on the following day, gangrene and mortification ensued, terminating fatally.

The next case, I witnessed in 1855. This occurred in a middle-aged
lady, of good constitution and plethoric habit. Five days before I was
called, a small pimple made its appearance on the under lip, to which she
called the attention of her physician, who was then treating a case of fever in the family. The nature of the disease was fully explained to her by
the doctor, who advised that immediate measures be taken to arrest it in
its present stage.

Feeling but little inconvenience from its presence, nothing was done until
the following day, by which time the swelling had greatly increased, and
the lip had assumed a purple aspect. The parts having put on a low grade
of inflammatory action, the patient was treated with active catharsis, and an
antiseptic cataplasm was applied to the lip. These, together with such remedies as appeared adapted to the most prominent symptoms, were used.
Still, the disease continued to advance, as in the foregoing cases. The lip
having assumed a gangrenous appearance, its fatal tendency too soon became alarmingly evident. Mortification ensuing, the patient died three
days afterward.

In the summer of 1856, a Miss G. consulted me in relation to a small
pimple which appeared the preceding day on the surface of the under lip,
attended with redness and swelling, but unaccompanied with any other
disturbance of the system whatever. With a view of discussing it thus
early, I gave her an antimonial emetic, and in due time followed with
twelve grains of submur. hyd., and in six hours thereafter with the black
dose. These evacuated the system freely. I applied, locally, a solution

of acet. plumbi. The following day there was no amendment, but, on the contrary, an increased tumefaction of the lip, with a deep purple appearance.

Having failed in arresting any one of these several cases with the ordinary remedies adapted to analogous diseases, it occurred to me that if suppuration could be established before the vital forces of the parts became exhausted, a more favorable result might be reasonably expected. With this in view, I passed an ordinary sized lancet from near the angle of the mouth, through the substance of the lip, transversely to a corresponding point on the opposite side. I then introduced a small strip of muslin, about three lines in width, to the extreme end of the puncture, and covered the parts with a cataplasm of yeast and Peruvian bark. A slight suppuration followed in thirty-six hours, and a speedy recovery took place in a few days.

It would be superfluous to give the details of five other similar cases which have occurred in my practice since the above mentioned. ·Suffice it to say that the latter is an index of each one. They severally exhibited the usual characteristics of the foregoing cases in their incipient stage, and were readily controlled and brought to a favorable termination by adopting this plan of treatment—free incision of the affected lip, introduction of a tent, and the local application of a cataplasm of yeast and Peruvian bark to the wound, with a view to the establishing of suppuration—so successfully pursued in the case of Miss G.

I practised here twenty years before I saw a case of this kind, and presume there are many physicians with an extensive business who have never met with one.

———•••———

LITHECTASY.

Lithectasy.—The removal of stone from the bladder, by the operation of lithectasy, as described by Dr. Willis, has hitherto attracted too little notice. The opinion seems to be gaining ground among our best surgeons, that the dangers of lithotomy consist in the too free use of the knife in the deep incisions, and that the most successful operators have been those who have made free external, and very small internal incisions, trusting more to a certain degree of stretching, or dilatation, in order to enter the bladder, and thus preserve that organ as free from injury as possible. It is probably for the same reason that lithectasy may some day prove a more useful improvement than is now generally acknowledged. It is well known that Sir Astley Cooper, in the year 1819, performed this operation, at the suggestion of Drs. Neil and James Arnott. It consists simply in opening the urethra upon a grooved staff, in the mesial line, behind the bulb, to the extent of a few lines, and then making gradual dilatation by means of the fluid pressure dilator of Dr. Arnott, " consisting of a cylindrical tube of silk, lined with the thin gut of a small animal to make it water-tight, and fixed upon a canula which traverses its axis, and having attached to its outer end a syringe guarded with a stop-cock, by which it may be forcibly distended with water or mucilage." This instrument, when empty, exceeds but little in size the bulk of the canula or catheter with which it is connected, and is therefore easily introduced along the groove of the staff into the bladder, and when there it can be gradually distended to its utmost limits. Mr. Elliot thinks it well, previously, to accustom the urethra to the presence of a foreign body, by the use of bougies, gradually increased in size, so as at the same time to produce a certain degree of preparatory dilatation. He also recommends that the external incision should be free, "since if the prostate were unfit to undergo the process of dilatation, either from great rigidity, as is frequently found in old subjects, or from morbid irritability, the operation could be at once completed by lithotomy." Mr. Elliot also suggests various improvements in the dilator, as, that it should be cylindrical and not tapering toward each end, as it will then preserve its situation more easily when introduced," etc.

He suggests that the dilatation should be not only gradual, but at intervals of a quarter of an hour at a time, instead of being continued for thirty or forty hours. It seems surprising that these parts can be dilated so completely, so easily, and so safely, and yet that surgeons have not tried the practice more generally. Mr. Elliot states, that although he continned the dilatation for twenty-five hours, he has no doubt that a sufficient degree of dilatation was accomplished in three hours, since no additional fluid was injected after that period, and he could easily introduce two fingers along with the scoop into the bladder, and if necessary could have extracted a stone as large as a hen's egg, or four and a half inches in circumference, the size of the instrument. Mr. Elliot remarks, that his patient, from beginning to end, was never in danger, that "the presence of the dilator effectually prevents any oozing, as well as the injurious contact of the urine with the raw wound. There was no chance of shock, no risk of peritonitis, infiltration of urine, inflammation of the veins of the neck of the bladder, or any of the grave sequelæ that too often supervene on the operation of lithotomy." *Part* vii. *p.* 102.

Calculi in the Female Bladder.—Experience appears to show, that the removal of a calculus from the female bladder, after the neck of the latter and the canal of the urethra have been gradually dilated by forceps constructed for the purpose, sponge tents or otherwise, is a preferable proceeding to its removal after the urethra has been incised. It also demonstrates, that dilatation can be carried on to an extent which, in the absence of well-authenticated facts, would appear almost incredible.

One of the most remarkable cases on record occurred in the practice of Mr. Okes, of Cambridge. The patient was eleven years old. Sponge tents, gradually increased in size, with string attached, were introduced into the urethra, opium, preceded by purging, being administered. The sponge was used morning and evening, for three successive days. The urethra was sufficiently dilated on the third day to allow of the calculus being withdrawn. It is stated, that the stone measured in circumference, at its major axis, $3\frac{3}{8}$ inches; in its minor, $3\frac{1}{4}$ inches. The calculus was seized in its long axis, and therefore the urethra must have been distended by the calculus and the thickness of the forceps to a circle of at least $3\frac{3}{4}$. Incontinence of urine lasted only three days.

This plan of treatment by dilatation is in imitation of that made use of in the natural efforts to get rid of a calculus from the female bladder, the stone itself acting as the dilating power; and numerous remarkable instances are on record of calculi thus voided, without any subsequent incontinence of urine. In far the greater number of cases, however, in which the calculi have been large, incontinence of urine, which was a marked antecedent symptom, has persisted; this, probably, arising from ulceration at the neck of the bladder, in consequence of the pressure of the foreign body. Thus, there is in the London Hospital Museum a calculus which was removed from a woman by the late Mr. Headington. Its anterior extremity was found sticking in the urethra, and the entire stone was removed easily by traction of the two index fingers. It measured $3\frac{1}{8}$ inches long, 2 inches broad, $1\frac{1}{8}$ inch thick, $7\frac{3}{4}$ inches round its larger, and $5\frac{1}{2}$ inches in its smaller circumference. Incontinence of urine lasted till death. The fact of incapability of retaining the urine usually following the natural method of expulsion, when the calculus has been large, suggests the propriety of operating without any unnecessary delay, in order to avoid this inconvenient and distressing sequence. *Part* xxvi., *p.* 249.

LITHOLIBY.

Litholiby.—Dr. Denamiel designates by this term an operation consisting in the crushing of the stone, as it lies in the trigon vesicæ, behind the prostate, between an instrument introduced by the urethra into the bladder, and the fore and middle finger of the left hand, introduced per anum. He affirms that some calculi are so friable as to break under the least pressure; that the trigon vesicæ, where free calculi generally lie, is accessible to the finger introduced into the rectum; and that a sound passed into the bladder may serve as the *point d'appui.* He also states that the action of alkaline fluids upon the mucus, which forms the common cement of the elements of calculi, leads to the disintegration of the mass, whatever may be the chemical composition of the layers which compose it.

The distance from the integument to the neck of the bladder is commonly $2\frac{1}{4}$ inches; it varies between 1 inch and 4 inches. The prostate gland and the trigon vesicæ are separated from the rectum by only a very thin layer of areolar tissue, in which fat is never deposited; consequently, any hard body may be easily felt and compressed.

The patient, having the bladder moderately distended, is put into the horizontal position, upon a properly constructed bed; the thighs separated and raised; and feet resting upon chairs. The left fore and middle fingers of the operator are then introduced into the rectum, and the stone is felt. A curved sound, grooved upon its convexity, as far as its vesical extremity, that it may the more readily hold the stone, is next passed into the bladder. Then pressure is made, until the calculus gives way. In many cases, a very slight amount will suffice. Should any difficulty arise, the pressure may be directed alternately toward the right or the left, that every part of the surface of the stone may be acted upon. In cases where the calculi are hard, several sittings are required, and the use of alkaline fluids becomes needed, to favor their disintegration. A quantity of warm water should be injected into the bladder after each operation, that the smaller fragments may be immediately washed away.

Part xxviii., *p.* 208.

LITHOTOMY

Treatment after Lithotomy.—These remarks were called forth by a case on which Mr. Sherwin operated, a child of nine years, the day following a journey of seventy miles; and although the operation was satisfactorily performed, the case soon assumed a dangerous aspect. On the second day, Mr. Sherwin says:

I now felt convinced that I should lose him; as, from the very onset of the attack the vital powers seemed unable to sustain any depleting measures, and though having most of the characteristics of peritonitis, the symptoms precluded the antiphlogistic treatment. On referring the same evening to Sir B. Brodie's published "Lectures," I felt impressed with the fidelity of his description of the untoward symptoms following lithotomy. I caught at a suggestion he offers in a similar case, which he rescued by laying open the rectum with the wound, so as to give exit to a quantity of sanies:

11th, 7 A M.—Found matters looking still worse; the boy had passed a wretched night, rolling from side to side in great pain; the belly hard and tympanitic; pulse feeble and fluttering, and hardly to be felt or counted, with more frequent intermissions; countenance of dusky leaden hue; occasional sighs and hiccoughs; tongue quite brown and dry. I now determined to open the wound, which was externally united: this was done with the handle of a scalpel, and having pushed up my finger to explore the parts, I gave exit to about two or three ounces of a pink colored sanies, having a fetid and ammoniacal odor.

I broke up the entire wound in the peritoneum, and had the patient raised out of the hollow of his bed into a more depending position; gave a little brandy and water with a teaspoonful of castor oil. 11 A.M.—Much improved in every respect; countenance calm; had slept a little, and parted with a good deal of flatus; the pulse settled to 100. 9 P.M.—Has slept well; looks happy; pulse slower; tongue moist; has asked for tea, and bread and butter. From this time the boy did well; and he returned to his home quite free from ailment in about three weeks after.

Remarks.—The urine was alkaline, with considerable deposit of lime and mucus; this (which ought to have been done before) was afterward corrected by mineral acids, with decoct. pareiræ bravæ, and quinine. If instead of giving a free vent to the sanies, I had treated the case as one of pure peritonitis, there can be no doubt but that he would have sunk in a few hours. Yet I committed an error in the first instance by operating so soon after a long journey. I relied too confidently on the youthfulness of the patient; time ought to have been allowed for the bladder and constitution to become tranquil before he incurred the additional risk of a formidable operation. Again, his bed was an inconvenient one; it allowed his pelvis to sink into a hollow, which, with my neglecting to leave a canula in the wound, allowed some of the urine to lodge between the rectum and bladder; a circumstance that has proved, probably, a more frequent source of mischief after lithotomy than is generally suspected.

Part viii., *p.* 94.

Lateral Operation of Lithotomy.—Dr. Keith thinks that in the first incision, many good operators commit an error in going too near the symphysis pubis, the consequence of which may be, that when the stone is grasped in the forceps, it is driven out of the hold of the operator by coming against the arch of the pubes, and he cannot, as he ought, draw downward, because the incision is not low enough. With this difficulty in view, most surgeons now make the first incision as far as is safe from the symphysis pubis ; and Dr. Keith seems to extend this incision quite as far as he is warranted past the side of the rectum.

But the most important incision is the deep one ; and in using his peculiar instrument, Dr. Keith was influenced by the fact, that the success of all the most fortunate lithotomists has depended upon the narrow limit to which they restricted themselves, in dividing the neck of the bladder. His instrument is " a gorget neither blunt nor sharp—an edge on it that behoved to cut through a substance so solid as a prostate gland, yet so blunt that such a tough elastic membrane as the bladder would stretch upon its edge." When the perineum is very shallow, this gorget will not be required, the bladder may be entered and the prostate notched by a knife, long in the handle and short in the blade, with its cutting edge limited to an inch and a quarter from the point; but in most cases it will be necessary to slit the neck of the bladder and prostatic urethra obliquely downward and outward to about half an inch, and then Dr. Keith brings his gorget into use to finish the operation. This instrument has its left edge quite rounded, the other ground to an edge, and then blunted with a file ; the point well rounded into a blunt bottom—a copy, in fact, of " Cheselden's Conductor." Dr. Keith says that by these means he insures a positive entrance into the bladder, " obviating the chance of merely dilating the *sphincter vesicæ*, as Cheselden and Martineau are alleged to have often only done ; and avoiding the cutting of parts that never should be cut." *Part* ix., *p.* 134.

Lithotomy.—Dr. Warren, of Boston, has practised the bilateral operation of lithotomy, and strongly recommends it, saying that he would feel disposed to employ it in most cases where lithotomy is required, in preference to the lateral operation. In his opinion, its simplicity, the comparatively small pain from the incision, the facility of seizing and removing the stone, the very slight loss of blood, and the absence of any severe consecutive symptoms, all concur in producing a favorable impression with regard to this mode of operating. The chief objection to this mode, arising from the great danger of wounding the rectum, he fully acknowledges, but thinks it will be found even less than in the lateral operation, if the staff, with the urethra and prostate gland be drawn toward the symphysis pubis, at the same time drawing out the rectum in the direction of the sacrum, with the left hand. *Part* xi., *p.* 138.

Remarks on Lithotomy.—[Much difficulty is sometimes experienced by the surgeon in seizing a calculus with the forceps, after the bladder has been opened. In two cases where this occurred at Guy's Hospital, under Mr. Key from the stone slipping up further into the fundus on every attempt to seize it, it was remedied by making considerable pressure externally on the fundus of the bladder ; when in each case it immediately slipped between the blades of the forceps, and was extracted.]

The two cases alluded to presented difficulties of a similar kind, the stone in each being lodged high up in the fundus of the bladder, so as to elude the grasp of the forceps, until it was dislodged by pressure made on the lower part of the abdomen. The cases elicited from Mr. Key, the following clinical remarks on the principle of obviating this not unfrequent occurrence in the operation of lithotomy. A calculus usually lies free in the bladder as long as the mucous coat of the organ preserves its healthy condition. The oxalate, urate, and even the phosphatic stones, are found in the base of the bladder, until the surface of the membrane becomes villous from inflammation, and its secretion becomes alkaline and viscous. The bladder, inflamed and irritated by the stone, contracts upon it with more force, and secretes an abundance of alkaline mucus, the phosphatic salts of which crystallize on the surface of the stone, and make it adhere often with considerable tenacity to the surface of the organ.

The part of the bladder usually occupied by a calculus under these circumstances is the fundus, which retains the stone with tenacity, while the lower part of the organ receives the urine as it passes from the ureters; and in sounding such a bladder, the calculus is felt either on the concave surface of the instrument, or by withdrawing it toward the pubes—a circumstance that always portends some difficulty in seizing it after the bladder is opened.

It has happened more than once that a patient has been removed from the operating table with the stone remaining in the bladder, after long and continued efforts made in vain to seize it; and the failure has arisen, not from the extraordinary size of the calculus, but from its peculiar position. The forceps, at first, though opened to their full extent, obtain but a slight hold of the stone, the extremity of it only is seized, and it soon escapes from the grasp of the operator. Repeated attempts are made to gain a firmer hold of it, and at each attempt the stone is pushed further from the opening, until the forceps are obliged to be buried nearly to the handles before the stone can be felt. It is in the retreat of the stone before the forceps that the difficulty of seizing it lies. The stone, instead of retreating in a direct line from the opening into the bladder, ascends behind the pubes, where the forceps cannot, without assistance, reach it, much less grasp it.

It is more than probable that in many of the cases recorded of insuperable difficulty in extracting calculi of ordinary size by lithotomy, the operator has not sufficiently borne in mind the impossibility of directing the blades of the forceps to the altered position of the stone, which, from the pressure of the forceps in the unsuccessful attempts to seize it, retires, not backward, but upward, so that it becomes placed in a line little less than perpendicular in relation to the external incision. In such a situation, even in very young children, it becomes difficult to seize it; and in the adult, especially when the prostate gland is enlarged, impossible to reach it. The advantage of pressure made above the pubes was forcibly shown in these cases.   *Part* xii., *p.* 208.

Lithotomy.—There are four steps (says B. B. Cooper) in the operation, as I perform it, viz.: open the perineum, open the pelvis, open the bladder, and take out the stone. Well, the first thing you do when the patient is laid on the table, is to sound him, and be sure that you feel the stone before you operate. Having ascertained the position of the stone, he is then to be tied up in the usual manner; and it is as well to tell the patient to practise the position, in order that he may become somewhat accustomed to one so unnatural; then pass the straight staff, and give it to an assistant to hold. Then, having examined the perineum, and ascertained the point of junction of the raphe of the perineum with that of the scrotum, place the tip of the fore-finger of your left hand upon it, and commence your incision about one finger's-breadth to the left of it, carrying your knife downward and outward to a point midway between the margin of the anus and left tuberosity of the ischium. By this incision you lay open the perineum; next pass your finger into the wound, and feel for the staff in the membranous portion of the urethra, and keeping the bulb out of the way, place the point of the knife in the groove of the staff, and make your second incision through the deep perineal fascia, in the same direction, and to the same extent, as the first. You have now completed the second step, and opened the pelvis: I know my anatomical friends will cavil at this, and say that I have not opened the pelvis; but there is only a slight fascia intervening.

Next commence your third step in the same place in which you did the second, by again placing the point of the knife in the groove of the staff; and, taking the handle of the latter in your left hand, from the assistant who has been holding it, depress it, till it is nearly parallel with the handle of the knife. Then push the knife along the groove in the staff, through the prostate, into the bladder, which you will know to have entered, by the resistance offered to its passage ceasing. This is a difficult part of the operation; for if you let the knife slip out of the groove, between the bladder and rectum, much mischief must accrue. You should have the groove of the staff turned a little to the left, in order that your incision through the prostate may correspond with the other incision. Next pass your left fore-finger into the bladder, and the staff being withdrawn, feel for the stone. In order that you may not make a larger incision through the prostate gland than is necessary, your lithotomy knife should be of the same breadth as your fore-finger, so that it may make an opening just big enough to admit it; and trust to enlarging the opening of the prostate by lacerating it with your finger: lacerating is an ugly word, gentlemen, but it is a safe one. You have now finished the third step, viz.: opened the bladder. All that you have hitherto done is what every good surgeon ought to do without difficulty; but the rest is beyond his control. I mean the fourth step—removing the stone. I have seen the very best lithotomists fail in seizing it, and the patient has been removed to bed with the stone still in his bladder. When you have your finger on the stone, and you introduce the lithotomy forceps along it into the bladder, with the blades of course shut, keep them so, until you have felt the stone with them. Then open them, and, seizing the stone, gently and gradually withdraw it. You should hold the forceps with their flat surfaces looking upward and downward, in order that you may be able to open them sufficiently, and also to protect the soft parts from injury in the abstracting of the stone.

They should also be of good length, so that the hinge may be in the perineum; then you will be able to open the handles. *Part* xii., *p.* 209.

Use of the Canula after Lithotomy.—The use of the canula after the operation of lithotomy, though practised by some, is by too many surgeons altogether neglected and despised. We say too many, because we believe that a neglect of this simple precaution is, from infiltration of urine, not unfrequently the cause of death.

The principal objection to the use of the canula is the fear of its causing inflammation of the lining membrane of the bladder, but this has been found by experience to be futile. And surely, if authority or precedent have any weight, its use by Dionis, Le Dran, Ambrose Paré, and in our own times by Sir B. Brodie and Mr. Liston, are enough to sanction its employment.

According to Dr. O'Ferrall, there is neither pain nor irritation, nor constitutional disturbance occasioned by the insertion of a properly made tube after the operation of lithotomy; and many sources of pain and danger are avoided by its use. 1st. The scalding pain, inseparable from the passage of urine through a fresh wound, is prevented. 2d. That insidious, but too surely destructive accident, infiltration of urine into the cellular tissue is rendered nearly impossible. 3d. If hemorrhage should occur, it may be, as is well known, generally arrested by its aid. 4th. The peritonitis and the diffuse inflammation, phlebitic or cellular, which might be supposed to spring from the alternate expansion and contraction of parts, newly subjected to operation, is, as far as the repose of the pelvic viscera is capable of effecting that desirable object, averted. *Part* xii., *p.* 210.

Lithotomy in the Female.—Mrs. ——, aged forty-five, was admitted upon the 10th of June, on account of stone in the bladder, from which she had suffered the usual symptoms for ten months. On the 12th, after dilating the urethra by the successive introduction of bougies, gradually increased in size, I passed my finger into the bladder, and divided the ring at its orifice outward and downward, by means of a straight bistoury. This incision was of very small extent, hardly exceeding the breadth of the blade, which was rather narrow. The textures then readily yielded, so as to allow me, without the use of violence, to introduce the forceps, and extract a stone about the size of a chestnut. Not the slightest inconvenience followed the operation. The patient regained the power of retaining urine in the course of eight days, and returned home quite well on the 23d.

Lithotomy in the female, continues Professor Syme, affords an instructive illustration of the principle on which this operation may be performed with safety on the male. However much the facility and rapidity of the operation may be promoted by cutting instead of tearing the textures thus far, it does not appear that the choice of these means materially affects the patient's chance of recovery, provided the opening from the skin to the prostate be made sufficiently free. But in both sexes there is still an obstacle remaining which admits of ready removal by incision, and cannot be overcome by tearing without almost certain death. This is the sensitive ring which surrounds the neck of the bladder, at the base of the prostate in the male, and at the corresponding part in the female.

In dilating the urethra, to accomplish any of the purposes which require its capacity to be temporarily increased, I find no means so convenient as the introduction of bougies. *Part* xii., *p.* 212.

Lithotomy with Albuminous Urine.—Mr. Phillips describes a case of lithotomy, performed upon a patient whose urine was so highly albuminous, that, on the application of heat, nearly one-fourth of the fluid in the tube became solid; there was also a slight excess of lithate of ammonia present. When the patient came under Mr. Phillips's care, he was much afflicted with the ordinary symptoms of stone; the bladder was very irritable; he was fifty-six years of age. A consultation was held on the case, and it was decided that the presence of the albumen was probably caused by the irritation excited in the kidney by the presence of the stone in the bladder, and an operation was decided upon. Before the operation, the albumen slightly decreased in quantity.

[In six weeks after the operation, this patient was discharged cured; the urine was quite free from albumen. Mr. Phillips observes:

This point is one of great interest in practice, and it has been laid down by an eminent authority, that under such circumstances it is imprudent to operate at all. Whatever may be the value of that rule in other cases, I am by no means satisfied of the propriety of its application in cases of stone in the bladder; and if it had been acted upon in the present case, the patient would still be suffering from his disease. The question is undoubtedly a very delicate one; does the albumen result from irritation within the bladder extending to the kidney, or is the irritation confined to the kidney itself?—in the one case removable by operation, in the other beyond its reach. I know no test by which we can distinguish between them, but the present case is a proof that such a distinction does really exist, though we are at present unable to detect it. *Part* xiii., *p.* 273.

Operation.—Mr. Liston observes the following rules: 1. Use the simplest instruments. 2. Interfere as little as possible with the ileo-vesical fascia. 3. Know well the exact position of the stone, for the use of the forceps is the most annoying part of the operation. 4. Dilate internally, if necessary, for a large stone; or make a bilateral incision, but it is very seldom necessary. 5. Introduce a gum-elastic tube through the track of the wound into the bladder, to secure the flow of urine from it, and keep it there, in children 20 hours, in adults 40 or 50. *Part* xiv., *p.* 207.

General Treatment of Lithotomy Patients.—The general treatment of lithotomy patients at St. Thomas's Hospital, is the following: Before the operation he is kept in a quiet ward for ten days or a fortnight, his diet attended to, and his bowels regulated; the day before the operation (for which, if possible, temperate weather is chosen) he has low diet, and a dose of castor-oil; and on the morning an enema of gruel, with or without castor-oil. After the operation he is put to bed with his legs straight and close together, and a napkin put on in the same way as a child's napkin; this is changed throughout the treatment, when it becomes wet. In the evening or next morning a piece of lint is pushed up the wound by the finger, and changed whenever the patient wets; and when all the urine comes per urethram, the wound is dressed with wax and oil spread on the lint, and introduced as before. If the urine does not flow through the wound at first, the finger is introduced to remove any obstruction; and if the discharge stop from swelling of the wound, no lint is introduced, but a bread poultice applied. Cold is not applied, and an opiate rarely given. For the first week or ten days the belly is fomented with chamomile. The diet is at first farinaceous, and is gradually improved; and castor-oil is given on the third day. *Part* xvi., *p.* 206.

Hint on Sounding.—When you sound for stone, use rather a short and straight instrument at first. Introduce it very slowly and cautiously, so that the point of the instrument sinks into the post-prostatic fossa, in which the stone is generally situated. If you do so, you will generally strike the stone at once; but if you sweep a sound, with a good full curve, into the bladder rapidly, you carry your instrument over the stone, and you may turn the point of it all round the bladder in vain.   *Part* xix., *p.* 171.

Incontinence of Urine after Lithotomy.—When *incontinence of urine* follows lithotomy, give the extract of nux vomica, beginning with an eighth of a grain thrice a day, and gradually increasing the dose.

Part xix., *p.* 172.

Diet after Lithotomy.—According to Bransby Cooper, patients should not be kept on spare diet after the operation of lithotomy, nor, indeed, after any severe ordeal of the kind. It should always be remembered that you cannot diminish constitutional power without increasing irritability; and that, consequently, support is generally requisite, and should be early prescribed.   *Part* xix., *p.* 173.

Extraction of large Calculus—Bilateral Operation with the double Lithotome of Dupuytren.—Prof. May gives the following: G. H., aged 18, entered the Washington Infirmary for stone in the bladder. On sounding him a few days after his entrance, a calculus was at once detected, and from several subsequent examinations, I believed the stone to be so large that I did not deem his case a favorable one for lithotrity. I therefore decided to cut him, and, on the 15th of April, performed the bilateral section before the medical class in the following way:

The patient having been etherized and placed in the usual position, a deeply-grooved staff was introduced into the bladder, and pressed firmly against the perineum, as near as possible in the median line. A crescentic incision was then made over the staff, which, commencing on the right side at a point equi-distant from the anus and the tuberosity of the ischium, was terminated at a similar point on the opposite side, the centre of the curve being three-fourths of an inch above the anus. The incision was, by a few strokes of the scalpel, deepened, the fascia and perineal muscles divided, and the membraneous portion of the urethra exposed, which was then opened upon the groove of the staff longitudinally, and to a sufficient degree to admit the beak of the double lithotome of Dupuytren, which being fairly placed in the groove, was introduced upon it into the bladder. The stone being felt with the end of the lithotome, the staff was extracted, and the instrument being reversed, the blades were sprung to No. 18 on the graduated scale, and it was withdrawn from the bladder, thus dividing the prostate equally, on both sides nine lines.

The calculus was then readily seized with the forceps, but, finding that from its size it would not pass through the incision that had been made in the prostate, the forceps were extracted, the lithotome again introduced, and the gland further divided by the blades being sprung to their maximum point of twenty-one lines. The stone was then seized with curved forceps, and extracted entire with not more than the usual force required in the extraction of a calculus of medium size by the lateral operation.

The following were its dimensions: Longest diameter, *two inches within a fraction;* shortest diameter, *one and five-eighths of an inch;* circumference, *five and five-eighths inches.* It was hard, being a triple phosphate, and round. The patient recovered from the operation in about the usual time, and being sufficiently strong to travel, left for his home in Virginia in about two months after the operation was performed.

The measurement of the several diameters of the prostate, from the urethra as the starting-point, to the periphery of the gland, is as follows:

and gives the average size of the gland in a healthy state in the adult. In old men and children there is, of course, considerable variation from it. The anterior face of the gland is considered. Transverse diameter, nine lines; oblique diameter, ten to eleven lines; inferior vertical diameter, seven lines; superior vertical diameter, three lines. The oblique diameter, the greatest, is the one divided in the lateral operation. This is eleven lines, or one line less than inch. Add to this the dimensions of the urethra, about four lines, and this section will give us but fifteen lines. Now, it is very certain that a calculus of over sixteen lines in its shortest diameter could scarcely be extracted through this opening without either tearing or incising beyond the limits of the gland, for although something must be allowed for the stretching and yielding of the parts, yet this is fully counterbalanced by the increased volume which the blades of the forceps would add in grasping the stone. The surgeon, therefore, is obliged either to tear the parts by main force, or to incise them freely beyond the prostate.

Now, in the bilateral division of the gland in which both the oblique diameters are incised, we have, allowing four lines for the urethra, a section of twenty-six lines; and if to this we allow for the stretching of the curve, approaching as it does toward a straight line during the passage of the calculus, it is evident that it will permit, without great difficulty, the passage of a stone of two inches in its short diameter, leaving, at the same time, intact the parts beyond the gland. None of the methods of perineal lithotomy, can, therefore, in its *free* and *safe* incision, be compared with the bilateral operation, permitting, as it does, the passage of a calculus of two inches in diameter and six inches in circumference, without causing any laceration.

In speaking of this operation, Velpeau remarks that " a calculus of twenty to twenty-four lines in thickness, and from five to six inches in circumference, might, *strictly* speaking, pass through the opening without causing any laceration."

If, says Prof. May, the stone be larger than this, it had better either be broken, if possible, through the wound; or extracted by the high operation. There are surgeons who prefer performing the bilateral section with a common scalpel, for the purpose of simplifying the operation, and from the belief also that the incision through the gland does not correspond to the expansion given to the blades of the lithotome, from the yielding of the latter on account of their length and slenderness. I do not think the last objection to be correct. If the instrument is made properly, and the blades are well and firmly articulated and sharp, I have not been able to discover any such defect. The operation can, no doubt, be very well performed with the common scalpel or bistoury, and if the lithotome of Dupuytren did not possess positive advantages over it, it ought to be preferred upon the ground of being the more simple instrument. But the lithotome, as Velpeau remarks, renders the parts more tense as it divides them, gives greater regularity to the wound, terminates the operation with a single cut, and especially makes " an actual curved, instead of a simple V incision, which latter is the only one which can reasonably be expected, if we use the bistoury or other lithotomes." It is an instrument, moreover, that can be safely used at all ages, as the blades can be sprung by the graduated scale on the handle from four to ten and a half lines on each side. I first used the double lithotome in 1842, and then on a child of three and a half years. The blades were set to four lines each, thus making an incision of eight lines through the prostate, and through this, with a pair of ordinary polypus forceps, I extracted a calculus one inch in its long, and five-eighths of an inch in its short diameter (about as large as a common sized almond in the shell) without the wound being even stretched by its passage. The child did not lose over ʒj. of blood, and the recovery was very rapid, the wound being nearly closed in two weeks after the operation was performed ; a fact which goes far to disprove the assertion made by some, that cicatrization is much slower after the bilateral than the lateral section.

There are, moreover, other reasons, besides those already mentioned, which, it appears to me, render this operation safer in many respects than the lateral method, and which I, therefore, think should cause it to be adopted, not only specially, for the removal of small calculi, but also as a general method.

In the first place, there are fewer vessels divided by it, and the bulb of the urethra is not touched, for the incision is made between the anus and the bulb, and the latter with its transverse artery can be always avoided. In the lateral operation, from the position and extent of the incision, I do not see how the bulb and artery can well escape, notwithstanding the directions in the books. Without attaching to their division great importance, it is yet undoubtedly preferable to avoid them when it can be done. If the double lithotome is used, the pudic artery cannot by any possibility, except anomalous distribution, be reached. Even the superficial artery, when in its usual position, is not usually divided ; so that the operator is incomparably less incommoded by hemorrhage, as the posterior branches of the transverse, and the anterior twigs of the hemorrhoidal artery are really the only arteries that are usually divided. Again, as the lithotome cuts *outward* and backward, there is less danger to the rectum. Indeed, I do not see how the intestine can be injured, unless it should be greatly distended from neglect, prior to the operation ; and lastly, the ejaculatory ducts and vesiculæ seminales are not exposed to risk, for it will be recollected that the membranous portion of the urethra is first opened, and then the blades of the lithotome are sprung. Their obliquity *outward*, from this point, is such that the ducts cannot be injured, while, the blades not passing the limits of the prostate, the vesiculæ cannot be reached.   *Part xxvi., p.* 246.

Causes of Death from Lithotomy.—The accidents which are of the most formidable nature after this operation are—hemorrhage, infiltration of urine into the cellular tissue with suppuration and abscess of this structure, inflammation of the bladder, peritonitis, purulent infection, and secondary disease of kidneys. Dangerous hemorrhage is stated to be of uncommon occurrence. Mr. Liston stated that he had lost but one patient from bleeding out of 100 operations.

Hemorrhage, properly so called, may arise from division of the superficial artery of the perineum, the transverse artery, or the artery of the bulb, and the internal pudic itself. In some cases the accident arises from the surgeon's making his incisions in an irregular manner ; but the most frequent cause is some irregularity in the origin, course, or relations of the numerous blood-vessels distributed to the perineum. The operator may, in making his incisions, err in three ways ; he may commence his incision too high, or he may incline it too much laterally toward the tuberosity of the ischium. Each error may bring its peculiar consequences after it.

When the incision is commenced very high up, the point of the knife is apt to fall on the bulbous portion of the urethra, or divide to one side of it the artery of the bulb.

By prolonging the incision too far downward, that is to say, carrying it much beyond the level of the tuber ischii, the superficial branches which the internal pudic sends to the margin of the anus are almost sure to be divided; but here again the superficial situation of the vessels, which are not usually large, enables the operator to secure them without difficulty.

The trunk of the pudic artery itself may be divided when the incision is lateralized too much, and its lower angle made to terminate very close to the ramus of the ischium. This accident has happened in the hands of the very best surgeons:

M. Blandin, and many other anatomists, think that it is impossible for it to occur, unless there be some irregularity which disturbs the normal relation of parts at the floor of the pelvis. Finally, the superficial artery of the perineum may be implicated, because, in some subjects, it is near to the median line; but the artery can be taken up without difficulty in this situation. Primary hemorrhage may occur during the external or internal incisions. In the latter case, the danger is proportionate to the extent of the incision through the prostate; in the former case, to the amount of its deviation from the median line.

Venous hemorrhage is another accident of lithotomy which occasionally occurs. A serious form occurs from division of the venous plexus about the neck of the bladder and prostate. In aged patients, and after long continued irritation of the urinary organs, these veins are apt to become abnormally developed, even to a varicose state. Besides this, they are enveloped in prolongations of the deep pelvic fascia, and thus prevented from retracting or becoming quickly closed after division. From these causes, troublesome venous hemorrhage may come on in old patients submitted to the operation. Sir B. Brodie lost a patient within a few hours from this cause, having been foiled in all his efforts to restrain the bleeding. It may take place in adults, or even in children, under peculiar circumstances. M. Robert witnessed two examples at the Hôtel Dieu of Paris. In one case, that of a young man, the venous plexus continued to pour forth blood until death ensued. No artery had been wounded. The second case was that of a child addicted to masturbation. The enlarged veins furnished a copious bleeding, which became suddenly fatal after an act of that vice. These are altogether exceptional cases, for we may lay it down as a rule that the danger of venous hemorrhage is in direct proportion to the age of the patient.

The period at which secondary hemorrhage sets in is very uncertain. You should make it an invariable rule to examine the patient's linen every day for any traces of blood, more especially if the pulse become feeble and the face pale. Secondary hemorrhage, however, usually commences about the fifth or sixth day—sometimes earlier, on the third or fourth—sometimes later, on the eighth or tenth day.

Infiltration of urine into the cellular tissue is one of the most frequent causes of death. It may take place under two different circumstances. It may occur whenever the internal incision is carried beyond the limits of the prostate, or when the neck of the bladder and prostate are injured and lacerated during the efforts made to extract a large calculus. In both these cases, the fibrous capsule of the prostate is divided or lacerated; the urine becomes infiltrated into the subjacent cellular tissue, inflammation sets in, and, according to its seat or extent, excites peritonitis or gives rise to sloughing and gangrene of the soft parts within the pelvis.

Infiltration, again, may occur, not from a too free internal incision, but because the external one has not been made on the same plane as the internal; because it has been too small, or the soft parts which constitute its walls have been lacerated and rendered irregular during the extraction of the stone; anything, in a word, which impedes the free discharge of urine through the external wound, may become an occasional cause of this infiltration, which takes place in the perineum, and not in the sub-peritoneal cellular tissue as in the former species. Simple inflammation of the pelvic cellular tissue, not caused by urinous infiltration, is a very rare accident.

The symptoms of urinary infiltration are extremely various, for the effects of the accident are modified by several circumstances. In some cases, the symptoms set in a few hours after the operation, and terminate fatally in a few hours more, or within a day or two; in other cases, the progress of the disease is slower, and the patient does not sink until after a considerable period.

The sub-peritoneal is, as might naturally be expected, the most rapid and dangerous. The patient complains of pain about the neck of the bladder, and from the very outset has a peculiarly unfavorable and anxious expression of countenance; the pulse is small, weak, and rapid; the tongue soon gets dry; and the lower part of the abdomen tumid and painful; often there is vomiting; prostration now rapidly ensues; there is low delirium, and the patient dies within forty-eight hours.

In other cases the typhoid symptoms and prostration are not so great; the fever at first is of a more irritative character, and is occasionally interrupted by rigors; still, as the urine continues to work its way between the layers of the fascia, and the inflammation ascends along the sides of the rectum, more unfavorable symptoms do not fail to present themselves.

Purulent infection is not often a cause of death in English surgery. Inflammation of the bladder is somewhat common; but we should estimate the inflammation caused by the stone, and that also of the operation. In alluding to the last cause of death after lithotomy, Mr. Gay, in his concluding remarks, says, that calculus vesicæ can never long exist without producing deterioration of the system and latent disease of the kidneys, and with such cases as these, he observes, lithotritists are very careful not to meddle.   *Part* xxvii., *p.* 150.

Lithotomy—New Method: (*Recto-Urethral.*)—This operation may be described briefly as follows: The rectum is cut into from the median line of the perineum, and thus freely dividing the commissure of the sphincter ani. From this dissect upward in the median line to the membranous urethra, which is slit up as far as the edge of the prostate, the knife being guided by a previously introduced staff. The prostatic urethra is then dilated until of sufficient size to allow of the introduction of the forceps and the extraction of the stone. The bladder and the prostate are therefore not wounded.   *Part* xxviii., *p.* 205.

Lithotomy.—If a patient be relieved by making water, says Prof.

Syme, the case is probably one of urinary irritatioι.. If the pain occurs during micturition only, there is probably stricture, but if the pain be slight *before* micturition, increases *during* the process, and becomes severe for a short time *afterward*, we have probably a case of stone. The success of lithotomy depends in a great measure on the manner in which the prostate is divided. There is one part which cannot bear injury, this is at the base of the gland where it joins the base of the bladder ; it is a dense texture, very tough and unyielding, forming a sort of ring around the urethra, endowed with an extraordinary degree of sensibility. Now, if this texture be torn, the patient will die, or if injured, the danger will be in proportion. The different success of different surgeons depends upon this ring being divided sufficiently by some and not by others: therefore, if on introducing your finger to dilate the deep part of the incision, you feel you have not cut enough, pass a straight probe-pointed bistoury along your finger, and, by a gentle sawing motion, carry the incision on to the extent you find necessary, in order to enable you to dilate with facility.

Part xxxi., *p.* 295.

Prevention of Hemorrhage after Lithotomy.—There are many objections to plugging the wound. It prevents the flow of urine, which creates much irritation, and on its removal fresh bleeding is often excited. To obviate this, attach to the common tube a conical bag of oiled silk, about an inch and a half from its inner extremity, pass the tube into the neck of the bladder, and then fill the oil-silk bag with sponge. The wound may in this way be most effectually plugged, and the escape of urine is secured by means of the tube. *Part* xxxi., *p.* 298.

Median Operation of Lithotomy.—In reference to the comparative mortality of the lateral and median operations of lithotomy, Dr. King having considered shock, hemorrhage, and infiltration of urine, which are less liable to occur in the latter than in the former operation—and purulent deposits and peritonitis which are accidents occasionally attendant on all operations, observes that the remaining source of danger, viz., inflammation of the neck of the bladder, is the most frequent cause of death after lithotomy, and we have to consider whether it is more likely to occur when the prostate is partly divided and partly lacerated, or when it is simply dilated. The prostate when once cut into very readily tears, and the inflammation excited by the urine getting into these fissures produces more fatal results in lithotomy than all the other sources of danger put together. But if the prostate be not incised at all, this condition of things is entirely altered. In the old Marian operation the prostate was actually torn asunder, by instruments, and there is no wonder that death so often resulted.

Mr. Allarton's proposal is of a very different nature. He recommends that the finger should be introduced, in the first place, and dilatation effected by careful pressure—that long-bladed forceps should next be passed into the bladder, and, the stone having been seized, should be carefully and steadily withdrawn—the length of the blades causing the instrument, with the stone in its grasp, to act as a wedge, and thus assist in the proces of dilatation. Even should the structure of the prostate tear under this gradual pressure, it is of little moment so long as the mucous membrane remains entire, the urine being thus prevented from having access to the lacerated portions, which access, and not the mere fact of laceration of the prostate, constitutes the grand danger in lithotomy.

Part xxxv., *p.* 118.

Rectangular Catheter-Staff for Lithotomy.—Mr. Hutchinson recommends the use of an instrument combining the advantages of both a grooved staff and a catheter. It is rectangular in form, and the groove commences only from the angle, being broader at that point to allow its being more readily found, and the angle being very prominent in the perinæum is more readily reached by the knife. There are also other important advantages : from the straight direction which the knife runs it does not readily leave the groove—from the groove only commencing at the angle, the urethra cannot be opened too far forward, or the artery of the bulb wounded. From its being a catheter as well as a staff, the surgeon may be quite certain it is in the bladder before commencing the operation, and the bladder can be injected without any change of instruments. There is no difficulty whatever in its introduction.

   *   *   *   *   *   *   *

One of the great advantages of this over the curved form of staff is, that the rectum is quite secure from being wounded if the finger be kept in the rectum whilst making the incisions.   *Part* xxxv., *p.* 120.

————•♦•————

LITHOTRITY.

Sir B. Brodie adverts to the inconveniences or dangers of lithotrity, as follows :

1. Hemorrhage. This may arise from the forcible passage of the lithotrity forceps through the neck of the bladder. Sir Benjamin has known it discolor the urine for two or three days. But it has never interfered with the operation.

2. Rigors may follow lithotrity. The rigor is usually produced by the stretching of the urethra by the withdrawal of the forceps: or it may be occasioned by a fragment of calculus sticking in the urethra. A dose of opium may prevent the rigor altogether, or defer it till the next day. Rigors do not appear to interfere materially with the patient's recovery.

3. Sir Benjamin refers to two cases in which fragments of calculus impacted in the urethra gave rise to urinous abscess in the perineum. One patient died two months after with symptoms of diseased kidney. The other patient got well.

4. Sometimes the patient suffers from pain in the whole canal of the urethra, from the simultaneous escape of many fragments. Sometimes he labors under great irritation of the bladder, apparently from a fragment lodged near its neck. He may have complete retention, but Sir Benjamin has never seen it last for any time.

The patient should partake plentifully of diluting drinks. If fragments lodge, a middle-sized catheter may be introduced into the bladder, when they may be either dislodged and come away, or pushed back and afterward crushed. Sir Benjamin has removed fragments from the anterior part of the urethra by long, slender forceps. It *might* be necessary to make an incision in the penis or the perinæum. Sir Benjamin, however, believes that if perfect repose is enjoined, after the operation, the passage of fragments will seldom occasion any serious inconvenience.

5. Inflammation of the mucous membrane of the bladder may occur. It generally subsides spontaneously in two or three days, or continues till a fragment is either discharged from the urethra, or pushed back into the bladder by the catheter. In one instance, Sir Benjamin saw this inflammation prove fatal. The stone had been large—perhaps the patient had not been kept quiet.

On the whole Sir Benjamin is of opinion that lithotrity has great advantages over lithotomy. He touches on the cases to which it is not applicable.

1. In boys, under the age of puberty, lithotomy is too successful to be abandoned. The urethra is not wide enough to be favorable to lithotrity.

2. Lithotomy is attended with little danger in the female, while her short and wide urethra admits too readily of the escape of the injected water by the side of the lithotrity forceps.

3. Large stones are not well adapted for lithotomy, but they are still worse adapted for lithotrity. Sir Benjamin inquires whether it would not be well to crush first and cut afterward.

4. Lithotomy is not well adapted for cases of enlargement of the prostate gland, where the patient cannot empty the bladder, unless the calculus is small; *then* the fragments may be washed out of the bladder through a large catheter. When the tumor of the prostate projects into the bladder, it is difficult to elevate the handle of the instrument sufficiently to catch the stone readily.

5. Lithotomy is very fatal where the kidney is diseased, especially Sir B. Brodie supposes from the loss of blood that it entails. Crushing he thinks *safer*. But any shock to the system must be hazardous, and it must, usually, be more advisable to palliate.

Sir Benjamin sums up what he has to say in favor of lithotrity in these words:

"With the exception of such cases as those which have been enumerated, there are few to which this method of treatment may not be advantageously applied. It may be said that the exceptions are numerous; but they are the result chiefly of delay. If a patient seeks the assistance of a competent surgeon within six or even twelve months after a calculus has descended from the kidney into the bladder, the urine having remained acid, it will rarely happen that he may not obtain a cure by a single operation, and with so small an amount of danger that it need scarcely enter into his calculations. As time advances the facility with which he can be relieved diminishes, and after the lapse of two or three years, especially if the urine has become alkaline, it is probable that the calculus will have attained such a size as to render the old operation preferable, and that the access of disease in the bladder or kidneys may render any operation hazardous. It would be absurd to say, and it would be unreasonable of human-kind to expect, that an operation that has for its object to relieve them of a disease so terrible as stone in the bladder, can be always free from inconvenience, and difficulty, and danger. Nevertheless, from what experience I have had, I am satisfied that the operation of lithotrity, if had recourse to only in proper cases, is not only much more successful than that of lithotomy, but that it is liable to fewer objections than almost any other of the principal operations of surgery." *Part* vi., *p.* 106.

Lithotrity.—The first case of lithotrity performed in Ireland, was by Sir Philip Crampton, in 1834, in the Meath County Hospital. The operation was only repeated once, and in less than a week's time the whole of the detritus had come away. Sir Philip asks what is the problem which lithotrity has to solve? According to Civiale it is as follows:

1st. The reducing of calculi within the bladder into fragments sufficiently small to be discharged or removed through the natural passage. 2dly. The effecting this by such means as shall excite no dangerous irritation in the urinary organs. 3dly. The freeing the bladder or urethra from the fragments which these organs may not have the power to expel.

The best instrument for performing the operation of lithotrity, is Baron Heurteloup's or Weiss's curved percuteur. The late Mr. Oldham improved this instrument by carrying out a suggestion by Sir Philip Crampton, by which fragments of the calculi are prevented from accumulating between its jaws. The invention of the screw is due to Mr. L'Estrange of Dublin. Sir Philip would prepare the patient for the operation by enjoining a light diet, abstinence from fermented liquors, clear out the bowels, and order the hip-bath: if the urine be acid, give alkalies combined with uva ursi or Peruvian bark; if alkaline, give the mineral acids; and if mucous deposits, infusion of Pareira brava; enjoin absolute rest, and use occasionally an anodyne enema. The urethra is to be gradually dilated, if necessary; when preternatural contraction of its orifice exists, divide it. Introduce the catheter frequently, as it allays the irritability of the bladder and urethra. The objects of the operation are to reduce calculi within the bladder to such a size that the portions may be removed or discharged through the natural passages, to effect this by such means as shall excite no dangerous irritation in the urinary organs, and to free the bladder from the small fragments which remain. Great care should be taken that the case be a suitable one for the operation, as in some cases cystotomy must be preferred. Lithotrity may be performed where the bladder is perfectly healthy and the stone is small; and it is decidedly advantageous where there is phthisis or albuminuria. It is a great and valuable addition to chirurgical therapeia, but cannot be considered as a substitute for cystotomy, since there are numerous cases in which the last operation will prove the safest and most effectual.

Cystotomy, for example, is preferable in boys before the age of puberty; it is so simple and the urethra is so small as not to admit of the lithotrite. Cystotomy is also preferable in the female; also where the calculus has attained a very large size; also where the prostate gland is enlarged, unless the calculus be of very small size. *Part* xiii., *p.* 266.

Lithotrity.—According to Mr. Liston, this operation is applicable, 1st, to patients above puberty, if the stone is not large, say $\frac{1}{2}$ to $\frac{3}{4}$ inch in diameter, or as large as a chestnut; 2nd, when the bladder and urethra are tolerably healthy, as shown by retaining the urine for hours, and being able to pass it in a good stream, and when the bladder will admit of injection and careful exploration. *Part* xiv., *p.* 207.

Treatment after the operation of Lithotrity.—Dr. Adams, of the London Hospital, says: In regard to the getting rid of the contents of the bladder, I am strongly of opinion that the less interference there is on the part of the surgeon the better. Let the patient drink freely of barley-water, and give him an alkaline mixture with tincture of hyoscyamus, and you will find the bladder relieve itself much better than you can relieve it by the aid of any instruments, however ingeniously contrived. I am averse to the exhibition of opium after the operation, unless the patient should have a shivering fit, and then it may be desirable to employ it; opium has the effect occasionally of inducing the retention of urine, and therefore I would not use it unnecessarily: a dose of castor-oil may also be given the morning after the operation, and the hip-bath is to be employed night and morning. *Part* xix., *p.* 171.

Lithotrity and Lithotomy.—In the course of his remarks on the Pathology and Surgery of urinary concretions, Mr. B. B. Cooper says: The choice between lithotrity and lithotomy is often one requiring considerable judgment on the part of the surgeon; and this is a question in which a knowledge of the chemical nature of the stone must always be of great service: not that the chemical composition of the stone has anything to do with either of these operations directly; but the physical character of the different kinds of stones varies as much as their composition, and that character can be judged of pretty correctly as soon as the composition of the calculus is known. Uric acid, for instance, often occurs in a form in which it easily breaks into pieces under a crushing force; and the crystallized variety of the triple phosphate also crumbles away completely under pressure. By means of the lithotrite it is easy to comminute such stones as these; but there are others which yield with great difficulty to the action of that instrument. The oxalate of lime calculus is of this nature; the tuberculated portions break off readily enough, but the mass of the calculus is crushed with great difficulty; and when it is broken, the fragments are so sharp that they are likely to produce extreme irritation in the bladder, and then a secondary action may be established, in which these fragments become the nuclei of other calculi, or at least cause the deposition of fresh quantities of earthy matter from the urine. Whatever may be the nature of the stone, I think it is always inadvisable to employ the crushing process if there be evidence of a tendency to the deposition of the earthy phosphates. Of course this must be judged of by the urine; and unless the tendency can be removed, it seems to me that the operation of lithotomy should be preferred; for I believe that the incision through the prostate gland causes less irritation than the use of the lithotrite, and the consequent presence of the calulous fragments. The advantage of lithotomy is, that the chief source of irritation is removed at once; and although there may remain the constitutional tendency to deposition from the urine, there would be no nuclei to promote that tendency, and it would be therefore the more likely to be counteracted by therapeutical agents.

Whenever, also, from the diathesis of the patient, the state of the urine, and the examination by the sound, the stone is believed to be of that kind which is crushed with difficulty, the operation of lithotomy is certainly indicated.

With regard to the constitutional condition of the patient, the same considerations would weigh with the surgeon in lithotomy as in lithotrity; and one of the chief points would be, to overcome, before the operation was performed, the constitutional tendency, if any still continued to exist, to further deposition. Generally speaking, the physical character of the stone bears little immediate relation to the operation of lithotomy; but I may say that the kind of stone most suitable to lithotrity is perhaps that most difficult to deal with in lithotomy. The more friable a stone, and the less the cohesion of its particles, the better suited it is to the lithotrite; but such a stone would be more likely to increase the difficulty of the operation in lithotomy, as it would probably crumble and break away when seized by the forceps, and so lead to the necessity of some modification of the operation, in order to get rid of the whole of the fragments. The hardness of the stone can be no objection in lithotomy, unless it be too large to be removed whole, in which case great irritation may be produced in the efforts of the surgeon to break it while in the bladder. I believe that the operations of lithotrity and lithotomy may, in a certain manner, be very advantageously combined. For instance, it sometimes happens that a stone is so large, that, although it may be removed without previous crushing, it requires a very extensive incision through the prostate. In such a case, I think that a strong kind of lithotrite may be introduced through the wound, and the stone easily broken down, without producing so much irritation as would arise from the extension of the wound by the forcible extraction of a large stone. *Part* xx., *p.* 158.

Lithotrity.—Mr. C. Hawkins says: No attempt to extract any portion of stone through the urethra should be made with the lithotrite; the operator should be content with crushing the stone in the bladder. If a portion of the stone should become impacted in the urethra, it is much safer to cut down upon it and remove it, than lacerate the urethra by efforts at extraction. *Part* xxiii., *p.* 200.

Lithotrity.—After the operation of lithotrity, it sometimes happens that a fragment of the stone becomes impacted in the membraneous part of the urethra. To ascertain the nature and seat of the fragment pass a soft bougie down the urethra; the fragment seldoms fails to leave a mark on the bougie, whereas a metal sound would pass over it and communicate no impression. Where impaction is to be apprehended, the patient should not be allowed to make water while on his knees, but must endeavor to do so while on his back. Immediately after the operation several injections of warm water should be thrown into the bladder by means of a large catheter, with large eyes, for the purpose of removing as much of the detritus as possible. If a fragment should be impacted, and if it should be near the neck of the bladder, it may be gently pushed back, but in all cases, if there is any resistance, injections of warm water should be used through the catheter. If it is impossible by these means to push back the fragment, there is only the choice between extraction and crushing, and whenever the former can be effected without much difficulty it is to be preferred. *Part* xxvi., *p.* 230.

Lithotrity.—In the choice of subjects for this operation, take care, if possible, 1st, to let the age be between thirty and sixty, with neither the irritability of youth, nor the debility of old age. 2d. The urethra should be large enough to admit instruments of considerable size. 3d. The bladder should be healthy, and capable of holding six or eight ounces of fluid. 4th. The kidneys should also be healthy. 5th. The calculus should be loose in the cavity of the bladder. 6th. The diameter of the stone oug it not to exceed an inch and a quarter, as near as can be calculated. Whe·e the above kind of case occurs, lithotrity and not lithotomy ought to be performed.

Simple enlargement of the prostate need not prevent the operation, but where there is inflammation or suppuration it is inapplicable, and lithotomy should be performed. Lithotrity should never be adopted, unless the bladder be free from inflammation, and one great means of knowing this is to ascertain the quantity of water which the bladder can hold. A bladder violently inflamed, is like a stomach inflamed, neither can contain much without parting with it. If the bladder can hold eight or ten ounces (other circumstances being favorable), lithotrity will generally succeed; but if it will contain only three or four ounces, this operation is not proper. As soon as the surgeon has filled the bladder, he should suddenly change the position of the patient backward, so as to throw the stone into the back of the bladder. The manipulations can be carried on better in this place than nearer the prostate and the anterior part of the bladder, which is always more irritable and sensitive than the back part. *Part* xxx., *p.* 163.

Lithotrity.—[In a case of lithotrity on a rather old patient, at St. Bartholomew's Hospital,] Mr. Skey, after carefully injecting the bladder with warm water, was observed to break the stone once, and then order the man to bed. Mr. Skey then explained to his class that this is a rule he adopts at the advice of Sir B. Brodie, never at the first sitting to break the stone more than once, so that the bladder may thus become accustomed as well to the instruments as the altered state of the stone.
Part xxxv., *p.* 122.

Lithotritic Instruments in Cases of Enlarged Prostate.—Supposing you have to perform *lithotrity* in a case of enlarged prostate, you must, in order to success, take into account the alterations which have taken place in consequence of the prostatic disease. The two principal are: first, elongation of the passage by an inch or more; second, formation of a sort of a pouch beneath the neck of the bladder, in which pouch the stone usually lies; to overcome the first, you require to have your instruments several inches longer than usual; you will best overcome the second by reversing the beak of the instrument when introduced into the bladder, or by tilting the pelvis of the patient backward, to execute which proceeding quickly, every lithotrity couch should be provided with some mechanical contrivance. *Part* xxxvii., *p.* 161.

Lithotrity.—According to Mr. F. C. Skey, cases should be rejected if there be—1. Manifest disease of the kidney. 2. The urethra so contracted as not to admit with facility a lithotrite of ample size. 3. The bladder so intolerant as to be incapable of retaining its urinous contents for three or four hours; and, on the other hand, a bladder of low nervous susceptibility. 4. Much enlargement of the prostate gland. Moreover, in performing the operation, the following cautions should be observed: The quantity of water injected should not exceed four or five ounces. No attempt should be made to open the instrument till it has been pushed thoroughly home into the bladder. In the act of separating the blades, pass the lower blade downward toward the bottom of the bladder, that the upper blade may not be painfully pressed against the neck. The instrument should retain the mesial line throughout the entire operation, there being neither necessity for, nor advantage in, directing the instrument to the right or left. At the first operation do as little as possible, breaking the stone only once. No advantage is gained by an abstemious diet. *Part* xl., *p.* 123.

LOBELIA INFLATA.

Uses of Lobelia Inflata.—In pertussis, combining the tinct. lobel., of which Professor Eberle speaks so highly, with the acid hydrocyan., extolled by Thompson and Roe, with equal propriety might I vaunt the recipe as a specific, as they do theirs, although such a thing as a *specific* probably does not exist, except it be sulphur for psora. In asthma, especially of a spasmodic kind, the most marked benefits result from the use of this plant singly, or combined as above—the existing disturbance of the nervous fibre of the bronchial surface, or the spasms of the mucous membrane of the bronchia are speedily allayed, and, by a short course, a cure, or a *suspension* of some length at least, is the sequence of its administration. For an adult, ℞ Tinct. lobel. inflat., ʒj.; acid hydrocyan., gtt. i–ii Ter quatuorve die. But if the paroxysm be severe, the tincture may be given in much larger doses, and repeated at short intervals, till entire relief is obtained. By this combination, I have enabled several *inveterate* cases of asthma (which had been repeatedly prescribed for by various physicians, quacks, and old women) to pass for several months with a complete suspension of all their sufferings.

In diphtheritic laryngo-tracheitis, continues Dr. Livezey, where the excitation of emesis cannot be readily accomplished, which frequently arises from the nature of the disease as well as the difficulty and unpleasantness of medicine to infants, this difficulty may be obviated by enemata, containing a portion of the tinct. lobel. or pulverized plant, which at once relaxes the system, removes the tension of the chest, changes the seat of excitement to a distant part, and emesis readily ensues; the bowels in the meanwhile are emptied of their contents, and recovery from every distressing symptom immediately follows.

In all cases of coughs, especially when inflammatory symptoms manifest themselves, as in catarrhal affections in children as well as in adults, I consider the tincture of this plant (or infusion, when the stimulus imparted by the alcohol might be objectionable) far preferable to ipecacuanha or the tartrate of antimony and potassa, being more decisive in its effects than the former, and a better and safer nauseant than the latter, without that fear of irritating the gastro-enteric mucous membrane, the pathological condition of which has been too much overlooked by earlier writers, but which is now claiming deserved attention.

In febrile disorders, incident to every section of country, more or less, in summer and autumn, when it is desirable (as in fact it is always so) to lessen vascular action, and as a febrifuge, the "nitrous powders" sink into utter insignificance in comparison with this plant, which is not liable to the same objection as the tartarized antimony used in combination with calomel and the nitrate of potassa by many of the older practitioners, which too frequently increases that tenderness and erethism already existing in the mucous membrane of the stomach and intestines. *Part* xvi., *p.* 134.

---•••---

LOCK-JAW.

Acupuncture in Protracted Lock-jaw.—[The patient, 25 years of age, unmarried, had for years been subject to attacks of suppurating sore throat, in which the jaw often became nearly immovable for two or three days before the discharge of the matter. In 1826 she had a severe attack, from which resulted complete lock-jaw, accompanied with hysterical symptoms, which attack yielded after six weeks of treatment so far that she could put a teaspoon into her mouth. After nearly a year the jaw again became completely fixed, without accompanying sore throat, and the same treatment, with galvanism, was tried without effect. Although unequivocally connected with hysteria, there was reason to think, from the inflammatory symptoms with which the disease set in, that the affection was not purely spasmodic, but was kept up by rigidity of the muscles closing the jaw, produced by inflammation, in consequence of which the antagonist muscles had become inadequate to the effort of opening the mouth, under the mere influence of volition.]

It was this view of the case which made Dr. Seller consider it more reasonable in making trial of the needles, to insert them into the muscles which open the jaw, in the expectation of exciting these to such a contraction as might overcome the rigidity of their antagonists.

On each of the two following days, two needles were inserted, one on each side of the mesial line, between the chin and the hyoid bone, the effect being short convulsive efforts, the teeth began to grate on each other, and the jaw was drawn from side to side, not by single alternate contractions, but by several convulsive movements on one side, followed by a nearly equal number toward the other side, interrupted occasionally by a momentary opening of the mouth to the extent of about two fingers' breadth.

The convulsion continued after the needles were withdrawn, ceased and became renewed again after a few minutes, and returned spontaneously in the evening on both occasions. Some increase of voluntary power over the jaw followed both applications of the remedy. After each trial of the acupuncture, some improvement was observable; but as the spontaneous convulsion was almost always followed by a slight loss of motion, the progress made was but slow.

The needles were usually inserted to the depth of half an inch, and sometimes to the depth of an inch.

[The acupuncture, together with the leeches, was used for ten days, by which time the patient could open the mouth two fingers' breadth, and chew soft substances. She then went into the country for five weeks, by which she derived great benefit, but being exposed to cold and wet on her return, had another severe attack, the consequence of which was the loss of much of the voluntary power over the muscles of the jaw. The needles were again resorted to with the same effects as before, but the pain produced by the convulsions were greater, and lasted longer, while the spontaneous convulsion recurred several times in the evenings, after each of the first trials. As leeching did not succeed in mitigating the convulsion, the temporal artery was opened with the desired result, and with the effect at the same time, of restoring, to a considerable extent, the sight of the right eye, which she almost lost with the first attack of lock-jaw. A second detraction of blood from the same vessel diminished the force of the convulsion so much as to permit the acupuncture to be used twice a day. Nine days after the renewal of the operation, the jaw had recovered its natural extent of motion. The aphonia, which had come on at the same time as the affection of the eye, was completely cured by a smart shock of electricity. So great was the effect produced by the recovery of her voice, and complete power over the jaw, that from a mere spectre, she reassumed her natural robust, ruddy appearance.]

Vide " Tetanus." *Part* xi., *p* 189.

———•♦•———

LOINS.

Pain of the Loins.—Dr. Oke says: Pain of the loins may be derived from the muscles, from the liver, from the duodenum, from the kidneys, from the colon, from the uterus, from the aorta, from the spine, or from matter collected on the psoas muscle independent of spinal disease. In order to arrive at its true cause, we must endeavor to ascertain what function is principally involved which will at once lead us to it.

If the pain be rheumatic, it will be increased by pressure, and by the slightest action of the muscles affected. There will probably be also rheumatism in other parts of the body, the system will not evince much disorder, the urine will be high colored, and deposit a lateritious sediment.

If derived from the hepatic function, the pain will shoot upward along the splanchnic nerves toward the scapulæ; the alvine evacuations will be either deficient in, or exuberant with, bile; or show a morbid quality of that secretion; the urine will have a bilous tinge; there may be congestion of the hemorrhoidal veins; and the spirits will be depressed.

If from the duodenal function, three or four hours after the meal the pain will be aggravated, shooting through toward the right side of the abdomen, and remaining till the food has passed into the jejunum. Dyspeptic symptoms will prevail, and there will frequently be painful pustules breaking out about the face. I have lately met with a case in which the boils were extremely annoying.

If from the kidneys, the pain will shoot down the course of the spermatic nerves toward the round ligament in the female, and toward the testis in the male, which will often be retracted by the action of the spermatic nerves upon the cremaster muscle. There will be more or less irritation communicated to the mucous membrane of the bladder. The urine also will be diagnostic in this instance; it may deposit mucus, calculous matter, blood, pus, or albumen, according to the nature of the case; or it may be otherwise morbid in its constitution.

If from the uterus, the pain of the back will arise either from disordered function or disease of that organ. In the former case the pain will be of a neuralgic character, will return in forcing paroxysms extending around the hips and hypogastric region, will be attended with hysteria, and often with increased quantity of the menstrual discharge. In the latter case the pains will be *constant* and severe, extending along the anterior crural nerve half way down the thighs. There will be a thin, offensive discharge from the vagina. The countenance will be wan and sallow, exhibiting the wear and tear of organic lesion.

If from the colon, there will be constipation, and inflation in the course of the bowel, or the fæcal discharges will be of small diameter, or there will be soreness of the intestine under pressure, especially at its ascending or descending portions, accompanied by mucus, or shreds of lymph in the form of boiled vermicelli, amongst the excretions.

If from arterial dilatation, an abnormal pulsation of the vessel involved —the aorta, for instance—may possibly be detected by auscultation in the incipient stage of the disease, *if such were suspected;* but in a large majority of cases such a cause may reasonably escape the attention of the ablest surgeon, from there being no tangible symptom that might lead him to suspect it; and even after the dilatation has considerably advanced, it may be sufficiently large to press upon and disturb the spermatic nerves, but not large enough to project and pulsate externally, and this may, at this stage, be confounded with disease of the renal function. A few years ago I met with a case of this kind in a man of middle age. The pain had been constant and wearing, shooting from the loins down the course of the spermatic nerves, and for a considerable time was reasonably attributed to the renal function, especially as there had been constant disturbance of this function. At length the aneurismal sac began to approach the surface, and then, of course, the cause became apparent.

If from disease of the spinal column, the pain will be aggravated by percussing the spinous processes at this part of the spine, or by suddenly striking the toes against an uneven surface. There will be involuntary action of the muscles, especially of the flexors of the legs, diminished temperature, abnormal feelings, and more or less loss of power of the lower limbs. Should there be at the same time any unnatural projection of the spinous processes, the disease will be confirmed.

If from a collection of matter upon the psoas muscle, unconnected with spinal disease, the pain will be continued, dull, and deep-seated, extending from the loins down the psoæ, or in whatever direction the matter may have taken its course. The pain will be aggravated by flexing the thigh toward the abdomen, and there will be difficulty in walking; moreover, there will be marks of a strumous habit, and more or less symptoms of hectic fever. Should any fluctuating tumor present at the groin, or at any other point where the matter may find its way out of the body, it will be conclusive as to the nature of the case. *Part* ix., *p.* 50.

LUMBAGO.

Nature and Treatment.—Lumbago is a very characteristic form of muscular rheumatism. It occupies the loins, and is often aggravated to torture by an unguarded movement implicating the muscles of the part; but if the patient remain perfectly quiet, he is comparatively free from suffering. When very severe, he may be obliged to remain in bed, and very often is confined to the sofa. Even when he is able to walk about, he often does so in a semi-bent position, being unable to raise his body into a complete erect posture for some time after he has risen; nay, in some cases he cannot straighten himself at all.

Purgatives are very frequently of great service in the different forms of muscular rheumatism, more particularly in lumbago, and as a general rule ought to precede the use of other remedies. The best plan, where there is nothing to contra-indicate its adoption, is to give from three to four grains of calomel at night, followed by a black dose next morning, and to repeat this once or twice during the first week, after which it is sufficient

to regulate the action of the bowels, and to give rather a brisk purgative
about once a week.   *Part* v., *p.* 77.

Treatment of Lumbago.—Dr. Macleod advises a brisk calomel purge
once or twice a week, and considers half a drachm to two drachms of the
compound tincture of guaiacum three times a day, with a grain of opium
at night, the best plan.   *Part* viii., *p.* 25.

Lumbago, Sciatica, Paralysis from Arsenic, etc., *vide* " Firing."

———•••———

MALARIA.

The active Principle of Malaria.—Dr. Gardner, Professor of Chemistry in Hampden Sidney College, submits the following propositions :
    1st. Sulphureted hydrogen gas exists in the stagnant waters and atmos-
phere of certain marshes.
    2d. The character of malarious regions is similar to that of those in
which sulphureted hydrogen is generated.
    3d. Certain agents have been supposed to give activity to the exhala-
tions arising from marshes, called malaria.
    4th. The properties of malaria are fully recognized by the profession.
    5th. Sulphureted hydrogen is the active agent in the production of
those forms of malarious fever met with on the sea coast, and the diseases
belonging to the same class found inland.
    He shows from carefully instituted experiments, that sulphureted hy-
drogen gas exists in the stagnant waters and atmosphere of certain marshes
where malarious diseases are prevalent, and that certain agents give activity to the exhalations arising from these marshes. On account of the
difficulty of procuring a sufficient quantity of atmospheric air to detect the
presence of the gas, he prepared pure surfaces of silver and brought them
into contact with the air and water in the suspected regions. Silver is
one of the most delicate tests for sulphur, and is not so liable to be attacked
by the agents which act upon lead, copper, etc., and so delicate a test of
sulphur is metallic silver, that it will detect it in a solution containing one
part in three millions of water ; and as a means of determining the amount
of sulphureted hydrogen in mineral waters, it is perhaps one of the best
tests which we possess.
    Dr. Gardner having prepared his silver plates (polished coins), exposed
them to the action of the air and water of marshes in different localities.
The polished coins were first perforated in a marked place so as to be recognized, next cleaned and dried, then carefully weighed, furnished with
strings, and lastly, suspended in the places fixed upon. Thirty different
coins were thus suspended in different places ; some were soon stained, and
others, as in the Buffalo River, were not affected for some time. Ultimately, however, most of them were more or less stained ; and it was
found that the shallow waters of marshes contained the most, and rivers
the least amount of gas, the coins suspended in the latter sometimes requiring a month, and those suspended in the air even more time for discoloration, while those suspended over the stagnant marshes, would be
affected in a week or even less.
    Sulphureted hydrogen has been discovered on the most deadly coasts.

It is produced in marshes where sulphates exist either in the vegetable matter, water, or soil. The destruction of the sources of the gas, by the exclusion of the sea, has annihilated the fatal malaria of some of the Italian marshes and given health to the pestiferous town of Viareggio.

The agents which decompose sulphureted hydrogen are also inimical to malaria. Fire is of this number, for by means of it the gas is converted, in the open air, into sulphurous acid and water. Chlorine destroys both malaria and sulphureted hydrogen, the latter by combining with its hydrogen and precipitating the inert element sulphur. The value of chlorine has been proved both in the American and British squadrons.

The existence of trees, by decomposing the organic compound, and appropriating its water, is calculated to destroy malaria.

Its weight, and the readiness with which water may be separated from it, preclude its rising to any altitude in the atmosphere.

It is produced in the autumnal months : because, then, the amount of moisture, the coolness of the nights over the temperature of the days, and the fresh deposition of leaves, furnish the most abundant materials for the formation of the organic compound.

The poisonous effects of sulphureted hydrogen are too well known to require comment. There is no agent, which marshes evolve, that is so destructive to life. Messrs. Thenard and Dupuytren killed birds in an atmosphere containing 1-1500th part of the gas. Nysten found that it was absorbed at once by the blood. Two or three cubic inches caused immediate death when injected into a vein, the cavity of the chest, or the cellular tissue of a dog. The same authority, with Lebkuchner, and Chausier, found that it was absorbed through the healthy skin, and produced dangerous effects. The gas is a narcotic poison, prostrating the nervous system, and destroying muscular energy. In small quantities it produces colic, and internal congestion.

Liebig states, that sulphureted hydrogen produces immediate decomposition of the blood. *Part* viii., *p.* 5.

Malaria.—For producing malaria it appears to be necessary that a surface should be flooded and soaked with water and then dried. The quicker the drying process, the more virulent is the poison that is evolved. For this reason Dr. A. T. Thompson recommended that the floor of a sick room should only be swept, never washed. An invalid might as well sleep in a swamp as in a room the floor of which is frequently washed. Dr. Alison has observed the more frequent occurrence of croup on Saturday night, the only day of the week on which the lower classes of Edinburgh wash their houses. *Part* xxxiv., *p.* 18.

MANGANESE.

Pharmaceutical Preparations of Manganese—Oxide of Manganese.— This is a very good preparation, especially when obtained by the humid method ; it should therefore be made only when it is wanted for use. The best mode of prescribing it is to add to an ounce of simple sirup, half a drachm or a drachm of the hydrated oxide, with some oily emulsion, to prevent the contact of the air.

· *Carbonate of Manganese* is best prepared by dissolving seventeen ounces of pure crystallized sulphate of manganese, and nineteen ounces of carbonate of soda, in a sufficient quantity of water. Double decomposition takes place ; one ounce of sirup is added to every seventeen ounces of the liquid, and the precipitate is allowed to settle in a well-stopped bottle. The supernatant fluid is then decanted off ; the precipitate is washed with sugared water, and allowed to drain on a cloth saturated with simple sirup ; it is then expressed, mixed with ten ounces of honey, and rapidly evaporated (the access of air being prevented) to a proper consistence for making pills. The dose is from four to ten pills, each four grains, every day in chlorotic cases, where iron has not succeeded. The hyperoxidation of the carbonate of manganese may be prevented by adding freshly prepared vegetable charcoal to the pills.

Neutral Malate of Manganese.—This is procured by treating carbonate of manganese with malic acid. It is an eligible preparation, as the base of the salt is in the form of protoxide, and the acid is easily digested. The dose is from two to four grains, in pills.

The preparations of manganese have this immense advantage over those of iron, that they can be combined with vegetable tonics and astringents, namely, tannin, and the substances which contain it, as gall-nuts, rhatany, catechu, dragon's blood, kino, monesia, canella, and cinchona. These can all be combined with malate of manganese. *Sirup of malate of manganese* consists of simple sirup, ℥xvj.; malate of manganese, ℥j.; essence of lemon, ℨij.: an ounce of sirup contains 29 grains of malate of manganese. *Pills of malate of manganese.*—Malate of manganese, gr. xv.; powder of cinchona, gr. xv.; honey, a sufficient quantity to make twenty pills. *Lozenges of malate of manganese.*—Malate of manganese, ℥j.; sugar, ℥xj.; mucilage of tragacanth, a sufficient quantity. To be formed into lozenges, each 12 grains in weight ; each of which contains a grain of the salt.

Tartrate of Manganese is prepared in the same way as the malate, tartaric acid being used. It may be substituted for the malate in all the above mentioned formulæ; and is used to prepare the following highly tonic sirup. Sirup of tolu, ℥xvij.; extract of rhatany, ℨiiss.; tartrate of manganese, ℨiiss. Dose, from four to five spoonfuls daily.

Phosphate of Manganese is best prepared by dropping a solution of phosphate of soda into a solution of sulphate of manganese. The precipitate is collected after filtration, dried, and preserved in well-stopped bottles.

This preparation may be employed, like the phosphate of iron, in cancerous affections. *Pills of phosphate of manganese.*—Phosphate of manganese, ℨiss.; powder of cinchona, ℨss.; sirup of catechu, a sufficient quantity. To be divided into four grain pills. *Sirup of phosphate of manganese.*—Phosphate of manganese ℨss.; sirup of tolu, ℥iij., ℨiij.; sirup of cinchona, ℥v.; essence of lemon, ℨiss.; powder of tragacanth, gr. x. This preparation must be made quickly, and preserved in a well stopped bottle. *Lozenges of phosphate of manganese.*—Phosphate of manganese, ℥j.; sugar, ℥xij. Mix and divide in twelve grain lozenges, each containing one grain of the phosphate.

Iodide of Manganese is prepared by digesting recently precipitated carbonate of manganese with fresh hydriodic acid; then filtering, and evaporating, the access of air being prevented. It may more conveniently be prepared extemporaneously, by mixing together an ounce of iodide of potassium, and the same quantity of sulphate of manganese, perfectly dried, and in the state of powder. It is then made into a pill-mass with honey, and divided into pills, each containing four grains of the iodide; which should be kept in a well-stopped bottle. The dose is at first one pill daily, gradually increased every three·days, to six pills; the medicine is then omitted for eight days, after which it is resumed again. *Sirup of iodide of manganese* is prepared by adding concentrated hydriodic acid to a drachm of perfectly pure hydrated carbonate of manganese, until it be entirely dissolved; then mixing with the solution 17 oz. of a sirup of guaiacum and sarsaparilla. Dose, from two to six spoonfuls daily.

In cases where iron has not succeeded, it is desirable not to make a sudden transition to manganese, but to combine the two remedies as in the following formula. Pure crystallized sulphate of iron, $\tilde{3}$xiij.; pure sulphate of manganese, $\tilde{3}$iiiss.; pure carbonate of soda, $\tilde{3}$xviiss.; honey, $\tilde{3}$x.; sirup as much as may be sufficient to make a mass to be divided into four-grain pills. Dose from two to ten pills daily. The insoluble preparations of manganese should be first used, as the carbonate, phosphate and oxide: then the more soluble preparations, the tartrate, malate, etc., may be employed. The use of this medicine should not be persevered in so long as that of iron, as its preparations are more rapidly assimilated. Manganese is not, like iron, found in the excrements of persons who take it—at least it is in very small quantity.

In the depraved state of the blood which succeeds intermittent fevers, manganese is useful; it is the most certain remedy for preventing a return of the attacks. Leucophlegmasia and engorged spleen, of long duration, are rapidly reduced by the use of iodide of manganese with sirup of cinchona. The preparations of manganese should also be used in urethro-vaginal catarrh in chlorotic patients, and in chronic blennorrhœa, especially in individuals weakened and rendered anæmic by excess. The salts of manganese with which we are acquainted, are powerfully astringent, and may be used as external applications, in all cases where other astringents are not indicated. In this respect they possess no other peculiarity. *Part* xx., *p.* 295.

Use of Manganese as an Adjuvant to Iron.—It is especially in *diseases of the blood* that ferro-manganic medicines are useful. They have a special action on the vascular apparatus, on the formation of the blood, and on the circulating fluid itself. They do not act merely as tonics or astringents; but are regenerators of the blood. They have succeeded admirably in anæmia following hemorrhage, operations, polypi, metrorrhagia, etc.; also in the chlorosis attending puberty, which is a more common disease than is generally supposed, and occurs even in males. M. Pétrequin has also frequently found the combinations of iron with manganese of benefit in the diseases of women at the critical period. He has often seen, in these subjects, *metrorrhagia*, accompanied with an aspect of the surface which would lead to the suspicion of organic· uterine disease; the hemorrhage, however, was but a complication, and the patients, apparently in a hopeless state, have recovered under the use of ferro-manganic preparations, conjoined with tonics and ergotine.

In *amenorrhœa* and *dysmenorrhœa*, the patients often imagine that they require to be bled; but care must generally be taken not to comply with this request.

These medicines are no less efficacious in the treatment of *anæmia* resulting from prolonged intermittent fevers, prolonged suppuration, strumous, syphilitic, or cancerous affections, phthisis, etc. Fills and the sirup of the iodide of manganese and iron are preferable in these cases.

In the *functional affections of the heart* connected with chlorosis and anæmia, and which must not be mistaken for organic disease, a combination of iron and manganese with digitalis and other moderators of the heart's action is advantageous. The same remark applies to the *functional disorders of the lungs*, attending the same constitutional states.

Disordered states of the nervous system are intimately connected with those of the blood. M. Pétrequin has found that the ferro-manganic preparations succeed well in these, even though uncomplicated with chlorosis.

He has also seen benefit from the use of iron with manganese in many cases of *dyspepsia, gastralgia*, and *gastro-enteralgia*.

In *nervous affections connected with exhaustion* from venereal excesses, onanism, rapid growth, etc., as well as in leucorrhœa, diabetes, etc., M. Pétrequin has a high opinion of these medicines.

It has been observed that manganese not only preserves water, but purifies that which has undergone change (Martin-Lauzer).

M. Pétrequin commences by giving the powder of iron and manganese, with some vinous drink; he then administers two pills daily, one before breakfast and one before dinner, replacing them soon by the lozenges. The sirups and chocolate complete the treatment. He gives the medicines at meal-time. The sirup he gives before breakfast, in doses of a teaspoonful; and he finds it useful to administer directly after it some infusion of centaury, or of chamomile flowers and orange.

Large doses are unnecessary and useless.

Preparations of Manganese and Iron.—M. Burin-Dubuisson, of Lyons, who prepared most of the ferro-manganic combinations used by M. Pétrequin, has published an interesting *brochure*, from which the following formulæ are extracted:

Powder for Effervescing Solution of Manganese and Iron.—Take of coarsely powdered bicarbonate of soda, 20 parts; tartaric acid, 25 parts; powdered sugar, 53 parts; finely powdered sulphate of iron, 1½ parts; finely powdered sulphate of manganese, ¾ part: mix carefully, and keep in well-stopped bottles. A teaspoonful is mixed with each glass of wine and water drank during meal time.

Pills of Carbonate of Iron and Manganese.—Take of pure crystallized sulphate of iron, 75 parts; pure crystallized sulphate of manganese, 25 parts; crystallized carbonate of soda, 120 parts; honey, 60 parts; water, sufficient quantity. Pills of 20 centigrammes (3 grains) are made; they keep easily, without becoming oxidized, in well-closed vessels. From two to four are given daily.

Ferro-Manganic Chocolate.—One part of carbonate of iron and manganese is first mixed with four of sugar, and divided into large lozenges; of these 100 parts (grammes) are mixed with 500 of chocolate paste, in the preparation of which 100 parts of sugar have been left out. This will make 800 lozenges, each of which contains about 3 centigrammes (nearly half a grain) of carbonate of iron and manganese. The chocolate decomposes the hydrated carbonate of manganese and iron of the saccharate into hydrated sesqui-oxide of iron and manganese; there is no metallic taste.

Sirup of Lactate of Iron and Manganese.—Take of lactate of iron and manganese, 4 parts; powdered sugar, 16 parts; rub together, and add of distilled water, 200 parts; dissolve rapidly, and pour into a matrass over a water-bath, containing 384 parts of broken sugar; filter the solution. This sirup contains about 15 parts of lactate of iron and 5 of lactate of manganese in 3,000 parts. One or two spoonfuls are taken daily.

Lozenges of lactate of iron and manganese are made by adding 20 parts of the lactate to 400 of fine sugar, with a sufficient quantity of water. The mass will make 840 lozenges; of which six or eight are taken daily.

Pills of Iodide of Iron and Manganese.—M. Burin-Dubuisson forms a solution of iodide of iron and manganese, in the proportion of one part by weight to two of water: the proportion of the salts is about three of iodide of iron to one of iodide of manganese. Six parts of this are mixed with 294 of simple sirup; of this, M. Pétrequin gives one or two spoonfuls daily.

Pills of Iodide of Iron and Manganese.—Take of the officinal solution prepared by M. Burin-Dubuisson, 16 parts (grammes); honey, 5 parts; some absorbent powder, 9½ parts. Divide into 100 pills. The honey and the solution are first mixed, and evaporated at first rapidly, then more slowly, to 10 parts. Then add the powder, and divide the mass into four parts, which must be rolled in powder of iron reduced by hydrogen; each of these must then be divided on an iron plate into 25 pills, and again rolled in the iron powder. Finally, they are covered with a layer of tolu, according to M. Blancard's process.

All these preparations must be made very carefully. M. Burin-Dubuisson has ascertained that the commercial salts of manganese frequently contain copper, and even arsenic; he hence insists on the necessity of calcining the sulphate of manganese twice, or more frequently, at a dark red heat, and of carefully testing the solution.   *Part* xxvii.,*p.* 337.

MANIA.

Antimony in Mania.—Dr. Sutherland states that the employment of antimony in the treatment of mania is of the highest value. A fourth of a grain of the potassio-tartrate may be given every fourth hour, or at the commencement of the paroxysms of furor. It is powerful as a means of controlling the action of the heart and arteries. In many cases in which it has been given, it has acted like a charm in instantly subduing the excitement and violence of the patient; and in some cases an alteration in the symptoms for the better has been traced from the commencement of its administration.   *Part* viii., *p.* 73.

Digitalis in Mania and Epilepsy.— *Vide* "Epilepsy."

Musk in Certain Cases of Delirium, Mania, etc.—Vide "Delirium."

Treatment of Mania and Nervous Excitement.—[Dr. J. Williams strongly recommends the use of narcotics and other remedies calculated to produce sleep, not only in order to put off, but even to cure an attack of mania. He observes that.]

Some of the mildest cases which occur, where there is preternatural excitement with vigilantia, are those of persons having over-fatigued the mental powers by continued application, more especially if confined to one subject; and the ill effects seem to be produced more frequently in those whose hopes and fears are in addition adding to the excitement, as is often noticed in junior barristers and students at our universities.

Now, in such instances, if a young man apply early, the case is usually cured very rapidly, sometimes even within twenty-four hours; if passed over for a few days, recovery is retarded, and if totally neglected, phrenitis or mania by no means unfrequently ensues. In such cases there is a great action, which is but too frequently mistaken for power; the pulse is quick, perhaps 100, 120, or even more, tongue white, face flushed, throbbing and heat of the temples, rolling, sparkling, and injected eye, rapidity of speech, and everything showing great excitement; now this description is not sufficient to guide us as to the treatment, for all these symptoms may depend on excessive nervous irritation, but more attention must be given to the pulse; if the pulse, in addition to being quick, is also full, hard, and bounding, and if the skin is dry and hot, then the abstraction of blood, both general and local, will usually be necessary, and often within an hour or two after depletion, the skin becomes moist, and the patient falls asleep. But what I am the more anxious to particularize, is the opposite condition, where bleeding is unnecessary and unsafe. Supposing the pulse to be quick, soft, and fluttering, weak or intermittent, the skin moist and clammy, and yet the excitement just as decided as in the other case, to bleed here is most improper, and many cases of insanity have arisen from such practice. The judicious administration of a narcotic will frequently act as a charm, and we have often found the following prescription very useful:

R Tr. hyoscyami, mxxx.; tr. humuli, ʒij.; camphoræ, gr. v. ad x. aut xv.; sir. auranti, ʒij.; mist. camphoræ, ʒvj.; M. et fiat haustus, h. s. s.

This has often caused calm and refreshing sleep; and the patient, who has previously passed two or three nights with great restlessness and watching, feels himself invigorated.

A very efficient way of relieving head symptoms, when dependent on visceral congestion, more especially of the liver, is applying leeches to the rectum, and if considered necessary, subsequently placing the patient in a warm bàth; a large quantity of blood may be lost in this way without producing much prostration. Many cases of insanity arise from extreme irritability dependent on prostrated power; and to support this power by good nutritious food, and sometimes even with brandy and wine, at the same time soothing the system by procuring refreshing sleep at night by morphia, will speedily evidence the advantages of such treatment.

* The great error originally was, allowing the power to sink; it is of the greatest importance that these powers should be supported—the nervous excitation must be calmed. In these cases, mistakes are but too frequently made; irritation is confounded with inflammation.

Purgatives may procure sleep, by diminishing vascular action, where bleeding is inadmissible. Narcotics, when given in insanity to procure sleep, should be administered in full doses.

Combining opium with camphor or henbane, or digitalis, will often be very judicious. With tartar emetic, calomel and opium in large doses will often calm the system when there is great restlessness and fever, especially if the head be kept cool. Opium should never be omitted where insanity has succeeded constant intoxication; and in those cases where the countenance is exsanguined, with cold, clammy skin, it is especially indicated, and

is no less useful in that anæmial state of the brain where there is great exhaustion, in whatever way produced.

Where there is constant vomiting, opium may be administered in an
effervescing draught.

The infusion of opium with a bitter, as recommended by Dr. Paris, will
secure the narcotic principle without interfering with the intestinal secretions.

It is impossible to limit the extent to which opium may be required;
but in stating that a full dose is necessary, from two to five grains may be
considered a large dose for most constitutions; where habit has impaired
its effect, one, and even two drachms of solid opium have been taken in a
very limited period. Pinel knew 120 grains of opium given in one dose
to a patient suffering with cancer of the uterus; and I have seen a wineglassful of laudanum taken at a draught, and this has been repeated three
times daily for months—such cases, however, necessarily form the exception.

When opium has disagreed with a patient, a strong cup of coffee will
often remove the unpleasant effects.

Administering an opiate in the form of enema renders it much milder,
and at the same time secures its sedative and narcotic influence, without
producing that headache, sickness, and dryness of the fauces, so often complained of when opium is taken by the mouth.

If narcotism be highly desirable, and neither of these modes seem practicable, rubbing the abdomen with laudanum and oil will sometimes be
found effectual. These narcotic frictions over the head will be often found
useful : even brushing the hair with a common hair brush for half an hour,
will frequently tranquillize a nervous and irritable patient. In some cases
it may be necessary to rub the scalp with liniments, or ointments, containing morphia, belladonna, veratria, or aconitine.

Antiperiodics.—Insanity is somewhat periodical : and it should be
remembered, that, when it is intermittent, it is not inflammatory, and in
such cases arsenic, tr. ferri sesquichloridi, the preparations of zinc, and
copper, with tonics, may be often usefully prescribed. Arsenic can be
strongly recommended in these cases, and has been given with the greatest
advantage; it appears to alter the sensibility and irritability of the brain.
Quinine is sometimes given with the same intention; thus, a case of in-
somnolence, was cured by giving gr. vj. of quinine at bed-time.

The douche, the author most properly remarks, should never be resorted
to, except when imperatively necessary; and the application of the ice-cap
will generally be found far more efficacious.

Our object is to keep the head cool—and not to make it suddenly cold.
Part xiii., *p.* 35.

Periodic Mania.—Large doses of tincture of henbane (one or two
drachms), preceded by an active purge, sometimes affords singular relief
in cases of periodic mania. *Vide* Art. "Testes." *Part* xviii., *p.* 214.

Cerebral Excitement—Mania.—In cases of violent cerebral excitement,
delirium tremens, and mania, everything points to the necessity of some
sure, speedy, and active mode of allaying excitement and procuring sleep
—yet the stomach is often highly irritable, or in such a state that it will
not absorb medicines, or the patient even refuses to swallow at all. Of all
cases, says Mr. C. Hunter, perhaps this is the one in which the value of

the hypodermic injection of morphia is most clearly seen. Inject one-third to half a grain of acetate of morphia beneath the subcutaneous cellular tissue of any part of the body, and in a few minutes sleep will be procured. *Part* xl., *p.* 279.

————•◦•————

MARASMUS.

Inspissated Ox-Gall.—[Dr. Clay has also found that the inspissated gall has a remarkable tendency to counteract the constipating effects of opium, which drug not only checks the secretion of bile, but almost all the other secretions of the body. The administration of gall, therefore, if this fact be further corroborated, will be a valuable addition to our list of remedies when we are wishful to give opium but dread its constipating effects. In the case alluded to by Dr. Clay, the patient was taking large doses of the pil. scillæ comp. c. opio at bed-time, for a constantly irritating, dry, asthmatic cough : eight grains of the inspissated gall were also given every night, which completely counteracted those constipating effects of the opium which had previously existed. Dr. Clay further states that,] In all cases of marasmus, whether of children or in the atrophy of adults, I have in ox-gall a valuable remedy. In acidity of the stomach, etc., of children, it is of most decided, effectual, and· immediate relief. The curdled vomitings, green motions, abdominal gripings, and restlessness immediately disappear, and a better-state of general health is substituted ; in all such cases there was a decided action on the kidneys, increasing the secretion. On looking at its effects upon children as just stated, partien-larly whilst at the breast, living almost entirely on milk, the result is not different to what we might suppose when considering the experiments of Bagliva, Lewis, etc. " *That it prevents milk from turning sour, and dissolves it when in a state of coagulation ;*" *an antacid preparation is indicated, which is one of the peculiar properties of this remedy.* To show its direct effect upon hardened fæces, a child of sixteen months old passed a very hard motion with very great difficulty, not having had one for three days. I poured a solution of ox-gall over it in a vessel, immediately its chalky appearance was changed to a more healthy bilious color, and reduced to a pulpy mass in half an hour; from this fact, I will suppose a case (one which has frequently occurred in my practice), an adult with hardened fæces in the rectum, almost, if not quite impossible, to pass without assistance ; under such circumstances, what could afford a better prospect of relief than two or three ounces of recent gall diluted with as much water, used as an injection. It is needless to observe I would pledge myself as to the result, viz., an immediate softening of the mass facilitating its propulsion.

The preparation I have been in the habit of giving, is simply the recent gall of the ox slowly evaporated to the consistence of an extract, and afterward made into pills.

I prefer the simple extract made into pills without any addition; and if the gall be *recent*, it has very little smell, but an intensely bitter taste. The gall-bladder of a moderate sized ox will afford as much extract as will make one hundred four grain pills, and is an article both cheap and easy to procure. *Part* vi., *p.* 68.

Iodide of Potassium.—Recommended in certain cases of, by Lisfranc. *Vide* " Iodic Preparations."

Mal-assimilation in Children.—Mr. Henry, surgeon to Middlesex Hospital, observes :

Sometimes a pallid cachectic emaciated child will in a few days gain some pounds in weight, after the operation of a brisk cathartic. What explanation can be offered of this fact ? If the intestines of such children be examined, the mucous absorbent surface will be found to be covered by a thick tenacious mucus, completely preventing assimilation of the chyle. A brisk cathartic, especially calomel, which may be combined with rhubarb and scammony, will wash this away, and the lacteals thus be left free to absorb the chyle, with which, for the first time they come in contact. *Part* xxxix., *p.* 264

MATICO.

Remarks on Matico.—When applied externally, Dr. Jeffreys recommends the inner side of the leaf as most powerful. "To leech-bites, and bleeding from cuts or other recent wounds, the inner side of the leaf should be pressed upon the bleeding part for a few minutes, when it will be found to possess not only an adhesive, but also a healing quality, not easily separated by washing the hands or other ordinary means." In bleeding from the nose, the powdered herb used as snuff has been found a very convenient mode of applying it. We subjoin the formulæ for preparing an infusion, a decoction, and a tincture :

Infusion of Matico.—Take of matico-leaves, one ounce. Boiling water, one pint. Macerate for two hours, or until cold. Dose— two tablespoonfuls for an adult, twice or three times daily, or oftener, if the case is a severe one or the symptoms urgent.

Decoction of Matico.—Take of matico-leaves, one ounce ; water, one pint. Boil for ten or fifteen minutes, and strain. Dose, the same as that of the infusion.

Tincture of Matico.—Take of matico-leaves, three ounces ; Proof spirit of wine, one pint. Digest for fourteen days, in the usual way, and filter for use. Dose—from thirty to sixty drops in water.

[By the term *inner* surface, Dr. Jeffreys means the under and reticulated surface of the leaf.] *Part* x , *p.* 165.

Use of Matico.—Dr. Ruschenberger says: In enlarging a burrowing bubo, I divided the arteria ad cutem abdominis, which bled freely. I directed that an attempt should be made to arrest the hemorrhage by lint and pressure. After a trial of ten minutes, which totally failed, I directed moistened matico leaves to be applied. The assistant reported in a few minutes that the matico exerted no influence, and proposed to secure the bleeding vessel by ligature. I now visited the patient, who had lost six or eight ounces of blood, and was still bleeding. After coarsely powdering some matico leaves in the palm of my hand, I formed the mass into a paste with cold water ; I then removed the clot, through which the arterial blood formed a passage of the size of a crow-quill : the blood flowed per saltem, forming a jet of at least three-fourths of an inch high. The paste was applied lightly with the fingers, and filled the wound. The surrounding skin was immediately sponged clean; the hemorrhage ceased instantly, and not a single drop of blood flowed afterward. No pressure was used, or dressing applied. In the first application the entire matico leaf had been simply dipped in water and then applied. It failed, as already stated.

I exhibited drachm doses of finely powdered matico in a case of profuse menorrhagia, repeated every two hours. The flow ceased after the third dose. The powder was simply mixed in about two ounces of water. The patient experienced no unpleasant effects from its use.

Part xvi., *p.* 319.

—•◦•—

MEASLES.

Iodide of Potássium.—M. Ricord observes: The iodide of potassium possesses the remarkable property of causing determination of diseased action to the skin. In cases of what may be termed "suppressed measles" and "scarlatina" it will frequently induce a healthful reaction under the most desperate circumstances. One or two grains, according to the age of the patient, under twelve years, may be dissolved in a quantity of sugared water, and administered, repeatedly, as an ordinary drink, the whole quantity being given in twenty-four hours, for three or four days. In measles, a small plaster to the chest assists the peculiar action of the iodine. In scarlatina, the compound tincture of iodine, diluted with three or four parts of water, may be frequently applied, by means of a camel-hair brush, to the front and sides of the throat and neck. Milk is injurious during the first two or three days, in cases either of measles or scarlatina.

Part vii., *p.* 43.

Turpentine in Collapse of.—In a case of collapse coming on in a boy three and a half years old, during an attack of measles, forty minims of turpentine, combined with two drachms of ipecacuanha wine, proved a most valuable diffusible stimulant. *Part* xxvi., *p.* 325.

Charcoal in Epidemics of Measles.—Dr. Wilson observes that throughout the course of the epidemic (measles) he has never observed diarrhœa to be beneficially critical, but otherwise, and has hence never hesitated to check it, for which purpose he has found no remedy so efficient as the ordinary wood charcoal in powder, and when assiduously and promptly exhibited, it has never failed, within his knowledge, to have a promptly beneficial effect. *Part* xxxv., *p.* 26.

—•◦•—

MEDICINES.

Liquor Hydriodatis Arsenici et Hydrargyri.—Of this *liquor hydriodatis arsenici et hydrargyri*, each drachm measure consists of—water, one drachm; protoxide of arsenic, one-eighth of a grain; protoxide of mercury, one-fourth of a grain: and iodine (converted into hydriodic acid) four-fifths of a grain. The color of the solution is yellow, with a pale tinge of green; its taste is slightly styptic. It cannot be properly conjoined with tincture of opium, or with sulphate, muriate, or acetate of morphia; for all these produce immediate and copious precipitates in it. Hence, if opiates are to be used during the exhibition of this arsenico-mercurial compound, they must be taken at different periods of the day. Tincture of ginger produces no bad effect.

The following formula is proper:

Liquoris hydriodatis arsenici et hydrargyri, ℨij.; aquæ destillatæ, ℥iiiss.; syrupi zingiberis, ℥ss. Misce. Divide in haustus quatuor. Sumatur unus mane nocteque.

Thus, one-sixteenth of a grain of protoxide mercury would be taken in each dose, along with two-fifths of a grain of iodine, which, being in the state of combined hydriodic acid, will be much diminished in energy of medical effect. This is no doubt the proper dose to begin the exhibition of arsenic with, but it will soon be necessary to increase it. The division into draughts is here necessary; first, to insure accuracy in the dose, so essential in the case of this active medicine; and, next, to prevent injury to the ingredients by the use of a metallic spoon as a measure—the general way in which, unfortunately, the dose of a medicine is determined. *Part* iv., *p.* 67.

New Classification of Medicines.—M. Mialhe, states that his researches have led him to conclude that the greater number of substances introduced into the economy act chemically either mediately or immediately on the serum of the blood, some *coagulating* and others *fluidifying* its albumen. In the class of coagulants are ranged all tonic, astringent, and styptic agents, as most of the mineral acids, a great many of the metallic salts, tannin, creasote, ergot of rye, etc. The class of fluidificants comprises all true diuretics, with many alteratives and general excitants, including most of the vegetable acids, ammonia and its salts, the iodides, sulphurets, and alkaline chlorides, etc. But some medicines, which at first act as coagulants, afterward become fluidifiant; this is the case with bichloride of mercury. Others, which have not any perceptible action on the albumen when first introduced into the circulation, become afterward coagulant in a high degree. Of this class is ergot of rye. This substance, according to Mialhe, having after a time effected a thickening of the albumen, ultimately produces a firm coagulation, " or rather a process of organization more than simple coagulation." By this action Mialhe explains all the known effects of the ergot; and he supposes the agaric used for stopping bleeding, the champignon, etc., to exert a similar coagulant agency. *Part* viii., *p.* 75.

Action of different Medicines on the Mental Faculties.—All stimulants and exciting medicines increase the quantity of blood that is sent to the brain. If this quantity exceeds a certain amount, then most of the faculties of the mind become over-excited. Nevertheless, the degrees of this action is observed to vary a good deal in different cerebral organizations; and it is also found that certain stimulants exercise a peculiar and characteristic influence upon special or individual faculties. Thus ammonia and its preparations, as well as musk, castor, wine, and ether, unquestionably enliven the imaginative powers, and thus serve to render the mind more fertile and creative. The empyreumatic oils are apt to induce a tendency to melancholy, and mental hallucinations. Phosphorus acts on the instinct of propagation, and increases sexual desire; hence, it has often been recommended in cases of impotence. Iodine seems to have a somewhat analogous influence; but then it often diminishes, at the same time, the energy of the intellectual powers. Cantharides, it is well known, are a direct stimulant of the sexual organs; while camphor tends to moderate and lull the irritability of these parts.

Of the metals, arsenic has a tendency to induce lowness and depression of the spirits; while the preparations of gold serve to elevate and excite them. Mercury is exceeding apt to bring on a morbid sensibility, and an inaptitude for all active occupation.

Of narcotics, opium is found to augment the erotic propensities, as well as the general powers of the intellect, but more especially the imagination. Those who take it in excess, are, it is well known, liable to priapism. In smaller doses, it enlivens the ideas and induces various hallucinations, so that it may be truly said that, during the stupor which it induces, the mind continues to be awake while the body is asleep. In some persons, opium excites inordinate loquacity; Dr. Gregory says, that this effect is observed more especially after the use of muriate of morphia. He noticed this effect in numerous patients, and he then tried the experiment on himself with a similar result. He felt, he tells us, while under its operation, an invincible desire to speak, and possessed, moreover, an unusual fluency of language.' Hence he recommends it to those who may be called upon to address any public assembly, and who have not sufficient confidence in their own unassisted powers.

Other narcotics are observed to act very differently on the brain and its faculties from opium. Belladonna usually impairs the intellectual energies; hyoscyamus renders the person violent, impetuous, and ill-mannered. Conium dulls and deadens the intellect; and digitalis is decidedly anti-aphrodisiac. Hemp will often induce an inextinguishable gaiety of spirits; it enters into the composition of the intoxicating drink which the Indians call *bauss.* The use of the *Amanita Muscaria* is said to have inspired the Scandinavian warriors with a wild and ferocious courage. Tobacco acts' in a very similar manner with opium, even in those persons who are accustomed to its use; almost all smokers assert that it stimulates the powers of the imagination.   *Part* ix., *p.* 82.

Pleasant substitute for Epsom Salts as a Purgative.—M. Garot recommends the following formula for the preparation of tasteless purgative salts (citrate magnesia)—Carbonate of magnesia 15 parts; citric acid 21 to 22; aromatic sirup 60 : water 300. The citric acid is separately dissolved and added to the carbonate of magnesia diffused in water. As thus prepared it is not effervescing; but it is easily rendered so by adding only half the quantity of acid, and reserving the addition of the other half, until the dose is taken. The above proportions in grains would constitute a dose.

Dr. Pereira long since suggested the use of citrate of magnesia in nearly similar proportions. He found that one scruple of crystallized citric acid saturated about fourteen grains of light or heavy carbonate of magnesia.
                                        Part xvi., *p.* 296.

How to mask the bitter taste of Epsom Salts.—Mr. Combes has found that *coffee* possesses the power of covering the nauseous taste of sulphate of magnesia; we are told that—

The following is his formula for an ordinary dose of about an ounce of the salt. Sulphate of magnesia 30 parts; ground coffee 10; water 700 or 800. Boil them briskly together for two minutes in an untinned vessel. Remove from the fire, and having allowed the mixture to infuse for a few minutes, strain it. Sugar it and drink it hot or cold, according to taste. To insure the effect, the coffee must be boiled with the salt as directed above; adding the latter to it afterward or to an infusion does not suffice.

If the quantity of the sulphate be much increased, and it is desired not yet to add more coffee than the above, that will suffice if, while the fluid is boiling, a grain or two of tannin be added. *Part* xvi., *p.* 296.

How to make Senna pleasant to the Taste.—The "Bulletin de Théra peutique" signalizes another use of *coffee* in disguising the taste of purga tives for children ; MM, Guersant and Blache frequently employing it for this purpose. A weak decotion of coffee is made, to which some milk and sugar are added, care having been taken while boiling the coffee, to put in a *few follicles of senna.* If it is given to the children with a little bread, they will generally take it with avidity. This medicine generally acts freely upon children, and thus administered does not induce the violent griping it sometimes does in the adult. (As a matter of taste, we think the senna tea and prunes of our grandmothers is a more delicious preparation). *Part* xvi., *p.* 297.

Formula for Frank's Solution of Copaiba.—Balsam ' of copaiba two parts, liquor of potassa (P. L.) three parts, water seven parts; boil it for two or three minutes, put it in a separator, and allow it to stand for five or six days, then draw it off from the bottom, avoiding the upper stratum of oil. To the clear liquid add one part, of sweet spirits of nitre, perfectly free from acid, to which a few drops of liquor of potassa has been added, until it slightly browns turmeric paper ; should it turn foul or milky a *very little* liquor of potassa will usually brighten it ; if not, place it in a clean separator, for a few days, and draw it off from the bottom as before, when it will be perfectly brilliant without filtering.
Part xvi., *p.* 297.

Medicines—To disguise the taste of.—We should prepare the mouth before instead of after swallowing nauseous medicines, in order that their taste may not be perceived ; aromatic substances chewed just before, as orange or lemon peel, etc., effectually prevent castor oil being tasted.
Part xxiv., *p.* 349.

Cod Liver Oil—Mode of taking.—Let it be taken in a simple weak infusion of quassia. This would seem the more valuable as it is in itself a mild and agreeable tonic bitter, assisting in improving the tone of the general system. *Part* xxvi., *p.* 327.

Administration of Phosphorus.—It has long been a desideratum in medicine, says Dr. Glover, to find some safe mode of administering phosphorus. I have given phosphorus lately in the following ways; first, in the form of a solution in chloroform ; secondly, in cod-liver oil. Chloroform dissolves about one-fourth of its weight of phosphorus ; and the solution is not inflammable. I have given four or five minims of this solution, shaken up with a drachm of ether, in a wineglassful of port wine, twice a day, with great benefit in rallying the forces of the patient, as I fancied at least, in cases of typhoid fever. The solution in the oil is made by cutting the phosphorus into chips, and putting it into a bottle of the oil, in the proportion of half a grain to the ounce, then immersing the bottle in hot water, and with a little shaking, solution is easily effected. I think I have seen this beneficial in strumous cases. *Part* xxvii., *p.* 246.

Wine—Medicinal Use of.—As a *diuretic*, Moselle may be as useful as gin or whisky. It contains an excess of salts, and may prove as energetic as, and less heating than, the essential oil in gin or whisky.

In *diabetes*, use the claret wines, which are free from sugar, and contain much tannic acid.

In *dyspepsia and gout*, use the wine most free from ultimate acidity and least stimulating. The best is the *least acid claret* wine; next, strong or perfectly dry champagne. Good Mansanilla will answer the purpose, and is much cheaper than Amontillado sherry. But, after all, weak brandy and water, or some pure spirit and water, is most free from acid and sugar, and answers best in dyspepsia. *Part* xxx., *p.* 298.

Phosphate of Lime.—Dr. Kuchenmeister recommends the following formula in cases in which phosphate of lime is indicated: Calcis phosphat., 3ij.; calcis carbon., 3j.; sacch. lactis, 3iij. M. 3ss. bis terve in die. Instead of the milk sugar, lactate of iron may be substituted, if iron be required. The especial use of the carbonate of lime appears to be that carbonic acid is liberated by the acid of the stomach, and dissolves the phosphate. Lactic acid also is formed from the sugar, or is set free from the lactate of iron, and dissolves the phosphate. The most ready way of absorption is, however, when the phosphate is given with food, especially with milk, with which it forms a soluble combination. *Part* xxxi., *p.* 234.

Employment of the Chlorate of Potash as a Topical Application.— The chlorate was used in solution in the proportion of from one drachm and a half to three drachms to one pint of water. He (Mr. Moore) had found it very useful in cases of indolent ulcer and phagedena, in cleansing cancerous sores, and as an application to the mucous membrane of the nose, mouth, and tongue in cases of ozena and secondary ulceration. The author suggested that the beneficial effects of the application were probably due to its setting free oxygen, and proposed its use in some forms of dysentery, with affections of the lower bowel.

Dr. Mayo said he believed Mr. Stanley used the same remedy (scruple doses every four hours) for phagedenic syphilitic ulceration.

Mr. C. Hawkins generally combined it in such cases with tincture of myrrh. The remedy was very useful in cases of cancer, in removing the odor, independently of its effect upon the sore itself. Scruple doses he thought scarcely sufficient to administer internally. *Part* xxxi., *p.* 310.

Selections from Favorite Prescriptions.—Dr. Horace Green gives the following prescriptions, many of which are the result of years of collecting from the most experienced and practical men who have visited the hospitals of New York:

Narcotics and Sedatives.—The narcotic principle in medicine differs from that of the sedative, in this, that its primary action is in some degree stimulant, whilst the sedative principle tends directly to depress the vital powers without inducing any previous excitement. The ultimate action of both narcotics and sedatives is to diminish the sensibility of the nervous system, thereby allaying pain and promoting sleep.

Among the direct sedatives *hydrocyanic acid* is one of the most prompt and efficient. Administered in appropriate doses, it tends directly to lower the sensibility of the nervous system, to diminish the frequency of the pulse, and to induce a sensation of quiet and calmness throughout the whole system. Alone, or in conjunction with other remedies, prussic acid constitutes one of our most valuable therapeutic agents.

The following combinations with this remedy have been proved to be of great service in the treatment of disease:

℞ Acidi hydrocyanici, medicinalis, gtt. lx ; morphiæ sulph., gr. iij.; tinct. sar.guinariæ, vini ipecacuanhæ, aa. f. ℥ss.; sir. pruni virginianæ, vel misturæ amygdalæ, f. ℥v. M. fiat mistura cujus sumat cochlearium parvum bis terve in die.

We have found the above a most valuable remedy in the treatment of *chronic bronchial disease;* in allaying the *cough* present in *tuberculosis,* and in all *pulmonary catarrhal diseases,* unattended with fever. As the acid is apt to floa: on the top of the liquid, the phial should be shaken on the administration of each dose.

℞ Acidi hydrocyanici, gtt. xl.; vini antimonii, f. ℥ss.; syrupi tolutan., f. ℥iss.; mucil. acaciæ, f. ℥ij. M. fiat mistura, capiat cochl. parvum ter quaterve die.

This may be used in the same cases as the former, when the cough is troublesome, and is attended with some degree of fever.

As a remedy in the treatment of *hooping-cough,* hydrocyanic acid surpasses in efficiency every other known general remedy. We have employed it for many years in this disease, and can fully substantiate the declaration of Dr. Hamilton Roe, that "Hydrocyanic acid of Scheele's strength will, if exhibited as soon as the whoop is heard, effect a cure in almost every case of simple hooping-cough." If the disease has been going on for many weeks, its effects are not so immediately felt, but nevertheless it will cure in most instances.

The following formula we are accustomed to employ:

℞ Acidi hydrocyanici, medicinalis, gtt. xxv.; vini ipecacuanhæ, f. ʒij.: syr. tolutan., f. ʒj.; aquæ destillatæ, f. ℥iij. Fiat mistura, cujus sumatur cochl. parv. quartâ quâque horâ.

It is important that its use be entered upon as soon as the presence of the characteristic whoop determines the nature of the disease. If the breathing is oppressed, or the symptoms present indicate the existence of bronchial inflammation, the administration of the sedative should be preceded by the exhibition of an emetic, and perhaps by the application of a few leeches to the chest.

If administered too freely, the acid will produce a greatly depressing effect on the vital powers. Should much debility, therefore, occur during its employment, the remedy should be omitted, and mild tonics, with a more stimulating expectorant, be exhibited for a few days, when the use of the hydrocyanic acid may be renewed.

"The dose of hydrocyanic acid for an infant," says Dr. Roe, "is about three-quarters of a minim of Scheele's strength, gradually increased to a minim, which may be given every fourth hour; for a child of three years of age, about one minim, gradually increased, if necessary, to a minim and a half every fourth hour; for children of ten or twelve years of age, a minim and a half, increased to two minims every fourth hour. It is safer to give this medicine in small doses at very short intervals, than to run any risk of producing too great depression by a large dose. The frequency of its exhibition must depend upon the strength of the patient and the severity of the attack. The dose should be repeated when the effects begin to subside, which in mild cases generally happens in three or four hours; but when much fever is present, its influence is felt but a very short time; under such circumstances, a larger quantity may be given and at shorter intervals, without any apprehension of danger, *so long as the fever lasts.*"

℞ Acidi hydrocyanici, medicinalis, f. ʒj.; liquor potassæ, f. ʒss.; infus. calumbæ, f. ʒij.; misturæ amygdal., f. ʒiv. Misce. capiat cochl. minim. ter die.

In cases of long-continued chronic bronchitis, the physician occasionally finds this disease complicated with a peculiar irritable condition of the gastric mucous membrane, manifested by tenderness of the epigastrium, a red tongue, frequent headache, and a feverish condition of the system. In such cases where the inflammation has extended to the mucous membrane of the stomach, producing this not uncommon form of *bronchogastritis*, the exhibition of the above combination with the hydrocyanic acid, the alkali, and the bitter vegetable infusion, will exert a prompt and a decidedly happy influence on this diseased action.

Combined with the extract of belladonna, hydrocyanic acid has also been found very useful in the treatment of *gastralgia* and in "*irritable gastric dyspepsia.*"

The following mixture prepared, and a teaspoonful of the medicine administered three or four times daily in these affections, will, by acting on the nerves of the stomach, greatly diminish their irritability.

℞ Extract belladonnæ, gr. x.; acidi hydrocyanici, medicinalis, gtt. lx.; tinct. calumbæ, sir. simp., aa. f. ʒj.; aquæ destillatæ, f. ʒij. Misce.

The above combination has likewise been employed with great benefit in the treatment of *spasmodic asthma.*

These, then, are some of the useful combinations of one of our most important therapeutic agents; and we can assure the practical physician that not only in these affections, to which allusions have been made, but in the treatment of many other diseases, he will find these remedies invaluable aids in controlling diseased action.

The *anhydrous*, or pure hydrocyanic acid, which consists of one equiv. of cyanogen, and one equiv. of hydrogen, is of a nature so exceedingly poisonous, that it cannot be employed with safety in medicine. The *medicinal* acid, which is the preparation that should always be directed to be used in our prescriptions, contains only 2.5 per cent. (United States Pharmacopœia) of the pure acid. That of the Apothecaries' Hall, London, contains 3.2 per cent.; whilst the medicinal acid of the French Apothecaries is nearly equal to that of the United States Pharmacopœia—namely 2.4 per cent. of the pure acid of Gay Lussac.

As the strength of the different medicinal acids cannot be depended on as being always of the same uniform power, it has been proposed that the cyanide of potassium be substituted in medicine for the hydrocyanic acid.

℞ Cyanidi potassii, gr. xxij.; alcohol. officinalis, f. ʒxj. Misce.

This preparation of cyanogen, which possesses the same medicinal qualities, and is of the same strength with the hydrocyanic acid, is greatly preferred by many practitioners as a therapeutic agent, inasmuch as it can be depended on as being always of a uniform strength. It may be used in the same doses and under the same circumstances in which the hydrocyanic acid is administered.

As palliatives in the treatment of all forms of *neuralgia*, the narcotics and sedatives are very generally resorted to by practitioners, especially during the paroxysms of the disease. When appropriately combined, their efficacy in these affections is more prompt and decided than when separately administered.

℞ Extracti hyoscyami, ʒss.; morphiæ sulphatis, gr. iij.;* strycnniæ, gr. ij.; capsici pulv., 3ss.; zinci sulphatis, gr. xv. **M.** Fiat massa, in pilulæ xxx. dividenda; capiat unam, ter quaterve in die.

In neuralgia, unattended by organic lesions, the above pills, exhibited every sixth or fourth hour; according to circumstances, will be found to be an excellent remedy. They have proved especially serviceable in that form of neuralgia in which the division of the fifth pair of nerves is so frequently involved. Not only in facial neuralgia, but in all cases where the disease has been caused by malaria, this combination may be administered with confidence that the result will be favorable. The valerianate of iron conjoined with the extract of hyoscyamus is an excellent antispasmodic and tonic, and may be employed with great advantage for the treatment of *chorea* and all the *neuralgic affections of anœmic and debilitated females.*

R. Extracti hyoscyami, 3ss.; ferri valerianatis, 3j. Fiat massa, et in pilulas triginta dividendas: quarum date unam ter in die.

The valerianate of iron and the valerianate of zinc are two highly valuable remedies, and were the therapeutic powers of these medicines better understood by the profession, they would be much more extensively employed than they now are for the treatment of disease. The valerianate of zinc, Dr. Neligan says, "is one of the most valuable modern additions to the Materia Medica."

R. Extracti hyoscyami, Ɖiss.; zinci valerianatis, Ɖj. Fiant pilulæ xxx. Capiat unam bis terve in die.

The above pill is a valuable remedy in the treatment of *facial neuralgia,* and, indeed, is equally serviceable in all the nervous and neuralgic affections for which the valerianate of iron has been advised.

R. Extracti belladonnæ, gr. viij.; camphori pulv., 3j.; quiniæ disulphatis, Ɖij. Misce; Fiant pilulæ triginti.

These pills are very effective in the treatment of *dysmenorrhœa.* One pill may be exhibited every hour or two hours till the pain ceases. In females of a nervous temperament, when painful menstruation occurs, independent of organic lesions, these pills, administered as above directed, seldom fail of affording relief. In those cases of dysmenorrhœa where a tonic is not particularly indicated, the following are more appropriate, and are equally efficacious.

R. Extracti belladonnæ, gr. viij.; ipecacuanhæ pulv., gr. x.; zinci sulphatis, 3ss. Misce; Fiant pilulæ xxx., quarum capiat unam quaque hora, donec leniatur dolor.

The following pills are highly recommended by an intelligent and experienced practitioner in the treatment of *leucorrhœa* occurring in anæmic and nervous females:

R. Extracti hyoscyami, 3j.; argenti nitratis, gr. x.; cantharidis pulv., gr. xij.; quiniæ disulphatis, Ɖij. Fiant pilulæ xl. Sumat unam mane et nocte.

The same physician advises the subjoined formula as a combination that may be employed with great advantage as a diuretic and alterative in the treatment of *cellular dropsy.*

R. Extracti conii, 3j.; cantharidis pul., Ɖij.; hydrarg. submur., 3ss.; ipecacuanhæ pulv., Ɖj. Misce; Fiat massa; in pilulæ xl. dividenda, cujus capiat unam ter quaterve in die.

A combination of the extract of belladonna with quinine has been employed very efficaciously in the treatment of *gastralgia.*

℞ Extracti belladonnæ, ℈ss.; quiniæ disulphatis, ʒj. M. Fiant pilulæ xxx. Sumat unam ter in die.

In that variety of gastralgia which is not unfrequently occurring in the course of *chronic gastritis*, we have derived the greatest benefit from the employment of the following pills.

℞ Extracti hyoscyami, ʒj.; argenti nitratis, gr. x.; bismuthi subnitratis, ʒiss. Fiant pilulæ xl.: quarum sumatur una mane ac nocte.

The nitrate of silver combined with some one of the sedative extracts may be employed advantageously in the treatment of almost all chronic gastric affections. In cases of obstinate, chronic gastritis, or long continued dyspepsia, we have found the following pills more efficacious than any other single remedy. They should be continued for several weeks:

℞ Extracti conii, *vel* lupuli, ʒj.; argenti nitratis, gr. x.; capsici pulv., quiniæ disulphatis, aa. ℈j. Misce; Fiat massa, in pilulas xl. dividenda. Capiat unam bis terve in die.

There is a troublesome and often an obstinate form of *gastric irritability*, denominated by the French *estomac glaireuse*, in which the patient occasionally ejects by eructation, a tasteless, watery fluid, and which is accompanied often by a severe burning pain in the epigastric region. This variety of the disease is arrested with great certainty by the exhibition of either the preceding, or the following pills.

℞ Extracti lupulinæ, ʒj.; argenti nitratis, gr. x.; bismuthi subnitratis, ʒiss.; quiniæ disulphatis, ℈ij. Fiant pilulæ xl.; cujus sumatur unam bis terve in die.

In *all forms of chronic disease, attended with acute pain*, as well as in all painful nervous affections, in the treatment of which, for any cause, full doses of opium are contra-indicated, the following combination may be administered with great advantage:

℞ Extracti hyoscyami, gr. xv.; extracti stramonii, gr. iv.; extracti humuli, ʒj.; morph. sulphatis, gr. iss. Misce. Divide in pilulas xxx.; quarum capiat unam omni semihora, donec leniatur dolor.

Of the therapeutic effects of muriate of ammonia, when internally administered, but little is known, as in this manner it is but rarely employed in this country. With the German physicians it has obtained a high reputation as a good alterative, and a promoter of healthy secretions in chronic diseases of the mucous and serous tissues. It not only promotes the mucous secretions, says Dr. Sunderlin, but the cutaneous exhalations, and improves also nutrition and assimilation. Combined with a sedative and narcotic, we have found it highly valuable in allaying irritation and in *promoting expectoration, in the early stage of phthisis*.

℞ Ammon. muriatis, ʒ ss.: opii pulv., gr. x.; digitalis pulv., scillæ pulv., aa. ℈j. Misce. Divide in pilulas triginti. Sumat unam quaque sexta hora.

Sleeplessness occurring in hypochondria, hysteria, and indeed in all nervous affections, may be overcome with great certainty by the administration of the following pills:

℞ Assafœtidæ, ʒj.; morphiæ sulphatis, gr. iij. M. Fiant pilulæ triginti, quarum exhibe unam vel duas hora decubitus.

The above pills—two to four exhibited daily—are very efficacious in arresting the dry cough which is occasionally consequent on disordered menstruation in nervous females.

Tonics and Stimulants.—The following combination of a chalybeate with a stimulant and a sedative has, for many years in our hands, proved a most valuable tonic, particularly when administered during convalescence from disease, and in all *debilitated and anæmic cases.*

℞ Extracti conii, ʒij.; sesqui-oxydi ferri, ʒiij.; tinct. calumbæ, ʒiss.; sir. toluta. ℥ss.; ol. gaultheriæ, gtt. x.; aquæ fontanæ, ℥ij. Fiat mistura; cujus sumat coch. parv. mane ac nocte.

Or the following may be substituted :

℞ Sesqui-oxydi ferri, extracti taraxaci, aa. ℥ss.; vini Xeris, ℥vj.; tinct. gaultheriæ, ℥ss.; aquæ font., ℥iv. M. capiat coch. magn. bis in die.

The following is a very excellent tonic, and may be exhibited whenever any of the ferruginous preparations are indicated.

℞ Ferri citratis, ʒij.; sir. citri, *vel* aurantiæ, aquæ menth. pip., aa. ℥ij.; aquæ puræ, ℥iv. M. exhibe cochlearium purum ter quaterve in die.

In *young anæmic females,* with indications of a chlorotic condition of the system; and also in *children of strumous habits,* the phosphate of iron, exhibited in combination with the sulphate of quinine, is a therapeutic agent of great value.

℞ Ferri phosphatis, ʒj.; quinæ disulphatis, gr. xij. M. Fiant pulv. xij., quarum capiat unam bis terve in die.

A physician of great experience, and celebrated for his successful treatment of diseases of females, has employed for many years, and with much advantage, the subjoined combination of an· alterative and a tonic in the management of *certain forms of uterine diseases.*

℞ Sirup. ferri iodidi, ℥j.; tinct. actææ racemosæ, ʒv.; tinct. rad. aconiti, ʒiij. Fiat mist. cujus cap. gtt. xx. ter in die.

We have seen engorgement of the os tincæ and non-malignant induration of this organ disappear rapidly under the persevering internal administration of the above tonic; while at the same time, the following ointment was applied once a week, by means of friction with the finger, to the indurated os.

℞ Extracti hyoscyami, extracti conii, extracti belladonnæ, aa. p. e.

To each ounce of which mixture add one drachm of iodide of potassa—mix thoroughly, and apply as above. `

℞ Ferri sulphatis, ʒij.; potassæ iodidi, ʒiss.; tinct. calumbæ, sirup zinziberis, aa. ℥ij. Fiat mist. capiat coch. parv. ter in die.

This mixture may be exhibited with advantage whenever we desire to promote the absorption of *glandular enlargements,* and in all cases where a tonic and an alterative are indicated.

Not unfrequently the general practitioner will encounter cases of obstinate intermittent; and of uncontrollable *neuralgic affections,* which will resist, altogether, the effects of the ordinary antispasmodics, when singly administered. In such instances, we have often succeeded perfectly, by the combination and exhibition of a vegetable and mineral tonic —as the following : .

℞ Liquor potassæ arsenitis, f. ʒiss.; tinct. cinchonæ, ℥iij.; sir. aurantiæ, ℥j. M. Hujns mist., sumat cochl. min. bis terve in die.

During the last two years, *intermittent fevers* have occurred more frequently, in some parts of this city, and in the vicinity of the city, than for many previous years. In some of these cases, where the disease has proved obstinate, not yielding to large doses of quinine, long continued, we have found it to be promptly arrested by the administration of a teaspoonful of the following mixture, twice or three times a day—the last dose being administered a short time before the period of the anticipated paroxysm.

℞ Quinæ sulp. ʒj.; liquor potassæ arsenitis, f. ʒlj.; acidi sulph. aromat., f. ʒj.; tinct. cinch. co., sir. zingiberis, aa. ʒij.

When the preparations of arsenic are employed, it is safest to give the medicine after a meal. When thus exhibited, larger, or more effectual doses may be given with more safety than when taken fasting. Should, however, gastric irritation arise, under its use, or swelling or stiffness of the eyelids occur, the medicine should be immediately discontinued.

Should it from any cause be desirable to administer these remedies in the form of a pill, we may employ the following formula:

℞ Acidi arseniosi, gr. ij.; quinæ disulphatis, ʒj.; conserv. rosæ, ʒss. Misce optime, et fiat massa, in pilulas xxx. dividenda; sumat unam bis quotidie.

We have had recently much experience in the use of the different preparations of manganese, and have become fully satisfied, that this mineral tonic, in its different combinations, will prove a most valuable addition to our pharmaceutic preparations.

The most important preparations of manganese for pharmaceutical purposes, are the *phosphate*, the *malate*, and the *iodide* of manganese.

After the subjoined formula, we have administered, in *tuberculosis*, to a large number of patients, the phosphate of manganese, with most favorable results.

℞ Manganesii phosphatis, ʒij.; tinct. cinchonæ, ʒiij.; sir. sarsæ, ʒiv.; mucil. acaciæ, ʒj.; ol. gaultheriæ, gtt. xx. Fiat mistura, cujus sumantur coch. duo vel tria minima bis terve in die.

Or we may administer, under similar circumstances, and to the same amount, the manganese combined with some of the preparations of iron; as in the following:

℞ Manganesii phosphatis, ʒiss.; ferri phosphatis, ʒiij.; tinct. calumbæ ʒij.: sir. tolutan. ʒiv.; ess. gaultheriæ, f. ʒj.

These mixtures should be kept in well-closed bottles, and as the manganese is not altogether soluble, the medicine should be shaken before being administered.

The malate of manganese is considered, by some practitioners, a more eligible preparation, inasmuch as it is quite soluble, and the base of the salt is in the form of proto-oxide, the acid being easily digested.

℞ Manganesii malat., ʒij.; tinct cinch., ʒij.; sir. simp. ʒiv.; ess. limon. f. ʒj. Fiat mistura, date coch, parv. mane ac nocte.

The iodide of manganese is an efficient remedy in the treatment of *glandular enlargements*, especially those of the neck, and of the spleen, in constitutional syphilis, and in the anemia arising from scrofula and from cancerous affections.

It may be administered in the form of pills; or as a mixture in the following formula:

℞ Manganesii iodid., ʒij.; tinct. cardamom., ʒj.; sir. sarsæ, ʒv. Misce. Sumat coch. parv. bis terve in die.

M. Petrequin has found manganese and iron, especially useful in blood diseases, such as the chloro-anæmia, after hemorrhage, operations, metror rhagia, etc. In the chlorosis which appears about puberty, in that also which occurs at the critical period of woman, especially when profuse hemorrhage prevails, and in the depraved state of the blood, which succeeds intermittent fevers, M. Petrequin has found the ferro-manganese preparations of remarkable efficacy. *Part* xxxii., *p.* 271.

Phosphate of Lime.—This substance may be rendered much more soluble, and therefore useful, by uniting it with carbonate of lime in the following proportions: phosphate of lime, 4 grammes; carbonate of lime, 8 grammes; sugar of milk 12 grammes. *Part* xxxiii., *p.* 284.

Muriate of Ammonia, internally.—It may be given in many chronic inflammatory diseases, as chronic bronchitis, enlargement of the lymphatic glands, chronic skin diseases, and chronic rheumatism. Dr. Watson testifies to its efficacy in certain forms of facial neuralgia, nervous headache, toothache, and sciatica. Its action is sometimes remarkably beneficial; when the secretion from the pulmonary mucous membrane is tough and tenacious, it speedily becomes altered in quality and consistence. In chronic periosteal inflammation, having a syphilitic origin, it seldom fails to give relief. In indolent bubo a strong solution (ʒij. to ʒj.) may be kept constantly applied, and five to ten grains may be given internally three or four times a day. In neuralgic affections, Dr. Ebden has given from 25 to 30 grains for a dose. *Part* xxxiii., *p.* 288.

Bichromate of Potash for Preservative Solutions.—This salt, in proportion of about four grains to an ounce of water, constitutes a solution quite equal to alcohol in its antiseptic powers, and which costs only about twopence a gallon. It will deprive a specimen already partially decomposed, of all odor, and preserve it for any length of time. As, instead of hardening, it a little softens tissues immersed in it, it has a great advantage over both alcohol and Goadby's solution, for all objects which are intended to be reëxamined, especially if the microscope is to be used. Preparations long kept in it become of a light olive green color externally, but retain most perfectly their natural appearance at a little depth from the surface. The change of color in the case of red structures such as muscle, may be prevented by the addition of a little nitrate of potash. In the same way, if it is desired, the softening may be prevented by the use of alum. Unless in combination with both the two last-named ingredients, it is scarcely adapted for a permanent solution. The great advantage over all others is, in respect to specimens intended to be kept for limited periods, either for private dissection or for exhibition. Those intended for the microscope are far less spoiled by it than by any other which I am acquainted with. The only odor which it gives to specimens is a very peculiar one, resembling that of new kid gloves. The cheapness and efficacy of this salt will, I think, make it quite a boon to pathologists.

Part xxxiii., *p.* 292.

Chlorodyne.—This agent given internally in doses of about twelve minims in a little water is a most pleasing anodyne. Its effects last for several days. It is particularly useful where opium cannot be tolerated.

Part xxxvi., *p.* 299.

Strychnia, Uses of.—In cases of organic lesion of the nervous centres, epilepsy, chorea, paralysis agitans, it is useless or even injurious. It is in cases of *functional derangement* where the *nervous powers* are wanting in vigor, where lassitude is a prominent symptom, as in dyspepsia of literary men and delicate females; chlorosis is perhaps the typical disease where it is of most use; if you substitute strychnia for quina in the usual prescription of quinine and iron in this disease, the effects will be truly aston-ishing. There is a double citrate of iron and strychnia analogous to the well-known preparation of iron and quina; this is particularly applicable; it contains one grain of strychnia to every hundred of the salt. Another convenient way of giving strychnia is to dissolve a grain in two minims of sulphuric acid, and add this to thirty ounces of water in which one drachm of ammonio-citrate of iron has been dissolved; the whole may be then placed in a gazogene and charged with carbonic acid. Give a wine-glass full of this daily, immediately before lunch. A very remarkable case of the efficacy of the above is related by Dr. De Ricci. *Part* xxxvii., *p.* 49.'

Pepsine.—This must not be expected to digest a large quantity of meat at once. A patient taking it must not eat more meat than a mutton chop at once. Pepsine loses its power in a week or ten days, by which time either the stomach has regained its tone, or some other remedy must be employed. About fifteen grains of Boudault's pepsine must be given about twice a-day, before meals, and spread between two thin slices of bread like a sandwich.   *Part* xxxvii., *p.* 78.

Prescriptions containing Henbane or Belladonna.—Never in any prescription combine any caustic-fixed alkali with tincture or extract of henbane, as the latter is thereby completely neutralized. Where it is desirable to administer an alkaline remedy with henbane, order either a carbonate or bicarbonate, which are quite as efficacious. The same pre-cautions apply to belladonna and stramonium.   *Part* xxxvii., *p.* 258.

Cocoa-Nut Oil Ointments.—The cocoa-nut oil is a more eligible body for the formation of ointments than lard, keeping much better, not staining the linen, and admitting of more complete absorption. To render the oil of commerce fit for pharmaceutical employment, it is in general sufficient to liquefy it at a moderate temperature, and strain it through linen. But if it retains its peculiar odor too strongly, and is of too yellow a color, it may be purified by digesting it for some hours in a water-bath, with some coarsely powdered vegetable charcoal, and filtering it while warm through paper. The following are some of the formulæ that have been tried with success:

R Iod. pot. ℨj., ol. cocos. ℨj.
R Ext. bellad. Ɗj., ol. coc. ℈iij.
R Veratrini, gr. iij., ol. coc. ℈iij.
R Sulph. quin. Ɗj, ol. coc. ℨj., ol. rosar. gtt. x. (very useful in pityriasis capitis.)
R Chlorof., ol. coc., aa. ℨj. (of great service in neuralgic and rheumatic pains, rendering the chloroform more fixed, and its action more durable.)
R Ol. terebinth., ol. coc., aa. ℨj.
R Hydr. ox. rub. gr. iv., ol. coc. ℨij.   *Part* xxxvii., *p.* 265.

Citrate of Iron and Strychnia.—The citrate of iron and strychnia is a preparation which has lately been used with considerable success at the Royal Free Hospital, by Dr. O'Connor. The dose is about three grains three times a day, and taken immediately after a meal. In cases of dys-pepsia of an atonic character, in atonic affections of the uterus, as an em-menagogue, and in chorea, it has chiefly proved useful.   *Part* xxxvii., *p.* 272.

Glonoine—Nitrate of Oxide of Glycil.—If nitric and sulphuric acids be added to glycerine, and the whole be kept at a freezing temperature, a compound is obtained, which is a nitrate of oxide of glycyl; this is possessed of the most powerful properties. For use, one drop diluted with ninety-nine of rectified spirit is the proper quantity, so energetic are its properties; of this, give a quarter of a drop in a dessertspoonful of water. In all spasmodic and painful affections, this will give instant relief; it has not been tried in tetanus and hydrophobia. If the pain or spasm be not simply neuralgic, but dependent on some deeper seated cause, it will of course only act as a palliative. Great caution must be exhibited in its use.

Part xxxvii., *p.* 295.

Opium and Sulphate of Quinine—Antagonistic Action.—M. Gubler, in a paper read before the Société Médicale des Hôpitaux, has attempted to establish a direct antagonistic action between the sulphate of quinine and opium. He states, that while opium causes cerebral congestion, quinine possesses a diametrically opposite influence.

In support of his theory, the author relates a case in which 30 grains of quinine and 5 grains of extract of opium simultaneously administered, failed to produce either the characteristic intoxication of quinine or the somnolency to be expected from opium. *Part* xxxviii., *p.* 248.

Imitation of Natural Spas.—Dr. Aldridge gives the following:

The spas that I have hitherto succeeded in imitating are the Rakoczy and Pandur Brunnens at Kissingen, and the Elizabethan Brunnen at Homberg. These are all so similar to each other—only varying in the proportions of their constituents—that it will be only necessary, at present, to give the formula for one of them. The one that I propose for this purpose is that of the Rakoczy:

Lime water, 3 wine pints; carbonated solution of magnesia, 11 ozs.; Bewley and Evans' soda water (No. 4), 12 drs.; sulphate of iron, 8 grs.; sulphate of manganese, 1 gr.; phosphate of soda, 2 grs.; chloride of sodium, 1 oz.; carbonate of potash, 10 grs.; muriatic acid (1160), 4 drs.; bicarbonate of soda, 5 grs.; silicate of soda, 30 grs.

Dissolve and filter the solution; divide into twelve equal parts; put each part into a bottle capable of holding a wine-pint; fill up with Bewley and Evans' soda water (No. 1), and cork rapidly.

The contents of one of the above bottles, taken in divided portions, about an hour before breakfast, will be found to possess all the physiological effects of the spa drank at the source. It will be found useful in cases of gout, dyspepsia, epigastric fullness, habitual constipation, neuralgia, obesity, etc. t is well not to continue its use for a longer period than nine days or a fortnight, and to follow the treatment by the exhibition of some mild tonic. Its employment is unsafe when there is weak action of the heart or where there is a tendency to cerebral congestion, or hemorrhage from any surface. *Part* xxxviii., *p.* 292.

Iodide of Calcium.—This salt is very valuable in cases in which the iodide of potassium is inadmissible. It does not occasion iodism, or resorption of the healthy tissues. It does not excite the circulation, nor irritate the stomach and bladder, by passing off too rapidly by the kidneys. Its solution in milk is perfectly tasteless. It is particularly useful in squamous diseases of the skin, and chronic metallic poisoning by mercury, lead, and copper.   *Part* xxxviii., *p.* 292.

New Method of Preparing the Phosphate of Lime of Bones.—On the ground of the necessity which exists for the administration of phosphate of lime in the molecular state which is best adapted for its incorporation into the living organs, M. Dannacy, of Bordeaux, proposes the following preparation of this salt: Beef-bones washed and powdered, common water, and pure carbonate of potash or soda, are boiled together for an hour, when a perfectly homogeneous substance is formed; this substance is thrown upon a paper filter, and the alkaline liquid flows out; the mass is washed at several intervals with hot water; it is then dried and passed through a silk sieve, when a powder of excessive tenacity is obtained, soft to the touch, and of a mobility equal to that of lycopodium. This powder contains all the natural elements of bones, but without the gelatine which holds them together; the disaggregation attains its utmost limit, and is truly molecular. The phosphate of lime of bones thus prepared is easily kept in suspension in potions and in cod-liver oil, and it is easily molded into different pharmaceutical forms, as pastilles, pills, etc.
                          Part xxxviii., *p.* 293.

Substitute for Human Milk.—[The human milk contains, besides salts of lime, chloride of potassium. Now, in common with carbonic acid, this salt enjoys the peculiar property of dissolving carbonate of lime or chalk. An absence of it in the food, as in wheat bread, is very injurious to a growing child. Hence a child fed on pap for a time grows fat, but the bones are soft; frequently it sickens, and severe symptoms supervene.]

Amongst the vegetable substances, that which comes closest to milk in its composition is, without doubt, lentil powder, or, as it is called for the purposes of obtaining a better sale, Revalenta Arabica, containing both phosphoric acid in abundance, and chloride of potassium; it also includes casein, the same principle which is found in milk in its constituent parts. Moreover, its nutritive matter is to its calorifiant matter in the proportion of 1 to $2\frac{1}{2}$, milk being in that of 1 to 2. No wonder, therefore, that under its influence many children affected with atrophy and marked debility have completely recovered.

Lentils have also a slightly laxative effect, and therefore, in many instances, where the child is of a constipated habit, they are to be recommended. Peas and beans in this respect resemble lentils; the former, however, are objectionable, on the ground that they produce much flatuleney. The latter is not generally obtainable; still the bakers take advantage of this fact in regard to beans, and usually, where wheat by partial germination has lost some of its nitrogenous aliment, or where the flour used is poor in quality, they add a proportionate quantity of white bean flour, to restore it to its proper nutritive value.   *Part* xxxviii., *p.* 294.

Tests for Adulterations of Medicinal Substances.—Dr. Squibb having had much practical experience in the preparation of officinal substances for the United States' navy, believes that advantage may attend the publication of a few simple tests of their purity, requiring little time, skill, or apparatus for their application.

Ether.—A strip of unsized paper, or a clean glass rod dipped into the ether and allowed to dry for a moment or two, will, by the odor it gives, afford evidence of the less volatile impurities it commonly contains. There usually remains a somewhat aromatic, slightly pungent odor, that is not hurtful in the more dilute ether used for common medicinal purposes, but the disagreeable oily odor often found is more objectionable, while really good ether should have no odor whatever. The ether used for inhalation should leave no foreign odor whatever. The strength of ether is less easily ascertained; but with a little practice, and having a good specimen for comparison, a very satisfactory estimate may be found in the slowness or rapidity of its evaporation from the palm of the hand. Ether for inhalation should give off bubbles of vapor rapidly at the temperature of the palm. A thin test tube, containing the specimen, should be grasped firmly for a minute or two, and then the ether should be stirred at the time of observation.

Hoffman's Anodyne.—Two drops of officinal compound spirit of ether, stirred into a pint of water, give to the mixture a distinct oily surface, and the peculiar fruity, aromatic odor of the heavy oil of wine free from the odor of ether and alcohol. Sixty drops render the water decidedly turbid: while, with four fluid drachms, a scanty precipitate of minute oil globules occurs after a few minutes standing. The fruity, apple-like odor is characteristic of the chief anodyne ingredient, the oil of wine, and is entirely wanting in the ordinary commercial article; and without this oil the preparation is a stimulant antispasmodic. With the oil it is a highly valuable anodyne antispasmodic, particularly adapted to nervous irritation and hysteria. The liquid universally sold is a residue of the ether-making process, containing varying proportions of ether and alcohol, with a little etherole or light oil of wine; but in no instance of the many examinations made by the writer, has any true heavy oil of wine been found.

Spirit of Nitric Ether.—Two or three fluid drachms of good sweet spirit of nitre, not more than seven or eight months old, plunged in an ordinary test tube, into water heated to 164°, will boil pretty actively; and, if fresh, or if well preserved from light and air, no matter what its age, it will boil actively in water at 156°. From the fact that this, among other liquids, may be heated far above its boiling point without ebullition, it becomes necessary to drop a few fragments of broken glass into the test tube with the spirit, after the latter has been heated and while still held in the water. Again, the formation of small gas bubbles around the fragments of glass, which occurs, as a fine effervescence, at any temperature above 140°, in any spirit that contains hyponitrous ether at all, must be distinguished from true ebullition, in which the bubbles are much larger, and form, as they successively reach the surface, beads around the edge of the liquid—this latter only occurring at the temperatures named. The preparation should not be quite colorless, but of a pale straw tint, and it should effervesce very slightly on the addition of carbonate of ammonia. When slightly acid the ammonia is the best corrigent, as the salts formed are therapeutically similar. The officinal preparation is a solution of five per cent. of hyponitrous ether in alcohol, while in commerce it is rare to find it containing more than three per cent., and in a great majority of cases it is below two per cent., and often in a proportion too small to be detected except by the odor. It thus happens that the physician who prescribes it for its diuretic or diaphoretic effects is disappointed, so much alcohol being substituted; and the preparation is falling into consequent disuse.

Choroform.—When equal volumes of chloroform and colorless concentrated sulphuric acid (or the strong commercial oil of vitriol) are shaken together in a glass-stoppered vial, there should be no color imparted to either liquor, or but a faint tinge of color, after twelve hours standing. Nor should there be any heat developed in the mixture at the time of shaking it first. All particles of dust, cork, or other organic matters must be excluded, or coloring will be produced; and if at the end of twelve hours the acid be only faintly tinged, it may be attributed to some such accidental cause. If, however, then or sooner it has become yellow, brown, or any dark color, the chloroform should be rejected. If warmth takes place on first shaking the mixture, it indicates an admixture of alcohol. One or two drachms of chloroform, spontaneously evaporated from a clean surface of glass or porcelain, or from clean, unsized paper, should leave no odor. Commercial chloroform will generally turn the acid brown in two or three hours, and will often render it black and tarry-looking within two or three days; while with chemically pure chloroform there is absolutely no reaction within many days.

Calomel.—The most common and injurious contamination is corrosive sublimate, which is easily detected by shaking a drachm or two in a test tube, with distilled water, and when the water has become clear, adding a drop or two of liquor ammonia. This will precipitate the sublimate, and render the water cloudy.

Iodide of mercury is often irritant and harsh in its action, owing to contamination with biniodide from faulty preparation. This is detected by rubbing a little of the iodide in a mortar with strong alcohol, and leaving it a few minutes to dry. The evaporation of the alcohol leaves the red iodide as a border to the iodide around the pestle, and in this way a minute contamination is detected.

Mercury with chalk has of late been often found harsh and irritating in its action, owing to faulty preparation, a portion of the mercury becoming oxidized, instead of being simply comminuted. To detect the peroxide a drachm or two should be treated with an excess of acetic acid, filtered, and then a few drops of hydrochloric acid added to the clear solution. If the preparation be good only a slight precipitate of insoluble subchloride will take place, from the small quantity of acetate of suboxide formed. If the preparation be old or badly kept, a pretty copious precipitate results. The clear solution is again filtered or decanted off this precipitate, and liquor ammonia is added. If the preparation is contaminated by the peroxide it will be thrown down in the form of white precipitate.

Blue pill may also contain the oxides of mercury, and thus lose its mild character. They may be detected in the same way as in the mercury with chalk.

Iodide of potassium is occasionally contaminated with carbonate of potassa, to the extent of impairing its medicinal power. This is easily detected, by adding lime-water to the solution of the iodide, when carbonate of lime will be precipitated, rendering the mixture cloudy.

Bitartrate of potassa frequently contains much tartrate of lime, which may be detected by stirring a few drops of liquor ammonia into a mixture of a few grains of the specimen in two or three drachms of cold water. The ammonia renders the otherwise insoluble potassa quite soluble, while it has no immediate effect on the tartrate of lime. If then a portion remain undissolved after the application of this test, it may be regarded as an impurity. *Part* xxxviii., *p.* 294.

Preserving Fluid for Microscopical Preparations.—M. Pacini strongly recommends the following fluid for the preservation of blood globules, nerves, ganglions, the retina, and all the soft tissues, which keep their form and appearance while they become hardened; perchloride of mercury 1, chloride of iodine (*chlorure iodique*) 2, glycerine (at 25° of Baumé) 3, and distilled water 113 parts. The mixture should stand for two months, and then one part of the liquid is to be diluted with three parts of distilled water and filtered. *Part* xxxviii., *p.* 296.

Iodate of Potash.—Messrs. Demarquay and Custin consider that the action of this salt is more powerful than that of the chlorate of the same base, and that it has yielded excellent results where the chlorate of potash had failed. The dose varies from five to twenty-two grains, and it has been used in diphtheritis, mercurial and gangrenous stomatitis, etc.
Part xxxviii., *p.* 296.

MELANCHOLIA.

Use of Seton.—In cases of obscure melancholia, a seton to the nucha, sometimes acts like a charm. It is particularly beneficial, in the shape of thin single filaments of gutta percha, or some other substance not permeable to pus. *Part* xxxiii., *p.* 237.

Vide " Insanity."

MELANOSIS.

Melanosis.—[There is an error in applying this term to all tumors and deposits of a dark color, no matter what their character or situation. Melanotic swellings appear to be pigment-colored morbid products, very variable in character, especially cancerous. Mr. Coote thinks the character of this affection, as described by Mr. S. Cooper, is calculated to put it in an improper light. He says:]

Chemical analysis by MM. Lassaigne and Foy, has shown that melanotic matter differs but little from blood in its ultimate elements. A solution of chlorine will bleach the black mass from a melanotic eye, consequently, it differs essentially from the carbonaceous deposits in the lungs of miners. This statement receives further confirmation from microscopical examination. Melanotic tumors do not consist of an unorganized deposit; the cells have their periods of growth, maturity, and decay; neither can they be regarded as mere accumulations of pigment, for the cells have a totally different form from those of healthy choroid.

In order to establish the view that melanosis, when fatal, is combined with the elements of cancer, it is necessary to define what these cancerous

elements are.   In the sooty-black non-vascular patch, characterizing cutaneous melanosis (an affection which Mr. Lawrence regards as malignant),
I never could discover any structural affinity with cancer, medullaris, or
fungoides.   It is true, that cancerous tumors may be sometimes colored
by pigment deposit, but that is no proof of the patient being affected with
melanosis.   The cavity of the globe may be occupied by a mass partially
black and partially white, or of reddish hue ; but it must be remembered
that diseases of different characters often manifest themselves in the same
tumor.   Melanotic tumors occasionally present a spotted appearance,
some parts being of a lighter color than others ; but this may depend upon
variations in the quantity of the pigment granules contained in the cells.
   The constant occurrence of primary melanosis in situations where, in the
healthy state, pigment is often deposited ; the chemical composition of
such tumors ; the appearances which they present both to the naked eye
and when placed under the microscope, warrant the inference that this is
a disease sui generis, manifesting itself by the accumulation of pigment
cells in a morbid state.   It is difficult exactly to define the meaning of the
term " malignant."   In man, however, melanosis is a rapidly fatal disease.
When once fairly established, whether the primary tumor be extirpated
or not, the patient dies, in the course of one or two years, of accumulations of similar character in all parts of the body.   In the horse the disease
is not so fatal.   Mr. Spencer has known an animal live for ten years after
the removal of the primary tumor, being fit for work the whole time.
   [In the human subject, melanosis is most frequently met with from the
40th to the 60th years.   Mr. Coote goes on to say :]
   Melanosis of the eye commences between the choroid and retina; the
former membrane remains of its natural consistence ; the latter is compressed, pushed to one side, or to the centre of the globe, but not otherwise altered.   In the earliest stage the eye becomes amaurotic, without
obvious cause ; frequent attacks of inflammation come on; but from five to
eight years may elapse without any morbid change being observable.
Then, if the growth proceeds from the posterior part of the eye, the retina
is pushed forward ; the vitreous humor is absorbed ; the posterior capsular vessels are destroyed, and the lens, rendered opaque, protrudes, together with the iris, into the anterior chamber.   The conjunctival vessels
become enlarged, tortuous, and distended with blood ; the sclerotic coat
yields unequally, and presents an irregular lobulated appearance, resembling staphyloma.   Sudden attacks of inflammation, attended with pain
and chemotic swelling, come on; the sclerotic coat gives way, either a
few lines from the margin of the cornea, or near the entrance of the optic
nerve; and the melanotic mass, freed from restraint, protrudes, covered
by conjunctiva, from the eyeball.   Primary melanotic tumors of the skin
are either cutaneous or subcutaneous.   The two commonly occur together.
   Cutaneous deposits (melanose membraniforme, Andral) appear as
smooth black spots, with a defined margin, varying in size from a pin's
head to a shilling, lying upon the cutis, and covered by the cuticle, which
is not raised.   Subcutaneous deposits (melanose tuberaforme, Andral)
exist as dark colored tubercles, varying in size from a pin's head to a
small orange.   Invisible when small, they distend the skin as they acquire
bulk, and appear as prominent bluish-black spots ; the color deepest in
the centre, gradually fading away to the circumference.   •

The integuments at last give way, and a black mass protrudes; the surrounding vessels pour forth some blood, and a dark-colored fluid flows from the open surface. If the mass be removed wholly, by the knife, or partially, by ligature, the wound will heal, but the disease inevitably returns, either in the cicatrix or some distant part.

The primary disease advances with unequal rapidity, but secondary accumulations generally form before the primary tumor has attained very considerable size. The absorbent glands are rarely affected. The development of internal disease is marked by general lassitude, and undefined pains over the trunk and limbs; the rest is disturbed; the appetite fails, and emaciation commences. The liver, rapidly increasing in size, projects with irregular surface from the lower margins of the ribs, and distends the abdomen; dark-colored matter is voided by the bowels or ejected from the stomach; the diarrhœa, if arrested, alternates with violent and uncontrollable pains in the head, and the patient dies exhausted, but retaining his faculties to the last.

Upon examining such a case after death, melanotic matter is found accumulated in every part of the body, except, perhaps, the cornea, synovial membranes, and tendinous structures. *Part* xiv., *p.* 128.

MELÆNA.

Acute Melœna cured by Gallic Acid.—Dr. Durrant, secretary to the Ipswich Medical Society, mentions the case of a cachectic young man with acute melæna, in which antiphlogistic remedies, acetate of lead, and turpentine with tincture of opium, were given without benefit. Four grains of gallic acid were then administered every four hours, with tincture of opium, and the discharge shortly ceased. *Part* xv., *p.* 120.

Treatment of Melœna.—Give oil of turpentine (which by its stimulant properties will excite the intestines to contract, and so mechanically check the bleeding) and small doses of gallic acid in the solid form. And let the diet be liquid, concentrated, cold, and given in very small quantities at a time. (Dr. Neligan.) *Part* xxi., *p.* 362.

MENINGITIS.

Tubercular—Case of.—A fine boy of nine months old, was suddenly attacked with convulsions. He recovered from these, and cut his first teeth shortly afterward; he was soon observed to fall away, to become listless, and to lose his appetite, without any condition of tongue which could indicate intestinal derangement. His bowels became constipated, his pulse irregular, and he began to vomit and to become torpid. Fever was soon added to his symptoms, and it was evident that he was the subject of meningitis. Leeches were applied, and calomel given, but in spite of treatment he lapsed into complete coma. As soon as the latter symptom became distinct, tartar emetic ointment was rubbed into the scalp every four hours over a space the size of a crown piece. Free suppuration ensued, and signs of amelioration were speedily witnessed. The child became gradually more sensible, his appetite returned, and in a fortnight all traces of his malady had vanished.　Dr. Hahn continues :

When there have been no previous symptoms indicative of tubercular diathesis, bleeding must be employed and calomel given.　The latter is chiefly to be relied on ; but we must not salivate unnecessarily.　Cold effusions will be found useful, sometimes availing to arouse the child after the supervention of complete coma.　But in the comatose condition, friction of the scalp with tartar emetic ointment, repeated every two hours till pustulation is established, will be of the greatest value.　When symptoms denoting general tubercular cachexia precede the cerebral affection, blood-letting, except loc lly and sparingly, is contra-indicated, and calomel cannot be pushed to the same extent.　But the counter-irritation may be employed as in the previous case.　　　　　　　　　　*Part* xxi., *p.* 73.

Meningitis, Tubercular.—By judicious management blood-letting may be almost dispensed with, in this as in most other diseases of infancy.　Its effects may be obtained by the use of the warm bath, antimonials, and diuretics, the latter medicines having a very striking antiphlogistic effect ; purgatives would serve the same end, but they cannot, except enemata, be safely used in many diseases of children.　In the more advanced stages, "calomel for the removal of lymph, and iodine (liq. potassæ iodidi comp.) for the absorption of effused fluid, are well known and trustworthy remedies."

It is very difficult in the cerebral affections of childhood, to distinguish cases which require antiphlogistic treatment from those requiring stimulants.　The occurrence of febrile disturbance will generally show that active treatment is required ; but if the fever is intermittent, leaving the patient depressed in the intervals, we must be very cautious how we use lowering measures.　(Dr. Copeman.)　　　　　　　　　*Part* xxi., *p.* 74.

Syphilitic Miningitis.—*Vide* Art. "Brain."

———•◦•———

MENORRHAGIA.

Ergot of Rye.—Speaking of the effects of ergot of rye in menorrhagia, Dr. Burne says:

，　I have heard persons express doubts of its efficacy ; but so many cases under my own care have been benefited or cured by it, that I cannot but regard it as a most valuable addition to the materia medica. . . . Cases in which an exhausting draining hemorrhage has persisted for five or six weeks after abortion, have yielded at once to the influence of the ergot.

It is very important that the ergot should not be at all in a state of decay.　　　　　　　　　　　　　　　　　　　　　*Part* ii., *p.* 33.

Gallic Acid in Menorrhagia.—In a paper read before the Medico-Chirurgical Society of Edinburgh, Professor Simpson stated that for the last year he had employed gallic acid in some cases of menorrhagia, with the most successful results.　Like all the other remedies directed against that disease, it had also occasionally failed in his hands.　Some of the cases which had completely yielded under its use were of an old standing, and aggravated description.　He gave it during the intervals, as well as during the discharge, in doses of from ten to twenty grains per day made into pills. It had this advantage over most other antihemorrhagic medicines, that it had no constipating effect upon the bowels. *Part* viii., *p.* 65.

Treatment of Menorrhagia.—Dr. Ditterich recommends the internal use of nitrate of silver as a remedy for this troublesome and obstinate complaint, as well as for the leucorrhœa which is present during the intervals and the nervous symptoms. The prescription is: R Nit. argenti, gr. iij.; aquæ destil. ʒij. solve. Of this solution ten drops are to be taken two or three times daily, and gradually increased to fifteen drops. The author affirms that the use of this solution, for a period of from four to six weeks, will perform a certain cure. After the lapse of about ten days, the leucorrhœa diminishes, and by the second menstrual period, the catamenial secretion is reduced to the proper quantity, and the nervous symptoms disappear. Koph has also recommended the nitrate of silver for the same disease in doses of one-tenth to one-twelfth of a grain every two hours. *Part* xiii., *p.* 361.

Treatment of Menorrhagia by Indian Hemp.—[It appears that the value of Indian hemp is not confined to neuralgic cases. Dr. Mitchell recommends it in uterine hemorrhage. Dr. M. says,] There are two tinctures in use, one of the herb, and the other made with the resin—the former is of little use, but the latter is a powerful medicine; when mixed with water it becomes milky, owing to the separation of the resin, to obviate which it is better to combine it with mucilage, or a small quantity of spirit: the dose that I have given of it is ten minims repeated every four hours; sometimes the first dose succeeds in checking a discharge which has lasted months, and that notwithstanding the employment of the most energetic means usually resorted to, including the whole range of astringents and plugging the vagina. In these cases it acts almost like magic. There is another form of hemorrhage which the practitioner will also find it of great value in; I allude to that distressing, debilitated sort of draining which occurs in some women when pregnant. In these cases the ordinary astringents frequently fail, and the ergot of rye, in consequence of inducing uterine contraction, is inadmissible. In these cases the tincture of hemp will be found peculiarly useful. *Part* xvi., *p.* 276.

Thlaspi Bursa Pastoris, in Menorrhagia.—Give decoction of thlaspi bursa pastoris (shepherd's purse); a handful of the fresh plant in three teacupfuls of water, boiled down to two—dose, a cupful twice a day.
Part xix., *p.* 270.

Oxide of Silver in Menorrhagia.—Give oxide of silver, in doses of half a grain or a grain three times a day, combined with a small quantity of morphia or opium. It is almost a specific for those cases in which there is no organic lesion. If there are high inflammatory symptoms, these must be subdued before beginning with the remedy. Oxide of silver blackens the stools. *Part* xx., *p.* 228.

Menorrhagia.—During an attack of the hemorrhage, let the patient take of ext. matico alcohol, gr. v.; plumbi diacet., gr. ij. M., ft. pil. ij. quartis horis. R Secalis cornuti, sodæ bib.orat., aa. Ðj.; mist. acaciæ, ʒss. aquæ cinnam., ʒiij. M. ft. haust. sumat demid. cum pilulis. Mr. Hooper.

prepares a combination of the diacetate of lead with the spirituous **ext.** of matico, than which no styptic appears more powerful.

Part xxvii., p. 354.

Profuse Menstruation, commonly termed Menorrhagia.—When Menorrhagia takes place in plethoric habits, says Dr. Oke, it is manifestly remedial, and ought not to be hastily restrained. In such a case the plethora is the object to be kept in view, rather than the discharge; and it will be best treated by a cooling diet, the recumbent position, and the mixture (*a*).

(*a*) ℞ Magnesiæ sulphatis, ʒvj.; infusi rosæ comp., ℥vss.; sirupi simplicis, ℥ss.; acidi sulphurici diluti, ℥ss. Misce. Fiat mistura, cujus capiatur fluiduncia ter quotidie.

But when the discharge has continued for a considerable length of time, producing an anæmic condition and great debility, the indication of cure will clearly be to restrain the uterine flux as speedily as possible by general and local means.

The system may be strengthened by (*b*).

(*b*) ℞ Confectionis rosæ, ℥ss.; infusi rosæ comp., ℥iij.; decocti cinchonæ, ℥iij. Misce et cola.

Colaturæ adde

Acidi sulphurici diluti, ʒj.; tincturæ opii, ♏xxx. Fiat mistura, cujus capiat quartam partem ter quotidie.

Opium, in menorrhagia, from this cause, is a valuable remedy, as it is found to increase the force of circular muscles; whilst henbane, hemlock, and belladonna relax them. Hence it is that the former contracts whilst the latter dilates the iris; and hence, also, the great use of opium in restraining profuse and dangerous hemorrhage after parturition, by causing contractions of the muscular walls of the uterus.

The bowels, if necessary, should be regulated by gentle aperients, such as the following:

℞ Pulveris rhei, balsami copaibæ, aa. ʒss. Misce; et divide in pilulas xij., quarum capiat duas horâ somni pro re natâ.

Turpentine and the secale cornutum have also been found efficacious in restraining menorrhagic discharge.

The best local remedy is the sulphate of alum hip-bath, which may be made in the proportion of twelve ounces of alum to two gallons of water. It may be used daily for about twenty minutes, first tepid, thence gradually reducing it to the normal temperature.

Should the discharge continue unabated, notwithstanding the use of the above remedies, a polypous growth or some morbid condition of the uterus is to be suspected; and the uterus must then be examined.

Part xxviii., p. 287.

Use of Cinnamon in certain Examples of Menorrhagia.—The symptoms usually presented are briefly these: the catamenia appear regularly every twenty-eight days, and are at first only of the proper quantity; but, instead of ceasing after a duration of three or four days, they continue unabated for ten or fourteen, and occasionally even for three weeks. The general symptoms which arise from this debilitating discharge are just such as might be expected. There is general weakness, languor, mental depression, with pains in the head, loins, and so on; the patient suffering, it is to be remembered, not from any diseased condition, giving rise to the hemorrhage, but merely from the loss of blood itself. In other instances the discharge continues a less time, but the flow is more abundant, clots being frequently discharged; this variety is generally followed by leucorrhœa.

Dr. Tanner was led to try the use of cinnamon, and having derived the most beneficial effects from its employment, recommends ʒj. doses of the tincture of cinnamon every six hours, to be continued for fourteen days after the symptoms have disappeared. If the case has been an obstinate one, continue the dose once daily for a month. *Part* xxviii., *p.* 288.

Menorrhagia.—A very common cause of menorrhagia is uterine polypus. *Vide* Art. "Polypi."

Use of Digitalis.—When unconnected with organic disease, it may be readily checked by infusion of digitalis. If there be organic disease, it will control the discharge, but its effects will not be permanent.
Part xxxiii., *p.* 265.

Obstinate Menorrhagia.—In two cases under the care of Dr. Henry Savage, of London, after all other remedies had failed, a cure was effected by injection into the uterine cavity, in one case, of three drachms of tincture of iodine of the London Pharmacopœia, and in the other of four ounces of a mixture (equal parts) of tincture of iodine and water. In the second case the injection was repeated every third day for a fortnight. Both cases were unconnected with pregnancy in any way. In both the uterus was rather increased in size, and softer than natural, the os being slightly open. Injections of alum and tannin had previously been productive of temporary benefit in one of these cases.
Part xxxvii., *p.* 209.

———•◦•———

MENSTRUATION.

In the Negress—Is not earlier than in the European. *Part* vi., *p.* 166.

Treatment of Remittent Menstruation.—Dr. Tilt says he uses the term remittent here in the same sense as in the pathology of fever. This variety of menstrual derangement being characterized by a change from the habitual type to some other, so that the menstrual periods are brought nearer, and tend to run into each other. The first case occurred in a tall, slender woman, aged twenty-nine. In this case menstruation commenced between fourteen and fifteen, and continued regular until six months since, when she left her native country, Lincolnshire, for town. For two months, although she menstruated as usual, she was troubled with leucorrhœa between each menstruation. The menstrual periods then came on every fortnight and lasted eight instead of five days. The patient was weak and exhausted, but not chlorotic; she had just passed a menstrual period; there was an absence of pain and of other symptoms of uterine disease; therefore, notwithstanding a discharge of which she complained, I omitted all *local* treatment, and ordered the following pills and mixture: sulphate of iron, two scruples; sulphate of quina, ten grains; extract of hyoscyamus, a scruple; mix for twenty pills, one to be taken night and morning. Camphor mixture, six ounces; liquor potassæ,

four drachms; tincture of hyoscyamus, six drachms; tincture of cardamoms, two drachms. Half an ounce to be taken thrice daily. An opium
plaster to be applied to the pit of the stomach.

The patient's general health improved, menstruation returned to its
wonted type, and from that time she only took one pill every night, until
the approach of the ensuing epoch, which passed on as it ought to do
and the patient was discharged.

Miss L——, aged sixteen, first menstruated between fourteen and fifteen; and regularly, for four months after its first appearance, did menstruation adopt the monthly type. Since seven or eight years of age she
had been subject to leucorrhœa, which for the last three months has preceded and followed the menstrual flow; the latter has made its appearance every fortnight. Still there was no intermediate leucorrhœa; there
were no pains in the back, none in front, and none were determined by
pressure on the abdomen; but the thighs were so painful that she could
scarcely walk, and her legs were at times much swollen. For this symptom my opinion was requested by her mother. The girl had very much
fallen· off, was much debilitated by loss of blood, and the undue influence
of the generative organ on her system had caused catamenial headache,
heaviness for sleep, momentary loss of her senses, and often fits of lowness
and shedding of tears. I ordered the following pills: Sulphate of quina,
ten grains; extract of gentian, a scruple; extract of aloes, ten grains;
extract of hyoscyamus, a scruple. Mix for ten pills, one to be taken night
and morning. I prescribed the compound camphorated mixture, and belladonna plasters to each of the ovarian regions.

The symptoms rapidly abated, and menstruation was forthwith brought
back to its original type.

The preceding cases are, in my opinion, samples of an idiopathic aber-
ration from the normal type of menstruation, and perfectly independent
of any *inflammatory* lesion of the ovaries or uterus. I strongly recommend this practice to the profession, premising that the treatment will not
be so rapidly effectual, and may even be attended by mischief if the
remittance of the menstrual flow depends, as it sometimes does, on ovarian
or uterine subacute inflammation, as in the following case:

· E. H——, aged twenty-one, of florid complexion, full habit, and of
middling stature; menstruation first appeared between thirteen and fourteen, became regular from the first, was very abundant, and lasted five
days at each period.

A few months ago the patient was attacked by a severe cold with fever,
which stopped menstruation for two months. When the latter returned
it was scanty, and accompanied by more than usual pain in the back, the
stomach, and head; and, attended by these symptoms, it made its appearance every three weeks instead of every month, giving rise also to sensations of weakness, trembling, and lowness of spirits, with which she had
previously been wholly unacquainted.

The patient localized her pains in the ovarian regions: pressure increased them, so did walking or any unusual exertion; she was slightly
feverish; the tongue was furred, and the bowels were costive.

I considered this case as one wherein the remittance of menstruation
was dependent on subacute inflammation of the ovaries, and I ordered six
leeches over each ovarian region; poultices to be kept to the same region
at night; and a flannel, sprinkled with camphorated liniment, to be ap-

plied over the abdomen during the day. Aloetic purgatives and a sedative mixture were also prescribed. The pain subsided; the patient felt well; but menstruation returned at the morbid period of three weeks, and was still painful, and left behind it a certain amount of abdominal pain. After giving a brisk purgative, I applied belladonna plasters to the ovarian regions, and gave pills similar to those taken by Miss L——. The patient now says she feels well, and as menstruation has resumed its physiological type, I believe her to be cured. *Part* xxiii., *p.* 246.

Management of Women after the Cessation of Menstruation.—[The superabundance of blood and nervous energy after the cessation of the menstrual flow may be safely and effectually kept down by the habitual use of small doses of purgatives; and as they may have to be continued for some length of time, it is best to consult the patient as to what medicine would be best tolerated. The purgative to be used depends upon the constitution of the patient. Perhaps the best is some mild purgative which has been found to agree with the patient. Dr. Tilt continues :]

I frequently prescribe the soap and aloes pill of the Edinburgh Ph. ordering five or ten grains to be taken with the first mouthful of food at dinner. Hemorrhoidal affections I have never seen *caused* by this frequent use of aloes, but I have seen them *relieved* by it. There must be some exaggeration as to the extraordinary property generally ascribed to this valuable drug, which can be associated with hyoscyamus, and is thus said to be less liable to induce piles. Kemp and Hufeland recommend the following powder to be given to those who are advanced in years, and who complain of a tendency to vertigo—Guaiacum resin, cream of tartar, of each half a drachm, to be taken at night. This, no doubt, will sometimes be found a useful laxative; so will the popular remedy called the Chelsea Pensioner, of which Dr. Paris has given the following formula in his excellent Pharmacologia: Of guaiacum resin, one drachm; of powdered rhubarb, two drachms; of cream of tartar and of flowers of sulphur, an ounce each; one nutmeg finely powdered, and the whole made into an electuary with one pound of clarified honey: a large spoonful to be taken at night. I generally administer the flowers of sulphur alone, or else to each ounce of it I add a drachm of sesquicarbonate or biborate of soda, and sometimes from five to ten grains of ipecacuanha powder. One to two scruples of these powders taken at night in a little milk, is generally sufficient to act mildly on the bowels, and I consider such combinations as very valuable when a continued action is required.

Whether sulphur cures by acting on the nerves or on the bloodvessels, or by modifying the composition of the blood itself, is difficult to tell, but it does certainly cure the diseases I have enumerated. It forms part of many popular remedies for the infirmities of old age, was recommended by Hufeland, and is lauded by Dr. Day in his work "On the Diseases of Old Age;" but its utility is not generally known in all derangements of the menstrual function, at whatever period of life they may occur, and particularly at the change of life, where, if required, its action may be continued with impunity for months and years. *Part* xxiv., *p.* 299.

Difficult Menstruation.—Dysmenorrhœa sometimes takes place from the very commencement of menstrual life, and there is good reason for believing that it depends on the small size or strictured condition of the os uteri. The menstrual fluid, after it is formed, or while forming, cannot readily escape; distention of the organ speedily follows, which, by exciting the contraction of the uterine fibres, produces pain almost simulating that of labor. Even the action of the abdominal muscles is called into play, and many cases of what are termed "spurious pregnancy" may be very possibly explained in this manner. It is believed, too, that women thus affected rarely, if ever, conceive or bear children, the normal healthy function of the uterus being interfered with, as well as the woman's health reduced by the constant suffering and pain. Of all the means of cure hitherto tried, dilatation of the canal of the cervix uteri seems to be the best, to which more recently has been added the introduction of a silver canula, as tried by Dr. Tyler Smith.

Part xxxii., *p.* 298.

Menstruation during Pregnancy.—That a discharge, more or less identical with the ordinary catamenial flow, may occur during pregnancy, is admitted by the majority of experienced observers. The following case, under the care of Dr. G. Hewitt, is an interesting example of this kind:

M. B., aged twenty-five, had been married six years. She became pregnant for the first time rather less than six years ago, and was delivered of a healthy child, now alive. During this first pregnancy, it is stated that every fourteen days a bloody discharge occurred, lasting three or four days, and this periodic discharge persisted during the *whole period of gestation*. The discharge was rather paler than that observed before she became pregnant. The child was suckled for six months, and during lactation no trace of bloody discharge was noticed. A second pregnancy, attended with precisely the same phenomena, terminated favorably three years ago. The second child, also now alive, was suckled for fifteen months, and the catamenial discharge is habitually rather excessive in quantity, continuing usually six to seven days; it occasionally extends over twelve or thirteen, and this has been the case since she was married only.

Part xxxviii., *p.* 203.

————•◦•————

MERCURY.

Mercury and Antimony—Methods of forming various Preparations of.—Vide "Antimony."

Ferruginated Pill of Mercury.—Vide Art. "Pills.'

Different Preparations of Mercury and best Modes of administering them.—Chlóride.—Calomel is chiefly useful when we wish to produce a speedy and powerful action on the constitution, as in venereal iritis or orchitis, but is less adapted to the ordinary symptoms. On the Continent it is extensively employed in tubercles of the labia, with or without ulceration, in various forms of creeping ulcers, and also in ulcerations of the throat and nasal fossæ. Desruelles says, that he cannot too much recommend this preparation, which, united to opium and an antiphlogistic regimen, may produce the most beneficial results. Ricord employs the following pills in the treatment of enlarged testicle, which remains after inflammation of that organ:

℞ Hyd. chlor. ℈j.; pulv. conii, sapon. hisp. aa. ℈ij. M. ft. pil. xxiv.

Bichloride.—M. Dupuytren ordered this remedy in small doses, one-sixth of a grain three times a day, in constitutional syphilis, and on the Continent it still continues to be extensively used for this purpose. In some chronic cases of syphilitic skin disease, I have seen it used with advantage; but as a general remedy in secondary syphilis it requires more care, is more dangerous, and altogether is a less eligible medicine than blue pill.

Pilula Hydrargyri.—This medicine is the form most used and relied on in England, and as it is one of the mildest, safest, most certain, and most manageable preparations of mercury, it justly deserves the preference given to it. In doses of five grains two or three times a day, it is applicable to nearly all those conditions which we have shown to be benefited by mercury.

Proto-ioduret.—MM. Cullerier, Biett, Ricord and others employ this remedy in many forms of constitutional syphilis, especially where secondary and tertiary symptoms are combined, and in primary sores in strumous habits. Cullerier says, that it is chiefly in constitutional syphilis that the proto-ioduret of mercury is administered with success. Its effects are principally evident in secondary ulcerations of the mucous membrane, cutaneous tubercles, exostoses, and chronic affections of the joints, where the other preparations of mercury have had little effect. It should always be guarded by opium, and given in half grain doses twice or thrice a day. The deuto-ioduret is more stimulating, and consequently its dose is smaller. Either of these may be employed in friction upon tumors and indolent buboes, after the removal of all acute inflammatory symptoms.

The cyanuret and deuto-phosphate of mercury are occasionally employed. The former is said to be preferable to the bichloride, being less apt to disagree, and less readily decomposed. It is an useful external application in some skin affections, allaying the violent itching and irritation of what M. Alibert terms *herpes squamosus*.

Inunction.—Inunction by the mercurial ointment was formerly employed to mercurialize the system more frequently than at the present day. In this way the mineral is less apt to disagree with the system, especially the alimentary canal, although, when used alone, it is less speedy in its effects. In buboes, I imagine that Hunter was correct in his opinion concerning the advantages of making mercury pass through the affected absorbents. The *ung. hydrarg.* is used in the quantity of half a drachm to a drachm night and morning, to be well rubbed in, before a fire, on the more delicate portions of skin. Cullerier prefers using mercury by friction in primary sores: he orders from a quarter of a drachm to a drachm and a half of mercurial ointment at each friction, leaving an interval between them of one, two, or three days, with the view of not irritating either the sore or the constitution, by bringing the latter suddenly under the influence of the remedy. Ricord frequently orders the frictions to the axillæ, and they are employed in this manner by Cullerier, in certain forms of ulcerations of the mouth and fauces. He narrates two cases cured by mercurial frictions in this situation, which had resisted its employment on other parts.

Fumigation.—Fumigation of the whole surface of the body is at present, rarely used as a method of affecting the system, but the apparatus formerly employed is still to be found in some of our hospitals. It is very speedy in its action. The remedy is, however, employed locally, and with

great advantage, in some affections of the throat and nasal fossæ, directed
to the part by a suitable apparatus, and more generally in some obstinate
diseases of the skin. For patients who have not strength to rub in mercury, and whose bowels will not bear the use of internal remedies, it has ·
been esteemed highly advantageous.

Topical Applications.—As mere local applications, calomel, black wash
(hydrarg. chlorid. x. vel xv. grs., aquæ calcis, ʒj.), yellow wash (hyd.
Bichlorid. j. vel ij. grs., aq. cal. ʒj.), solutions of the bichloride in distilled water, the nitric oxide ointment, the nitrate ointment, the simple
blue ointment, and the *ung. hyd. c. ammoniaco*, are all of them occasionally applied. We select from these in proportion to their stimulating
properties, adapting to the condition of the symptoms we treat.

Part ix., *p.* 20.

Mercurial Ointment—Use of "Prepared Sevum."—Under this title a
very elegant and valuable preparation has been for some time before the
public. It is employed in the manufacture of mercurial ointment (unguentum hydrargyri), and possesses the singular property of *immediately* extinguishing the globules of metallic quicksilver, and producing the necessary degree of oxidation, without at all interfering with the *intentions* of
the Pharmacopœia. It resembles in every point very pure suet, as its
name implies, and produces a finer article of ointment, both as to color
and quality, than by the old and laborious process of patient trituration.

Strong Mercurial Ointment.—℞ Prepared sevum, 1 oz. or part; quicksilver 7 do.; mix in a warm mortar, then add lard (softened with heat).
13 ounces or parts; mix well.

Weak Mercurial Ointment.—℞ Prepared sevum 1 oz. or part; quicksilver 7 do.; lard (softened) 3½ lbs., or 56 do., as before. *Part* ix., *p.* 84.

Mercury, Administration of.—After mercury has been given for some
time, a portion of it would seem to be retained in the system in the form
of some insoluble compound. If iodide of potassium is now given, it combines with the mercury, forming a new and soluble salt, dissolving out the
mercury, and setting it once more afloat in the circulation. This new salt,
a double iodide of mercury and potassium, is eliminated from the system
along with the excess of iodide of potassium, so that the cure would then
seem to be radical and complete. ·

Mercurial Poisoning.—It is important to know that iodide of potassium
renders medical treatment in poisoning by certain salts of mercury more
active, and may, therefore, occasion accidents. M. Dumas recommends,
that when calomel (the chloride of mercury) is taken, and is wished to
remain as such, common salt (chloride of sodium) should not be taken.
When corrosive sublimate is taken (the bichloride), to prevent its being
decomposed, sal ammoniac (the hydro-chlorate of ammonia) is to be
given with it. If doses of calomel are given to two dogs, and at the same
time iodide of potassium is given to one of them, the dog so treated will
die first.

Chloride of sodium (common salt) would seem to be of value in preventing the attacks of mercurial poisoning. Those workmen who are exposed to its influence, and who are fond of salt, resisting the contamination longer than those who are not.   *Part* xxvii., *p.* 240.

Mercurial Fumigations.—A very simple and effectual plan is to have
the patient seated on a caned chair; underneath this you must have a

spirit lamp so placed that the flame impinges on a thin metallic plate, which contains the mercury to be volatilized; this may be from one to three drachms of calomel for each fumigation, or if the patient inhale the mercury according to Mr. Lee's practice, fifteen grains will be sufficient. The chair and patient must be closely surrounded with a blanket.

Part xxxiv., *p.* 222.

Rapid Mercurialization.—Pass ten or fifteen grains of the ung. hyd. fort. within the sphincter ani three times a day, and in twenty-four or thirty-six hours ptyalism will be established. The patient must be carefully watched lest it run too far. *Part* xxxiv., *p.* 274.

Mercurial Fumigation.—The efficacy of calomel fumes is much enhanced when combined with the vapor of hot water. For this purpose, two separate processes have been had recourse to, one to volatilize the calomel, and the other to give off steam; but by a very ingenious lamp, made by Mr. Blaise, both these processes are combined into one. Mr. Pollok, who had used it at St. George's Hospital, finds that it is very useful in private practice for volatilizing sulphur, iodine, etc.

Part xxxv., *p.* 187.

———•◦•———

MILK.

Extemporaneous Production of Milk.—M. Dichost, a Russian chemist, proposed the following plan for the preservation and extemporaneous preparation of milk. He evaporates newly drawn milk, at a very gentle heat, till it is all brought into a state of fine powder. It is then put into small glass bottles, which are completely filled and hermetically sealed, with ground glass stoppers. A small quantity of the powder thus obtained, dissolved in an appropriate quantity of water, affords on the instant a milk of a very good quality. The powder will remain good for a great length of time. *Part* vi., *p.* 85.

Artificial Maternal Milk.—The maternal milk differs from the cow's, principally in containing less caseine or curd, and more lactine, or sugar of milk, and from ass's milk in containing a little more curd and butter. Therefore a very perfect substitute for maternal milk may be made by adding about two and a half per cent. of cream to ass's milk, or by removing a portion of curd from cow's milk, and adding a little sugar.

Part xxxvi., *p.* 238.

Substitute for Human Milk.—Lentil powder, or, as it is called, Revelenta Arabica, contains phosphoric acid, chloride of potassium, and casein. Its nutritive is to its calorifiant matter in the proportion of 1 to 2½, milk being in that of 1 to 2. Of all vegetable substances it forms the best substitute for human milk, being far preferable to pap, or pulp of wheat bread, which, from the absence of chloride of potassium and the too frequent presence of alum (the former of which is necessary to the solution of carbonate of lime, and the latter of which forms with phosphate of lime an insoluble salt,) is totally unfit for this purpose. As a food for children with atrophy and debility lentil powder is invaluable.

Part xxxviii., *p.* 294.

MOLES.

Tattooing of Moles on the Skin.—The part should be washed with soap and water, and rubbed till the blood is introduced into the most delicate branches of the erectile tissue; the skin is then made tight and covered with color similar to the natural color of the skin, which is formed of white lead and carmine. Three needles, sunk into a cork pad, so that their points project, are then thrust into the skin, and their points from time to time dipped in the paint. In extensive spots, we must proceed gradually, so as not to produce too great swelling. The most difficult part is the choice of color corresponding to that of the skin.   *Part* xiv., *p.* 190.

Treatment of Moles by Acid Nitrate of Mercury.—Small moles on the face, if superficial and not too thick, may be readily destroyed by the acid nitrate. A cicatrix of course results, but it is small, and far less unsightly than the original disease. Small cutaneous nævi are often treated at the various London hospitals, by means of the nitric acid. Unless the disease be of very small extent, the employment of a ligature appears to be a much more certain means of effecting the end desired. If there be a subcutaneous base to the morbid structure it often persists in growing, despite frequent applications of escharotics. There is a mild form of dilated cutaneous capillaries which produces the marks known as "port-wine stains," "spiders," etc., in the treatment of which much benefit may be obtained by the dexterous application of fluid caustics. With a finely-pointed glass brush, charged either with nitric acid or the acid nitrate of mercury, the tortuous vascular trunks should be severally painted, a minute streak of the caustic being thus left along the whole course. In this way, by repeated applications, the whole of the larger vessels may be destroyed, and the disfigurement, to a large extent, diminished. The "port-wine stain" is of course very much more difficult to remove than the less diffused forms of this condition, such, for instance, as are of frequent occurrence on the cheeks or nose; even in it, however, much benefit may, by patient treatment, be gained.   *Part* xxxi., *p.* 241.

MORBUS COXARIUS.

When warranted in Removing the Carious Bone.—According to Mr. H. Smith: When the head of the femur is carious, and is acting as a source of irritation and wearing the patient down, when we are satisfied that nature cannot accomplish a spontaneous cure, and when at the same time the caries is *confined, or nearly so,* to the femur, and there is no disease of other and internal organs, we are warranted in removing the carious bone. The operation consists in making a longitudinal incision over the head and for a convenient distance down the shaft of the femur, and another transverse one; clearing away the tissues down to the bone, turning it out, and sawing off the diseased portion; lastly, in uniting the edges of the wound by suture.   *Part* xix., *p.* 115.

MORTIFICATION.

Treatment of Mortification.—In the *treatment* of mortification, according to Prof. Cooper, three primary indications are concerned : 1. To stop the progress of mortification. 2. To promote the separation of the dead part from the living. 3. To heal the wound, if an operation has been necessary, or otherwise the ulcer resulting from loss of substance. These indications are common to all species of mortification. In fulfilling the first of these —in endeavoring to arrest the progress of mortification, supposing it to be acute—you will seek to remove the exciting cause.

Where mortification is evidently the result of inflammation—where inflammatory fever and an excited action of the blood-vessels surrounding the mortified part exist—a moderate antiphlogistic treatment is indicated. The excessive action of the sanguiferous system should be cautiously reduced by leeching, purgative, diaphoretic, diluent medicines, and abstinence from animal diet; but this treatment is only to be continued so long as the local inflammation and inflammatory fever exist concurrently with mortification, since by the mortification of any large portion of the body the system itself is greatly shocked, and rendered unable to stand against violent treatment. In such cases too much circumspection cannot be employed, since frequently immediately upon the subsidence of the inflammatory fever, the patient sinks into a state of prostration and nervous agitation; and in every case there is more or less of weakness, and, if the system has been too much reduced, the consequences are likely to be disastrous.

After the abatement of the inflammatory or symptomatic fever, which usually takes place in the transition from gangrene to sphacelus, the opposite system of treatment must be pursued : stimulants, anodynes, and a more generous diet are to be given.

At one time, bark was considered by the surgeons of this country as almost a specific in resisting the progress of this disorder ; without denying, however, its usefulness in particular cases, this opinion is altogether untenable, and is now rejected by men of experience. So far from being valuable in all cases, its exhibition would frequently be very injurious. After the first stage of mortification, when the inflammation surrounding the mortified part has abated, it will often be advisable to employ it as a tonic, especially if the appetite is bad and the patient low ; it should then be administered with wine and light diet. Also, when the constitutional disturbance is of the typhoid kind, bark and quinine may be useful. As stimulants, however, ammonia and wines—those of Spain or Madrid—are far preferable. Opium is also very serviceable where severe pain or nervous symptoms are present; the best forms of it are the muriate and acetate of morphia ; and they should be given frequently in the day, in order to keep the constitution under their influence during the whole of the twenty-four hours.

Surgeons trust now more to common means, such as linseed poultices and fomentations for stopping the progress of mortification.

The second indication I named was to promote the separation of the slough. Although the slough is dead, and may be cut, pricked, or scratched, without pain, and no functional connection exists, there remains the attachment of cohesion, from which it cannot forcibly be wrested without pain or danger.

Where amputation is not strictly indicated, the parts should be left as much as possible to nature, only applying moist and emollient applications. In the derangement and prostration of the system, always implied in mortification, a little violence will bring on an extension of the evil; and therefore, besides the use of the emollient poultice, with or without a solution of chloruret of soda, or with a small proportion of finely-powdered charcoal, it is to a general treatment that we are to look as the most efficient method of expediting the removal of the slough. Let the patient have the benefit of the fresh air; let his linen be frequently changed, and his chamber be well sprinkled with chloride of lime, and his constitution be supported in the manner I have described, and he will then be in the most favorable circumstances for losing the slough. Sometimes you will find one half of the slough healing much better after the other half has been cut away; and, as this proceeding involves no injury of living textures, it is, under some circumstances, advisable to adopt it. I ought to mention that when a slough separates no hemorrhage generally takes place; the blood-vessels are loaded with coagulum; and this will explain why, when amputation in mortification is performed a little above the line of separation, there is often no hemorrhage of importance.

The third indication—to heal the ulcer, or wound, if amputation has been necessary—need not to be dwelt on, as it will be considered when we come to speak of the treatment of ulcers, wounds, and amputations.

Part xvi., *p.* 301.

Chronic Mortification, or Dry Gangrene.—[The causes of this state are often diseases of the valves of the heart, ossification of the large arteries, and obstruction of the smaller ones by fibrin. Mr. Cooper observes :]

The first example of chronic mortification, or dry gangrene, is the gangrena senilis, or mortification of old persons. This kind of mortification differs in many respects from any other example; it is peculiar in the discoloration which takes place being always preceded by severe burning sensation in the parts. It commonly occurs in elderly persons—in nineteen cases out of twenty. Not that you may not have similar cases in youth. Dupuytren relates several instances of young persons suffering from this disorder. It commences at the greatest distance from the centre of the circulation, generally one of the toes, in the form of a dark purple spot at the side of one of the small toes. Previously, however, you find the patient has been suffering pain about the toe, which is often supposed to be gout; and you find that the extension of the disease is preceded by burning sensation. Its progress is variously marked in different cases: you find that the foot is gradually, sometimes quickly, affected as far as the ankle, and has a dark livid color; the leg higher up presents a reddish-brown color, and the whole limb has a mottled appearance. When the surgeon examines the part of the leg higher up, he finds the temperature of the limb much lower than natural, and this loss of heat is found to extend along the limb.

Although this is called dry gangrene, in most cases there is a separation of the cuticle, and a dark bloody serum effused into vesicles, as in acute mortification, and at the bottom of the vesicles is seen the cutis, dark-colored and livid. Whether you are to have much swelling depends on the rapidity with which the disease extends: when it advances rapidly there is much swelling, but where the progress is slow the swelling is gene-rally very slight.

The patient sometimes suffers a good deal of disturbance in the sto-mach; he suffers from eructations, and delirium and coma come on early in severe cases. Where the disturbance is great in the beginning, the patient often dies before the mortification has reached to the ankle, about the tenth or twelfth day, from constitutional disturbance.

Now, what are the causes of gangrena senilis? It has been generally supposed that there is ossification of arterial trunks, and sometimes we can feel very distinctly that the artery is ossified. The larger arteries are not invariably ossified in this disease.

Cruveilhier always referred gangrena senilis to ossification. There must be some unfavorable circumstances combined with the ossification, as impaired health, diseases of the heart or its valves, producing disorder of the circulation. Then the venous blood cannot pass freely, and accumu-lates in the lower extremities, impeding the circulation; and this will ex-plain to you the cause of gangrena senilis. It is doubted by many good surgeons whether ossification of the arteries alone is capable of producing gangrena senilis. I think it is not. No doubt in a broken constitution, joined with ossification, it may act as the exciting cause. Dupuytren thought the cause was arteritis, by which the arteries became blocked up by fibrin. It was observed that the blood was buffy; in consequence of his view, he tried venesection, and three-fourths of his patients were saved. This mode of treatment, when tried in this country, did not give such favorable results.

We found that bark was insufficient in this disease, and that opium was a much more available remedy; and the opinion is retained by the best surgeons that opium is better than bark in the treatment of gangrena senilis. If opium or its preparations be used, half-grain doses of hydro-chlorate of morphia should be given every four hours.

Musk, too, has been tried, and was found to be a most useful medicine. Stimulants, brandy and wine, ought not to be forgotten. With respect to the local treatment, fomentations and emollient poultices are the most em-ployed. I have seen other applications tried; I have seen Laburruque's solution of chloruret of soda, and this, in one case I attended, had the effect of diminishing the fetid smell, but did no other good.

Applications of charcoal were also tried, but these were no better than the other. A new practice of late has been introduced; in Chelsea Hos-pital, where gangrena senilis is very common among the pensioners, it was suggested that it would be a very rational plan to maintain the tempera-ture of the limb by enveloping the whole in carded wool. This was tried in a case by Sir Benjamin Brodie; the patient got better, and recovered with the loss of two toes.   *Part* xvi., *p.* 302.

————•◆•————

MOUTH.

Cancrum Oris, and Phagedæna of the Cheek.—Dr. Hunt describes these diseases as being identical, varying only in the degree of severity—both commencing by ulceration of the mucous membrane of the cheek, or where it joins the gums, and that the external eschar is the consequence of the internal ulceration. He considers them to proceed from a cachectic state of the system; that they occur more commonly in cold and wet weather—sometimes attacking several members of the same family simultaneously, and occasionally prevailing almost like an epidemic. The author has treated them very successfully by a free exhibition of the chlorate of potash, the beneficial influence of that salt being generally apparent within forty-eight hours of its being given, that it seldom fails to arrest the progress and to effect a cure, if administered prior to the patient being very much exhausted. The quantity of the salt he has been in the habit of prescribing, varies from Ðj. to Ðij. in twelve hours, according to the age of the child.   *Part* vii., *p.* 87.

Aphthous Ulcers of—Use of Pure Tannin.—Mr. Druitt says : In one or two cases of lingering atonic phagedæna, I have found it of some service, sprinkled thickly on the sore; but more particularly so in those aphthous ulcers which sometimes occur in the mouths of adults, from acidity of the stomach, and congestion of the liver.   *Part* x., *p.* 139.

Treatment of Aphthæ by Sulphuric Acid.—Professor Lippich, of Padua, has recommended the following liniment in the treatment of aphthæ : honey, 15 parts; diluted sulphuric acid, 1 part by weight. The ulcerated surfaces should be occasionally brushed over with this liniment by means of a camel's-hair pencil. The proportion of sulphuric acid may be increased if the case is obstinate.   *Part* xiv., *p.* 90.

Aphthous Ulcerations of the Mouth and Tongue.—*Vide* Art. " Gallic Acid."

Aphtha.—Apply solution of the sub-carbonate of soda, or of borax, of varying strength. (When the aphthous crusts have a disposition to fall off, it is only necessary to pencil them with a soft brush dipped in water.) A long continued use of alkaline applications is inadvisable; change them therefore for astringents and the mineral acids. Or apply a solution of nitrate of silver, eight grains to the ounce. Internally give soda, aqua calcis, or magnesia usta. If there is a vomiting of the milk, give an emetic; if the stools are cheesy-looking, give purgatives, especially castor-oil, or if there is much secretion of mucus, rhubarb or jalap. To relieve the colicky pains give rhubarb and magnesia, or liq. succin. ammon. by the mouth or rectum. Avoid giving medicines in *sugar*, which being changed into lactic acid, favors the growth of the aphtha. Take care that the milk is of good quality, and that the child is exposed to a free and pure atmosphere.
Part xvi., *p.* 144.

Ulcerative Stomatitis or Noma.—[By this name, Dr. West describes an affection of the mouth, distinct from follicular or aphthous stomatitis on the one hand, and from cancrum oris or gangrenous stomatitis on the other. It attacks the gums, and destroys them extensively by a process, not of gangrene, but of ulceration. It occurs chiefly in children who have had deficient food and have lived in damp, unhealthy places: but is not preceded by any special derangement of the general system. The symptoms are as follows:]

On opening the mouth, the gums are seen to be red, swollen, and spongy, and their edge is covered with a dirty white or greyish pultaceous deposit, on removing which their surface is exposed, raw and bleeding. At first only the front of the gum is thus affected; but as the disease advances. it creeps round between the teeth to their posterior surface, and then, destroying the gum both in front and behind them, leaves them denuded, and very loose in their sockets, but it is not often that they actually fall out. The gums of the incisor teeth are usually first affected ; those of the lower jaw more frequently and more extensively than those of the upper ; but if the disease be severe, the gums at the side of the mouth become likewise involved, though it is seldom that the two sides suffer equally. Sometimes aphthous ulcers, like those of follicular stomatitis, are seen on the inside of the mouth in connection with this state of the gums ; but oftener it exists alone. On those parts of the lips and cheeks, however, which are opposite to, and consequently in contact with, the ulcerated gums, irregular ulcerations form, which are covered with a pultaceous pseudo-membranous deposit, similar to that which exists on the gums them-selves. Sometimes, too, deposits of false membrane take place on other parts of the inside of the mouth, the surface beneath being red and spon-gy, and bleeding, though not distintly ulcerated. If the disease be severe and long-continued, the tongue assumes a sodden appearance, and is indent-ed by the teeth, and the cheek on one or other side is somewhat swollen, while the saliva, though rather less abundantly secreted than at the com-mencement of the affection, continues horribly fetid, and is often streaked with blood, the gums themselves bleeding on the slightest touch. But even if left alone, the affection usually subsides in the course of time, though it may continue almost stationary for days or weeks together, and this notwithstanding that the general health is tolerably good. It would be too much to say, that this unhealthy ulceration never degenerates into gangrene ; but though a very large number of cases of ulcerative stoma-titis have come under my notice, I have seen only one instance in which it was succeeded by true gangrene of the mouth. When recovery has commenced, the disease ceases to spread ; the drivelling of fetid saliva diminishes ; the white pultaceous deposit on the gums, or on the ulcera-tions of the cheek or lips, becomes less abundant ; the ulcers themselves grow less ; and finally, the gums become firm, and their edges of a bright red, though still for a long time showing a disposition to become once more the seat of the ulcerative process, and continuing for a still longer . time to cover the teeth but very imperfectly.

Various internal remedies and local applications have been at different times recommended for the *cure of this affection*. Tonics have been much employed, and the supposed analogy between this state of the gums and that which exists in scurvy, has led practitioners to give the preference to remedies supposed to be possessed of antiscorbutic properties. Lotions of alum, or burnt alum in substance, or the chloride of lime in powder, have all been used locally with more or less benefit. It was my custom also to prescribe these remedies in cases of ulcerative stomatitis ; but since the chlorate of potash was introduced to the notice of the profession by Dr. Hunt, I have learned to rely upon it almost exclusively. It appears, in-deed, almost to deserve the name of a specific in this affection ; for a marked improvement seldom fails to be observed in the patient's condition after it has been administered for two or three days, and in a week or ten days the cure is generally complete. Three grains every four hours, dissolved in water, and sweetened, is a sufficient dose for a child three years old, and five grains every four hours is the largest quantity that I have administered to a child eight or nine. If the bowels be constipated, a purgative should be previously administered ; but there seems to be no form nor any stage of the affection in which the chlorate of potash is not useful. The diet should be light but nutritious, and quinine and other tonics are sometimes serviceable if the child's health should continue feeble after the local malady has been cured. *Part* xviii., *p.* 111.

Gangrenous Stomatitis, or Cancrum Oris.—[Ulcerative stomatitis is an affection of such frequent occurrence that many instances of it come under my notice every year, especially during the damp autumnal months; while it is attended with so little danger, that the only case in which I have known it prove fatal was one in which gangrene of the mouth supervened upon it. *Gangrenous stomatitis*, on the other hand, is a disease so rare that I have only five times had the opportunity of witnessing it: but so fatal, that in four out of these five cases the patients died.

Dr. West proceeds to the treatment. He says:]

The arrest of the sloughing is the one point to which in the *treatment* of this affection the attention of all practitioners has been directed. The small amount of success which has attended their efforts is partly attributable to the circumstance that the affection has frequently been overlooked, until it has already made considerable progress; in part also to the fact that when recognized, the local remedies employed in order to check the gangrene have either been too mild, or have been applied with too timorous a hand. Unfortunately, too, there is considerable difficulty in applying any caustic effectually to the interior of the mouth—for not only does the tense and swollen condition of the cheek prevent our obtaining easy access to the gangrenous parts, but the child naturally resists an operation which cannot but occasion it most severe pain. Ineffectual cauterization, however, is useless, or worse than useless; and though every endeavor should be made to prevent the needless destruction of healthy parts, yet of the two evils, that of doing too much is unquestionably less than that of doing too little. It is of importance, moreover, not only that the cauterization should be done effectually, but also that it should be practised early.

When once the mortification has extended through the substance of the cheek, the chances of arresting its progress must be very few. As the slough-ing advances from within outward, it is to the interior of the mouth that our remedies must be applied, and since the advance of the disease is too rapid to allow of our trying mild means at first, and afterward resorting, if neces-sary, to such as are more powerful, we must employ an agent sufficiently energetic at once to arrest its progress. Various caustics have been re-commended for this purpose, but none appear to be so well fitted to accom-plish it as the strong hydrochloric or nitric acid. I am accustomed to employ the latter, applying it by means of a bit of sponge, or of soft lint or tow, fastened to a quill, while I endeavor, by means of a spoon or spatula, to guard the tongue, and other healthy parts, as far as possible, from the action of the acid. In the only case that I saw recover, the arrest of the disease appeared to be entirely owing to this agent, and though the alveo-lar processes of the left side of the lower jaw, from the first molar tooth backward, died and exfoliated apparently from having been destroyed by the acid, yet it must be owned that life was cheaply saved even at that cost. Some increase of the swelling of the cheek almost invariably follows the application of this agent—a circumstance which may at first occasion unfounded apprehensions lest the disease be worse. Twelve hours, how-ever, must not be allowed to elapse, without the mouth being carefully examined, in order to ascertain whether the disease has really been checked, or whether there is any appearance of mortification in the parts beyond the yellow eschar left by the first application of the acid. The cauterization may now be repeated, if it appears necessary, and even though the disease had seemed completely checked, ; yet reliance must not be placed on the improvement continuing, but the mouth must be examined every twelve hours, for fear the mortification should spread unobserved. During the whole progress of the case the mouth must be syringed frequently with warm water, or with chamomile tea mixed with a small quantity of the solution of chloride of lime, in order to free it from putrid matters that collect within it, and to diminish, as much as possible, their offensive odor. Should the case go on well, the frequent repetition of the strong acid will be unnecessary, but the surface may still require its application in a diluted form, or it may suffice to syringe the mouth frequently with chloride of lime lotion, or to apply the chloride in powder once or twice a day, according to the suggestion of MM. Rilliet and Barthez. In the last two cases of this affection that came under my notice, I likewise employed the chlorate of potash internally, as recommended by Dr. Hunt, but it did not appear to exert any influence over it; and valuable though the remedy is in ulcerative stomatitis, it would, I think, be merely trifling with your patient's chances of recovery to trust to it in true gangrene of the mouth.

During the whole course of treatment you have another indication to fulfill—namely, to support your patient's strength by nutritious diet, and by the employment of wine and other stimulants, and the administration of quinine, or of the extract or tincture of bark, or whatever form of tonic might seem best suited to the peculiarities of the case.

In conclusion let me remind you, that during the whole progress of the case, your prognosis must be regulated by the state of the local disease, rather than by the urgency of the general symptoms. So long as the sloughing is unchecked, the affection is tending rapidly to a fatal issue, and this even though the pulse be not very feeble, though the appetite be good, and the child still retain some show of cheerfulness.   *Part* xviii., *p.* 113.

"*Nurses' Sore Mouth*."—Dr. Holt states that every case he has treated of this disease " has yielded within forty-eight hours to the use of iodide of potassium, in gr. v. doses three times a day."   *Part* xviii., *p.* 303.

Cancrum Oris.—Apply strong nitric acid freely to the edges of the slough, all around, taking care that the little patient takes a full inspiration previous to the application of the acid, so as to obviate the danger of the vapor getting into the lungs ; and repeat the application every day, as long as it may be necessary. Put on a linseed poultice, which should be changed twice a day; and detach each slough as soon as it can be done. Let the patient have meat diet, and wine. And give chlorate of potash, fifteen grains and upward (for children of six or eight years old) daily, in divided doses.   *Part* xxi., *p.* 223.

" *Stomatitis Ulcerosa* " *of Children*.—[These ulcerative affections in the mouths of infants and young children are often exceedingly troublesome. They may not depend upon any specific cause, but chiefly on debility, with possibly some trivial local affection superadded. Mr. Mackenzie has employed the following simple method of treating the disease with much success :]

The term "stomatitis ulcerosa " sufficiently and accurately expresses the nature of this affection ; but in its mode of origin, situation and extent, it presents many varieties. Thus, in one form, it commences as a small inflammatory spot, either on the frenum of the tongue, the outer surface of the gums, or the mucous membrane of the cheek or lip; but wherever it commences, ulceration speedily supervenes, attended with febrile disturbance, a coated tongue, profuse salivation, and a disordered state of the tomach and digestive organs. In another form, it is found to be connected with the passage of some of the larger teeth through the gum, more especially when several are about to make their appearance together. In this case, the gum becomes swollen, painful, and dark-colored; and, after a few days, the portion over the protruding teeth gives way by ulceration, which, in some cases, extends considerably, attended with tumefaction of the mouth and cheeks, increased salivary discharge, and febrile disturbance. More frequently, however, it commences with a general swelling and irritation of the gums, together with much fetor of the breath, a coated tongue, and much gastric disorder. Along the upper margin of the gum, or rather that which is in contact with the teeth, a line of ulceration now soon becomes developed; and this, when once begun, rapidly spreads, the gums, at the same time, being spongy, swollen, and very painful. Unless excited by some local cause, such as the irritation of a decayed tooth, it usually commences in the lower jaw, and from thence is communicated to the mucous membrane of the corresponding cheek. The irritation attending it affects the salivary and cervical glands in a remarkable manner; both become swollen, and the former secrete so profusely that the child appears to be constantly dribbling. In this form there is generally some febrile disturbance, and much gastro-intestinal disorder. If severe, it may not only cause destruction of the gums, but loosening of the teeth, suppuration of their sockets, and partial necrosis of the jaw. Its intensity, however, varies very considerably in different cases; in some it is so slight as to require little or no special treatment, whilst in others it can only be controlled by very prompt and energetic mensures.

In the general management of these cases, we are directed to employ, locally, strong solutions of the nitrate of silver, or of the sulphate of copper or zinc, with or without astringent, stimulating, or detergent gargles, and to administer, at the same time, quinine, tonics, and a liberal diet. I formerly followed these instructions closely, but sometimes with equivocal success ; and I am now, after repeated trials, disposed to give the preference to the following method of treatment. It consists in removing, in the first place, any apparent cause of irritation, such as a decayed tooth, should it exist, and applying, daily, the dilute nitric acid of the pharmacopœia, to the whole of the ulcerated surfaces, by means of a sponge, or camel's-hair pencil; whilst, at the same time, the sesquicarbonate of ammonia is given in full doses, combined with citrate of iron. When the tongue is coated, and the alvine discharges are unhealthy, it is necessary to premise an emetic of ipecacuanha and squills, as well as a purgative of calomel and rhubarb. It is also necessary that the patient should be well supported by a nutritious diet, an adequate allowance of malt liquor, or wine.

I will briefly add, that the employment of ammonia in these cases was first suggested to me from observing its beneficial effects in the ulcerative affections of the mouth and throat, which occur in children in connection with scarlet fever.   *Part* xxvi., *p.* 95.

Stomatitis (Ulcerated) and Cancrum Oris.—In a severe epidemic of this disease, the cases were treated by a mild aperient of magnesia and rhubarb, and by chlorate of potash dissolved in water sweetened with sirup, in doses of 4 grains every fourth hour. The mouth was also washed with a weak solution of chloride of sodium. They all recovered in about six days. *Part* xxvii., *p.* 83.

Thrush.—Dr. Jenner says this disease depends upon the presence of a parasite. It is speedily removed by applying a solution of sulphite of soda, 3j. to the 3j. of water. The secretions of the mouth, being acid, combine with the alkali and set the sulphurous acid free, which is the active agent in destroying the parasite. *Part* xxviii., *p.* 227.

Cancrum Oris.—According to Dr. Fleming, this disease is generally preceded by some other malady, as measles, croup, etc., followed by bilious diarrhœa, which induces a state of the system in which there is a deficiency of sulphur. The treatment must consist in the local application of a solution of the biborate of soda. The constitutional remedies are Fleming's tincture of aconite, six drops to two ounces of water; a teaspoonful to be given every three hours. This will subdue the vascular excitement. The tincture of nux vomica must afterward be given to stimulate the secreting vessels of the liver, and also sulphur to supply the deficiency of this element in the system.

* * * * * * * *

If you meet with the case before it has spread far, remove the slough with the knife, apply the strong solution of the nitrate of copper freely to the exposed surface, and paint the surrounding cheek with collodion.

Part xxxiv., *p.* 80.

Mouth—Congelation in Operations on.—It will be very difficult to produce the required benumbing effect, says Mr. Quinton, except with great care. It is necessary that the cold be applied equally and with some pressure. It is much better to inclose the freezing mixture in a thin India-rubber bag, to prevent the ingredients escaping and irritating the mouth. It will also be necessary repeatedly to change or mix the fluid so as to maintain the desired cold. *Part* xxxiv., *p.* 137.

Ulcerous Stomatitis in the Army.—M. Bergeron writes that during the Crimean war, ulcerous stomatitis, amongst the young soldiers, assumed an " endemo-epidemic " form. The most rapidly efficacious method of treatment was found to consist in the exhibition of chlorate of potash, preceded or not by an emetic. If, after some little time, no benefit followed this treatment, the dry chloride of lime was substituted for the chlorate of potash. In most instances, however, speedy cure resulted from the use of the chlorate alone. *Part* xl., *p.* 58.

MOXA.

Lime Moxa.—When it is recommended to apply a moxa to any part of the body, Dr. Osborne, of Dublin, has found quicklime to answer the purpose admirably. The quicklime is to be placed on the skin, inside a , *porte moxa*, or a strip of card bent together and tied so as to form a circle; some water is then dropped on and mixed with it. "In about two minutes the mixture swells and becomes dry, and at the same time a high degree of heat is produced, which, according to some experiments, may amount to 500° Fahr." This is certainly a very convenient and cheap mode of applying the moxa, and may be useful in making issues of any depth. Dr. Osborne thinks "that the heat produces a contraction and change in the action of the vessels of the parts over which it is applied, with great excitement of the absorbents, enabling them to return to a state of health after the failure of all other means," as is well known and acted upon by veterinary surgeons when they use the actual cautery.

Part v., *p.* 129.

New Method of Applying Counter-Irritation—" Electric Moxa."—Dr. Bird has proposed a novel method of producing a persistent discharge from the skin by means of galvanism. The making an issue, the insertion of a seton, the application of a moxa or cautery-iron, all appear formidable operations to timid patients.

Apply a blister the size of a shilling to the part where you wish to establish a counter-irritation, and another of the same size a few inches from it; when the cuticle is raised, snip it, and apply to the first one a piece of zinc foil, and to the other a piece of silver; connect them by a copper wire, and cover with wet lint and oiled silk. In forty-eight hours an eschar will appear under the zinc plate. Keep the plates on until the eschar separates, and then apply a poultice to the sore that remains.

Part xvi., *p.* 293.

———•◦•———

MUSCLES.

Affections of Voluntary Muscles—Some of the Consequences of Blows and the like Injuries of Muscles.—A blow on a muscle or on its nerve may be followed by complete wasting. Total atrophy of the abductor indicis and adductor minimi digiti has followed a sharp and very severe blow in front of the anterior annular ligament.

After a severe injury to a joint, the muscles acting on it may pass into a state of fixed contraction, or may start into contraction at any effort to move them, whether actively or passively. The joint thus stiffened is likely to be regarded as one that has been wrongly treated; the fracture or the dislocation, if either have occurred, may be thought to have been left unreduced, and an incurable anchylosis may be talked of. But the stiffness of the joint is due to the muscles alone; and if, by giving the patient chloroform, they be relaxed and put beyond the influence of his will, the joint becomes at once naturally movable, or nearly so. This condition has been noticed at the elbow, the knee, and the hip. Chloroform, which may first serve as a test of the state of the joint and muscles, may afterward be used, to give opportunity for painless and free motion of the joint while the muscles are recovering. And their recovery may be accelerated by friction, warmth, passive motion to any extent that they will allow, and (which is far better) every possible effort of the patient's own will to move them. *Part* xxxvii., *p.* 245.

Myalgia, or Muscular Pain.—Dr. Inman has written an article on myalgia or muscular pains. The importance of this affection does not arise from it, *per se*, but from its great resemblance to other painful affections, as hysteria, neuralgia, pleurisy, peritonitis, disease of the liver, kidney, bladder, or uterus; for all which affections the author has seen it mistaken, of course causing needless alarm to both patient and physician. It is generally attended with want of power of the system; the fleshy parts of the muscles, or their tendinous prolongations, will not bear the least stretching, and in many cases the pain arises solely from this cause, from over fatigue, etc. The pain is independent entirely of the course of nerves, is hot and aching, and attended commonly with tenderness on the least pressure. This affection will be aggravated by antiphlogistic treatment, but relieved by measures calculated to raise the tone of the system, as stimulants, tonics, generous diet, etc.   *Part* xxxix., *p.* 77.

Hysterical Muscular Hyperæsthesia.—In addition to general treatment, M. Briquet recommends faradization of the skin, as performed by M. Duchenne. By his apparatus the electrical current is limited to the skin. The hyperæsthesia is usually at once dissipated. Stimulant applications, as very hot cataplasms, dry heat, chloroform, and acetic ether, locally applied (which act more as irritants than narcotics,) sinapisms, and blisters will also be of the greatest use in the relief of the local symptoms.
                                                      Part xxxix., *p.* 87.

N Æ V I .

Treatment by Caustics.—Speaking of caustics, Sir B. Brodie says, Caustics may be used with advantage in congenital tumors, nævi, etc. Little vascular spots on children's faces are an object of anxiety frequently in the upper classes; if you look at these you will see one large vessel and several branches supplying them. You may destroy these in the following manner: Take a glass pen (pointed glass made into the shape of a pen), which will hold nitric acid, and apply it to the principal vessel; or, in this way, look for the principal vessel, puncture it, and insert into the puncture a fine point of potassa fusa; a moment's touch will be sufficient to destroy the vessel; if the potassa extend further than you intended, apply vinegar. You may thus obliterate the vessel without leaving a scar. There are some congenital nævi abounding in the skin, formed by a very intricate mesh of vessels; the skin is elevated and of a mulberry color. If these are of large size, they must be destroyed by ligature or the knife; if of smaller size, you may use caustics not unprofitably. The nitric acid is the best application; this makes a slough, the blood coagulates, and the parts become indurated. This is only applied when nævi are of small size. In subcutaneous nævi, which are not of the same color, but purple, caustics may be applied to effect their destruction, whether of a large or small size; the great object is to destroy them with caustic rather than ligature. These nævi have been cured by the application of vaccine matter, which acts by producing a slough, but I cannot depend upon it, not having tried the matter myself. You may cure these subcutaneous nævi on the same principle; by this method puncture them with a finely-pointed lancet, then, having a probe armed with nitrate of silver by dipping it into fused nitrate of silver, introduce it into the puncture, the caustic presently causes sloughing, and the vessels are obliterated. If the tumor be of a large size, the application must be repeated. I have used this plan with great advantage, when it was necessary to save the skin.

I was called to see a child with nævus of the nose; to have cut it out, would have disfigured her for life; so I used a narrow instrument for dividing the skin, and inserted the caustic-armed probe into the wound; the operation, after having been performed a few times, succeeded perfectly, and a scarcely observable mark only was left. I have destroyed extensive nævi in this way, without leaving a scar. The nitrate of silver is the best caustic for such tumors, and when you apply it, use olive oil to prevent it excoriating the skin. I may observe once for all, that it is necessary to use this precaution. If you are employing caustic potass, have vinegar by you; if chloride of zinc, bicarbonate of potass, and so with the other caustics. *Part* iii., *p.* 72.

Treatment of Nœvus—Operation by Prof. Pattison.—An assistant, by means of a spirit lamp, made the needles red-hot, and they were passed in rapid succession about twenty times into the tumor in all directions. There was no hemorrhage, and the child apparently suffered very little pain. The operation was repeated twice afterward, after intervals of a week, and in the course of a month the tumor had entirely sloughed away, and the part healed. *Part* vi., *p.* 157.

Treatment of Vascular Nœvus.—Prof. Smith, of Baltimore, has devised the following method of treating vascular nævus. He saturates a thread with a saturated solution of caustic potash. This is dried by a fire, and a needle being armed with it, the base of the tumor is transfixed with the needle, and the thread quietly drawn through the part. This is repeated in different parts of the tumor. Dr. S. states that he has now under care a case treated by this plan, and the tumor is rapidly wasting, without any distressing symptoms having occurred. *Part* viii., *p.* 160.

Blepharoplastie.—Dr. Baumgarten was consulted about a child, six months old, which had a large oval nævus maternus on the lower eyelid of the right eye, extending down to the cheek. Pulsations isochronous with the pulse could be both seen and felt, and as the period of its bursting could not be far distant, to judge from its appearance, Dr. Baumgarten determined to remove it by extirpation, and to replace the loss of substance by blepharoplastie. In effecting the extirpation of the nævus, it was found that the vascular dilatations extended so deeply, that the orbiculus muscle was cut across, and the incisions penetrated into the cavity of the orbit. The hemorrhage was less than might have been expected. The flap to cover in the large wound that had thus been made was taken from the temple and united to the vicinal parts by four sutures. In spite of the continual application of cold water, some swelling of the face followed, but soon subsided. Union by the first intention took place throughout the part operated on by the third day, and by the fourth the last suture was removed. The wound by the temple suppurated freely, the edges, however, being drawn together, and the bottom filled with healthy granulations. In another week the loss of substance on the temple was replaced, and the cicatrices of the eyelid were scarcely visible. *Part* viii., *p.* 165.

Cure of Nœvi by Croton Oil.—M. Lafarque states his method of curing nævi, by inoculating with croton oil, as follows: Five or six punctures should be made on and around the tumor, with a lancet dipped in the oil, just as in vaccination.

Each of the punctures causes immediately a pimple, which in thirty-six hours is developed into a little boil. These boils unite and form a red, hot, painful tumor, covered with white crusts, and resembling a small car-bunele. Two days afterward the scabs separate, and in lieu of the nævus is seen an ulcer, which is to be treated on general principles. It would be dangerous to make more than six punctures on a very young infant, as the irritation and fever are considerable. *Part* ix., *p.* 179.

Creasote in Nævus Maternus.—Dr. Thornton informs us that of all the applications he has tried against nævus, the most effectual is creasote. He had treated three cases in the course of the year successfully with this substance. It is applied two or three times daily, more or less diluted. Excoriation, ulceration, and gradual disappearance of the nævus ensues; the cicatrix had always been smooth and sound. *Part* xi., *p.* 186.

Aneurism by Anastomosis.—Aneurism by anastomosis, or nævus ma-ternus, as it is termed, when congenital, consists, as is well known, of a congeries of enlarged and dilated arteries and veins, which can be emptied of their contents by pressure, and gradually refill when the pressure is re-moved. Mr. Cooper considers the disease to be of an *atonic* character, dependent, not upon excessive action, but upon a defective condition of the coats of the vessel, arising from arrest of nutrition; so that the dis-ease may be said to originate in the vasa vasorum.

When the tumor is small, it is often sufficient to keep the surface con-stantly wetted with a strong solution of alum; or a saturated solution of alum may be injected into the tumor with a very fine syringe, but this must not be done if the tumor is large. Pressure, by means of a plaster-cast bound upon the part is only applicable when the disease is situated over bone, and is not always successful; neither is vaccination. The ap-plication of nitric acid is objectionable, from the hemorrhage which re-sults when the slough separates; the same danger, that of hemorrhage, attends the practice of excision. The ligature is the most generally appli-cable mode of treatment, and may be applied, if the tumor is small, by passing two needles through its base at right angles to each other, tying the ligature tightly round them, and replacing it by another when it be-comes loose. *Part* xx, *p.* 124.

Treatment of Nævus by a Solution of Iodine.—[Dr. Bulteel has used with the most satisfactory result, a solution of iodine ℈j., in sp. vin. rect. ℥ss. He says:]

The preparation was applied freely once every day, not exciting the slightest constitutional derangement, and the disease every two or three days scaling itself, if I may use the expression, and thus disappearing *gra-datim* till nothing more could be seen but two little spots of the size of a pin's head. The application at once arrests the growth of the nævus and nothing but a regular daily application is needed for its final removal.

Part xx., *p.* 126.

Use of Collodion in Nævus.—Dr. Brainard. of Chicago, struck with the contractile power possessed by the etherial solution of gun-cotton, was induced to test its application to the surface of erectile tumors. The first case which he treated in this way was an erectile tumor, the size of a strawberry, situated over the anterior fontanelle of a very young infant. Although the tumor was considerably elevated above the general surface

of the scalp, it was at once reduced when the solution had dried, and, after a second application, at the end of six weeks, seemed to be cured.
Part xxi., *p.* 197.

Use of Nitric Acid.—Apply a drop of strong fuming nitric acid, by means of a glass rod, and let it dry on. If the nævus is very small, not even a scar will be left. *Part* xxi., *p.* 261.

Use of the Actual Cautery.—Pass a flat platinum needle, heated to whiteness, through the substance of the nævus. *Part* xxi., *p.* 261.

Treatment of Nævi.—The following methods of treatment for the cure of nævi have each their advocates, and are more or less benficial, according as the nævus may be of the cutaneous, subcutaneous, or mixed variety.

They may be severally arranged under the three following heads:

1. To induce atrophy of the new growth, by—
   a. Compression.
   b. Astringents or refrigerants.
   c. Ligature of the vessels of supply.
2. To excite inflammation in the tissue of the nævus, and thus obliterate the cells of the new tissue, by—
   a. Seton.
   b. Acupuncture.
   c. Laceration of the tissue by punctures.
   d. Incision and the insertion of sponge.
   e. Cauterization with potassa fusa, chloride of zinc, etc.
   f. Injections of stimulating solutions.
   g. Punctures with a probe coated with argenti nitras.
   h. Vaccination.
   i. Punctures, with a lancet's point covered with croton oil.
3. The entire removal of the new growth, by—
   a. Excision of the disease only.
   b. Amputation of the part affected, as of lips, prepuce, labium pudendi, fingers, etc.
   c. Ligature in various ways.
   d. Complete destruction with caustics. *Part* xxiv., *p.* 196.

Removal of a Nævus by Platinum Wire, heated by a Galvanic Current.—[Cases of fistula in ano and hemorrhoids having been successfully cured in this manner, in University College Hospital:]

Mr. Hilton has been trying this plan of cutting and searing at the same time upon a nævus of the flat kind, situated in front of the ear of a child two months old. The operation was performed with Cruikshank's battery and a very thin wire, which was first intended to tie around half the tumor, which was about the size of a crown piece. But the wire ran so easily through it, that the whole was completely removed, and the parts are now fast cicatrizing. This is rather a quicker measure than the ligature, and just as secure, since hemorrhage is so rare. *Part* xxv., *p.* 195.

Treatment of Nævi.—Mr. Lloyd destroys nævi slightly raised above the surface with potassa fusa, and there is hardly ever a return of the growth. We have seen him use the caustic upon very young children, and the latter did not seem to suffer much pain. With erectile tumors, Mr. Lloyd excites the sloughing action, by injecting into the substance of the growth the aromatic spirit of ammonia, by means of a small syringe, with a long and delicate pipe. The nævi seldom resist the action of the caustic fluid, and generally become obliterated in a few weeks.

Part xxv., *p.* 196.

New Instrument for injecting the Perchloride of Iron in Cases of Nœvus, etc.—In several cases in which this remedy had been employed in cases of nævus, two circumstances proved unfavorable to its success. In the first place, by its being in some too freely used, inflammation and sloughing had been produced ; and, in the second, the flow of blood had prevented the defective instrument acting efficiently. To remedy this latter defect, Mr. Furgusson has invented the following:

It consists of a very small glass syringe, the point of which terminates in a fine platinum tube. This tube is incased in another one, about a quarter of an inch longer than the first, ending in a sharp trocar-like point, and having, near its extremity, an oblique opening in one side. By rotating the outer tube on the contained one, their apertures may be made to correspond or otherwise, at the will of the operator. Thus, then, the necessity for two instruments is quite done away with. The syringe having been charged, the operator rotates the outer tube, so as to conceal the orifice of the inner one entirely, and protect it from the ingress of blood. In this state the instrument is passed into the centre of the tumor, and, having been stirred about as much as may be thought desirable, the tube is turned back so as to expose the orifice ; and the piston being at the same moment depressed, a drop or two of the solution is squeezed out.

Part xxviii., *p.* 172.

Erectile Tumor of the Orbit.—The following mode of treatment was quite successful. A solution of lactate of iron (eight grains to one drachm of distilled water) was injected into the centre of the tumor. Violent pain in the head and vomiting succeeded, but these gradually disappeared, and the recovery was perfect. Dr. Brainard, the author of this paper, believes the injection of the perchloride of iron into the blood to be exceedingly dangerous, because it is a substance abnormal to the constitution of the blood, and because it produces instant coagulation. In the case of the lactate of iron, its components already exist in the blood, and its effects are not sudden coagulation, but a thickening of the coats with deposition of coagulable lymph from subacute inflammation being induced.

Part xxviii., *p.* 174.

Treatment of Nœvus by Tartar Emetic.—Apply on a piece of thin leather, cut accurately to the size of the tumor, a compound of fifteen grains of tartar emetic to ʒj. of galbanum plaster. Inflammatory action is set up and the vessels obliterated. *Part* xxix., *p.* 207.

Use of Acid Nitrate of Mercury.—In moles and nævi of the face, if superficial, apply a solution of the nitrate of mercury in strong nitric acid. There is a mild form of dilated cutaneous capillaries which produces the marks known as "port-wine stains," "spiders," etc., in the treatment of which much benefit may be obtained by the dexterous application of fluid caustics. With a finely-pointed glass brush, charged either with nitric acid, or the acid nitrate of mercury, the tortuous vascular trunks should be severally painted, a minute streak of the caustic being thus left along the whole course. In this way, by repeated applications, the whole of the larger vessels may be destroyed, and the disfigurement to a large extent, diminished.

Vide Art. " Boils." *Part* xxxi., *p.* 240.

Nævus—Caustic Collodion.—In cases where excision is impracticable, there is no better caustic, when it is desired that they should disappear quickly and certainly, than a solution of four parts of deuto-chloride of mercury in thirty of collodion. It should be applied with a camel's-hair brush. *Part* xxxiv., *p.* 277.

More than a Hundred Nævi on the same Infant.—A case lately occurred to Mr. Hutchinson of the Metropolitan Free Hospital where there were more than a hundred distinct nævi of the most superficial character on the same child ; all were cured, except about twelve on the scalp, by the continued application of the compound iodine ointment. To the remainder it is proposed to apply nitric acid should they not diminish under a continuance of the former treatment. *Part* xxxvii., *p.* 138.

Treatment of Nævus by Injections with Tannic Acid.—Mr. Haynes Walton has recently treated several cases of nævus in the following manner : A small tendon knife having first been pushed into the base of the tumor and moved about slightly, to break up the tissue, a solution of tannin, a drachm to an ounce of water, is injected by means of a syringe with a small nozzle. This must be slowly performed, and must be given up directly the tension of the tumor becomes apparent ; by this means the blood coagulates, and after the lapse of some weeks the tumor disappears. There is no risk of sloughing taking place as when the muriated tincture of iron is used. *Part* xxxvii., *p.* 269.

Subcutaneous Nævus over the Anterior Fontanelle.—Mr. Erichsen treated a congenital nævus over the anterior fontanelle of an infant a few weeks old, at University College Hospital in the following manner : A puncture was made through the scalp on one side of the nævus, and a blunt needle-eyed probe armed with a ligature was passed through the base of the nævus to the opposite side, which emerged through another opening made with a knife. This was repeated at right angles to the first thread, and the four double cords were firmly tied, through fissures made in the skin, around the tumor, and complete strangulation effected. No cerebral symptom was manifested during the process. In such cases as these Mr. Erichsen does not use needles in the usual way, because the membranes of the brain might be punctured, and death might ensue. But when performed in the manner described, there is not the same risk, and in about half a dozen cases thus treated by him no accident or untoward symptom occurred, and the nævus was got rid of. When a nævus is situated over a bone, of course the sharp needles may be employed, as is commonly witnessed.

A nævus over the anterior fontanelle, common prudence would teach us requires to be managed differently fro` a ` nævi in ordinary and less important situations. *Part* xxxviii., *p.* 147.

NECRÆMIA.

Necræmia.—This term is applied by Dr. Williams to that condition of the blood, in which it appears to be itself primarily and specially affected, and to lose its vital properties. It is, in fact, death beginning with the blood. The appearance of petechiæ and vibices on the external surface, the occurrence of more extensive hemorrhages in the internal parts, the general fluidity of the blood, and frequently its unusually dark or otherwise altered aspect, its poisonous properties, as exhibited in its deleterious operations on other animals, and its proneness to pass into decomposition, point out the blood as the first seat of disorder; and, by the failure of its natural properties and functions, as the vivifier of all structure and function, it is plainly the medium by which death begins in the body. The blood, the natural source of life to the whole body, is itself dead, and spreads death instead of life. The heart's action is faltering and feeble; the atonic vessels become the seat of congestions, and readily permit extravasations. The brain, insufficiently stimulated, after slight delirium, lapses into stupor; the medulla no longer regularly responds to the *besoin de respirer;* and the respiratory movements become irregular. Muscular strength is utterly lost; offensive colliquative diarrhœa, or passive intestinal hemorrhage often occurs; sloughing sores, or actual gangrene of various parts are easily produced; and putrefaction commences almost as soon as life is extinct. The track of the superficial veins is marked by bloody stains; hypostatic congestion takes place to a great extent; the blood remains fluid, and stains the lining membranes of the vessels. Rokitansky describes the blood as often foamy, from the development of gas, and of a dirty red raspberry-jelly color; its serum dark from exuded hematine; and its globules swollen up by endosmosis. Coagula are either totally absent, or are very soft and small. The exudations are of a dirty red—turbid, thin. There is scarcely any rigor mortis; the tissue of the heart and of other organs is flaccid and softened, and stained by imbibition of the serum. Gas is quickly formed in the vessels and in the areolar tissue, giving rise to a kind of emphysema. It is very remarkable that this necræmic condition, or one closely resembling it, may be brought on by violent shocks inflicted on the nervous system, as well as by the introduction of miasmatic or animal poisons into the circulation. Violent convulsions, overwhelming emotions, the shock of an amputation, a stroke of lightning, even a severe exhausting labor, are mentioned by the German pathologists as having produced this effect. More common causes are, however, malignant scarlatina and typhus, yellow fever, the plague, and the disease called glanders. It may be said, generally, that the early appearance of sinking and prostration in any fever, indicates that the blood is thus seriously affected. We are ignorant what is the exact nature of the changes which take place in this condition of the blood. Probably they are more of a vital than merely chemical kind—that is, they affect the properties of the blood more than its composition. The blood globules do not appear to be destroyed; but they circulate probably some time before death, as so many dead particles prove to be enlarged and to stagnate in the capillaries, and to part with their contained hematine. The fibrin is in great part destroyed; but how this comes to pass we are ignorant. We can perceive, on the whole, scarce anything more than that the powers of vital chemistry rapidly decay, and those of ordinary chemical affinity supply their place. *Part* xxxi., *p.* 52.

NECROSIS.

Chloride of Zinc in Necrosis.—The difficulty of penetrating the hard-ened case of new bone when long formed, is too well known to require any comment; and it not unfrequently happens that any attempt to reach the sequestrum is either rendered abortive thereby, or occasions such a degree of disturbance to the whole shaft, as to produce more harm than good. Mr. Guthrie, has availed himself of the peculiar properties of the chloride of zinc, which, attacking the animal tissue of the bone, destroys it, and thus causes the earthy matter to soften and become detached. The sequestrum is by this means exposed, with little pain or disturbance of the part, and may be dealt with according to circumstances. *Part* ii., *p.* 137.

Necrosis.—The opinions of medical men, as to the source from which bones are repaired after necrosis, have been divided between the soft parts and periosteum on the one hand and the bone on the other. Bone may be deposited in most parts of the body, and also by the periosteum and soft parts in the neighborhood of bone; but it does not seem probable that these are the efficient agents in the process when any extensive form-ation of bone is required. It seems more probable that this is accom-plished by bone, and especially by the epiphyses in the long bones, after certain dead portions have been extracted. Hence when no epiphysis is present, as in the cranial and other flat bones, we percieve little effort to be made for the renewal of any displaced portions. So great is this power of reformation in the long bones of young people that in a very interesting case related by Dr. Lawrie, of Glasgow, almost the entire tibia, with the exception of the epiphyses, was removed and completely renewed, the leg becoming as useful as ever.

In the treatment of extensive necrosis, two practical difficulties present themselves: first, in supporting the constitution, and preventing hectic; and second, in the very tedious process of production of new bone, and the ultimate cure, by discharge of the dead portion. The latter is known to consist in the deposit of new bone around the old and dead bone, in-casing it, and subjecting it to the very doubtful process of absorption, or of separation, and escape, through the cloacæ in the new bone, and the ulcers in the soft parts.

How soon may the dead bone be removed by operation? The answer appears to be: As soon as the inflammatory stage has passed, suppuration been fairly established, and the constitutional symptoms will permit. The nature of the operation to be performed must depend on the extent of the disease. When the entire thickness is involved, the necrosed part should be exposed and a portion cut out, and occasional attempts made to extract the portions connected with the epiphyses. There is little risk in hurrying them away too soon, provided violence is not used in the attempt; they will become loose when the natural process of separation is complete, and then comparatively little force will be required for their extraction. When the surface of a bone only is exposed and necrosed, it seldom happens that the dead part is incased in a new bone. It generally scales off, and finds its way through the ulcer in the soft part, or through an abscess. Should the dead portion be extensive, and the position of the bone admit of it, it would save time to lay open the sinuses, expose the bone, and remove with a sharp chisel all the dead portion.   *Part* viii., *p.* 103.

Iodide of Potassium.—Recommended in cases of Necrosis, by Lis-franc.—Vide "Iodic Preparations."

Observation on Necrosis.—Never attempt any operation until the sequestrum is completely detached; and even then, do not interfere, if the extrusion of the dead bone is going on favorably.   *Part* xix., *p.* 133.

Necrosis, caused by Exposure to Phosphorus Vapors.—[Mr. Stanley recently had a patient at St. Bartholomew's Hospital, who had lost the whole of his lower jaw by necrosis. The affection was ascribed to the influence of phosphorus vapor, to which the man was exposed in his trade of a *lucifer-match maker.* It appears, however, that means are now adopted to prevent such disastrous effects occurring in this occupation.' We are told that]

Workmen in lucifer-match manufactories have now a chance of escaping the baneful effects of the evolution of phosphorous acid, by placing saucers filled with oil of turpentine about their work-rooms. As oil of turpentine is a solvent of phosphorus, it is expected that it will absorb the vapors which do so much mischief. This precaution is taken at a large lucifer-match manufactory in the neighborhood of the London Hospital, and the very best results are expected from it.   *Part* xxi., *p.* 189.

Necrosis.—Whenever tendons pass over newly developing bone, it is of the greatest importance that union should be averted between them, by commencing passive motion as soon as it may safely be done.

Part xxxiii., *p.* 326.

———•◦•———

NEEDLES.

Detection of Needles, etc., imbedded in the Body.—[Portions of iron or steel are extremely liable to be introduced into the body, frequently proving very injurious. There are means, however, by which their presence may be readily determined. Mr. Smee, after some remarks on a case which came under his care, where a needle was introduced into one of the joints of the finger, and caused suppuration and subsequent anchylosis, which' might have been prevented could it have been shown that the needle was actually present, and its exact spot demonstrated, says :]

You are all acquainted with the curious condition which steel assumes under certain circumstances, whereby it evinces properties which are called magnetic; you know, moreover, that magnetic poles repel, and opposite attract, each other. You have, therefore, but to render a piece of inclosed steel a magnet, and you will be able not only to ascertain its presence, but to determine by its polarity its general direction; and by the amount of magnetism it evinces, you may even infer its probable bulk. When you suspect the presence of a piece of needle, or other steel instrument, you must subject the suspected part to a treatment calculated to render the needle magnetic; and there are two principal methods by which this object may be effected. The first, by transmitting a galvanic current at right angles, to the suspected part; the second, by placing a large magnet near the part affected, so that the object may be magnetized by induction.

For my own part, I should use the second plan, or the plan of magnetizing by induction, to render the needle magnetic. For this purpose, I have employed a temporary electro-magnet, which I magnetized by the voltaic battery, and you will find, that by keeping the part affected as close as possible to the instrument, for about half an hour, you will sufficiently obtain the desired object. To test the existence of a magnet within the body, we may take a magnetized sewing needle, and suspend it by a piece of silkworm's silk, when it will exhibit certain phenomena upon the approach of the suspected part, provided it contain a piece of magnetized steel. Although this simple contrivance will amply suffice, I, myself, possess a needle, which was made for me, and which is well adapted for the purpose. It consists of a delicate needle, about six inches long, centred upon a small agate cup, resting upon a steel point, so that the smallest possible amount of resistance is offered to its free play. When a part, containing magnetic steel, is brought near the needle, it may be attracted or repelled, it may move upward or downward, or it may exhibit disquietude according to the position in which the new magnet is held. We may detect the position of the foreign body, when it is of any size, by ascertaining where its north and south poles lie, and these are determined by their repelling and attracting the opposite poles of the magnetic needle. The disquietude or motion upward and downward, merely indicates magnetism, but not the direction of the magnet.

You will doubtless be surprised when I tell you, that, in this manner, I have detected a piece of needle impacted in the finger of a young woman, although it weighed but the seventh of a grain.   *Part* xi., *p.* 184.

Exploring Needle—Use of, in Pelvic Abscess.—Prof. Simpson states that the exploring needle is never used to more advantage than when employed for the exploration of pelvic abscesses, when they happen to be unusually difficult or doubtful in their diagnosis. The best exploring needle is a long, slender thread-like trocar, with a wire stylet passing through it, and this instrument may with safety be passed into the most important organs, and the most malignant tumors. Inflammatory pelvic tumors feel fixed and immovable to a degree seen in the case of no other morbid growth, and more particularly when occurring in the broad ligament—their most common seat—and lying close to the ilium, they feel so hard and adherent that they might almost be mistaken for an osseous tumor.
          Part xl., *p.* 205.

----•♦•----

NERVOUS DISORDERS.

Croton Oil in Nervous Disorders.—Mr. Cochrane of Edinburgh relates the following:

Some time ago I was called to attend a patient aged about 30, of a strong and robust constitution. When I first saw him, he was outrageous, and could not easily be managed by four strong individuals. His gestures, deportment, and violence were such as would have induced many practitioners to have had recourse at once to the strait jacket, but to me they occasioned little alarm, as I well knew the certainty of my remedial agent speedily producing an effect, at once useful to the patient, and gratifying to those around him. I prescribed as follows:

℞ Ol. tiglii gtt. x. ; mucilag. gum. arab.; sirup simp. aa. ℥j. Misce. Sign. Give a teaspoonful every ten minutes until he become calm.

Half an hour had scarcely passed when he became quiet, and at the end of an hour, he had so far recovered as to be able to sit up in bed, and give rational replies to every question.

I was called to attend a female patient, whom I found in bed completely prostrate, and apparently insensible to everything around her. In fact she was completely comatose, her pupils were greatly contracted, her pulse could scarcely be felt, and, in fine, she seemed all but sunk into the sleep of death. The remedy which I employed in this case, was the croton oil, in combination with mucilage and castor oil, thus proportioned:

R Ol. tiglii, gtt. viij.; ol. ricini, ℥iij.; mucil. G. arab. ℥j. Misce bene. Sign. enema. To be administered in a quart of gruel.

Though I scarcely expected any good to result from the above potent remedy, I must say, it had a most beneficial effect upon the patient, not by producing an alvine torrent, but by occasioning a very copious discharge from the bowels per anum, as well as from the stomach, by vomiting, together with a return of sensation and motion, and the use of her mental faculties. *Part* iv., *p.* 36.

Diseases of the Nervous System with the same Symptoms, but arising from different Causes.—[We cannot be too frequently reminded how important it is in practice to treat each case according to its own merits, without being influenced by the *name* affixed to the disease. Dr. Chambers judiciously points out the following instances, in which similar symptoms arise from totally opposite causes, and therefore require very different treatment:]

In apoplexy we have a suspension of the functions of the brain, dependent upon an excess of blood in that organ. In syncope we have a similar state of the cerebral functions from a deficiency of blood. We have convulsions dependent upon an excess of blood in the brain, as in cerebritis; and, *per contra*, we have convulsions dependent upon a deficiency of blood; as in excessive hemorrhage. In the varieties of delirium tremens, in the varieties of puerperal convulsions, and in continued fever, as contrasted with inflammation of the brain, we have a similar type of symptoms, arising under opposite conditions of the system, and requiring opposite modes of treatment.

The delirium tremens which attacks the habitual drunkard, who becomes suddenly deprived of his drink, is in appearance similar to the delirium that attacks the individual of usually temperate habits, during an excessive debauch. But experience tells us that in the one case we have to deal with exhaustion; and in the other, with a state closely bordering upon (if not actually), inflammation of the brain. The puerperal convulsions that arise during the efforts of parturition, are in appearance the same as the convulsions that come on after the birth of the child, which merely depend upon fatigue, combined, it may be, with too great a loss of blood; and the delirium of fever has so close a resemblance to the delirium of cerebritis, that writers of no mean authority have been induced to view the two diseases as identical, or more properly speaking, to consider the former disease as the consequence of the latter, and to regulate the treatment accordingly. There is not, I am convinced, in the whole range of practical medicine, a more fatal error than this; it induces its disciples (and they are numerous) to have recourse to blood-letting at a period when their efforts should be directed to the increase and restoration of the vital fluid. I have alluded to blood-letting because it generally stands first on the list of remedies; but it is quite possible to do an equal or even greater amount of mischief by the improper use of purgatives and mercurials.

Part xv., *p.* 45.

Effects Produced on the Blood by Mental Labor.—Intellectual, like muscular action, probably involves an expenditure of living material, and introduces a changing series of particles, those which have been used giving place to others which come with the energy of new life to perpetuate the action. Stagnation may induce decay, but undue persistency, haste. or intensity, especially in creative efforts, may occasion waste. The author proceeded to adduce examples. One instance was an account-keeper, who, after being for some weeks engaged twelve hours daily at the desk, lost the power of fixing his attention, and became affected with such sensitiveness of the nervous system as to be frequently kept awake at night by tingling of the skin, and, when he fell asleep, disturbed by frightful dreams. There was no emaciation, loss of appetite, or disturbed digestion, and the urine was natural with the exception of a few oxalate-of-lime-crystals; but there was a strong venous hum in the jugular veins, a slight cut bled freely, and the blood under the microscope exhibited a remarkable deficiency of pale corpuscles, the proportion not being more than a fourth of the average in health, or a twentieth of what is common in phthisis. This patient, with better regulated habits, and the use of cod-liver oil and nitro-hydrochloric acid, has rapidly improved. The author observed, that the clergy, being specially exposed to the wear of thought and sympathy, are peculiarly liable to this disordered condition of the blood, their nervous system becoming unduly susceptible, and their minds rendered too easily accessible to the delusions of pseudo-science and quackery. He described the case of a popular clergyman, who, without impairment of digestive or muscular power, became affected with sleeplessness and disturbed continuity of thought, the principal physical symptom being jugular murmur. Nitro-hydrochloric acid, cod-liver oil, and subsequently phosphate of iron, with phosphoric acid, were employed with most satisfactory results. Dr. Thompson was disposed to think, that the wear of inordinate and anxious work acted as a succession of shocks through the nervous system on the blood, and he illustrated his views hy histories of effects produced by sudden and violent shocks physical and mental, showing that railway collisions occasionally produced results analogous to those depending on intellectual causes, and adducing an instance from the practice of Sir Henry Marsh, of death from entire change in the condition of the blood, without any other organic disease, induced by the mental shock occasioned in a young lady by having accidentally administered poison to her father. After relating instances illustrative of the exhausting effects of exclusive attention to one object, and remarking on the varying phenomena resulting from differences of temperament, or from association with indigestion and other collateral ailments, the author proceeded to show, that in addition to measures directed to regulation of the mental habits, medicines calculated to enrich the blood were most important auxiliaries, and that oils could often be employed when chalybeates proved too exciting. The class of cases referred to pointed to the conclusion, that over-work of the brain may often occasion deterioration of the blood before the condition of other organs disturbs the brain.

Part xxxv., *p.* 30.

NEURALGIA.

Abstracts from the best Writings on Neuralgia.—The following is th, formula of Rauque's celebrated liniment, and we have found it in several instances a valuable and powerful application:

R Extract of belladonna, two scruples: laurel water, two ounces; sulphuric ether, one ounce. Mix.

Let it be rubbed on the part, and a flannel moistened with it left applied.

Dr. Johnson says, that steeping two or three folds of lint or rag in the liquor ammoniacæ, and inclosing them in the top of a wooden pill-box, and applying it to the skin from one to two minutes, is a very valuable means of counter-irritation, producing a crop of vesicles, and requiring no subsequent dressing.

The endermic application of morphine is very strongly recommended by Dr. A. T. Thomson, in all cases where pain is the prominent symptom. Dr. T. employs the hydrochlorate, mixing one or two grains with six of sugar, and sprinkling it on the denuded blistered surface twice a-day. To affect the *general system*, the nearer it is applied to the head the better. Smaller doses may be used at first. A pustular eruption, often of some severity, usually follows, and is itself a source of relief.

Dr. Richah, of Strasburg, attributes great good to one grain of quinine and two of common snuff, introduced into the nostril of the affected side. It has been found to act as a charm, and may at all events be safely tried. Perhaps errhines are too much forgotten in affections of the fifth pair. Frictions with the veratria ointment, or by the endermic method, are doubtless of value, and perhaps failure not unfrequently depends on their imperfect mode of application.

Dr. Churchill advises the following form of plaster:

R Carbonate of ammonia, one drachm; extract of belladonna, three drachms.

Pareira speaks favorably of the tincture of aconite rubbed in with a sponge attached to a stick, till the pain ceases. One to three drachms were used at each application. Three minims may be given internally for a dose.

Mr. Jeston after giving one or two doses of calomel and rhubarb, gave—

R Narcotine, two grains; dilute sulphuric acid twenty minims; infusion of roses, one ounce and a half. Every two hours during the intermission. It frequently arrested the disease at once. The same observer advises colchicum, especially in rheumatic and intermitting pains.

Mr. Baily, of Harwich, obtained much credit from the following preparation of belladonna: Macerate for twenty days, two ounces of the dried leaves in a pint of proof spirit. Dose from twenty to forty drops.

M. Valleix, in his elaborate treatise on neuralgia, in addition to fly blisters, quinine, steel, etc., states that much benefit resulted from pills composed of equal parts of henbane, valerian, and oxide of zinc, given in increasing doses of from one to thirty per day.

The hydrochlorate of ammonia, in doses of a scruple to half a drachm, three times a day, is recommended by the German and some British practitioners, as of great value in cases of facial neuralgia and hemicrania.

A pound of quicksilver laid on the affected eye in oil silk, pencilling the part with Gourlard extract, equal parts of eau de cologne and sulphuric

· ether poured on the cheek and forehead, a plaster of opium and bella-donna, were also the means of temporary relief.

Dr. Baillie was very partial to three or four grains of the extract of henbane twice or three time a-day in facial neuralgia ; and Dr. Warren placed his chief reliance on small doses of blue pill and belladonna. Shaving the head, and washing it with cold water, and the use of the cold douche for two or three minutes on alternate days, has at times succeeded.

In the " Bulletin Gén. de Thérapeutique," it is stated that the principle of treatment is to check or mitigate the paroxysm by a full dose of opium and ether, given immediately before the paroxysm, and to administer large and frequent doses of bark during the remission. Ten to fifteen grains of quinine, exhibited after the pain has ceased, will at once make an impression, and often abridge the next paroxysm.

Many very obstinate cases were cured by giving opium until narcotism was produced. Some were bled during its continuance, and the pain ceased in the majority.

Dr. Christin speaks highly of the following plan :

℞ Acetate of morphia, one grain ; distilled water, four ounces ; sirup of acacia, one ounce. Mix. A tablespoonful every hour.

When the pain is relieved, and sleep commencing, every two hours, suspending if narcotism is induced ; the patients to avoid fluids during its administration. It often caused perspiration, diarrhœa, and diuresis.

We think well ourselves of small and repeated doses of opium. Dr. Bardsley, in his Hospital Reports, relates several successful cases from the free use of morphine.

Mr. Greenhow read a paper at the meeting of the British Association at Newcastle, insisting upon the value of inducing *rapid but moderate salivation*, and relates several cases of success. It would, no doubt, prove useful in many cases where the visceral health was principally disturbed. The suggestion is worth remembering.

Dr. Burgess strongly advises ten grains of the extract of aconite made into 12 pills with liquorice powder, and one to be given every two hours, repeating it till the pain was relieved.

Croton oil, has also lately been much recommended by Sir Charles Bell and Drs. Newbigging and Allnat, as possessing some specific influence on the ganglionic nerves, apart from its purgative action.

Dr. Bennett has found the iodide of potass of great use in cases of nervous headache, when the circulation was not affected.

Dr. Martinet, particularly in cases of crural and sciatic neuralgia, advises he use of turpentine as follows :

℞ White of egg, No. 1 ; turpentine, three drachms ; sirup of peppermint, two ounces ; sirup of orange, two ounces. Mix. A tablespoonful three times a-day, adding laudanum if sickness is present. In most instances the pain has ceased in a week.

A drachm of creasote to the ounce of lard has been strongly recommended as a local application.

Magendie has found great benefit from inserting two platinum needles in the nerve, and passing the current from Clark's electro-magnetic machine, connecting the positive pole with the needle nearest the origin of the nerve. If the pain shifts, we must follow it in the affected branch. •

The following is Dr. Graves' neuralgic plaster :

℞ Powder of opium, two scruples; camphor, half a drachm; Burgundy pitch, and plaster of lead, of each as much as may be necessary. Mix. This is enough for the largest plaster. Steep the part with warm water before applying it. *Part* viii., *p.* 28.

Neuralgia of the Urethra.—A woman thirty-two years of age, mother of four children, suffered for eight months from pain at the lower part of the abdomen, with scalding on making water, and a constant sense of titillation at the orifice of the meatus. The pain became so severe as to prevent the patient from sleeping. The bladder was examined, but no sign of calculus found. Various remedies were tried without effect. Two issues, with the Vienna caustic, were now made over the hypogastric region. The patient had tepid baths, containing two drachms of the sulphate of potass, and some pills composed of hyoscyamus and extract of lettuce. This mode of treatment effected a cure. *Part* viii., *p.* 168.

Extract of Tobacco in Neuralgia.—Extractum nicotianæ will cure neuralgia so that it shall not return again, and this with once using. It has been known to cure toothache speedily with one rubbing on the face.
Part xii., *p.* 43.

Periodic Neuralgia.—Sir B. Brodie recommends in those cases of neuralgia assuming an intermitting character, large doses of sulphate of quinine, from a scruple to half a drachm daily. Combine it if necessary with Fowler's solution of arsenic; but omit the arsenic unless unsuccessful with quinine and other remedies. *Part* xiii., *p.* 62.

Aconitum Napellus in Neuralgia.—It is of the greatest importance that it be used with caution, or serious mischief will be the result. Dr. Kirby directs a liniment made with one drachm of tincture of aconite of the shops, and seven drachms of fresh palm oil, or with two ounces of camphor liniment. Rub half a drachm or a drachm of the former, or double the quantity of the latter, into the part affected, twice or thrice a-day, according to its effects. It must be watched attentively, as the medicine is cumulative. If its poisonous effects appear, give a stimulant, as wine, or get the patient into the fresh air. *Part* xiii., *p.* 65.

Intermittent Facial Neuralgia—Mr. Hargrave recommends three grains of sulphate of quinine, with one-eighth of a grain of sulphate of morphia, an hour before each expected attack, and then give five drops of tincture of Indian hemp three times a day, and rub some cajeput oil on the part affected. Continue the quinine three times a day, and increase the Indian hemp to seven and ten drops three times a day till relieved.
Part xiii., *p.* 66.

Cardiac Neuralgia treated by Colchicum.—In cardiac neuralgia, according to Dr. Fife, colchicum was especially useful, either with or without a few drops of the tincture of digitalis with each dose, when the action of the heart was much increased as well as irregular. A local application in these cases, of great efficacy in relieving both the inordinate action and intense pain, was the tobacco-leaf, slightly moistened and placed over the region of the heart, care always being taken to remove it so soon as any feeling of giddiness, faintness, or sinking, was experienced by the patient.
Part xiii., *p.* 67.

Valerianate of Zinc.—Recommended in most of the protean forms of hysterical neuralgia. Dose, three-fourths of a grain to one grain twice or three times a day, made into pills with mucilage or conserve of red roses, or in a solution in orange-flower water, or in distilled water flavored with sirup of orange-flowers. The compounder must bear in mind that the crystals of valerianate of zinc do not dissolve readily in cold water, floating on the surface in consequence of their lightness; they should, therefore, be first incorporated with a few drops of water in a mortar.

Incompatibles.—All acids; the solid carbonates; most metallic salts; and astringent vegetable infusions or decoctions. *Part* xv., *p.* 64.

Facial Neuralgia from Uterine Disease.—May depend upon ulceration of the os uteri; if so, cauterize the ulcer with nitrate of silver, or the acid nitrate of mercury; as the ulcer heals the facial affection will probably cease. *Part* xv., *p.* 65.

Tic Douloureux.—Cautiously apply an atropine lotion to the side of the face, night and morning: R Atropinæ sulphat, gr. ij.; aquæ rosa, ʒss. M. fiat lotio; and give the following pills: R Ext. belladonnæ, gr. one-fourth; fel. tauris, inspis. gr. iv.; pulv. scammon. gr. iij.; sodæ sesquicarb. gr. iij.; assafœtidæ gr. ss. M. ft. pil. ij. horâ somni sumend. Give an alkaline warm bath twice a-week, and insist upon abstinence from stimulating food and drink, and upon the patient taking plenty of exercise. Or try etherization. Put two drachms of ether into a water jug with a mouth wide enough to receive the face, and place this in a hand-basin containing a little hot water. Direct the patient to breathe into and out of the jug, placing a towel over his face to prevent the escape of the vapor. To prevent the recurrence of the attacks give 5 minims of turpentine three or four times a-day, and let the alkaline baths, and the effervescing Pitville waters be used. *Part* xvi., *p.* 88.

Morphine in Frontal Neuralgia.—Let from a quarter of a grain to a grain of muriate of morphia be snuffed up the nostril of the affected side, daily, having previously cleansed the mucous membrane by an emollient application. *Part* xvi., *p.* 89.

Neuralgia.—Rub in fifteen or twenty drops of chloroform, and repeat the application if necessary. *Part* xix., *p.* 67.

Sciatica, Chronic.—Where all the usual remedies have failed, electro-galvanism may be safely recommended, with every chance of success.

* * * * * * *

In severe cases, put the patient under the influence of chloroform, and with a red-hot iron make an eschar along the outer part of the dorsum of the foot. *Part* xix., *p.* 308.

* * * * * * * *

Neuralgia accompanying Herpes Zoster.—Apply a blister near or over the affected part; and when the blistered surface has healed, apply a belladonna plaster.

Give grain doses of oxide of silver, combined with compound galbanum pill and extract of hyoscyamus; and use a liniment containing tincture of arnica montana, tincture of opium, and soap liniment. *Part* xxi., *p.* 79.

Tic Douloureux remedied by Operation.—A young woman, aged 25, was brought to Dr. Allan, a perfect martyr from tic, beginning over the right eyebrow and extending over the face. Her complaint had been of six years' duration, and was gradually becoming more severe. It commenced with characteristic exactness at a certain hour in the morning, at times changing its time of visit until night. On feeling the pained eyebrow, the cellular substance on both sides seemed very thick. A hard body was detected ; and on cutting down, a calcareous concretion was dislodged from its position immediately over the supra-orbital foramen, where it was attached to the nerve. Since its extraction, the girl has been comparatively free from pain. Dr. Allan asks: "*May not inveterate tic be often caused by similar deposits in inaccessible portions of nervous channels ?*" *Part* xxv., *p.* 73.

Neuralgia, Facial.—M. Cazenave rubs the following pomade over the affected nerve, renewing the application according to circumstances:— Pure chloroform, 4 drachms; cyanide of potassium, 3½ drachms; axunge, 3 ounces; wax sufficient to give consistence. If the neuralgia is in the scalp, a piece of the ointment the size of a pigeon's egg is to be rubbed over the part, and the head is then to be covered with an oilskin cap.
Part xxvi., *p.* 43.

Use of Strychnia.—Dissolve two grains of strychnia in ʒj. of phosphoric acid (P. L.), and give five minims three or four times daily, either alone or combined with some other remedy adapted to the nature of the case. *Part* xxix., *p.* 54.

Neuralgia.—Where the simple carbonate of iron fails to give relief, give the saccharine carbonate of iron and manganese. *Part* xxix., *p.* 315.

Hypodermic Injections.—In Edinburgh the use of narcotic injections by means of a small glass syringe, with a sharp hollow needle, like the sting of a wasp, has become almost universal; if, in a case of neuralgia, it be introduced at the point where there is most pain on pressure, and a few drops of narcotic fluid be injected, instantaneous relief will often be afforded. In the case of elderly people caution is required, as the injection is apt to take a strong effect.

For the relief of a localized pain, it is not necessary to confine the injection to the painful part : the injection may be inserted with quite as striking results in any other part of the body, and thus the tendency to abscess in the part, from repeated injection, is avoided.
Part xxxviii., *p.* 31.

Dental Neuralgia.—Place in the ear, on the side on which the neuralgia prevails, a little of the following, on cotton wool : acetate of morphia, one and a half grains, acetic acid, two drops, and eau de cologne, ʒij.
Part xxxix., *p.* 76.

*   *   *   *   *   *   *   *

Vide Art. "Medicines."

———•◆•———

NIPPLES.

Treatment of sore Nipples.—The tincture of catechu holds a high place, and has been found a very excellent astringent ; like the other remedies of this class, it is best adapted for the simply excoriated or abraded nipple. Nearly similar to it is the solution of pure tannin, so highly recommended by Mr. Druitt. It is made by dissolving five grains in an ounce of distilled water. The following is a favorite lotion with Dr. Johnson, who has been in the habit of using it for many years:

R Sub-borat. sodæ, 3ij.; cretæ precipitat, ʒj.; spiritus vini, aquæ rosæ, aa. ʒiij. M. fiat lotio.

This may be applied alternately with the following ointment, or the latter may be used alone:

R Ceræ albæ, ʒivss.; ol. amygdal. dulc. ʒj.; mellis despumat. ʒss.; dissolve ope caloris, dein adde gradatim, bals. peruviani, 3iiss. M. fiat unguentum.

In some cases we have seen benefit result from the use of tincture of galls and compound tincture of benzoin (Friar's balsam), in equal proportions.

It is always well to have in mind a number of these different preparations, for it not unfrequently happens that one will answer our purpose when others have failed. For fissured nipples some authors strongly advise the application of solid nitrate of silver; Dr. Johnson thinks it sometimes a good remedy in such cases, at a remote period from delivery; but that during the puerperal state its use is not advantageous, as it is apt to be followed by mammary abscess. *Part* xviii., *p.* 303.

Treatment of sore Nipples by Collodion.—The following observations are quoted from Professor Simpson's paper on gun-cotton solution: It has been proposed to use the ethereal solution of gun-cotton for other purposes than the dressing and curing of wounds—for example, as a substitute for the starch bandage in fractures; as an application and dressing to ulcers, etc. In abrasions, and slight injuries of the skin about the fingers, it forms an excellent and adhesive dressing. There is one extremely painful and unmanagable form of ulcer in which I applied it eight or ten days ago, at the Maternity Hospital, with perfect success. I allude to fissures at the base of the nipple.

It acted successfully by maintaining the edges so firmly together that they were not again re-opened by the infant: the gun-cotton dressing was not, like other dressings, affected by the moisture of the child's mouth; and as a dressing, and at the same time, by securing rest to the part, it allowed complete adhesion and cicatrization speedily to take place. I have applied it also repeatedly to ulcers of the cervix uteri and over various cutaneous eruptions. Its application relieves at once the smarting of slight burns. *Part* xix., *p.* 272.

Sore Nipple.—Apply lycopodium powder mixed with a little oxide of zinc. It must be powdered well over the part after every time the child sucks. *Part* xxi., *p.* 260.

Chapped Nipples, M. Cazenave's Balm for.—Olive oil, ʒx.; Venice turpentine, ʒij.; yellow wax, ʒj.; alkanet root, ʒss.; boil together, strain, and add of balsam of Peru, 3iis.; camphor, 9¼ gr.; stir constantly until cold. *Part* xxvii., *p.* 161.

Sore Nipples.—M. Bourdel recommends the application of a piece of lint dipped in the tincture of benzoin placed over the part, then removed, wetted with the tincture, and replaced so as to cover the ulcer with a layer of liquid. The first application is painful, but the pain seldom lasts more than fifteen minutes; the tincture forms a coating, which the action of sucking does not displace. *Part* xxx., *p.* 228.

t Sore Nipples.—M. Legroux has found the following treatment very efficacious. Collodion is rendered elastic by the addition of half a part of
castor oil, and 1½ parts of turpentine to 20 of collodion. It is applied by
means of a pencil over a radius of some centimetres around but not on the
nipple. Over this is applied a piece of gold-beater's skin, having some pin-
holes opposite the nipple to allow of the passage of the milk. This, by the
drying of the collodion, becomes rapidly agglutinated. Before suckling,
the gold-beater's skin is moistened with a little sugar and water, and
becoming soft and supple, easily admits of sucking. If it is cracked it
must be replaced. *Part* xxxv., *p.* 255.

Sore Nipples.—An excellent application is a mixture of equal parts by
weight, of glycerine and tannin ; the tannin readily dissolves in the glycerine. *Part* xxxvii., *p.* 239.

———•••———

NITRIC ACID.

Nitric Acid in Diseases dependent on Vascular Debility.—[Mr. Wil-
kinson acknowledges that mercury is the only remedy to be relied on in
cases truly venereal, but contends that nitric acid acts almost as a specific
in many diseases dependent upon vascular debility. The remedy, he remarks, is by no means new, but it has not been properly understood ; that
it has cured many cases for which he recommends it, there is abundance
of testimony on record.

The first case in which he tried it, was one of dropsy of the abdomen,
with diseased liver.]

His countenance was sallow and shrunken, his abdomen and legs swelled
to an enormous size, the latter resembling in shape the limbs of an elephant. His scrotum hung half way down his thighs, and the skin of his
penis was distended to the thickness of a man's arm. His pulse was small
and weak, and beat not more than thirty strokes in a minute. His history
was soon told. He had been a constant frequenter of a public house, had
been ill about two years with diseased liver, and then dropsy had supervened about ten months before paying me his first visit.

[He was ordered six grains of calomel and ten of colocynth at bed-time,
which brought away two motions, resembling melted pitch. The dose
was repeated ; two motions like the former followed, a third was brown
and looser. From his uneasy state and difficulty of breathing, a trocar
was passed, and a pail and a half of highly albuminous fluid drawn off.
Hyd. c. cret., cream of tartar and jalap, at bed-time, produced a watery
evacuation, containing yellow bile.]

I now determined to give the nitric acid, beginning with thirty drops
of the dilute every four hours, in a glass of decoction of cinchona. This
was increased ten drops per diem, till he took 250 daily, and continued it
for two months. The dropsy had entirely disappeared, and his pulse risen
to 90 in a minute, and full. The secretion of bile and urine had returned ;
he could eat a beef-steak for breakfast, and was ready for another before
his accustomed hour of dining, which was one o'clock. In less than six
months he was as fat and well as ever he had been during his life. The
most singular part of this case is, that my patient afterward returned to
his old habits of drinking, but, I believe not to his former excess. I saw

this person three years afterward; he had no return of his complaint whatever. He took the nitric acid nearly three months. There is one thing here I wish to point out, viz., that in all cases of obstinate obstruotion of the liver, a large dose of calomel must be given; small doses are worse than useless.

I make it a practice of giving the nitric acid and bark before and after operations for scirrhous breast, in chronic erysipelas, and immediately after the acute stage of that disease; in debility, after an attack of gout, and in most nervous diseases; in extreme old age I have found it increase the appetite, raise the spirits, and induce sleep, where opium and other narcotics have tended to keep up the disorder they were intended to remove. In.valvular affections and enlargement of the heart by dilatation, I have found the most decided benefit, especially if the liver perform its office tolerably. Of course, in such cases as the last, a cure could not be expected, or even looked for, and I have seen quite enough of digitalis to discard it in toto. If the nitric acid is taken for some time, it raises the pulse, it renders it fuller, but deprives it of its wiry hardness. It does not destroy the teeth, like the other mineral acids, nor turn them black. I have never seen it produce salivation, but it will cause great redness of the mucous passages, the tongue and fauces. *Part* xii., *p.* 139.

NOSE.

Cure of Crooked Nose by Subcutaneous division of the Cartilages.— [Dr. Dieffenbach remarks that the wrynose is either a natural deformity, or is caused by accident. He has operated in two cases with complete success: in one, the deformity was congenital, and in the other, it was caused by a fall. He thus describes the operation:]

With a small curved bistoury I made a puncture by the side of the bridge of the nose, at the point of union between the cartilage and the bone, the bistoury was then carried under the skin, so as to separate tho cartilage of the side and bridge of the nose from the bone. By a second puncture, on the other side, the middle partition of the nose and the cartilage of that side were divided.

The nostrils were then stuffed with lint, and the nose retained in its proper position with strips of plaster. The parts healed quickly, without inflammation or suppuration. *Part* iv.,*p.* 107.

Case of Nasal Enlargement successfully treated.—This was a case of peculiar enlargement of the nose, in a young lady, unaccompanied with pain or any other inconvenience than the size. Besides constitutional treatment, Dr. Clay made pressure on the organ, by means of a mold made of plaster of Paris, which was useful not only by pressing uniformly, but also by its mere weight. The mold was secured to the head by different tapes, which were applied so as to increase the pressure. In a week the mold was found too large, and a second one was made; a third, fourth, and fifth were obliged to be made, as the nose diminished in size till it regained its natural dimensions. *Part* v., *p.* 143.

Suggestions for the improvement of the Rhinoplastic operation. — It often happens that when a lost nose is restored by this operation, it becomes a skinny, shrivelled appendage, and out of all proportion, small. This may be owing to the circumstance that when union of the transplanted portion has taken place, the connecting slip between the nose-flap and the forehead is divided. This proceeding would cause inadequate nourishment to be communicated to the new nose, which would only be kept alive by the new vessels that inosculated in the cicatrix all round: whereas if the connecting slip were allowed to remain for a much longer time than is often done, it would assist materially in keeping up the life and vigor of the transplanted nose. Dr. Keith therefore recommends that the connecting slip be allowed to remain undivided for a much longer time than is generally done, and even left undivided altogether.

Part ix., *p.* 176.

Enlargement of the Nose.—[This often consists, according to Mr. Lis ton, of a kind of hypertrophy of the skin.]

There is a great enlargement of the follicles, some of them are so larg that on opening them you can insert the point of the finger—in fact, they may often be described as a series of small encysted tumors, containing a quantity of sebaceous matter, and of different sizes.

Where these tumors only involve a portion of the skin they can be easily removed; and even where they are of a large size the whole may be taken away.

The tumor is of the simplest possible character, and if you take it away entirely there will be no reproduction of it, and if this is properly gone about there is no risk from bleeding, or from any other cause. If the tumor is extensive, involves the apex and both alæ, an incision must be made right down the median line of the nose, through the whole thickness of the diseased skin; your assistant puts his finger in the nostril and with a pair of hooked forceps and a knife you dissect the tumor from one side, and make the nose as like as possible, in size and shape, as it was before. There is often a good deal of bleeding, but you need not stop on that account. Having completed the operation on one side, you proceed with the other, and make the two sides as nearly as you can of the same shape. This may occupy some few minutes. In this peculiar tissue you cannot expect to pull the vessels out and tie them, so that if they continue to bleed very profusely, small sewing needles must be put through the bleeding points and threads tied round them, the ends of the needles are then cut short off. In general, stuffing the nostril with lint and putting on a compress and bandage will completely arrest the flow of blood.

Part x., *p.* 163.

Case of Aneurism by Anastomosis in the anterior Nares.—[The subject of this remarkable case was a woman aged thirty, who became a patient at Steevens' Hospital, Dublin. Dr. Wilmot says.]

About four years and a half ago she observed a small tumor, not larger than a pea, situated on the inside of the left ala nasi. The formation of this tumor was preceded and accompanied by a good deal of pain, which was not confined to that spot, but occupied the entire left side of the nose; she also experienced a sense of fullness and tension about that side of the head, and in a few months the tumor increased so much as to attract the notice of her friends. She was now sent to me from the country by a friend, who conceived the tumor to be a polypus. Upon examination, I found the tumor, which was about the size of a small olive, attached to-the inner surface of the ala of the left nostril. It was of a dark blue color, soft, smooth, and equal on its surface, and upon pressing it, an obsure pulsation could be felt in it. The coronary artery of the lip and the lateralis nasi pulsated strongly, and appeared to feed the tumor.

In consultation with Mr Cusack and Mr. Colles, it was agreed to try the effect of nitrate of silver applied to the interior of the tumor : to accomplish this the tumor was punctured with a cataract needle, and through the punctures a small probe, coated with the nitrate of silver, was introduced. A rapid flow of blood followed each operation, but was soon stopped by pressure. The caustic was applied in this manner three or four times, and during the intervals astringent lotions and pressure were employed. This plan brought about some reduction in the size of the tumor, but it was not of long duration; in a very short time it acquired its former size, or perhaps became rather larger ; the headache, also, became very great with intense throbbing, not only in the tumor, but round the entire left side of the head and face.

In this unrelieved state she was obliged to leave the hospital ; but she returned, after an absence of nearly half a year. The tumor was now observed to have undergone a remarkable change in size and shape. It was much larger, and had altered its oval shape to a round form. It now bore some resemblance to a large hemorrhoid ; it filled the anterior cavity of the left nostril, and extended a little beyond its margin; its free surface lay against the septum, and completely blocked up its passage. The tumor preserved the same bluish color and smoothness on its surface, and its pulsation could now be seen as well as felt. All the circumjacent arteries were enlarged, the lateralis nasi was dilated to the size of a crow-quill, the coronary artery of the same side was also greatly enlarged, and pressure on either of these arteries commanded the pulsation in the tumor. She complained at this time of want of sleep from the pain and throbbing in the head ; she also stated that vision had been rather dull in the left eye for some short time back.

Finding that all the symptoms were rapidly increasing, and that the several plans of treatment adopted were unsuccessful, we resolved on perforating the tumor with the actual cautery. The operation consisted in perforating the tumor in two distinct places with a nail-shaped cautery iron. This operation was repeated six times, at intervals of 14 days between each. After every application the tumor swelled, became painful, and in about three days pus was observed to ooze through the openings. By following up this plan the tumor gradually diminished, and the enlarged arteries lessened. At the expiration of three months she was discharged from hospital perfectly well. There was then no trace of the tumor, the lateralis nasi artery could not be felt, and the other arteries which had been enlarged, were restored to their natural size.

Part xv., *p.* 194.

Operation for Restoration of the Nose.—[In this case the loss of the nose was due to a blow, received a long time previously ; the patient was now forty years of age. We are told that]

Mr. Ferguson gave, in this instance, the preference to the Indian method ; and the patient having been placed under the influence of chloroform, a triangular piece of leather, cut into the shape of the new organ, and made to suit the irregularities of the stump, was spread flat upon the

...., with its base uppermost; deep incisions, with subsequent parings, were then made along the margins of the deformed nose, following the line, where the sides of the flap, to be presently cut from the forehead, were to be implanted. When the paring had been carefully and regularly done on both sides, Mr. Ferguson cut out the skin and cellular tissue of the forehead, down to the periosteum, according to the shape above mentioned, and this being carefully dissected from above, downward, to the root of the nose, where the dissection was carried deep, to render the vascular connection more extensive; the flap was twisted on itself, and its edges were brought into contact with the grooves previously made. The hemorrhage was rather considerable, and somewhat increased the already great amount of trouble which this operation entails upon the surgeon; the sutures were, however, very neatly applied, three each side; they kept the transplanted structure very steadily in situ, and the angles of the raw surface on the forehead were likewise approximated by sutures. The cavity of the new nose, which was partly supported by the shrivelled remains of the old, was borne up by a small quantity of lint; the same was likewise put on the raw surface of the forehead; the parts were carefully and warmly wrapped up, and the patient removed.

Part xxi., *p.* 197.

Mode of Extracting Foreign Bodies from the Nostrils.—Dr. Homans for many years has practised the following: Closing the nostril which is free, he blows forcibly with his own mouth into the mouth of the patient, and the result is the discharge of the body. He states that in no case where such substance completely obstructed the passage, as beans, peas, grains of corn, etc., had this method failed of success; but when the substance introduced was so shaped as not entirely to obstruct the passage, as a button, the air blown in might pass through and not remove the body. *Part* xxi., *p.* 199.

Ozæna; or Fetid Discharge from the Nostrils.—Dr. Druitt of London, gives the following:

[The fetid odor in ozæna is dependent on putrid or decomposing organic matter; there are several diseased conditions of the nose attended with these symptoms: in *all*, our local treatment must be calculated to remove or destroy putrescent matter, and unless this be attended to, the disease, no matter what its original cause, may be prolonged to an almost indefinite period.]

What the local treatment should be may be seen from the following case which I have lately treated:

A young lady, aged 20, consulted me for an offensive discharge from the left nostril, of twelve months' duration. It followed a cold in the head, which had been unusually severe, and attended with much pain in the bones of the face. Since that time she had been infested with nauseous taste in the mouth, stuffiness and obstruction in the nostril, and profuse yellow, offensive discharge, sometimes streaked with blood. The stench of her breath was most unbearable. There was no tenderness of the nose nor any other outward sign of disease. Her appetite was bad, and spirits low, inasmuch as she felt herself a nuisance to her friends, and her family doctor had pronounced the case one of disease of the bones, and had prescribed some zinc ointment, which had done no good.

· I immediately caused the affected nostril to be syringed by means of a large brass syringe, with warm water, to which a few drops of Condy's disinfecting fluid had been added. Several syringefuls were used without any effect or any decrease of the odor; but after persevering a little longer, the patient blew her nose, and expelled a small fragment of yellow putty-like stuff—consisting evidently of pus, in that state of decay to which the name yellow, or cheesy-tubercular matter is applied. The syringing was proceeded with, and in the course of half an hour the nostril was completely emptied of quite a large quantity of this yellow stuff, the fetor of which was so terrible that it clung to the clothes of those present for some hours. The result was, that the nostril was entirely freed from smell, and although there was great irritation, and the eye was rendered very vascular and swelled, the patient expressed herself greatly relieved, and quite comfortable by comparison.

On the following day the irritation had subsided, and there had been no return of ill odor. There appeared some swelling and excoriation at the anterior extremity of the turbinated bone. A small quantity of very dilute citrine ointment was directed to be put up the nostril with a hair pencil every night.

On the eighth day she called, and reported that there had been no return of the ill odor. This case is a good example of its kind; accumulation of muco-purulent matter, following catarrhal suppuration, and keeping up a diseased suppurating state of membrane by its presence.

Slighter and earlier cases of the same class are very common. An ordinary "cold," i. e., catarrhal mucous discharge from nose, throat, and internal ear, is aggravated by a feeble condition of health, or by residence in a damp situation, and is followed by suppuration of one or both nostrils. If the health improves, the malady gets well of itself; or if it comes under treatment early, it is effectually treated without any troublesome local applications, as in the following example:

A lady, aged 38, of consumptive family and appearance, consulted me for offensive discharge from the nostrils, the consequence of a cold that she could not get rid of. There was an immense discharge of yellow muco-purulent offensive matter, and great general debility. She was speedily relieved by bark and nitric acid, ten minims of dilute nitric acid, and an ounce and a half of decoction of yellow bark twice daily; and a visit to Tunbridge Wells completed the cure. Moreover, she inhaled every night the vapor of creasote, ten drops of which were dropped into a large basin of boiling water, so that she might snuff up the steam.

The sum of the matter is this:

Ozæna is an accidental complication of any suppurating or ulcerative disease of the nose.

It is the tendency of muco pus to accumulate; and it is the tendency of the mucous membrane of the nose, if ulcerated, to exude flakes and clots of lymph or false membranes, which matters putrefy, and cause the smell.

If these putrefying substances be washed away, and the cavity kept clean, there can be no smell; and this process carried out, as I have described it, makes the patient at once more comfortable, and conduces to the radical cure of the ulcer, no matter what the first origin of that ulcer may have been.

As auxiliary measures the citrine ointment diluted, the vapor of creasote, and other astringents may be of use; and of course such constitutional remedies as may be adapted to relieve any existing cachexia. Bark and nitric acid are my favorite remedies; but the iodide of potassium, cod-liver oil, etc., have their uses. *Part* xxxviii., *p.* 324.

NYMPHOMANIA.

Anaphrodisiac Properties of Bromide of Potassium.—Thielman recommends this remedy as an excellent anaphrodisiac in satyriasis, in the frequent and painful erections during gonorrhœa, in spermatorrhœa, and in nymphomania. He administered it in doses of from 2 to 3 grains every two or three hours; and, at the same time, enjoins a mixed vegetable and milk diet, and forbids all acid substances. *Part* xxxi., *p.* 222.

· ŒDEMA.

Acute Œdema of the Lungs.—It occasionally happens, says Dr. West, that children are attacked with intense dyspnœa, and other symptoms of disorder of the respiratory organs, which terminate rapidly in death; while it is discovered, on an examination of the body, that the thoracic viscera generally are free from disease, but that the cellular tissue of the lungs is loaded with serous fluid. This *œdema of the lungs*, however, though it sometimes destroys life very speedily, is seldom, if ever, a purely idiopathic affection, but occurs generally as one of the complications of that acute anasarca which not unfrequently succeeds to scarlatina, and even then is not of common occurrence.

Bleed freely, and give large doses of tartar emetic. If the extremities are very cold, and the surface livid, apply a large mustard poultice over the chest, and give a large dose of nitrous ether every two hours, till the patient rallies sufficiently to bear bleeding. Afterward treat the general dropsy. *Part* xvii., *p.* 92.

Œdema of the Glottis from swallowing Boiling Water.—Dr. Jameson says: In all cases where boiling water has been taken, or attempted to have been taken, into the mouth, the danger at all times is imminent; for, although the little patients seem to suffer comparatively very little for the first few hours, still symptoms of grave importance set in, sooner or later, which, if not combated by appropriate treatment, will either kill the patient, or call for the operation of tracheotomy. The operation is, therefore, I think, imperatively called for, when the usual remedies, such as emetics, leeches, and the application of heat to the surface, etc., fail in allaying the urgent symptoms. But when the breathing becomes stridulous and croupy, or amounting to a mere pant, from spasm of the glottis, the pulse quick and small, the temperature of the body diminished, the head drawn back, face congested, eyes half open, inclination to coma, and difficult deglutition, I should, on the first accession of these symptoms, at once be inclined to operate; but when these have lasted a sufficient length of time to cause complete coma, or if bronchitis or laryngitis has set in, then, I think, it will be found useless; for when patients under such circumstances die after operation, provided it is not produced by the shock inflicted on the nervous system, it is from the accession of bronchitis, laryngitis, or pneumonia; consequently, if any of these exist before we operate, we can entertain but small hopes of recovery.   *Part* xvii., *p.* 147.

Œdematous Glottis—Apply a solution of nitrate of silver, where it arises from a sub-acutely inflamed mucous membrane.   *Part* xxvi., *p.* 69.

———•••———

ŒSOPHAGUS.

Extraction of Foreign Bodies from the Œsophagus.—To extract foreign bodies from the œsophagus, use a slender piece of whalebone to the end of which a thread is attached. When the instrument is passed beyond the obstruction, the thread is to be drawn tense, so as to bring the whalebone into the form of a V, and it is then withdrawn, bringing up the foreign body.   *Part* xvi., *p.* 186.

Extraction of a Fish Hook from the Œsophagus.—Two children amused themselves by playing at angling, the younger taking the part of the fish. After several endeavors to catch the hook in his mouth, the child succeeded too well, and, determining, it appeared, to play his part to perfection, swallowed the hook. The consequence was, that his brother drew the line, and fixed it at once in the œsophagus. All attempts to extract it proved futile, till the surgeon took a pistol bullet, and having pierced it, put it on the line, and allowed it to slip down to the impacted hook. The weight removed the latter, the point of which, sticking into the lead, it was safely returned.   *Part* xvii., *p.* 300.

Stricture of the Œsophagus.—In some of those cases where no food can be taken, employ transfusion of blood, to give the patient time to rally, so as to admit the introduction of bougies subsequently.   *Part* xx., *p.* 130.

Vide "Transfusion."

Extraction of Foreign Bodies from the Œsophagus.—If the body be small and sharp, as a needle or fish-bone, use a large goose or swan quill feather, with the barbed portion ruffled, and imbued with oil. The patient's head being supported against the breast of an assistant, lower the tongue, introduce the feather, with its concave side downward, into the throat, turn it rapidly round, and draw it out. If the body be large, use a rather straight lithotrite with an imperforate scoop. Introduce it with the blades closed, down to the foreign body, separate the blades sufficiently to grasp the substance, and after a few gentle turns, withdraw it. If the substance is a piece of flesh, and near the cardiac orifice, propel it onward to the stomach with a probang. For extracting coins, use the double ring of Graefe, attached to the end of a rod of whalebone, with a steel spring.   *Part* xx., *p.* 132.

Œsophagus—Foreign Bodies in the.—Do not use the probang indiscriminately, to push down everything into the stomach. If the substance impacted be meat, or any soft, non-irritating and digestible substance, it is proper to use the probang. But all sharp and pointed bodies should be extracted; and the best instrument for the purpose is a whalebone rod, having at one end a piece of watch-spring, which is connected securely to a flat hook, having a hole in the centre for the attachment of some loops of silk which may aid in entangling the foreign body. If the attempt at extraction is not successful, give an emetic of speedy opeiation, in the hope that the foreign body may be either expelled completely, or so altered in position that it may now be easily caught hold of. *Part* xxi., *p.* 220.

Œsophagus—Stricture of.—According to Dr. R. Bennet, If caused by aneurism pressing on the trachea and nerve-trunks, the voice will be *stridulous*, and paroxysmal attacks of suffocative dyspnœa will occur. If caused by an abscess, the voice will not be lost; if caused by malignant disease, the recurrent laryngeal nerves will soon be involved, and *paralytic aphonia* will result, although the larynx may not be affected.
Part xxx., *p.* 135.

OIL.

Local Application of Cod-Liver Oil.—The class of cases for which it appears most applicable, is that of chronic eczematous eruptions, unattended by acute inflammation of the skin or general pyrexia. In abating the troublesome itching which frequently accompanies this disease, especially in old people, it has manifested powers decidedly superior to those of any other application with which we are acquainted. In the majority of instances it can, of course, only be expected to assist constitutional treatment, not to supersede it. We are inclined to recommend the practice of exhibiting it *simultaneously with tonics*, as iron, quinine, etc.; which is now adopted with great success at several hospitals. The digestion and assimilation of the oil appears to be much aided by such combination. In the treatment of cutaneous struma and lupus at the Hospital for skin diseases, it is usual to administer along with the oil small doses of mercurials, which are often continued for many months. The success attending this practice is very great, and appears to much exceed that which results from the administration of either drug alone. *Part* xxvii., *p.* 76.

Substitute for Cod Liver Oil.—Cocoa-nut oil seems to possess the same valuable properties as cod-liver oil, and in some cases was efficacious where the latter had been useless. *Part* xxix., *p.* 92.

Cod-Liver Oil.—1. *When too nauseous for the patient,* give it floating on some bitter menstrum, in coffee, ginger wine, infusion of quassia, or, better still, in a solution of quinine, with a drachm of the tincture of orange peel, or give it in very hot milk, or smear the mouth with marmalade or black currant preserve, and having thus absorbed the attention of the gustatory nerve, immediately swallow the oil. 2. *When the oil excites sickness.* Prepare the stomach by hydrocyanic acid and bismuth three times a-day. Give first a little dry biscuit or bread crumb, and then float the oil on the coldest spring water, and give it immediately; give it in the recumbent posture, an hour or two before getting up or after going to bed. 3. *When the oil cannot be digested,* the following is useful: ℞ Rad. rhei, ʒiij.; rad. zingiberis, ʒij.; rad. gentian, ʒiss.; sodæ carbon. ʒiij; aquæ lbs. viij. The roots to be cut into small pieces; the infusion to be made with cold water, and to stand twelve hours. Take a wine-glassful thrice a-day for a week before beginning the oil, and then give it with the oil.
Part xxix., *p.* 325.

Cod-Liver Oil, Test for.—Drop a little sulphuric acid, *guttatim*, into the oil. It causes a centrifugal movement, and a beautiful violet color, which changes to purple on agitation, and ultimately to a rich sienna brown. This is best seen by adding one or two drops of the acid to half a teaspoonful of the oil spread out on a white porcelain plate. Sulphuric acid when added to olive oil causes a dirty grey color—to poppy-oil a deep yellow color—to ordinary fish-oil a deep brown color.

Part xxx., *p.* 236.

New Mode of Giving.—Take the yolk of one egg; sugar, two ounces; orange-flower water, one ounce; cod-liver oil, three ounces; essence of bitter almonds, one drop. Either the sixth or eighth part will be a dose, according to the quantity of oil which is intended for the patient.

Part xxx., *p.* 319.

Cod-Liver Oil Oleine.—When cod-liver oil is constantly vomited, give oleine prepared from the same oil in the same dose; it will have all the beneficial without any of the disagreeable effects of the oil itself.

Part xxxii., *p.* 77.

Glycerine as a Substitute for Cod-Liver Oil.—Give one to three drachms of glycerine in an ounce of water daily as a substitute for cod-liver oil; it is quite as efficacious, much less disagreeable, does not disorder digestion, and may be combined with any other remedy.

Part xxxii., *p.* 79.

Cod-Liver Oil Solidified with Gelatine.—Take of pure gelatine, half an ounce; water, simple sirup, of each four ounces; cod-liver oil, eight ounces; aromatic essence, as much as may be sufficient. Dissolve the gelatine in the boiling water, and add successively the sirup, the oil, and the aromatic essence; place the vessel containing the entire in a bath of cold water; whip the jelly for five minutes at most, and then pour it, while still fluid, into a wide-mouthed glass bottle, furnished with a cork, or with a pewter cap, or if a bottle be not at hand, into a porcelain or earthenware pot, which should be carefully closed. *Cod-liver oil gelatinized with Carrageen or Irish Moss.*—Take of fucus crispus half an ounce; water, eighteen ounces; simple sirup, eight ounces; cod-liver oil, eight ounces; any aromatic, according to taste. Boil the carrageen in the water for twenty minutes; pass the decoction through flannel; concentrate it until it is reduced to four ounces by weight; add the sirup, the oil, and the aromatic; whip the mixture briskly, having first placed it in a cold bath, and pour it, while still a little warm, into the vessel intended to receive it. The sirup may be replaced by an equal quantity of Garus' elixir, mint or vanilla cream or rum, etc.

Part xxxvi., *p.* 291.

———•◦•———

OMENTUM.

Returning the Omentum in cases of its protrusion.—[A young man was pushing open a door with a gardener's knife, the point of which was toward himself. As the door was shut he thrust himself against the point, which entered the abdomen close to the left side of the umbilicus. About three inches of the omentum protruded, which, as the surgeon was unable to return, was pushed back with a bougie. Mr. Cooper says:]

Now I have to make some remarks about returning the omentum in cases of its protrusion; in this instance, a concentrated force was employed in order to effect its reduction, but I think some little precaution is necessary in handling so delicate a tissue as a serous membrane. If it has protruded through an opening too small for it to be returned, the usual method is to enlarge the wound sufficiently to allow of its being replaced; but if it has been so long exposed to external agents as to be altered in its character, and be unfit to be returned into the abdomen, it should be allowed to remain to slough away, or, perhaps, in order to avoid the inconveniences attending upon a large slough, it may be cut off, and any vessels that may bleed tied, but do not push the ligatures in that ease into the abdomen. It might be a question whether any means for the prevention of symptoms were to be adopted in apparently so simple a case; if so, what should be the means? Some may say bleed, but in my opinion, you only disturb the natural functions by abstraction of blood, and render the patient irritable, and therefore more prone to inflammation. In this case, perfect quietude, and regulation of diet, were the means adopted, and they have proved sufficient. Purging is certainly wrong; for, by increasing the peristaltic motion of the bowels, you interrupt nature in her process of cure, by uniting the omentum to the cut edges of the wound of the peritoneum lining the abdominal walls. This patient, you observe, was four days without a motion and even then I ordered only a small dose of castor-oil, but it proved sufficient. *Part* xii., *p.* 197.

ONYCHIA.

Onychia.—Mr. Hamilton gives the following: Sometimes, in consequence of a tight shoe, the flesh of the side of the nail of the great toe is pressed against the side and upper angle or corner of the nail. Now, Dupuytren observed very truly, that in consequence of this corner of the nail being a little overlapped by a fleshy prominence, the scissors in cutting the nail are prevented from going far enough to cut this part of the nail completely, so that the angle projects in a sharp little point, which irritates the flesh pressed against it, and finally ulcerates a way into it. This is further accomplished by the pressure from above on the arch of the nail; which being flattened and straightened, the sides are forced out. The flesh, therefore, irritated and inflamed, swells, reddens, and ulcerates, and there is a thin fetid discharge from the corner of the nail; standing or walking is painful; and the pressure of a shoe can scarcely be borne; the whole foot, when the irritation runs high, gets swollen and red, and even the lymphatics up the leg are inflamed. This is called the onychia simplex. Sometimes only one side is affected, and if so, it is generally the outside; at other times, both sides of a nail, and in some instances, both great toes, suffer from this painful disease. I am inclined to think that, besides the local cause I have mentioned, the constitution has something to do with it. I have observed so many cases in delicate strumous people and in those who labor under other diseases. I operated on a gentleman who was paralytic of the whole side of the body and of speech, who had it in both great toes. There is also a young lady who is at present, and has been for the last three years, laboring under paraplegia, with cataleptic attacks, and who has been bed-ridden for that period, and, consequently, never wore a shoe, yet for a year and a half has had onychia simplex of the right great toe nail at the outside. The onychia simplex is not a disease that gets well of itself; its progress is usually from bad to worse; the swelling of the toe becomes very great, so much so, that a case is given by Dupuytren, where from the size and redness of the toe, the patient was for a long period treated for gout—a mistake, however, scarcely credible. The more the flesh swells, the greater is the pressure on the toe nail, the deeper and more extensive the ulceration, from which fungoid granulations are seen to rise.

If you see this disease early, when the upper end at the side of the nail is alone engaged, you may stop it in this way: Let the patient lay up, and poultice the toe with bread and water; this lessens the irritation and inflammation, and you will find that you will be able to insinuate, by means of a small lachrymal probe, a minute shred of lint under the angle and side of the nail, and between it and the flesh; after it is fixed in, wet it with a solution of nitrate of silver, ʒj. to the ounce; if the lint remains in, it need not be removed for forty-eight hours. You will then find the irritation and its consequences lessened, and by renewing the application two or three times the disease will be cured; and to avoid a return, you should caution the patient when cutting his nails, to cut them straight across, to be sure there is no little projecting point at the angle, but also most particularly against rounding off the angle, which allows the flesh to be pressed over it the more readily. I cured in this way a large, heavy man, who had been previously treated by caustics, poultices, and ointments, without any good.

When, however, the disease is more advanced, the pain and irritation excessive, it is better, after rest and poultice, and a purgative if required, to proceed with an operation, one of the most painful in surgery, though happily of short duration, by slitting up the nail and removing it. It is done in this way: the blade of a strong, short-bladed, sharp-pointed scissors is passed under the nail, quite to the root, the nail is slit up in the centre, one side is seized at its middle angle with a strong forceps, and torn out by turning it over on itself. If both sides are diseased, then the other half of the nail is served in the same manner, a poultice is applied, and in a few days the part will be well. It is quite remarkable how soon a case of a year's standing is thus cured in so short a time.

Chloroform happily enables us to perform this painful operation without the consciousness of the operation.   •

Sometimes the toe is bruised by a heavy body falling on the nail; blood is effused under the nail, inflammation, suppuration, and ulceration of more or less of the matrix ensue, with a loosening and separation of part of the nail from its bed. In this case the nail acts as a foreign body, and no relief is afforded until it is torn out. You have an instance of this in a boy formerly in the house, on whose toe the edge of a pail fell; also in a young woman, a patient of Mr. Adams, to whom a nearly similar cause originated the injury, a bucket having crushed her toe, and with so much subsequent inflammation, that it extended to the periosteum, matter formed between it and the bone, with death of the last phalanx, which had to be removed.

In an unhealthy constitution onychia simplex may run into the second variety, which has been called onychia maligna, from the severity of its symptoms, not from any cancerous character it possesses: it is a disease of the matrix which secretes the nail. This diseased action may be caused by an injury which crushes or tears the root of the nail in its bed, or by disease originally commencing at the root of the nail, with inflammation and ulceration, and finally an alteration in the nail itself, as we might expect from its secreting structure being diseased.

The toe is very much swollen, of a deep red color, the nail is either gone, and its whole matrix converted into a large, unhealthy looking ulcer, the surface greenish or black looking, with raised white callous edges, and profuse, thin, fetid, oily, and often bloody discharge; or if there is a nail, it is quite altered, dark, thin, and even shrivelled like wet parchment, and is evidently not the cause of the state of the toe, as in onychia simplex. The swelling and redness very constantly affect the foot, and I have even seen them extend some distance up the leg. Sometimes there will be a fungoid granulation springing up from the centre of the ulcerated matrix, even from the bone itself; after the nail is gone and the disease is lessening in violence, an attempt at a new nail will be seen to be made by some white horny prominences here and there.

It is not always confined to the great toes, as I have seen it affect some of the smaller toes at the same time.

The pain is very great, and the least touch of the part gives exquisite pain; wearing a shoe is out of the question, unless the leather over the toe is cut out. There is great irritation in the system: and from that and restless nights, and want of exercise, the patient gets pale, and thin, and low-spirited. The fetor of the discharge, in spite of every care on the part of the patient, is most offensive.

It is a disease of youth rather than age: I have seen á girl ten years old affected with it.

The treatment that Dupuytren was the first to propose, is very severe, indeed, though certainly very effectual; it was to remove the entire matrix of the nail; he made a deep incision with a sharp straight bistoury, in a semi-circular form, a little above the root of the matrix, and carried it round the sides; he raised with a forceps the edge of the integument next the matrix, and cut under it toward the end of the toe, keeping close to the bone, so as to remove the diseased matrix entirely. The part was to be examined closely, to see if there was any portion of the nail remaining, which was to be removed; it was then to be covered with a pledget of lint, with holes in it and smeared with cerate, and dry lint outside it, and not opened for five days.

In about a fortnight it had generally healed. You will sometimes have to perform this operation, but not often. Mr. Wardrop found that mercury given to salivation effected a cure; and the late Mr. Colles was in the habit of treating such cases very effectually with mercurial fumigation. You may combine these, giving three grains of blue pill three times a day, and apply mercurial fumigation daily till the sore assumes a healthy granulating surface, and the surrounding inflammation and swelling subside; the simple applications, bread and water poultice, or simple cerate dressing, may be used; sprinkling the ulcerated surface with red precipitate powder nearly answers as well as the fumigation.

Part xxxii., *p.* 191.

OOPHORITIS, OR OVARITIS.

Oophoritis—Sterility dependent on.—[As this affection is not well known, Dr. Rigby relates a ease:]

C. C., aged 31, brunette; tall; married six years. One child born about a year after her marriage.

Complains of constant and severe pain of both groins, especially the left, with severe dragging pain in the loins and lower part of the abdomen, both of which are increased by stooping, but relieved by standing. The . catamenia come regularly and last three or four days; they are preceded for nearly a week by much suffering, which also continues during the whole period; the discharge is very profuse with clots and exudations; constant urging to pass water, which is turbid; bowels unhealthy; tongue red and dry; has had profuse and painful menstruation from her youth. Since the birth of the child, the pain has been considerably relieved, although the discharge has been increased.

Examination per Vaginam.—Nothing wrong about the os or cervix uteri; the uterine sound passes easily to the full distance (2¼ inches) without pain, but is followed by profuse discharge of blood.

Examination per Rectum.—High up in the direction of the left ovary a hard body can just be reached, which is acutely sensitive to the touch, and which she describes as the centre of her pain.

The following remedies comprised the principal treatment of this protracted case, and were varied from time to time, pro re nata.

℞ Ung. antimonii pot. tart. inguini sinistro omni nocte applicand.

℞ Pil. hydrarg. chlorid. co. gr. v., alternis noctibus.

℞ Sodæ potassio tart. ʒj. o.m.

℞ Acidi nitr. dil. mxv. ex infus. gentianæ comp., ter die. Hirudines vj. ovario sinistro.

℞ Aquæ menthæ viridis, aquæ destillatæ, aa. ʒvss.; acidi sulph. dil., mx; sirupi rhædos, ʒss. M. ft. haustus ter die sumendus.

It is difficult, and sometimes impossible, to trace the history of these cases to their origin; but from the fact of her having suffered from dysmenorrhœa up to the time of her marriage or pregnancy, and never afterward, we have reason to conclude that the canal of the cervix, or os uteri, had been unusually small, and produced considerable resistance to the free discharge of the catamenial fluid. That this form of dysmenorrhœa is not necessarily a barrier to conception is a well-known fact, although it is equally certain that sterility is the more frequent result; but when pregnancy does occur under these circumstances, the expulsion of the fœtus, even when very premature, produces such an amount of dilatation in the contracted canal as effectually to remove the cause of dysmenorrhœa. I have long since pointed out the fact, that obstructive dysmenorrhœa, when of sufficient severity and duration, is frequently attended with ovarian inflammation, which may be reasonably accounted for by the severe struggle and painful efforts which the uterus is excited to make at the menstrual periods, for the purpose of expelling the catamenial fluid which has accumulated within its cavity. This state of uterine excitement must be a source of considerable irritation to the ovaries, occurring at a time when they are known to be highly congested, and their vessels in a condition near akin to that of inflammation.. That the uterus suffers great distention from the menstrual fluid accumulated within its cavity is known by the fact that the patient herself will frequently feel it like a hard painful ball behind the symphysis pubis, which disappears as soon as the discharge comes on. In a great many instances I have reason to know that the uterus never entirely clears itself of the catamenial fluid, but remains full for many days afterward, and probably retains a certain quantity until it is expelled at the next period, as in many of these cases the moment a dilator is introduced, a quantity of brownish-red shiny discharge comes away, the characters of which are also evident from its peculiar smell. ·I may also add that, in almost all cases of long-standing obstructive dysmenorrhœa, the cavity of the uterus is considerably enlarged, being frequently half and sometimes a whole inch longer than natural, and allowing the sound to move about with an unusual degree of freedom.

[One of the most prominent symptoms in another case was *profuse and long continued menorrhagia*. Dr. Rigby observes :]

I know no form of menorrhagia where the discharge is more profuse or the disease more obstinate, than when it is dependent on an inflamed state of one or both ovaries ; and here again I may observe that in by far the majority of cases, it is the left ovary which is affected—indeed, it is quite an exception to the rule when we find that it is the right one. It is difficult always to account for these peculiarities, and we are apt to theorize in attempting their explanation ; but it has frequently struck me that a loaded state of the sigmoid flexure of the colon, from the pressure which it must exert on the neighboring parts, would render the left ovary more liable to congestion by obstructing its returning circulation. As in the case above alluded to, which had also been for many years of her life one of obstructive dysmenorrhœa, the history of the symptoms and the examinations distinctly prove the existence of ovarian inflammation ; and its relief by appropriate treatment also shows that this affection was the cause of the menorrhagia, which ceased as soon as the oophoritis was relieved.

The symptoms of oophoritis varied somewhat in this case from the ordinary course, and depended upon the position of the ovary, being much more backward than usual, and almost approaching the hollow of the sacrum ; hence she had none of the inguinal pain which is so frequently observed in these cases, but it was confined to the region of the sacrum, as is usually seen in cases of retroversion, and was necessarily greatly increased by the passage of fæces down the rectum. This displacement of the ovary downward and backward into the recto-vaginal pouch, when in a more marked degree, forms one of the most agonizing affections with which I am acquainted ; the paroxysms of suffering are really frightful, and whilst they last the patient is nearly wild with torture. In three or four cases which I have seen the ovary has been found lower than usual, and approaching very nearly to the central line of the sacrum.

The slightest touch produces severe pain, of that sickening and intolerable character which pressure on the corresponding organ of the male produces, especially when inflamed. In the present case, no movement of the ovary was produced by pressure in the left groin, while the finger of the other hand was examining per rectum, but the anterior wall of the uterus was felt inclining more than usual toward the bladder, as in anteversion, from the uterus being probably pushed somewhat forward by the ovary behind. The attacks of heat and swelling of the vagina, and the great tenderness of the os externum, were connected with considerable derangement of the assimilating organs, and form a part of a series of affections which I have endeavored to describe under the term of uterine gout—the general state of the circulation indicating a close resemblance to that of it in a gouty diathesis, but the affection localizing itself on the uterus and organs belonging to it.

[In the next case reported by Dr. Rigby the sterility appeared to be owing to a *contracted state of the os and cervix uteri*, attended, as this state often is, with ovarian irritation or inflammation. The principal symtoms were irritability of the bladder, and severe pain in the right groin and front of the right thigh, with exacerbations at the menstrual periods.]

· Oophoritis, or, at least, ovarian irritation is a frequent attendant upon that form of dysmenorrhœa which arises from a contracted os and cervix uteri; the continued repetition of uterine irritation, at the catamenial periods, arising from the efforts which the uterus is excited to make for the purpose of expelling the fluid which has been secreted into its cavity, after a time brings on an irritable state of that organ (the ovary), which is so closely connected with the process of menstruation.

Part xviii., *p.* 259.

———•◆•———

OPERATIONS.

Necessity of Preparatory Treatment, before Operation.—[Mr. Cooper strongly insists upon the necessity of well ascertaining the state of a patient's health, as to the absence of organic disease, the condition of the bowels, state of the urine, etc., before undertaking an operation. We are often tempted to perform slight operations at the moment, but it is dangerous to do so, especially as to operations on the head and face—encysted tumors of the scalp, for instance. On this subject, Mr. Cooper says:]

A lady applied to an eminent surgeon, to ascertain from him whether a small encysted tumor could be removed with perfect safety from her head; to which he replied, "certainly;" the operation was immediately performed, but seven days afterward she was dead from an attack of erysipelas.

A short time ago, an individual came under my care with an external pile and a fissure in the mucous membrane of the rectum; he was considerably out of health and attributed all his ailments to the sufferings he experienced in the passing of his motions, owing to the local disease: he urged me to relieve him by operation. I kept him, however, a week or ten days under my care before I operated, and by soothing remedies had somewhat improved his condition, when I removed the external pile, and drew the bistoury across the fissure, the whole time of the operation not exceeding half a minute. The patient felt immediate relief after the operation, he had little or no pain in passing his motions, but in the course of four or five days he was seized with symptoms of subacute peritonitis: calomel and opium, and leeches, were ordered; but four days afterward he died.

Upon examination of the body, he was found to be the subject of granular kidneys (the morbus Brightii), which no doubt had caused his death. It had been ascertained, during life, by my dresser, that his urine was albuminous; but I considered the severity of his suffering demanded the performance of this slight operation: although the sequel renders it a matter for consideration whether I was right, under these circumstances, in subjecting him to a fresh source of irritation.

From such cases as these you must be impressed with the necessity of doing everything which the science of surgery can insure, so far as lies in your power, to place your patient in the greatest state of security before you subject him to any surgical operation, and even then never promise that any operation, however simple, will be perfectly free from danger, for depend upon it, it is as unwise to treat slightly the most trifling incisions of the skin, as it is dishonest to attach to an operation more importance than it justly deserves.

Some surgeons suppose that it is better to perform what are usually considered simple operations at the moment than to allow the dread of anticipation to remain on the mind of the patient, and then proceed to act upon this opinion without any preliminary precaution. There are, however, I believe, but few patients who will not duly appreciate the cautious recommendation of a surgeon to submit to some little preparatory discipline, and he will gain much more confidence from the patient by this display of judgment, than from the hasty recklessness which evinces boldness and self-reliance, rather than judicious precaution.

Part xvii., *p.* 140.

Plastic Surgery—Hints on.—A transplanted flap of skin will not unite readily to the denuded edges of a defective part, such as an old cicatrix. Even if it did unite, it would become raised and thickened. The whole of the epidermoid surface of the old cicatrix should, therefore, be pared away, so that two raw surfaces may be brought into contact. Before applying the transplanted flap, the pared edges of the defective part should be loosened from their attachments to the extent of two or three lines, by *flat strokes* of the knife. If this be not done, it is probable that the two edges will not be on the same level, the transplanted part will be raised. *Part* xxxi., *p.* 181.

Contributions to Operative Surgery.—Dr. Knox remarks:

Systematic writers on surgical anatomy and operative surgery usually devote a considerable section of their works to what they term " simple operations," practised indifferently on all, or nearly all parts of the body; such as division, cauterization, compression, dilatation, extraction, reduction, reunion, etc. But it seems to me superfluous to speak of such operations at any length. The student can only acquire a knowledge of them by seeing them put in practice by others, and by practising them himself. The reunion of divided parts by needles, stitches, adhesive and other plasters; the reduction of dislocations; the extraction of foreign bodies; dilatation by means of the fingers or by instruments; the application of the heated iron; compression by bandages; and division with the knife or scissors, constitute nearly the whole of the surgeon's manipulative education. Should he neglect practising it on the dead, he will have to learn it on the living; sometimes at his own cost, sometimes at that of his patients.

In the selection of instruments the young surgeon should follow the example of the best operators of his day, selecting the form they prefer. Let him remember always that an operation is not a dissection, but a series of incisions and steps taken agreeably to a plan previously laid down toward accomplishing a clearly understood object. Where the fingers can be used, they are preferable to knives or forceps. Never press on inflamed or suppurating parts, lest the pressure cause sloughing. To employ caustics advantageously merely requires judgment and a little dexterity. Rust, of Vienna, made the actual cautery fashionable for a time, and with Baron Larrey the moxa was a universal remedy. A sounder pathology has greatly diminished the frequency of appeal to these violent remedies. Nevertheless they are of easy application, and prove sometimes successful.

Hemorrhage is the accident which the surgeon most dreads, whether occurring in consequence of accidental wounds, or caused by operations. In whatever way it happens, the surgeon must look carefully to it, and ascertain its source. Be in no hurry, but lose no time. If the bleeding come from a vessel of any appreciable size, seize it carefully and steadily with the forceps used in dissection, and request an assistant to place a ligature around the vessel, *clear of the points of the forceps.* If the bleeding come from a vessel or vessels which cannot be discovered, the surface may be exposed for some time to the air, or moistened with cold water and vinegar, or a thin linen rag dipped in these, and kept moist, may be laid over the part. Occasionally simple pressure applied for a time by the fingers of an assistant will arrest a hemorrhage; the elevation of the limb, should the bleeding occur there, is at times very successful. Other means for arresting hemorrhage occurring from the division of small vessels have been recommended, such as torsion or twisting, which may be done with the common forceps, touching the part with lunar caustic, applying turpentine, tincture of the muriate of iron, etc. I have followed Mr. Abernethy's mode of treating certain hemorrhages with marked success.

In the terrible hand-to-hand conflicts which took place on the memorable 18th of June between the French and English cavalry, a young soldier of the English received a wound in the parotid region, immediately below the ear. I did not see this soldier until about three weeks after the accident, when it fell to my lot to bring to England the first ship-load of those who, though wounded, but not yet recovered, had escaped the terrible field. These wounded men, about ninety in number, embarked at Ostend, and were placed ultimately by me in Haslar Hospital. The first object which caught my attention, on gaining the upper deck of the vessel, was this young man. He lay extended on the deck, pale, exhausted, almost exsanguineous, and seemingly dying. He spoke with difficulty. The wound below the ear had never closed, and it bled daily, so that he could no longer sit upright. As usual, a pile of rags, lint, portions of bandages, etc., steeped in blood, and now hardened, concealed the wound, and kept the danger out of sight. The sergeant, my only assistant, cautioned me not to remove this pile, as he had seen dangerous results repeatedly in this case, whilst on their route from Brussels to Ostend. Regardless of this, I put Mr. Abernethy's plan in force, removed all pressure, exposed the wound to the air, applied a rag loosely to the wound, directing it to be constantly wetted with vinegar, and directed his head to be raised on pillows. The hemorrhage never returned, and he rapidly recovered.

In some persons there exists a hemorrhagic constitution, amounting to a serious disease.

A retired officer of the Cape Regiment of Infantry had been for some years subject to this hemorrhagic tendency. The slightest wound of the skin occasioned a considerable loss of blood, which flowed all the more that he continued to wash the wounded part with cold water. I found that pressure with the fingers, employed for but a short time, closed the wound uniformly, and arrested the hemorrhage.

In unhealthy sores, whether originating in wounds or otherwise, great caution is required in the avoiding incisions into such diseased structures.

A soldier in the Royal African Regiment of Infantry had for some time suffered from a corroding, ill-conditioned ulceration of the fingers and back of one of his hands. The surgeon under whose care he was wrote to me to come to head quarters, to assist him in amputating this hand.

On examining the disease, I found that the bones of one finger were carious, and at least contributed to maintain the disease. I recommended, therefore, that instead of amputating in the forearm, the three phalanges of this finger should be removed; but the surgeon, aware of the alarming hemorrhages which had followed all incisions, however slight, made into the semi-putrescent fingers and hand, declined attempting it. Persisting in my opinion, the case was handed over to me, to act as I thought fit. A straight probe-pointed bistoury was passed close to the bone, as high as the lateral ligaments connecting the first phalanx to the metacarpal bone, and these ligaments were cautiously divided successively, and the three phalanges withdrawn from the ulcerating mass. No bleeding followed, and the hand recovered under the use of lotions and nitrate of silver.

In general, the common dissecting-forceps is the best instrument for seizing hold of the divided artery, and securing it until a ligature can be applied, but the surgeon should also be provided with a tenaculum. When the tongue is wounded, for example, by a tooth accidentally driven into it, the closeness of the tissue renders the forceps useless. You must transfix the bleeding orifice of the vessel with the tenaculum, and tie in a small portion of the surrounding texture. The arteries in the palm of the hand are difficult to be secured, and may require the use of a tenaculum. They must be tied where divided, and, if possible, a ligature put upon both orifices, lest the freedom of anastomosis render your ligature of no avail.

Lastly, when a large trunk, such as the bronchial, femoral, etc., has been accidentally punctured or wounded, the vessel must be secured *where wounded*, by placing a ligature above, and another below, the wounded part. In my younger days, surgeons mistook wounded arteries for aneurism, and to the tumor caused by the effused blood they gave the name of traumatic aneurism. One error naturally produces another; they mis-applied Mr. Hunter's ingenious treatment of aneurism by employing it in cases of wounded arteries. I denounced this extraordinary practice in my earliest lectures on anatomy, but it continued to be in vogue for a long time. When the brachial artery was wounded at the bend of the elbow, the hospital surgeons of the day persisted in making another wound higher up, and tying the artery where it was not wounded, but sound. This practice, beneficial only to the student, as it afforded him generally an opportunity of witnessing several operations instead of one, has at last, I believe, been reluctantly abandoned. I am at a loss to comprehend how it ever got a footing amongst surgeons.   *Part* xxxiv., *p.* 265.

Painful Cicatrix after Amputation.—Mr. Hancock thinks that this is not so much induced by the nerve or its bulb being implicated with the cicatrix, as by the adhesion and connection of the cicatrix by firm, unyielding, cartilaginous structure to the periosteum or bone. Separate the cicatrix from the periosteum by a subcutaneous incision, and prevent reunion by from day to day moving the skin backward and forward. It is no use excising the cicatrix ; in the end matters are only made worse.

Part xl., *p.* 96.

————•••————

OPIUM.

Tests for Opium.—Where opium cannot be detected by the smell, Mr. Taylor prefers the sesquichloride of iron as a test, discovering as it does meconic acid in one hundred and sixtieth of a gr. of opium. It might be supposed, says he, that if, on adding strong nitric acid to a portion of the liquid, a bright red color resulted, this would be a sufficient indication of the presence of morphia, and therefore of opium ; but a serious mistake might be committed in such a case, unless the operator had previously employed the iron test, and determined the presence of meconic acid in the liquid. It is worthy of remark, that the nitric acid test, while it destroys the color given by the meconate of iron (a dark red), will bring out, when added to excess to the same portion of liquid, the peculiar bright amber-red tint which it is known to give in a solution of morphia. The tests for meconic acid and morphia may be thus applied to one quantity of liquid.

Mr. Taylor found that nitric acid detected one-fifteenth gr. of muriate of morphia, diluted in 300 parts by weight of water ; sesquichlor. iron detected the one-eleventh gr. in 231 parts of water ; and iodic acid the one hundredth grain in 1300 parts of water. Thus, *iodic acid* is by far the most delicate test, discovering as it does morphia in less than one-fifth of a grain of opium ; but it is also the one most open to fallacy, and cannot be employed in colored organic liquids, containing these small quantities. Practically its utility is far less than would be anticipated from the result of experiments upon the pure salts of morphia. Other experiments were performed for the purpose of ascertaining how small a quantity of *meconic acid* need be present in a fluid to admit of its separation by acetate of lead, and subsequent identification by sesquichlor. of iron. No precipitate of meconate of lead occurred when the proportion of meconic acid was less than one-forty-eight gr., *i. e.*, about 0.34 gr. common opium. Unless, indeed, soluble matter of several grains of opium exists in the liquid for analysis, it will be difficult to obtain meconic acid and morphia separately. The *iron test* for *meconic acid* is far more delicate than any of the tests for morphia, and is much less liable to be interfered with. The one-fiftieth gr. or smallest visible portion of solid meconic acid is easily detected when free, while in solution, in a small quantity of liquid, even one-five hundredth gr. may be discovered. Thus, the presence of this acid may be determined in a liquid from a much smaller quantity than would suffice to form a separable precipitate of meconate of lead ; for, while for this latter one-third of a grain of opium is required, less than one-hundredth of a grain suffices for the exhibition of the acid by the direct application of the iron test. The procural of the precipitate of meconate of lead does not increase the certainty of the iron test, but merely enables us to obtain the meconic acid in a concentrated and solid form. *Part* xi., *p.* 100.

Opium.—In reference to the employment of opium generally, the constipation which it causes renders it obnoxious to some constitutions. If this (as is believed) arises from an arrest of the biliary secretions, the combination with mercury, rhubarb, or colchicum, will obviate it. In cases where any of these are not admissible, the ox-gall comes to our aid; and whether it is by directly stimulating the secretion of bile, or acting as a substitute for it, there can be no question of its being able to counteract the constipating tendency of opium. But this power of causing constipation becomes available in the treatment of a very formidable disease—namely, in peritonitis from perforation of a portion of the intestinal canal; and as our object here is to arrest the action of the intestines, to enable the opening to be sealed up with organized lymph, it is evident, that to effect this object, the *uncombined* use of opium can only be relied on. Should the aid of mercury be required to combat the consequences of the inflammation, its administration must be postponed to an after-period.

Part xv., *p.* 87.

Muriate of Opium.—The following is Dr. Nicol's formula: Take of the best powdered opium, ʒj.; muriatic acid, ʒj.; distilled water, ʒxx. Mix. Shake this mixture very frequently every day, during fourteen days, then strain and filter. The dose is from twenty to forty drops, according to circumstances.

Dr. N. says: I have found by experience, that this is the best anodyne I am acquainted with. I may mention that I prepared solutions of opium with acetic, nitric, sulphuric, citric, tartaric, and muriatic acids, and also prescribed them, but the muriatic solution was vastly superior to any one in every respect. All of them produced headache, with the exception of the muriatic. I prefer muriate of opium to the tincture, wine, or powder of opium, and also to the muriate and acetate of morphia; in fact, to any other preparation of opium. It never makes my head ache, but all other preparations do. *Part* xvii., *p.* 303.

Opium—Nausea from.—To counteract the nausea from opium, combine with it 30 minims of dilute sulphuric acid. The nausea from hydrochlorate of morphia is best controlled by dilute hydrochloric acid.

Part xxix., *p.* 326.

Opium in the Treatment of Chronic Ulceration of the Legs, etc.—Mr. Skey of St. Bartholomew's Hospital, says: I venture to attribute to this remarkable drug the property of promoting the formation of healthy granulations on a surface that, notwithstanding all the previous appliances of surgery, is yet flat, pale, and ungranulating. Now, there is no example of the power of opium to effect this object, more conclusive, or in which there is more work to be done, than that form of disease of which I am speaking, —which consists of a gap formed on the surface of the body, of greater or less depth and diameter, and in which there exists not even a trace of a curative action,—and yet the object is accomplished by means of this agent, and often with remarkable celerity. We call opium a stimulant and a sedative. As a stimulant, it is not very often employed in practice: while its properties, as a sedative, are well known, and are in daily requisition. Its property of mitigating pain and of promoting sleep, is that for which it is almost exclusively employed, and so completely is its action associated with this sedative principle, that its occasional influence as a stimulant is almost entirely lost sight of, and the stimulating property has merged in the supposed sedative.

. I believe that its sedative properties have little concern with the result. In truth, opium is a most valuable stimulant of the vital powers, and whether its action originate with the centre or the periphery of the circulation, whether primarily on the heart or on the capillary vessels, I do not pretend to know; but there is no drug, simple or composite, known to our pharmacologists that possesses an equal power with opium, of giving energy to the capillary system of arteries, of promoting animal warmth, and thus maintaining an equable balance of the circulation throughout the body. To maintain the balance of the circulation! How much of meaning is attached to these words! How many affections of the bodily frame may not be brought within the range of this definition! Take the common chilblain; what is it but a local congestion of blood caused by defective capillary power?—there is no better remedy than opium; cold feet, as characterizing a person or a constitution, equally relieved; senile gangrene, the result of arrest of the capillary circulation, or its apparent opposite, local hyperemia—these diseases, one and all, manifest a loss of local power, a failure in the balance of the circulation. The term "inflammation," a word formerly in the mouths of our professional brethren on all occasions, is now limited in its application, and should be yet more limited, and I believe, in a yet more advanced state of medical science, will be restricted to an actually rare condition of the system. The influence of opium in such conditions is that of promoting a genial warmth over the system, a glow exactly resembling, and in fact identical with, that produced by the reaction on the system which is caused by the cold-bath. *It is local health,* and the sensation is most agreeable. The benefit derived from opium, when administered for the purpose of arresting inflammatory action of the vessels, admits, I think, of much doubt, and should be resorted to with some hesitation as a remedial agent, though I am quite persuaded that the evil of its administration is greatly overrated. But who will profess ignorance in these days of the inestimable value of this agent when resorted to immediately after an attack of inflammation has been subdued by a local or general bleeding? Here we can imagine that, the activity of the disease being checked, the diffusing influence of opium on the circulation may act as a simple derivative, operating on the vessels at the moment they are not indisposed to yield up their blood, and to which indeed they are compelled by the diffusive power of the general stimulus.

Many years ago, and before the introduction of railway travelling, I was summoned late one afternoon to see a patient some eighty miles from London. I travelled outside the mail. This occurred in the month of December, and the night was extremely cold. By some mistake I omitted to bring my great-coat; and, for the first hour, I suffered a good deal. On reaching a town at some ten miles' distance from London, I took the opportunity, while changing horses, to run across the street to a druggist's shop, where I ordered a draught, containing twenty-five drops of tincture of opium. I believe I was the only person outside the coach that night who did not suffer the slightest sensation from cold.

But it will be urged by many, who have experimented on, and who have observed less than I have done, the medical properties of opium, the infinite importance of studying the reactive effects of this daily poison, and they would inquire into the condition of a person so treated on the following day. You may be assured that it amounts to *nil*. You will, I am sure, readily understand what I mean when I say the cold and the opium mutually balanced and mutually neutralized each other. There could be no reaction, because the influence of the depressing agent—viz., the cold, rather than otherwise, exceeded in duration that of the stimulant. If the period of prostration were brief, and limited to one or two hours, the argument might hold; but it is but a sorry objection to be urged after all.

I wish I could impress on the minds of the medical authorities in the Crimea the real benefit that might be derived to our troops, beaten down by intense cold and suffering in its various forms, from the judicious administration of opium. If twenty-five or thirty drops of tincture of opium, in addition to his ordinary quantum of rum, were administered to each soldier whose nightly services are required in the trenches or on guard, you would hear little complaint of cold for that night, neither would it produce the smallest tendency to sleep.

If cold beget suffering, opium is the antidote to that suffering, and the one will assuredly neutralize the other.

Notwithstanding the prejudices and the bigotry that have long beset the public mind on this subject, and from which our profession is not totally exempt, there is no comparison to be drawn between the practice of dram-drinking and the excessive indulgence in the use of opium.

The man who indulges in spirituous liquors makes daily inroads on his digestive powers not less than on his brain. His appetite is destroyed, and the pabulum for his blood is withheld from his circulation. He is stamped for life, and his perfect health is irrecoverable. The influence of opium, when taken as a means of indulgence, though deleterious, is not permanently injurious. It exercises no serious influence on his digestion or on his cerebral organs, and, the practice once controlled, leaves him in a condition to regain, without difficulty, the fullest vigor of both bodily and mental health.

I have related to you the particulars of several cases of chronic ulcer in which recovery was attributable to the medicinal properties of opium, and almost to opium alone. The character of these ulcers strongly marks the inactivity of their nature, and hence the class of society to which they belong. They are marked by a flat base, which indicates, by its pale, flabby uniformity of surface, that no reparatory action has approached it. It is often surrounded by a thick, high ridge of lymph, covered by unhealthy integuments. The depth of the ulcer, which may be seven or eight lines, is caused partly by the ridge, and partly by the excavation of the ulcer below the natural level of the healthy integuments. So long as this ridge exists, although granulations may form, and will form, from the date of the employment of the opium, yet cicatrization will never complete the process of cure unless the wound or ridge be absorbed. Now the action of opium is not alone exhibited in the development of healthy granulations, but in the entire complement of such actions as are required by the sore, viz., the formation of new material, and the absorption of the old.

The influence of the stimulant is exhibited therefore not on one partienlar function. It does not merely promote secretion, but it stimulates the healthy vital actions in their entirety—viz., secretion, organization, and absorption contemporaneously; the granulations are secreted and organized, while the circumvallation of unsound material, the product of years of growth, is gradually absorbed and reduced to the level of the surround-ing integument; for the removal of this wall is quite as indispensable to the ultimate result as the obliteration of the cavity by granulation. With-out the two surfaces be brought to the same level, the process of cicatri-zation, or skinning over, will never be perfected.

If, therefore, we find that a disease like that I have described, and which exhibits so palpably a dormant condition of the remote capillaries, is amenable to this form of stimulant, which can only accomplish the cure by the substitution of healthy for morbid actions, why should we restrict its employment to this class of diseases? Why, as I have elsewhere in-quired, may we not experiment with success on any local disease depen-dent on the same cause—viz., an inert condition of the remote vascular system?

In claiming for opium the merit of rousing into healthy action the dor-mant capillary system, to the end of accomplishing the permanent cure of ulcer of the legs in old persons, I by no means wish you to infer that I consider all other modes of treatment unworthy of trial. Indeed, I attach great value to that recommended by Mr. Baynton, of Bristol, and others; but, having tested their value, I have no hesitation in pronouncing that which I have recommended, so far as I am competent to judge, as by far the most certain and efficacious.   *Part* xxxi., *p.* 192.

———•◆•———

ORCHITIS.

Treatment of Diseases of the Testicle by compression.—Mr. Langston Parker states that in common swelled testicle compression may be em-ployed as soon as the patient is able to bear the application of the plasters; and this is generally much sooner than might be supposed, however acute the disease may be. The great advantages possessed by compression, are almost immediate relief to pain; the patient can usually pursue his ordi-nary duties. Compression is also advised in chronic enlargement and in-flammation of the testis—the result of constitutional syphilis.

Compression of the testis is to be practised by surrounding the organ by straps of plaster, applied as closely and tight as the patient can bear. The plasters I generally use are those of ammoniacum, with mercury, or iodine and belladonna. These are to be smoothly spread upon thick wash-leather and cut into thin straps; an assistant then grasps the testicle, and draws it as far downward as he can in the scrotum, which should previously be washed with a little spirits of wine. The first strap should be placed at the upper part, circularly round the testis, and succeeded by others, placed in the same direction, till the whole is covered: a second series of straps is then to be placed in an opposite direction to the former, crossing them at right angles, from behind forward. One or two long ones may then be placed over these where they appear to be most needed, to keep the whole in place. The parts should be supported by a well-fitting sus-pensory bandage, although the plasters at once relieve any inconvenience or pain that may have been occasioned by the dragging or weight of the testicle.   *Part* ii., *p.* 109.

Pressure by Condensed air as a Surgical Remedy.—Pressure applied to diseased parts, when judiciously employed, has long been regarded as a valuable remedy in particular diseases, in some cases of diseased testicle for example; this has generally been applied by means of straps of plaster, or some such application, which, however, cannot be properly or durably applied. Dr. Krauss suggests the adoption of compression by condensed air, in Mackintosh bags, variously shaped, so as to fit the different parts of the body which are most liable to require such applications. He would surround a diseased testicle with one of these air cushions, consisting of two bags, one hanging in the other, and both narrow on the top, to surround the spermatic cord. Each bag is open on one side, from the top to the bottom, and they are attached to each other by their corresponding edges, so as to leave between them an air-tight space, accessible only by means of an air-tight screw, fixed to the bottom of the outer bag. Along the side opening are holes to lace the double bag, previously to its being inflated, around the testicle, and it is subsequently filled with air, by means of a simple air pump. The inside bag is thus uniformly pressed against the whole of the scrotum contained in the air bag. On the swelling of the testicle decreasing, more air can easily be introduced, or, on the other hand, if necessary, the degree of pressure can be reduced by allowing part of the air to escape.

Dr. Krauss proposes an air bag, made in the shape of a cylinder, to replace the solid bougie for dilatation of strictures, also an *air pessary*, on the same principle, for the support of prolapsions of the womb, and an air bag, for the purpose of *Tamponnement* in hemorrhage of the uterus.

He further suggests the application of pressure by condensed air, as a curative means in certain diseases of the joints—in perforation of the roof of the palate—for the cure of ulcers, and for the dispersion of tumors. Dr. Krauss concludes by directing attention to the application of air and water-cushions to diminish the pressure that artificial legs frequently produce upon the stumps to which they are applied.

Part viii., *p.* 146.

Acute Orchitis.—Mr. T. B. Curling strongly recommends *tartarized antimony.* "A quarter of a grain of tartar emetic may be exhibited every three or four hours, and the dose, if necessary, increased until nausea is produced. This is one of the most valuable remedies that can be employed in acute orchitis; and when patients are desirous of avoiding the trouble, mess, and exposure consequent upon the application of leeches, the exhibition of tartar emetic will generally render local depletion unnecessary, whilst its depressing influence being only temporary, the patient quickly regains his health and strength. I have seen most acute orchitis arrested and subdued in thirty hours by keeping up constant nausea by means of this remedy. When there is much pain or constitutional derangement, two or three grains of calomel, combined with eight or ten grains of Dover's powder, or with small doses of morphia, may be given at bedtime. In consecutive orchitis, in which the tunica vaginalis is so generally affected, considerable benefit is derived from mercury. In acute cases, after the bowels have been freely acted on, and the pulse has been lowered by tartar emetic, I usually prescribe mercury, and continue it until the gums become slightly affected. I am confident that by this treatment the duration of this form of the disease is often materially abridged, and, what is of some importance, it is succeeded by much less induration and thickening of the epididymis than when the exhibition of mercury has been ·deferred to a later period." *Part* viii., *p.* 207.

Enlarged Testicle.—Ricord employs the following pills in the treatment of enlarged testicle, which remains after inflammation of that organ:
Hyd. chlor. ɘj.; pulv. conii; sapon. hisp. aa. ɘij. M. ft. pil. xxiv.
Part ix., *p.* 20.

Treatment of Hernia Humoralis, or Gonorrhœal Orchitis, by Opium. —In the reports of cases of this description under Mr. Gay, in the Royal Free Hospital, London, we find that the gonorrhœal inflammation of the testicles and appendages were speedily and completely cured, by purgatives and opium. Hyoscyamus has been given with equally good effects. The full and free purgation was always necessary before giving the opium. Fifteen minims of laudanum may be given every four hours, and the previous purgative may be composed of five grains of calomel with twenty-five grains of jalap, or a strong black draught. *Part* ix., *p.* 186.

Orchitis—Incision into the Tunica Albuginea.—M. Velpeau considers that the excruciating pain experienced in orchitis depends on a species of strangulation; the tunica albuginea, not yielding, compresses the swollen and inflamed testicle, and thus gives rise to the intense pain. He accordingly, acting on these views, recommends an incision into the tunica albuginea. He has performed it with success fifteen times, nor did permanent injury of the testicle occur in any one case. *Part* xii., *p.* 302.

Treatment of Gonorrhœal Orchitis.—In taking a review of the method of treatment usually employed in this disease, Mr. Phillips states that *punctures, frictions,* and *compressions,* are of limited application; *purgatives* are not of use except in moderation, to keep the bowels open; *local bloodletting* produces as much inconvenience as it does good; and *general bleeding* is usually uncalled for. The plan of treatment which Mr. Phillips prefers, is that by nauseants.

Give a mixture containing epsom salts, and a sufficient quantity of tartar emetic to produce decided nausea from the first; say half a grain for the first dose, and then a fourth or a sixth of a grain every four or six hours, so as to keep up the nausea for two or three days. *Part* xviii., *p.* 215.

Treatment of Orchitis.—Mr. Cooper advises active antiphlogistic treatment. Thus, in persons of plethoric habit, bleed from the arm; in others, in addition to the application of leeches to the affected organs, cup from the loins to about eight ounces. Give also a pill containing a grain and a half of calomel, one-third of a grain of tartarized antimony, and half a grain of opium; and the following mixture: ℞ Magu. sulph. ʒiij.; liq. ammon. acet., ʒj.; liq. antim. tart., ʒiss.; tinct. hyoscy., ʒiss.; aq. menth., ʒvij. M. capt. ʒj. 3tis horis donec alvus bene responderit. Keep the patient on low diet, and in the recumbent position. And as a local application use a lotion containing a drachm and a half of muriate of ammonia, two ounces each of rectified spirit and liq. ammon. acet., and four ounces of water. If the inflammation does not abate, open the congested vessels of the scrotum, and promote bleeding from them by warm fomentations. If enlargement and harshness of the testicle remain after the subsidence of the inflammatory symptoms, apply strips of lint spread with the following ointment: ℞ Ung. hydrarg.; cerat. saponis, aa. ʒij.; camphoræ, gr. v. M.; and over this, apply adhesive plaster, so as to make considerable pressure. Do not, however use pressure in the early and acute stage.

Rheumatic and Gouty.—Give alkalies, and a small dose of colchicum at bedtime.

Gonorrhœal.—Apply warm fomentations to the scrotum, perineum, and penis, so as to reëstablish the discharge, and then give calomel and opium every night. *Part* xix., *p.* 174.

Collodion in Orchitis.—Prof. Costes relates cases of this disease in which, after covering the scrotum with a mixture of 20 parts of collodion and 6 of ol. ricini, the swelling and pain were quickly relieved, and a rapid and complete cure was obtained. *Part* xxxii., *p.* 293.

----•••----

OVARIAN AFFECTIONS.

Ovarian Tumors—Diagnosis.—It has occasionally happened that solid growths or tumors of the ovaries, whether of a malignant or non-malig. nant character, are attended with an effusion into the peritoneum, or an ascites, and may thus be mistaken for the more usual form of the ovarian disease, viz., the encysted dropsy. Dr. Kilgour furnishes us with some valuable hints on the diagnosis of these affections.

The non-malignant, solid enlargement or tumor of the ovary, and which sometimes attains a very great size, is, generally speaking, of the same character as the fibrous tumor of the uterus, and unless improperly inter-fered with, may exist for many years without giving more disturbance than is occasioned by its bulk. The malignant disease is similar to that met with in the mamma, and sometimes is of the hard form ; in other cases it presents the characters of soft scirrhus, or encephaloid disease. The non-malignant disease is not attended with pain—the malignant one is so generally, but not always. The latter is almost invariably attended with much constitutional disturbance ; it is much more rapid in its course ; and, whilst it indicates almost its nature by this quickness in its fatal pace, it frequently still further demonstrates itself by attacking the mammæ, the uterus, or the pylorus.

The fibrous and the scirrhous tumors, when felt through the abdominal wall, are smooth or rough, or knobbed or tuberose, on the surface ; and no diagnosis of the two diseases can be made by this means ; but the semi-solid or gelatinous cyst is almost always smooth, and invariably to a practised hand, gives more a feeling of elasticity than solidity, whilst traces of fluid, perhaps faint, will be discovered in partial spots of the ab-domen, viz., in some of the other cysts. The semi-solid or gelatiniform and elastic cyst is always fixed, but the solid tumor is often movable, and, when attended with effusion, it moves about by slight pressure in the fluid.

Now, are there any accurate means of distinguishing solid ovarian dis-ease with ascites, from encysted dropsy of the ovarium ? But, first, how is encysted dropsy itself known from ascites ?

Cruveilhier furnishes us with two very important diagnostics. 1st. In ascites the liquid always occupies the most dependent parts, viz., the pelvis and lumbar region ; whilst the small intestines floating in the fluid, corres-pond to the umbilical region, and the arch of the colon and stomach occupy the epigastrium. Percussion, therefore, elicits a dull sound over the hypogastric and lumbar regions; whereas, in encysted dropsy, the cyst develops itself anteriorly to the intestines which it pushes back, so that here the tympanitic sound does not exist. In ascites the fluctuation is more decided than in encysted ovarian dropsy. 2d. In ascites the neck of the womb is in its proper place, while in encysted ovarian dropsy it is actually drawn upward, so that it is difficult to reach it; the pelvic cavity being also in some measure filled by the tumor; and the general health is often good; while in ascites this is not the case, anasarca also often accompanying it. If a solid ovarian tumor co-exist with ascites, it may generally be known by its *mobility;* it moves up and down in the fluid, striking the finger exactly like a child in utero, in what is termed the *ballotement.* In the encysted dropsy, if a solid tumor is present, it is fixed; it is outside the cyst of the bag of water, or forms part of the wall of the cyst, and cannot readily move about. But we apprehend that in these as well as in most, if not all the diseases of the womb and the contiguous parts, we shall find Dr. Simpson's *uterine sound* or *bougie* one of the most important means of diagnosis which has lately been brought before the public. *Part* viii., *p.* 95.

Treatment of Ovarian Cysts.—Mr. Phillips states it as his opinion, " that we have not the means of determining with absolute certainty whether a tumor be an ovarian cyst or not; and that we have no sure means of ascertaining the contents and connections of tumors presumed to be ovarian." There have been numerous cases, however, in which it may have been perfectly correct to operate, but we suspect that these form the exceptions rather than the rule. Mr. Isaac Brown brings forward cases of ovarian tumors which were dispersed without these severe proceedings. He made use of mercurials, diuretics, tonics, *tight bandaging*, and tapping. These cases, however, were of young unmarried women, in whom the reparative powers of nature may have been more vigorous, or in whom the disease may not have been so obstinate.

The treatment was adopted at the suggestion of Mr. Gibson, of Halstead. It consisted of mercurial friction over the abdomen, with flannel bandages tightly applied, mercurial alteratives, and steel medicines, varied by diuretics, such as acetate of potash, spirit of juniper, and squills. When the health was improved, and the size of the abdomen somewhat diminished, showing that the cause of mischief was somewhat arrested, tapping was resorted to; and after this a pad was made of napkins, and tightly bandaged, so as to produce a good deal of pressure in the situation of the tumor : this pad was increased in thickness next day, and firm compression continued. The mercurial friction was continued on the inside of the thighs, and the diuretics again commenced. The pad was continued, and the compression increased as the patient could bear it. Several cases are related in which this treatment was successful. It will be necessary, however, to continue the treatment for a considerable time after the tumor seems to have been dispersed, otherwise it will be likely to return. *Part* x., *p.* 124.

Case of Ovariotomy.—The following case of extirpation of an ovarian tumor seems to have been one of the most successful yet recorded. Much credit is due to Mr. Southam for having added to our capabilities of forming a true diagnosis in these formidable diseases. [Having determined on extirpation, the room being heated to 75°, and the bladder emptied, etc., it was performed in the presence of Drs. Radford, Clay, Watson, and several surgeons, as follows] :

An exploratory incision, midway between the umbilicus and pubes, was first made, and the peritoneal cavity opened sufficiently to admit the finger, A characteristic membrane of a bluish white and shining surface appearing at the opening at once satisfied me of the existence of a cyst, and the finger introduced between it and the peritoneum, discovering no adhesions in the immediate neighborhood, I punctured it with a full-sized trocar. After from sixteen to eighteen pints of clear, lemon-colored slightly mucilaginous fluid had been evacuated, pressure on the parietes being well sustained during its escape, the canula was withdrawn, and using the index finger as a director, the opening was enlarged above and below with a probe-pointed bistoury, to the extent of between six and seven inches. Having ascertained by the hand introduced into the abdominal cavity, that there were no impediments to the extraction of the tumor, it was carefully drawn out, gentle pressure being continued on the abdomen. Finding that it was attached to the uterine extremity of the left broad ligament by a short and slightly vascular pedicle, I tied it firmly with a single ligature of the strongest dentist's silk. The pedicle was now divided, and the tumor being removed, the margins of the wound were immediately approximated to prevent the ingress of air. After a brief interval, the wound was again opened to remove what blood had escaped internally, and to ascertain that the vessels of the broad ligament were firmly secured. The uterus and opposite ovary were also examined and found healthy. One end of the ligature being cut off, the other was left dependent at the lowest point of the wound, the edges of which were brought together by four interrupted sutures and straps of transparent tissue plaster. Upon these a broad pad was applied, and the whole being adjusted by a bandage, the patient was lifted into bed, within twenty-five minutes from the commencement of the operation.

[The case proceeded uninterruptedly to a favorable termination; the ligature came away on the forty-ninth day, and the fistulous opening then closed. After remarking that the difficulty in making a correct diagnosis forms the chief objection to the operation, which must continue so long as mere examination of the abdomen, and the history of the case alone, are relied on in forming it—we are told that in the present case, though the enlargement was uniform and fluctuation distinct in every part—]

An examination per vaginam et rectum, cleared up all doubts, not only of the existence of an ovarian tumor, but of its exact nature. The absence of any protrusion of the vaginal parietes, the elevated position of the uterus in the pelvic cavity, and the inability to cause it to bound away from the finger, proved that the fluid could not be ascitic, whilst the projection of the swelling on the left side, the decided influence which raising and depressing the abdomen produced on the position of the uterus, with its inclination to one side more than the other, evidently indicated that the disease was connected with the left uterine appendages. The uniformity in the abdominal distention, the distinct fluctuation in every part of it, and the inability to discover any solid matter encroaching on the pelvic cavity, led me to infer that it consisted of one or two cysts only; and the comparative immunity from any great degree of suffering until within the last twelve or eighteen months, the absence in the history of any previous attacks of peritonitis, together with the slight impediment to the action of the bowels, rendered the existence of adhesions doubtful.

Though somewhat emaciated, her general health did not appear impaired; appetite good; tongue clean; pulse natural; bowels occasionally constipated, but easily acted on by medicine; catamenia regular, though in less quantity than formerly; felt pain at times in the left inguinal region, or whenever she lay on the left side, and in consequence of the pressure of the tumor upward, she has been unable to lie on her back, or in any other position, excepting on the right side, for the last twelve months. The symptoms clearly indicating encysted dropsy of the left uterine appendages, advanced to such a stage as to render surgical interference necessary, and her constitution not being much affected, I considered the case was peculiarly favorable for the operation. In the operation, the evils of both the major and minor incisions were guarded against, by making the opening no larger than was necessary to ascertain the nature and connections of the disease, and to admit of its removal after reducing it by paracentesis, without occasioning the least violence or displacement of any of the neighboring parts. Had the slightest obstacle occurred previous to the successful termination to the operation, this plan would also have enabled me to have receded without much danger to the patient. *Part* xii., *p. 247.*

New Operation for Ovarian Dropsy.—Prof. Kiwish relates the case of a peasant, æt. thirty, mother of four children, who was received into the hospital at Prague on account of obstinate ischuria and constipation. The cause of these affections was found to be a tumor, the size of a head, lying between the rectum and the vagina. By careful examination the operator was satisfied that this tumor was not formed by the uterus, but by an enlarged ovary containing fluid.

With a curved trocar a puncture was made in it, through the vaginal parietes. Through this about nine pounds of a chocolate-colored fluid was drawn off, upon which the sac completely collapsed, and the uterus, which had been pushed high upward and forward on the brim of the pelvis, returned to its natural situation. The canula was left for thirty hours in the wound, to permit all the fluid to drain off. In ten days it was necessary to repeat the operation, and on this occasion the opening made by the trocar was so far dilated with a bistoury that a finger could be introduced into the sac; several pounds of fetid bloody pus and numerous flakes of lymph were removed. Water was injected into the sac with considerable force, and in order to keep the opening pervious, a thick curved uterine tube of tin was introduced into it, and fastened in front of the external genitals. During the ten days following the operation there was considerable fever and a good deal of fetid discharge; but at the end of a fortnight the discharge improved in quality, and diminished in quantity; the tube was then removed for some hours daily, so that the patient was permitted to take some exercise, and from this time she gradually recovered. In four weeks the wound had contracted so much that the tube could not be again introduced; and in about six weeks from the date of the second operation, the patient was dismissed cured. A year after this the author again saw the patient; she was then in perfect health; the uterus was in its normal condition and situation, and behind it the remains of the sac could be felt as a small, hard and easily mobile ·body, causing not the slightest inconvenience.

The author states that the following conditions are necessary to insure success : 1st. That there be no other complication, and that the tumor be unilocular ; this is to be proved by its being entirely emptied by an exploratory puncture with a trocar. 2d. That the cyst contain not more than fifteen pounds of fluid. 3d. That the opening made be large enough to permit the easy introduction of the finger. 4th. That the injections of water be of such a temperature as shall be agreeable to the patient, and that they be thrown deep into the sac. 5th. That the tube introduced into the opening be withdrawn at intervals, and that its use be not entirely laid aside until the opening has become contracted, and the discharge has become solely purulent ; if the opening contracts prior to this, it must be again enlarged with the knife. *Part* xiv., *p.* 319.

Ovarian Dropsy.—As *palliatives*, Dr. Allison advises iodide of potassum with squill and juniper. After tapping, introduce a small silk cord as a *tent*, by which the water may be occasionally evacuated. *For a radical cure*, inject a solution of iodine into the sac. *Part* xv., *p.* 307.

* * * * * * * * *

If the tumor is solid, says Dr. Locock, do not meddle with it. If an unilocular cyst, tap *once*, and apply pressure for several months ; mercury and diuretics do harm. If the tumor is malignant or many-cysted, tapping and pressure will do no good : in these cases alone is extirpation indicated, and in these is it *least* likely to do good. *Part* xv., *p.* 308.

Case of Ovarian Disease.—[A lady with all the symptoms of ovarian dropsy, having a large and tense abdomen, and distinct fluctuation, was tapped ; no fluid issued from the canula, nor did any follow its withdrawal. The symptoms were not aggravated by the operation, but in a few weeks she died ; and post mortem, the trocar was again passed without giving exit to fluid.]

On opening the abdomen, the cavity of the peritoneum was found full of a gelatinous substance like glue, which could be drawn out in long strings, and would not drop. This tenacious fluid could with difficulty be removed, though a bucketful was taken out. There was then found a cyst of the right ovary, not capable of holding a quarter of the fluid taken out. The cyst appeared to have burst, then lessened in size, while the secretion still went on from its lining membrane into the cavity of the abdomen, causing the sense of fluctuation.

[A case similar to the above in the character of the fluid occurred in the practice of S. Smith, Esq., of Leeds. On tapping, the contents of the cavity were found of such a consistence that they could only be evacuated by taking hold of the portion which protruded through the canula, and drawing it out by winding it over the hands, as one would wind a rope. In this manner many gallons were evacuated.] *Part* xv., *p.* 311.

New Plan of treating Ovarian Dropsy.—It is proposed by Dr. Tilt to treat certain cases of ovarian disease by establishing solid adhesions between the tumor and the abdominal walls ; effecting a very small ulcerative opening of the cyst through the centre of these adhesions ; and so inducing gradual discharge of the fluid, and contraction of the walls of the cyst. The cases to which this method is applicable, are those where the cyst is monolocular, and without any amount of solid deposit. These points may be ascertained by a preliminary tapping, by which we may judge also of the degree of tendency to peritonitis. If, after tapping, the case is thought to be a suitable one, the cyst is to be allowed to refill to half its previous size, and the treatment is then to be commenced. It consists in applying a portion of Vienna paste, so as to produce an eschar of the size of a half-crown, at some part of the abdomen; either at the spot where the fluctuation is most superficial, or, if there be no such spot, in the mesial line, an inch or two below the umbilicus. The eschar is to be left to separate of its own accord, and then, if the thickness of the abdominal walls requires it, another portion of caustic applied to the abraded surface. The second step in the treatment, the formation of a valvular opening into the cyst, is not to be attempted by surgical interference; it will take place by ulceration spontaneously, a few days or weeks after the separation of the eschar. When the contents of the cyst begin to escape, abdominal pressure must be used; at first, moderate, with a view, not of emptying the cyst, but of giving support: afterward gradually increased, with a view of diminishing the size of the cyst, now become too large for the quantity of fluid secreted by its lining membrane. The contraction of the cyst will necessarily be slow, and it is of great importance to keep it quite full. For this purpose injections should be used, and their employment should commence when the secretion becomes very fetid. The point of an india-rubber tube, eight inches long, and funnel-like in shape at its other extremity, is to be gently passed through the opening, into the cyst, and tepid water gradually and gently injected in sufficient quantity, care being taken to exclude air; the patient is then told to strain, when the overplus of the fluid will trickle out through the tube. When the use of injections has been commenced, they should be used regularly, every day before breakfast; and oftener, if the fetidity of the secretion requires it. As to the other modes of treatment—small tumors may be cured by giving large doses of the preparations of iodine internally, and using them externally. When the cyst is voluminous, and bulges into the vagina, it may be punctured *per vaginam*, and an india-rubber sound left in its cavity, and moderate pressure applied to the abdomen. Subcutaneous incision into a monolocular cyst is sometimes warrantable. Tapping, as a palliative, is to be deferred as long as possible; and ovariotomy is to be reserved for multilocular cysts, and those monolocular ones which contain much solid deposit.

Part xviii., *p.* 289.

Case of Ovarian Tumor containing Teeth and Hair.—The patient was an unmarried woman, fifty-eight years of age, who had had a tumor in the abdomen, presumed to be ovarian, for twenty-eight years. The swelling having latterly increased very rapidly, so that respiration was impeded by the distention of the abdomen and pressure on the diaphragm, she was tapped, and about seven quarts of serum withdrawn. She died forty-eight hours afterward, with symptoms of exhaustion and peritonitis. The tumor, on being removed, proved to be a cyst varying in thickness in parts, but generally about that of a shilling: its contents consisted of teeth, hair, bony deposit, some transparent masses of a cellular structure (as examined by the microscope), serum, sebaceous matter, and granular fat; which were contained in numerous small cysts. Teeth were found in all parts of the tumor, and were counted to the number of forty-three: some were contained in cysts; others imbedded in the semi-transparent masses, and two or three were growing from the walls of the parent cyst.

In one part a few were imbedded in a mass of bone, bearing a strong resemblance to an upper jaw ununited in the mesial line. *Part* xx., *p.* 235.

   ' *Ovarian Dropsy* is liable to be confounded with, 1. Retroflexion and retroversion of the uterus. 2. Tumors of the uterus. 3. Ascites. 4. Pregnancy. 5. Pregnancy complicated with ovarian dropsy. 6. Cystic tumors of the abdomen. 7. Distended bladder. 8. Accumulation of air in the intestines, especially if there has been chronic peritonitis leaving some ascitic fluid. 9. Enlargement of the solid viscera of the abdomen, the liver, spleen and kidney. 10. Accumulation of fæces in the intestines.

Part xxii., *p.* 289.

Mr. I. B. Brown's new operation for treating ovarian dropsy consists of excising a portion of the sac, returning the remaining portion into the peritoneal cavity, and closing the wound by sutures, allowing any fresh portion of the fluid secreted by the remainder of the cyst to escape into the peritoneal cavity, and to be there taken up by absorption, and discharged by the kidneys. This plan was brought to Mr. Brown's mind by reflecting upon the numerous cases in which a spontaneous cure followed an accidental rupture of the cyst, succeeded by a copious discharge of urine. Mr. Brown relates three cases thus treated, which, though followed by severe peritonitis, ultimately did well. *Part* xxvi., *p.* 347.

Diagnosis of Chronic Ovarian Tumors.—According to Dr. Tilt, *ovarian tumors many be confounded with tumors of the unimpregnated womb.* Retroversion and retroflexion of the womb have been mistaken for incipient ovarian tumors, fallen into the recto-vaginal pouch, or confined there by false membranes. The mobility of the tumor, by the uterine sound previously introduced, will show whether or not it be uterine.

Retroflexion of the womb is more likely to simulate incipient ovarian cysts:

Ovarian Tumors may be confounded with Abscess of the Walls of the Womb — Case.—Some years since Professor Recamier was consulted by a medical man for his wife, who had long suffered from what was called ovarian dropsy. On making a very careful examination, Recamier discovered a round tumor about the size of a pigeon's egg, situated between the rectum and the uterus. On exploring the rectum with the index of the left hand, while that of the right remained in the neck of the womb, more than usually dilated, he felt fluctuation, and as the pus seemed nearest to the posterior wall of thè neck of the uterus, Recamier determined on making an incision there. To perform this operation he placed the index of the left hand in the neck of the uterus, and guiding a convex bistoury on the pulp of the finger, he plunged the extremity of the bistoury into the abscess; a few teaspoonfuls of pus came out, and to facilitate its egress he enlarged the inferior angle of the wound, by completely cutting through the posterior lip of the os uteri, the index of the left hand placed in the rectum serving to guide the bistoury, and preventing too deep an incision. During the following day a small quantity of pus was voided. Frequent injections were made, and the patient soon got well. This case shows how to detect and to cure similar instances of disease.

Ovarian Tumors may be confounded with Abscess of the Cavity of the Womb.—Husson presented to the Anatomical Society of Paris a case of this description, the neck of the womb was completely obliterated, and its dilated cavity contained two tumblers of pus.

Ovarian Cysts may be confounded with Hydrometra or a Collection of Water in the Womb, and we do not doubt but that some of the cases described as cases of spontaneous cure of ovarian cysts are to be referred to the rupture of such uterine tumors.

After fully ascertaining the impossibility of the womb being distended by a child, it would be well to imitate Lisfranc, who in one of his cases introduced a sound into the womb, and cured the patient in a month.

Ovarian Tumors may be confounded with Cystic Tumors in the substance of the Uterus.—By means of the sound such a tumor might be shown to be uterine, before it attained to a considerable size, or after it had been emptied.

Ovarian Tumors may be confounded with the Uterus distended by the Menstrual Secretion.—Dr. Williams had such a case in St. Thomas's Hospital. Examination per vaginam detected a fluctuating tumor, which was freely opened with an abscess-lancet, and a large washhand basin was filled with the retained menstrual fluid.

The uterus, distended by retained menses, is not always regularly developed, but may increase to the right or the left, and give that obscure perception of fluctuation which is frequently found in a malignant mass. On each side of a central tumor may also be found smaller elongated tumors, formed by proportionally-distended oviducts, with obliterated abdominal ends, as in the case related by Dr. Jackson, in the "American Journal of Medical Sciences."

Ovarian Tumors may be confounded with an Accumulation of Gas in the Womb.—Mauriceau, Schmitt, M. Lefevre, and many other authors, have seen examples of this singular occurrence.

The obliteration of the os uteri on the one side, and the clear sound furnished by the distended womb, will point to a correct diagnosis.

Ovarian Tumors may be mistaken for Uterine Fibrous Tumors.—This mistake is much more liable to occur than any of the preceding, because the frequency of such tumors is great.

The absence of fluctuation, the hardness of the tumor, the very gradual progress of the disease, may indeed allow one to affirm that the tumor is solid; but were it not for the uterine sound, it would be difficult to affirm that it is not ovarian.

If we find that the uterine sound passes, as it were, into the morbid mass, if there is no possibility of separating the womb from the tumor, and if every movement given to the tumor conveys similar movements to the sound, we may consider the tumor uterine; but if we find the uterus small and movable, if the sound passes anteriorly to the tumor, and can be separated from it, and when thrown upon the rectum it appears healthy, then we may confidently affirm the tumor to be ovarian. The cavity of the womb may be lengthened, and the sound will indicate the modification of structure; but although the sound may only penetrate the womb to its normal depth, or two inches and a half, still the uterus may not be normal, for its enlarged cavity may be filled with a fibrous tumor.

Part xxvii., *p.* 292.

Differential Diagnosis of Ovarian Dropsy and Ascites.—The diagnosis of these two diseases, the one from the other, is in some cases a matter of considerable difficulty. There is, says Mr. I. B. Brown, one symptom of great value, which is not generally known. In a case of ascites in which the distention is so great, that the hydrostatic line of level in front is not changed by posture, the lumbo-lateral regions of both sides will be found *equally* dull on percussion, owing to the intestines floating as far forward and upward as their attachment will permit. In an ovarian case, no matter how great the distention, one loin will be found clear, and the other quite dull, owing to the intestines being pushed over to the healthy side. Thus is indicated also, and with unfailing accuracy, on which side the ovarian cyst, if it exist, has originated. *Part* xxxviii., *p.* 221.

OX-GALL.

Flatulence.—Administration of ox-gall recommended. *Part* vii., *p.* 92.

Ox-Gall.—Dr. Allnatt gives the following among other cases :

I was summoned hastily into the country to see a lady, seventy-seven years of age, who was apparently sinking from the effects of unrelieved constipation. Excrementitious vomiting had taken place, and the powers of life seemed waning. The question was, whether or not, from the violence of the inverted action of the intestines, intus-susception had occurred. On examination, I thought I could detect a hardened mass, impacted about the head of the colon, and evidences of accumulation below that point. I therefore advised, as a last resort, an enema of ox-gall and turpentine (the latter ingredient more as a stimulant to the inactive bowel than for any specific effect), with thin gruel, to be vigorously injected, warm, as far as possible into the intestine. In less than half an hour, a mass of scybala was expelled, the exterior portions of which had been imperfectly softened by the action of the gall, covered with a coating of thick mucus. Other portions speedily followed, and convalescence ensued, with no other unfavorable symptom than that of slight pain, which might have been produced by the action of the turpentine in immediate contact with the mucous membrane of the bowel. There is one point, in connection with the present subject, of considerable importance, and that is, the destruction of the narcotizing property of opium, when combined with ox-gall. The constipating effect of opium is principally produced by its action upon the liver, the secretion of which it arrests, and renders insufficient for the due stimulation of the alimentary canal. In many cases, this is a serious drawback to the exhibition of opium, for we often require its sedative, when its constipating effects would be sufficiently injurious to preclude its use. Five or eight grains of inspissated ox-gall will neutralize the effect of a grain of opium, without destroying its sedative efficacy. It also prevents, in a great measure, its injurious action upon the brain.

[In another communication, Dr. Allnatt recommends the following process for the preparation of the inspissated ox-gall :]

An open vessel, containing any quantity of perfectly recent ox-gall, should be plunged into a saucepan of boiling water, and simmered until the bile is of sufficient consistence to be formed into pills. It should be frequently stirred during the operation to prevent an unequal hardening of the mass. The addition of a little calcined magnesia will expedite the process. If carefully prepared, it will keep for years, and when required for use should be gently warmed before the fire. Two drachms dissolved

in a pint of hot water, or thin gruel, will be of sufficient strength for ena-
mata. One or two five-grain pills may be given twice or thrice daily,
according to the exigency of the case. *Part* xii., *p.* 91.

PALATE.

Perforating Ulcer of the Palate.—The patient, under the care of Dr. J.
Ross, was a girl, aged 22: the opening was of the size of a goose quill in
the soft palate, a little to the left of the mesial line, just behind the edge
of the osseous palatal arch; no bone could be detected by the probe; her
speech was considerably affected, and a portion of everything she attempted to swallow escaped by the nose. There was no reason to suspect
syphilitic affection. On the 19th March the opening was touched with a
red-hot wire; on the 23d the eschar came away, and the raw surface was
now touched every second day with tincture of iodine. By the 13th April
the opening had become much less; she spoke better and could also swallow better; very little escaping by the nose, and that only of any thin
liquid, such as water. The cautery was reapplied: on the 16th of April
the tincture of iodine was resumed as before; on the 25th the opening had
still further diminished, and on the 13th of May it was closed so that nothing came through it; the powers of speech and deglutition being also
quite restored. In this case, after a raw surface had been produced by
the separation of the eschar, consequent upon the application of the
cautery, the tincture of iodine seemed powerfully to excite the granulating
or reparative action. It might also, perhaps, be used in a similar manner
in fistulous openings in other situations. *Part* vi., *p.* 119.

Cleft Palate—Bead Suture.—The operation for cleft palate has been
improved by an ingenious suggestion of Mr. Maclean, of Dublin, and
carried into effect by Sir P. Crampton and Dr. Cusack. It consists in the
mode of tying the ligatures, a part of the operation of acknowledged difficulty. After the ligatures are passed through the edges of the fissure and
brought out at the mouth, their ends are to be passed through a small perforated metallic bead, such as are used in making purses; the bead is then
to be pushed down along the ligatures, closing them as it descends, until it
touches the approximated edges of the wound; it is then to be compressed
by a pair of strong blunt-pointed forceps, and the ligatures are thus firmly
secured, without a knot at the required degree of tension. This ingenious
method of securing the ligatures might be extended to other surgical operations where a knot would be difficult to tie, such as applying a ligature
to hemorrhoidal tumors and polypous masses, which are situated in parts
difficult of access; in short, with some modifications, we have no doubt the
principle might be made exceedingly useful in many surgical operations
where parts to be tied are deep-seated, in the same way as we should
apply the double canula in polypi of the womb. *Part* vii., *p.* 115.

Treatment of the over-large Openings of the soft Palate.—Very small
openings in the soft palate, that either remain after a partially successful
stitching, or are caused by penetrating sores, may be closed by exciting
inflammation in the borders. For this purpose concentrated tinct. of cantharides is the most effectual: lapis infernalis causes the loss of a layer of

the organized mass, and the process of inflammation that follows produces an insufficient granulation, so that the hole generally increases in size. The concentrated acids recommended by many surgeons for exciting inflamma- tions, only produce a superficial corrosion of the borders; nor does such a quick granulation follow their use as that of the cantharides. If the opening is large and oval, and the palate soft, the edges are cut evenly to fit to each other, leaden sutures are then put through the edges with a small-cared hook, and twisted.   *Part* xii., *p.* 191.

Cleft Palate and Staphyloraphy.—The observations of Graefe and Roux in Europe, and Warren in America, first showed that this congeni- tal deformity may be treated on the same principles as the management of hare-lip. Mr. Ferguson observes that:

The fissure in cleft palate may be such as only to divide the uvula, or it may extend forward through the soft and hard parts as far as the lips, in which latter instance there is generally a hare-lip as well. In the uvula, soft palate, and even through the palate bones, as also a portion of the superior maxillæ, the fissure is invariably in the medial line, but when the alveoli in front participate in the malformation, it is somewhat to one side. In certain instances the fissure is double in front, when the whole of it may be likened to the letter Y; the two lines in front leaving between them the intermaxillary bone.

The soft velum ought to remain in a state of perfect repose, and for this purpose the levator palati, the palato-pharyngeus, and the palato-glossus muscles should be divided. This cuts off all motor influence in an outward, upward, or downward direction. For this purpose use a knife with a blade like the point of a lancet, the cutting edge being about a quarter of an inch in extent, and the flat surface being bent semi-circularly. Make an incision half an inch long on each side of the posterior nares, and divide the levator palati muscle on both sides, just above its attachments to the palate; then pare the edges of the fissure, and with a pair of long blunt- pointed scissors, divide the posterior pillar of the fauces, and, if it seems necessary, the anterior pillar too, the wound in each part being a quarter of an inch in extent; then introduce stitches by means of a curved needle set in a handle, the threads being tied so as to keep the cut edge of the fissure in exact contact. The first incision, that for the division of the leva- tor palati, should be made midway between the hard palate and the pos- terior margin of the soft flap, just above the thickest and most prominent part of the margin of the cleft. You may commence cutting either at the end nearest you, as you stand behind the patient, or that furthest off, as may seem most convenient. For ligatures, those of stout silk, or flaxen thread, are the best; and it is of great importance that a stitch be used close to the lower end of the uvula, as there is a great tendency to separa- tion there. The after treatment the same as after ordinary operations, except that the parts are to be kept at rest as much as possible; and nutri- ment to be given by means of enemata of gruel and soups.

It is only of late that it has been thought possible to remedy the cleft in the hard palate, except by plastic operations, succeeding the union of the soft parts. Dr. Warren says it may be closed in the same way as the soft velum: dissect the soft tissues from each side of the fissure in the palate, to such an extent as to make a flap broad enough to join its fellow of the opposite side in the mesial line, and stitch the whole between the uvula and the anterior extremity. Reunion to a considerable extent, takes place and toward the inner margin of the bones, and also on the upper surface of the soft portion in the middle, there will be a cicatrix analogous to mucous membrane.   *Part* xiii., *p.* 240.

Dieffenbach's Operations on the Palate.—In cases of small holes in the soft or hard palate, pencil their borders several times a day with a coneentrated tincture of cantharides. Inflammation and granulation come on and close the opening. Large openings are to be closed by suture, after paring the edges; and leaden wire is said to be preferable to silk, for ligatures, as it keeps the edges close together, and does not cut through the textures.

When there is adhesion between the velum palati and posterior wall of the pharynx occasioning deafness, and stopping the communication between the nares and air-passages, the adhesion must be divided transversely, by means of a long scalpel, about half an inch below the adherent border of the velum. The edge must be fixed by a hook, and drawn from the wall of the pharynx, then, with a lancet-formed knife, the surface of which is curved, directed upward, the velum is to be loosened, and the separation completed by scissors, also curved upon their flat surface. The upper adhesions are to be destroyed by passing a blunt curved iron instrument, like a very small spatula, along the inferior nares. Next prepare a ligature with a small curved needle at each end; with one of the needles transfix the velum, a few lines from its edge, and bring it out at a high point on the anterior surface of the palate; the other needle must be used in same manner, a short distance from the side of the other; and the edge of the velum must be brought about half an inch from the palate, All mechanical means for closing the fissured palate, are not only injurious but dangerous; but if the size of the cleft, or other circumstances, render an operation unadvisable, then it may be covered with a gold palate, fixed to the teeth. In cases of holes in the palate, the edges of which are so callous that an operation would be unsuccessful, the opening may be stopped by wearing a double piece of India rubber, without fear of its being enlarged. Two pieces of India rubber, the thickness of pasteboard, are cut about four or five times larger than the opening, and between them a small round piece, and they are to be transfixed by waxed thread: thus, one plate lies on the anterior, the other on the posterior side of the palate, and the small middle strip in the opening. The patient can apply it himself, and it should be taken out to be cleaned once a week.

                          Part xiii., *p.* 244.

Removal of Scirrhous Tubercle from the Soft Palate.—[Mr. Adams records a very successful case of recovery from the application of ligature in this rare disease. A man applied at the London Hospital in consequence of a tumor on the left side of the velum palati. He first perceived it three years ago, and since that time it had gradually increased in size, but was unattended with pain or inconvenience until lately.]

The tumor, when examined, appeared about the size of a small walnut, was somewhat oval in shape, the long axis being from above downward, and was evidently situated in the substance of the velum palati between its interior and posterior mucous surfaces. It presented a somewhat whitish aspect from the stretching of the anterior layer of the velum over its surface, to which it was formerly adherent. The velum was perfectly movable, and the tumor was drawn up at every movment of the palate, and a bent probe could be introduced behind it. It had a remarkably hard feel, and on running the finger over it, it gave the idea of true scirrhus.

Mr. A. proceeded to strangulate the tumor by ligature. This was accomplished with some difficulty by the introduction of armed needles, and with an instrument of firm, though inflexible silver, having a steel point, armed with a long ligature, and let into an ivory handle. By these means the whole of the tumor was encircled, and the ligatures being tightened, it was at once apparent that its complete strangulation had been effected. Very slight constitutional disturbance ensued, and on examination on the following day the tumor was evidently sloughing. Five days after the operation he removed the greater part of the mass, leaving a large sloughy-looking wound: the slough, however, had no tendency to spread. By the frequent gargling with a solution of chloride of lime, a healthy grann-lating action was induced, and it began to heal rapidly. In the course, however, of a few days a warty vegetation sprang up from its surface; this was gradually destroyed by the repeated application of solid nitrate of silver, and the disease was perfectly cured.] *Part* xv., *p* 211.

Cheap kind of Artificial Palate.—[An anonymous correspondent of the " Lancet " says:]

I have found the substance, gutta percha, suitable for making artificial palates, very easily molded on a cast of the mouth into the necessary shape, and retaining its firmness and smoothness unimpaired by the temperature to which it is there subjected. Kneaded out into a smooth sheet, about the thickness of a sixpence or a shilling, and pressed into the proper form—the edges accurately following the sinuosities of the teeth, and a hooked process or two of the same material adjusted in the usual way—it will be found to answer very well, being smooth, light, and firm. If required, a slight rim of gold, fitted to a few of the teeth, may be fixed to the edge of the gutta percha. If care be used to mold the material equally and smoothly, it will be more agreeable in the mouth than a metallic body.

Part xviii., *p.* 174.

Operation for Cleft Palate.—According to Prof. Syme the best way of proceeding is to place the patient on a chair in a good light, then to seize one edge of the fissure at its middle by sharply pointed forceps, and introduce the knife, which should be thin and lancet-shaped like the one of this form used for the extraction of cataract, a little above the commencement of the cleft, and cut evenly down from this point to the extremity of the uvula so as to detach a slice of sufficient thickness to expose the submucous textures. The same process being repeated on the other side of the fissure, nothing remains but to introduce the stitches, which is best done by means of a slightly curved needle with fixed handle, which should be directed from without inward, first on one side of the fissure, and then on the other. The two inner ends of the threads being then tied together, one of the other ends is to be pulled until the knot is drawn through the edge of the palate, and sufficiently far out of the mouth for the purpose in view. Two stitches are sufficient, one being placed at the root of the uvula, and the other midway between this point and the angle of the edges of the fissure. The threads should be tied with the " reef knot," and, in doing so, resiliency of the textures may be counteracted by keeping the threads in a state of tension. For at least two days the patient should subsist entirely upon fluids, and of these even have a very sparing allowance. He should also, of course, avoid talking, coughing, sneezing, and all other actions calculated to disturb the uniting process :

Prof. Syme objects to Mr. Fergusson's advice to take out the sutures on the second or third day—since the union, however perfect in the first instance, can then have little power of resisting pressure, either from food or the tongue, independently of the disturbing influence of the pharyngeal muscles. The threads should penetrate the whole thickness of the palate, and be tied with no more force than is sufficient to retain the edges in contact, so that in the event of union taking place, they may neither cause sloughing of the portion included nor cut their way out by ulcerative absorption.   *Part* xxix., *p.* 209.

PANCREAS.

Use of the Pancreatic Juice.—The experiments of Dr. Bernard go to show an error which has been long entertained by physiologists, namely : That the bile is the fluid by which fatty matters are acted upon—a property clearly proved by M. Bernard to belong *most exclusively* to the pancreatic juice, which must, therefore, now be regarded as the true agent by which fatty bodies are digested.

When fat is introduced into the stomach of the rabbit, the contact of the gastric juice produces no alteration, nor is it in any degree changed in its passage along the intestinal canal, until it arrives at that portion where it is brought into immediate contact with the pancreatic juice : and it is exactly at the mouth of the pancreatic canal that the lacteals convey chyle of a white color ; *higher up they contain only chyle of a transparent hue.*

No one can read these details, and not arrive at the same conclusion as Dr. Bernard, that the pancreatic juice, hitherto considered as the abdominal saliva, the use of which was to soften the food, is in reality charged with the important office in the exhibition of the cod-liver oil, already alluded to. We know, also, that the best time to give it to the patient, is one or two hours after breakfast, after dinner, and after tea. If given at these times it does not occasion those disagreeable eructations which are apt to occur when it is taken either with, or immediately before food ; by taking it at this time we can now see how these eructations are avoided by the newly discovered and peculiar action of the pancreatic juice. In no disease is cod-liver oil more valuable than in scrofula mesenterica. *Part* xix., *p.* 98.

PARACENTESIS.

Paracentesis Thoracis.—Dr. Hughes, advises, not to allow air to be admitted through the canula if it can be avoided. It may rekindle inflammation, or convert the adhesive into the suppurative inflammation. Unless the lung is capable of free and full expansion, do not attempt to draw off all the fluid ; remove only so much as the expanding lung and the surrounding compressed organs are capable of replacing. Watch the opening carefully, especially during inspiration and coughing, and when the stream begins to fail, turn the patient on his punctured side till there is an alternate flow and stoppage of the stream during inspiration and expiration, then immediately withdraw the canula. Apply a flannel bandage with moderate firmness around the chest. *Precautions.*—1. Always introduce an exploring needle first, to know if the diagnosis be correct. 2. Do not puncture one side before it is presumed that the other is sound enough to carry on respiration. 3. Draw off the fluid slowly through as small a canula as the density of the fluid will admit. 4. Only draw off the fluid till the air seems to threaten to be admitted.   *Part* xiii., *p.* 86.

Paracentesis of the Scrotum.—[The subject of these remarks, by Mr. Skey, was a publican, about 55 years of age, who was laboring under an advanced stage of ascites and anasarca.]

The legs and the scrotum were both largely distended with fluid. Before operating, my attention was directed by Dr. Lobb to the fact, that pressure on the scrotum entirely emptied that appendage, when steadily persisted in for some short time, and on removing the pressure and placing the man in the upright posture, the fluid again gravitated into the bag, which became distended as before. It was obvious that the continued pressure caused by the water had broken down or elongated the fibrous and cellular tissues about the cord, and thus opened the communication between the abdomen and the tunica vaginalis.

Under these circumstances, I determined to evacuate the serous contents of the abdomen through the scrotum, and with this view I introduced a full-sized hydrocele trocar into its lower and most pendulous part. The fluid flowed readily and continuously till some quarts had escaped.

Practically this case affords matter for more than a passing observation. Anasarca of the scrotum is a common attendant on ascites in the male subject. As a general rule, it commands but little attention, the interest which would otherwise attach to it being merged in the larger evil. If the question were now asked of the surgical world, how often does the relation that existed in the above case prevail in other cases? I doubt whether a very positive, or even a satisfactory reply could be obtained. The fact of the communication is curious, if it be nothing more. It is very true that the operation of paracentesis abdominis is neither a difficult nor a dangerous operation, but it will hardly be denied, that simple as it is, paracentesis of the scrotum is yet more so.   *Part* xxxiii., *p.* 213.

Paracentesis Abdominis.—Use neither pressure nor bandage; allow as much of the fluid to flow out gradually as the natural elasticity of the cyst or abdominal parietes will expel; when the flow has quite ceased of itself, close up the orifice, keeping the patient recumbent.   *Part* xxxiii., *p.* 272.

Paracentesis Thoracis.—The best point for the operation is close on the upper edge of the sixth rib, midway between the sternum and spine. The chief danger is from the admission of air into the chest after the operation; this may be very much obviated by having an India-rubber apparatus fixed to the instrument, which, by its elasticity, sucks, as it were, the purulent secretion from the pleura, and at the same time allows the lung ample time to expand.   *Part* xxxiv., *p.* 284.

PARAPHIMOSIS.

Extract of Belladonna in the Reduction of Paraphimosis.—A child, three years and a half old, was the subject of severe paraphimosis; the glans red, swollen, and tender; the prepuce strongly drawn back, forming a thick and apparently adherent ring, the constriction of which completely stopped the circulation. This state had lasted eight days, and the sufferings were excessive.

The strangulation became more menacing, and all the symptoms were aggravated; the glans was bluish and gangrene was threatened, when M. Mignot employed frictions around the glans, with an ointment composed of thirty parts of simple cerate to twelve parts of extract of belladonna. Under the influence of this remedy the circle of constriction relaxed, dilated, and the tissues gradually recovered their normal condition, without loss of substance or suppuration following.

The second patient had acute balanitis, brought on by a severe gonorrhœa, and followed by paraphimosis. The patient refused operation, although gangrene was threatened, when the belladonna was applied, which induced relaxation and rapid amendment. *Part* iv., *p.* 105.

Reduction of Paraphimosis.—It is necessary to reduce the swelling of the prepuce as well as that of the glans. Prof. South advises, to squeeze the prepuce gently but steadily for a few minutes, and if this does not suffice, make a few punctures to let out the serum. Then press the glans with the thumbs of both hands while the two forefingers grasp the penis behind the prepuce; or grasp the whole penis with the left hand, and with thumb and forefinger of the other hand, empty the glans. As soon as ever a little of the glans gets beneath the constricting band, continue the pressure until the whole is returned. After the reduction keep the penis in cold wet cloths for some hours, and afterward apply a warm poultice. *Part* xvi., *p.* 216.

PARALYSIS.

In no Case of Paralysis or Apoplexy should a careful examination of the heart's action be omitted. *Part* i., *p.* 69.

Aphorism of Practical Surgery.—No disease is more difficult of cure than paralysis of the arm induced by dislocation of the humerus. The paralysis seems to arise from the stretching, compression, and perhaps also partial rupture of the nerves, which form the brachial plexus. Often no remedial means are of any avail. *Part* iii., *p.* 115.

Paralysis of the Seventh Pair of Nerves.—The patient, a young female, presented herself to M. Magendie, having a complete paralysis of all the facial muscles supplied by the seventh pair, on the left side, with great exaltation of sensibility in the auditory nerve. The whole face was drawn toward the right side. Sensibility continued perfect in the face, tongue, etc. Galvanism was prescribed, one needle being placed over the parotid gland, the second successively over the supraorbital, infraorbital, and mental foramina. The patient was cured. *Part* iv., *p.* 63.

Paralysis treated with Cantharides.—The tincture of cantharides is given, by Dr. Seymour, in very large doses, in cases where the paralysis cannot be traced to any affection of the sensorium, and where there is no trace of organic disease. In the case which was commented upon by Dr. Seymour in one of his clinical lectures, the patient had entirely lost the use of the upper limbs and had a weakness of one leg. In a great majority of such cases, we should find a disease of the vertebræ above the seat of the injury, and there would be pain on pressure or on percussion; but in this case this symptom was entirely absent, and if there had been any actual disease of the spinal marrow, we might have expected to find the diseased action continued to the lower extremities, as well as to the upper: but such was not the case, as every part below the upper extremities appeared perfectly sound and healthy. In such a case as this Dr. Seymour ventures to give 40 minims of the tincture of cantharides twice a day. *Part* v., *p.* 52.

Strychnine in Paralysis of the Face.—Although paralysis of the muscles, those of the face, for example, seldom exist without some organic lesion, yet we sometimes have reason to believe that it is truly functional, and unattended with any particular disease. In such cases we shall find strychnine of value; and we think that its powers have been miscalculated, on account of the indiscriminate use which has been made of it. Even when the paralysis is originally owing to some lesion or effusion, that cause may have been remedied, and nothing remains but a continued inability on the part of the muscles to regain their powers. Here, then, is a case in which strychnine would be of great use, as well as when the paralysis is strictly functional. When the face is the seat of the affection, the strychnine may be applied to the cuticle in the following way: About one drachm of a solution containing about three grains of strychnine to an ounce of alcohol, may be applied to each side (when both sides are affected), three times a day, and the absorption assisted by friction; when only one side is affected, it will be sufficient to confine the application to the muscles implicated. In a case reported by Dr. Joslin, of New York, this was persevered in for about two months, with success. A blistered surface renders the effects of the application more powerful. *Part* vii. *p.* 46.

Paralysis from Exostosis of the Spine.—Exostosis, or bony vegetations, arising from the bodies of the vertebræ (independent of any disorganization of these bones) are by no means of rare occurrence; most pathological collections contain numerous examples of their different stages, especially of what seems their natural termination, viz., perfect anchylosis of the affected bones. This anchylosis may be more or less extended, affecting but two neighboring vertebræ, or perhaps the greater part, more rarely the entire of the vertebral column, while the new bony material is found to vary from a thin lamina to a prominent and rough projection, occupying the situation of, or more properly covering, the subjacent intervertebral cartilage.

[Although the affection may have advanced to complete anchylosis, there may be an absence of all severe pain when the bone is handled; which is remarkable, considering the displacement and injury those important nerves must undergo which are so closely connected with the front of the spine, more particularly in the lower part of the dorsal and lumbar regions. Dr. Battersby relates some interesting cases to prove that these nerves do occasionally suffer from the disease giving rise to a train of most painful symptoms which have baffled the diagnosis of the most skillful practitioners. One case particularly is related which proves this. A train of the most painful symptoms terminated in the death of the patient.]

On displacing the abdominal viscera, the inter-vertebral spaces of the lumbar region were at once observed to be singularly prominent, the cartilages being partially faced with irregular bony protuberances, so as nearly to unite the adjoining bones. A section of the vertebræ was removed, and a large nervous twig was discovered lying stretched over the most prominent of the new formations which engaged the sides of the vertebræ. The anterior vertebral ligament had a marked glistening appearance, and on dissection proved to be very much thickened, while underneath it was formed a new dense structure of a fibrous nature, in which all the characteristics of the periosteum were lost, and the surface of the bones, to which it was intimately adherent, was rough and irregular. There was no distinction between the fine cancelled structure of these and their new processes. The bones were quite healthy, as also the cartilages. The spinal canal was opened from the sacrum to the middle of the dorsal region. There was about an ounce of clear fluid in the interior of the sheath of the cord, which, like its membranes, were perfectly natural. The only irregularity here discovered was two little points of bone on the posterior aspect of the bodies of the dorsal vertebræ, which felt through the dura mater, which was unremoved, about the size of pins' heads. The opening for the nerves were perfect.

This gentleman's sufferings, for the space of nearly two months, could not be surpassed; toward the conclusion, he used to consume more than a scruple of the muriate of morphia daily, and that merely with the effect of mitigating the pain. The new bone, in occupying the situation of the lumbar ganglia of the sympathetic, gave rise to the symptoms of visceral neuralgia, by irritating these and their branches, while the same irritation communicated through the lumbar nerves (which are in direct connection with the former) to the spinal cord, its functions became deranged both above and below the point of irritation, exhibiting what Dr. Marshall Hall denominates the morbid, direct and retrograde action of that part.

The progress of the paralysis was very remarkable as pointing to the spinal origin of the symptoms. It first appeared over the upper part of the abdomen, then attacked the lower extremities, and lastly, the integuments of the chest and arms. *Part* viii., *p.* 53.

Diagnosis in Cases of Paralysis of the Face.—[It is of the greatest consequence in practice that we distinguish between hemiplegia of the face and paralysis of the facial nerve, and of this latter as it occurs *within* and *without* the cranium.]

I had recently, says Dr. Hall, an urgent summons in such a case. The patient was situated in a lunatic asylum, a circumstance which rather disposed the mind to expect *cerebral* disease. Beside, the patient complained of pain of the head at one time, and was apparently drowsy at another. The face was drawn exceedingly to the right side. In the first place I desired the patient to close the eyelids; the right eye remained open. In the second place I inquired whether the arm or leg were affected, and found that they were not. In the third place I begged the patient to put out the tongue; it was protruded in the direct mesial plane. In the fourth place, I inquired where the patient had been sitting, and we went upstairs and placed the chair near the window, precisely as it had been occupied the day before; it was so placed as to expose the right side of the face to the draught from the window.

Taking these facts together, I did not hesitate to declare that the case was one of paralysis of the facial nerve : in hemiplegia the eyelids of the affected side can always be closed, though not so firmly as those of the other side. In so severe a case of facial hemiplegia the limbs are almost certainly paralyzed, and the tongue is generally affected and protruded to the affected side. Still a question was raised, whether this nerve was affected *within* or *without* the cranium ; there was pain of the head and drowsiness.

Now, the portio dura and the portio mollis of the seventh pair (the facial and the auditory) are placed so immediately together within the cranium that it is scarcely possible for one of these nerves to be affected without the other ; *yet there was no deafness.*

I remained therefore of opinion that the case was one of paralysis of the facial nerve, external to the cranium, confirmed, as it had been, by the fact which I had almost anticipated, of the special position and exposure of the patient, as she had sat sewing in her bedroom. The issue has proved my opinion to be the just one. No affection of the cerebrum has occurred, and the facial paralysis is gradually subsiding under the usual local remedies, viz., leeches, fomentations, sinapisms, etc.   *Part* ix., *p.* 40.

Paralysis.—Sir Benj. Brodie gives cases of the different forms of paralysis, with the morbid appearances in the brain or spinal column, which he detected ; but after most careful examination of these cases during life, he acknowledges that their treatment is often exceedingly difficult, as we have not yet sufficiently advanced in our knowledge of this complaint, to be able to state positively whether the disease is of one kind or another. If the disease be an inflammatory affection of the membranes, we may distinguish it tolerably well ; but if it be of a chronic character, it is difficult to discriminate between softening of the spinal marrow, tubercles in the spinal cord, and effusion of fluid in the theca vertebralis ; besides, these three affections may be combined together, or there may be one first and the others may supervene.

However, let us suppose that there is a case of inflammation of the membranes of the spinal marrow. The patient comes to you with a severe attack of dreadful lumbago, and by and by he states that there is numbness in his legs, and then difficulty in moving them. In this case you may be pretty sure that there is inflammation of the membranes of the lower part of the cervical cord. How is that to be treated ? In the first place take blood by cupping from the loins, and repeat it according to circumstances. Begin by purging the patient, clearing the bowels well out—a right plan to pursue in all cases of inflammatory disease. Then put the patient under the influence of mercury, exhibit calomel and opium, and treat him as you would a patient laboring under pleuritis or iritis.

But if you are called in at a late period, when the inflammation has subsided, and the paralysis consequent on it remains, even then you cannot do better than put the patient under a course of mercury, a mere alterative course—five grains of Plummer's pill, night and morning—the eighth of a grain of bichloride of mercury, twice a day, in addition to which you may apply blisters to the lower part of the back.

The treatment of a chronic affection of the spinal cord producing paralysis must be, to a great extent, empirical, because you cannot make a certain diagnosis. Let me repeat what I just now observed, that I have never seen any beneficial results arise from the use of counter-irritation.

Probably the bowels are very torpid—they will require to be kept open, and it is very difficult to effect it. The stools will be black, like tar, and the lodgment of the black secretion in the intestinal canal appears to be productive of great mischief to the system. Calomel and a black draught may be exhibited every now and then, but a patient cannot take them from day to day. Sometimes the comp. ext. colocynth will be sufficient, but simple purgatives often fail. The pills which I am about to mention, I have found to be convenient in cases of this kind. Two scruples and a half of comp. ext. colocynth; half a scruple of soap; one drop of croton oil. Let these be well rubbed up and carefully mixed, and divided into a dozen pills, one or two of which may be taken every night, or every other night, when wanted. These are excellent pills; they cause nothing like the inconvenience produced by a large dose of croton oil, and are very efficient indeed.

The treatment which I have found to be the most successful, and under which I have seen the greatest benefit arise, is a grain of zinc made into a pill and given three times a day, and then a draught of twenty minims of tincture of cantharides, to wash it down.

It is from the continued use of the zinc, and not from the exhibition of large quantities, that benefit is to be derived.

In other cases I have thought that benefit has arisen from the long-continued use of very small doses of bichloride of mercury, combined with tincture of cantharides. Small doses do not seem to act as mercury on the system. I apprehend it acts much in the same way as the sulphate of zinc. Exhibit the sixteenth of a grain of bichloride of mercury in a certain quantity of tincture of cantharides, in a draught three times daily, and such plan of treatment will sometimes be useful. But it is right to state, that in a great number of cases of chronic paraplegia, the disease is incurable. The disease, however, may go on for years before it ascends to the brain and destroys life.   *Part* ix., *p.* 100.

Brucine in Obstinate Paralysis.—Brucine is substituted by M. Bricheteau for strychnine, in the treatment of obstinate paralysis remaining after an attack of apoplexy, with equally good effect, and with the additional advantage over strychnine of being able to employ it in larger doses without danger of fatal accidents.

Dose.—A centigramme (1·154 gr. Fr.,=1-6th gr. avoir.) in infusion of arnica; increase the dose one centigramme daily, until its effects are evident, and then proceed discretionally.   *Part* xiv., *p.* 59.

Paralysis of Sensation.—This form of paralysis is less dangerous than that of motion, inasmuch as it is cured with less difficulty. In fact it is almost always curable, and generally follows hysterical affections.
                                                      Part xv., *p.* 45.

Facial Paralysis cured by Quinine.—Dr. Durant, of Ipswich, mentions a case of paralysis of the side of the face occurring after a course of mercury, which was cured by the administration of quinine. *Part* xv., *p.* 62.

Electricity in Paralysis.—In the use of electricity, says Prof. Matteucci, we must remember that the excitability of the nerves appears to be lost. Now though the *contractions* excited by an electric current passed down a nerve in the direction of its ramifications, i. e. a *direct* current, are more powerful than those produced by the passage of a current in the *inverse* direction, yet the *direct* current weakens and destroys the excitability of a nerve, while the inverse current augments it. The best form of electricity that can be used in paralysis is that from the electro-magnetic machine. Apply the interrupted current, and at first a very feeble one; and after twenty or thirty shocks, let the patient rest for some seconds.

Paralysis following Local Injury.—In paralysis following local injury, as concussion of the nerves, Dr. G. Bird would apply electro-magnetism from the *single current* machine, taking care to transmit it in the direction of the vis nervosa, or in other words, in the direction of the nervous ramifications.

From Lead (Dropped Hands).—Take electric sparks from the cervical and dorsal vertebræ thrice a week; also from the paralyzed parts, and in recent cases transmit *small shocks* along the course of the affected nerves.

Hysterical.—Employ electricity either in the form of shock, or the interrupted current from the electro-magnetic machine. If the paralysis is simulated, it will rarely resist the pain and surprise of the shock; and if the affection, however excited at first, is now uninfluenced by the patient's will, the electro-magnetic current is a most valuable therapeutic measure.

Of the Portio Dura.—Use electricity: any form will do, as it is merely the stimulus which is required, acting on the paralyzed muscular fibres, and arousing their normal irritability.

Rheumatic.—(Following the sudden application of cold, independently of any evidence of central spinal lesion.) Take electric sparks thrice a week from the spine and the paralyzed muscles.

From Effusions, etc.—When the *primary cause* is removed, and the paralysis is still persistent, apply electro-magnetism, the *single current* transmitted in the course of the nervous ramifications, and patiently continued for some time. Be very careful not to use this agent where rigid arteries are suspected, or ramollissement of the brain exists. Fatal apoplexy has been known to follow the use of electricity in such cases.

When it continues, after the disease in the brain is removed, the muscles must be artificially excited to action, by electricity or otherwise, to insure their nutrition. *Part* xvi., *p.* 103.

Paralysis—Cerebral.—Dr. Todd says: It is important to notice the state of the muscles of a paralyzed limb; for if rigidity of the muscles exists at an early period, local depletion and counter-irritation will be attended with benefit, whereas such measures are not applicable when complete relaxation exists. *Part* xviii., *p.* 80.

Paralysis of the Portio Dura.—[As facial paralysis, Dr. Todd observes, is to a patient and his friends a very alarming disease, it is important for the practitioner to be well acquainted with the various kinds of palsy affecting the face, so that a favorable prognosis, when the case will admit of it, may be at once given. The case which formed the subject of the following observations by Dr. Todd, was one of paralysis of the facial portion of the seventh pair of nerves, accompanied by severe pain behind the right ear. Dr. Todd observes:]

The leading character of these cases of facial palsy is the inability to close the eyelids, from paralysis of the *orbicularis palpebrarum* muscle; this is the pathognomonic sign which determines the peculiar nature of the palsy, and distinguishes it from the more serious form of facial palsy which is dependent on disease of the brain and palsy of the fifth nerve. It is remarkable how seldom the seventh pair of nerves is affected by disease of the brain. I cannot say that I ever saw a single instance of paralysis of the orbicular muscle of the eyelids due distinctly to diseased brain; and I have only seen a few in which the power of the muscle appeared to be enfeebled from that cause. Thus we have a point favorable and consolatory to a patient affected with *portio dura* paralysis; namely, that the affection being seated in that nerve affords a strong probability that he is free from disease of the brain; for diseased brain would give rise to a different form of facial palsy, and very rarely, if ever, cause this.

You have only to examine this patient with care, and you will find that he has almost every sign which indicates that the paralysis has its seat in the portio dura nerve. He cannot close his right eyelids; in making the attempt, however, he seems not to have lost the power altogether, for the upper lid is slightly depressed; yet if you put your finger on the orbicular muscle you do not find the slightest contraction of it.

Our patient is unable to frown on the right side, while he does so distinctly on the left; neither can he move his scalp on the right side; the corrugator supercilii, and the frontal portion of the occipito-frontalis muscles, are paralyzed—and hence these movements cannot be effected. The levatores alæ nasi, and the zygomatic muscles, are likewise, paralyzed on the right side, and therefore, the right nostril is motionless, and the angle of the mouth hangs on that side. The orbicularis oris muscle is paralyzed as to its right half; the patient is consequently unable to purse up his mouth, and if you ask him to whistle, he will afford you indications of his inability to perform this as well as other actions. The act of smiling or laughing is exaggerated on the left side, and the reason is because the left muscles have lost completely the resistance of those of the right side, which remain perfectly motionless, and which from disease have lost their tone, and have suffered much in their nutrition. For the same reason all the movements of the features which act in symmetry, and which at the same time counterbalance each other, are found to take place to an exaggerated extent on the healthy side. Hence in smiling, laughing, and speaking, the face is drawn more or less to the right side: the distortion takes place on the healthy side, the paralyzed side remaining unmoved. The popular notion, in cases of this kind, is that the disease is on the side to which the mouth is drawn. No medical man, however, can fall into this mistake if he be at all acquainted with the real condition of the patient.

Another muscle which is paralyzed in this case, and in all cases of the same kind, is the buccinator. Hence the cheek hangs loose, and as the patient speaks, it flaps to and fro. This extreme looseness of the cheek is not an early symptom of this form of paralysis; it manifests itself more and more, the longer the duration of the disease, and ultimately becomes the cause of symptoms very troublesome to the patient. It interferes not only with articulation, from its looseness and flapping movements while the patient is speaking, but mastication likewise. The palsied muscle allows the food to accumulate between the teeth and the jaw, and fails in its functions of supplying the mill with its proper amount of material to be ground. After a little time, patients learn to remedy the defect of articulation which the paralytic condition of the buccinator muscle causes, by supporting the cheek with the hand; and a similar kind of support serves to remove the inconveniences of mastication.

You will observe that all the muscles paralyzed in this affection are *superficial:* they are all muscles more or less concerned in the expression of the countenance. The deep-seated muscles are not affected—these are muscles of mastication—the only muscle paralyzed, which is concerned in mastication, being the buccinator, which is, however, only accessory to that function, and is as much or more a muscle of expression.

[As the buccinator receives a motor branch from the fifth, in addition to its supply from the seventh, the circumstance of its being paralyzed, when the disease or disorder is confined to the seventh pair, is very curious, and has not as yet, Dr. Todd remarks, received an adequate explanation. As to the treatment of this affection, much treatment is not generally required when it has arisen from cold or from constitutional causes; mild purgatives, alkalies or sudorifics, or iodide of potassium, and locally warm fomentations. Leeching or blistering are not so distinctly useful; and strychnine, Dr. Todd remarks, *is of no use* in these cases. If recent otitis be the cause of the attack, more antiphlogistic treatment will be needed, and sometimes even salivation will be beneficial.] *Part* xviii., *p.* 83.

Treatment of Paralysis from Lead.—Prevent the further introduction of the poison by cleanliness and frequent washings; stimulate the skin by friction and exercise ; Dr. Todd would also give baths containing sulphuret of potassium, in the proportion of one, two, or three ounces, to as many gallons of water ; let the patient have good food, and breathe pure air ; and apply galvanism as a local stimulant, for ten or fifteen minutes at a time, three times a day. *Part* xviii., *p.* 88.

Paralysis, Facial.—In paralytic affections of the facial muscles, when the antagonist muscles distort the features, the distortion may be remedied by the application of collodion; the parts being adjusted to their normal position before the solution is applied, and being held in that position with the finger until the solution is dry. (Dr. J. Starlin.) *Part* xix., *p.* 319.

Paralysis Facial.—In facial paralysis from exposure to cold, apply the "heated hammer," a modification of the iron recommended by Dr. Corrigan, which is to be heated for fifteen or twenty seconds in the flame of a spirit lamp, and then run lightly, being alternately raised and depressed, over the affected surface. *Part* xx., *p.* 54.

Paralysis Agitans.—Paralysis agitans, says Dr. Swan, is emphatically a disease of emotion. Emotion is its first and last cause; without emotion it would never be called into existence, or, being once induced, it would never manifest itself. This at least is true, of its first phase ; whether any physical lesion may supervene in its protracted course, remains a deeply interesting question.

Alone, reposing, asleep, the agitation is absent. It is renewed when cause of emotion comes into operation. It frequently subsides in the society of the patient's immediate relatives or friends, as his wife and children, and is reëxerted on the appearance of a visitor or a stranger.

The peculiar shaking, and the equally peculiar powerlessness, or shall I call it paralysis, cease on giving *confidence* to the patient. I may here adduce an anecdote: A gentleman, a magistrate, confined to his chair by paralysis agitans, wished to consult a legal book. He asked for it, and his servant gave it to him, as he supposed. On opening it, he found it the wrong book. In his anger he rose from his chair, and reached it himself. Surprised at discovering his power of walking, he endeavored to repeat the experiment, and remembering that before he had risen from his chair, he had rather violently closed his book, he repeated this manœuvre, and ever since, on doing this—but only on doing this—he regains his power of walking.

One patient could walk whenever he pleased, with the tips of his fingers merely on his wife's arm, but not otherwise.

It is essential to replace a (unfounded?) conviction in the patient's mind, that he is powerless, by another, viz., that he really possesses power, the circumstances being changed. The prepossession—the depressing emotion must be removed, and replaced by an emotion of the opposite kind.

In speaking of emotion as the cause of paralysis agitans, we ought to notice that this emotion is of the painful and agitating kind, and not unallied to fear and vexation. The elevating emotions or mental states, as hope, confidence, energy, have a marked beneficial effect. The movements made with firmness and resolution are always least attended by agitation.

There is, in consequence, a disposition in this malady, to rapid movement. The patient is apt to *run* instead of walking deliberately. An energetic volition overcomes the influence of emotion; volition of less energy is more or less defeated by emotion in its turn.

The paralysis agitans has hitherto made an exceedingly slow, but not the less fatal, progress.

Unfortunately, we possess no *post-mortem* examinations of this disease. I suspect no morbid lesion would be detected. No such lesion, hitherto known, would lead to the peculiar phenomena of this malady, except toward its close, when a sort of general paralysis takes place, which may be the effect of effusion and consequent pressure.

As emotion is the original and continued cause of this trying malady, an important question arises—What would be the effect of a sustained removal of all sources of emotion, if, and when this may be possible?

Seclusion in a cottage, a judicious companion, books of quiet interest, repose in the nearly recumbent position (the head especially being supported), free exposure to the open air, the gentlest exercises, the farm, the fields, the garden—the plants, the corn, the cattle, the poultry (not his own). It becomes an important question also, whether the shower-bath, douche along the spine, etc., may be useful; various sedative or narcotic medicines long given to subdue emotions, as we would give them to subdue pain, in stated forms and doses, regularly and systematically.

The bichloride of mercury, quinine, strychnine, etc., should be put to a cautious trial by competent judges. *Part* xxiii., *p.* 83.

Rheumatic and Local Paralysis, treated by Pulvermacher's Chain Battery.—Mr. Vallance highly recommends this chain battery in preference to the same strength of currents from the ordinary machine, believing that the current from the hydro-electric chain of Pulvermacher has a much greater effect. *Part* xxv., *p.* 57.

Paralysis of the Lower Limbs.—M. Gerard recommends the ergot of rye in daily doses of from 8 to 40 grains. *Part* xxv., *p.* 59.

Lead Palsy.—The state of lead cachexia, according to Dr. Todd, is very greatly improved by the long continued use of sulphur baths.
Part xxv., *p.* 69.

Incomplete Paralysis of the Lower Extremities, connected with Diseases of the Urinary Organs.—Mr. Wells, surgeon to Samaritan Hospital, says : There is a form of incomplete paraplegia—mere weakness and loss of control over the muscles of the limbs—the effect of disease of the bladder, kidneys, or urinary passages, and only cured by the relief of this primary disease. There may be no pain in the dorsal region on pressure, but cases have occurred where the pain, on pressure in the dorsal region, led to the diagnosis of spinal disease, and after death the spine and its contents were found perfectly healthy and the kidneys diseased. The intimate nervous connection between the urinary organs and the cord by means of the sympathetic, is probably the cause. Some impediment to the discharge of urine is one of the earliest symptoms. There is generally obstinate gastric derangement. The sensibility of the limbs is not impaired, or very slightly, and they do not become atrophied or lower in temperature than natural. The sphincter ani is not paralyzed. The bladder, to a great extent loses its contractility, but not entirely. There is no history of violent neuralgic symptoms at the commencement of the disease. Great amendment will often follow catheterism and the removal of any obstruction to the free discharge of urine. Exercise, warm clothing, bathing, and change of air, are important. Avoid aloes and saline aperients, as they tend to increase the urinary irritation. Gregory's powder is the best aperient. The patient may wear an elastic belt to support the lax abdominal parietes. A mixture of cantharides and iron tends much to restore the contractile power of the bladder, and relieve the urinary irritation. Opium relieves irritability very much. That which is productive of most good effects is a complete change of life, as a long sea voyage. Paraplegia is a common result of frequent seminal emissions, voluntary or involuntary; it is undeniable that the frequent agitation of the nervous system, so caused, leads to chronic inflammation and softening of the cord, with paraplegia as a necessary consequence. *Part* xxxvii., *p.* 37.

Paralysis.—Dr. Althaus states that in cerebral paralysis, the excitability of the muscles in the paralyzed limb is often, but not always, increased. In lead palsy and traumatic paralysis, the muscular excitability is almost lost. In hysterical rheumatic, and spontaneous paralysis, the paralyzed muscles respond normally to the electric current. *Part* xl., *p.* 314.

PARAPLEGIA.

The Use of Setons in Paraplegia.—Dr. Marshall Hall strongly recommends the use of setons in preference to issues, on the course of the spine in paraplegia, and in acute or chronic local or limited inflammation of different parts, as in hepatitis or nephritis. In cases of diseases of the spinal marrow, with paraplegia or paraplegic spasm, setons are more especially valuable; but Dr. Hall looks upon the usual seat of application of these setons as improper. He thinks the great error committed by medical men is the applying the seton *below* the seat of the disease. "The spinal nerves proceed for some distance, from above, directly rather than obliquely, downward, and the seat of the disease is *at* or *above* their junction (insertion or origin) with the spinal marrow." *Part* iv., *p.* 46.

Ergot of Rye.—M. Payan states that we may find ergot of rye very useful in paraplegia. When we consider its effects, not on the uterus only, but also on the rectum, bladder, and lower extremities, and, indeed, occasionally on the whole system, causing the patient to feel universally *benumbed*, as she frequently expresses herself, followed by powerful ex-citement, we must suppose that it acts primarily and especially on the spinal cord; and we may consequently believe that in some cases of para-plegia it will be found useful. *Part* vi., *p.* 88.

Paraplegia from Ascarides.—In the proceedings of the Ipswich Medi-cal Society, there is recorded the case of a child, twelve months old, which was attacked with sudden loss of power in the lower extremities, while the sensibility of those parts was exhausted. After purgatives had been given without advantage, the administration of sesquioxide of iron was followed by the expulsion of a " firm ball of ascarides," and the relief of all the symptoms. *Part* xv., *p.* 68.

Paraplegia.—The alkaline and phosphatic condition of the urine, says Dr. Garrod, may be remedied by the administration of benzoic acid in large doses, two scruples four times a day. *Part* xix., *p.* 28.

Reflex Paraplegia.—Dr. Brown-Séquard remarks, that if strychnia be administered in the reflex form of paralysis, it will be advantageous. This is well illustrated in a case of paraplegia produced by exposure to cold and wet. But, given in cases of paraplegia consequent on congestion or actual inflammation of the cord, strychnia will only aggravate the affection.
Part xl., *p.* 40.

—•◦•—

PARASITES.

Benzin or Benzole, as a Remedy for Animal Parasites.—Our readers are probably aware that benzin or benzole is a clear, colorless fluid, pos-sessed of a pungent etherial odor, which is produced by the decom-position of benzoic acid, or other organic substances, at a light tempe-rature. It was long ago ascertained by Milne Edwards that its vapor was very fatal to insects. This property has led M. Reynal, of the veterinary school at Alfort, to employ it for the treatment of pedicular maladies among animals. He has found that it destroys the parasites in these dis-eases, more surely, and with more safety to the animal, than tobacco-juice, mercurial ointment, or any other of the many remedies used. It destroys the epizoa without at all injuring the skin.

It is proposed to use this fluid in the parasitical diseases of the human skin, especially in phtheiriasis or morbus pedicularis, and in scabies, etc.
Part xxxi., *p.* 196.

PARONYCHIA.

Lotions and Medicated Poultices in Phlegmonous and Erysipelatous Inflammations, and especially in Paronychia.—In all these cases Dr. F. J. Brown urgently recommends the employment of astringent and sedative lotions, and poultices made with these instead of water, for not only, he says, may the disease by these means be sometimes checked before suppuration takes place, but when matter is formed the inflammation is not so great, and the parts are much sooner healed. He says:

The astringents that I employ are the sulphate of zinc and burnt alum mixed with acetate of lead. This is an unchemical mixture, but its use is satisfactory. I am indebted to my father, an old staff surgeon, for the prescription, which is, for each ounce of water three grains of burnt alum, two grains of zinc, and two grains of lead. The lotion should be used warm. It is advisable to omit the lead after the disease has been subdued, for fear of its effects on the muscular system, although I have never seen ill effects from perseverance in its application for many weeks. These ingredients, placed in paper as a powder, in sufficient quantity for a wine-bottleful of water, enable a patient to use the lotion both freely and cheaply.

I have no doubt but that many surgeons use lotions for the affections mentioned, and I must therefore apologize for bringing forward this mode of treatment; but I have seen so many fingers crippled by the persistence of inflammation under the water-poultice treatment, that I consider the subject worthy of attention. Surgeons can see the improvement that occurs in many diseases of the eye, ear and throat, from the use of astringent lotions, yet they commonly neglect such applications in phlegmonous inflammation occuring in the trunk and limbs.

Nitrate of silver is sometimes applied over surfaces affected by erysipelatous inflammation, but I am not aware that astringent lotions are usually applied by means of cloths laid upon the parts. I recollect reading in one of the periodicals of sulphate of iron lotion for erysipelas, and I have employed it with advantage.

I presume that the astringents diminish the calibre of the bloodvessels, and effect some change upon the nutritive process by which the profuso formation of cells is restricted. Certain it is that the inflamed part becomes diminished in size and whitened; and suppurating parts yield secretion in greatly diminished quantity (without becoming hot and dry, as might be anticipated), whilst their bulk is reduced.

The internal treatment that exerts most influence on paronychial inflammation is sulphate of quina in Epsom salts mixture, preceded (in severe cases) by a few doses of tartrate of antimony in Epsom salts mixture. The same internal treatment is peculiarly efficacious in erysipelas and phlebitis, and in the unhealthy inflammations generally, as they are termed.

In concluding these few remarks, I would mention that the ancient lapis divinus (alum, nitre, and sulphate of copper) constitutes a gargle that will quickly remove inflammation of the throat; and the same (with the omission of the nitre) forms a lotion under the use of which sores on the penis heal with rapidity.

The medication of poultices by means of ointments is advantageous in certain cases. Resinous ointment mixed with a poultice considerably hastens the suppuration and cure of a boil, and it will cause the skin **to** yield much sooner in abscesses of the breast and neck than occurs under simple poulticing. Red oxide of mercury ointment mixed with a poultice cleanses foul sores, and expedites their healing. Medicated fomentations and poultices were in great esteem formerly, but they have fallen into a neglect which I consider to be unmerited.   *Part* xxviii., *p.* 23ε.

PEDICULI.

Pediculi Pubis. — Dr. Haural recommends the following treatment; Wash the parts thoroughly, first with soap and water, then with pure water; dry them, then pour chloroform on drop by drop, and rub it in: then cover the parts with a folded handkerchief for half an hour, when another washing with soap and water should be performed, in order to detach the debris of the pediculi.   *Part* xxxvii., *p.* 182.

Pediculi Pubis.—Dr. Ryding, of Oakham, uses the following lotion: Bichloride of mercury, twelve grains; rectified spirit, two ounces; distilled water, two ounces. Apply this carefully for ten minutes with a flannel, and immediately afterward well dust the parts with ammonio-chloride of mercury. Repeat this night and morning for two days, then use a warm bath and soap. The ova will be destroyed effectually by this process. . . . .
Apply the following liniment for forty-eight hours: Finely levigated nitric oxide of mercury, two drachms; olive oil, one ounce; mix. . . . .
Apply an ointment containing half a drachm of iodide of potassium to an ounce of lard. . . . .
Rub in a large quantity of calomel at bed-time. One application will usually be sufficient.   *Part* xxxviii., *p.* 176.

PENIS.

Amputation of the Penis.—[Mr. Barnes publishes an account of the mode in which M. Ricord avails himself of the process of contraction after amputation of the penis to keep the urethra open. The principle of most surgeons in this operation is to counteract contraction.]
M. Ricord's principle is to avail himself of this process of contraction, and turn it to account in preserving the orifice of the urethra patent. The proceeding is this: having performed the amputation, with the precaution of preserving sufficient skin, and no more, to sheathe the corpora cavernosa, and secured the vessels, the surgeon seizes with the forceps the mucous membrane of the urethra, and with a pair of scissors makes four slight incisions, so as to form four equal flaps; then using a fine needle, carrying a silk ligature, he unites each flap to the skin by a suture. The wound unites by the first intention; adhesion being formed between the skin and mucous membrane, which become continuous, a condition analogous to what is

observed at the other natural outlets of the body. The cicatrix then contracting, instead of operating prejudicially, as in the old methods, tends, on the contrary, constantly to open the urethra, whilst a perfect covering is provided for the ends of the corpora cavernosa. The difficulty of directing the stream of urine, is one which becomes troublesome in proportion to the shortness of the stump. The patient must provide himself with a funnel-shaped canula, made of box, ivory, or metal, the base of which being applied over the stump, and resting on the pubes, the other end will serve to carry the urine clear of the person. *Part* xi., *p.* 170.

Penis—Cancer of.—M. Bonnet employs the actual cautery to execute the amputation. The patient being put under the influence of chloroform, and wet compresses disposed round the penis, the organ is held by means of forceps, and the heated iron applied perpendicularly to the back of the penis. When the fibrous structure is divided, the iron is to be passed into the corpora cavernosa, and so through the penis. Four or five applications will be wanted in all. When the cancer extends to the scrotum or abdomen, the operation is more tedious, as the ramifications must be followed by the cautery, though the pubis itself has to be reached. If the inguinal glands are affected, they should be removed by a bistoury, and the cautery applied. There is generally far less reaction than after ordinary amputations of the penis. In about a week the eschars begin to be detached in fragments, and they have all fallen in fifteen or twenty days. By this operation, then, we can much more readily act on healthy tissue, we are enabled to attack cases the knife could not reach, and we prevent hemorrhage. *Part* xx., *p.* 165.

Case of Considerable Sprouting of Warts on the Glans Penis.—[Ricord believed that warts upon the penis were non-syphilitic, other eminent surgeons think they are; but there can be no question that these excrescences may be implanted on the organs of generation in the same way as they are present upon the fingers. From the narrow space in which they grow, they are liable to produce great irritation and inflammation, and their removal rendered a matter of anxiety. The patient in the case of Mr. Hancock, was a married man, aged 35, and stated positively that he had never had any venereal affection whatever. He had never noticed anything the matter with the penis until four months before admission, when the warts began to grow.]

The patient has congenital phimosis, and noticed at the time just mentioned, that some tumor was developing between the glans and the prepuce in the neighborhood of the corona. The pressure from within soon caused slight pain in the prepuce, and inflammation ensued, marked with a vivid redness on its external surface near the corona glandis. The patient applied poultices; ulceration and perforation took place, and the mass of warts, which had been the exciting cause of all these symptoms, protruded through the ulcerated opening in the prepuce.

The verrucæ having thus obtained room, seemed to grow more rapidly than before; the aperture just mentioned became larger, and the warts grew to such an extent as to cover the glans almost completely, and to double its size. The extremity of the prepuce was, in the meanwhile, almost separated by ulceration from the rest of that process, abundant suppuration had set in, and the parts looked, to an unpractised eye, as if the organ had been suffering from carcinoma. Very little or no pain accompanied these changes.

The patient was brought into the operating theatre, and when he had been rendered insensible with chloroform, Mr. Hancock began to remove with the scissors the enormous crop of warts which had sprung up about the part, as also the thickened semi-detached pieces of prepuce which were giving to the organ a misshapen aspect. When the whole mass of verrucæ had been excised, the penis was surrounded with lint dipped in cold water, and the patient placed in bed. The progress has been most satisfactory since the operation, and the parts are now quite cicatrized.

Part xxix., *p.* 241.

———•••———

PERICARDITIS.

Treatment of.—On account of the frequent occurrence of pericarditis, its dangerous nature, and the numerous important diseases—endocarditis, valvular disease, atrophy, hypertrophy, dilatation—which are frequently its consequences, it is highly important that its detection should be easy, and its treatment simple and straightforward. Although the pericardium is composed of two distinct kinds of tissue, yet as they are intimately connected, and supplied by the same vessels, the character and products of the inflammation depend more upon the condition of the blood than upon the nature of the tissue primarily affected.

Dr. Shearman would bleed, first generally, and then locally, to such an extent as to cut off part of blood to the part, and to decrease the quantity of fibrin in the blood; give opium to diminish irritability and vascular excitement, and to relieve pain; give purgatives moderately; and blister. But all these remedies combined will be inefficient for good, except mercury be given. Get the patient, therefore, as *quickly as possible* under the specific action of mercury; and for this purpose the best method is to give calomel with opium, and to use frequent frictions with strong mercurial ointment. Colchicum, emetic tartar, and aconite may sometimes be useful in allaying excessive action; but must be given with great caution.

Part xvi., *p.* 113.

Ptyalism in Pericarditis.—Dr. Taylor's eases seem to show that our opinions on the powers of mercury in pericarditis require revision. In *twelve* cases, ptyalism was not followed by any abatement of the disease; and in six cases pericarditis followed upon the ptyalism.

Part xvi., *p.* 116.

Rheumatic Pericarditis.—The treatment of pericarditis, says Dr. C. Kidd, has recently undergone considerable modification. Taking blood by venesection, which would first suggest itself, though necessary in some cases, in others is all but inadmissible. It has been recently shown by Bouchardat, that rheumatism may even be induced by the coagulable state of the blood, the result of repeated bleedings. Every particular case, of course, will require a different line of action. Venesection after the middle of the first week, as a general rule, will lengthen the period of recovery, and many cases will not require bleeding at all.

The local abstraction of blood in rheumatic pericarditis will be always found the most beneficial. The treatment must vary, as we have to treat patients ill fed and etiolated in cities, or healthy and full of red blood in the country. Antimony, alkalies, nitre, and colchicum, are very valuable. The exhibition of mercury has been lately dwelt upon, the general impression being that its beneficial effect will, in a great measure, depend on the period at which it is given. If early in the disease, it will prove much more satisfactory than later, its action being more properly directed to prevent the deposition of organizable matter in the pericardium than to remove it afterward. Indeed, our late statistics would go to prove that salivation has no very marked effect on the disease at all, the ceasing of the friction sound, according to Taylor, being more of a coincidence than really brought about through the agency of the mineral. As to the use of tartar emetic to remove inflammation, perhaps there is no difference of opinion; the dangerous effects of this valuable medicine having little or no existence except in the estimate of those who have not studied its effects.

Case.—Margaret B., aged 20, single, had suffered formerly from rheumatism, and lately very much from debility, and irregular menstruation. She complained, on admission into Guy's Hospital, of burning hot pains in the joints, and all the accompanying symptoms of rheumatic fever. The heart's action was found to be quite normal, as well as the impulse, a very feeble bruit being perceptible with the first sound, particularly over the valves. The second sound free. Ordered pills with antim. tart. and calomel, and a draught for the morning, with senna and vin. colchici, to be kept very quiet, and to get simple drinks, without food. As the symptoms of pericarditis gradually came on, with acute pain below the left nipple, between the fifth and sixth ribs, a rubbing sound was detected with the systole, and occasionally of a "to and fro" character. Cupping glasses were now put on, and ℥vj. of blood drawn from the cardiac region, the former medicines being continued. Although the "rubbing sound" continued for six days longer, the general symptoms began to improve; but the bruit began to be traceable along the aorta. She was now, in addition to the same medicines, ordered a blister to the region of the heart. In a week after this, the pericarditic symptoms had entirely disappeared, although she had suffered some little relapse. *Part* xxii., *p.* 116.

Pericarditis.—Dr. Stokes says that whenever the fever present is of a typhus character wine is required. *Part* xxix., *p.* 21.

----•♦•----

PERINEUM.

Ruptured Perineum—Operation.—After dwelling on the difficulty of accomplishing the re-union of the parts in ruptured perineum, Mr. Fergusson says, that "it is generally allowed that in cases which do not heal up soon after delivery, the parts being kept in perfect rest, it is better to wait, before attempting any surgical means, until the primary inflammation has subsided. Mr. Fergusson has chosen the interrupted suture, certain objections to them being removed by precautionary measures. This patient, 18 years of age, had been delivered of her first child by the forceps six months previous to her admission, and ever since had been suffering from the effects of a lacerated perineum, extending from the fourchette to the margin of the anus, the fæces involuntarily passing through the recto-vaginal aperture.

After this young woman had been duly prepared for the operation, by rest and opening medicine, she was brought into the theatre and placed under the influence of chloroform. The patient being secured in the position for the operation of lithotomy, Mr. Fergusson began by paring the whole length of the margins of the perineal gap, from above downward, and brought them in exact apposition, by three interrupted sutures. The next step of the operation consisted in making a longitudinal incision on each side of the line of sutures, in order to take off the tension which the neighboring parts would naturally exercise upon the sutures. These lateral wounds were filled with dry lint, cold compresses applied to the perineum, and the patient removed to a bed, with her knees kept together by a roller.

Much care was subsequently used in keeping her quiet and regulating the action of the bowels by enemata; and about eleven days after the operation Mr. Fergusson was enabled to remove the three sutures, as pretty firm adhesion had taken place. The bowels now became regular, without the necessity of the injections which had hitherto been systematically administered, and about one month after the operation, both the perineal wound and the lateral incisions were completely healed. The further progress of the patient has been satisfactory, the rectum has regained the faculty of retaining its contents, and the poor woman is delivered from a very distressing infirmity.   *Part* xxii., *p.* 305.

Rupture of the Perineum.—The plan of Mr. Brown's operation is as follows: Having made a clean incision into the vagina, so as to separate from each side of the rent any portion of mucous membrane, three or four sutures were passed deeply through the parts, and attached to a piece of quill or elastic bougie on each side. Three or four smaller sutures might be passed also through the edges of the wound, so as to bring them into more certain apposition. To prevent the inner edges of the wound being drawn separate by the sphincter, and the lochia allowed to penetrate into the wound, Mr. Brown divides this muscle; and this he considers one of the most essential features of his operation. In all cases he administers opium, which allays the irritability of the nervous system, and exercises a most salutary influence over the patient. He has never seen any harm arise from its constipating effects.   *Part* xxvii., *p.* 196.

Abscesses in the Perineum and Neighborhood of the Anus.—[According to Prof. Syme, the explanation of the origin of abscesses in this situation which is usually given and received, is very erroneous, so far as the rectum is concerned. They are said to be from ulceration in the mucous membrane, allowing intestinal matters to enter the cellular texture. But such an occurrence never does take place, since ulcers in this situation are always attended with an induration of the subjacent texture; and]—

It is this firmness of base that renders ulcers at the rectum recognizable by touch, which from long and large experience, I may confidently assert, is sufficient for the diagnosis of all derangements in this part of the body, while speculums are not only painful and useless, but calculated to mislead. If further evidence were required to disprove the agency of ulceration in giving rise to the abscesses in question, it would be afforded by the effect of wounds penetrating the mucous membrane, which give rise to abscesses, it is true, but totally different in their nature and character from those of the ordinary purulent collections met with in this situation. The most frequent instances of such an injury are produced in a way that would not readily occur to you, viz., the administration of enemata. Many years ago, on making my daily visit to this hospital, I was told that a patient, who had been admitted with retention, was suffering from extravasation of urine. Upon examination, I found much swelling of the nates and neighboring part of the perineum, but no difficulty in passing a full-sized catheter, through which a large quantity of healthy urine was evacuated. Having then ascertained that an injection into the rectum had been employed as a substitute for more efficient relief, I suspected the truth, and introducing my finger into the anus, at once felt an aperture on the anterior surface of the bowel, through which the fluid injected had no doubt passed, so as to simulate the appearance of urinary extravasation. In those days, the instrument employed for throwing injections into the rectum, was the old metal syringe with a straight pipe, which, when introduced behind the patient, as it generally was, could hardly fail to encounter resistance from the opposite surface, requiring force which was sometimes employed so strenuously as to make the fluid escape in a wrong direction into the operator's face. Impressed with the danger of such a procedure, as manifested by the case just mentioned, and others that came to my knowledge from the inquiries which it suggested, I recommended that the old injecting apparatus should be abolished, and that Read's syringe should be employed in its stead. But even from his more safe and apparently harmless mode of administration, I have known perforation of the mucous membrane produced ; and in order to put you still further on your guard, I may mention that a most kind and attentive practitioner asked me to see a gentleman, in whose case he felt so much interested, as to administer an injection by the apparently innocuous means of a bag and pipe, or in other words, a bladder, with an ivory tube attached to it, with the effect of perforating the bowels, and distending the hip with the usual mixture of gruel, salt and oil.

The fluid injected excites inflammation of a very violent character. attended with a corresponding degree of constitutional disturbance, the local result being very speedily a large collection of extremely fetid fluid and air. These characters of the abscess may be supposed to depend upon the peculiar nature of the matters allowed to issue from the bowel, but are more probably connected with the sort of inflammatory action which is excited by the wound.

The abscesses which, under all ordinary circumstances, occur at the verge of the anus, differ entirely from those which we have been considering. Instead of being large and diffused, they are small and circumscribed ; instead of being preceded by intense inflammation, and attended with violent constitutional disturbance, they take place without either one or the other of these conditions ; instead of being rapidly they are slowly formed ; and instead of dark-colored fetid matter, they contain merely a little of what used to be called well-conditioned pus. It is such abscesses which lay the foundation of fistula in ano. When allowed to open spontaneously, they almost invariably do so on the external surface—that is, through the skin ; and if, when this has happened, or the contents have been evacuated by an incision, a finger is introduced into the rectum, while a probe is employed to explore the cavity formed by suppuration, it will be found that the mucous membrane, although to a considerable extent completely denuded, still remains entire. Sooner or later an aperture is formed by ulceration, through this detached portion of the lining membrane, and then the fistula becomes complete or open on both the external and internal surface with which it is connected.

Then, as to the urethra, it has long been taught that abscesses connected with it in general proceed from ulceration of this membrane, allowing urine to escape into the cellular texture. But whenever urine can be positively ascertained thus to issue from its proper channel, the local and constitutional effects are so violent and characteristic as to prevent the possibility of overlooking them; while the abscesses that usually precede the formation of a fistula in perineo take place slowly and insidiously so as frequently to escape observation until they discharge their contents, which in the first instance are almost always simply purulent, the urine finding its way through them only by a secondary process of ulceration in the denuded mucous lining of the urethra, which, like that of the rectum, remains entire for a time. It is true that strictures frequently give rise to abscesses of the perineum, but not by impeding the flow of urine so as to cause the extravasation, their real agency in producing this effect being through the excitement of irritation, which gradually leads to the result in question. *Part* xxxiii., *p.* 187.

Ruptured Perineum.—In the Vienna Lying-in Hospital, Vidal's serresfine seem to have superseded every other means of approximation. It may be necessary to pare the edges a little; then, as soon as the bleeding has ceased, two or three may be applied according to the extent of laceration. Allow them to remain two hours, keep the parts clean, and, above all, keep the patient on her side till the termination of the case.
Part xxxiv., *p.* 246.

Perineo-Plastic Operation.—Dr. Savage, of Samaritan Hospital, states that one great element of success in this operation is to remove the *entire thickness* of the vagina as far as the perineal fascia. *Part* xxxvii., *p.* 217.

—•◦•—

PERIOSTEAL AFFECTIONS.

Treatment of Periostitis.—Mr. Ferrall has tried the three principal modes of treatment usually adopted in this disease, viz.: 1st, by incision; 2d, by mercury; and thirdly, by hydriodate of potass. By the first the cure was completed in twenty-eight days, and by the last in thirteen days: relief was more *immediately* procured by incision, that is, by cutting down upon the bone through the periosteum for the space of about two inches, but the cure was, nevertheless, protracted.

He gives from eight to twenty grains of hydriodate of potass three times a day in the third mode of treatment, to which he gives the preference, since the iodine treatment avoids a painful, though brief operation, and is not followed by an open sore.

The second ground of preference, namely, the earlier period at which the patient can resume his occupation, is clearly on the side of the iodine, for the case treated by mercury occupied thirty-seven days, that by incision twenty-eight days, and that by the hydriodate of potass thirteen days.

Sarsaparilla is also spoken of as a medicine of great efficacy in sub-acute and chronic periostitis. *Part* i., *p.* 120.

Periosteal Disease.—Dr Oke gives the following case:

J. C., aged 40, a baker by trade, consulted me for an agonizing pain of a rheumatic character in the right tibia, which was considerably enlarged, and its periosteum thickened along the upper half of its anterior and inner surface. This pain had existed for *eight years!* It attacked him every night as soon as he was warm in bed, and had in a great measure long deprived him of sleep. He is a married man; and solemnly assures me that he has contracted no syphilitic disease for the last twenty years, when he had a swelling of the groin. He told me he had spent in vain almost all he possessed in medical advice, and had been once in a hospital with no better success; that he could bear his sufferings no longer; and, that in the event of my treatment being also unsuccessful, he had decided on submitting to amputation as a last resource. I at once put him under the use of the iodide, of which he took five grains in solution three times a day, and continued the treatment for six weeks; at the end of a week the pains left him and never returned; the enlargement of the tibia diminished, and he speedily recovered. *Part* ix., *p.* 61.

Periosteal Thickening cured by Iodide of Potassium.—Mr. Alexander Ure relates a case of periosteal inflammation of left ulna, about its middle third, of two months' standing, which, after blisters, leeching, etc., had been tried, was cured by taking two grains of iodide potass. twice daily, in infus. gent. co., and a grain of opium at bedtime, for a fortnight; bran poultices applied to the arm. *Part* xi., *p.* 186.

Treatment of Periostitis.—In obstinate cases, says Prof. Miller, where aggravation and suppuration seem imminent, direct incision is unwarrantable, but it may be done as follows: Insert a fine bistoury or tenotomy needle, at a little distance from the tense part, passing it over, cautiously, beneath the integument; then turning and pressing its edge, divide the tense membrane wholly to the desired extent; now cautiously withdraw the instrument, making a valvular, oblique, subintegumental wound; finally, close the single puncture immediately; with isinglass plaster or collodion. *Part* xxiii., *p.* 275.

Syphilitic Periostitis.—Iodide of potassium for this disease, says Dr. Todd, certainly deserves the name of a specific, the chief drawback to it is, that its effects are so evanescent. To obviate this, mercury may be given with it, or a short alternate course of each, and then using only tonic means, resume the mercurial and iodine treatment if necessary. *Part* xxiii., *p.* 87.

Periosteal Disease affecting the Dura Mater.—The dura mater, says Dr. R. H. Goolden, is supposed to be very little liable to disease, except as the result of injury, or in connection with strumous softening of the petrous portion of the temporal bone, or with abscesses about the ear, or as the effect of syphilitic poison; and this poison, supported by some of our best authorities, seems to have diverted attention from a very common affection of this membrane, of the same character as the periostitis which gives rise to nodes on the tibia or cranial bones.

This partial affection of the dura mater may or may not coëxist with general periosteal disease. It is part of the same morbid state, and it has no necessary connection either with syphilis or with mercury, though these poisons, and especially the latter, greatly favor its development. Indeed, the worst cases have been those who, in the tropics, have taken large quantities of mercury for fevers or hepatic disease, often many years previously, and have been afterward exposed to cold and damp in our more northern latitudes. They give way, at least for the time, to very simple treatment, viz.: iodide of potassa, with sarsaparilla, blisters or issues to the head, and full doses of opium every night, with a good nutritious diet—in the same way as periosteal nodes are known to do. When the pericranium is the seat of the disease, it is at once recognized by the presence of great tenderness, as well as unevenness to the touch; but when the dura mater is affected, this morbid condition is not so palpable; it is, however, evinced by unmistakable symptoms. The patients are often free from pain during the day, but at eight or nine o'clock at night the pain sets in, and is so agonizing that they are willing to submit to any measure for relief. It lasts till three or four o'clock in the morning, followed by a profuse perspiration, when the patient gets some sleep. The intermittent character, and the time and duration of the paroxysms, are very remarkable. For some time the cerebral functions are not impaired, but at length the sufferer complains of a constant headache, though not so severe as during the paroxysms; he holds his head forward, with his brows knit; then follow occasionally epileptic fits, weakness of the lower limbs, paralysis, and the patient becomes greatly emaciated, despondent, and suffers colliquative perspirations.

Some years ago, a sailor, who had frequently been a patient for such attacks, was accidentally killed. This afforded an opportunity of examining the head, when it was found that the inner table of the skull was greatly thickened, and also the dura mater.

Such is the most marked and aggravated form of the disease occurring in patients debilitated by climate, mercury, purpura, or syphilis, which no one would fail to recognize as identical (except in situation) with periosteal disease, when it attacks the tibia, ulna, cranial bones, crest of the ilium, etc., in the form of nodes, and for which the iodide of potassium seems to be the appropriate, if not specific remedy.

Although this aggravated form of periosteal disease of the dura mater is most common in sea-port hospitals, where the patients have been for the most part exposed to *all* the predisposing causes, yet it occurs also in a milder form, and therefore more likely to escape recognition, as the cause of many distressing headaches, ultimately leading to epilepsy or paralysis, or at all events reducing the sufferer to the most distressing state of debility.

These cases are marked by headache, having its regular nightly paroxysms, morning perspirations, and gradual emaciation. The patients have mostly been treated for dyspepsia, rheumatism, gout, neuralgia, brow ague, and often for supposed obscure cases of phthisis, having, in addition to the above symptoms, some cough and bronchial murmurs; but by the peculiar expression of countenance, the pain and wakefulness during the first part of the night, the true nature of the disorder has been recognized.

Part xxiv., *p.* 54.

Periosteal Disease Affecting the Humerus and Femur.—This disease often affects the upper end of the humerus, and the lower end of the femur, and is often overlooked. The shoulder is aching, tender, and cannot be used on account of the pain, the muscles being inserted into the periosteum. The pain is more severe at night; there is no perceptible swelling. There soon follows a state of permanent congestion, or subacute inflammation. The hip joint is liable to a similar affection, but is more rare. In these cases the iodide of potassa must be given three times a day. If of long standing, blisters or issues must be employed. The nitric acid issue is the best. A piece of lint is to be applied the size required, not too wet with the acid, to the tender part anterior to the joint, as it is generally under the covering of the deltoid and biceps, near the joint. It should then be covered over with a piece of lint, dipped in a solution of carbonate of soda. A linseed poultice should be then applied. The slough usually comes away in five or seven days, and the discharge will continue till the pain is removed.

Periosteal Deposits.—Dr. Goolden also alludes to some painful swellings of the tarsal and metatarsal, as well as carpal and, metacarpal bones, often observed to remain after attacks of gout, when all active signs of gout have subsided—and sometimes mistaken for gout—and to the known success of the iodide of potassa in relieving the pain. These swellings of the fingers and wrists are very different from chalkstone deposits, though they disfigure the hands. They are very common in advanced life, and then they rarely subside so as entirely to restore symmetry of form. But the same observation holds good in all other forms of periosteal deposit; that is to say, although the activity of the disease may be arrested by iodide of potassa and blisters, the absorption of earthy matter in old age is much more difficult; the pain will subside, but the tibia and frontal bone still retain the swelling and unevenness.

Another set of periosteal deposits is on the fangs of the teeth, causing the most agonizing toothache, without any apparent decay of the teeth. The fang of the tooth becomes thickened, too large for the alveolar cell, and, when drawn, the membrane shows unusual vascularity, and there is a deposit of dentine, softer than the fang of the tooth, and may be cut with a penknife between the membrane and the fang, giving it bulbous form, and rendering it difficult to extract without breaking. This is not uncommon after mercurial salivation; and in ladies who have taken metallic remedies for a continuance—especially salts of iron—given for the relief of headache, and remittent pains about the chest and other parts—sometimes for neuralgia—all dependent upon this state of the system.

Part xxiv., *p.* 57.

Periosteal Disease affecting the Dura Mater.—[In previous notices of this disease, Dr. Goolden has shown some important, but not generally recognized forms of its development, and its independence of syphilis. In considering its remedial treatment, he says:]

No more valuable remedy has been introduced into medicine than the iodide of potassa, but its precise value is scarcely generally recognized. Some practitioners give it in eight-grain doses, three times a day; and give it with calomel or blue-pill, and colchicum; others never venture beyond two grains, and even then fear the results; yet no one ventures to dispute its almost general efficacy in nodal periostitis.

As far as I can draw any inference from my own cases, I should say that smaller doses produce the specific effect quite as soon as the larger; and I have often known two-grain doses act readily on the system, when larger doses have failed; but I think it necessary to combine the salt with liquor potassa, as any acid on the stomach will decompose the salt, and the free iodide will thus be very likely to act as an irritant. I may also observe, that it is not well borne where there is any considerable gastric irritation, indicated by a foul tongue, dry skin, precordial pains after food, etc., attended with acid eructations, and especially where there is urine turbid with lithates or lithic acid; and yet we may have all these, as well as periosteal nodes, to contend with; and I am quite sure, that during the active forms of gout and rheumatism, the medicine is never well borne; yet it is often very useful in relieving pains which are still existing after all constitutional traces of specific disease have subsided. It is therefore necessary to relieve the dyspeptic symptoms by appropriate remedies, before using the iodide of potassa; or not to set down our failure to the inefficacy of the salt. The disagreement of the medicine is soon detected by the excessively nauseous, metallic taste in the mouth, before the gums are affected, or the catarrhal symptoms so severe as to oblige us to discontinue it; and when that taste distressingly prevails, the salt rarely produces any beneficial effect.

But I will even go further in asserting, that in some instances periosteal nodes have been the result of the very medicine we are giving for their cure.

I have met with cases of periosteal nodes, which have appeared during a course of iodide of potassium and sarsaparilla, taken for secondary skin eruptions, and which have subsided on substituting mercurial medicines for the iodide.

It will be found that the different preparations of iron with quinine, sometimes gentian and ammonia, sometimes nitric acid, and decoction of sarsaparilla, may be given with advantage; but the relief is very different in degree and kind from that produced by the iodide of potassa or by mercury in the cases to which they are respectively applicable. I have occasionally observed some benefit to accrue from the use of the phosphate of ammonia, where the iodide of potassa could not be persevered in. I must first refer to iron as a remedial agent. I have not lately used iron in any form as a remedy until satisfied that the patient was intolerant of iodide of potassa, or else as a tonic during such intervals as it has been found desirable to intermit the use of that salt; but amongst those who have applied to me as private patients, I have been able to collect facts relative to the effects of iron which had been previously recommended.

Of all remedies, next to the iodide of potassa, iron has certainly been generally the most serviceable; but the form in which it is exhibited does not appear to me at least to be of much consequence. A lady, near Dorking, consulted me for neuralgic pains on the right side of the face, from which she had suffered for six years. She had at different times consulted some of our most eminent physicians and surgeons, and derived some benefit from carbonate of iron, prescribed for her by Sir B. Brodie; but it never quite relieved her. The tic occurred in paroxysms in the evening; and on questioning her, I learned that she had also headache, pains in the crest of the ilium, and tibial nodes. She had the appearance of one who had been much stouter, but was emaciating and anæmic. Small feeble pulse; clean tongue, and had no sleep for pain. She took iodide of potassium, five grains; liquor potassæ, half a drachm; compound decoction of sarsaparilla, an ounce and a half; thrice a day. An opium pill at night.

Under this treatment she gradually lost all pain. The opium was soon discontinued, but she slept well, and the medicine was at length omitted, in consequence of the disagreeable metallic taste. Her medical attendant, Mr. Curtis, favored me with a favorable report of her since, and she is now taking quinine and iron under his direction.

The carbonate of iron was considered to have a kind of specific action in such neuralgic cases, and was prescribed in spoonfuls; but I think it a clumsy way of giving medicine; being nearly an insoluble powder, and any quantity of course may be given that will pass off by the bowels. The more soluble salts are certainly the most effective, and none more so, or more agreeable, than the vinum ferri as prepared at Apothecaries' Hall; but the sulphate or hydrochlorate, or the ammoniated tincture, will answer equally well. The chalybeate waters are even more certain in their effects than any of our medicinal potions, and this is a fact not so generally recognized as it should be. It matters not whether the water be natural or artificial. Small doses largely diluted are more readily absorbed and diffused than larger and more concentrated doses.

The anæmic appearance usually observed in periosteal disease would seem to point naturally to iron preparations, and though they do not seem directly to control the morbid action going on during the activity of nodal deposit, as both iodide of potassa and mercury, in their appropriate cases, are observed to do, yet their indirect influence is very decided, and when the acute symptoms are relieved, it is most desirable to alternate the iodide of potassa with iron preparations; and there is one form of iron which is especially applicable, viz. the iodide, which is best given in the form of sirup.

Quinine is an important agent in the treatment of this disease. Periosteal disease is rife in the aguish districts of Kent and Essex, and although the iodide of potassa will control the paroxysms, the relief must be followed up by such remedies as restore the constitution to a normal state, which the iodide will not do, and without which the relief can only be temporary.

The anasarcous swellings indicate an obstruction in the chylopoietic vessels, whether in the liver, spleen, or kidneys, and Bright's disease is no unfrequent attendant, evinced by albuminous urine. Without hoping to restore the kidney to its normal function, when that is evidently degenerated, much good accrued from the exhibition of quinine, either alone, or in combination with sulphate of iron, dissolved in dilute sulphuric acid.

Where a simple tonic is required, quinine is not the most efficacious, and is often observed rather to oppress than invigorate the digestive functions (I am acquainted with two persons in whom severe inflammation of cellular tissue is the result of a grain dose of quinine); but some of the simple bitters, with ammonia, are often found more useful. This holds good mostly in tipplers—I do not mean absolute drunkards, but those who are constantly drinking small quantities of wine, dilute spirits, or even beer, at all times and seasons, and in cases where constitutions have been debilitated by residence in the tropics, or by the exhausting passions. I have not been able to satisfy myself that there is any reason for preferring one bitter rather than another. I have prescribed gentian, quassia, cascarilla, cusparia, and simarouba, each for a stated time, in order to watch their comparative effects, and I am inclined to think that any preference is rather a matter of fashion than founded on any carefully and extensively watched clinical observation; but taking our Pharmacopœia preparations, I think I may safely say that the dose should never exceed half an ounce in an ounce and a half draught.

Concerning topical applications: I have already referred to the efficacy of issues and blisters, and in the severer forms of cephalalgia arising from the disease of the dura mater, I prefer them; but I may also recommend the application of spirit of wine, the most convenient mode of using which, is, to wet some lint with the spirit, and having applied it over the head or other painful part, to prevent evaporation by covering it over with oil-silk: it produces a copious sweat in the part, and with very great relief. I need hardly mention, that eau de Cologne, or any strong spirit most readily procurable, will answer the purpose. Old nodes may be painted with the tincture of iodine, or rubbed with the iodine ointment, but these are not convenient applications to the scalp, and the latter is objectionable where there is much tenderness.

There is only one more remedy which I must not omit to mention—that is, guaiacum. It is by no means universally applicable, but in some cases most decidedly useful, and especially where there is a cold, dry surface, and languid pulse, and where the iodide too readily produces catarrh. Lest I should confound such cases with the catarrh rheumatism affecting the head or other parts, I have been cautious to draw my inferences only from cases in which tibial or other easily recognized nodes are seen and felt.

Part xxv., *p.* 59.

Acute Periostitis.—Mr. Curling says: The chief difficulty in diagnosis lies in its great resemblance to acute rheumatism. In both there is high inflammatory fever, with swelling of the limb and great pain, increased by pressure; but the point of difference is here—that in periostitis little or no pain is caused by pressure, unless it be made over, or in the course of, the affected bone. The swelling is not limited to the larger joints, to the ankle or to the knee, but occupies a wider range, and is œdematous in character. The conclusion in favor of periostitis will be much strengthened if it be found that the attack of inflammation succeeded an injury. In the treatment, do not rely on local depletion, with calomel and opium; make an early and free incision down to the inflamed periosteum, not waiting even for evidence of matter, for the mischief is then done, the periosteum is already separated from the bone, and the bone will die.

Part xl., *p.* 95.

———•••———

PERITONITIS.

Opium in Peritonitis.—The pamphlet published by Mr. Bates, of Sudbury, some years ago, on the treatment of severe peritonitis by opium, made a strong impression on the minds of some medical men. He recommended opium both by the mouth and rectum; and insisted on a rigid adherence to the horizontal posture, till all pain had subsided. Mr. Bates's practice, however, may be considered as chiefly valuable in those severe cases where, either from ulceration or injury, perforation of the intestine has taken place, and which have been supposed to be almost invariably fatal. Some very striking cases, however, are related by Dr. W. Stokes in the second number of the "Dublin Journal of Medical and Chemical Science," which strongly confirm the opinions of Mr. Bates in cases where perforation is supposed to have taken place. Dr. Stokes truly remarks, that in many of these cases the patient sinks with awful rapidity, and gives no time to pursue the active treatment which is adopted in other cases. Mercury and purgatives would in such cases probably increase the evil, by *tearing asunder* recent adhesions, and thereby preventing nature closing the communications between the mucous and peritoneal cavities. One of Dr. Stokes's cases is related as follows:

"The well-known symptoms of perforation of the intestines had existed for two days; The exhibition of sixty drops, in the twenty-four hours, of the preparation called the *black drop* was followed by the most signal improvement. The pulse regained its fullness and softness, the extremities became warm, and the countenance had lost the hippocratic expression. The patient could bear pressure on the abdomen, which the day before was exquisitely painful. The same treatment was continued for twenty-four hours longer; and by the end of that time every symptom of abdominal inflammation had completely subsided. The belly felt natural, there was no tenderness, the pulse was good, and the patient declared himself well." At this period of the case, Dr. Stokes omitted the opium, and gave the mildest possible saline laxative, as there had been no stool for 48 hours. Four evacuations took place, followed by the immediate return of the symptoms of peritonitis, under which the patient rapidly sunk.

Dr. Watson remarks:

This example puts in a very strong light the *good* effects of *opium;* the *dangerous* effects of *purgatives;* and the *mode* in which recovery from these frightful accidents *may* sometimes be brought about.

Dr. Stokes gives another instance in which the patient *did* recover; after taking 105 grains of opium, besides what was administered in injections: and he alludes to a third case, in which the employment of opium was successful, when peritonitis had supervened upon the bursting of a hepatic abscess into the cavity of the abdomen.

Dr. Watson recommends applying the same principle of treatment, as an auxiliary, *in all cases of peritonitis.* The opium is not to supersede the bleeding, nor the mercury; it is not incompatible with either of those remedies; and it may be most advantageously adopted in conjunction with them both. *Part* v., *p.* 28.

Treatment of Peritonitis.—[The constipation which occurs in cases of peritonitis should never be treated by giving acrid purgatives. Dr. Corrigan observes:]

Relieve the serous inflammation, and permit the peristaltic action of the intestines to return, but do not force it; look upon the constipation as effect, not as cause.

Let the first object be, therefore, to look upon inflammation as the cause of the constipation in peritonitis, and to endeavor to remove it by the application of leeches, by blistering, and putting your patient under the influence of mercury; and recollect what I told you of the danger of a relapse from the use of stimulants of any kind.

Where accumulations occur in the colon, their removal may be advantageously obtained by the introduction once or twice of the long tube, as recommended by Dr. O'Beirne; but it is worse than useless to repeat this process after, and so attempt to force a discharge of the contents of the intestine.   *Part* xiv., *p.* 90.

Peritonitis.—Apply a layer of collodion over the whole surface of the abdomen. (M. Latour.)   *Part.* xxv., *p.* 325.

Acute Peritonitis after Abortion.— Chloroform.— Chloroform, when given in full doses, either by inhalation or swallowing, depresses and brings down the rate of the pulse from 90 or 80 to 70, 60, or less. This may be taken advantage of in some instances of disease, especially acute serous inflammations. Dr. Simpson relates a case of acute peritonitis after abortion: the pulse was weak and scarcely perceptible, ranging above 150, and there was little hope of the patient surviving. Chloroform was given to relieve the intense pain, when the pulse was found to sink down to 100, or less, and became stronger and steadier; and as long as the action of the chloroform continued, the pulse continued thus greatly lowered in rate and improved in power. The patient was kept for sixty consecutive hours under its influence, and the great abdominal tenderness and tympanitis were then almost entirely reduced, the patient being in a much more satisfactory state. The pulse never rose again to any very high rate, and she recovered nicely.   *Part* xl., *p.* 180.

———•♦•———

PERSPIRATION.

Pure Tannin, a remedy for Excessive Perspiration.— Dr. Charvet relates several cases in support of the anti-sudorific property which he attributes to tannin. He prescribed it in doses of from half a grain, to two grains, in the form of pill, in the evening, with or without opium, which neither checks nor favors its action. The cases occurred among consumptive patients who had arrived at the last stage of the disease.

They are additional examples of the activity with which tannin suppresses sweating, even when the disease from which it arises is beyond the resources of our art.   *Part.* iii., *p.* 53.

Night Perspiration of Phthisis. Dr. T. Thompson recommends four grains of oxide of zinc, and four grains of extract of hyoscyamus, made into two pills, every night for a time.   *Part.* xxix. *p.* 92.

Colliquative Sweating.— In the "Dublin Hospital Gazette" it is stated that tannin dissolved in the aromatic sulphuric acid, or dilute sulphuric acid, forms a good combinatiom in cases of colliquative sweating and chronic diarrhœa.   *Part.* xxxiv. *p.* 277.

Vide Art. "Phthisis Pulmonalis."

———•♦•———

PESSARIES.

New kind of Pessary.—The great advantage of a pessary of the kind described and recommended by Mr. Clay, would no doubt be, as he says, to support the womb, and, at the same time, would not so distend the vagina as to render the evil of prolapsion even greater than ever, the moment the instrument is withdrawn. It is described as follows:

It consists of a small shield of wood, ivory, etc., of a peculiar shape, secured to the vaginal entrance by bandages attached to a belt applied around the body. To the inner surface of the shield is fitted a strong coil of steel wire, plated over with gold or silver, the dimensions of the coil being such, that, when worn, the vaginal canal will not be in the least extended, but with every facility assume its original dimensions. At the end of the coil is a caoutchouc ring, a little larger in dimension than the coil on which the os uteri rests when applied; *when it is weighed with the uterine mass, it should be about the length of the vaginal canal in a healthy state.* I think a coil, varying from three and a half to four and a half inches, will be found sufficient. To prevent any folds of the vaginal coats from getting entangled in the coil, a thin slip of caoutchouc is proposed to stretch along the under and outer surface of the coil.

Advantages over the old Pessaries.—First, The elasticity of the coil allows of the free motion of the body in every possible direction, with perfect ease. Second, The vaginal canal not being obstructed, the catamenia can flow through the caoutchouc ring and along the coil without any hindrance. Third, The dimensions of the coil and ring being so moderate, no undue pressure can prevent discharges either from the bladder or rectum. Fourth, The laxity of the vaginal canal may be removed, and its original dimensions restored (*the measurements of the coil being not larger than the vaginal canal in a healthy condition*). Fifth, Local applications for improving the tone of the parts are facilitated by the opening in front of the shield through which injections can be thrown, and retained at pleasure, by introducing a small piece of sponge, or plug, into the opening; and the same plan might be a protective to females in heated or crowded rooms, for sudden appearances of the catamenia. *Part* iv., *p.* 119.

Medicated Pessaries.—Dr. Simpson has been in the habit of applying a variety of substances in the form of medicated pessaries, particularly zinc and lead ointment, as simple emollients; mercury and iodine as discutients (and particularly the iodide of lead); tannin, alum, and catechu, as astringents; opium, belladonna, etc., as anodynes. The pessaries were made of the size of walnuts, and could be easily introduced by the patients themselves—one or two in the twenty-four hours. By their use, for instance, we could keep the cervix uteri, when ulcerated and indurated, constantly imbedded in mercurial or iodine ointment for weeks, and sometimes with the most marked benefit and success. They fulfilled another indication in cases of irritation and inflammation of the mucous membrane of the cervix uteri and vagina. They kept the opposed diseased surfaces from coming in contact; and it was well known how important a matter this was in the pathology of mucous and cutaneous surfaces. They were composed of the medicine used, mixed up in the form of an ointment, and brought to a requisite degree of consistence with one or two drachms of yellow wax to the ounce of ointment. After being made up in the proper form, they were usually coated by the druggists with a firmer covering, by dipping them into an ointment made up with wax and resin, kept liquid by heat. About an ounce of the different ointments made four balls.

1. *Zinc Pessaries.*—℞ oxidi zinci, ℨj.; ceræ albæ, ℨj.; axungiæ, ℨvj.; misce, et divide in pessos quatuor.

2. *Lead Pessaries.*—℞ Acet. plumbi, ℨss.; ceræ albæ, ℨiss.; axungiæ, ℨvj.; misce.

3. *Mercurial Pessaries.*—℞ Unguent. hydrarg. fort., ʒij. ; ceræ flavæ, ʒij. ; axungiæ, ʒss. ; misce.

4. *Iodide of Lead Pessaries.*—℞ Iodidi plumbi, ʒj. ; ceræ flavæ, ʒv. ; ax ungiæ ʒvj. ; misce.

5. *Tannin Pessaries.*—℞ Tanninæ, ʒij. ; ceræ albæ, ʒv. ; axungiæ, ʒvj. misce.

6. *Alum and Catechu Pessaries.*—℞ Sulph. aluminis, ʒj. ; pulv. catechu, ʒj. ; ceræ flavæ, ʒj. ; axungiæ ʒvss. ; misce.

7. *Belladonna Pessaries.*—℞ Extr. belladonnæ, ʒij. ; ceræ flavæ, ʒiss. ; axungiæ, ʒv. ; misce. *Part xviii., p.* 302.

Caoutchouc Air-Bags.—One bag may be used either as a pessary in displacement of the uterus, as a plug in uterine hemorrhage, or as a dilator of the os uteri. On the same principle, M. Gariel treats strictures of the urethra, œsophagus, cervix uteri, etc. ; and similarly the nasal fossæ might be plugged in epistaxis. In all cases the bags are introduced collapsed, and, when introduced, are inflated either by a bag-insufflator or syringe.

Part xl., p. 240.

———•✦•———

PHLEBITIS.

Actual and Potential Cautery as Means of Preventing and Curing Phlebitis.—The cauteries employed by Mr. Bonnet are the *potassa cum calce,* the chloride of zinc, and the red-hot iron. The red-hot iron rapidly applied produces a very superficial eschar; the potassa cum calce acts much more deeply; the pain in regard to either is sharp, but speedily at an end, and the inflammation that succeeds is trifling. The chloride of zinc produces much deeper eschars than either the red-hot iron or the potash and lime. The author quotes a case of phlebitis following venesection, and four cases of severe constitutional disturbance following wounds received in dissection, which were treated by the hot-iron with immediate and complete success. As many as ten cauterizing irons were used at once in the case of phlebitis, the subcutaneous cellular tissue being found in a semigangrenous state. In the dissection wounds, the seat of the injury alone was deeply seared; the iron was elsewhere carried superficially along the course of the red lines. The author has applied the same method to the treatment of hemmorhoidal tumors and prolapsus ani. Of these diseases existing together, he gives four cases which were successfully treated— one, in part, by means of the potassa cum calce, the rest by the chloride of zinc. He has also found the caustic an effectual agent in treating varicocele. *Part viii., p.* 165.

Treatment of Phlebitis.—The principles of treatment, says Mr. Cooper, are to promote the secretions without lowering the strength, and to allay irritation. For these purposes give a combination of calomel, antimony, and opium, and a mixture containing liq. ammon. acet., tinct. of hyoscyamus, and camphor mixture. Keep the limb elevated, apply fomentations and poultices over the whole limb, and make punctures through the skin wherever it has become tense from effusion ; but do not apply leeches. When the local irritation has been thus subdued, give bark, mineral acids, porter and nutritious food, and continue them without fear so long as the natural secretions are duly performed. *Part xx., p.* 65.

PHLEGMASIA DOLENS.

Phlegmasia Dolens.—In the treatment of this affection, says Professor Simpson, which depends essentially on a toxæmic state of the blood, the first and most important indication of general treatment is, depuration of blood by exciting the various organs of elimination to increased activity, by their appropriate stimulants. An emetic, or a mercurial purgative combined with ipecacuanha or antimony, may be given at first, but not so as to produce debilitating effects. Perhaps small and repeated doses of alkaline salts, are, as a general rule, the safest and most efficient remedies to fulfill this indication. Tonics and stimulants are rather required than any antiphlogistic measures, and of these iron and quinine are the best. The best local treatment is, to wrap the limb up in cotton wool, and then incase the whole in oil silk, to prevent the escape of the insensible perspiration ; the limb should be slightly raised in bed. Toward the end of the case, a flannel bandage, neatly applied from the toes upward, will greatly favor resorption. *Part* xl., *p.* 198.

PHTHISIS PULMONALIS.

Employment of Sea Salt (*Chloride of Sodium*) *in Pulmonary Consumption.*—M. Latour relates three cases in the human subject, in which the administration of salt appears to have been followed by the happiest results. In one of the cases, the disease had gone so far that there was distinct cavernous rattle with pectoriloque, muco-purulent and purulent expectoration streaked with blood, great emaciation, hectic fever, etc., and yet the patient made a perfect recovery at the end of a few months, the sea salt having been given uninterruptedly for sixty days.

The aliment should consist almost exclusively of beef or mutton grilled or roasted, of good rich soups, or animal jellies. Every fine day, when the sun shines, and during its warmest period, the patient should take gentle exercise in the open air ; and his chamber should be well aired twice or thrice a day. Flannel is recommended to be worn next the skin.

Half a drachm to a drachm of the chloride of sodium is administered daily, either in a glass of beef-tea or in some pectoral infusion, or if this should excite cough, it may be given in divided doses made up into bread pills, drinking a little beef-tea afterward. It is best to commence with small doses. In general, some thirst is at first caused by the administration of the sea salt, and for this M. Latour directs a weak infusion of gentian flavored with orange-peel. *Part* i., *p.* 21.

Inhalation of Conium and Iodine.—Advised in the treatment of phthisis, by Sir. C. Scudamore:

℞ Iodinii puri, iodid. potassii, aa. gr. vj. ; aquæ destillat. ℥v. ʒvj. ; Alcoholis, ʒij. M. fiat mistura, in inhalationem adhibenda.

"I now always prefer to add the conium at the time of mixing the iodine solution with the water; and it should be a *saturated* tincture, prepared with the genuine dried leaves. In the commencement of the treatment, I advise very small proportions of the iodine mixture ; for example, only from half a drachm to a drachm for an inhaling of eight or ten minutes, to be repeated two or three times a day. Of the soothing tincture, I direct half a drachm—which I usually find sufficient; but it may be increased if the cough be very troublesome." *Part.* i., *p.* 30.

Prevention of Tubercles.—M. Coster recommends ferruginous bread, containing half an ounce of carbonate of iron, to the pound.

Part i., *p.* 32.

Lime Moxa.—Dr. Osborne of Dublin states that in a case of commencing softening of tubercles, and in another apparently of purulent infiltration after pneumonia the effect of lime moxa in putting a stop to the ulcerative process was most decided. *Part.* v., *p.* 129.

Phthisis induced by the inhalation of Gritty and Metallic particles.— Dr. Holland draws attention to an ingenious contrivance to prevent the inhalation of that large quantity of gritty and metallic particles which cause so much pulmonary disease among the grinders in Sheffield. Many years ago a magnetic apparatus was contrived which attracted the metallic particles before entering the nose and mouth ; but this was of no avail in attracting the non-metallic substances, and moreover the grinders would not be at the trouble to make use of it. Since that time another plan has been suggested and brought into practice, which seems likely to save the lives of thousands of these tradesmen not only in Sheffield, but also in all large towns where grinding or filing is carried on, especially among those mechanics who prepare the different kinds of machinery for cotton, flax and woollen manufactories. "A wooden funnel, from ten to twelve inches square, is placed a little above the surface of the revolving stone, on the side the furthest from the grinder, and this funnel terminates in a channel immediately under the surface of the floor ; *or we may consider the channel simply as the continuation of the funnel,* in order to avoid any confusion in the explanation. The channel varies in length, according to the situation of the grinder, in reference to the point where it is most convenient to get quit of the dust. If we suppose that eight or ten grinders work in the same room, each has his own funnel and channel, *and they all terminate in one common channel, the capacity of which is perhaps twice or three times as great as each of the subordinate or branch channels.* The point where they terminate is always close to an external wall. At this point, within the general channel, a fan is placed, somewhat in form like that used in winnowing corn, and to this is attached a strap which passes under and over a pulley, so that whatever puts the pulley in motion, causes the fan also to revolve. The pulley is placed in connection with the machinery which turns the stone, so that whenever the grinder adjusts his machinery to work, he necessarily sets the pulley and the fan in motion. The fan acting at this point, whatever may be the length of any of the subordinate channels, causes a strong current to flow through the mouth of each funnel, which carries along with it all the gritty and metallic particles evolved, leaving the room in which the operations are pursued free from any perceptible dust.—When the whole apparatus is perfect and in excellent condition, the atmosphere of the place is almost as healthy as that of a drawing-room. *Part.* viii., *p.* 32.

Vomiting, a cure for Phthisis.—It is stated that 176 patients under consumption, 47 in the incipient, and 129 in the advanced stage, admitted during a period of four years into the military hospital at Capua, were ultimately discharged perfectly cured, their treatment having consisted in the administration of a tablespoonful, night and morning, of the following mixture : Tartarized antimony, three grains ; sirup of cloves, an ounce ; decoction of marsh mallows, six ounces; mix. The dose was to be repeated until vomiting ensued. *Part.* viii., *p.* 80.

Miner's Phthisis.—[It is well known that, besides the diseases to which we are all liable, miner's are, from their occupation, peculiarly subject to affections of the respiratory and circulatory organs. From a very instructive paper by Dr. Makellar on a peculiar form of lung disease, which may be termed BLACK PHTHISIS, we extract as follows ; premising that it is caused by small particles of coal inhaled, accumulating in the lungs, and giving rise to irritation, and finally ulceration. It is thus closely analogous to the " grinder's disease," "mason's disease," etc., which commit such fearful havoc amongst certain of the operative classes, and have all a common origin.]

The rise and progress of the malady may be thus sketched : A robust young man, engaged as a miner, after being for a short time so occupied, becomes affected with cough, inky expectoration, rapidly decreasing pulse, and general exhaustion. In the course of a few years, he sinks under the disease ; and, on examination of the chest after death, the lungs are found excavated, and several of the cavities filled with a solid or fluid carbonaceous matter.

[Dr. M.'s remarks are upon the disease as it appears among the colliers in the Lothians, but we believe that they will apply to others generally. In the district above named, the ventilation of the mines is, on account of their immunity from explosive gas, very much neglected. Hence a large accumulation of carbonic acid and other pernicious gases. After working some time in these ill-ventilated places, the lungs inspire more of the impure air, in order to make up for the deficiency of oxygen ; and every now and then a deep and sustained inspiration is taken, during which the floating particles are drawn in. When the mine becomes so impure as to be actually unable to support a light, the men are necessitated to leave it, until by the gradual accumulation of purer air, it again becomes capable of supporting respiration and combustion.]

It is now known, that this disease originates in two principal causes, viz., First, The inhalation of lamp smoke with the carbonic acid gas generated in the pit, and that expired from the lungs ; Second, Carbon, and the carburetted gases which float in the heated air after the ever-recurring explosions of gunpowder, which the occurrence of trap-dykes renders necessary.

[It was long supposed that the change in color of the lungs was a form of melanosis, a systemic disease, properly so called. It has been lately proved, however, that the black color is not from any change in the system, but is produced by the infiltration of particles of coal, and chemical analysis confirms the fact. The minute bronchial ramifications are first filled, and the disorganization gradually extends until the whole lobe is infiltrated, softening going on in the meanwhile, from the irritation produced by the foreign substance.]

The first indication of cure, is change of work, and a lengthened sojourn in pure air. The following indications should also be attended to : To add oxygen artificially to the hyper-carbonized blood : To remove the overplus of carbon in the blood, either directly or indirectly. In regard to the former of these, I have never ventured on the direct application of oxygen to

the lungs, because these organs have generally been in an irritable condition, and have contented myself with recommending the free use of pure
atmospheric air, and bathing.   I have also endeavored to increase its
amount therapeutically, by the exhibition of oxydized preparations of iron,
which I have found most beneficial in this complaint; nor has their use
been followed by any bad effects, as frequently happens in other diseases of
the lungs. I endeavored to accomplish the second indication, chiefly by
alkalies, especially the carbonate of soda, but the results were by no means
satisfactory.   Small doses of calomel had no better effect.   It appeared,
however, to act beneficially when combined with jalap, especially in the
first stage of the disease.   The treatment is modified according to the different stages as follows: In the first, although the physician is seldom
consulted, I recommend, besides the already mentioned hygienic measures,
especially warm or cold baths, according as they are borne, and, under certain circumstances, an emetic, and a purge of calomel or jalap.   In the
second, the same treatment on a more extensive scale; and, in addition,
carbonate of soda, and other alkaline remedies, but more especially the
extract. aloes. aquos ; rhubarb, cort. rhamni frangulæ (especially extolled) ;
and in summer, the use, four times a week, of the artificial Carlsbad water,
in so far as the strength of the patient permits.   In the third, I have seen
the most astonishing effects from the continuous use of warm baths, and
the artificial Carlsbad water, and after the cure, and the continued use of
one of the above-named extracts, chosen according to the individual peculiarity of the case, I have frequently, after a time, had the felicity to see
before me a renovated man.   Preparations of iron are often here of the
most decided service.   Bleeding, and the so-called expectorants, on the
other hand, are never of the least use.   Derivative measures are only useful
in relieving the rheumatic pains of the chest.   The severe fits of coughing
sometimes also require palliative measures.   In the last stage nothing can
be done, but by mild restoratives, and a strict attention to diet, to endeavor
somewhat to prolong life, and strengthen digestion by bitters.   At this
period iron is especially useful, particularly the ferrum iodatum.   The
tinct. ferri pomat. and the tinct. nervin. bestusch., are also of signal
benefit, and prolong life for a considerable period.   The painful symptoms
at this period, often require numerous remedies, and the daily use of
opium or morphia.   Anasarca generally disappears speedily under digitalis,
squill and other diuretics, which act by producing smart diarrhœa.   When
structural change of the lungs occurs along with the melanosis, little
relief can be afforded.   All that can be done, is to alleviate some of the
more distressing sympathetic sufferings ; the dyspnœa, however, continues most obstinate, and slowly destroys the patient.   *Part* xii., *p.* 64.

Use of Naphtha in Phthisis.—Dr. Hastings ascribes the failure of those
medical men who have been less successful than himself in the treatment
of phthisis by naphtha, to one or all of the following causes.   First, From
a deleterious agent being employed for a medicinal one.   Second, From
its use in cases where it was contraindicated.   Third, From patients being
treated in unfavorable situations.

He proceeds to say, that cases are continually occurring in which oily,
milky, and coal-tar naphtha are administered, and most prejudicial results
ensue.   The preparation recommended by Dr. Hastings is the pyroacetic
spirit, which is obtained by the destructive distillation of an acetate gene-

rally of lead or lime, and in its natural form is scarcely distinguished from pyroxylic spirit.

The author's test was its colorless and transparent character, and its agreeable ethereal alcoholic odor; its increase of temperature consequent upon admixture with water ; its preservation of appearance on the addition of nitric acid ; and its taste being warm, without the least sensation of burning. Dr. Ure has recently suggested an easy method of effecting this object, which is founded on the following facts. If nitric acid of specific gravity 1.45 be added to pyroxylic spirit, the mixture assumes a red color, but no effervescence takes place. If the same acid be added to pyro-acetic spirit, there will be no change of color, but an effervescence will slowly be formed, accompanied by an elevation of temperature, and copious evolution of gas, resembling in appearance the action resulting from the mixture of alcohol with nitric acid, but with an acetic instead of an ethereal odor. Pyro-acetic spirit may also be generally distinguished from pyroxylic spirit, by its causing no appearance of milkiness on mixing with water, in the state in which it is met with in commerce.

Dr. Hocken states that "the most ready test is to be found in litmus paper, which is reddened by the non-medical, but is unaffected by the medicinal compound."

In stating the cases in which he recommends the use of naphtha, Dr. Hastings observes, that the less phthisis is complicated with other affections, the more suitable it is for this treatment, where the pulse is at the ordinary standard, or thereabouts, where the hectic is slight, laryngeal and peritoneal disease absent, the functions of the stomach and bowels not much impaired, the constitutional disturbance inconsiderable, and the physical signs denoting only a slight deposit of tubercles in one lung—the prognosis is favorable, and a speedy recovery may be anticipated. In many cases this mild character of the disease is never witnessed, however early they may be seen; at the same time, for want of close observance, this period frequently altogether escapes notice ; hence success often depends upon an early diagnosis of disease. If naphtha is employed in acute phthisis, where the cough is very harassing, with slight frothy expectoration, respirations thirty to forty per minute, pulse a hundred and twenty to a hundred and forty, hot skin, profuse night sweats, great thirst, appetite deficient, or altogether wanting, and the physical signs denoting an extensive crop of tubercles in both lungs, it will be found injurious rather than beneficial. If it be employed in chronic phthisis, coexisting with disease in other organs, its value is diminished, in proportion to the extent of the complications and their vitiating influence on the constitutional powers ; if it be continued in certain cases where improvement had followed its use, after the appearance of intercurrent pneumonia, bronchitis, or pleurisy, it would do great mischief. Many such cases give way to a short course of treatment with antimony, digitalis, etc., and then the pyro-acetic spirit may be again employed with the greatest advantage. Where hemoptysis is present, or where it has recently existed, naphtha is generally contraindicated. When complicated with dyspepsia, little or no benefit will accrue from its use until that affection is removed. The author has also found that the disease is not amenable to this plan of treatment when the patients are in crowded hospitals, or in other situations where the atmosphere is impure.

The dose in which the author appears generally to administer the naphtha

is from ten to twenty drops in a small quantity of water three times a
day.   *Part* xii., *p.* 70

Treatment of Incipient Phthisis.—[The following remarks were made
by Dr. Graves, in an obscure case of pulmonary disease, subsequent to an
attack of fever, and are applicable to numerous cases in general practice.
This fever soon subsided under ordinary treatment, but a troublesome and
increasing cough was left behind, which began to keep the patient awake
at night.   This raised suspicion, and an accurate stethoscopic examination
was made of the chest, when on the right side, below the clavicle, respiration was found feeble, and mixed with crepital and bronchial râles.
There was nothing to point out whether this was an unexpected deposition
of tubercles, or mere bronchitis, with effusion ; and therefore the safe side
was taken, and the patient treated as if the former were the case.]

I immediately ordered leeches to be applied under the clavicle, to be
repeated as the exigency of the case might require, and prescribed the
hydrocyanic acid in the form recommended by M. Magendie.   He recommends a drachm of the cyanuret of potash to be dissolved in an ounce of
distilled water.   This solution is stated by him to be equal in efficacy, and
capable of producing all the advantageous effects of hydrocyanic acid, at
the same time that it is less volatile, less liable to undergo change, and can
be always prescribed of the same strength.   He says that it possesses all
the beneficial properties of hydrocyanic acid, in relieving the irritative
cough of phthisis, or the excitement which accompanies gastric derangement.   Of this solution I ordered the patient to take one drop in half an
ounce of water every fourth hour, to be increased in the course of three or
four days to double the quantity.   On making an examination this morning, I find that his symptoms are improved ; there is less dullness on percussion, respiration is clearer, and the crepitus is diminished.   On the
whole, his condition authorizes us to entertain hopes of being able to bring
about a cure.   If phthisis be curable, or if tubercular deposition admit of
being resolved, it is only at the very commencement of the disease, and
before that state of constitution is established in which there is a tendency
to the formation of tubercular productions.   If we happen to be so fortunate as to detect phthisis at this early period, I think that it is possible for
us not only to palliate, but also to remove it.   By free and repeated leeching, the use of blisters, a mild diet, and the insertion of one or two setons
over the part dull on percussion, we shall often be able to remove any
threatening symptoms, and perhaps save the patient's life. *Part* xii., *p.* 71.

*Use of the Seeds of Phellandrium Aquaticum in Phthisis and Chronic
Bronchitis.—Recommended as a Palliative.*—M. Sandras has published
the results of a careful investigation into its merits, conducted during eight
years at the Beaujon.   He speaks of it in the highest terms of praise as a
palliative of the most distressing symptoms of phthisis ; and believes that
occasionally it even exerts a curative agency, and at all events, indefinitely
postpones the progress of cases which furnish all the symptoms of incipient
tubercle.   He is, however, fully aware how deceptive these symptoms often
are, and speaks with due caution on this point.   The important agency of
the seeds, however, in relieving suffering in undoubted and advanced cases
of the disease seems certain ; the days of the sufferer not only being considerably prolonged, but his path to the grave materially smoothened.
The good effects generally manifest themselves in from a week to a fort·

night, by a diminution of fever and diarrhœa, a return of appetite and sleep, less dyspnœa, and an easier cough, so that the patient often supposes himself nearly well. The strength is supported in this way for a considerable longer period than it otherwise would be; and when at last it finally gives way, the course of the disease then becomes very rapid. *Chronic bronchitis* is obviously and speedily modified advantageously by this medicine. It is especially indicated in that form which comes on in aged persons in cold damp weather, and persists until this changes; and in young lymphatic subjects, deficient in reactive power, it cuts short the tedious cough left by colds. M. Sandras has found it of no avail in emphysema and nervous asthma, except inasmuch as these were connected with chronic bronchitis. *Part* xix., *p.* 89.

Phthisis Pulmonalis.—Manganese has appeared to M. Hannon to be very useful. The sirup of the iodide seems to be the best form of administration in these cases, but the carbonate, phosphate, or sulphate may also be given. *Part* xx., *p.* 35.

Hemoptysis, as a Symptom of Phthisis.—The diagnostic value of hemoptysis, as a symptom of tubercle, is estimated very highly by Dr. Walshe. It appears that, with the exception of cancer of the lung, aortic aneurism, and disease of the heart, there are very few cases in which a material hemorrhage takes place from the lung independently of tubercles. Neither those cases of apparently simple chronic bronchitis, nor those of irregular menstruation, in which blood is voided from the lungs to any extent, appear to be exceptions to this proposition, although the tubercles may remain for a considerable period latent after the occurrence of the hemoptysis. *Part* xx., *p.* 79.

Intercostal Neuralgia as a Sign of Phthisis—This symptom is almost constant in phthisis pulmonalis. Among fifteen cases under M. Beau's observation at the time of writing, it was not absent in more than one; and only one of these cases presented the symptom of *spontaneous* pain. The author, therefore, thinks it will prove a useful diagnostic mark in cases where the physical signs of phthisis are marked by bronchitis. The predominance of the pain in the anterior part of the spaces, where the alteration of the nerves is least considerable, is ascribed by M. Beau to the circumstance that when a nerve is diseased in any part of its course, the morbid sensibility is always referred to its peripheric extremity.

Another form of the intercostal neuralgia of phthisical patients is the pain between the shoulders which has been so frequently described as characteristic of phthisis. *Part* xx., *p.* 79.

Treatment of Phthisis.—According to Prof. Bennett, faulty nutrition is the first element in the production of the disease; and this faultiness consists in an inability of transforming the carbonaceous constituents of vegetable food into fat, or of acting upon the fatty matters introduced into the system so as to render them easily assimilable. The first indication of treatment, then, is to cause a large amount of fatty matter to be assimilated, by giving food rich in fat. In most cases, however, the powers of the stomach and alimentary canal are much enfeebled, and unable to separate this fat from the food. It therefore becomes necessary to give the animal oils themselves, which will readily enter the system, and become assimilated: and this is the rationale of the good effects of cod-liver oil, which can be digested when no other kind of animal food can be taken in sufficient quantity to furnish the requisite amount of fat. The ordinary dose of cod-liver oil should be a tablespoonful thrice a day, but it may be advantageously increased to four, five, or even six. The kind of oil is of no importance except as regards the palate.   *Part* xxi., *p.* 127.

Use of Tannin.—Dr. Alison, of London, would give tannic acid in any stage of this disease, but especially in the third, when there are cavities. The dose may be one, two, or three grains, twice or thrice a day, dissolved in water or any simple vehicle, flavored with sirup, which will cover the taste. If there is much sweating, add a little dilute nitric acid. Tannin may be given at the same time as iron, cod-liver oil, or any such means.
Part xxi., *p.* 326.

Phthisis Pulmonalis.—Do not let the patient breathe an atmosphere warmed by stove-heat, even although equable in its temperature; it is stated by Dr. J. Hutchinson, to be extremely prejudicial. If the patient cannot rest at night for coughing, give gr. iv. of the ext. of hemlock, with gr. ss. of ipecac., and one-eighth gr. of muriate of morphia, at bed-time. Immediately on the first suspicion of pulmonary consumption, give the cod-liver oil, commencing with ʒj. for a dose, three times a day, and seldom exceeding ʒiv. Counter-irritation is of essential importance; employ a solution of ʒj. of iodine and iodide of potass. to ʒij. of spirits of wine. Use it first on one side and then on the other, even if one lung only is affected. By these measures the cough is allayed, the weight is increased, rest is procured, and counter-irritation is set up. Collateral symptoms must be met as they arise; if hectic fever or hemoptysis appear, we must suspend the oil.   *Part* xxiii., *p.* 105.

Use of Cod Liver Oil.—Thinking it owing to its non-absorption, that the oil sometimes appeared to lose its efficacy, M. Loze, a naval surgeon, combined it with a mucilage containing pancreatic juice, which thus forms an artificial chyle. He states it to be thus completely and readily absorbed, and in phthisis its effect more directly obtained.   *Part* xxiii., *p.* 299.

Diagnosis of Phthisis.—In speaking of the diagnosis of phthisis, Dr. Walshe lays down the following highly practical and useful propositions:
" (*a.*) A young adult who has an obstinate cough, which commenced without coryza, and without any obvious cause, a cough at first dry, and subsequently attended for a time with watery or mucilaginous looking expectoration, and who has wandering pains about the chest, and loses flesh, even slightly, is, in all probability, phthisical. (*b.*) If there be hemoptysis, to the amount of a drachm even, the diagnosis becomes, if the patient be a male, and positively free from aneurism or mitral disease, almost positive. (*c.*) If, in addition, there be slight dullness under percussion at one apex, with jerking, or divided and harsh respiration, while the resonance of the sternal notch is natural, the diagnosis of the first stage of phthisis becomes next to absolutely certain. (*d.*) But not absolutely certain; for I have known every one of the conditions in *a*, *b*, and *c*, exist (except hemoptysis, the deficiency of which was purely accidental) when one apex was infiltrated with encephaloid cancer, and no cancer had been discovered elsewhere to suggest to the physician its presence in the lung. (*e.*) If there be cough such as described, and permanent weakness and hoarseness of the voice, the chances are very strong (provided he be non-syphilitic) that the patient is phthisical. (*f.*) If decidedly harsh respiration exists at the left apex, or at the right apex behind: if the rhythm of the act be what I have called

cogged-wheel, and there be dullness, so slight, even, as to require the dynamic test for its discovery, there can be little doubt of the existence of phthisis. (*g.*) If, with the same combination of circumstances, deep inspiration evokes a few clicks of dry crackling rhonchus, the diagnosis of phthisis, as far as I have observed, is absolutely certain. (*h.*) If these clicks, on subsequent examination, grow more liquid, the transition from the first to the second stage may be positively announced. (*i.*) If there be slight flattening under one clavicle, with deficiency of expansion movement, harsh respiration, and slight dullness under percussion, without the local or general symptoms of phthisis, the first stage of tuberculization cannot be diagnosed with any surety, unless there be incipient signs at the left apex also; the conditions in question, limited to one side, might depend on chronic pneumonia or on thick induration matter in the pleura (*k:*) The existence of limited though marked dullness under one clavicle, with bronchial respiration and pectoriloquy, so powerful as to be painful to the ear, the other apex giving natural results, will not justify the diagnosis of phthisis. I have known this combination when the apex of the lung was of model health, and a fibrous mass, the size of a walnut, lay between the two laminæ of the pleura. I would even go further, and say, that the combination in question is rather hostile than otherwise to the admission of phthisis, as, had tuberculous excavation formed at one side, the other lung would, in infinite probability, have been affected in an earlier stage. (*l.*) Pneumonia limited to the supra and infra-clavicular region on one side, and not extending backward, is commonly, but not always tuberculous. (*m.*) Subcrepitant rhonchus, limited to one base posteriorly, is not, as has been said, peculiar to tubercle; it may exist in emphysema, and in mitral disease. (*n.*) Chronic peritonitis, in a person aged more than fifteen years, provided cancer can be excluded, involves as a necessity, the existence of tubercles in the lungs. To this law of Louis it is necessary to add the qualification, provided Bright's disease be also absent. (*o.*) Pleurisy with effusion, which runs a chronic course in spite of ordinary treatment, is, in the majority of cases, tuberculous or cancerous: the character of the symptoms, previously to the pleurisy, will generally decide between the two. (*p.*) Double pleurisy, with effusion, is not, as has been said, significant of tubercle; for it may depend on Bright's disease. If the latter disease can be excluded, carcinoma and pyohæmia remain as other possible causes. (*q.*) If a young adult, free from secondary syphilis and spermatorrhœa, and not dissolute in his habits, speedily lose flesh without clear cause, he is, in all probability, phthisical, even though no subjective chest-symptoms exist. (*s.*) But he is not by any means certainly so, for he may have latent cancer in some important organs, or he may have chronic pneumonia. (*t.*) Nay, more, he may steadily lose weight, have dry cough, occasional diarrhœa, and night sweats, and present dullness under percussion, and bronchial respiration under both clavicles, and yet be non-phthisical. I have known all this occur in cases, both when the lungs were infiltrated superiorly with primary encephaloid cancer, and when they contained secondary nodules of the same kind. (*u.*) Failure of weight becomes less valuable as a sign of phthisis, the longer the thirtieth year has been passed. (*v.*) The discovery of cardiac disease with marked symptoms, deposes against, but does not exclude the existence of active tuberculization. (*w.*) The existence of cancer in any organ is unfavorable to the presence of tuberculous disease, but tubercle and cancer *may* coexist, even in the same lung." *Part* xxiv. *p.,* 68.

Expectoration as a Means of Diagnosis in Diseases of the Chest.—If a person with some severe chest complaint coughs frequently, and expectorates only frothy, salivary-looking fluid, says Dr. Theophilus Thompson, we suspect pleurisy; if a glairy fluid like the white of egg, we suspect bronchitis; if it has a rusty tinge, and resembles gum water colored with blood, we are likely to find pneumonia. If there is a sudden gush of pus in considerable quantity, we expect to find that matter accumulated in the cavity of the pleura has found its way into the bronchial tubes. In consumption the expectoration assumes four characters : 1st, salivary or frothy; 2d, mucous; 3d, flocculent; 4th, purulent or porraceous. The first may proceed from irritation or slight tubercular deposit. The 2d may proceed from a more confirmed affection of the bronchial tubes. The 3d is peculiarly characteristic of secretion from a vomica modified by the absorption of its thinner constituents; and the 4th is indicative of phthisis far advanced, and (if mixed with froth) usually involving both lungs. The black matter often expectorated is not carbon, as commonly supposed; it is rather a pigment known to be formed under slight or not severe forms of bronchial inflammation. On a little heat being applied to this expectoration, and the microscope used, crystals of apparently triple phosphate may be seen, the proportion of the salts being in an inverse ratio to the degree of inflammation present. The 3d form of expectoration mentioned above, viz., the flocculent, is stated to be almost a pathognomonic symptom of phthisis. When spat into water it assumes the form of globular masses, like little balls of wool or cotton. Some of these masses have subsided, some are suspended at different depths, others float on the surface, sustained by bubbles of air, entangled in the surrounding mucus. If the process of contraction is going on in a vomica, a diminished quantity of expectoration is a favorable symptom. This is promoted by the use of appropriate regimen, the administration of cod-liver oil, and by the inhalation of turpentine. When the bronchial tubes contribute much to the supply, the skin being moist and the appetite defective, naphtha may sometimes be useful, but generally speaking, tannic acid will probably be found a more appropriate remedy. *Part* xxiv., *p.* 78.

Cod-Liver Oil.—Combine liq. potassæ with the cod-liver oil, especially in the early stage of phthisis. Where cod-liver oil cannot be administered internally, says Dr. T. Thompson, it may be rubbed into the chest, night and morning, combined with a little oil of lavender. If diarrhœa be produced, one ounce and a half of cod-liver oil, four drops of creasote, two drachms of compound tragacanth powder, and four and a half drachms of aniseed water, form a suitable mixture, of which an ounce may be taken thrice daily. If vomiting is produced, the addition of creasote often makes the stomach more tolerant of the remedy. The taste of the oil may be covered by eating dried orange peel, or by introducing a little dinner salt into the mouth before or after taking the oil. *Part* xxiv., *p.* 80.

Hepatic Congestion attending Cases of Incipient Phthisis.—Dr. T. Thompson gives a combination of chalybeates and saline aperients. The natural springs may be imitated by administering two grains of sulphate of iron, a drachm of sulphate of soda, a scruple of carbonate of soda, and ten grains of dinner salt, in half a pint or a pint of warm water, every morning. Use at the same time exercise in the open air, the shower-bath and friction of the skin. *Part* xxv., *p.* 104.

Treatment of Cough in Phthisis.—Perhaps there is no symptom of which consumptive patients complain so urgently as of cough, and there is scarcely any which so often baffles our efforts for its relief. Dr. T. Thompson says: If any degree of bronchial inflammation be present, small doses of antimony are indicated, and in some instances the application of a few leeches over the windpipe affords much relief. In allaying cough in irritable subjects, much advantage is often derived from the administration of four minim doses of tincture of aconite in spermaceti mixture; and counter-irritation may often be resorted to with advantage. When the urgency of the cough has more relation to the character of the expectoration than to nervous irritability, lemon-juice has sometimes seemed to me to be a useful remedy. In other similar cases the solution of potash does good, especially in combination with squill; although this latter remedy, in cases complicated with any degree of bronchial inflammation, would probably aggravate the symptoms.

Anodynes, such as hemlock, henbane, Indian hemp, are occasionally useful, and there can be no doubt of the value of hydrocyanic acid. A draught containing an eighth of a grain of cyanide of potassium, an ounce of aniseed water, and some sirup of lemons, is perhaps more trustworthy than prussic acid in the usual form of administration. In a great number of instances, however, we are obliged to place our chief reliance on opium, or on some of the salts of morphia. An agreeable linctus may be composed of an ounce of conserve of roses, half an ounce of lemon-juice, half an ounce of sirup of poppies; or a drachm of tincture of opium and a drachm of diluted sulphuric acid may be mixed with an ounce and a half of treacle or honey, and a teaspoonful given occasionally.

You have had an opportunity of observing the relief often derived by inhalation: an ounce and a half of the strobiles of hop in a pint of hot water sometimes proves very soothing. Some of our patients have derived still greater advantage from inhaling two grains of extract of opium, by means of the apparatus introduced by Dr. Snow. On the whole, however, no remedy has acted so promptly and satisfactorily in allaying cough, as the inhalation of fifteen or twenty minims of chloroform.

Part xxv., *p.* 106.

Lungs, Affections of—Iodide of Potassium.—Mr. Molloy says that when the period of acute inflammation has subsided in broncho-pneumonia, pneumo-bronchitis, chronic bronchitis, pituitous catarrh, and in dry asthma, iodide of potassium is an exceedingly valuable remedy, although the theory of its beneficial influence is somewhat obscure. *Part* xxv., *p.* 108.

Urate of Ammonia Ointment in Phthisis.—*Vide* Art. " Ammonia."

Tannate of Quinine in the Night-Sweats of Phthisis.—M. Delioux has administered tannate of quinine with the effect of arresting night-sweats in cases of pulmonary consumption. He says that, though it is sometimes inferior to pure tannin, it is superior to disulphate of quinine; and that it combines the action of a tonic and antiperiodic. He gives it in powder, the quantity taken daily being from half a *gramme* to a *gramme* (seven and a half to fifteen grains), in three or four doses, taken at intervals during the afternoon or evening, so that the last may be administered three or four hours before sleep. *Part* xxviii., *p.* 90.

Creasote Inhalation.—To relieve the cough, Dr. Inman, of Liverpool, places from four to ten drops of creasote in the bottom of an old teapot and then pours a small quantity of boiling water over it. The vapor must be inhaled through the spout, which must be protected by being covered with a little flannel. *Part* xxviii., *p.* 92.

Appearance of the Gums in Consumption.—Dr. Thompson remarks : "Considerable attention to this inquiry has impressed me with a conviction of the frequent existence in consumptive subjects, of a mark at the reflected edge of the gums, usually deeper in color than the adjoining surface, and producing a festooned appearance ; this mark is in some persons a mere streak ; in others, a margin, sometimes more than a line in breadth. In the most decided cases, this margin is of a vermilion tint, inclining to lake."

[This streak on the gums, Dr. Thompson states, is often among the earliest signs of pulmonary consumption. In reference to the value of this sign as an aid to diagnosis, Dr. T. observes:

" When in either sex it coincides with a pulse not materially altered in frequency by change from the sitting to the standing posture, the presence of phthisis may, with high probability be assumed, even before having recourse to auscultation."

Cocoa-Nut Oil as a Substitute for Cod-Liver Oil.—Dr. Thompson says: "Among the patients to whom cocoa-nut oil was given, there were some instances of arrested phthisis, as decided as any I have been accustomed to attribute to the use of cod-liver oil, over which it possesses advantages in reference to economy and palatableness; and it is interesting to remark that its efficacy was experienced by some who had previously taken cod oil uselessly, and by others who had discontinued it on account of nausea."

Treatment of the Diarrhœa of Phthisis.—In the diarrhœa of phthisis, Dr. Thompson employs trisnitrate of bismuth in doses of five grains, combined with three grains of gum arabic and two of magnesia, every four or six hours.

Night Perspirations of.—Give four grains of oxide of zinc, and four grains of extract of hyoscyamus, made into two pills, every night for a time. *Part* xxix., *p.* 92.

Palliative Treatment of Phthisis.—Profuse expectoration of.—To check this give creasote, pyro-acetic spirit, infusion of pitch, or balsam of tolu ; but by far the best remedy, says Dr. T. Thompson, is petroleum or Barbadoes tar, which often moderates the cough and expectoration remarkably.

Diarrhœa of.—Give the trisnitrate of bismuth, combined with gum and magnesia, or with Dover's powder.

Cough of.—Mix one part of chloroform with three parts of spirits of wine, and let the patient inhale when necessary, but with caution, and under medical direction. The inhalation of camphorated spirit is often sufficient, or even the vapor of hot water, or infusion of hops. Sometimes frequent deglutition, as the swallowing of a little oil, will relieve the cough. Sometimes four minims of tincture of aconite is a good palliative.

Night Sweats of.—Give gallic or acetic acid. Dip the night dress in sea-water, or salt and water, and dry it before using. But the best remedy is four grains of oxide of zinc at bed-time, combined with a little henbane or hemlock. *Part* xxx., *p.* 45.

Night Sweats in Phthisis.—Mr. Hutchinson, of the City Hospital for

Chest Diseases, shows that night sweats in this disease may be checked with impunity.

Under the usual treatment of phthisis (full diet, cod-liver oil, and tonics), the tendency to night perspiration often ceases spontaneously. If it becomes desirable to expedite the process, it may be done by the sesquichloride of iron, the mineral acids, or, best of all, by the gallic acid. The following is the prescription for a night-draught containing the latter:

R Acidi gallici, gr. vij.; morph. acet., gr. ¼; alcohol q. s. (a few drops); syr. tolutan., ʒss.; aquæ, ʒj.

The night-pill, as we find it in the Pharmacopœia of the Brompton Hospital for Consumption is:

R Acid. gallic., gr. v.; morph. hydrochl., g. ¼; mist. acac. q. s. Ft. pil. ij.

It is also of advantage to adopt an astringent regimen as far as convenient. The patient should be directed to sleep on a mattress, alone, and not heavily clothed; he should wear no flannel in bed; as dry a diet should be taken as conveniently can be borne, and fluid should be especially avoided in the latter half of the day, none whatever being allowed later than several hours before bed-time. *Part* xxx., *p.* 49.

Remedies in Phthisis.—[In a visit to the Brompton Hospital, the writer notices some of the remedies which are there used. He says:]

Among a few of the medical novelties we noticed, and which are found useful at Brompton, are divers forms of inhalations: one an inhalation of hydrocyanic acid vapors, of course in small quantities; inhalations of chlorine and inhalations of the chemical substance chloroformyl, inhalations also found very useful of conium and creasote.

A mixture of tannin, nitric acid, and lupulin is very valuable in the *night sweats* of the worst cases; the oxide of zinc also is found to answer wonderfully in some cases which will even resist acids and tannin; as practical facts not generally known, these valuable results cannot be too generally made public.

A mixture of decoct. hematoxyli and aqua calcis, not very chemical but very valuable, is used in *diarrhœa.* A solution of iodine as a caustic, now general in hospitals, is also found most useful for painting the chest; it is simply one part each of iodine and the iodide of potassium and two of rectified spirit. Dr. Quain also finds a solution of nitrate of silver to act almost "like a charm," when applied in some cases with a probang to the top of the larynx and to the vocal chords.

    *   *   *   *   *   *   *   *

Treatment of Irritable Stomach in Phthisis.—Give hydrocyanic acid and trisnitrate of bismuth, as in the following formula: Hydrocyanic acid three minims; trisnitrate of bismuth ten grains. Make this into a draught with mucilage and green mint tea, and give it three times a day. *Part* xxxi., *p.* 84.

Tubercular Infiltration.—According to Dr. C.R. Hall, greyness indicates that the exudation is chronic; yellowness, that it is acute; jelly-like consistence, that it is recent. The grey infiltration takes place while there is yet a fit state of blood to pour out contracted plasma; the yellow points to a deteriorated condition of the blood when the disease has injured the constitution; the jelly is a still later exudation, and takes place toward the close of life, when the blood is very poor and unable to furnish a coagulated lymph. *Part* xxxii., *p.* 70.

Dyspepsia preceding and attending Phthisis.—Mr. Hutchinson, surgeon to Metropolitan Free Hospital, says: The severity of the tubercular dyscrasia, may be measured by the facility with which fats, oils, sugar, etc., are relished and digested. If a patient has acquired a liking for cod-liver-oil and other kinds of fat, the disease is in abeyance; and the most ominous symptom of all is when the patient quickly loses all relish for such things. In all cases accustom the patient to oils and other fats; if the stomach will not bear them, give tonics, with an alkali or mercury in small doses and with great caution, until the stomach is improved; then give freely hydrocarbons, such as pork chops, bacon, butter, cream, sugar, dried fruits, alcohol in various combinations, etc. *Part* xxxii., *p.* 94.

Phthisis.—*Vide* Selections from Favorite Prescriptions, Art. "Medicines."

Phthisis.—Dr. Addison believes it to be nothing more than the acute stage of strumous pneumonia. Mere tubercles may lie dormant for years, if inflammation of an active kind be not set up. *Part* xxxiii., *p.* 96.

Phthisis.—Dr. Bullar states that we may often very materially soothe the passage to the grave by the cautious administration of small doses of opium. If the patient be anxious, restless, tossing about, and breathing very bad, etc., by giving a few drops of the liquor opii sedativus every ten minutes, the patient will become calm, tranquil, and will die quietly.
Part xxxiv., *p.* 272.

Tuberculosis.—The proximate cause of the tubercular diathesis, according to Dr. J. F. Churchill, is the decrease in the system of the phosphorus which it contains in an oxygenizable state. Therefore give some preparation of phosphorus in the lowest possible degree of oxidation, and, at the same time, one which may be directly assimilated: such a remedy is the hypophosphite of soda, or lime, which should be given in doses of from ten grains to a drachm to adults in the twenty-four hours. The general symptoms will rapidly disappear. *Part* xxxvi., *p.* 55.

Chronic Phthisis.—Dr. E. Smith, of Brompton Hospital for Consumption, says: There are various conditions of the throat met with in phthisis. In the earlier stages the patient complains of dryness of the throat and cough, and, on examination, the throat is found smooth and shining, and the parts attenuated. It is a state of lessened tonicity without inflammatory action. A useful means of treatment here is the application of a mixture of equal parts of chloroform and olive oil, by means of a large brush; the patient should also frequently swallow about a tablespoonful of a strong solution of suet in milk; great relief is obtained from the application of a strong solution of nitrate of silver to the fauces by means of a large brush. When the case is more advanced, an inflammatory state appears, with distended vessels and enlarged mucous follicles, chiefly upon the pharynx, but also on the uvula. This state, and also where there is ulceration and fibrinous exudation, is best treated by the nitrate of silver. When the inflammation runs high and extends down the larynx, the application of nitrate of silver often causes alarming symptoms of choking; the best topical application is then equal parts of oil and liquor potassæ well laid on with a large brush. *Part* xxxvii., *p.* 68.

Use of Ergot of Rye.—A case is related by Dr. B. P. Staats, of Albany,

New York, in which the expectoration, the diarrhœa, and other symptoms of relaxed fibre of atonic sympathetic nervine system, seemed to be considerably relieved by the administration of small doses of ergot of rye. This was continued with small doses of ipecacuanha and morphia.

Part xxxix., *p.* 93.

Carbonate of Lead.—M. Beau observes, that it is extremely rare that a case of phthisis is found amongst workers in lead, and accordingly recommends a trial of this mineral in cases of threatened phthisis. He administers from two to sixteen grains of carbonate each day in pill, suspending the use of it as soon as the patient appears to be sufficiently impregnated. The patient must be supported by nourishing food, wine, tonics, and causing him to observe all the rules of a rational hygiene.

Part xl., *p.* 55.

Ozonized Oil.—It is found, says Dr. T. Thompson, that the administration of *ozonized oils* has a remarkable tendency to reduce the frequency of the pulse. It was administered to fourteen patients. In two no such effect was observed ; but in the larger proportion of the remainder the effect was very considerable, in some cases to the amount of twenty beats. Oils may be ozonized by exposure for a considerable time to the direct rays of the sun, after previous saturation with oxygen gas.

Part xl., *p.* 294.

PHIMOSIS.

Treatment.—Mr. Key considers it unadvisable to cut away a portion of prepuce in a state of active phagedæna, or even when ulceration has stopped and has left the surface covered with a white slough.

[In many cases] the excessive action seems to have nothing of a specific nature : it appears to be a common attack of inflammation, ending in gangrene, the poisoned sore acting merely as an exciting cause; for as soon as the slough is cast away, the sore puts on a healthy appearance, and heals quickly under the application of astringent dressings.

When the inflamed part is under the influence of the specific poison, the operation of dividing the prepuce, instead of staying it, as it does in the case of simple gangrene, seems for a time to increase it, by adding to the inflammation. Exposure of the sore, however, is indispensable for the preservation of the glans, and should be performed as soon as the unhealthy nature of the sore is ascertained. This can be known by observing the nature of the discharge, which changes from the common secretion of chancre to a dirty reddish or brown fluid, mixed with fine shreds of white slough. The nature of the secretion may of itself determine the propriety of dividing the prepuce; but more especially will it be required, if there be also much inflammation proceeding beneath the skin. The best dressing for sores of this phagedænic character are the balsams, or turpentine, with the addition of opium if severe pain or extreme irritability demand it. When they are disposed to bleed, warm olive-oil, mixed with an equal part of turpentine, checks the hemorrhagic tendency, without increasing the inflammation or irritation of the part. This application is most efficient when the specific action does not predominate, and agrees best with a sore in which the action approaches to the black slough. When the phagedænic action is maintained by a high degree of local and general **irrita-** bility, equal parts of Peruvian balsam and the sedative solution of opium form a most effective application. When the part can bear it, lint steeped in equal parts of port-wine and tincture of opium will sometimes check the ulceration, and induce a healthy surface.

The operation for phimosis presents but little choice: the mode of ex- posing the glans must be regulated by the state of the prepuce, and by the situation of the sore that is required to be exposed.

The main point in practising is to extend far enough the division of the inner layer of skin ; and, when circumcision is first performed, advantages will be obtained by turning back the angles of the divided inner layer, and uniting them by means of very fine sutures to the edge of the outer layer of skin. This proceeding shortens the process of cicatrization, and lessens the deformity. 　　　　　　　 . 　　　　　　　 *Part* ii., *p.* 100.

Aphorisms of Practical Surgery.—It is not prudent to divide the fræ- num for phimosis during the existence of a gonorrhœal discharge, as the wound is then apt to degenerate into a troublesome ulcer. (Dupytren.)
Part iii., *p.* 116.

Belladonna.—In cases of phimosis and paraphimosis, it has been suggested to use an application of belladonna to the part, before resorting to the knife. An ointment, composed of thirty parts of cerate and twelve parts of extract of belladonna, should be rubbed hourly on the prepuce in cases of phimosis, and on the glands in cases of paraphimosis. If great inflammation exists, a little opium may be added, and less belladonna.
Part vii., *p.* 215.

Operation for Phimosis.—M. Ricord's plan. The penis is allowed to remain in its natural position, and no traction is used. A circular mark is made with ink upon the prepuce, about two lines anterior to the base of the glans, and parallel to the corona : a long and strong needle, its point covered with a wax bead, is then introduced between the glans and prepuce, and made to pierce the whole thickness of the latter, on the mesial line, and a little in front of the circular mark. The mucous mem- brane and skin of the prepuce are thus fixed, and the needle is allowed to remain. Behind it, and in a longitudinal direction, a fenestrated forceps, with notched edges, is then firmly applied. The fenestræ of the instru- ment correspond to the circular mark and the glans : at this stage of the operation the latter is to be pushed backward. The next step is to pass sutures, five or six in number, through the fenestræ ; and, when all the threads are applied, the prepuce is shaved off with a bistoury made to glide between the needle and forceps. The latter is then withdrawn care- fully, so as not to disturb the ligatures. The assistant should be desired to press the forceps very tightly when the prepuce is being shaved off : if this be neglected, the prepuce will yield, and the sutures will be cut. When the forceps is removed, the arteries which are noticed to bleed should be tied or subjected to torsion ; the threads which pass above and below the glans are then divided in their centre, and the respective ends of each half resulting from this section are tied, to bring the mucous mem- brane in contact with the skin. Of course there will be twice as many sutures as there were threads passed. 　　　　 / 　　 •

Treatment.—We should, after this operation, enforce rest, low diet, as- persions of cold water, and camphorated pills ; union by first intention rarely takes place completely. The submucous cellular tissue will generally be found infiltrated with serosity on the next day, but it is gradually re-absorbed. The sutures ought to be removed on the fourth day; they might, if left longer, lacerate the tissues. The parts are usually healed up by the tenth or fifteenth day, excepting in those cases where the union by first intention takes place as early as the fourth or fifth. *Part* xvii., *p.* 187.

Operation of Phimosis.—Mr. Colles' plan. I seize the edge of the prepuce, at its fold forming the narrow band, in the left hand, and holding the scalpel in the right, and at right angles with the penis, I remove a circular portion of skin about a quarter of an inch wide. The outer fold of skin being loose, is then drawn back on the penis, leaving the glans covered by the inner and tighter fold. I then divide this layer about half way back, more or less, slitting it up exactly in the centre, by passing a sharp-pointed bistoury under it. We have now the outer fold of skin loose, with a large circular orifice; the inner, or more contracted portion, presenting also an orifice, but larger by double the perpendicular. incision, which forms two angular flaps. I then turn these flaps outward, and by a suture attach each angle to the edge of the external skin, at about a quarter of its circumference from the frænum; a slight suture at the frænum completes the operation. I then draw all forward so as to cover the glans. In two or three days I remove the sutures, and generally find the wound healed, leaving a covering for the glans differing in no respect from the natural and perfect prepuce. *Part* xix., *p.* 173.

——•••——

PILLS.

Pilula Hydrg. Protoxydi.—*Vide* Art. "Antimony."

New mode of making a Ferruginated Pill of Mercury.—In Dr. Collier's second edition of the "London Pharmacopœia," he gives the outline of a formula for preparing blue pill with sesqui-oxide of iron. It is as follows:

℞ Ferri sesqui-oxydi, ʒj.; hydrargyri, ʒij.; confect. rosæ Gallicæ, ʒiij. Contere donec globuli non amplius conspiciantur.

It is made in five minutes; common blue pill demands a week. The globules are not visible, even by the microscope. It is uniform in its appearance and effects. It makes a smoother pill, retaining its form more permanently. It salivates in a few days in the usual doses. The presence of the iron prevents the wear and tear of the human body under the effects of the mercury. It is particularly eligible for the strumous, the irritable, and for reduced anemial constitutions requiring mercury. The powers of life are not so much (scarcely at all) prostrated under its use. Its resolvent power is greater than that of mercury alone, especially with respect to buboes. Practitioners will at all events know what they are using; at present they have for blue pill all manner of alloys and sulphurets-. mercurial-zinc pill, mercurial-sulphur pill, etc. *Part* vii., *p.* 89.

To cover Pills or Extract of Copaiba with Gelatine.—The process M. Garot adopts, is as follows: Fix the pills on long fine pins; plunge them into thick purified glue placed in a hot-water bath; then remove them by a rotatory motion, and stick the pins in paste spread out on a slab, so that the pills may remain elevated in the air; as soon as fifty are thus treated, rotate them individually in the heat of a taper, to harden the external pellicle; pull out the point of the pin, and the process is complete.

It is applicable to every substance capable of a pilular consistence; such as balsam, camphor, musk, assafœtida, mercurial and ferruginous preparations, etc. Two hundred pills can be coated with gelatine in an hour, and will be ready for use after the lapse of two hours. The pilular mass so coated remains soft for a much longer time than according to any other plan.

Part xiv., *p.* 138.

Preparation of Blue Pill.—Mr. Stoddart gives the following directions for the easy and rapid preparation of blue pill. By this process, he states, that a pound of the pill mass may be obtained in an hour, so perfectly prepared, that no metallic globules are visible, even with a Coddington lens : " Triturate the mercury with the *powdered liquorice* (adding a small quantity of distilled or rose water), till the globules are quite imperceptible ; the confection of roses is *next* added, and all well mixed. The rapidity with which the liquorice ' kills ' the mercury is really astonishing to one accustomed to the old way of rubbing the metal with the conserve." *Part* xxxiii., *p.* 294.

Honey as an Excipient for Pills.—M. Thibault believes that much of the disappointment following the employment of pills arises from their, as ordinarily prepared, acquiring a degree of induration that prevents their solution, and enables them to traverse the alimentary canal unchanged. To prevent this he recommends the employment of honey ; pills prepared with it always remaining soft, however long they may be kept.

Part xxxv., *p.* 307.

Excipient for Pills.— Mr. Martin suggests, as preferable to honey, which has been recently recommended as an excipient for pills, the employment of treacle, which is far easier of manipulation, a much less quantity being required. Pills so prepared last soft and flexible for years.

Part xxxvii., *p.* 250.

———•◦•———

PLACENTA.

Incarcerated Placenta—Incision of the Os Uteri in Cases of.—It sometimes happens that the placenta is separated from the uterine parietes, but is confined within its cavity, in consequence of the os being *firmly and rigidly contracted.* This state is what is termed *incarcerated* placenta, and differs from the ordinary forms of irregular contraction of the uterus, in the contraction being more limited to the os and cervix.

The result of these cases is most generally fatal, the patient dying from the effects of typhoid fever, probably excited by the putrescent mass retained in the system. When a portion of the placenta only is retained, a purulent discharge consequent upon inflammation is sometimes secreted, by the living membrane of the uterus, and by which the particles of the intruding body are carried off.

In such cases *after all the ordinary means have been tried in vain,* and death seems certain, as a last resource, before the powers of life were too far exhausted, would this operation be admissible ?

Mr. Power gives the following directions for the performance of this operation. The patient should be placed on her left side, close to the edge of the bed, as in the ordinary obstetric position, the forefinger of the left hand should then be carried to that part of the os or cervix intended to be cut, and a probe-pointed knife or bistoury conveyed cautiously along the finger in the vagina to the point mentioned, at which the os or cervix may be divided. This is done by gently insinuating the point of the instrument within the os, and pressing its cutting edge against the rim on each side, in the direction in which it is intended to be incised, the parts will give way readily before it: and then cautiously giving the blade a withdrawing motion, the openings may be enlarged as much as may be deemed advisable. The bladder should be previously emptied, and if the incision be brought forward great care should be taken to avoid its neck. The liquor amnii will escape after the first incision, and if the uterus act, the case may then be left to nature. *Part* ii., *p.* 151.

Placenta retained Eleven Weeks.—This case is interesting in connection with the question which has been much debated, of the occurrence or non-occurrence of absorption of the placenta in cases where it is retained for a considerable time in the uterus.

A poor woman, 37 years old, having overexerted herself, was taken in labor in the fifth month of her second pregnancy. A midwife who was summoned tore the funis in her endeavor to remove the placenta, and an accoucheur who was then sent for could not succeed in extracting it. The woman now resumed her usual occupation till she was compelled to seek medical advice by the occurrence of hemorrhage from the uterus.

Ten weeks after her miscarraige she applied to Dr. Scholler, who on making a vaginal examination found the cervix uteri thick, the os sufficiently open to admit the finger, and the uterus itself felt large and as though it contained a foreign body. The woman was ordered to remain in bed, and to take gr. x. of ergot of rye every two hours. After the administration of twelve doses, pains like those of labor came on, and were followed by the expulsion of coagula mixed with fibrous and membranous matters, and having a very offensive odor.

Dr. Scholler now fancied that the case was at an end, and supposed that this was an instance of real absorption of the placenta, but after the lapse of some days, having adminstered a purgative, pains came on in the abdomen and recurred periodically for some hours, until a thick mass was expelled from the uterus. This mass was ascertained to be the placenta, which had not undergone the slightest decomposition, was hard, surrounded by a coating of fibrin, and shrunk to the size of half a goose's egg. On a section it presented the peculiar structure of the placenta. The patient did well. *Part* vi., *p.* 167.

Placenta Prœviu.—*Vide* Art. "Labor."

PLASTERS.

Isinglass Plasters.—Mr. Liston has for many years been in the habit of using, after operations, and for other surgical purposes, a plaster consisting of oiled silk covered with a coating of isinglass.

The following is the method of preparing it: Moisten an ounce of isinglass with two ounces of water, and allow it to stand for an hour or two until quite soft; then add three ounces and a half of rectified spirit, previously mixed with one ounce and a half of water. Plunge the vessel into a saucepan of boiling water, and the solution will be complete in a few minutes.

Having stretched the oil silk on a board, by nailing it round the edges, apply the solution of isinglass with a brush, taking care to move the brush evenly, and in the same direction, making it smooth as you proceed—as in varnishing a picture. When quite hard and dry, apply another layer, in the same manner, but moving the brush in the opposite direction, in one case horizontally, and the other perpendicularly. In this manner apply four coats of the solution, or even a fifth, if the surface be not entirely smooth. The last layer should be reduced in strength by the addition of a little more water and spirit. An ounce of isinglass is sufficient for about a square yard of the plaster.

The following precautions should be preserved: The distance between the nails should not be more than an inch and a half, otherwise the oil silk will shrink in festoons, and will not remain flat. The isinglass must be well soaked in water before the spirit is added, otherwise it will not make a complete solution : and the spirit, when added, must be diluted with a portion of the water, to prevent precipitation of the isinglass. The brush must be a flat " hog tool," such as is used for spirit varnish, and well made, otherwise the hairs will be found to come out, and this is an inconvenience, as the operation must be performed quickly, while the solution is warm. The solution, when cold, should be of the consistency of blanc-mange.

The oil silk has been in a great measure superseded by the use of a membrane, consisting of the peritoneal covering of the *cæcum* of the ox. rubbed down, and carefully polished in the manner in which the common goldbeater's skin is prepared. The following is the report of this plaster :

From the extreme thinness of the plaster, the wounds can be examined without its removal. It adheres much better than plaster made with isinglass spread on silk ; and in the first instance of its application becomes firmly fixed. It is difficult to fix the isinglass plaster spread on silk, unless it is very good. From the extreme tenuity of the membrane plaster, it is equally unirritating with goldbeater's skin ; and when once applied it remains so accurately adherent, that it does not require to be changed for many days. Altogether, after a good deal of experience in all the different plasters, we find it the best uniting material that has ever been produced.

In applying the isinglass to the membrane plaster, the directions already mentioned, with reference to the oil silk, may be observed, but a layer of drying oil is spread on the other side of the membrane. *Part* iv., *p.* 106.

India-rubber Court Plaster.—Mr. Rowland submits the following as the best method of making india-rubber court plaster, *which does not wash off*:

A stout frame of wood must be made, about three yards long (or any length that would be most convenient), and about one yard and a quarter wide. Within this frame must be placed two sides of another frame, running longitudinally and across, so fixed in the outer frame that the two pieces may slide, independently of each other, backward and forward about six inches. Tapes of canvas must be tacked around the inside of the inner frame, and the corresponding sides of the outer frame, so as to form a square for the material to be sewed in; which, when done, the two loose frames must be drawn tightly to the outer, by means of a twine passed round each, in order to stretch, perfectly free from irregularities, the silk or satin previous to laying on the composition.

To make india-rubber plaster: Dissolve india-rubber in naphtha, or naphtha and turpentine, and lay it on with a brush, on the opposite side of that which is intended for the plaster, and when perfectly dry, and the smell in a great measure dissipated, it will be ready for the adhesive material; to make which, take equal parts of Salisbury glue, or fine Russian glue, and the best isinglass, dissolved in a sufficient quantity of water over a water-bath, and laid on with a " flat hog tool " while warm. It is requisite to use great caution in spreading the plaster evenly, and in one direction, and a sufficient number of coatings must be given to form a smooth surface, through which the texture of the fabric is not perceptible. Each coating should be perfectly dry before the succeeding one is given, and placed in a situation free from dust, and where a draught of air would facilitate the drying. The quantity of water used, and the weight of the two materials, must be a little varied according to the season, and the gelatine strength they possess.

Lastly, the plaster being ready to receive the polishing coat, which gives also the balsamic effect to it, a preparation is made in nearly the same manner as the tinctura benzoini composita of the pharmacopœia, with the addition of more gums; this preparation must be laid on once only, and with a brush kept for the purpose. For making plasters on colored silk, it is only necessary to select the silk a shade deeper than the color required, as the plaster causes it to appear a little lighter. The process being finished, the plaster must be cut out of the frame with a pair of scissors, as near to the canvas to which it is sewed as it will admit. For sale, it is cut up in squares, which is best done by means of a compass and rule. I have tried various solvents for india-rubber, and find none answer so well as those above mentioned. Ether dissolves it with facility, and possesses the advantage of cleanliness, but it is much more expensive, and evaporates so rapidly that it is almost impossible to spread the solution smoothly on the silk; naphtha evaporates more slowly, and is, therefore, preferable, but the quality requires attention, as it may be obtained almost free from that creasote smell which is the only objection to its use. The addition of a small quantity of turpentine facilitates the solution of some specimens of india-rubber. The white india-rubber is better than that which has assumed a black color.

The grand arcanum in making court-plaster is *glue* and *isinglass*. The polishing coat is not absolutely necessary, but it improves the appearance of the plaster, and the gums may probably increase its healing property, and by giving it a more even surface, cause it to adhere more closely. It has occurred to me, that a similar plaster might be made for common use, with calico instead of silk, which might, in some cases, supersede the use of strapping; and also that the adhesive material might be made the vehicle for cantharadine or other stimulants. The isinglass plaster is apt to crack in warm, dry weather, but this does not occur if it is kept in a cellar in an earthenware jar. *Part* vii., *p.* 169.

An Elegant Sticking Plaster.—Black silk is strained and brushed over

ten or twelve times with the following preparation: Dissolve ℥ss. of benzoin in f. ℥vi. of rectified spirit; in a separate vessel dissolve ℥j. of isinglass
in water; strain each solution, mix them, and let the mixture rest, so that
the grosser parts may subside; when the clear liquor is cold, it will
form a jelly, which must be warmed before it is applied to the silk.
When the plaster is quite dry, in order to prevent its cracking, it is finished
off with a solution of terebinth. chia. ℥iv. in tinct. benzoes f. ℥vj.

Part vii., *p.* 169.

Prestat's Adhesive Plaster.—The following composition is said never to
crack, and not to inflame the skin: Empi. diachyl. gum., 400 grs., purified rosin, 50 grs., tereb. venet., 38 grs., are mixed together at a gentle
heat, and then 12 grs. of gum mastic, and 12 grains of gum ammoniac
incorporated, and the mass spread on linen. In winter it is advisable
to add 10 grs. more turpentine, and 12 grs. of ol. amygdal.

Part x., *p.* 176.

Adhesive Plaster.—An excellent adhesive plaster, unirritating to the
skin, not acted on by water, or the discharges from the wound, and possessing all the good properties of collodion except its want of color, with
the additional advantage of being cheaper, is made by dissolving, with the
aid of a moderate heat, gum lac in spirit of wine, in sufficient quantity to
make it of the consistence of jelly. It can be kept in a wide-mouthed bottle, and spread with a spatula as required.   *Part* xxi., *p.* 357.

Addition of Tannate of Lead to Adhesive Plaster.—M. Herpin states,
that his own experience teaches him that Baynton's treatment, by strapping, may be extended to every branch of surface, whether resulting from
wound or ulcer; and the only inconvenience he has found attending it is,
the production of eczematous eruptions, or vesications in irritable skins.
After having tried various means of obviating this, he remembered the
great advantage that accrued from the treatment of bed-sores, by means
of plasters powdered with the *tannate of lead*. He caused some of this
substance to be combined with adhesive plaster, which henceforth produced
no irritation. As the addition of the tannate diminishes the adhesiveness,
the proportion may vary accordingly, as this quality is desired or not. It
is retained when 1-20th of the tannate is added, and when not much required the proportion may be raised to 1-12.   *Part* xxxi., *p.* 235.

Scott's Plaster.—In some affections of joints (of the knee particularly)
it is very useful sometimes to get the part into as quiet a state as possible.
The best plan yet known is that called Scott's plan, much used in London
hospitals, viz.: sponge the skin of the part (the knee for instance) with
spirits of camphor till the skin smarts and looks red. Then spread an
ointment composed of equal parts of the ung. hydrargyri fort. cum cam-
phorâ and plain ceratum saponis, on lint; cut the lint into narrow strips,
and apply them freely round the knee to the part, fully four inches above and
below the condyles of the femur: over this next apply soap plaster, spread
on calico, cut also in strips; this may be applied for a fortnight or longer,
if no pain ensues in the knee; while over the whole is rolled a bandage or
roller, steeped in gum and chalk. The effect of this plan in removing pain
and swelling is sometimes very remarkable.   *Part* xxxiv., *p.* 284.

Improved Adhesive Plaster.—M. Colson, as the result of twenty years' trial, recommends the following plaster in place of the ordinary diachylon, as it never gives rise to irritation or erythema.

R Olive oil 500, minium 250, yellow wax 185 parts.

These are to be heated together and stirred round with a spatula until the mixture assumes a black color, when it is to be taken off the fire, and stirred until quite thick. It is then to be formed into rolls on a marble table. *Part* xxxviii., *p.* 294.

---◦◦•---

PLEURISY.

Treatment of Chronic Pleurisy with Effusion.—The following was dictated by Dr. Hope during his last illness, and concluded on his deathbed:

"Show that I used mercury in all degrees of intensity, so as to ascertain what quantity was the most effectual, but at the same time, least injurious. Show that I always used opium, in full proportion, with the mercury, and that I used the milder and the external forms when the others could not be borne—thus taking *especial* care to protect the mucous membrane.—Add that I found prompt and free salivation by calomel and opium, and the use of one or two drachms of cintment on each groin and axilla, night and morning for forty-eight hours (in conjunction with the other remedies presently to be specified), produce the most rapid and satisfactory effects of absorption, in cases where the dyspnœa and faintness seemed to be most urgent and dangerous. It was quite common, and, in fact, occurred in the majority of cases, that the fluid descended one-third, and still oftener one-half, down the chest, within the space of forty-eight to sixty hours, carrying with it the extreme dyspnœa and faintness, to the great relief of the patient.

"Say that blisters were used from the first, and that the following became my settled plan of managing them. One blister six inches long, 3½ broad, exclusive of margin, was placed longitudinally over, and a little to the outside of the angles of the ribs, leaving space for another of similar size between the first and the spine. Great care was taken to not remove the cuticle (one means of which was to cover the surface of the blister with silver paper), as this forms by far the quickest healing plaster; but after about forty-eight hours, during which the running was absorbed by dry napkins, carefully prevented from adhering, it became necessary to cover the whole with the mildest soap plaster, spread on soft calico, to prevent the cuticle from being accidentally abraded. In this way all irritation promptly subsided, that is, in the course of from two to three days, and the patient was ready for the second blister, which was placed between the first and the spine. It was similarly treated; and, at an equal interval, a third was placed in front of the original one; that is, rather forward in the axilla. When pain indicated the possibility of a pleuritic stitch in any part of the side, it is needless to say that the first blister was placed over that. Say that diuretics are conjoined: viz., squill; sp. æth. nit.; juniper; iodide of potassium, and, when there is no irritation of the mucous membrane, the various other preparations of potass. Digitalis, by creating faintness, is apt to confuse the symptoms; I do not therefore use it till later. Where all these remedies had failed for two or three days, and dyspnœa continued as urgent as ever, I have occasionally used a powerful hydragogue, as half a grain to a grain of elaterium, combined with calomel and capsicum to prevent nausea; or the pulv. jalap. comp. 3j.; so as to produce ten or twelve copious watery evacuations per day, stimulants being at hand in case of any sinking tendency.

" The patient is better in bed, both because it favors gentle transpiration and obviates faintness.

" Remind that, hitherto, I have been treating a case in which the dyspnœa seemed imminently dangerous, and the most vigorous use of remedies consequently indispensable; but now explain that inconvenience sometimes resulted from hypersalivation; for, notwithstanding an immediate suspension of the mercury either on the first appearance of tenderness of the gums, or of amelioration of the symptoms—especially the dyspnœa and obvious commencement of absorption, untoward salivation would occasionally occur and greatly retard the convalescence. Explain that, on several times observing this, and having reason to believe that the patient could bear the dyspnœa with safety for some hours longer, provided he were prevented from rising, which creates faintness, I used more moderate quantities of mercury, being content to affect the gums within three or four days. In this way, the action of the remedy was easily controlled, either by omitting the mercury for two or three days, if its action threatened to be considerable, or by merely diminishing it according to the evidence of the mouth and of the symptoms. I found, however, that t did not answer to suspend it altogether, but that a continuation of it lrely in a mild form, as a blue-pill night and morning, or at night only, for the purpose of maintaining the first impressions for a period of two or three weeks, or in short, until all the disagreeable symptoms had disappeared, was attended with far better success. Explain, further, that the great acceleration of pulse, which rises commonly to 120 or 130, and in young persons, even to 150 or 160, and which is attended with what the patient calls ' internal fever,' thirst, craving for cold drinks, and dryness and heat of skin, is not necessarily a result of fever, but it *is* necessarily a result of anæmia, occasioned by the deficiency of oxygenation from the total incapacity of one lung at least. Here was the error made by Broussais, who supposed this to be fever, and put his patient on the lowest diet. On the contrary, acting on the opposite principle, I always supply my patients with at least one or two pints of concentrated beef-tea, or plain ox-tail soup; and if the state of the tongue and the alimentary canal fully authorizes it, I permit them tender old mutton or beef for dinner. On this treatment the pulse and ' internal fever' rapidly fall in proportion as the anæmia disappears.

" Next proceed to those cases in which hectic is established, resulting, for the most part, I should imagine, from the fluids being of a puriform character—for, after a month or six weeks, and sometimes much earlier, if the inflammation have been very intense, it assumes this character. Allude to the opinion pretty prevalent, that mercury is injurious in such cases, and say that I have not found it so, but that its use was still indispensable; for I have noticed that where it has been omitted, contrary to my wishes and instructions, a recurrence of the effusion has taken place, notwithstanding the use of mineral acids and the various other remedies usually considered available against hectic; whereas, on resuming mercury with opium, and giving the mineral acids for hectic, I have been enabled to restore matters to their former condition, though not without an extra shake to the patient."

Dr. Hope suggests that sulphate of iron may be added to the sulphuric acid mixture, in order to coöperate with the animal food in removing all remains of anæmia. *Part* iv., *p.* 68.

Pleuritic Stitch.—Rheumatism of the intercostal muscles may be confounded with the genuine pleuritic stitch. Treatment same as in ordinary rheumatism. *Part* v., *p.* 77.

Pleurisy.—In young and healthy adults, Mr. Guthrie advises to bleed in a very " determined manner and with an unsparing hand, until an impression is made on the system, until the pain and difficulty of breathing are removed, until the patient can draw a full breath, or faints ;" and repeat it every three or four hours, according to the symptoms, not placing, however, much dependence upon the pulse. And give mercury to affect the gums ; three grains of calomel with a third or half a grain of opium, every two or three hours. In the later stages, when the pulse is becoming weak, and there is much dyspnœa, or when the disease is becoming chronic, apply a blister. *Part* xvii., *p.* 90.

A new Sign of Pleuritic Effusion.—Dr. Roy, of Lyons, mentions, in the " Revue Médicale," the following sign of pleuritic effusion when the fluid has much diminished : Put the left hand on the affected side of the chest, the patient sitting up in bed ; then percuss the ribs with the right hand. This will give rise to fluctuation, which will be easily perceived by the left hand. Dullness on percussion, absence of vesicular murmur, bronchial respiration, and ægophony, will of course remain the characteristic symptoms when the fluid is abundant. *Part* xxv., *p.* 109.

Iodine Injections in Pleuritic Effusion.—Dr. Atlee relates the case of a gentleman (age not given) from whose side nine pints of pus were discharged on the 16th December, through a trocar passed into the left side of the chest between the seventh and eighth ribs, midway between the spine and the sternum. No further discharge took place until the 2d of January, but the closed wound then reopened, and from that time about a pint of pus continued to be discharged daily, with the effect, in spite of restoratives, of rapidly wasting the patient's strength. On February 2d, 3½ of liq. iodin. c. (U. S. Disp.) diluted with ℥j. of tepid water, was thrown in without inducing any ill effect, no precaution against the admission of air being taken ; and next day the amount of discharge was diminished by one-half. Each day the strength of injection was increased, and on the 7th February the iodine was used undiluted. The amount of matter discharged rapidly decreased, and by the end of February the flow had ceased, the patient daily recovering strength, and in a few weeks later being able to go to business. When seen three years later he was quite well.

Part xxxi., *p.* 87.

PNEUMONIA.

Pneumonia Treated with Spirits of Turpentine.—Mr. Martin relates the case in which he was so successful by means of this remedy, as follows: I was called to visit M— S——, aged twenty-five. I found her in an advanced state of pneumonia, severe dyspnœa, respiration 40, pulse 120, a short hard cough accompanied by dark brick-colored sputa, tongue white (loaded), bowels confined, dull sound on percussion over the entire of the thorax (excepting a small space, of two inches in diameter, beneath each clavicle). Here the respiratory murmur, which was elsewhere absent, was of a loud mucous character. She had been attacked, six days before, with rigors and pains in her chest; and, having been treated solely with whisky-punch *to drive out the cold*, her present state was extremely alarming. Bleeding and calomel were of no avail in arresting the disease, the pulse rose to 140, the lips and cheeks were livid, and eyes sunken, with slight tracheal râle. Thinking the patient so near death that it would be fruitless to wait for the action of mercury, I determined to have recourse to brisk doses of turpentine, which I had seen used with success in cases of pneumonia which resisted mercury. I therefore prescribed the following mixture :

R Spt. terebinthinæ rect., ʒij.; vitelli ovi dimidium.; áquæ rosarum, ʒvss.; tinct. opii, ʒj.; Fiat mistura cujus coch. duo magna sumantur 3tia q.q. hora. Emplast. lyttæ sterno.   .

Next day I found the patient much easier: respiration 40, less labored ; the cheeks have lost their livid hue, but the lips are still of a dark purple; pulse 118, softer and fuller; tongue still loaded; she had six copious watery stools during the night, with a copious secretion of urine; two inches below the clavicle there is an audible and distinct crepitating râle; sputa still dark-colored; blister vesicated well; she has finished the mixture; complains of slight strangury. To have the mixture repeated, camphor mixture being substituted for the rose-water. The patient recovered rapidly, and without relapse.   *Part* ii., *p.* 53.

Bleeding in Sthenic Pneumonia.—Dr. Kennedy, in his *Observations on Blood-Letting*, goes on to say: In sthenic pneumonia, it frequently happens, that in spite of treatment the lung becomes solid; or, it may be, the patient does not present himself till this has occurred. A good deal of difficulty often exists in deciding on the propriety of general bleeding in such cases: the extremities may be cold, and the surface covered with clammy perspiration; the pulse, too, may be weak; and yet there are few cases in which general bleeding will be found more beneficial. Reaction will be found to establish itself, and the lung will become much more rapidly clear than if less energetic means had been used. There is still another case connected with pneumonia, and which presents itself to the medical man by no means unfrequently. A person gets a slight cold, which is neglected; after some time he asks advice, and, on examination, a portion of the lung is found solid. All fever has subsided: the necessity for bringing back the lung to its healthy state need not here be insisted on. Now, this cannot be better done than by following up a plan of treatment which has been already spoken of by Dr. Stokes for the cure of empyema, only with a little more vigor. In place of local bleedings, or possibly in conjunction with them, one or two general bleedings will be followed by the most decisive results. It may be recollected, among the details of the treatment alluded to above, that the lowest diet is enjoined : hence, the *modus operandi* of this plan appears to me sufficiently obvious, by keeping in mind the principle I am endeavoring to establish. The system is deprived of a quantity of its blood, and the food taken is not sufficient to supply the deficiency. Under these circumstances, the system is, I believe, actually forced as it were to take back whatever may have previously been poured out—such as serum, lymph, or, possibly, even pus. It is curious to observe, in some cases, with what great rapidity this may be effected. *Part* ii., *p.* 72.

Colchicum Autumnale.—Suggested as an auxiliary in the treatment of pulmonary inflammations, uncomplicated with abdominal affections.
Part iv., *p.* 11.

Treatment of Pneumonia.—[Blood-letting, tartarized antimony, and mercury, are stated by Dr. Watson to be the three great remedies in this dangerous disease; and this opinion accords with that of most other eminent men—for, although every one may not use the tartarized antimony and mercury in the same way, yet the general principles of treatment will be found nearly to correspond. However much we depend upon bleeding in the early stages of the treatment, a time arrives when it is no longer admissible, and is even positively hurtful.]

We want some remedy, therefore, to assist the lancet, or to employ alone when the lancet can do no more; and we have two such, in *tartarized antimony* and in *mercury*. The tartar-emetic plan I believe to be the best adapted to the first degree of the inflammation—that of engorgement; and the mercurial plan to the second—to that of hepatization.

I need not tell you that the tartarized antimony is not given in this disorder with the object of producing vomiting. Dr. Thomas Davis states that it always acts best when it produces no effect except upon the inflammation itself, i. e., when neither vomiting, purging, nor general depression are produced. The first dose may produce all these effects; but the second and third doses may be *tolerated*, and it is during this *tolerance* of the drug that its beneficial effects are chiefly perceived: if the vomiting and purging be excessive, it is well to combine a small dose of laudanum. Dr. Thomas Davis first bleeds freely in pneumonia; he then begins with one-third of a grain of tartarized antimony in a little water, with a few drops of laudanum or sirup of poppies: he repeats this dose every hour for twice; he then doubles the dose for the next two hours; and goes on thus, adding one-third of a grain every two hours until he reaches two grains every hour. He has not exceeded this last dose, and has occasionally continued it for many days without injurious effects. Whatever be the *modus operandi* of this medicine, there can be no doubt that this treatment is both judicious and safe.

When the dyspnœa has been put an end to by antimony thus exhibited, the medicine may be intermitted; and if the inflammation show any disposition to rekindle, it must be again extinguished by a repetition of the tartar emetic.

When, however, the inflammation has reached the second stage, that of solidification, mercury is more worthy of confidence, in my opinion, than tartarized antimony. The object of giving it is to make the gums tender; and it is expedient to do this as speedily as may be. Small doses of calomel repeated at short intervals—a grain every hour, or two grains every two hours, or three grains every three hours—combined with so much of laudanum or of opium as may be requisite to prevent it from running off by the bowels—offer the most certain way of accomplishing our object. If the bowels are irritable under the calomel, blue pill, or the hydrargyrum cum creta, may be substituted for it with advantage; and if the internal use of the mercury be anyhow contra-indicated, or if it appears slow in occasioning its specific effect, the linimentum hydrargyri may be rubbed in, or the strong mercurial ointment.

Many persons, I am persuaded, are saved by treatment of this kind, pushed to slight ptyalism; the effusion of lymph, tending to spoil the texture of the lung, is arrested, and the lymph already effused begins to be again absorbed; and the ease and comfort of the patient, as well as the alteration for the better of the physical sounds, attest the healing qualities of the remedy.   *Part* iv., *p.* 45.

Counter Irritation.—By means of the ung. ipecacuanhæ, or ung. emetinæ, is preferred by Dr. Turnbull to other rubefacients in pulmonary affections, on account of producing little or no pain, or inconvenience to the patient.   *Part* v., *p.* 84.

Bloody Expectoration.—Dr. Graves states, that when we find in pneumonia that the expectoration is tinged with dark venous instead of arterial blood, we may conclude that it is of a more dangerous nature (originating from effusion of blood from branches of the pulmonary artery, which ramify on the air-cells,) than when the bronchial vessels only are implicated.— *Vide* Art. " Hemoptysis."   *Part* viii., *p.* 54.

Complicated with Cerebral Disturbance.—When pneumonia, as in certain constitutions and in certain epidemics, is accompanied with marked symptoms of cerebral disturbance—a very embarrassing complication— the use of *musk*, either alone or in combination with *calomel*, has been found by Recamier to be often of decided advantage.   *Part* ix., *p.* 77.

Lotion of Tartar Emetic in Pulmonary Diseases.—Mr. Duncan M'Diarmid, an American surgeon, has found great benefit from a solution of emetic tartar applied externally in some pulmonary and other complaints.

Dr. Hannay, in 1823, recommended this form of application, and in 1843 writes, " I still regard this lotion as a highly valuable application to the chest in pulmonary diseases." Dr. H. finds that the addition of gr. v. of hydr. oxymur. to the ounce of solution increases its power and efficacy.
                                          Part xii., *p.* 302.

Treatment of Pneumonia.—[The indications to be fulfilled in treating inflammation of the lungs, are, 1st, To subdue inflammatory action; 2d, To prevent deposition; and, 3d, To guard against relapse. · With the first intention, moderate bleeding, at the commencement of the attack, will be useful, and if the crepitant râle remains after this, it will be a safer criterion for the repetition of the bleeding than the beef-fed appearance of the blood. Dr. A. T. Thomson considers that the use of tartar emetic, as a contra-stimulant, in full doses, is far more advantageous than repeated bleeding. He observes:]

My practice, as soon as I have fully satisfied myself of the existence of the disease, and if the attack has not run on to the second stage, is to order one bleeding to the amount of sixteen or twenty ounces; to follow this, immediately, with three or four grains of calomel and one grain of opium, with the view of preventing that nervous irritability which often succeeds the use of the lancet, and of sustaining the beneficial impression made on the system by the bloodletting.

In two hours afterward, I give one grain of potassio-tartrate of antimony in a fluid ounce and a half of emulsion of bitter almonds, and repeat this dose every third or fourth hour, until a decided diminution of inflammatory action takes place—that is, until the crepitation has nearly disappeared, and the sputa are no longer rusty and tenacious. The intervals between the doses of the tartar emetic are then extended to six hours, and afterward to eight hours, and so continued until convalescence is confirmed. I prefer the bitter almond emulsion, on account of its containing hydrocyanic acid, which has a sedative quality, and a more decided influence in quieting the nervous system, and abating the cough, than small doses of opium. When the pneumonia is uncomplicated, this plan, with the occasional aid of some mild aperient, has, in my hands, seldom failed to carry the case to a successful termination. When the attack has passed beyond the first stage, when dullness on percussion indicates hepatization, then the object of the second indication—namely, to excite the capillaries and prevent further depositions—requires attention ; and, in order to fulfill this indication, I order four or five grains of mercury with chalk, or one grain of calomel, to be given in each interval of the administration of the tartar emetic. *Part* xiv., *p.* 71.

Treatment of Pneumonia in Children.—According to Dr. West, in *idiopathic* pneumonia occurring in previously healthy children, depletion is as important as in the adult ; and is to be followed up by tartar emetic, given in doses of one-eighth of a grain every ten minutes (to a child two years old), till vomiting is produced, and continued every hour or two afterward for twenty-four or thirty-six hours. Then if the physical condition of the lungs, and the general state of the patient, are found greatly improved, persevere with the medicine at longer intervals ; but if the signs of inflammation are advancing, give mercury with small doses of antimony, and use larger doses of the latter to combat any sudden increase of fever or dyspnœa. If under any circumstances bronchial breathing is distinctly audible, the mercurial treatment is indicated ; give, to a child two years old, a grain of calomel every three or four hours, and a little tartar emetic, except contraindicated by sickness or debility; if the stomach and bowels are very irritable, use mercurial inunction. Do not blister, but employ stimulating liniments, by which there is no risk of those unhealthy sores which often follow a breach of the surface. If at the outset, large doses of antimony do not seem to be required, give two-thirds of a grain or a grain of calomel with two or three of James' powders every six hours. It is difficult to know when to give stimulants ; but they are plainly indicated when there is much diarrhœa, the pulse becoming more frequent, and above all smaller and smaller, and the respiration, though slower, more labored, and irregular. Then give wine, even to a child at the breast, and ammonia in decoction of senega, or dissolved in milk, which conceals its pungency. If there is diarrhœa, let the nutriment be arrow root, or the *decoction blanche* of the French ; otherwise give strong beef tea, or veal broth. In *secondary* pneumonia, especially if preceded by well marked bronchitic symptoms, antimony may sometimes be given at once, without bleeding.

General Management.—It is desirable, in all cases of pneumonia at all severe, that infants should be taken from the breast, and that the mother's milk should for a time be given them from a spoon. This is of importance on two accounts—partly because the thirst they experience induces them to suck overmuch (hence it is well that barley-water or some other diluent be given them frequently instead of the milk, in order that they may quench thirst without overloading their stomach); partly because the act of sucking is in itself mischievous, since, as must at once be perceived, it taxes the respiratory functions to the utmost. A second important point is never to allow the children to lie flat in bed or in the nurse's arms, but to place them in a semi-recumbent posture in the arms, or propped up in bed.

When pneumonia has reached an advanced stage, or has involved a considerable extent of the lungs, the children should be moved only with the greatest care and gentleness, lest convulsions should be brought on.

Part xvii., *p.* 88.

Treatment of Pneumonia.—Dr. Todd asserts that all cases of pneumonia have, independently of this or that mode of treatment, a decided tendency to depress the general powers of life—some more, some less; and that, with all, a very decided direct antiphlogistic treatment is hazardous—with some, extremely so—and that in none is it absolutely necessary; but, with others, there is no safety for the patient, unless the treatment from the beginning be of a decidedly supporting and stimulating nature.

Apply flannels soaked in warm spirits of turpentine over the regions of the dullness, and keep them on for half an hour. Let these be applied three times a day for three or four days. Give the liq. ammon. acetatis as a diaphoretic, in doses of six drachms every three or four hours. An occasional dose of a mild aperient may be given, and the patient allowed a pint of beef tea, with a little milk and bread, daily. *Part* xxvi., *p.* 52.

Lungs, Inflammatory Affections of.—In a paper upon the different sounds of the respiratory apparatus, Dr. T. Thompson observes, that in proportion as sounds are confined to inspiration, they afford reason for depletion; in proportion as the rhonchi become bubbling they indicate secretion, and suggest a discontinuance of antiphlogistic treatment.

Part xxviii., *p.* 79.

Typhoid Pneumonia.—Take care how you confound pneumonia occurring in the course of typhus, with a pure inflammatory attack. The symptoms may easily lead you astray, but to treat a case of typhoid pneumonia on the antiphlogistic plan would probably be destructive. Too great weight is placed on physical signs in typhoid pneumonia. The successive signs of crepitus, dullness, cessation of vesicular breathing, and its replacement by bronchial respiration, are too often mistaken for the effects of inflammation, whereas the same signs are seen in typhus. They are, in fact, often symptoms of typhus, and of all other forms of fever, whether these be variola, erysipelas, purulent poisoning of the blood, glanders, scarlatina, or measles. One of the greatest modern improvements of medical practice consists in treating these cases on the plan recommended by Dr. Stokes. Look attentively to the antecedents of a case of this kind when called upon to treat it; examine its history. The editor has been guided by one simple index in most of these cases—viz., the brown tongue. If the tongue be ever so slightly brown at the back, take care how you deplete; on the contrary, begin in good time with broth, ammonia, and wine or good brandy. Don't be afraid of the physical signs of pneumonia, if the history of the case and the tongue indicate coming typhus. It is truly surprising how these physical signs vanish by the timely exhibition of stimulants. The blood is decomposing, the coloring matter is acting on the tongue, the stimulating properties are disappearing, and the functions of life will soon cease, unless you compensate for a time for this loss of stimulation, by an artificial one, till the poison has been exhausted or eliminated. These views are also fully supported in some of Dr. Todd's late lectures. *Part* xxxi., *p.* 17.

Pneumonia, Chronic.—Dr. Cotton, of Brompton Hospital, for con-sumption, etc., believes that counter-irritation is of the greatest benefit. Apply one or two blisters, and follow these by Croton oil liniment, or iodine, or a combination of both. If there be no tubercular tendency, you may employ mercury carefully combined with a more tonic plan of treat-ment. *Part* xxx., *p.* 72.

Absence of Chlorides 'from the Urine as Diagnostic of the onward Progress of Pneumonia.—Dr. Bennett states that in several cases of pneumonia, the absence of chlorides from the urine marked precisely the onward march of the pneumonia, whilst their presence indicated its cessa-tion, and was generally accompanied by the returning crepitation and com-mencing absorption of the exudation. It still remains to be determined whether the absence of these salts is a cause or a result of exudation into the lungs—whether the interference to the respiratory function, by dimin-ishing the amount of oxygen absorbed, gives rise to those chemical changes in the blood which react on the urinary secretion.

Dr. Bennett looks upon this chemical fact as an important diagnostic sign. Therefore, in cases of pleurisy and pneumonia always *test the urine for chlorides*, as follows: Add a few drops of nitric acid to a portion of urine in a test-tube, and then a few drops of a solution of nitrate of silver. If chlorides be present, a dense white precipitate of chloride of silver, which is insoluble in acids, will fall. If chloride of sodium be altogether absent, no precipitate will occur. *Part* xxxi., *p.* 78.

Treatment of Pneumonia.—[There are but few diseases which are treated more differently by different practitioners, than pneumonia. The methods and remedies vary from the most simple to the most heroic. In the General Hospital in Vienna, the treatment is almost entirely dietetic, they are simply left to nature. Dr. Todd, of King's College Hospital, dis-courages blood-letting and even tartar-emetic; he gives large doses of liq. ammon. acet. or citrat., and supports the patient from the first with animal broths, given frequently in small quantities, with a small amount of stimulus. From the statistics which we have been able to collect, we find that the treatment by blood-letting, conjoined with tartar-emetic, is in the present type of disease, the worst, and the dietetic the best, especially in severe cases. The indications to be fulfilled are:

1. To diminish the general fever.
2. To relieve the local symptoms.
3. To check the tendency to death by depression.]

Dr. Routh says: The surest remedy to reduce the frequency of the pulse is aconite. The tincture of the P. L. should be avoided as uncertain. It is most to be depended upon when made from the alcoholic extract of the root, say one grain of the extract to twenty drops of alcohol; the dose of this tincture would be from half a drop to three minims (one drop is about equivalent to one grain of opium). For children one or two drops may be added to eight ounces of water, and half an ounce given every two hours; for an adult, half a drop every two hours will very soon reduce the feverish excitement. Its action must be carefully watched lest an overdose be given. To relieve local symptoms the patient may be placed in water as warm as can possibly be borne, until the patient faints, which will usually be in about twenty minutes ; or instead of this, Junod's exhausting apparatus may be used, which will draw the blood from the affected part to the extremity. As a counter-irritant, the acetum lyttæ with chloroform vesicates very speedily, especially if covered with cotton-wadding immediately after the application. This produces comparatively little discomfort to the patient, and, if repeated occasionally, a vast quantity of serum may be got rid off. The next best application to the chest is flannel dipped in turpentine. At the commencement, promote expectoration by small doses of emetic tartar, and afterward support your patient by mild emollient diet, broths, and gentle stimulants.   *Part* xxxii., *p.* 80.

Treatment of Consolidated Lungs from Pneumonia.—One of the most interesting features we have recently noticed in Dr. Todd's practice at the King's College Hospital is a plan of treating solidified lungs and strumous pneumonia by turpentine—a mode not new possibly, but eminently valuable, and one in which Dr. Todd seems to gain greater confidence at every session.

J. B., aged 21, was admitted into King's College Hospital, October 2d, suffering under various symptoms of chest disease, the result of a severe attack of pneumonia. Dr. Todd pointed out to his class that the entire lung of one side was completely solidified. This lung had, in all probability, gone through the three stages of pneumonia so familiar in practice, but often so very unmanageable in their results, the first and second stages of pneumonic inflammation usually merging into one another, and leaving the lung quite solid.

The chief practical point, to Dr. Todd, being, that the consolidation of pneumonia does not necessarily destroy the vesicular structure of the lung, any more than effusion into the iris, in iritis, removable by mercury, destroys the structure of that delicate part ; the inflammatory effusion, in pneumonia, occurring almost universally through the lung-tissue, as well as *into* the air-cells and inter-vesicular tissue. In a very advanced stage of pneumonia, it is true, we may have pulmonary abscess. This was evidently not the case in the present instance. The treatment adopted by Dr. Todd, and which he finds the most effectual, was the following : Wine, six ounces, daily ; a draught every third hour, composed of julep of acetate of ammonia, with aromatic spirits of ammonia in excess ; and strong turpentine stupes, carefully applied, every night and morning, over the back of the chest and site of the consolidated lung. Diet moderately stimulating.

25th. This man is quite well. The right lung, as will have been observed, is most usually that affected. Dr. Todd has great faith in the stimulant action of turpentine—a remedy not often used, but which in this and numerous other cases has proved almost specific in its action. In phthisical cases also it may be used combined with strong acetic acid, when its action becomes even still more beneficial.   *Part* xxxiii., *p.* 99.

Asthenic Pneumonia—Treatment by Quinine.—In the first stage of an attack in a healthy constitution, says Dr. Corrigan, the capillaries of the lungs become distended, but they preserve their sthenic condition ; in such a case, of course, you would bleed and give tartar emetic to act upon the whole vascular system. But if the capillaries have passed from this sthenic condition, or if from the state of the constitution, the type of the disease, or long-continued depressing influences, they have lost their sthenic power from the very commencement of the attack, then we have to deal with a contrary state of things, in which bleeding would be injurious and dangerous. You must meet these cases by large doses of quinine, five grains every three hours. Quinine appears to possess the same power in giving contractile action to the capillaries of the lungs which we know it possesses in so marked a degree over the capillaries and venous radicles in the spleen. The large proportion of venous capillaries in both the lungs and spleen seems to support this view. *Part* xxxiv., *p.* 33.

Pneumonia—Bleeding.—What-are the comparative effects of practising or abstaining from bleeding in a case of pneumonia? Is one or the other practice indiscriminately to be adopted? The answer to these questions, abstracted from the evidence of Profs. Alison, Bennett, Drs. Watson, Gairdner, Jos. Bell, etc., may be given thus: The non-bleeding plan has a demonstrable advantage over that of indiscriminate and repeated bleedings. The judicious practice of *moderate early bleedings,* general or local, in cases of more or less sthenic pneumonia, and of refraining from it altogether in asthenic pneumonia, whether as regards the character of the disease or the constitution of the patient, is pressed upon us both by experience and science. *Part* xxxviii., *p.* 69.

Pneumonia, Secondary, of Rheumatism.—Opium and ammonia, says Dr. E. L. Ormerod, are preferable to wine for the support of the exhausted nervous system, when this demands especial attention in rheumatic pneumonia. Depletion done judiciously may be borne, but it requires great judgment—if done wrongly it will tend to produce or increase the secondary inflammation. As a general rule you may use blisters, slight cupping, and watery evacuations from the bowels and kidneys. *Part* xxxix., *p.* 88.

Syphilitic Pneumonia.—There is an inflammatory consolidation of the lung which owes its origin to the poison of syphilis. A case is recorded, under the care of Dr. O'Connor, at the Royal Free Hospital, in which it was associated with a papular eruption, and enlargement of one of the testicles. The treatment consisted of blisterings all over the chest, five grain doses of iodide of potassium, and four grains mercury with chalk, and conium, twice a week. Subsequently the iodide of mercury with chalk, were given, till the gums became tender. *Part* xl., *p.* 54.

POISONING.

Poisoning by Aconite.—[Mr. Sayle relates the case of a man who died in consequence of taking decoction of aconite. He saw him an hour after he had taken it, when he was quite insensible, pupils widely dilated, and pulse scarcely perceptible; he was foaming at the mouth, and throwing his arms about. A teacupful of brandy was administered, which, for a time revived him, but while the contents of the stomach were being evacuated by means of the pump, he suddenly expired.]

The plant was the aconitum napellus, stalks and leaves quite fresh. Of these, six were cut up and boiled in half a pint of beer down to a quarter, half of which he drank.

Remarks.—The case in itself presents nothing remarkable; but as they are rarely met with, I think it behooves the medical man to publish these symptoms carefully for the information of others. Dr. Fleming, in his prize dissertation, speaks of four degrees of operation in man, and finishes his remarks on the fourth degree with these words: "When the action of the drug is carried to a fatal extent, the individual becomes entirely blind, deaf, and speechless. He either retains his consciousness to the last, or is affected with slight wandering delirium; the pupils are dilated; general muscular tremors, or even slight convulsions supervene; the pulse becomes imperceptible both at the wrist and heart; the temperature of the surface sinks still lower than before, and at length, after a few hurried gasps, death by syncope takes place." It will be seen that this case and Dr. Fleming's description admirably agree, and that death takes place by syncope is proved by all the organs examined post-mortem being enormously distended with blood.

The stimulating plan of treatment will probably succeed, when employed early after the evacuation of the poison from the stomach.

Part xiii., *p.* 149.

Poisoning by Aconite Root.—This has not unfrequently been mistaken and eaten for horse-radish; it may be known by the acid taste of the aconite parings, and the pinkish color which they assume when exposed to the air.

With regard to the treatment of such cases of poisoning, Dr. Headland recommended the immediate and free administration of animal charcoal, mixed with water. This to be followed by a zinc emetic, then by brandy and ammonia. The charcoal has the power of retaining and separating the poisonous alkaloid, and if we have rendered help in time, the patient may perhaps be saved.   *Part* xxxiii., *p.* 308.

ACONITINA.

Recovery from a Large Dose of Aconitina.—[No case of poisoning by this deadly alkaloid has hitherto been published, and consequently the description given by Dr. Bird is highly important. The patient was a highly educated gentleman, and obtained the aconitina by means of a prescription of his own writing. It is supposed that almost immediately after taking the poison he fell, and struck his head a severe blow against a piece of furniture, and that the poison, or the blow, or both, produced immediate and violent vomiting; but how long it may have been before he was discovered, cannot be stated.]

An excellent surgeon, and shortly after, a physician, were called to him; and about two o'clock in the afternoon, which must at least have been eight hours after taking the poison, Dr. G. Bird met these gentlemen. The patient was then fearfully collapsed; the surface cold and sweating; quite pale; the heart's action scarcely perceptible; pupils acting to light; no paralysis whatever, either of sensation or motion. Notwithstanding the intense exhaustion, the intellect was unimpaired. The most prominent symptom was the repeated and terrific vomiting of a brownish fluid. This vomiting was, however, peculiar, and perhaps hardly deserved that title.

the patient really being seized with a kind of general spasm, during which he convulsively turned on his abdomen, and with an intense contraction of the abdominal muscles, he jerked out, as it were, the contents of his stomach, with a loud shout, depending, apparently, on the sudden contraction of the diaphragm. These exhausting and distressing symptoms had occurred every minute or two. On attempting to make him swallow any fluid, a fearful spasm of the throat took place, producing the distressing effects so well known in the hydrophobia from the bites of rabid animals: this was not produced by the sight of water, but the convulsive movements of the body, and the emptying of the stomach, were excited by abruptly touching him. He was placed in a hot bath, afterward removed to bed, covered with blankets, a large mustard poultice applied to the scrobiculus cordis, and an enema of turpentine administered. He remained in much the same state, the sedative effects of the poison on the heart gradually lessening, so that at nine o'clock the pulse was easily perceptible, although weak; the hydrophobic spasms were, however, then produced by every attempt to swallow, so that none of the medicines suggested for him could be made use of. It was therefore determined merely to administer enemata of beef-tea, with the yolk of an egg, and ten grains of laudanum, chiefly with the intention of procuring rest and giving support. He had a fearful night of exhaustion and spasm; intellect perfect, and even vivid, so as to enable him, whenever he recovered a little from his exhaustion, to carry on a conversation.

After this hard struggle with death, this man emerged from the effects of the poison; and at two o'clock on the following day, when another consultation was held, he was regarded as convalescent. Dr. Golding Bird drew attention to the fact, that although at least *two grains and a half* of aconitina had been swallowed, yet that the majority of the poison must have been got rid of during the vomiting which followed the injury to the head, resulting from the fall. He also pointed out the remarkable train of symptoms developed, especially the convulsive vomiting and imperfect hydrophobia, as possibly being characteristic of the effects of the poison. For although they differed importantly from the effects of aconite root, with the exception of the sedative influence on the heart, still such a difference becomes intelligible when it is recollected that a pure alkaloid often differs materially in its physiological action from that of the plant from which it is an extract, as shown remarkably in the case of the alkaloid conia. *Part* xvii., *p.* 290.

ARSENIC.

Action of the Hydrated Sesqui-oxide of Iron on Arsenic.—Dr. Maclagan concludes:

That the hydrated oxide of iron is a real chemical antidote to arsenious acid, and that when it removes arsenic from solution and soluble combinations it acts by chemically uniting with it.

That it appears much better fitted for removing arsenic, when it has been precipitated by ammonia than when precipitated by potash; and that it answers better when in the state of a moist magma, than when dried at 180°, even though, when thus dried, it still retains a considerable per centage of combined water.

That thus there appears to be good grounds for believing that in the ex-

periments on animals, and the cases in the human subject, in which it has
been found to arrest the action of the poison, that it acted as a chemical
antidote and not as a mechanical protection to the stomach; that the large
quantities which have been found necessary are required not to protect the
stomach mechanically, but to render the poison chemically inert. That, as
far as chemical evidence goes, at least twelve parts of oxide prepared by
ammonia, and moist, are required for each part of arsenic, and that when
the oxide has either been precipitated by potash, or been dried even at a
low temperature, that about three or four times larger quantities are requisite.   *Part* ii., *p.* 43.

Antidote to Arsenic.—Dr. G. Bird recommends the following ready
preparation of the hydrosesqui-oxide of iron as one of the best antidotes to
arsenic: Half an ounce of the tincture of the sesqui-oxide of iron; one oz.
of liquor potassa.   Mix.   *Part* vi., *p.* 149.

By White Arsenic—Liq. Kali Carbonici.—D. Emsmann, of Eckarts-
berge, was called to a young woman who had been poisoned by means of
white arsenic.   She was in great pain, was vomiting, purging, and suffering
great thirst, etc.   He gave, every half hour, a spoonful of a mixture composed of half an ounce of the liq. kali carb. in two ounces of sir. altheæ.
The effect was immediate, the vomiting ceased, the pain was relieved, and
the other symptoms gradually disappeared.   *Part* vi., *p.* 149.

Arsenic as a Poison—Its Tests and Antidotes.—In order to prove the
existence of arsenic, in a court of justice, says Dr. Shearman, we should be
enabled to show the following facts so satisfactorily, that a jury may not
only see, but perfectly understand them.

1st. The metal should be produced either from the contents of the stomach, intestines, or urine, if the patient should survive; or, if dead, from
these and some part of the body.

2d. We should be able to prove that the animal substances experimented
upon were the excretions and parts of the patient's body only, unmixed
with any other matter.

3d. We must also prove that the tests we use to show the existence of
arsenic have not a particle of arsenic in themselves. And this requires
great caution, because a skillful advocate might make a guilty prisoner appear innocent, owing to this omission.

4th. As antimony, bismuth, tin, zinc, lead, tellurium, cadmium, selenium,
and potassium, sublime in a somewhat similar manner to arsenic, and
may be mistaken for it, it is absolutely necessary to guard against such a
mistake.

The most common mode of obtaining arsenic from an organic solution,
is that of Dr. Christison, in which he gets rid of the animal matter by
boiling for half an hour in distilled water with strong acetic acid, which
often precipitates the casein, and renders it sufficiently pure; if not, the
solution should be neutralized by potash or ammonia, slowly evaporated to
dryness, redissolved in distilled water, filtered when cold, and then evaporated several times again. This eventually produces a solution free from
animal matter. With the ammoniacal nitrate of silver this gives a lively
yellow precipitate, the arsenite of silver; with the ammoniacal sulphate of
copper, an apple, or grass-green precipitate, the arsenite of copper; and
with sulphureted hydrogen gas (previously acidulated with acetic acid),
it throws down an abundant sulphur yellow precipitate, the sulphuret of

arsenic. This sulphuret should be collected on a filter, dried, mixed with black flux, or freshly ignited charcoal, introduced into a bulbed tube, and properly heated by a spirit lamp, when a brilliant polished metallic ring of metallic arsenic will be sublimed all round the tube. This is called the reduction test. This metallic ring of arsenic should then be oxidized by exposure to the heat of a spirit-lamp in atmospheric air, when octohedral crystals of arsenious acid, with triangular facettes, will be deposited on the upper part of the tube, which may be easily seen with a tolerably good microscope.

In Marsh's test, where hydrogen gas is generated from zinc, sulphuric acid and water, and the suspected substance is added in solution, arsenic having such an affinity for hydrogen quickly combines what that gas and forms arsenietted hydrogen, which being ignited, metallic arsenic is deposited on porcelain or glass, and may be seen in *rhomboidal crystals* with a powerful microscope. The objection to the test is, that we are obliged · to use zinc, which often contains arsenic; and although it shows the most minute quantity, how can we swear, after the first layer of zinc is oxidized, that there may not be arsenic in the next? for arsenic runs in the veins of the ore.

In Professor Reinsch's test, modified by Christison, we mix the suspected matter with distilled water, add ℥ij. of pure hydrochloric acid to every eight ounces of fluid, immerse a very thin and bright copper plate, and boil for half an our, when the whole of the copper plate will be coated with arsenic. By cutting these plates into chips, and exposing them in a tube at a low red heat over a spirit lamp, arsenious acid will be sublimed in *octohedral crystals with triangular facettes*, which may be rendered more distinct by turning out the chips, covering the tube with the finger, and chasing the oxide up and down the tube over the lamp.

A most ingenious, scientific, and elegant method of obtaining arsenic has been introduced by Robert Ellis, of University College. He has discovered that the oxides of copper have such an affinity for arsenic, that by merely passing arsenietted hydrogen over them, a double decomposition takes place: caloric is given out; the oxygen of the copper uniting with part of the hydrogen forms water, which is seen in the process; the arsenic of the arsenietted hydrogen uniting with the copper forms arseniuret of copper—the remaining hydrogen being set free. This arseniuret of copper may be easily sublimed in a glass tube, when the whole of the arsenious acid will be deposited in *thick brilliant clusters of octohedral crystals on the tube.* The objection urged against Marsh's apparatus will equally apply to this—that of being obliged to use zinc for the generation of hydrogen. The cleanest and safest mode of detecting arsenic is by decomposing distilled water by galvanism, to which is added the suspected solution, and pure sulphuric acid: collecting the hydrogen from the negative pole or zincode of Smee's battery, igniting it, and examining the stain left in a glass tube, open at both ends. If there is the smallest particle of arsenic, the hydrogen will unite with it; and you then have a stain of metallic arsenic with *rhomboidal crystals* which you may then oxidize into *octohedral crystals;* collect, dissolve in water, go through the fluid tests, reduce the sulphuret in a tube, and sublime into arsenious acid again. This is the most delicate test known, and perfectly free from the charge of using any substance in which arsenic can exist.

The most likely substance to be mistaken for arsenic by any of these tests is antimony, because antimony sublimes into the same kind of crystals as arsenic.   But by attending to the following rules the two substances may easily be distinguished.   Metallic arsenic sublimes into rhomboidal crystals at a heat of 356° without liquefying.   Arsenious acid sublimes at 380° into octohedral crystals.   Metallic antimony sublimes not under 810°, and on cooling, acquires a highly lamellated texture, and *yields octohedral crystals like arsenic*, which are *insoluble in water ;* whereas the octohedral crystals of arsenious acid are very soluble, and which solution may be tested by the three fluid tests.   In the reduction tests with sulphureted hydrogen gas, it should be carefully remembered that the sulphurets of antimony, tin, selenium, cadmium, and tellurium, have nearly the same yellow color, and are deposited in the same manner as arsenic, and when reduced to their metallic state with black flux, they not only give an appearance so much like arsenic, that it requires a very practised eye to distinguish each, if even that be possible; and tellurium and cadmium also exhale a garlic odor like arsenic.

The question then comes—how can a witness swear most positively, that a substance is arsenic and nothing else ; and how can he convince an unscientific jury of that fact ?   I think only in the following manner :

1st. By producing the metal, and showing its crystals.
2nd. Reducing it to oxide, and showing its crystals.
3rd. From these crystals going through all the fluid tests.
4th. Reducing the sulphuret again to its metallic state, then to the oxide and again going through the fluid tests.

If this be shown clearly with all the before-mentioned tests, it will be impossible for any advocate to mislead a jury.   The only antidotes which have been discovered for arsenic are the moist hydrated peroxide of iron, and the moist hydrated persulphuret of iron.   I have lately given dogs and rabbits large doses of arsenious acid in solution and powder, and immediately afterward large doses of the moist hydrated peroxide of iron, and then killed them within a short time.   The stomachs have shown minute patches of inflammation, but no arsenious acid could be detected by Reinsch's method, the copper plates having merely a scaly deposit of iron upon them ; nor could arsenious acid be detected in any other way.   This is a strong presumption that the whole of the arsenic was reduced to its metallic state.

Dr. Golding Bird suggests that hydrated per-oxide of iron may be extemporaneously prepared by adding one ounce of liquor potassæ to half an ounce of tincture of sesquichloride of iron.   *Part* ix., *p.* 55.

Magnesia in the Treatment of Poison by Arsenic. — Magnesia, not strongly calcined, is recommended by M. Bussy as an excellent antidote to arsenious acid ; it removes it entirely from a state of solution in water, and forms an insoluble compound.   Magnesia in a gelatinous state answers best.   Magnesia decomposes emetic tartar, the salts of copper, and corrosive sublimate, also the organic alkalies, morphia and strychnia.

Dr. Christison recommends the light pure magnesia, which may be obtained in a gelatinous pulpy state, by adding a solution of caustic potash to a cold saturated solution of sulphate of magnesia, and washed afterward with cold water.   The dense magnesia has very little action on arsenic in solution.   When the gelatinous cannot be obtained, then use the light calcined, in proportion of between thirty and fifty parts to one of arsenic taken.

As in the hurry of these cases it is frequently difficult to know what quantity of arsenic has been taken, it must be left to the discretion of each practitioner to judge what quantity of the magnesia he shall administer as the antidote. · *Part* xiv., *p.* 117.

Poisoning by King's Yellow.—King's Yellow, according to Dr. Christison, contains sulphuret of arsenic, caustic lime, and free sulphur, and in all probability, the lime exists in the form of a triple sulphuret of lime and arsenic.

The hydrated peroxide of iron acts as the best chemical antidote, combining with the arsenic in the stomach to form an arsenite of iron which has little solubility, and therefore little energy as a poison. As the arsenic may be again set free by the secretions of the stomach, take care to give the peroxide in excess, and repeatedly until all effects subside.

Part xiv., *p.* 119.

Poisoning by Arsenic.—[In a paper read before Guy's Hospital Physical Society, Mr. Odling states it as his opinion that the only plan of treatment to be depended upon is the removal of the poison physically from the stomach, and that this is best effected by using the double-action stomach-pump. He next considers the remedies to be used in cases of arsenical poisoning, and first, of the hydrated ferric oxide, or sesqui-oxide of iron. This, by being administered in the state of a moist magma, suspends the poison, but its power is extremely weak, and the compound formed with it is perfectly soluble in the gastric juice, and has been found to possess poisonous properties. Magnesia, so much vaunted at one time, is even less fitted to act as a chemical antidote.]

Mr. O. would at once wash out the stomach by means of the double action stomach-pump, with a solution of chromate of iron or alumina, or a mixture of permanganate of potassa solution, or with hydrate and acetate of ferric oxide, or with hydrate and acetate of alumina. By these compounds the soluble arsenious acid is immediately converted into insoluble arsenic acid or into the insoluble sesqui-arseniate of alumina, iron, or chrome. Ten grains of the permanganate of potassa may be mixed with half a pint of the aluminous emulsion, under which circumstances, its irritant action would be very trifling, not more than that of an ordinary sulphate of zinc emetic. *Part* xxiii., *p.* 317.

Arsenic—Test for.—Give magnesia mixed to the consistence of cream, in doses of two or three tablespoonfuls. In a case reported by Dr. Maclagan, the patient took four ounces in three quarters of an hour, and, no doubt, vomited it nearly all up again. Reinsch's test is a most valuable and convenient one in cases of poisoning by arsenic. All that is required is a little muriatic acid, a bit of copper wire, and some vessel as a test tube, in which they can be heated together. These articles are so common that it must be rare when they cannot be supplied. If the piece of copper be crusted black during the boiling, and when heated in a candle-flame loses its crust, and gives off alliaceous fumes, the evidence will be sufficiently precise. *Part* xxv., *p.* 322.

Electro-Chemical Mode of Testing for Arsenic.—Dr. Davy's process is adapted to detect arsenic in all its states of combination, and in various organic mixtures; and it is a strong recommendation of it, that it obviates in many instances, any troublesome or tedious manipulations. It essentially consists in depositing the arsenic in a metallic state upon a surface of platinum (as a platinum capsule or a sheet of that metal), by touching the spot with a rod or thin slip of zinc, and maintaining the contact for a few seconds, when the metal arsenic falls as a film, more or less thick in pro-portion to its amount, and adhering firmly to the platinum, whence it can be removed by heat or acids, and subjected to any further tests that are desirable.

To prepare the solution for testing, some pure muriatic acid must be previously added ; and when the fluid is very dilute it is then concentrated by boiling before using the electro-chemical test. After the concentration, which may be carried to a considerable extent with advantage, it is well to add some more muriatic acid before testing. Sulphuric acid appears, from some experiments, not to interfere with the result, but nitric acid did. "There was some difficulty in exhibiting the arsenic."

In testing such arsenical compounds as realgar and orpiment, arsenical pyrites, etc., they require first to be acted on by nitric acid to dissolve them, and then all excess of this acid, either exhaled by heat or neutralized previous to adding muriatic acid and testing, as a minute quantity of nitric acid retards the reduction of the arsenic or redissolves it.

Part xxxiv., *p.* 299.

BELLADONNA.

Belladonna Poisoning.—Dr. Jenner, of University Col. Hospital, re-commends to apply a blister to the back of the neck, and give an aperient with five grains of the sesquicarbonate of ammonia every hour or half-hour, according to the severity of the symptoms.   *Part* xxxv., *p.* 279.

Animal Charcoal an Antidote to Vegetable Alkaloids.—Dr. Garrod, of University Col. Hospital, says that if to the solutions of the poisons of hen-bane, belladonna, stramonium, or morphia, a little animal charcoal be added, the poison is completely neutralized. This property makes animal charcoal of the greatest use as an antidote to these substances ; common black bone will do very well ; vegetable charcoal does not possess these properties.   *Part* xxxvii., *p.* 259.

Poisoning by Belladonna.—Use of Opium recommended. *Vide* "Poisoning by Opium."

COLCHCUM.

Poisoning by— Case.—The subject of the following case was ordered in a public institution six drachms of tincture of colchicum in a half pint mixture of Epsom salts, of which he took one ounce every six hours. It was ascertained that a larger quantity (six ounces) of the colchicum had been put into the bottle than was prescribed. Vomiting soon commenced after the first dose, and after the third the nose began to bleed profusely, accompanied with violent purging. Notwithstanding these violent symp-toms, the medicine was continued. His medical attendant found him sitting up in bed, with his back reclined against the wall, his arms hanging listlessly beside him, his head bent forward upon his breast, and his shirt drenched with blood from his nostrils. His mouth was open, his eyes were staring, full, and turgid ; the vessels of the adnata congested and the pupils dilated ; pulse 170, full, bounding, and incompressible, and respi-ration short and hurried. Thirty ounces of blood were taken from the arm, and a mixture containing potass. carb. and liq. opii sed. was prescribed, followed by port wine and cinchona bark. This treatment seemed to rally the patient, but he ultimately relapsed and died.

Dr. Thompson makes the following practical remarks:

On reviewing the treatment of this important case, I have little to remark, except that it is probable, had my assistance been sooner demanded, I should have opened the temporal artery, instead of bleeding from the arm. I am of opinion, that in the early stage of poisoning by an *acrid*, or a *narcotico-acrid poison*, the poison is circulating in the brain, and that much benefit would result from rapidly abstracting a large portion of it from the vicinity of that organ, upon which much of its energy is exerted. By such a practice, also, the sympathetic irritation would have been greatly lessened, and time would have been thus afforded for providing against the collapse, which, in all these cases, is the result to be dreaded.

Part viii., *p.* 48.

COPPER.

By the salts of Copper— Treatment by Solution of Carbonate of Soda.—Liquid albumen is generally administered as an antidote in cases of poisoning with the salts of copper, but it has this disadvantage, that as we are unacquainted with the exact quantity necessary to neutralize the copper, if we employ too great a quantity, the poison is dissolved in the excess of albumen. To remedy this inconvenience M. Benoist proposes to substitute for albumen, a solution of carbonate of soda, which forms with the salts of copper an insoluble carbonate, having no deleterious action on the economy. *Part.* v., *p.* 84.

Hydrated Protosulphuret of Iron—Suggested as an antidote in poisoning by the *Salts of Copper. Vide* Art. "Poisoning by Corrosive Sublimate."

CORROSIVE SUBLIMATE.

Gold Leaf and Iron-filings, as a Galvanic Antidote to Corrosive Sublimate.—All the compounds of mercury are more or less poisonous, but none more likely to be so than the corrosive sublimate or bichloride, on account of its being introduced so much in the process of tanning and to prevent the decay of timber, as well as in the destruction of insects; thus exposing individuals to the danger of introducing it accidentally into the stomach. Gluten and albumen have hitherto been our chief antidotes, especially albumen, which changes the corrosive sublimate into calomel, and thus renders the patient liable to very severe salivation, which, of itself, is attended with inconvenience and even danger. Dr. Buckler, amongst other experiments, found, "that by throwing gold dust into a solution of mercury, no action took place till iron-filings were added, when the metallic mercury was at once revived, and was seen to precipitate in a state of amalgam with the gold; at the same time, the oxygen from the corrosive sublimate goes over to the iron, and forms an oxide of that metal with which the chlorine combines, leaving a hydrochlorate of iron in solution."

The result is a complete decomposition of the poison. Two grains of gold and two of iron are sufficient to decompose five grains of corrosive sublimate.

The proposed antidote should be kept by the druggists in papers containing each,

Finely-divided gold, ditto iron, aa. Ɖij; gum acacia, ℥ss. M.

free from dampness, to prevent oxidation to the iron. In poisoning with any compound of mercury, one powder is to be stirred in a tumbler of water, and swallowed; if any of it is rejected, another powder should be given. If a solution of mercury were swallowed, we could not expect much benefit to arise from the use of gold and iron, in any other state than that of dust. In case of poisoning with the insoluble compounds of mercury, if the dust cannot be obtained, then use the metals in the form of beads, fine chains, or any other shape in which they can be swallowed. Dr. B believes that they would decompose the soluble salt with as much rapidity, at least, as it could be formed in the stomach.

Mr. Barry thinks that Dr. Buckler's discovery may prove exceedingly important; but seems to disagree with him on some parts of the question. He is of opinion that the decomposition is owing " to the thin stratum of fluid immediately enveloping the two contiguous particles of iron and gold;" and, therefore, that "it is essential that these metals should be in a state of division so exceedingly minute, as to remain a short time in *suspension throughout the whole fluid of the stomach.* Every drop of that fluid must be made to contain a multitude of these particles, and yet the entire weight administered be very small." The chief difficulty in this case will be, not in the minute division of the gold, but in that of the iron. It is probable, however, that in this combination of gold and iron, we shall possess, when properly managed, a complete antidote to one of our commonest and strongest poisons.   *Part.* v., *p.* 34.

Hydrated Protosulphuret of Iron as an Antidote to Corrosive Sublimate.
—M. Mialhe has discovered that hydrated protosulphuret of iron, a perfectly inert substance, instantly decomposes corrosive sublimate; protochloride of iron and bisulphuret of mercury, two inert substances are formed. This preparation will probably also be found equally efficacious as an antidote to other poisonous salts, as those of copper and lead.

The following is the mode of preparing the hydrated protosulphuret of iron: Dissolve any quantity of pure protosulphate of iron in at least twenty times its weight of distilled water, deprived of air by boiling, and precipitate the iron with a sufficient quantity of sulphuret of sodium, dissolved also in distilled water, deprived of air. Wash the protosulphuret thus obtained, with distilled water, and preserve it in stoppered bottles, filled with boiled distilled water.

Although the preparation of this sulphuret of iron is very simple, and may be effected in a few minutes, yet it would be desirable to keep it always prepared, that no time may be unnecessarily lost in any case of poisoning.

The precaution of preserving this sulphuret out of contact of the air, must be strictly observed, as it has a great tendency to pass into the state of sulphate.   *Part.* vii., *p.* 83.

Antidotes of Corrosive Sublimate, Copper, Lead and Arsenic.—By means of numerous experiments, first made in the laboratory and then repeated on dogs, MM. Bouchardat and Sandras have arrived at many interesting results relative to the antidotes of corrosive sublimate, copper, lead and arsenic.

Their conclusions were, that the following substances may be regarded as antidotes, and employed as such in medicine :

As Antidotes for Corrosive Sublimate.—A mixture of zinc and iron filings ; or powder of iron reduced by hydrogen ; or the moist persulphuret of the hydrated peroxide of iron.

As Antidotes for Copper.—A mixture of zinc and iron filings ; iron reduced by hydrogen ; porphyrized iron ; zinc filings ; or the persulphuret of the hydrated peroxide of iron.

As an Antidote for Lead.—The moist persulphuret of the hydrated peroxide of iron.

As Antidotes for Arsenic.—The moist hydrated peroxide of iron ; the dry hydrated peroxide of iron ; and the moist persulphuret of the hydrated peroxide of iron.

These experienced chemists add the following reflections : This last preparation, the persulphuret of the hydrated peroxide of iron, possesses this superior advantage over all the rest, that it changes the nature of all the four poisons above noticed, and is especially applicable in those cases where we have not had time to find which of the poisons has been taken. As to the manner of administering these antidotes, and the doses which it is necessary to administer, the simplest means appear the best. The powders of zinc and iron may be suspended in any electuary, or they may be swallowed in wafer paper. The magma of the hydrated preparations of iron may be swallowed in the form of jelly, in which they are procured from the druggists. Several draughts of lukewarm water ought to follow the antidote, and the fauces be tickled with a feather, to excite vomiting and the expulsion of the poison. The efforts at vomiting scatter more effectually over the stomach the antidote which is administered. As to dose, the experiments proved that 100 grains of the powder of iron or of zinc sufficed to prevent any bad effects from 15 grains of the acetate of copper. Fifteen drachms of the moist magma of the persulphuret were required to produce the same effect with the same dose (15 grains) of the acetate of copper. To act as an antidote to $4\frac{1}{2}$ grains of arsenious acid, 15 drachms of the moist magma of the persulphuret, or 30 drachms of the moist hydrated peroxide of iron, or 20 drachms of the dry hydrated peroxide of iron, were required. With regard to the time when these antidotes can be administered with advantage, in so far as the acetate of copper is concerned, the lapse of 40 minutes from the time of swallowing the poison ought not to be regarded as a sufficient reason for not administering the antidote ; but arsenic is more quickly absorbed. Nevertheless, the antidote should always be administered, because, though it will not neutralize what is absorbed, it will prevent its further absorption, by decomposing what remains in the stomach. *Part ix., p.* 78.

Mineral Poisons.—MM. Sandras and Bouchardat recommend a universal antidote for the mineral poisons, the persulphuret of iron in such quantities as to be always in excess in the intestines, to prevent the reabsorption of the poisonous matter. They administer first a purgative, and order a soap-bath, then give the patient a mixture of sirup and persulphuret of iron night and morning. Opium, strychnia, or belladonna may be employed at the same time. Two cases only proved fatal out of 122 with lead colic thus treated, and the others were rapidly cured.

Part xiv., p. 324.

New Process for the Detection of Metals in Medico-Legal Researches.—
M. H. Gaultier de Claubry gives the following: "Process by which all
Metals can be obtained by a single operation, in chemico-legal researches."
His objects are,—1, to obtain in all cases a solution of the metal; 2, to
collect the metal from the solution; and 3, to present it in solution, in as
concentrated a form as possible, to the action of chemical reagents. He
says:

With this intention (that of obtaining a perfect solution of the metallic
substances), hydrochloric acid or chlorine have been employed, with more
or less advantage. Without stopping to discuss the advantages or inconveniences arising from their employment, we may say, that the alteration
desired to be affected by them is always more or less difficult, and that a
great proportion of the organic matter resists their action. We know,
from numerous facts, how much more readily a body enters into a new
combination when in a nascent state, than when in the form under which
we see it; and it is precisely in this state that chlorine may be made available for the object which occupies our attention. If we introduce any
organic matter into fuming hydrochloric acid, and, after having removed
the fatty matters, which are altered with difficulty, gradually add concentrated nitric acid to the fluid, either cold or slightly warmed, a complete
solution is obtained of everything, with the exception of fatty matters.
The solution is almost colorless, transparent, and can be afterward tested
with the greatest facility.

The stomach, intestines, liver, products of vomiting, excrements, blood,
urine, wine, milk, earth from burying-grounds, etc., can all be treated after
this method, which requires no particular care, so that the operation is
performed as easily as the solution of a metal in an acid. Where the poisonous agent is arsenic, if the operation be conducted slowly, the metal
does not pass off by evaporation; however, as a portion of chloride of
arsenic may be volatilized, and as the chlorine and acid require some
means to prevent them from passing off, and incommoding the operator
by filling the laboratory with their vapors, it is always best to use a retort
furnished with a tubular receiver. When the operation is finished, the
condensed liquor is to be treated in the manner to be presently described.
A tubular retort, into which are introduced in succession, first, the hydrochloric acid, then the suspected materials, and finally the nitric acid, is
thus sufficient for the operation. If it be known that arsenic do not exist,
and there be no necessity for guarding against the escape of acid vapors
and of chlorine, the operation may be performed in a matrass. By this
process the difficulties are prevented which arise from the employment of
sulphuric acid for the destruction of the organic materials, and a perfectly
liquid product is obtained.

When the materials are much disorganized, the nitric acid is to be introduced gradually, and gentle heat is to be applied. When, after successive
additions of the acid, the organic matters have disappeared, leaving only
fatty matters, the liquor is to be decanted, and the residuum washed several
times in distilled water. This is to be poured off, and mixed with the acid
solution. After this, the detection of the metals becomes extremely easy,
and may be effected in various ways.

If it be desired to use hydrosulphuric acid, the nitric acid must be
driven off, by boiling the liquor with an excess of hydrochloric acid, until
chlorine ceases to escape; after this, the liquor will only have to be tested

for zinc, which may be present accidentally, or for those metals which are not precipitable by hydrosulphuric acid. If Marsh's test is to be employed, the liquor must be saturated with pure potash; and, after decomposition has taken place, sulphuric acid must be added, till the last traces of nitric acid are removed. The operation may then proceed in the ordinary manner.

I have employed another process, which seems to offer important advantages, and is easy to be performed; it depends on the precipitation, by a galvanic current, of the metals in solution. After having concentrated the liquors, as far as experience may determine to be necessary for driving off an excess of acid, there are to be placed in the solution two plates of platinum, or a single plate of that metal, forming the cathode of a permanent battery; and another of zinc (if that metal be not sought for), of tin, or platinum, forming the anode. After an interval of greater or less duration, according to circumstances, but never exceeding, in the most unfavorable conditions, eight or ten hours, the platinum is covered by a deposit of the metal, or metals, which were in solution. This deposit is to be washed, and treated with hot or cold nitric acid; a solution of the metal or metals is thus obtained, which, from the small quantity of liquid, can be operated on with the greatest facility. In this way, almost infinitesimal quantities of the various metals may be detected, and it is obvious that the same proceeding is applicable to all, with the exception of silver, which is rarely to be tested for in cases of poisoning, and zinc, which necessitates the employment of tin or platinum, as the anode of the pile.

Although sparingly soluble, chloride of lead dissolves in an excess of hydrochloric acid easily enough for all the lead to be detected in the liquor.

If the presence of arsenic be suspected in the matters to be examined, the liquid procured by the treatment with nitric acid, must be saturated with potash and after the solution has been conveniently concentrated, it must be mixed with the solution of the organic products. In no other case have volatile products to be dealt with.

It is well known that bakers have sometimes fraudulently introduced extremely small proportions of sulphate of copper into paste. The combustion of the charcoal from bread is very tedious, but an examination is performed with ease and rapidity by the process which I have described. It permits a large quantity of bread to be operated on, and a repetition of the experiments, with a degree of exactitude, which leaves nothing to be desired.

When, in testing for zinc in bread, or in other organic matters, recourse is had to carbonization, there is always danger of a portion of the metal being volatilized; by treating it with aqua regia, the operation is rendered easy, and no part of the metal is lost. It is not necessary to mention all the other circumstances to which this new method may be applied. I have met with no case in which I have not been able to employ it; and hence I may consider its adoption will render great services to chemists, when called on to make researches of the kind under consideration.

It may be objected to this method, as to many others in which hydrochloric acid has been used, that this acid may contain arsenic. There is but one answer to this objection, viz., that as hydrochloric acid can be obtained free from arsenic, such must be procured, and alone employed. Sulphuric acid, also, often contains a greater or less quantity of this metal; that only which is free from it is to be used. *Part xix., p. 215.*

Animal Charcoal an Antidote to Poisons.—Fresh animal charcoal, when used in sufficient quantity, has the property of withdrawing from their solutions most, if not all, known vegetable and animal poisonous principles, and some mineral poisons. It should therefore be immediately administered in all cases; whilst, in the case of mineral poisons, the usual antidotes should also be given.　　　　　*Part* xx., *p.* 298.

CUBEBS.

Use of Electro-Magnetism.—Dr. Page, of Valparaiso, has used this means in a case of poisoning by a large dose of powdered cubebs. The patient took half an ounce of this drug on going to bed, and was found next morning with his face red and swollen, lips dark purple, veins of the forehead and temples turgid, eyes rolling upward and injected, with the pupils contracted to a point, respiration very slow, short, and gasping, and with all the other symptoms of comatose sleep. Every method that could be thought of to rouse him was tried in vain; he soon returned to the same state of insensibility, and death seemed to be inevitable. In this case, Dr. Page tried the electro-magnetic battery with success. With an assistant rapidly rotating the wheel, he applied the balls at first to each side of the neck, and ran them down behind the clavicles. The arms and body now moved convulsively, but the patient lay as unconsciously as before: but on applying one ball over the region of the heart, and the other to a corresponding point on the right side, the patient opened his eyes widely, his head and body were thrown convulsively forward, and he groaned. He again sank back into his former state; but on applying the balls to the same regions, he became conscious, and ultimately recovered. Dr. Page in this case used a large horse-shoe magnet mounted upon a stand, in a vertical position, with an *armature*, fixed upon an axis between the poles, so as to revolve in front by means of a wheel; but a much more portable machine is now made by most surgical-instrument makers, and which ought to be in the possession of every general practitioner.
　　　　　Part vii., *p.* 32.

PRUSSIC ACID.

The Liquor Oxysulphatis Ferri—Thought to be an antidote to poison-ing by prussic (hydrocyanic) acid.　　　　　*Part* v., *p.* 68.

Cold Douche.—In cases where prussic acid has been administered, and the frame is influenced by that deadly poison, a valuable auxiliary will be found in cold affusion, to chlorine, ammonia, artificial respiration, etc. Herbst, Orfila, and others, speak highly of its powers. It occasionally happens that a sudden alternation from cold to hot applications, and from hot to cold, will be more beneficial than a continuance in the one or the other, exemplifying what Dr. Marshall Hall says, "that it is not the mere application of cold, but the sudden application of *cold* to a *warm* surface, which is the effectual means of exciting respiration. It is the *sudden alternation.*" In the cases of persons to all appearance dead, heat and cold are powerful measures in arousing the respiratory system; but they are not to be regarded as substitutes for other methods of resuscitation, so much as allies to them. The value of temperature in congenital asphyxia is admitted universally: one dash of cold water will suffice sometimes to excite breathing where it is delayed.　　　　　*Part* viii., *p.* 45.

* *Sulphate of Iron, with an Alkaline Carbonate, an Antidote for Prussic Acid.*—[Messrs. Smith recommend, that in cases of poisoning by prussic acid, the first thing to be done should be to give a large dose of either caustic or carbonated magnesia, in order to neutralize the effects of the free acid, which is almost invariably to be found in the stomach, and which interferes with the action of the remedy they propose. This consists of two substances: the first, a salt of iron, of the same constitution as Prussian blue, and which is readily prepared by the following process:]

Seven parts of proto-sulphate of iron, say seven half-drachms are required, four of which are to be formed into persulphate. This is done by adding to the solution a quantity of sulphuric acid equal to the half of what it already contains; which, for two drachms, would be twenty-three grains of acid of the density of 1.845, and at a boiling heat; adding, at short intervals, small quantities of nitric acid, till red nitrous fumes cease to be given off. The liquid is then to be evaporated in a porcelain basin of perfect dryness, by the heat of a water-bath, stirring constantly with a glass rod, till the excess of acid is thoroughly driven off. The operations will be more quickly finished in a bath of a saturated solution of salt. The perfectly dry salt is then to be dissolved in distilled water, along with one and a half drachms of proto-sulphate of iron, so that the solution may amount to two ounces. This solution will not of itself precipitate prussic acid, but if a solution of an alkaline carbonate be previously added, containing a quantity just sufficient to take all the sulphuric acid from the iron salt, the prussic acid combines instantaneously with the iron, forming the very permanent and insoluble compound Prussian blue. As the solution of the sulphate of iron contains in all nine equivalents of sulphuric acid, the same number of equivalents of carbonate of potash—the alkaline carbonate we use—will be required to seize upon these and produce complete decomposition. The relative quantities are 910 grains of proto-sulphate of iron, and 623.43 grains of carbonate of potash. Now, as the quantity of sulphate of iron given in our formula was seven half drachms, or 210 grains, the correct quantity of carbonated alkali can be found by the following proportion — 910 : 622.43 : : 210 : : 144. Therefore 144 grains is the proper quantity for the exact decomposition of the iron salt; and for the sake of simplicity, we dissolve this in the same quantity of water as the sulphate of iron. As each of the solutions contains exactly 961 minims, which, by calculation, should throw down 56.8 grains of red prussic acid, between 17 and 18 minims of each should separate the grain; and as the hydrocyanic acid of the London Pharmacopœia contains two per cent. of real acid, 35 minims of each would be required to precipitate 100 grains of such an acid. The acid of the Edinburgh Pharmacopœia, on the other hand, containing about three per cent., a third more, or about 52 minims of each of the solutions, would be necessary to separate all the prussic acid from 100 grains. It is probably unnecessary to carry the calculation higher, as we suspect, that if a larger quantity than 100 grains should be taken, the fatal effect would be so rapid, as completely to exclude the possibility of rendering any available assistance. These are the quantities theoretically necessary, and, when pure materials are used, will be found very nearly correct, as tested in an open vessel; but when given as an antidote for the poison, we would recommend not less than three times the theoretical quantity to be given, as from the presence of food, mucus, etc., in the stomach, it is improbable that the antidote would mix immediately with the poison at every point, so that, to render the action more certain, a large excess is advisable, more especially as this can be attended with no evil consequences, as the only effect that could follow an excess would be the formation of sulphate of potash and an insoluble mixture of proto-carbonate and peroxide of iron, which, if active in any way, would, by producing sickness and vomiting, be really in the direction most to be desired.   *Part* xi., *p.* 99.

Poisoning by Prussic Acid.—*What ought a practitioner to do in so fearful an emergency?*

According to Dr. Christison, he ought, in the first place, to dash cold water on the face, the naked anterior part of the chest, and dorsal spine. Care must be taken not to soak the clothes of the patient. The object is not to chill the patient, but to produce a sudden shock on the external respiratory nerves, for the purpose of inducing a sudden expansion of the thoracic walls, and the full inflation of the lungs as a consequence thereof: and further, by getting the lungs thus expanded, we enable the right side of the heart to unload itself. 2. Diffusible stimuli may be given. 3. A small, but sudden abstraction of blood, *pleno rivo*, from the jugular vein, must be practised if the heart has ceased to beat, or beats very feebly, 4. If the cold affusion, diffusible stimuli, and bleeding from the jugular, are not sufficient to restore the action of the heart and lungs, then artificial respiration must be resorted to. We need say nothing in favor of the cold affusion, as every one believes its employment in poisoning with prussic acid to be orthodox. The same remark will apply to the exhibition of diffusible stimuli and trying artificial respiration.

Part xii., *p.* 118.

Poisoning by Prussic Acid—Treatment.—Of all remedies, says Mr. Hicks, chlorine, ammonia, and the cold effusion, appear to be most generally relied on; and as ammonia is most readily to be obtained, this is resorted to in the greater number of instances. Should I be called to a case, I would on no account lose time by endeavoring to pour fluids into the stomach, but would at once put in practice a suggestion, for which I have to thank Mr. Taylor, which, he states, is of much service in many cases of asphyxia. It is merely to saturate a handkerchief with the liquid ammonia, and then to wave it over the face of the patient, by which means the individual being as it were enveloped in an atmosphere of ammonia, there is every chance of its vapor passing into the lungs; and this has been found even of more service than where the ammonia has been given internally. There is, however, another remedy mentioned by authors, but which I think has been spoken of too lightly; I allude to venesection. I would by no means neglect to adopt venesection in any future case, in combination with cold affusion, ammonia and artificial respiration. I would, however, observe, that in advocating bleeding, I do not mean to say that it is to be performed indiscriminately, but merely in those cases where congestion of the brain and lungs is evident from the bloated and livid appearance of the face. With respect to the treatment, I cannot do better than conclude with the words of Dr. Christison, who says, it is right to remember that on account of the dreadful rapidity of this poison, it will rarely be in the physician's power to resort to any treatment soon. enough for success; and further, that his chance of success must generally be feeble, even when the case is taken in time, because, when hydrocyanic acid ·is swallowed by man, the dose is generally so large as not to be counteracted by any remedies. *Part* xii., *p.* 121.

Poisoning by Prussic Acid.—[Mr. Bishop waº sent for to a man who was stated to have taken poison. He found him in bed, senseless, with ghastly pale countenance; face swollen and covered with perspiration; breathing slow, labored, and accompanied by a hissing sound; the corner of the sheet was between his teeth; along the sides of which quantities of thick white foam issued at each expiration; the eyes were wide open, fixed and glazed, and the pupils widely dilated; the pulse slow and scarcely perceptible, heart's action weak, and the whole body in a rigid state, with the respiration becoming at each instant more laborious. His wife thought he had taken prussic acid, from finding a bottle so labelled, and Mr. B. accordingly decided on instantly trying the effects of cold water dashed on the body.]

. I then prepared him for the cold douche, by tearing away his shirt and flannel waistcoat, and directing two assistants to hold him off the side of the bed. A bucket of cold water was soon brought, and with a vessel holding about a quart, I commenced pouring the water upon him, so that it might flow over his face, chest, and abdomen. It produced a decided shock; he gave a start, after which the muscular system became relaxed; the sheet dropped from his teeth, and the hands opened; respiration was more quickly performed, and he sobbed violently. I applied it a second time; he again started, sobbed, began to roll his eyes about and utter the most agonizing cries. He evidently knew me, and in a second or two begged of me not to douche him again; but as respiration was still slow, and the pulse weak, I continued, and found that after each application of the water he breathed quicker, and the pulse also became quicker and stronger. I now dissolved two scruples of the sulphate of zinc in a tea-cupful of warm water, and asked him to drink it, which he did very well. As soon as he had swallowed the emetic, ammonia, which I had sent for, on ascertaining that hydrocyanic acid had been takèn, was brought to me; it was very strong, and I applied it to the nostrils, and rubbed the temples and the palms of the hands with it. The pulse rose, and the face became red, and at each inspiration of the ammonia, the patient said, "Oh, I am better now; this has done me good;" indeed, he became very loquacious, and it was with difficulty he could be restrained. In about ten minutes, vomiting took place, and the ejected matter smelt so strongly of prussic acid, that it was almost impossible to remain near it. The pulse was now 90, and full; the countenance bloated, with redness of face; and he occasionally complained with crampy pain in his arms and legs, and said, "It is coming on again." I continued the application of the ammonia, and every minute or two caused him to inhale it. A vein was next opened in the arm, and sixteen or eighteen ounces of blood extracted, *pleno rivo.* It was of a dark color, and I thought at the time emitted the odor of prussic acid. Afterward I was convinced that it was an error, and that it arose from the room being so impregnate with the smell from the vomited matter. He occasionally complained of cramp in different parts of his body, but no other unfavorable symptoms followed. The patient had taken about 40 minims of prussic acid. *Part* xii., *p.* 124.

Poisoning by Prussic Acid.—[From an account of a case of poisoning by ·prussic acid, we extract the following, as being most interesting to the toxicologist.] A Jewess, aged 22, of generally good health, was ordered a mixture, to take a fourth part twice a day, for a pain in her side: and a lotion for chilblains was also given to her at the same time, which contained nearly four grains of anhydrous prussic acid. By mistake the labels were reversed, and a quarter of the lotion, containing little less than one grain of the pure poison, was taken. Death ensued in from fifteen to twenty minutes. Mr. Letheby obtained from the remainder of the lotion, amounting to about two ounces, 9.2 grains of cyanide of silver; this would indicate 1.85 grains of anhydrous prussic acid; and as half this quantity was taken, a dose equal to 45 or 50 drops of the medicinal acid, or 23 to 25 drops of Scheele's strength, were swallowed.

The principal points for consideration are the following: *The Dose.*— Here a little less than one grain of absolute hydrocyanic acid, diluted with one ounce of water, occasioned death in from fifteen to twenty minutes. It is the smallest fatal dose upon record; for although the Parisian epileptics are reported, in most of our works upon medical jurisprudence, to have been killed by about two-thirds of a grain of prussic acid, yet it is now proved beyond all doubt that they are in error, and that the quantity of anhydrous acid which each patient took was five and a half troy grains. We learn this from a letter recently received from Professor Guibort, and published in the "Pharmaceutical Journal" for May. How so egregious an error could have crept into our English works is past my comprehension. In reasoning, however, upon the present case, it does not appear to me that we are warranted in supposing that one grain of pure hydrocyanic acid would, under all circumstances, be sufficient to cause death; on the contrary, the experience of almost every one, to say nothing of the cases which are upon record against this conclusion, would suggest that, in this instance, it was an unusually small dose for such a fatal event; and I am led to think that its potency was increased by the empty condition of deceased's stomach. All that we can say, therefore, upon this case, is, that one grain of hydrocyanic acid may occasion death; we go beyond our warrant when we say it will.

[The immediate cause of death seems to be stoppage of respiration by the spasmodic condition of the muscles concerned in that act. The slow, laborious breathing, turgescence of the face and venous system generally, as well as the foaming at the mouth, support this opinion; and these symptoms so simulated epilepsy in the above that it was at first supposed she was laboring under such an attack.] *Part xii., p. 125.*

Poisoning by Hydrocyanic Acid.—Dash cold water on the patient; apply ammonia to the nostrils, and heat to the spine and feet; give an injection containing tincture of assafœtida, use friction with a flesh-brush to the skin; and as soon as the jaws become relaxed, and the patient can swallow, give an emetic, and afterward some weak brandy and water, and strong coffee. Mr. Gray would also cause the patient to inhale the fumes of ammonia, when he has ceased to be able to swallow.

Part xiii., p. 145.

Poisoning by Prussic Acid.—The rapidity of death does not always appear to be in proportion to the largeness of the dose, but modified by circumstances, such as idiosyncrasy, bodily strength, and the quantity of food in the stomach. There are some grounds even for thinking that beyond a certain dose the effects are not increased, that is to say, a dose far greater than a merely fatal dose does not produce more violent symptoms or speedy death than the exact poisonous dose. The medico-legal question of how long a person, after a poisonous dose, may have power and consciousness to perform acts of volition and motion, is of the highest importance, as from these acts principally can it be inferred whether death has been the result of suicide or murder. In the case of the trial of Belany for the murder of his wife, the medical opinions were strong that all volition would cease after the scream which has been considered as characteristic of poisoning by this substance. This may be quite correct where a scream does take place, but it is by no means so frequent a symptom as is commonly supposed. It does not appear to have been heard in the case of Sarah Hart; it did not occur in two cases reported by Mr. Hicks (Med. Gaz., 1845); nor in a case given by Mr. Nunneley (Prov. Med. and Surg. Jour., 1845).

A sufficient number of cases, however, are now on record, to prove that after large doses, viz.: from two drachms to four ounces of the medicinal acid of different countries, and consequently of a variety of strengths, relevant remarks may be made, and acts of volition and motion deliberately performed.

A gentleman at Bristol (1843), after swallowing half an ounce (Lon. Phar.)=five grains anhydrous acid, walked about sixty yards, articulated to an acquaintance several words distinctly and relevantly, and did not die for ten or twelve minutes. He gave no scream. A case is reported by Sobernheim of a young gentleman who took four ounces from two vials. He was found dead in bed, the clothes drawn up to his breast, his arms beneath the clothes, and on each side an empty two-ounce vial. In Mr. Nunneley's case, already referred to, a gentleman, after taking an ounce, appears to have walked or rather ran up a stair, was quite sensible, and spoke rationally for about five minutes, and lived three quarters of an hour.

There are no post-mortem appearances universally found after poisoning with prussic acid. The odor of the acid should be sought for both externally and internally; but it is not always appreciable externally as is shown by Sarah Hart's case. Internally, however, it can generally be detected within three or four days; occasionally it is altogether wanting, but these cases are rare. Among the most characteristic signs of poisoning by this drug should also be noticed, the calm and life-like appearance of the countenance, and the bright state of the eyes. There is also extreme fluidity of the blood, the veins being full and the arteries empty. The left auricle and ventricle of the heart are generally found empty, and sometimes all its cavities; but, in cases recorded by Mr. Nunneley, of Leeds, the heart was completely distended with dark fluid blood. The action of this powerful poison seems now generally acknowledged to be directly on the nervous system, to what tissue soever it be applied. Dr. Lonsdale's experiments have led him to conclude that, the immediate effects of the poison are exerted on the brain and spinal cord, and that the contractility of the heart is indirectly enfeebled, according to the dose, or whether the acid be in a pure or diluted state.

Part xiv., p. 115.

New Test for Prussic Acid.—The following method of testing for hydrocyanic acid is proposed by Mr. Austin, of Dublin. The precipitate of cyanide of silver, say half a grain, obtained in the usual manner, is mixed with a small quantity of oxide of iron and carbonate of potash, and the whole fused together in an iron or plantinum capsule. The fused mass is then dissolved in half an ounce of distilled water, filtered, and rendered slightly acid by the addition of a few drops of hydrochloric acid. The liquid thus treated is next divided into two portions, to one of which a few drops of a solution of sulphate of copper is added, which immediately causes the evolution of the chocolate-brown color, so characteristic of the ferrocyanide of copper; and to the other a few drops of the muriate tincture of iron, or any persalt of iron, when the solution becomes intensely blue by the formation of the ferrocyanide of iron, the ordinary prussian blue.

In Mr. Austin's opinion, "these two tests, with the well-known odor of prussic acid, are, independent of all others, sufficient to convince the medical jurist of the presence of free prussic acid."

The precipitates above mentioned are very distinctly obtained with half a grain of cyanide of silver.   *Part* xiv., *p.* 117.

LEAD.

By Salts of Lead.—*Hydrated Proto-Sulphuret of Iron*—suggested as an antidote in poisoning by the salts of lead. *Vide* Art. "Poisoning by Corrosive Sublimate."

Lead Poisoning.—In addition to the acid. sulph. aromat., mercury is exceedingly valuable in controlling the effects of, or removing this and other latent poisons from the body.   *Part* xxvi., *p.* 348.

Poisoning by Lead.—Dr. Goolden states that iodide of potassium in doses of 10 grains acts as a curative agent in lead poisoning, by converting the lead into a more soluble form, which can be readily taken up by the blood. It acts more rapidly in conjunction with galvanism.

In a case of aggravated paralysis from lead poisoning, but in which there was absence of colic, the following prescription was completely successful; Iodide of potassium, 5 grains; liquor of potassium, $\frac{1}{4}$ drachm; peppermint water, $1\frac{1}{2}$ ounces; three times a day. As the recovery progressed, it was observed that the blue margin of the gums gradually disappeared.

Part xxix., *p.* 326.

Poisoning by Lead, Mercury, Gold, Silver, or any other Metal—*MM. Poey and Vergnes' Electro-Chemical Bath.*—Place the patient on a wooden bench, in a metallic bathing-tub, isolated from the ground, and filled with water up to his neck. The water is made slightly acid with nitric or hydrochloric acid, if mercury, silver, or gold is in the system; and with sulphuric acid, if lead is suspected. The negative pole of a pile is then brought into contact with the sides of the bathing-tub, and the positive pole placed in the hands of the patient. The work of purification is now in full activity. The electrical current precipitates itself through the body of the sufferer, penetrates into the depth of his bones, pursues in all the tissues every particle of metal, seizes it, restores its primitive form, and chasing it out of the organism, deposits it on the sides of the tub, where it becomes apparent to the naked eye.   *Part* xxxi., *p.* 227.

Lead Poisoning.—Dr. Tunstall states, that when we have loss of power of the superior extremities, with corresponding loss of substance, without diminished sensation, if there be no evidence of cerebral mischief, we should suspect lead as the cause of the disease. The term paralysis should be restricted to those cases which have their origin in the brain or spinal cord; in lead atrophy the loss of power is dependent on loss of muscular substance, and differs from true paralysis in being gradual instead of sudden in its invasion. The treatment should consist of warm baths, electricity and friction. *Part* xxxiv., *p.* 298.

Drop-Wrist from Lead-Poisoning.—A case lately occurred at Charing-Cross Hospital, of a printer who had been the subject of this affection for only two days, resulting from absorption of lead, owing to the tips of the fingers being denuded by constantly handling new type. This case was cured completely in a week, by the patient sitting with his hand in a solution of sulphuret of potassium (ʒj..to ʒx.) for three hours three times a day. This acted from the great chemical affinities of sulphur and lead.

Part xxxvi., *p.* 46.

Lead Poisoning—Disease of the Sheffield File-Cutters.—During the process of cutlery, the file is placed upon a bed of lead, which rests upon an anvil. This lead is gradually worn away, and may be collected in considerable quantities in the form of fine black powder. The file-cutters' disease results from the absorption of a portion of this lead, as is common to file-cutters, painters, lead smelters, shot manufacturers, sheet-lead rollers, sugar-of-lead, red-lead, white-lead and litharge workers, compositors, plumbers, potters, sealing-wax makers, enamellers of German cards, color grinders, lead miners, etc.

Dr. J. C. Hall, says, that persons who work much in lead should use the bath daily, or if this be not obtainable, they should wash thoroughly the whole of the upper part of the body. The addition of about four ounces of sulphide of potassium to thirty gallons of water much increases the efficiency of the warm bath, causing a formation of sulphuret of lead. The habitual costiveness must be overcome by attention to diet, by the frequent use of injections, and by the administration of doses of sulphate of magnesia in infusion of roses. Iodide of potassium exerts a most powerful influence on the poison of lead; it should be taken fasting, that it may not be decomposed by acids, and it should be largely diluted. There is no evidence to show that sulphuric acid is an antidote to slow lead poisoning. The best means of purifying water from the contamination of lead, is by filtering it through sand and animal charcoal. *Part* xxxvi., *p.* 56.

OPIUM.

Poisoning by Laudanum—Novel Treatment.—A young female, aged 22, swallowed an ounce of laudanum. The ordinary symptoms soon succeeded. There was a state of almost perfect insensibility, the face livid and swollen, pulse slow, not exceeding 45 in a minute, and the jaws firmly shut. Dr. Buck saw her in about half an hour, and prying the mouth open, put into it 40 grains of ipecac., and as much of sulphate of zinc, in half a gill of water. He repeated this dose at intervals of ten or fifteen minutes, five times, using 200 grains of ipecac., and as much sulphate of zinc. It is doubtful, however, whether any was swallowed. In half an hour, as no change had occurred, he injected into the stomach, through an elastic catheter, twelve grains of tartar emetic dissolved in half a gill of water. After waiting half an hour, and perceiving no symptoms of an operation, he threw down 24 grains of tartar emetic. This in a short time induced a very feeble effort to vomit, and about half a gill of fluid was thrown up. But the symptoms became more alarming; the pulse was slower, and the face extremely livid, while respiration was nearly extinct. He now threw down sixty grains of sulphate of zinc dissolved in half a pint of water, but without any sensible effect.

"Under these circumstances, seeing that there was no prospect of making her vomit by any ordinary means, I was resolved to make an experiment. I injected a pint of vinegar into the stomach, and immediately after it, a large teaspoon four times heaped full of salæratus, dissolved in half a pint of warm water. The effect was instantaneous. It broke forth foaming from the mouth in a stream of the full size of that orifice, with such a force as to be projected a yard or more. The quantity thrown up I judged to be at least a quart, in a state of complete effervescence. In about fifteen minutes, as there was no further vomiting, I repeated the operation, using but half the quantity of vinegar with the same quantity of salæratus and water, with the same immediate effect, and then left her for the night, with directions to give her freely strong green tea, if she should recover sufficiently to drink.

"Next morning found her much prostrated, had vomited several times during the night, but was perfectly rational. She gradually recovered."

Part v., *p.* 75.

Poisoning by Morphia.— Coffee as an Antidote.—To relieve himself of a severe attack of toothache, Dr. Fosgate swallowed in solution one and a quarter grain of the sulphate of morphia, equal to about seven and a half grains of solid opium. In about half an hour, a sensation of thickening and rigidity of the muscles of the back of the neck came on, and gradually extended itself to all the flexors of the limbs. In about five hours severe nausea succeeded, accompanied by efforts to vomit. Tea and sour cider increased the efforts to vomit so much that the stomach rejected fluids the moment they reached it, so that the second mouthful could not be swallowed before the first was rejected. Prostration of strength and apathy, with full slow pulse, and pricking sensation of the skin, were added to the other symptoms which were continually increasing in severity, when coffee was proposed. One gill of cold strong infusion of coffee was swallowed, and was retained about five minutes; the distressing symptoms, however, were by it abated, the nausea in part subdued, as was also the sensation of rigidity of the muscles; and the occasional repetition of this simple remedy during the course of the night completely removed all the distressing symptoms. Dr. Fosgate states, that whilst suffering from the severe nausea, but previous to the exhibition of the coffee, his mind was depressed, and he felt considerable anxiety, no pleasurable sensations or reveries having been felt. But after the draughts of coffee, the depression of mind and all anxiety vanished, and there succeeded that exquisite revelling of the imagination so much sought after by the opium eater. This state continued for five or six hours, and was succeeded by sound sleep, on awaking from which he experienced a few hours of lassitude. The morphia had been taken after eighteen hours' fasting. *Part* v., *p.* 62.

Poisoning by Opium or Belladonna.—Opium and belladonna are mutually remedial, when either has entered the circulation in a poisonous dose. From this cause, if both be prescribed together, as with a view to lull cerebral excitement, the effect desired will not be produced, whilst if either be given separately it will. In cases of poisoning by opium, give a solution of belladonna—say a drachm of the tincture every half-hour, or, if it cannot be swallowed, inject it subcutaneously. Conversely, in a case of poisoning by belladonna, opium may be used. Several cases are recorded in a paper by Benjamin Bell, illustrating this subject.

Part xxxviii., *p.* 244.

Narcotic Poisoning—Cold Douche.—In narcotic poisoning, this application is indicated urgently, but here it must be perseveringly repeated, not relinquished on a little trial. The great source of danger clearly consists in the blood being no longer duly oxygenated, through deficient or temporarily suspended breathing. The brain, therefore, becomes doubly influenced—primarily, by the narcotic, secondly, by venous blood. In an instance witnessed under the care of Mr. West, of Turnbridge, occurring in an infant who had accidentally swallowed a large quantity of opium, and was so affected by it that there was the completest coma, a pallid countenance, livid lips, and fearful pauses in the respiration and circulation, this remedy was given a fair trial. No sooner was it used than inspiration followed, and scarcely was it desisted from ere it became needful to resort to it again. Friction was had recourse to at intervals, that the warmth of the surface might be preserved. A sort of artificial respiration was kept up until natural breathing returned, and the cerebrum awoke from its lethargy. The nerves of the skin were made to play that part, which under ordinary circumstances the vagi nerves perform (through the stimulus of carbonic acid), and so life was continued, and a perfect recovery ensued.

Part viii., *p.* 45.

Electricity in Poisoning by Laudanum.—A case of this description is recorded by Mr. Corfe. The patient had taken an ounce and a half of laudanum the preceding evening, and on his admittance into the Middlesex Hospital, was to all appearance a lifeless corpse; and after all the more ordinary remedies had been tried in vain, Mr. Corfe thought of the electromagnetic battery, conjointly with electricity. After this had been acting upon him for a time the pulse became more steady, firm, and frequent, and the respirations more indicative of resuscitation. A powerful electrical machine was also got into full play before a large fire: brilliant sparks and strong shocks were occasionally passed through the head, spine, thorax, and abdomen. By these means the whole body was thrown into violent and convulsive succussions and muscular contortions. The patient recovered.

Part ix., *p.* 78.

By Opium.—Dr. Lancaster advises, after the use of the stomach-pump, to give coffee, and pass currents from the electro-magnetic apparatus through the shoulders, chest, abdomen, arms, and legs. In some cases, cold affusion will be beneficial. Such remedies as ammonia should not be given but under the most urgent circumstances. *Part* xix., *p.* 218.

Laudanum, Poisoning by.—In a case of poisoning by laudanum, in an infant, Dr. Herapath excited respiration by galvanism, by placing the zinc or positive wire on the mucous membrane of the mouth, and the negative or copper wire just below the ensiform cartilage. The current seemed to enter by the fifth nerve, from this to the medulla oblongata, then along the phrenic and external respiratory and spinal nerves to the diaphragm, and the inter-

costal and other accessory muscles of the respiratory apparatus. If the positive or zinc wire slipped from the cheek to the tongue, the movements became more gasping and convulsive—another set of nerves becoming
influenced. *Part* xxv., *p.* 317.

Poisoning by Laudanum.—To evacuate the stomach speedily and
effectually, introduce into it a quantity of carbonate of soda, followed by
vinegar. The effervescence is so powerful that all the contents of the
viscus are discharged. If emetics have before been taken ineffectually, they
begin now to act. *Part* xxvi., *p.* 348.

Poisoning by Opium—Use of Belladonna.—Belladonna has been found
useful in poisoning by opium. When the patient is comatose and other
remedies fail, try the following: tincture of belladonna, six drachms in five
and a half ounces of water. Take an ounce of this every half hour, till
the coma begins to disappear, or till the pupils dilate. In another severe
case, one ounce of the tincture of belladonna was given at once, in three
ounces of water ; in half an hour two drachms more were given.
Part xxix., *p.* 326.

Use of Belladonna in Poisoning by Opium.—Dr. Graves first suggested, that in continued fever, with contracted pupils and coma, if an
agent administered internally would occasion dilatation of the pupils, it
might also relieve the other symptoms of cerebral derangement.

For cases of Poisoning by Opium.—Always have ready the following
preparation of belladonna : take four ounces of the leaves of belladonna,
and two pints of rectified spirit, and percolate. Of this give six drachms
in doses of about one drachm every half hour.

In one case, ten drachms of the above tincture of belladonna were given
in the course of one hour with success. *Part* xxx., *p.* 301.

Narcotic Poisoning.—Dr. Marshall Hall's " Ready Method."—When
from the degree of narcotism all ordinary remedies fail in inducing vomiting, and the stomach pump is not at hand, place the patient on a table,
with the head projecting beyond its edge, if possible ; if not, on the floor ;
and being placed on the *side*, the finger of one person is to be introduced
into the fauces, whilst the body is briskly and repeatedly rolled into the
prone position by another ; thus mechanical vomiting will be produced,
and the poison expelled. But supposing the narcotism is too deep for the
success of this manœuvre, volition has ceased, and that the patient can no
longer be made to move or walk about—that all physiological respiration
has ceased—we must long and perseveringly employ the " Ready Method "
to continue respiratory movements till the poison is eliminated from the
blood.—*Vide* Art. "Drowning." *Part* xxxv., *p.* 49.

ŒNANTHE CROCATA.

[Several melancholy cases of poisoning by this plant (hemlock dropwort)
are related by Mr. Bossey. Several convicts were at work in the Royal Ar-
senal at Woolwich, and mistook the plant for celery. They ate a considerable
quantity, and were soon attacked with the most violent symptoms, strong convulsions in paroxysms, with insensibility. In the more violent cases the face
was bloated and livid, the foam about the mouth was sanguineous, the breathing stertorous and convulsive, pupils dilated and insensible, with most of
the other symptoms of apoplexy. These cases died. In others, the symp-

toms were milder, and recovery took place. These were able to swallow emetics of salt and mustard with warm water, by means of which they vomited freely and ejected a large quantity of imperfectly masticated root, and were thereby greatly relieved. The convulsions ceased, sensation and reason were restored, but there remained giddiness, pallor of the face, dilated pupils, coldness of the extremities, much weakness, severe rigors, and a slow feeble pulse.]

Further vomiting was promoted, and more of the root discharged. Friction and warmth were applied to the extremities, whilst ammonia and rum, with thin gruel and other drinks, were administered internally, till reaction was more fully established.

Emetic doses of the sulphate of zinc and copper, and also mustard and water, were given without effect to the patients lying on the deck of the vessel. They were also bled very largely both from the arms and jugular veins. The introduction into and removal of warm water from the stomach by the pump, brought away small portions of the noxious roots. Cold affusions upon the head being perseveringly used, lessened the struggling, and produced some exhaustion. In three cases the subsequent fits became less violent; they passed into a state of maniacal delirium, with much jactitation of the limbs, and after some hours were removed into the hospital. But in one more patient all these remedies were ineffectual: he died convulsed, at a quarter before one o'clock. As a last effort, the trachea was carefully opened by an incision, and artificial respiration kept up, but life was quite extinct.

Several of the men who had eaten the root, seeing the others suffer, took the salt water emetic with success, and had no symptoms of being poisoned.

The first indication of treatment was doubtless to evacuate the stomach; but, as its sensibility was destroyed, and the poison was taken in the solid form, this could not readily be accomplished. Large and immediate depletion seemed to be essentially useful, by removing the imminent danger of extravasation from over-distention of the vessels; the cold affusion was also beneficial in rousing the patient, so as to make him sensible to the emetics, and so were purgatives during the after-treatment.

Called thus in a moment to so many urgent cases of poisoning, it became needful to use such remedies as were at hand; but, upon reflection, it seems to me proper, in similar circumstances, to rely chiefly on emetics given early, on large blood-letting *immediately* employed, and the cold affusion. *Part* x., *p.* 90.

STRYCHNIA.

Tannin, as an Antidote. — In a case where strychnia had been incautiously taken by the patient to the amount of half a grain in six hours, and where the symptoms were becoming exceedingly dangerons, Dr. Ludicke ordered ice to be applied to the head, and half a grain of tannic acid to be given every hour, either in an effervescing draught or in distilled water. After twelve grains had been taken, he substituted for it a decoction of two ounces of oak bark in six ounces of water, with an ounce of sirup of cinnamon and a scruple of sulphuric ether. The symptoms of poisoning entirely disappeared. Mesner, in Dresden, recommends as an antidote for strychnine, decoction of galls or of oak bark; five ounces of which precipitate two grains of nitrate of strychnine. *Part* vi., *p.* 85.

Electricity in Poisoning by Strychnine.—The following statement is deserving of further investigation: M. Duclos has instituted a series of experiments on rabbits, dogs, and guinea-pigs. He poisoned these animals with strychnine and brucine, and then electrified them, and found that, on application of the negative electricity excited by means of an electrical machine, the symptoms of poisoning subsided, and the animals were saved; the positive electricity, on the contrary, increased the muscular contraction produced by the poison, and hastened death. Animals which had been poisoned with arsenious acid could not only not be saved by electrifying them, but were killed sooner, whether positive or negative electricity was employed.   *Part* ix., *p.* 83.

Purified Animal Charcoal as an Antidote to all Vegetable and some Mineral Poisons.—This substance, says Dr. Garrod, may be used as an antidote to opium and its active principles, morphia, etc.; nux vomica and its active principles, strychnia and brucia; henbane, deadly nightshade, bitter sweet, thorn apple, tobacco, hemlock, bitter almonds, prussic acid, the aconites, etc.; in fact, to all vegetable poisons—to animal also, as cantharides. The carbo animalis purificatus of the pharmacopœia should be used, and in the proportion of half an ounce to a grain of morphia, strychnia, etc. It combines with and renders inert vegetable and animal substances, and absorbs some mineral poisons, especially arsenic, and renders them harmless, and exerts no injurious effects on the body.

It should be rubbed in lukewarm water, so as to form a fluid of slight consistency, and thus given in quantities of from one to four ounces. Emetics also should be given: ipecacuanha, however, will not do, as the charcoal renders it inert. Give sulphate of zinc in scruple or half drachm doses, or use the stomach-pump, and then give more of the charcoal.

Might not this substance be tried to prevent the injurious effects of animal poisons, such as rabies, syphilis, poison of serpents, etc., applied in the form of poultice to the parts?   *Part* xiii., *p.* 142.

Chloroform in Poisoning by Strychnine.—A case, under the care of Dr. Munson, in which all the symptoms of poisoning by strychnine were present, was very successfully treated by the inhalation of chloroform.
                                                      Part xxii., *p.* 329.

Poisoning by Strychnine.—In a case of poisonous symptoms being induced from an over-dose of strychnine given in mistake, the following prescription gave immediate relief: Twenty-four grains of camphor were dissolved in six ounces of almond mixture, one-fourth to be taken every two hours.   *Part* xxvi., *p.* 348.

Test for Strychnia.—Mr. Maxwell Simpson, in a note to the editor of the "Dublin Hospital Gazette," says: I think it right to make it publicly known that strychnia is not the only substance that will produce a purple color when brought into contact with a mixture of bichromate of potash and oil of vitriol, the test usually relied on for the detection of this poison. I have found that naphthalidam, an organic base derived from naphthalin, will produce, as might have been expected, an exactly similar color when tested with the same mixture. The color is best brought out by making a mixture of equal volumes of oil of vitriol and a cold saturated solution of bichromate of potash, and bringing it, while still warm, into momentary contact with a particle of the naphthalidam.   *Part* xxxiii., *p.* 309.

Strychnia and Woorali.—These two poisons, according to Dr. Pavy, of Guy's Hospital, have the effect of reciprocally neutralizing the action of each other, according as the one or the other is in excess. Frogs poisoned with woorali, when flaccid and insensible, very soon become tetanic if strychnia be injected; and on the other hand, if poisoned with strychnia and afterward punctured with woorali, the tetanus speedily disappears. When treated in this way, they will recover from a larger dose of each than would be sufficient to destroy life, if either were given alone. Thus it would appear that the one might be used as an antidote for the other.

Part xxxiv., *p.* 301.

Strychnia, Tests for.—Dr. Harley, of University College, London, says: The physiological test is the most reliable. If 1-8000th of a grain be injected into the thoracic cavity of a frog, it will become tetanic in ten or fifteen minutes. In order to apply any of the tests, we must first have the strychnia in a pure state. Suppose an animal has been poisoned with the smallest possible quantity, take the blood from the heart and large vessels, mix it with twice its bulk of water, coagulate by boiling, acidify with acetic acid, decolorize by filtering through crystals of sulphate of soda or animal charcoal, concentrate the filtrate, add potash to precipitate the strychnia, purify and apply the tests. Strychnia seems to produce death by destroying muscular irritability, and rendering the tissues unable to absorb oxygen and exhale carbonic acid. . . . . . One part of bichromate of potash dissolved in fourteen parts of water, to which two parts of sulphuric acid are afterward added, is the most delicate and certain test for strychnia. When added to a suspected solution, if strychnia be present, it will be precipitated in the form of a beautiful golden-colored insoluble chromate. The crystals are immediately formed. A single half grain of strychnia, although divided into millions of atoms of crystals each, will demonstrate the presence of strychnia as well as if a pound weight of it were operated upon. (Mr. Horsley.)

To do away with all possible sources of fallacy from the action of external re-agents, you must put a little strychnia, with sulphuric acid, on a piece of platinum foil, and then connect the foil with the positive pole of a single cell of a Grove's or Smee's battery, and, by touching the acid with the negative pole terminating in a piece of platinum wire, the characteristic violet color is instantly produced. In operating on the contents of the stomach, acidify them with acetic acid, dilute if necessary with water, and filter; evaporate this on a water-bath to the consistence of a thin paste, add eight or ten times its bulk of cold alcohol, filter and distill so that the spirit may not be lost. The residue, after the evaporation of all the spirit, must be diluted with water, filtered again, and super-saturated with liq. potassæ. Shake this with its own bulk of ether, and allow the two solutions to separate, decant the clear ethereal solution, and treat the aqueous residue with a fresh quantity of ether, and so a third time, if necessary. The ethereal solution must be distilled to remove the ether, and the residue dissolved out of the retort with a small quantity of diluted acetic acid and filtered; treat again with potash and ether, and after the spontaneous evaporation of the ether, the alkaloid will be sufficiently pure to be identified. (Prof. Letheby.) *Part* xxxiv. *p.* 305–315.

Poisoning by Strychnine.—Professor Haughton of Dublin, is of opinion that nicotine and strychnine are mutually antidotes to each other's action.

He has performed some very interesting experiments on this subject. The nicotine is always easily procurable in the form of tobacco leaf infusion.

Part xxxv., *p.* 277.

Tests for Strychnine.—It is known that peroxide of lead, peroxide of manganese and chromate of potassa will each of them produce a red color when added to a mixture of strychnine and sulphuric acid.

Mr. Lindo considers the red color produced by these three tests is in every instance referable to the same cause—namely, the separation of the hydrogen from the strychnine; that, when the metallic peroxides are used, they are converted into protoxides, which combine with sulphuric acid when the chromate of potassa is employed; that the chromic acid is converted into oxide of chrome, which combines with sulphuric acid; and that the oxygen liberated in each case takes hydrogen from the strychnine, forming water, the reaction being partly induced by the affinity of sulphuric acid for water.   *Part* xxxv., *p.* 280.

Camphor, in poisoning by Strychnine.—Give two grains of powdered camphor, with half a teaspoonful of tincture of camphor, every quarter of an hour, if necessary, a little morphia may be added. Two cases are reported by Dr. Rochester, which were successfully treated in this way.

*   *   *   *   *   *   *   *

A case of poisoning by strychnia, is related by Dr. Pritchard of Filey, Yorkshire, in which from three to five grain lumps of camphor were successfully administered. Emetics and the stomach pump were employed, and artificial respiration by Dr. Marshall Hall's ready method was necessary at one part of the tetanic spasms. Toward the decline of the tetanic movements, which lasted about twenty minutes, the camphor was continued with opium.   *Part* xxxv., *p.* 342.

Strychnine— Dectection of.—Messrs. Rodgers and Girdwood, from a carefully conducted series of experiments, have come to the following conclusions: That strychnine can be detected even when it has not been given in excess; that it is not decomposed in the body; that it is found unchanged in the urine; and can be detected in the blood, organs, and tissues of the body, quite independently of the contents of the stomach. It is more easily detected than any other poison, from the delicacy of its reactions, and from its extraordinary stable qualities.

The process itself is as follows: The substance to be operated upon is digested with dilute hydrochloric acid, 1 to 10, until it is apparently fluid; the liquid is then filtered and evaporated to dryness over a water-bath; what remains, treated with spirit as long as anything can be dissolved, and the filtered tincture evaporated as before. The residue must now be dissolved in water and filtered.

This aqueous solution is to be rendered alkaline by ammonia and agitated in a bottle, or long tube, with about $\frac{1}{2}$ an ounce of chloroform. After subsidence, the chloroform is drawn off by means of a pipette, transferred to an evaporating basin, and expelled over a water-bath; the residue left on the basin must then be moistened with concentrated sulphuric acid, and exposed for some hours to the temperature of a water-bath, by which proceeding, all organic matter except the strychnine is destroyed. The charred mass is then treated with water, and the solution filtered to separate the carbon; excess of ammonia is added and the solution again agitated with about 1 drachm of chloroform. If, on evaporating a small portion of this chloroform solution, and acting upon the residue with concentrated sulphuric acid, any charring takes place, the foregoing process must be repeated.

The chloroform solution will afford strychnine sufficiently pure for conclusive testing. For this purpose, a small quantity is taken up in a capillary tube, and evaporated by adding successive drops, on the smallest possible space of a warm porcelain capsule. If the quantity of strychnine in the solution is large, say the 1-2000th of a grain or more, the method pursued in using the reagent is similar to that adopted by others, viz. moistening the spot, when the capsule is quite cold, with concentrated sulphuric acid, and then adding a minute fragment of bichromate of potash. When, however, the quantity is very small, no color will be perceived by this mode of testing. Under such circumstances, sulphuric acid, rendered slightly yellow by chromic acid, is said to be found successful.

We may, in conclusion, enjoin a caution against two sources of failure in conducting this test. The common recommendation to stir the spot moistened with sulphuric acid, with a glass rod before the addition of bichromate is to be avoided, because the acid sulphate of strychnine may so be removed altogether; and the operator must be careful not to expose the matter under examination to an intense light, as in his anxiety to watch the color changes he is too apt to do, the effect of light, in more than moderate amount, being to suspend the chemical reactions.

Part xxxvi., *p.* 282.

Poisoning by Strychnia—Inhalation of Chloroform.—A case occurred lately in Boston in which violent tetanic spasms, produced by swallowing two grains of strychnia, were completely subdued in ten minutes by Dr. Jewett, by the administration of chloroform. The patient recovered rapidly. *Part* xxxvii., *p.* 257.

Poisoning by Strychnia.—The poison of strychnia is completely neutralized by nicotine. In a case of poisoning by the former, Dr. O'Reilly of St. Louis, U. S. recommends to take a cigar and infuse it in half a pint of water, which give in doses of one tablespoonful every five minutes. Probably, when half the quantity is taken a favorable change will be noticed the muscles will have become relaxed, the spasms less severe, and the intervals between them longer. The infusion may then be given less frequently. Of course, in a healthy person, such quantities of tobacco internally administered would produce serious effects; but in this case its effects are antagonized. *Part* xxxviii., *p.* 238.

Antidote to.—Dr. Bewley, wishing to kill a mangy cur, and having read in Magendie's "Report on Strychnia," that the sixteenth of a grain will kill the largest dog, determined to make sure of this very little animal by giving it about half a grain. But either Magendie's statement was incorrect, or the drug was adulterated, for at the end of ten minutes the dog, though suffering frightfully, was not dead. Dr. Bewley resolved to put him out of his misery at once, and accordingly mixed half a drachm of prussic acid with a little milk, and put it under the dog's snout. He lapped the milk with avidity, and in less than a minute vomited, got upon his legs, ran away, and recovered. *Part* xl., *p.* 278.

Poisoning by Strychnine.—Action of wourali poison. *Vide* Art. "Tetanus."

Poisoning by Strychnine.—A case of poisoning by strychnine is related by Dr. Bennett, of Sydney, in which apparently iodine conduced toward recovery. He explains its action by its forming an insoluble hydriodate of strychnine.   *Part* xl., *p.* 315.

UPAS ANTIAR.

Poison of the.—[This energetic poison has not been examined since the beginning of the present century. It is obtained from Borneo and Java.]

The following are the principal results obtained by Professor Albert Kölliker, in his experiments with frogs.

1. That antiar is a paralyzing poison.

2. It acts in the first instance and with great rapidity (in 5 to 10 minutes) upon the heart, and stops its action.

3. The consequences of this paralysis of the heart are the cessation of the voluntary and reflex movements in the first and second hour after the introduction of the poison.

4. The antiar paralyzes in the second place the voluntary muscles.

5. In the third place it causes the loss of excitability of the great nervous trunks.

6. The heart and muscles of frogs poisoned with urali may be paralyzed by antiar.

7. From all this it may be deduced, that the antiar principally acts upon the muscular fibre and causes paralysis of it.   *Part* xxxvii., *p.* 256.

YEW–BERRIES.

Poisoning by.—[As cases of poisoning by the berries of the yew (taxus baccata) are rare, and as some writers have denied the poisonous nature of the tree altogether, the following case by Dr. James Taylor, of Castle Cary, becomes interesting.]

October 28th, 1838. Mary Baker, a fine healthy child, between five and six years of age, ate freely of yew-berries just before going into church. About an hour after, during divine service, she fell from her seat and was instantly removed in an insensible state to her home. I saw her immediately; the surface of the body was cold; the countenance pale; breathing laborious and frequent; pupils very dilated; pulse feeble; convulsions and vomiting. Having carefully examined the head, and finding that it was not injured by the fall, I gave an emetic, and from what was ejected it was evident she had eaten a considerable quantity of the berries; not the mucous part only, but the seeds, wherein I believe is the most active principle of the berry, for the mucous or fleshy part of the berry has been frequently eaten with impunity. As soon as it appeared the stomach had been freed of its contents, a purgative was given, and had the desired effect, but the child never rallied from the first. She continued in a comatose state, and died in *four hours* after eating the berries. An inquest was held, but no post-mortem examination allowed. I stated, in my evidence, I considered yew-berries poisonous, and that the child's death had been occasioned by them, but I remember several of the jury were very skeptical on the point.   *Part* xix., *p.* 218.

ZINC.

Poisoning with Chloride of.—Dr. Thomas Stratton relates two cases of poisoning with chloride of zinc. In both cases a wine-glassful of solution was swallowed, containing in one case about twelve grains of the salt, and in the other about two hundred grains. In the latter case, burning pain in the gullet, burning and griping pain in the stomach, great nausea, and sense of coldness were instantly felt. Vomiting followed in a few minutes. Dr. Stratton saw this patient twenty minutes after the accident, and instantly made a strong solution of home-made brownish soap, of which he made the patient swallow at intervals, three or four pints. Afterward olive oil was given, and the patient recovered. The other case was not seen by any medical man; but it also terminated favorably. Dr. Stratton suggests either soap or carbonate of soda or of potash, as antidotes to chloride of zinc.   *Part* xix., *p.* 218.

POLYPI.

OF THE EAR.

Mr. Wilde, in his treatise on the "Causes and Treatment of Otorrhœa," observes:

The last cause and complication of otorrhœa is what I have throughout this paper denominated polypus. Fleshy, pedunculated, morbid growths in the ear, nearly colorless, having a thin cuticular covering, unattended by pain, not appearing as the result of inflammation, and unaccompanied by discharge, I have seen, but such cases, in comparison with those to which I have so frequently alluded, and now refer, are extremely rare. Throughout this essay I have constantly employed the terms fungus and polypus as indicative of these morbid growths, the product of inflammatory action, and long-continued otorrhœa. By fungus, however, I particularly allude to those vascular and granular masses which generally grow either from diseased bone, or upon the destruction, in the whole or in part, of the membrana tympani, and whose attachments are to be found p   p   in the very bottom of the auditory passage; while polypi are, for the most part, confined to the glandulo-ceruminous portion of the tube, and are attached by narrower roots than the fungi. It is stated in books that polypi are smooth on their surface, while fungi are lobulated. Here, however, is a very good specimen of a polypus removed from the posterior wall of the glandular portion of the meatus, presenting such characters. In many instances polypi may be coexisting with granular tympani or fungous masses proceeding from the middle ear. Generally the polypus grows more externally, that is, appears at the external orifice, while the fungus is mostly confined to the bottom of the tube. The latter may, however, appear externally.

The instrument of greatest value for the removal of aural polypus from any portion of the meatus, is the small snare-like apparatus consisting of a fine steel stem, five inches in length, with a movable bar sliding on the.

square portion toward the handle; in a properly-constructed instrument the small upper extremity, flattened out and perforated with holes running parallel with the stem, should not exceed the fourteenth of an inch in its greatest diameter. A fine silver, or what is much better, from its greater flexibility and strength, a fine platina wire, with its extremities fastened to the cross bar at the handle, passes through the holes in the flattened end of the small extremity of the instrument, and allowed to be of such a length as, that when the bar is drawn back close to the handle, this ligature is put fully on the stretch, and drawn tight through the holes at the small extremity. In using it, the cross bar is pushed forward and a noose made of the wire at the small extremity, of sufficient size to include the morbid growth, which it is then made to surround, and toward the root of which it is pressed by means of the stem; the cross bar is then drawn up smartly to the handle, and it never fails of either cutting across, or of drawing with it whatever was included in the noose. Some bleeding generally follows, which should be allowed to subside, then syringe the parts with slightly tepid water, and again examine the ear, and if possible discover what portion of the polypus may remain, which, whether it may be the mere point of attachment, or a portion unaccessible to instruments, should be invariably touched with the armed *port-caustic,* and the same application applied from day to day, until all traces of the morbid growth are vanished. Unless this latter point of practice be strictly and perseveringly adhered to, it is in vain that we can expect a total eradication of the disease; no more, however, of the auditory apparatus should be submitted to the action of the caustic than the actually vascular, granulating, or fungous surface. I have frequently witnessed the whole canal in a state of ulceration, and an erysipelatous inflammation extending over the entire auricle, from a large stick of lunar caustic having been inserted into, and rolled round in the meatus to remove a polypus or fungus growth, the eradication of which had already been frequently attemped by instruments; a practice as cruel as it was ineffectual. *Part* ix., *p.* 162.

Ear Polypi.—For the removal of these growths Mr. Toynbee uses a kind of ringed forceps, each blade of the forceps having a ring at the extremity instead of teeth. By this the structure is not broken up, and the growth has a better chance of being removed by the roots.
Part xxix., *p.* 257

Polypus of the External Meatus.—In all cases of discharge occurring from the external meatus, says Dr. Toynbee, the first step is to use a syringe so as thoroughly to cleanse the meatus. When this has been done, there is no difficulty in determining whether a polypus be present, although it may be situated close to the membrana tympani. Polypi occurring in the external meatus may be divided into three classes.

1. The one of most frequent occurrence, which may be called the raspberry polypus.
2. That which has been termed the gelatinous polypus.
3. The globular polypus.

The cellular raspberry polypus is most frequently met with, and consists of numbers of round beads, somewhat similar in appearance to the free surface of the raspberry. These beads are attached by means of small filaments, to a central stem, which forms the root. It is frequently covered by ciliated epithelium, and when examined microscopically its interior is found to be composed of small rounded cells. It is usually so soft that, upon being taken hold of by the ordinary dressing forceps, it breaks up and bleeds freely. The raspberry polypus varies much in size ; sometimes it is not larger than a grain or two of mustard seed, at others it fills the whole of the meatus and projects from the orifice. The parts of the meatus to which this kind of polypus is attached are very various ; as a general rule they are attached to the inner half of the tube, and frequently close to the membrana tympani. When small, their color is usually a deep red ; but when they increase in size they become more pale, and the rounded masses considerably increase in size. The formation of these polypi is often attended with considerable pain and by a discharge of blood. It is not uncommon for this polypus to remain undisturbed during several years, the whole of which time it throws off a most offensive secretion without producing symptoms sufficiently urgent to induce the patient to apply for relief ; in other cases the head symptoms arc so distressing as to cause serious alarm. These polypi are usually the result of irritation in the tympanic cavity and they are frequently symptomatic of obstruction of the eustachian tube.

The treatment of polypi by astringent applications, has no beneficial effect ; the same remark applies to the use of the nitrate of silver, whether solid or in solution. The potassa cum calce answers the best of anything, and if made to contain a small quantity of iron, it is firmer, much less deliquescent, and may be more readily applied than the usual form. The first step in the proceeding is, to syringe out the meatus with tepid water, and dry it with cotton wool ; then place the patient in a strong light, pass a glass tube down to the polypus to protect the meatus, and press the end gently against the polypus, so that it may fully occupy the distal part of the tube, the potass cum calce must then be introduced and kept in contact with the polypus for half a minute; this will scarcely give any pain, but if it should happen to touch the surface of the meatus, the pain will be very acute, the tube must therefore be allowed to remain for a few minutes, the meatus must then be syringed out, to wash away the little oozing of blood, etc. On inspecting the polypus, it will be seen to present a pulpy, uneven mass of a dark livid color. As a general rule, the potass may be applied daily in the same manner until the whole of the mass is destroyed. *Part* xxxv., *p.* 147.

OF THE NOSE.

Gelatinous Polypus.—If Dr. Lewis Shaw's method of removing the gelatinous polypus from the nose be found efficacious, it will certainly be an improvement on the more ordinary methods of excision, extraction, ligature and caustics. He powders very finely the sanguinaria canadensis, and causes it to be snuffed up the nostril, and the throat to be gargled with a strong infusion. In one case, by repeatedly using these means, the polypus broke in twenty-four hours, and discharged a considerable quantity of gelatinous fluid. The remedy was continued till the whole inner surface of the nose was made raw, and occasionally afterward. As the case, however, has not been watched a sufficient time, we could not depend upon the treatment. The sanguinaria canadensis is one of the best known acronarcotics of the poppy tribe. *Part* vii., *p.* 215.

Polypus of the Nose.—In the higher classes of society polypus of the nose is not an uncommon affection. It is frequently nothing more than a peculiar excrescence of the Schneiderian membrane, which is not malignant. It is a tumor connected generally by a thin neck to this membrane, or by a narrow pedicle, or a long thin membrane continuous with Schneiderian, but less vascular.

The polypus is very smooth, and but little vascular, though sometimes vessels burrow into it. It is gelatinous in density, and appears to consist of coagulated albumen. In a few instances there is but one polypus ; but commonly there are two or three, and frequently clusters, so that we can scarcely count them. The color, which it is essential to notice, is pearl-like or white, mixed with brown, of an opal appearance. Soft polypi of this kind, Sir B. Brodie has never seen attached to the septum nasi, the inferior turbinated bone, or any part of the nostril, but almost always to the cells of the ethmoid bone, though occasionally to the superior turbinated bone.

There is at first merely an unnatural secretion of mucus, often without pain—the smell is affected or even disappears, and even the taste may become considerably impaired. The symptoms may go on for years, while the polypus may go on increasing and become more solid, the base being at last almost cartilaginous. It may increase even to come down outside the nostril, or may descend down to the pharynx, behind the soft palate, of the size of the fist.

What is the best way of removing a polypus from the nose ? A ligature can seldom be applied properly ; neither can the operation be safely done with the knife, and seldom with the scissors. The forceps, made for this purpose, is no doubt. the best instrument. The whole of the opposite surfaces of the blades ought to be quite rough, convex above, concave below, opening laterally ; sometimes opening from above downward. The forceps should be oiled and warmed, the polypus caught by the base, and the instrument cautiously closed. The part should then be not only pulled forward, but twisted a little to each side and then pushed backward—again twisted a few times, first in one direction and then another, and at last it should be pulled forward with some force, when it will generally come away entire. It is too often the case that when the neck of the polypus is laid hold of by the forceps, the surgeon suddenly extracts, without the repeated twistings in all directions so strongly recommended by Sir B. Brodie. It is owing to the neglect of this simple procedure that a great portion of the polypus is often left behind. When the diseased part has been removed, Sir B. Brodie recommends that the parts should be painted over every day, by means of a camel's hair brush, with white precipitate ointment. The unguent, hydrarg. nitrat. diluted may also be used, but this causes more irritation than the white precipitate, and does not answer so well. The white precipitate ointment should be applied regularly, not for a few days or weeks, but for years. This should be done effectually ; not by just brushing over the parts which are most external, but by smearing the whole surface of the nostril both upward and backward, even as far as the pharynx. Astringent lotions may also be used, as zinc or alum. Sometimes the polypus is of a more fleshy nature and attached to the nose by a narrow neck, like those of the uterus and rectum. When this is the case it may be snipped off with a pair of probe-pointed scissors, slightly curved. Nitrate of silver may be applied to the part, and it is probable that it may never reappear. Some polypi, however, it is absolutely necessary to remove by ligature; as in a case related by Sir B. Brodie, in which there was an enormous tumor projecting the velum pendulum palati forward to the mouth, so that the finger could only just reach its lower margin.

In such a case there would be great difficulty in applying a ligature, and it would be evident at once that it would be almost impossible to remove the mass either by the forceps or the scissors. Sir Benjamin Brodie recommends that a bougie be passed into that nostril from which the polypus is supposed to rise, and pushed forward into the pharynx. The finger is then to be passed to the back of the throat, and the bougie bent so as to bring one end out at the mouth, to which is to be fastened a double ligature. The bougie is then withdrawn from the nose, and of course the ligature follows its course. The ligature is then cut off from the bougie, and the two cut ends hang out of the anterior nostril over the upper lip, the loop at the opposite end hanging out of the mouth. The next step is to get the ligature over the tumor. "For this purpose you cut through the loop hanging from the mouth, so that there are now two single ligatures. One end of the single ligature is to be passed through a silver tube, and putting the tube into the mouth and pharynx, you carry one end of the ligature under the base of the tumor on one side of it. You leave that out of the mouth, and your assistant holds both ends of the ligature, to prevent it from slipping; then with the same silver tube you are to take hold of the other loose ligature at the mouth, and carry that on the other side of the polypus, and there your assistant is to hold it. A knot that will not slip must then be made of the two ends of the ligature that hang from the mouth. You have now a ligature on each side of the polypus, and then, by carefully drawing the ligatures out at the end of the nose, you have got hold of the polypus at its base. A silver tube is then to be introduced into the nostril, and you tighten the ligature upon the shoulder of the tube in the same manner as you tighten a ligature on the polypus of the uterus. It must be tightened every day till you have completely cut through the polypus." The polypus, however, should be secured by a ligature, so that when loose, the patient may draw it out, instead of being in danger of choking. But the method adopted by Dessault is perhaps still more convenient. "You require a silver tube by which the ligature is to be directed into the mouth, a short silver tube to be introduced into the nostril for tightening the ligature, and two pretty long ligatures. You introduce a bougie into the nostril, and bring out one end at the mouth. To this you fasten a single and a double ligature; the single one must be very long. This being done, the bougie is to be drawn out at the nose, and of course the ligatures follow it. You then cut off the bougie, and you have the two ends of the double ligature hanging out of the nose, and the loop hanging out of the mouth; one end of the single ligature also hangs out of the nose and one end out of the mouth. The single and the double ligature always pass on one side of the polypus; but by means of a silver canula you draw the single ligature to the other side of the polypus. The ligature being held in its place by an assistant, the end of the single ligature projecting from the mouth is passed through the loop of the double ligature, and the ends of the double ligature being drawn out of the nose, the single end follows, and you make a ligature which you fasten by means of a canula introduced into the nose." This method of Dessault is certainly preferable to the one first described.

Other tumors of a malignant nature may grow from the nostrils which may be confounded with the two kinds of polypus just referred to. No good has hitherto resulted from interfering with them, and therefore Sir B. Brodie thinks it better to let them alone, as "they have generally so broad a base that any operation for their removal is out of the question."

There are some non-malignant affections which are sometimes mistaken for polypi : for example, a scrofulous child may have difficulty of breathing through the nostrils, and on examination the membrane is found turgid and vascular, with an excrescence upon it. This, however, will frequently be nothing more than a thickening of the mucous membrane of the nostril at the anterior extremity of the inferior turbinated bone. The mucous membrane may not be more thickened than elsewhere, but it is more apparent in that situation on account of the projection of the bone.

In some cases in which the mucous membrane has been sufficiently thickened to obstruct the respiration through the nostril, I have introduced a pair of probe-pointed scissors, slightly curved, and snipped off a portion of the projecting mucous membrane. There is no harm whatever in its excision. You may suppose this to be a very simple operation ; and so it is, for it is done in an instant, but yet it requires some care in order that it may be done properly. In the dead body you might snip off a bit, and if you had not completed it by one incision you could make another. But in the living subject the mucous membrane is full of vessels, and the part must be snipped off at once ; for the moment one division is made with the scissors, the hemorrhage is so great that you cannot see a bit of the remaining part which requires to be divided.

Delicate children who are liable to this disease of the Schneiderian membrane are always benefited by the exhibition of steel; it should, however, be given not in large doses, for a short time, but in small ones long continued. Where the constitution is weak, you may sometimes cure the disease in three weeks, but the rectifying of the constitution is a work of years. Some good may be done by local treatment. Dissolve two grains of sulphate of zinc in an ounce of rose-water, and inject a portion into the nostrils two or three times a day ; or paint the inside of the nostril with diluted ung. hydrarg. nitratis by means of a camel-hair brush.

I have seen some cases in which a small abscess had formed in the tumor that I have just described. Suppuration has taken place in the substance of the Schneiderian membrane, just where it projects in front of the inferior turbinated bone, and the best plan to adopt is to cut off, with a pair of scissors, membrane and abscess altogether. When an abscess forms in a pile, that is best relieved, not by laying open the abscess, but by snipping off the pile. *Part* ix., *p.* 93.

Removal of Nasal Polypi.—Dr. D. McRuer has been in the habit, for some years, of employing the following method for the removal of the gelatinous and soft polypi of the nasal passages.

A piece of catgut is passed from the nostrils to the mouth, to which is fastened a piece of soft and dry sponge, corresponding in size, when firmly compressed, to the narrowest part of the nasal passage ; it is then gently drawn forward by the posterior fauces through the nose, and in Dr. McRuer's experience of at least ten cases it has never failed to bring with it all the morbid growths much more effectually and easily than could possibly be accomplished by the old methods of forceps, ligature, etc. *Part* xxiii., *p.* 157.

Polypus of the Nose.—In a clinical lecture on this subject, Mr. Syme remarks as follows : When you are going to remove a polypus remember that non-malignant diseases of this description are generally very limited in the seat of their origin from within the nose. They never proceed from the *floor, septum,* or *external wall,* but *always from the roof,* or that part which is formed by the turbinated plates of the ethmoid bone, so that the growth always *descends* and fills up the lower parts of the nose, even extending into the throat. Never, therefore, attempt to extract it *low down,* but *high up.* Select forceps of a very small size; introduce the instrument gently along the upper passage of the nose, with the blades separated as much as possible, till you come to the neck of the polypus— then compress the handles, and by combination of traction and torsion in one uniform direction, break through the connecting textures. If the growth does not follow the instrument, try again and again. The mucous polypus, always originating from the small extent of surface that has been thus defined, whether it does so singly or, as more frequently happens, in groups, descends so as to occupy first the higher and then the lower channel of the nose, but cannot attain any great size so long as it is limited to these situations ; and not possessing sufficient vigor of expansion to enlarge the osseous space, in order to attain any considerable bulk, must therefore proceed backward toward the pharynx. Keeping these things in mind, you will at once perceive that the plan of removing polypus by means of a thread or wire, whether simply put up the nose, or passed through it into the throat, cannot possibly extirpate the growth, or do more than remove a portion of its substance. You will also require no arguments to prove the inutility and inexpediency of trying to accomplish the object in view by scissors, knives, or caustic; so that our choice is thus limited to evulsion by forceps.

[Mr. Syme then proceeded in the way that has been described, and after several introductions of the forceps, succeeded in removing a large round polypus quite entire, immediately after which the patient breathed with perfect freedom through both nostrils.]

It seems not unworthy of notice that in this case there are some points of resemblance to that remarkable tumor named the fibrous polypus, of which the characters are unity of growth, ligamentous toughness of consistence, extreme firmness of attachment, and disposition to bleed. Several cases have occurred here in which the patients had nearly died of hemorrhage, and all the strength that I could exert was hardly sufficient to effect extraction, while blood streamed in torrents from the nose and mouth. But as this disease is not malignant, the operation, however formidable, proves satisfactory in its result. Now, you may have remarked, that the tumor which has just been removed was solitary, and confined to one nostril, instead of occurring in both, as the mucous polypus almost always does ; also that its connections were very firm, and that the bleeding was considerable. It would seem as if there may be conditions intermediate between the two sorts of growth, in which the respective characters more or less closely approach those of each other. For instance, some years ago, a nobleman returned from public service in one of the colonies, on account of complete obstruction to breathing through his nose, with a constant discharge of watery fluid from it, and occasionally alarming hemorrhage, of which the amount was estimated not by ounces but by pints. He remained in London for two months under the care of several practitioners, who regarded the disease as incurable; and finding himself thus given up as hopeless, he applied to me, bringing with him a letter from the late Mr. Bransby Cooper, which stated that the result of repeated consultations with Sir B. Brodie, Mr. Travers, Mr. Cæsar Hawkins, and himself, was a decision against interfering with the disease, which they seemed to regard as a tumor of the throat. Seeing no sign of malignant disposition in the aspect of the patient, who was about thirty-four years of age, and recognizing in the tumor the characters which were familiar to me as those of a nasal growth stretching backward into the pharynx, I at once undertook to remove the source of complaint. The patient and his friends at a distance having given their consent, I introduced the forceps, and at the very first pull extracted the whole growth, with immediate, complete, and permanent relief. Four years have now elapsed, and there has not been the slightest symptom of relapse to interfere with the enjoyment of perfect health, or the vigorous exertion of an active life. *Part* xxxi., *p.* 223.

Nasal Polypus—New Forceps.—Mr. Gant has recently invented a pair of forceps for the removal of nasal polypi which *cut* and hold at the same time. "One edge of either blade is finished off somewhat like that of an ordinary pair of scissors; the other edge is broad and rasped. This combination of scissors and rasped forceps is a modification of the grape or flower scissors of the conservatories." *Part* xxxviii., *p.* 148.

RECTUM.

Polypus of.—[In his lectures on Surgery, Sir A. Cooper stated that he had only met with ten cases of polypus of the rectum. Mr. Syme states that he once saw five in the course of a fortnight, and thinks it not so rare as is generally supposed. Mr. Syme says:]

It presents itself in three different forms, of which one usually occurs in childhood, and does not appear much beyond puberty. It is extremely soft and vascular, of a florid red color, and assumes the form either of a worm from two to four inches in length, or of a strawberry with a connecting foot stalk two or three inches long. The tumor seldom protrudes except when the bowels are evacuated, and then admits of ready replacement, though not without occasional hemorrhage, which may be of considerable amount. The vascularity of this growth, and its attachment above the sphincter, made me averse from removing it by incision; and Sir A. Cooper has mentioned the alarm that was on one occasion excited in his practice by doing so. I have always employed the ligature; and though the soft texture readily gives way when the thread is drawn, bleeding has never occurred in a single instance, or any other symptom in the least degree disagreeable resulted from this mode of removal. I am therefore induced to regard it as the best that can be employed.

The disease appears in adults in two very distinct forms. In one of these, the growth is soft, vascular, prone to bleed, lobulated or shreddy, and malignant-looking, so as on the whole to resemble very much the cauliflower excrescence of the os uteri, but possesses a peduncle or foot-stalk of firm texture, capable of sound cicatrization after being divided. The profuse, frequent, and protracted bleeding which proceeds from this sort of growth, renders its removal an object of great consequence; and this may be effected very easily, with perfect safety, by transfixing the radical cord of connection with a double ligature, tying the threads so as to include a half of it in each, and then cutting it across a little below the constricted part. In a patient of Mr. Craig, of Ratho (who detected the disease from the great hemorrhage it occasioned), I could not accomplish protrusion of the tumor, but guided a ligature on my finger, and tied it on the neck within the rectum. It is more satisfactory to force or draw the swelling beyond the sphincter, so that the sound and morbid parts may be distinguished with certainty, and this can usually be done with great facility, although the growth has attained a large size. In a hospital case recommended by Mr. Anderson, of Castle-Douglas, I brought into view and removed a tumor not less than an orange, which had a most malignant aspect, and had nearly exhausted the patient by hemorrhage.

In the other form which polypus of the rectum assumes in adults, the tumor is of a firmer consistence, smoother surface, and more regularly spherical or oval form, so as to resemble the growth which in general constitutes polypus uteri. The symptoms resulting from this simple swelling are rather annoying than seriously alarming; and the patient, therefore, is apt to delay requiring assistance for a long while. In the case of an old lady, whom I saw with Mr. Hillson, of Jedburgh, the tumor was about the size of a cherry, with a long stalk, and we were assured had protruded every time the bowels moved for twenty years. In another case, a gentleman whom I saw with Dr. Johnson, of Cumnock, the tumor was nearly as large as an egg, had a cuticular covering, and appeared to have existed for a period equally long. I have always removed these growths in the way that has been already described, and never met with the slightest consequence of a disagreeable kind. *Part* xii., *p.* 207.

Polypus of the Rectum.—[A little girl, five years old, had been subject for two or three years to great distress in defecation, accompanied by the protrusion of a polypus. She was considerably reduced by sanguineous discharge. Dr. Burns says:]

On examination of the anus, I found a polypus protruding as large as a small seckel pear, being considerably diminished at the time from frequent bleedings. On dilating the anus as much as possible, by traction in opposite directions, I found the pedicle to be somewhat elongated from the mucous membrane of the rectum above the sphincter; to this I immediately applied a ligature of silk thread, allowing the ends to remain long, which were secured externally by a strip of adhesive plaster; about twenty-four hours after its application the polypus separated, and two days after, the ligature came away. She suffered some pain while the ligature remained, which did not demand special attention. Since its removal about eight months have passed away, and there has been no return of the disease; no hemorrhage, the function of the part is normal, and the child's health and appearance very much improved. *Part* xvi., *p.* 194.

Polypus of the Rectum.—*Vide* "Use of the *Ecraseur.*"

UTERUS.

Polypus of, expelled by the Action of Secale Cornutum.—[Mr. Moyle was requested to attend without delay a Mrs. W., who had suddenly lost a large quantity of blood from the womb, and had just recovered from a long state of syncope. The blood was lost in about two or three minutes. She had frequently had small hemorrhages previously, and was becoming weaker in consequence. Her legs and thighs were swollen almost to bursting, her countenance pallid, respiration difficult, and general health declining. After she had recovered greatly from her fainting, and after Mr. Moyle had satisfied himself that the flooding was owing to polypus of the uterus, he proceeded as follows :]

A fresh appearance of hemorrhage induced me to give her at once two drachms of the tincture of secale cornutum. I also applied a bandage firmly round the abdomen, and applied cloths, wetted with cold vinegar and water, to the pudendum. The discharge proved to be little, and no faintness followed. In twenty minutes after the first dose, the tincture was repeated, and in a few minutes she complained of being griped. Suspecting this griping to be a slight contraction of the uterus, I ventured an examination by the vagina. The vagina was full of coagula ; the os uteri was flabby and dilated to the size of half-a-crown piece, immediately within which I found a substance of somewhat firmer texture than the coagula, and around which my finger passed freely. During the examination there was a pain of sufficient force of the os uteri to embrace the finger firmly, and I now felt confident of being able to subdue the hemorrhage for the present, and was not without hopes that I might, by a perseverance of the remedy, enable the uterus to throw off the extraneous substance within it. A third dose was now administered, which kept up the pains at short intervals, but they were weak and feeble. Finding this the case, the supposition was, that she was too much reduced from the disease and the recent loss of blood for the medicine to have its full effect. A cup of gruel, with a small quantity of brandy in it, was given her, and in half an hour after, another similar potion, which had the effect of reviving her to a great degree. I now took my leave about eight o'clock P.M., giving directions for a repetition of the food, together with some beef-tea, at intervals of an hour or every second hour, leaving with her four doses of the secale, to be taken at intervals of half an hour ; in case there should be the slightest appearance of flooding, I was to be sent for immediately.

Early on the following morning, I found her laboring under sharp contractile pains of the uterus, from having taken, two hours previously, two doses of the secale. Examination discovered the mass of polypus filling the vagina. The patient was very cheerful, and expressing herself convinced that the mass was coming away. The pains were by this time not so severe as they had been, and consequently I now gave her three drachms of the tincture in a little brandy. This had the effect, in about twenty minutes, of producing a severe pain, which brought the mass to the os externum. It was now grasped with the hand, and, on the recurrence of the pain, the whole was discharged. Slight hemorrhage only followed the expulsion of the polypus, which equalled in size two large placentæ. From this moment she recovered with great rapidity. There was a slight appearance of the menses at the end of six weeks, succeeded by a more abundant appearance at the termination of another similar period. She daily improved in health, the œdema gradually subsided, and although she was for many months unable to put the whole weight of her body on her right leg, yet from bandaging, the use of tonics, etc., she is now, in all respects, a perfectly healthy, robust woman.

The successful result of this case induced Mr. Moyle to try the use of the ergot in another patient who had previously been under his care. He gave her four doses of the tincture of secale cornutum, 3ij. in each dose. Two or three slight pains were now experienced, nausea and vomiting followed. Shortly afterward she had a severe labor pain. She then took 3iij. more of the tincture, and the pains increasing, the polypus mass was felt at the os uteri. By the further use of the medicine the substance was completely expelled. It was about the size of an average placenta.

Part iv., *p.* 120.

Polypus of Womb.—A polypus descending from the womb is said to be insensible, whilst an inverted uterus is very sensible. If, however, a polypus descend with a covering from the inner surface of the womb, it is evident that its sensibility will be more or less retained.

In partial inversion of the uterus, M. Lisfranc thinks favorably of the mode of examination proposed by M. Malgaigne, which we shall describe. In this affection the bladder and a portion of the intestines are lodged in the concavity formed by the depression of the fundus of the uterus; if, then, a curved catheter is passed into the bladder with its concavity downward, and the beak of the instrument is directed to the most depending part of the bladder, its extremity will be readily felt by the finger in the vagina, if the case is one of inversion, unless, indeed, the intestines have become adherent to the womb in such a way as to prevent the catheter penetrating into the depression formed by the inverted organ, a circumstance of very rare occurrence. But M. Lisfranc thinks that the best way of discriminating between polypus and inversion of the uterus, is by a mode of examination similar to that above recommended, in the case of an intra-uterine polypus or of a commencing inversion. If we seize and depress the tumor with two fingers passed into the vagina, and then introduce the index-finger of the other hand into the rectum, no tumor can be felt through the gut above the one which is grasped in the vagina, if the case is one of inverted uterus. But if, on the contrary, we feel through the rectum, a second tumor similar in shape to the uterus, above the vaginal tumor, then this latter tumor is a polypus. In one instance, indeed, M. Lisfranc was misled by this mode of examination; he diagnosticated inversion of the uterus, but the patient having died, a small fibrous tumor was discovered implanted on the uterus, which was flattened and reduced to the tenth part of its natural size.

M. Lisfranc has on several occasions removed by *enucleation* both polypi and fibrous tumors which were not pedunculated, whether situated completely within the cavity of the uterus, or having partly (or in the case of polypi entirely) made their way into the vagina.

In one case having drawn a fibrous polypus almost entirely through the vulva, he perceived that its envelope, which consisted of a thin layer of the tissue of the uterus, was lacerated, and passing the index finger through the rent, enucleated the tumor with the greatest facility. In another case enucleation was effected almost accidentally : M. Lisfranc, while examining a polypus, found the envelope give way beneath the nail of the index-finger, and by an easy manipulation enucleated the tumor in a few seconds. On examining the uterus immediately afterward, he found that the part of that organ to which the polypus had been attached, had singularly contracted, that the depression caused by the tumor had diminished greatly in depth, and at least two-thirds in breadth, it seemed to be diminishing while the finger was in contact with it, and in ten hours the uterus had regained its natural size, and the cervix would not admit the finger. We mention these latter facts, as we conceive they have an important bearing on the question of hemorrhage after excision of polypi. M. Lisfranc has also frequently enucleated, with the nail of the index-finger, small cellulo-vascular polypi occupying the neck of the womb. In a case where a fibrous tumor as large as the clenched hand projected into the vagina, its envelope was lacerated with the nails, and the contained tumor turned out. But enucleation must generally be preceded by an exploratory incision: and by this combination of means, M. Lisfranc has removed fibrous tumors while still completely included within the cavity of the uterus. A lady was reduced almost to extremity, by protracted uterine hemorrhage caused by a fibrous tumor, which could be felt through the dilated cervix uteri. The neck of the uterus was seized with Museaux's hook, depressed almost to the vulva, and a more perfect examination being then practicable, the tumor was found to extend from the middle of the body of the uterus almost to its lower extremity, and to be lodged in its posterior wall, from which it was commencing to disengage itself. A straight, blunt-pointed bistoury was passed along the fore-finger, a vertical incision slowly and cautiously made over the tumor until the finger was enabled to be insinuated beneath the envelope and complete the enucleation, which was not accomplished without some difficulty. Occasionally, enucleation may be more easily achieved by substituting a spatula for the finger. If it is necessary to enlarge the incision in order to effect the removal of the tumor, a grooved director will often guide the knife more conveniently and safely than the finger. In some cases where the cervix uteri was insufficiently dilated, M. Lisfranc divided it anteriorly. Whenever the peduncle of a polypus is very broad, we should incise the envelope, and endeavor to enucleate the tumor; in this, however, we cannot always succeed. If the tumor is removed, the envelope sometimes contracts and cicatrizes, sometimes sloughs in whole or in part.

Lisfranc, in common with many other French writers, disapproves altogether of removing polypi by the ligature; and the Reviewer agrees with this opinion in general, although there may be cases in which it is necessary to use the ligature: "Thus, if a polypus of moderate size is completely included within the uterus, and is implanted high up, especially at the summit of the organ, and if the symptoms imperatively demand an operation, a ligature should be applied, if its application is possible, as it occasionally is when a sufficiently small peduncle can be detected; or if a patient is so exsanguine that the smallest loss of blood is to be dreaded, we should employ the ligature, unless the peduncle is too thick, or unless we are unable to bring it, when bulky, fairly within our reach, and pierce it with several needles, each armed with a double ligature and thus tie it in two or more separate portions."

How should we proceed if we felt an artery pulsating in the peduncle? Dupuytren recommended excision, having previously placed a ligature of reserve in case of hemorrhage: Lisfranc disapproves of this, inasmuch as it would certainly lose its place; and instead he would at once place a ligature on the peduncle, and then excise the tumor at once, leaving the ligature on the peduncle for about eight or ten hours, and then removing it. If hemorrhage should come on, he is convinced that plugging would be sufficient. If the artery felt in the peduncle was only a small one, he would not even apply a ligature, but excise the polypus at once, trusting to plugging, if required. *Part* x., *p.* 151.

Uterine Polypi and Ulceration.—Dr. Montgomery directs if small, to remove them by twisting with a forceps, consisting of a straight stem, eight inches long, having two short spring blades, with serrated tips, upon which slide a brace movable from the handle, by which they are easily pressed firmly together, and made to grasp very securely, any object caught between them. Apply nitrate of silver to restrain bleeding. Where it is necessary, in a larger pedunculated polypus, apply a ligature; Niessen's double canula is recommended, and with it, silk salmon fishing-line soaked in linseed oil, which combines strength, perfect pliability, and softness, and is unaffected by moisture. N.B. In persons of a high habit, and who are subject to indulgences in dietary, be careful not suddenly to suppress menorrhagic discharges, because of the dangers of determination to cerebral congestion. *Part* xiv., *p.* 301.

Polypus Uteri.—Very small polypi situated high up in the cervix, says Dr. Locock, may be removed by an instrument made for the purpose, consisting of a very small, sharp scoop, like a carpenter's gouge, inclosed in a canula from which it is made to protrude by turning a screw. Larger polypi should be excised; but should first be twisted round several times so as to produce torsion of the arteries; or, if they are very large, a ligature should be applied for two or three days, and when the circulation has become well strangulated, the neck of the polypus should be cut through above the noose. *Part* xvii., *p.* 277.

Polypus Uteri, Intra-uterine—When the symptoms afford reason to suspect the existence of a polypus concealed within the uterus, says Prof. Simpson, the diagnosis may be rendered certain by the dilatation of the os and cervix uteri, by means of sponge-tents. The tents recommended are of a conical form, and are introduced by the aid of a director resembling the uterine sound. Usually a single tent, applied for twenty or thirty hours, opens the os and cavity of the cervix sufficiently to allow an examination of this part by the finger. In order to examine the cavity of the body of the uterus, it is necessary to employ a series of tents for several days, taking care to pass them within the os internum. When the presence of a polypus is ascertained, if it be gradually but certainly making its way downward, and the hemorrhage and other symptoms are not urgent, wait for its descent through the os, before attempting its removal; facilitating its passage by the dilatation of the os and cervix with sponge-tents, and by the internal use of ergot. But if there is too much hemorrhage to wait, or if there is no likelihood of the tumor's descent, proceed forthwith to remove it With this object, first dilate the os uteri further; then if the polypus is large, divide the pedicle with very curved blunt-pointed scissors, or with a silver wire passed around it and tightened by means of a screw; or if these means are inapplicable, contuse and crush the tumor by a pair of lithotomy forceps, or similar instrument. Or, if the polypi are small and vesicular (in which case they are generally numerous, and situated in the cavity of the cervix), remove those that are fully formed and pedunculated, by the scissors, or by scratching them off with the nail; and destroy those that are not completely developed, but are imbedded like peas in the mucous membrane of the cervix, by the application of potassa fusa. *Part* xxi., *p.* 275.

Polypus Uteri—Intra-Uterine.—When the womb remains large and bulky after delivery, says Dr. Oldham, and when we are satisfied there is not another ovum, although we may suspect the presence of a polypus, we are decidedly not justified, so long as no alarming symptoms occur, in endeavoring to make out exactly by manual interference, whether such is the case or not, or in arousing the uterus to contraction by the exhibition of the ergot of rye. The system of non-interference must be pursued ; the safety of the patient consists in the quiescence of the uterus. To insure this, strict rest, mild sedatives, and the avoidance of all local irritation should be enforced. But if, in spite of all endeavors, it be necessary to remove the polypus, the best plan is, if the pedicle is small, to twist it off. If, however, it occur at a time when physical injury to the uterus may be hazardous, the ligature should be applied to the pedicle to prevent hemorrhage, and then the body of the polypus removed with the knife.
Part xxvi., *p.* 316.

Polypus Uteri—Varieties.—The term " polypus uteri," says Dr. Ramsbotham, has been given at different times to organic diseases of the uterine structure, as well as to formations, within the uterine cavity, of very various and dissimilar kinds ; and even now, though it is restricted to tumors attached by vascular connection to the uterine substance, the phrase is applied to more than one variety of morbid growths. Some are dense, firm, and compact, in their structure ; some soft and cellular ; some of a florid scarlet ; some of a deep peony color; and some, when removed, almost white. They take their origin also from different parts of the organ,—the fundus, the body, the internal channel of the neck, or the outer circle of the mouth itself.

Dr. Lee has noted four distinct species of polypus uteri, none of them malignant in their nature :—the fibrous ;—the follicular or glandular, which he describes as a morbid enlargement of the *Glandulæ Nabothi ;* and which, consequently, are situated only at the mouth or neck ;—the cystic or cellular, made up of a congeries of small vesicles or cysts, containing a fluid more or less transparent, and yellowish in color. This variety is formed just beneath the lining membrane of the uterus, and springs from every part of the cavity. The tumor is highly vascular ; and the cysts composing its chief bulk are bound together by fine fibrous tissues ;—and, lastly, the mucus, which does not grow to so large a size as either of the others, and which seems to be produced by a morbid change in the mucous membrane itself, and to be analogous to the polypous tumors sometimes formed within the nose and other mucous cavities. *Part* xxvii., *p.* 201.

Ligature in Polypus Uteri—In applying a ligature upon a polypus of the uterus, says Dr. Ramsbotham, we might grasp some of the structure of the uterus itself. To obviate this, the neck of the polypus must be tied some distance below its attachment ; for that portion of the stem left in connection with the uterus will wither and come away in shreds, or be absorbed after the main bulk has been removed. The sensation of pain must, to a great extent, be our guide. If the patient complains much, the noose should be relaxed and again drawn tight over the lower portion of the neck or body of the tumor. *Part* xxvii., *p.* 203.

Polypus Uteri.—Galvanism applied to the uterus has brought these growths into view where ergot had failed. *Part* xxix., *p.* 266.

Extraction of Polyi 'from the Uterus.—Mr. Canney recommends *excision* rather than the ligature when the polypi are not large. Dr. Tyler Smith prefers *ligature ;* Mr. Hodgson says the *torsion* is sometimes both better and safer than either excision or the ligature. Dr. Copland gives us an interesting case to show the effects of *biborate of soda.* He says:

Polypi, or fibrous tumors, on the inner surface of the uterus, were occasionally thrown off without resorting to the ligature, or any other operation. Some years ago he had been called in consultation to the case of a lady suffering from constantly recurring uterine hemorrhage. A tumor was protruding from the os uteri. The question of removal was discussed, and it was decided that biborate of soda should be given, with a view of producing the contraction of the uterus, by which the growth might be thrown off. The medicine was given in large doses, and continued for two or three days. The uterus contracted powerfully, and the tumor was expelled. All the symptoms abated for three or four days, when a second tumor presented itself. Dr. R. Lee then joined the consultation, and it was determined that the use of the soda should be persevered in. The result was that this second tumor, like the first, was thrown off, and the patient recovered. He could speak from his own knowledge, that she was alive and well 13 or 14 years afterward. This might not have been a case, strictly speaking, of polypus of the uterus, but it was certainly one of a tumor under the villous coat of that organ, which was thrown off by the contractions of the uterus.

Part xxix., *p.* 304.

Polypus Uteri—Detection of.—The polypus will be best detected during the relaxation and forcing down, attendant on an attack of flooding. The bi-valved speculum assists by expanding and opening the os. Dr. Locock particularly points out that. the tumor is always best found out *during hemorrhage,* and indeed it cannot be detected at all when very small, and only in the cervix, in the intervals of the attacks of hemorrhage.

For bringing a polypus into view, the ergot of rye may sometimes succeed, but *galvanism* is more safe and more efficacious. The os and cervix uteri may be dilated by means of sponge-tents—use two or three graduated sponge-tents in succession so as to open the canal for inspection. M. Jobert de Lamballe has recently contrived an *intra-uterine* speculum.

In those cases which indicate the necessity of exploration beyond the uterus, first bring the polypus in view, if you can, by dilating the os uteri by sponge-tents, and giving repeated doses of ergot of rye, assisted by the application of galvanism. If you cannot get hold of the tumor so as to encircle the neck, pull it lower down by the aid of a tenaculum, if this operation be not particularly resisted—and now try again to ligature the neck of the tumor. *Part* xxx., *p.* 212.

Excision of Large Pedunculated Uterine Polypi.—Prof. Simpson prefers to remove large uterine polypi by excision, rather than by ligature. You can always arrest hemorrhage by well plugging the vagina. For excision use a polypus-knife (called a *polyptome*). First reach the peduncle by the apex of the fore-finger of the right hand introduced along the pubic surface of the vagina. Then push the instrument along this finger, and by hooking down the peduncle it is divided by the knife, which is placed in the concavity of the instrument, something like the lately improved hernia-knife.   *Part* xxxi., *p.* 210.

Waterproof Ligatures.—In cases of polypus, etc., the ligature sometimes breaks abruptly from the corrosive effects of the discharges. If the ligature be previously rendered waterproof by a solution of caoutchouc it answers beautifully, and comes away as sound as when applied.
                                                 Part xxxii. *p.* 318.

Uterine Polypi.—These, when pendent from within the os uteri by a narrow peduncle, may be readily removed without any hemorrhage by the écraseur. Slip the loop of the chain around it, and by tightening slowly and steadily, the stem will easily be cut through.
                                                 Part xxxv., *p.* 253.

Uterine Polypi.—For the removal of these tumors an instrument lately invented by Dr. Aveling, of Sheffield, will be found very useful. It consists of a long curved stem, at one end of which is a hook, and fitting into the concavity of this is a plate of metal, which by a screw in the handle is capable of being withdrawn lower down the stem. When used the plate is screwed half way down the stem, and the instrument is passed up so that the hook may be round the peduncle of the tumor : by means of the screw the plate of metal is now forced up into the concavity of the hook. Thus the tumor is removed, without the disadvantages of either the knife or the ligature ; viz. of the former, hemorrhage, which is here avoided, as the peduncle is not divided by a cutting but by a *crushing* action, and of the latter, the fetid discharge caused by the putrefaction of the polypus.
                                                 Part xxxvi., *p.* 246.

Removal of Large Uterine Polypus, by the Curved Ecraseur.—Dr. Savage of the Samaritan Hospital, lately removed a vascular uterine polypus, without pain or hemorrhage, by means of an écraseur the curve of which can be made to fall into the hollow of the sacrum and the point to pass up into the uterus. When removed by this instrument, the polypus is first seized by a pair of ring forceps, and the chain is passed over these, and drawn tight, precisely as the cord in the ordinary operation by ligature.   *Part* xxxvii., *p.* 214.

Polypus Uteri.—Mr. I. B. Brown is of the opinion that the best mode of removing these growths, is to seize them with a pair of long vulsellum forceps, and having dragged them into sight to pass a needle armed with a strong double ligature through the base, which can now be tied in two parts, then cut off the polypus just anterior to the ligature, and plug the vagina with oiled lint. This plan is infinitely preferable to that of either simply cutting off the polypus, or the more tedious process with Gooch's apparatus, where the sloughing of the polypus within the vagina generally causes serious constitutional disturbance, not unfrequently pyæmia, and sometimes death.   *Part* xxxvii., *p* 217.

—•••—

PREGNANCY.

Nux Vomica, in the Vomiting of Pregnant Women.—Dr..Croyher, of Presburg, assures us that minute doses of the nux vomica, given in some aromatic or in cherry-laurel water, are a *specific* remedy against the troublesome vomiting to which many women are subject during the early months of pregnancy. In order to insure success, the bowels must be kept in a gently open condition, but neither purged nor constipated. The author says, that the effects of this remedy are certain, provided the vomiting is the result of pregnancy alone, and is not dependent on any morbid state, either of the stomach or of any other organ. The dose recommended is from two to four drops of the tincture—the strength of this is not stated—to be gradually increased to ten, twelve, or eighteen drops every morning in bed, and again in the evening. In many cases it proves quite successful within a week or even a shorter time ; in other cases its use must be continued longer. *Part* iii., *p.* 125.

Gravidine as a sign of Pregnancy.—The fluid portion of the urine of pregnant women being drawn off, there appears a "natural sediment," which, whether held in solution, or separated by ether, has a striking resemblance to the serous globule, but, when in a sedimentary state, bears an equally strong resemblance to the milk globule in recent milk. This substance differs from albumen and caseum, the two animal substances most analogous to it : from the former, in being soluble in water by means of heat ; from the latter, in being soluble by sulphuric and nitric acids. From gelatine it also differs : first, in being precipitated from its solution in water on cooling ; secondly, though partially precipitated by tannin, the precipitate was soluble in water on boiling. The author calls it " gravidine," both from *gravidus*, big with young, occurring as it does in pregnant women ; and also from *gravis*, heavy, seeing that it falls to the bottom of the vessel. Kiestein is but the pellicle which results from the decomposition of gravidine. As the globules forming the latter substance are decomposed, urates and purpurates are developed in the urine ; and when these have broken up and assumed new combinations, the triple phosphates appear, with that beautiful crystalline appearance described by Dr. Bird as one of the characteristics of kiestein.

Part v., *p.* 162.

Severe Gastric Irritation in Pregnancy.—Whenever in a pregnant woman, in any stage of her gestation, severe vomiting, wearing away the strength of the patient, and preventing proper nutrition, shall have for several days resisted all the usual remedies, whilst the fever continues unabated, and the vital forces are failing, we ought not to delay a moment, says Dr. Edwards, in procuring the expulsion of the fœtus.

Part xiv., *p.* 284.

Diagnostic Sign.—A good diagnostic is the enlargement of the *anterior* wall of the womb, its ordinary flatness becoming effaced by the fourth or fifth week. *In congestion* of the womb, it is the *posterior* wall which is chiefly enlarged. *Part* xv., *p.* 315.

Appearance of the Os Uteri during Pregnancy.—Dr. Whitehead says : In order to ascertain the existence of pregnancy from a few days after conception to the middle or end of the fourth month, examine the os uteri with the speculum. Immediately after the conception, as during menstruation, the labia uteri are in a state of great vascular turgescence, and the os closed and linear. In from ten to twenty days the whole uterus is found enlarged, and the circulation in it augmented ; the labia are thickened and apparently elongated, the commissures less distinct, and the os apparently sunk in or dimpled. In the fourth week the os tineæ; which was before a mere chink with parallel boundaries, now an elliptical or rounded aperture, separating the labia to the extent of a line or two, and occupied by a plug of mucus. At six or eight weeks it becomes decidedly oval or circular, with a puckered or indented boundary. *Part* xvi., *p.* 239.

Menstruation in Relation to Pregnancy. — Conception, says Prof. Dubois, may take place in a woman not yet arrived at the age at which she ought to menstruate. There are, in fact, many women who do not menstruate till the seventeenth, eighteenth, or nineteenth year. Such women may become pregnant at that time of life, although they have never menstruated. M. Dubois has known a woman become pregnant two years after the cessation of the menses. The woman finding her abdomen enlarging, entered the medical department of an hospital. The physician under whose charge she was, had so little idea of the woman's being pregnant, that he delivered a clinical lecture on the case, as one of ovarian dropsy. On making an examination of the case, M. Dubois easily made out the pulsation of the fœtal heart. In fact, labor very soon supervened.

The menses may be suppressed physiologically, and yet pregnancy take place. Thus, it is not rare to see nurses become pregnant before menstruation has reappeared. We find also, that women who are extremely irregular, who, for example, menstruate only once or twice a year, become pregnant; although, in general, this state is one very unfavorable for conception.

Various diseases and changes in habits may derange the menstruation, and give rise to the idea of pregnancy. This error occurs frequently, chiefly to persons anxious to become in the family way. Nothing is more common than to find the menses suppressed for some time after marriage. It is also very frequently observed, that women leaving the country to reside in the town suffer from suppression. This may be said to occur habitually in young women coming from the country into domestic service in Paris.

In other cases, the menses, after having been suppressed for three or four months, re-appear suddenly, with some profuseness. This is sometimes taken for the occurrence of abortion, when it is merely the recurrence of the menses after they have been suppressed, in consequence of some change in the habits of the female. *Part* xxii., *p.* 272.

Nausea and Vomiting of Pregnancy.—You must first try to get the secretions into a healthy state. One of the most serviceable remedies in these cases, according to Dr. Tyler Smith, is the infusion of calumba with soda and hydrocyanic acid, or you may give this in an effervescing form with citric acid—in some patients opium answers better, and perhaps the solution of the bimeconate of morphia is the best form in which an opiate can be given. Salicine, in doses of three to five grains, three times a day, is a valuable medicine. Creasote, in one or two drop doses made into pills with bread, is an efficient remedy. Professor Simpson particularly recommends the nitrate of cerium in doses of one to two grains in water, and also the inhalation of the vapor of laudanum. *Part* xxxiii., *p.* 251.

Molar Pregnancy.—If the life of the mother should be threatened, the ovum should be detached by the catheter or the uterine sound without hesitation. Ergot of rye must also be given to excite contractions, but in ordinary cases, as in simple abortions, we must wait until the ovum can be reached with the finger before we attempt to remove it. In hydatid degeneration, the treatment may be more positive—give ergot, and if the os uteri be dilatable, introduce the hand to detach and remove the hydatid mass. *Part* xxxiii., *p.* 270.

Pregnancy—Diagnosis of, from Abdominal Tumors.—Dr. Oldham says: By applying the hand, the tumor at first feels soft and ill-defined, but by pressure it rapidly assumes a tense rounded form, becoming firm and resisting. This may be taken as a trustworthy characteristic of a pregnant uterus, since there is no other tumor which possesses any power of altering its form when irritated by palpation. *Part* xxxiii., *p.* 270.

Pregnancy—Duration of.—To ascertain the most probable day of a woman's confinement, add 278 days to the last menstruation.
Part xxxv., *p.* 209.

Vomiting of Pregnancy.—In a case which occurred to Dr. Clay, of Manchester, where the induction of premature labor seemed absolutely necessary, from the failure of all other means, for relieving the incessant vomiting—on introducing the finger to guide an instrument for this purpose, the os and cervix uteri were found very tender and painful when touched, and violent efforts of vomiting caused. Considering this state to be produced by pressure on the os uteri, instead of proceeding with the operation, he caused the patient to be laid quite prostrate on the back, with the head very low and hips considerably raised. In about 24 hours the tendency to vomit was considerably less, and small portions of food could be retained : she continued to improve, and ultimately safely completed the period of utero-gestation, but at any time the slightest attempt to resume the upright position was followed by violent retching and distressing vomiting. Dr. Clay was convinced that there is pretty generally, if not always, considerable congestive inflammation and great tenderness about the os and cervix uteri which are best treated by local bleeding at the seat of mischief. That the irritable state of the stomach is purely symptomatic of that condition of the os and cervix uteri (that is) in these obstinate cases of the latter months: That these cases differ widely from, and must not be confounded with, those of nausea and sickness of the early months, however severe; and where the stomach itself particularly, and in some measure the entire digestive functions are much deranged ; and attention to the condition of the stomach will, in most, if not in all cases, be remedied by medicine and diet. That diet or medicine have little or no effect in the severer cases above described, *in the latter months ;* but that a position of the body calculated to relieve the os and cervix from pressure against the pelvic viscera, is best accomplished by lying on the back with the hips raised and head low, with food in very small quantities given at long intervals. Lastly, and mainly, Dr. Clay places much reliance on the application of a few leeches, by means of the speculum, directly to the os and cervix uteri—the seat of congestive inflammation, and consequently the cause of general irritation and sympathetic action of the stomach and its consequences. The leeches are to be repeated if any tenderness remains, and the position strictly observed until the symptoms are entirely conquered. *Part* xxxvii., *p.* 202.

Pseudocyesis.—Diagnosis.—There is a form of spurious pregnancy, says Prof. Simpson, in which there is a firm unyielding swelling of the abdomen, often supposed to be due to the enlargement of a gravid uterus, but which is in reality due to a tympanitic state of the bowels and a peculiarly tonic condition of the abdominal muscles; and the abdominal walls are so firm and tense, and resist the pressure of the hand so effectually as to render an adequate examination utterly impossible. In such cases as this give chloroform; under its influence, if deep enough, the abdominal muscles will become perfectly relaxed, and on pressing on the abdomen the walls will give way before your hand, and sink backward until you can feel the spinal column quite distinctly. This curious affection is probably owing to some affection of the diaphragm, which is thrown into a state of contraction, and pushes the bowels downward in the abdominal cavity.   *Part* xl., *p.* 180.

— • • • —

PROLAPSIONS.

PROLAPSUS ANI.

Prolapsus Ani.—Bransby Cooper makes the following remarks on prolapsus ani, which so frequently accompanies piles: Under ordinary circumstances, you will cure the prolapsus by palliative means, and by curing the piles which have caused it, but if the mucous membrane and the muscles have been so much relaxed as to render a large prolapsus permanent, you must take up two or three folds of the mucous membrane which covers it, and surround each fold with a ligature, then return the prolapsed gut into the pelvis. The patient will be disappointed at first as he is not relieved; it is the case that there will be no great relief till the ligatures come away, but after that the cure is permanent, at least so it has proved in three or four cases in which I have employed this method.   *Part* iii., *p.* 88.

Prolapsus Ani — New Mode of Treating.—Dupuytren's method of curing a prolapsus ani in the adult was at first by excising a portion of the mucous membrane of the bowel, and afterward by cutting away only the folds of the skin at the margin of the anus. The anus in these cases being immoderately dilatable, this process causes a degree of consolidation and contraction. It is seldom that this is required in the child. Sir Benjamin Brodie's plan will generally succeed by injecting every morning 2 or 3 ounces of a lotion composed of ʒj. of tinct. ferri muriatis and a pint of water: at the same time giving occasional gentle aperients, and not too much vegetable food. Dr. McCormac, reflecting on the method of Dupuytren, applies the same principle to cases of children in the following simple way: When the child goes to stool, the skin anterior to the anus is to be drawn to one side by means of the fingers extended around. At first the child may not be able to evacuate its bowel, but when encouraged to persevere it will do so, and will often, in this simple way, be entirely cured.
                                        Part viii., *p.* 162.

Prolapsus Ani.—Five different means of treating this affection are mentioned by M. Dieffenbach in his operative surgery. 1st. By diminishing the anal opening by excision of folds around it. 2d. By excision of wedge-shaped pieces from the anus. 3d. By excision of parts of the anal ring, and of the callous prolapsus. 4th. By extirpation of the spongy prolapsus. And 5thly. By cauterization.   *Part* xxii., *p.* 218.

Pelvic Viscera, Prolapsus of.—In these cases, with lacerated perineum, the object must be to remove the actions of the sphincter ani and the levatores ani, by removing their points of attachment to the coccyx. Mr. Hilton describes his plan of operating in these cases as follows : A narrow, sharp-pointed knife was introduced through the skin on one side of the point or free extremity of the coccyx, about half or three quarters of an inch from its end ; it was then passed into the pelvis between the concave surface of the coccyx and the rectum, special care being taken not to puncture the intestine. The cutting edge of the knife was now made to sweep over the sides and ends of the coccyx, so as to separate from it the coccygeal attachments of the sphincter and levatores ani. The knife was then withdrawn through the same small opening by which it had been introduced, scarcely any blood escaped at the wound, but a compress of lint, supported by adhesive plaster, was applied over it to keep the parts quiet, and to intercept the flow of blood. *Part* xxix., *p.* 277.

Nitric Acid.—Apply nitric acid as follows : Wipe the acid down the protruded part in separate streaks or tracts vertically from the sphincter down to the lowest portion of the gut; then replace the protrusion and allow no motion for two days. Dr. M'Dowel says : You may re-apply the acid at intervals of seven or ten days if necessary. *Part* xxx., *p.* 154.

Strychnine.—Dupuytren's method of treating prolapsus ani, was by excising radiating folds of the skin round the anus, while Guersant used the actual cautery. Duchaussay thinks these acted only by stimulating the sphincter muscle, and therefore he applies strychnine. Apply one-sixth to one third of a grain of strychnine to a blistered surface in the neighborhood of the anus. Repeat this occasionally according to its effects.
Part xxx., *p.* 155.

Treatment of Prolapsus Ani by Strychnia and by the Actual Cautery. —Dr. A. Johnson says : If the child be about two years old, apply a blister to the cleft between the nates, and dress the blistered surface with one-twentieth of a grain of strychnia—on the fourth day one-sixteenth of a grain may be applied on a second blistered surface, the cuticle, of course, being removed. Five or six days afterward this may be repeated if necessary. In a child of four years old, one-eighth of a grain may be used each time. If this fail, apply the actual cautery in three or four places at the junction of the skin with the mucous membrane. This may be repeated in a few weeks, if necessary, but less extensively. Strychnia may do for very mild cases, but the actual cautery is the most certain remedy.
Part xxxi., *p.* 156.

Prolapsus Ani treated with Nitrate of Silver.—Dr. Lloyd says : Smear the whole surface of the protruded bowel with solid nitrate of silver, and then return it. Repeat this once a week or fortnight. This need not be confined to simple prolapsion, but may be used in cases of hemorrhoidal congestion and thickening of the mucous membrane about the verge of the anus. *Part* xxxi., *p.* 158.

Prolapsus Ani and Hemorrhoids—The Ecraseur.—The écraseur is not so frequently used in these cases as it deserves. Two cases are related by Dr. R. Davies, in which a speedy and safe cure was effected, and that after the nitric acid plan had failed. *Part* xl., *p.* 111.

PROLAPSUS UTERI.

Use of Nitric Acid.—Mr. Benj. Phillips, in one case of prolapsus uteri, treated by him at the St. Marylebone Infirmary, succeeded in effecting a cure, or, at least, in affording complete relief by destroying a portion of the mucous lining of the vagina by means of nitric acid. The contraction consequent on the separation of the sloughs reduced the size of the vagina so much as effectually to retain the uterus *in situ.* *Part* i., *p.* 95.

Use of the Actual Cautery in Procidentia Uteri.—Almost every remedy has been in vain tried in many of these cases. The actual cautery, though a severe remedy, will often be successful when all other applications have failed. Cases where this was successfully applied are brought forward by Dr. Lowrie, of the Glasgow infirmary.

The following case shows the efficacy of this valuable remedy in procidentia uteri. C. M'L., aged 18, a servant, while carrying a heavy tub, felt something give way in the pelvis, and as if the vagina immediately afterward was unusually distended. Some days after this, the uterus distended the vagina, and rapidly descended so as completely to prolapse. It could easily be returned by pressure, but again descended almost immediately. She derived no benefit from the free application of the nitrate of silver, astringent injections, pessaries, bandages, and the ordinary treatment. Strips of the mucous membrane of the vagina were dissected off from the lateral and posterior parts of the vagina, without any benefit. Weiss's three-pronged speculum was introduced and dilated, and the actual cautery freely applied to both lateral surfaces of the vagina, nearly as high as the uterus. Great pain was of course experienced, followed by other severe symptoms ; the patient was kept recumbent for about six weeks.

Nine weeks after the operation the following report was entered in the journal : " Not the slightest tendency to renewal of the procidentia ; she has no feeling of prolapsus. Uterus felt nearly in its natural position, with a circular contraction of the vagina a little below os uteri. The contraction firm, but quite elastic." We need hardly mention that the contraction of the vagina is here made to support the womb ; and this must occasionally give way, especially when previously over-distended by the use of large pessaries ; and therefore in all cases of procidentia it will be well to make use of some kind of support, such as that recommended by Mr. Clay, previously noticed, (*Vide* Article " *Pessaries,*") which will not produce this relaxation of the vaginal parietes. *Part* iv., *p.* 129.

Prolapsus Uteri.—[Mr. Whitehead says that prolapsus is most frequently a consequence of inflammation and ulceration of the lower part of the uterus. He thinks that pessaries only aggravate the disease, and remarks, that in addition to attention of the general health,]

The local treatment should consist in applications of nitrate of silver, or other suitable remedies to the diseased surface, and in the insertion of medicated tents by the aid of the *prolapsus tube.* This latter procedure may be practised immediately after the nitrate has been employed, although the remedy with which the tent is charged be of a very different nature from that of the caustic. The manner of using the *prolapsus tube*—which will be found of equal service in the management of prolapsed displacement of the uterus, as in most other forms of uterine disease, and enables the patient safely and efficiently to apply the remedies herself, without the interference of the practitioner—is extremely simple. The charged tent, to which a length of thread has been previously attached, must be placed in the tube, the upper orifice of which is to be applied against the protruded portion of the uterus, in such a manner as to receive the os uteri within it. The instrument, previously smeared with some unctuous material, and having its curved arm placed anteriorly, in a direction toward the abdomen, is now to be forced gently and steadily backward, until the whole, or greater portion of it, has passed within the canal, or until a moderate degree of resistance is felt to oppose its further ingress.

The uterus being thus restored to its natural position, the tent or pledget must be passed upward against the cervix, and held in that situation by means of a skewer or other suitable instrument, the tube at the same time being gently withdrawn. The recumbent posture should be strictly maintained for several days, and very little exercise taken for some weeks afterward. The lotions, used for moistening the lint-tent, are strong solutions of nitrate of silver, sulphate of zinc, sulphate of copper, matico, opium, and tannin. The metallic preparations should not be employed oftener than every third or fourth day, the vegetable applications being used intermediately. An emollient injection should be made use of after the removal of each tent. *Part* xvi., p. 277.

Prolapsus Uteri—Galvanic Cautery.—In a case of long continued prolapsus, and in which the vagina was very lax and distensible, Mr. Marshall determined to apply the galvanic cautery to produce a series of eschars upon the walls of the vagina. A peculiar speculum made for the purpose, consisting of two large blades, and inclosing double rows of fenestræ about an inch in length and half an inch in breadth, having been introduced and the blades separated, the mucous membrane was seen to bulge through the apertures. The coil of heated wire· was now applied, and eight eschars rapidly made on each side of the vagina. For the first fortnight the patient was confined to bed, and detergent injections used twice daily; as the sloughs separated, mildly stimulating ones were applied. The capacity of the vagina was considerably diminished, and on moving about no prolapsion was found to take place. It is important to observe that if the vagina is protruded, it must be first returned, as, although under these circumstances, it may be easier to apply the cautery, yet it is most difficult and dangerous to return the mass afterward. *Part* xxviii., p. 273.

Prolapsus Uteri.—Having made the usual horse-shoe denudation in the operation for the cure of this disease, Mr. Fergusson applies the common interrupted suture instead of the quill suture, which is generally used. Mr. Fergusson believes that the quill suture sometimes causes tendency to sloughing from over pressure. *Part* xxxvi., p. 238.

Prolapsus Uteri—Plastic operation.—In this operation, says Dr. Hutchinson, the great element of success is to denude a sufficient portion of the back part of the vagina, to get contraction of at least the lower two inches. To this end do not denude two narrow slips, but a portion extending from an inch to two inches on each side, commencing at the anal commissure, and extending an inch and a half upward into the vagina.
Part xxxvii., p. 221.

PROLAPSUS VESICÆ.

Cured by Operation.—[This patient first observed a small tumor to protrude from the vagina, which gradually increased to the size of an orange, and then to the size of the fist, hanging between the thighs: the greater part was formed by the bladder and anterior paries of the vagina. After remaining in bed twenty-four hours, the tumor could be easily reduced, but owing to the capacity of the vagina it soon prolapsed again in the erect posture, and was then accompanied, on making exertion, with an involuntary dribbling of urine. Mr. Lightfoot performed the operation for episcorraphie, as recommended by Dr. Fricke, of Hamburg, in the following way:]

The bowels having been previously evacuated, and the hair removed from the parts, the patient was placed on a table, in the same position as for lithotomy, without, however, tying the hands and feet. The thighs being well separated by two assistants, I took hold of the left labium and transfixed it obliquely about the middle with a narrow bistoury three quarters of an inch from the edge, and in such a manner as to include more of the skin than of the mucous membrane; the knife was then carried rapidly downward in the same direction to the raphe, half an inch or so in front of the anus: the superior attachment of this flap was next divided, by carrying the incision upward as high as on a level with the meatus urinarius. The same was repeated on the opposite side, after which the frenulum, and other parts included within the angle formed by the union of the two incisions in front of the anus, were carefully dissected off. The two surfaces thus formed extended from opposite the urethra to within half an inch of the anus, each being about two inches long, and varying in breadth from an inch posteriorly to half an inch anteriorly. The hemorrhage was so trifling, as merely to require the torsion of one small vessel: the oozing having ceased, six strong hempen sutures were passed through the entire thickness of the denuded surfaces, and tied moderately firm. The first one was applied a few lines in front of the anus, and the last one immediately below the meatus urinarius.

A gum elastic catheter was introduced into the bladder, and the knees were bound together, after which the patient was placed in bed on her left side. The antiphlogistic regimen was strictly adhered to for four or five days, during which cold water was constantly applied to the parts, and the vagina occasionally washed out and cleared of coagulated blood, by means of cold water injections. An anodyne was given at bed-time, and repeated for three or four nights, to allay irritation and confine the bowels. Two of the sutures were removed on the fourth day, and the other four on the sixth; at the expiration of which, union by the first intention had taken place throughout the whole extent. The bowels were moved on the eighth day, and an occasional dose of aperient medicine was afterward given.

In the course of three weeks she was allowed to leave her bed, and walk about a little. The bond of union is very firm, and appears like an elongated perineum, extending from the anus to within a quarter of an inch of the urethra.

. In performing this operation, I think it would be better not to attempt the union of the posterior part of the labia, but to leave an opening into the vagina between the bond of union and the frenulum sufficiently large to allow of the discharge of the vaginal, mucous and menstrual secretion. By adopting this method the operation would be much facilitated; the most troublesome part of it, and, at the same time, the most painful to the patient, being the dissection required for the removal of the frenulum and the parts in front of the anus. During the treatment, likewise, coagulated blood, and the secretions from the vagina and wounds, could be more easily removed; and in case of considerable inflammation occurring after the operation, cold water could be more readily and continuously applied by means of a syringe. By this modification of the operation, the union of the labia would form a kind of bridge, with two communications into the vagina; care, however, must be taken to make the bond of union of sufficient extent, so as to allow for the subsequent contraction of the cicatrix, otherwise one or other of the openings might become so large as to allow the inverted mucous membrane gradually to be insinuated through it, and any unusual effort would expose the patient to a return of the complaint. *Part* v., *p.* 125.

PROSTATIC AFFECTIONS.

Iodine as applied to reduce Enlargement of the third Lobe of the Prostate Gland.—After alluding to the difficulty he had in applying the iodine on the third lobe of the prostate, without touching any other part of the urethra, Mr. Stafford proceeds:

"I at length thought of a very simple mode of applying it, which is by charging a bougie at its point with the *iodine, iodide of potassium,* or any other substance you may wish, and then dipping it into melted tallow so that a coating may be formed upon it. By such method I have been enabled to introduce any application I might desire up to the prostate gland, without touching the surface of any other part of the urethra. The bougie having reached the desired spot, its point is allowed to rest upon the diseased part, when the tallow gradually melts and brings the iodine or iodide of potassium into contact with it, and by drawing the bougie gently backward and forward the necessary friction is produced. I have found it advisable to be very cautious as to the strength of the application, for the prostate gland will not bear a strong preparation either of the iodine or iodide of potassium at first. It is usually in an irritable or inflamed state; consequently, even the mechanical pressure of the bougie will give pain. The preparations I have used, therefore, have been very mild. At first I have found it necessary to employ even anodynes, such as belladonna, opium, hyoscyamus, etc., to quiet irritation and pain. When these have subsided, I have begun carefully by introducing the iodide of potassium in the proportion of *one grain to the drachm of unguentum cetacei,* and increasing it as the patient could bear it. I have then gone on with two, three, four, five, and even as far as ten grains, or a scruple to the drachm, according as the case required it. After this I have added iodine to it; half a grain, one, two, three, four, or even more grains in the same manner. The surgeon who applies it can alone judge of its effects. When the swelling is so great that the neck of the bladder is completely blocked up, and no catheter can be passed onward into the interior, the patient must be relieved at all hazards, else the bladder will slough or urinary coma will succeed. Under these circumstances the surgeon is reduced to the alternative of either puncturing the distended organ, or carrying an instrument through the seat of obstruction."

By the use of a small elastic catheter without a stilette, we have succeeded in relieving retention of urine under the most urgent circumstances. We should say, as a general rule, that the greater the swelling, the less chance there is of passing a stiff, curved instrument. If, after the trial of all ordinary expedients, the bladder still remains unrelieved, then the best and safest plan unquestionably is to perforate the obstruction. The perforation is easily accomplished, and is never followed by disagreeable effects.

Part ii., *p.* 128.

Hemorrhage from Diseased Prostate Gland—Ruspini's Styptic.—Sir B. Brodie, speaking of hematuria dependent upon disease of the prostate gland, says:

" Those medicines which operate as styptics when taken internally, and which are useful in cases of hemorrhage from the lungs, are also useful in hemorrhage from the prostate. I had a patient with very diseased prostate. A frightful hemorrhage took place. The usual methods of treatment were adopted, but were of no avail. The skin became pale, the pulse became weak, and the patient was exhausted ; yet the bleeding continued. Large quantities of blood were drawn off with the catheter : nevertheless, the bladder continued to become more and more distended with blood, and was felt prominent in the belly as high as the navel. All other remedies having failed, I gave the patient a dose of the nostrum known by the name of Ruspini's styptic, and repeated the dose two or three times in the course of the next twelve hours. In about half an hour after the first dose was taken the hemorrhage ceased, and it never returned. The patient lived a year and half afterward, and there was no reason to believe that any ultimate harm arose from the bleeding."

Part vi., *p.* 50.

Treatment of Diseased Prostate—There is a description of enlarged prostate, says Mr. Colles, in which surgery can render essential benefit to the sufferer, and that by a very simple operation. When we find a patient in advanced life, complaining of unusual frequency of micturition, with more than ordinary straining, his urine depositing a good deal of muco-purulent sediment, and possibly a muco-purulent discharge from the urethra, we should make a very careful examination of the state of the prostate. If, under these circumstances, we introduce the finger into the rectum, and find the gland enlarged in either lobe, and upon pressing on one particular spot, we feel the point of the finger sink, as into a cavity ; and particularly if we find this pressure to cause the discharge, per urethram, of a quantity of thin purulent fluid, to the amount, varying from a few drops to a teaspoonful ; here we may hope to render an essential service. The operation to which I allude, is simply that of striking a lancet into this hollow, soft spot, which will generally be found to contain some matter. Now, as such an operation cannot be conveniently or securely performed by the common lancet, I have employed the pharyngotome, having previously adjusted the instrument, so as to allow the lance to project only to a length, varying from one-eighth to one-half an inch, according to the apparent thickness of this soft part, our object being to open into this cavity. The operation will be found to cause very slight pain indeed, and that confined to the region of the wound ; not even extending (as we might have anticipated) to the glans penis. So trifling and so momentary is the pain, that I have at different times performed the operation, and the patient merely imagined I had pressed a little more rudely on the gland. We are guided to the spot where the puncture is to be made, by holding the point of the forefinger of the left hand gently pressed on the soft part, and introducing the instrument on this as on a director.

In some of these operations I have had incontestable proof that some pus had been contained in the cavity, for I have found it on the blade, and in the sheath of the instrument, yet in no instance have I been able to discover, afterward, any trace of matter discharged by stool, so small has been the collection of this fluid; in some of the patients a few drops of blood have passed afterward through the urethra. In one or two, some urine has passed for a time by the rectum; the quantity, however, was, in general, very inconsiderable, but often sufficient, by its presence in, and irritation of, the rectum, to cause the patient to go to stool, though no fæces were in the rectum. This occasional watery stool was at once the only proof and inconvenience attending on such cases. This escape of urine, however, gradually ceases in the course of a week or two, never to return.

In one instance only have I seen hemorrhage follow this operation, and in that it was easily commanded by laying on the orifice a small compress of lint, and retaining it for some minutes, firmly pressed against it by the forefinger introduced into the rectum. *Part* xii., *p.* 214.

Senile Enlargement of the Prostate.—The symptoms in enlargement of the prostate gland depend with respect to their urgency upon the size it has acquired; they are, sense of weight in the perineum, intolerance of pressure from the hardness of a seat; difficulty in passing the urine, and also in voiding the fæces, which will be found flattened by the encroachment of the hypertrophied gland on the rectum. Mr. Cooper says:

At this stage of the complaint, the retention of urine occasionally supervenes, rendering the introduction of a catheter necessary. This operation should be performed with the utmost gentleness, as the slightest flow of blood would cause decomposition of the urine, and consequent aggravation of all the symptoms. An elastic gum catheter should always be used for drawing off the water, and, if possible, it should be introduced without a stilette; leeches should be applied to the perineum; the rectum emptied by means of enemata; and suppositories, recumbent position, and soothing remedies employed. I have also found colchicum of great use in such cases, and I believe that its beneficial influence arises from the circumstance that this disease frequently attacks subjects of a gouty diathesis. I usually prescribe the colchicum in the following form.

R Ext. colchici acet., gr. j.; pil. hydrarg., gr. j.; pulv. Doveri, gr. v.; ext. colocynth. co., gr. iij. M. Ft. pil. bis quotidie sumenda.

It does not always happen that the whole of the prostate gland becomes hypertrophied in old age; but very frequently the third lobe only is affected, or perhaps it may more properly be said that a new development arises; for in a state of health, at the adult period, the third lobe is scarcely perceptible. When this third lobe enlarges, it presses the inferior region of the bladder or " trigone " upward above the commencement of the urethra in the bladder, preventing the evacuation of the urine, and consequently producing retention. Nor is this the only inconvenience; for by the raising of the bladder immediately behind the prostate, a kind of reservoir is established below the entrance to the urethra; and, in the effort to empty the bladder, a portion of its contents is always left; this becomes specifically heavier than the newly-secreted urine, which does not intermix with it; and, after a time, the retained urine undergoes decom-position, which gives rise to very urgent symptoms—such as frequent desire to make water, tenesmus, deep-seated pain in the perineum, and liability to positive retention. It is quite clear that these symptoms can-not be removed while the exciting cause remains; the fetid urine must therefore be immediately drawn off by means of the catheter.

The mode of introducing the catheter in such cases is similar to that in ordinary practice, until it arrives at the point of obstruction, when the penis and instrument are both to be drawn forward for the purpose of straightening the urethra; the handle of the catheter is then to be con-siderably depressed, so as to tilt up the point, and it is then pressed onward into the bladder.

The cleansing of the bladder may be effected by injecting it with tepid water by means of a syringe; and an improved instrument has been invented for this purpose, by which a continuous current is kept, the same stroke of the piston removing one quantity and supplying a fresh one. Constitutional remedies must not be neglected; and when an alkaline state of the urine exists, medicines of an acid character are generally indicated. Among the most efficacious of these is the following:
R Nitro-hydrochlor. acid. gtt. iij.; sir. papav., ʒiij.; inf. colom., ʒiss. M. Ft. haustus ter quotidie sumendus.

In addition to this an opiate suppository at bed-time will often be found of great advantage; but if an acid condition of the urine be not thus restored, liq. potassæ will frequently be found capable of reëstablishing the normal acid state; this anomaly has been accounted for by Dr. G. O. Rees, on the supposition that the alkali renders the secreted urluc less irritating to the mucous membrane of the bladder, and prevents the secretion of alkaline mucus, from which the urine had acquired its abundant preponderance of alkali.

I must again direct your attention to the propriety of employing the prostatic catheter in cases of enlarged prostate; for I have frequently known great mischief arise from a perseverance in the attempt to relieve a patient by the ordinary instrument.   *Part* xix., *p.* 183.

Prostate, Enlarged.—M. Vanoye recommends the administration of sal ammoniac in large doses, commencing with 15 grains every two hours; we may double or treble this quantity, so that ʒss. is taken per diem. Mucilaginous vehicles, bitter extracts or aromatics, and a good animal diet, should be employed at the same time. This plan should not be fol-lowed in hemorrhagic dispositions, or in affections-due to poverty of the blood.   *Part* xxvi., *p.* 111.

Fibrous Tumors connected with the Prostate.—Prof. Fergusson states that an important circumstance connected with lithotomy is, that not unfrequently, in extracting the stone, and without any undue violence having been used, a portion of prostate gland would protrude before it. Formerly he had been in the habit of attempting to avoid the removal of such portions, but finding that no inconvenience resulted from the practice, he had latterly adopted the plan of always removing them. He thought they were probably tumors connected with the prostate, and not parts of the gland itself. *Part* xxxiii. *p.* 283.

Enlarged Prostate.—Amongst other means of treatment the following, by Dr. H. Thompson, are particularly worthy of note. Let the patient sit every morning for about twenty minutes in a tepid hip bath (90° or 94°, or warmer), to which the bittern or mother lye of the Kreuznach springs has been added in varied proportions, beginning with half a pint, or pound, according to the form in which it is obtained, to four gallons of plain water.

Local application may be made either by enema or suppository; if by the former method the following formula may be depended upon as not too irritating to the rectum. It should be retained there as long as the patient can conveniently do so. The best instrument for injecting it is an india-rubber bottle with ivory tube, as the constituents of the Kreuznach water will rapidly injure metallic apparatus.

R Potass. iodidi, gr. v. Kreuznacher bittern, ʒij.; dec. hordei vel lini, ʒiij. Misce pro enema, quotidie utendum.

To this a little opium may be added if necessary, in order to enable the bowel to retain it.

The suppository, which, on the whole, is perhaps more easily adminis-tered and borne than the enema, may be used after the following form :

R Potass. iodidi, gr. ii.–v., vel, potass. iodidi, potass. bromidi, aa. gr. ii.–iij.; cerati, gr. viij. Misce, fiat suppositorium.

This should be employed at the time of going to bed, and may be repeated every night for a considerable period.

The iodide and bromide of potassium may also be given internally, three to ten grains of the former, to one of the latter, twice a day.

The bromide of potassium given internally in these cases, has a very beneficial effect on the enlarged organ, it may be given week by week alternately with the muriated tincture of iron, for a period of several months. *Part* xxxvii., *p.* 163.

———•◦•———

PUERPERAL AFFECTIONS.

Treatment of Puerperal Convulsions.—According to the views of Dr. W. Tyler Smith, the spinal system is chiefly concerned in the production of this form of convulsion, and therefore all our remedies must be such as affect the nervous system. "Remedies affecting the spinal system," says Dr. S., "very naturally divide themselves into those which act on the central organ, the spinal marrow, and those which affect the extremi-ties of incident spinal nerves."

The action of bloodletting on the spinal marrow, is greatly modified by the condition of the circulation. In fullness of the vascular system, it is the most powerful sedative of spinal action we possess. Hence, vene-section is the grand remedy in the simpler form of puerperal convulsion, where the disease chiefly depends on stimulation of the spinal marrow by excess of blood, on the mechanical pressure exerted by the blood on that organ, together with the counter-pressure of the distended brain on the medulla oblongata. In such cases, bleeding should be performed with a view to its sedative action on the spinal marrow, and to avert the mechanical effects of vascular pressure upon this organ. Alone, it will be sufficient to subdue the disease, particularly when the fits come on before the beginning of the labor, or after delivery. But another most important intention of bloodletting should never be lost sight of—namely, that of preserving the brain from injury during the convulsion. Besides the primary cerebral congestion, which has been the cause of the attack by its counterpressure on the medulla, the convulsive action itself, with the glottis closed, exerting great muscular pressure on the whole vascular system, and causing, as it does, the great turgidity of the vessels of the head, is a dangerous source of fatal cerebral congestion, or of serous or sanguineous effusion. As in the case of epileptics, women in puerperal convulsions frequently die of apoplexy, produced by the immense pressure exerted on the cerebral column of blood during the fits. It is in a great measure the effect of bloodletting in warding off the accident from the brain that bleeding is so universal in this disease. The due recognition of distinct operation of bloodletting on the cerebral and spinal systems is of the utmost consequence. In plethoric states of the circulation, it is in this disease, curative in its action on the spinal marrow, preventive in its action on the brain.

In the absence of definite ideas regarding the effects of bloodletting in this malady, it has been often pushed to excess, or practised where it should have been altogether avoided. In the numerous cases where, besides vascular excitement of the spinal marrow, some irritation of spinal excitor nerves exists as a conjoined cause of convulsion, repeated bleedings will often fail to subdue the disease, unless the eccentric irritation be at the same time removed. When irritation of the uterus, the rectum, or the stomach, is in part excitor of the convulsion, bleeding alone cannot be relied on. It may at first diminish the impressibility of the central organ, rendering it less susceptible of the incident irritation, but if persisted in to a large extent without the removal of the eccentric irritation, it becomes in the end positively injurious, by increasing instead of diminishing the excitability of the spinal marrow.

[The propriety and extent of venesection are to be estimated, not by the violence of the disease, but by the state of the circulation in the intervals of the fits. After noticing that patients not rightly bled at first are frequently subjected to successive depletion till the loss of blood itself becomes the cause of the final seizure, he says:]

Similar remarks would apply with almost equal force to the other parts of the common antiphlogistic regimen. Nearly allied to the modus operandi of bleeding are the effects of nauseating doses of emetic tartar, which have been found so serviceable in the treatment of puerperal convulsions by Dr. Collins. It is extremely probable that this remedy acts on the spinal system through the medium of its effects on the circulation.

[During the attack of convulsion the glottis is in great part, or wholly, closed, and Dr. M. Hall questions if a true convulsion ever occurs without this symptom, and the cerebral and spinal congestion it occasions. Cold water must be dashed over the face or chest, to excite sudden inspiration and dilatation of the glottis. Excitation of the incident nerves in this way has been known to prevent a convulsion.

Harvey mentions the case of a woman who became comatose during labor, and was recovered by stimulation of the trifacial nerve in the nostrils. Denman also relates a case, where a woman had a convulsion at every labor pain, but he kept off the attacks, till delivery was completed, by sprinkling cold water over the face on every accession of pain. Cold applied to the head by napkins, iced water, ice itself, and cold water poured from a height, are approved remedies in puerperal convulsions. Does the cold act as a sedative on the cerebral portion of the spinal marrow, or does it lessen the distended state of the cerebral circulation? It probably acts in both these ways. When used in the form of continuous douche it would tend to excite acts of inspiration, and thus dilate the glottis.]

The application of cold to the spine as well as to the head may hereafter be found beneficial in puerperal convulsions. Whenever cold in any form is resorted to, its use, except for the purpose of exciting the respiration, must be continuous, as the intermittent application of cold, locally or generally, would excite instead of allay the spinal system. The benefit derivable from cold must arise from its local action on the nervous centres, because in tetanus, the purest form of increased morbid spinal action, cold applied to the spine is serviceable, whereas when applied to the whole surface of the body, it is extremely dangerous, and even fatal.

[It is important that we should learn precisely the true action of opium on the spinal system. Thus, some give opium to allay after-pains; others say, you increase their energy; some say it excites contraction in uterine hemorrhage; others maintain that it produces inertia, etc. There is a great discrepancy of opinion with regard to the propriety of its administration in puerperal convulsions. When a frog is narcotized by opium, a slight touch produces universal convulsions. Reasoning from this fact, we should judge opium to be an excitor of the spinal system; its absolute failure of arresting spasms in tetanus confirms this. Belladonna, on the contrary, acts as a sedative to the spinal marrow. Mr. Bonny suggests that it stimulates indirectly the reflex actions. Besides this, Mr. Smith thinks there are good reasons for believing it to be a direct excitant of the spinal system.]

Some striking distinctions may be made respecting the administration of opium under different circumstances, particularly in puerperal convulsions. If a dose of opium be given in this disease in a full state of the circulation, before bleeding, there is an aggravation of the disorder; while if it be given in puerperal convulsions in an anæmic subject, or after excessive depletion, it is of great service. If in a case of convulsions opium be given at the commencement, it is dangerous in its effects; but the same medicine is frequently valuable in the advanced stage of the same, when the vascular system has been powerfully depleted. Thus it would appear evident, that in convulsions with a full state of the circulation, opium is a stimulant to the spinal marrow, while in convulsions, with anæmia, it is distinctly sedative. It is certainly an important point in practice, that the effects of opium in puerperal convulsions depend on the state of the circulation; that in plethoric or inflammatory conditions it is always dangerous, while in anæmia and debility it may always be used beneficially.

[A case is related by Mr. Charles Vines, of Reading, which illustrates some important points in the pathology of puerperal convulsions, and seems to confirm the above views on their nature. The patient, twenty years of age, when eight months advanced in her first pregnancy, was suddenly seized with convulsions. When Mr. Vines first saw her, the symptoms were : Face and whole body livid, features distorted, frothy mucus about the mouth, œdema of the upper extremities, frequent and violent convulsions, and perfect unconsciousness ; there was also inordinate and tumultuous action of the heart, and a quick, feeble fluttering pulse. On examining the abdomen, the lower part was found greatly distended, and retention of urine was suspected. The catheter was passed, and five and a half pints of urine withdrawn. Great improvement of the symptoms followed. There was no return of the convulsions after this evacuation of the bladder. The patient had had for some weeks, œdema of the hands and feet, which, when recurring in these cases, has lately been shown to indicate albuminuria. The cause of the fits seems to have been the continual irritation of the vesical nerves ; at all events they were kept up by it.]

It appears clear that the irritation of the vesical nerves was conveyed to the spinal centre, and reflected upon the motor nerves and the muscular system in the form of convulsions ; how, otherwise, can we account for the cessation of the fits, and the speedy return of consciousness, when the local irritation was removed. *Part* xii., *p.* 293.

Puerperal Convulsions—Use of Galvanism.—In those cases where there is a cold skin, congested countenance, and slow pulse, galvanism, Dr. Wardell says, will be useful. One wire should be placed behind the neck, and the other over the last lumbar vertebra. *Part* xviii., *p.* 286.

Puerperal Convulsions.—Puerperal convulsions may seize the patient either before, in the progress of labor, or after it has concluded. Those that occur before or in the commencement of labor generally depend upon the irritation of some other organ than the uterus, and hence are much more fatal than those which are the result of labor ; you have in fact two sources of irritation acting upon the spinal system in place of one. Dr. R. Lee relates the case of a lady who " returned home after midnight from a large dinner party, at which she had partaken of a variety of dishes and wines, and had been seated before a large fire." Labor came on soon after, and with it violent convulsions. Another patient " being in the eighth month of her pregnancy, dined on curry and rice, and ate bacon and eggs at tea ;" the following day she had convulsions and premature labor. Both these were fatal cases, and in both the stomach was a primary, the uterus a secondary source of nervous irritation. Violent mental emotions act precisely in the same manner. More commonly, however, these are not the cases that induce the paroxysm ; on the contrary, labor proceeds to a certain point without interruption ; the action of the uterus is perhaps powerful, the head large, and the resistance to its advance great. A severe struggle arises, congestion takes place in the uterus, the pains are interrupted, a morbid irritability is excited in the uterus, which is communicated to the spinal centre, and thence reflected over all the muscles in violent convulsions. The uterus alone is the source of irritation here, and therefore the cause of the attack is more easily removed.

Dr. Murphy sums up his remarks upon the nature and causes of puerperal convulsions, as follows :

1st. Puerperal convulsions should not be confounded with epilepsy, nor with apoplexy. They agree with the epileptic attack in their physiological, but not in their pathological characters. Apoplexy is an effect of the paroxysms, which may or may not follow from them.

2d. The predisposing causes of puerperal convulsions, are either an excess of blood (hyperæmia), a deficiency of blood (anæmia), or impure blood.

3d. The proximate causes of convulsions are chiefly eccentric causes, being the morbid irritation of the afferent nerves supplying the different vital organs.

4th. *Morbid irritation of the uterus* is the 'most common proximate cause of puerperal convulsions, the result either of hyperæmia or anæmia. Hence the division into sthenic or hyperæmic convulsions, and asthenic or anæmic convulsions. Under the latter head we include not merely loss of blood, but poverty of blood, and impure blood, because the effect seems to be similar, only differing in degree.

5th. *Morbid irritation of other organs* also causes puerperal convulsions, because, during pregnancy, and at the time of labor, the nervous system is more excitable than at any other time ; and hence any organ may easily be rendered morbidly irritable. Puerperal convulsions so caused are much more fatal than the former, because the nervous centre is exposed to a two-fold source of irritation—the organ primarily affected, and the uterus that is secondarily excited.

6th. In the whole of these phenomena we must perceive a beautiful illustration of the reflex nervous function ; the peripheral nerves that supply the affected organ rapidly communicating their irritation to the spinal system, which, as an excito-motor centre, radiates the irritation over the whole of the voluntary muscles, and the muscles of respiration, in violent convulsive paroxysms. Even the involuntary muscles, as the uterus and heart, do not escape, but give every evidence of greatly increased muscular contractions.

In cases of *hyperæmic* convulsions, bleed largely and promptly, at the very commencement of the paroxysm, or indeed as soon as the premonitory symptoms are sufficiently well marked. Give also a terebinthinate enema, and if the stomach is loaded, an emetic ; or ten grains of calomel, followed by a saline senna draught containing a little tartarized antimony. And keep up the good effect of the depletion by repeated doses of tartarized antimony. Keep cloths wrung out of iced water applied to the head, and especially to the back of the neck ; being careful, at the same time, to keep the lower extremities warm. When the paroxysm comes on, dash a basin of cold water rapidly in the face ; and if this does not arrest it, take care that the patient does not injure herself during the fit, but do not hold her down, as if with the expectation of stopping the convulsion. Some recommend immediate delivery of the child, but it is not right to adopt this practice indiscriminately. If the head has descended within reach of the forceps, apply them ; but do not use the forceps if the paroxysms have subsided, for fear of again inducing them. If the head is impacted, and the child is dead, remove it by the crotchet. In other cases trust to the uterine action for effecting the delivery. *Never turn*, except the turning be otherwise necessary, as for a preternatural presentation.

Asthenic, or Anæmic convulsions require a different mode of treatment. Get the bowels freely evacuated by the use of warm stimulating cathartics, such as aloes with assafœtida, turpentine, etc. ; and then give opium, stim-

ulants, as camphor, ammonia, wine, and brandy, and nutritious food.
During the paroxysm, dash cold water in the face. If venous congestion
of the head results from the convulsions, cup from the back of the neck,
and then apply a sinapism ; taking care at the same time to support the
patient's strength, and to keep the surface warm.

The treatment of *hysterical* convulsions consists in the use of stimulating purgative enemata, followed by diffusible stimulants with opium,
and in dashing cold water in the face during the paroxysm.

Part xix., *p.* 264.

Puerperal Convulsions, Anœmic.—While stimulants are given, and the
contraction of the uterus is secured, give opium, which Dr. Lever says,
will act like a charm.

Hysterical.—In this form of convulsions, which occurs chiefly during
pregnancy, great benefit will result from the administration of a mild
opiate as soon as the paroxysm is over.   *Part* xxi., *p.* 305.

Puerperal Convulsions.—In fullness of the vascular system, says Dr.
Steele, blood-letting is the most powerful sedative of spinal action. Hence,
when the convulsions depend on the stimulation of the spinal marrow, by
excess of blood, or on mechanical pressure exerted by the blood on that
organ, or on the medulla-oblongata, we must bleed. Remove, also, if
possible, the *eccentric* cause of irritation, whether it exists in the womb,
the rectum, or the stomach. The blood-letting must be regulated, not by
the violence of the disease, but by the state of the circulation *in the interval of the fits.* Evacuate the liquor amnii, which, by relieving the distention, diminishes the size of the womb, and the quantity of blood circulating
in it, and also makes the organ less irritating to the general system.
Evacuating the liquor amnii, is to the womb what an emetic or an enema
may be to the stomach or bowels. Do not trust to chloroform, as, "when
the function of the true cerebral or sentient portion of the nervous system
are diminished or abolished, as is the case in anæsthesia, the irritability of
the excito-motory, or true spinal system of nerves, is increased."

Part xxx., *p.* 196.

Puerperal Convulsions.—After the more common remedies have failed,
the administration of turpentine conjoined with castor oil by the mouth
has been found by Dr. Woodhouse, of the Royal Berkshire Hospital, to
be very efficacious.   *Part* xxxiv., *p.* 236.

Puerperal Coma.—A middle aged, stout multipara was seized suddenly
after her last confinement with loss of consciousness ; the labor was natural
and had not been preceded nor followed by convulsions. The friends,
imagining the case to be one of apoplexy, were much alarmed. Dr. Winn
being called to the case, says : "I found her in a condition closely resembling that induced by pressure on the brain. She was in a perfectly
unconscious state, from which no impression made on the senses could
rouse her. As the breathing, however, was not stertorous, the heart not
much depressed, and the countenance tranquil, I was induced to refer the
affection to a class of phenomena which I have termed puerperal coma, to
prevent its being confounded with puerperal apoplexy, a disease of infinitely graver importance, and for which a totally different treatment is
required. In the above instance, I was glad to have it in my power to
assure the relatives of my patient that the complaint would in all probabi-

lity terminate safely. The only remedies employed were a mercurial aperient, an ammonia draught every four hours, and the frequent administration of small quantities of fluid nourishment. The result justified my diagnosis: on the following day the comatose state had passed away, and the patient was free from any alarming symptoms.

This affection, in most cases, appears to owe its origin to one or more of the following causes: nervous shock, a loaded portal system, uterine hemorrhage, and the too frequent administration of cordials and narcotics. A variety of this disorder frequently ensues after convulsions, and requires equally mild treatment. *Part* xxxvii., *p.* 205.

PUERPERAL FEVER.

Contagiousness of.—Mr. Storrs thinks that medical men do not go far enough in considering this disease to be propagated by medical men and nurses from one puerperal patient to another. He thinks that it is quite as frequently carried by the medical attendant to each fresh labor-case from some original infectious case, whether of gangrenous erysipelas, or typhus fever, or of whatever animal poison besides may hereafter be found to pro- duce it. In some cases which occurred in his own practice, he has no doubt that he took it to each patient from a case of gangrenous erysipelas with subsequent abscess, which he was attending at the time of these unfortunate occurrences. And such may be the case of other practitioners. They think that they convey the contagion from one puerperal patient to another, instead of from one common source. They probably lose a puerperal case and immediately take every precaution to prevent a similar occurrence, by careful ablution, and a complete change of dress. Nevertheless, the next case of labor is attended with the same fatal result; simply because the practition- er is still in attendance on the case which originally gave rise to the mischief.

Mr. Storrs enumerates cases recorded by different practitioners, all of which prove that each disease had a common origin from some case of erysi- pelas or sloughing ulcer. He concludes his paper with the following advice.

As it is well to be always guarded against such a misfortune, I think it desirable for midwifery practitioners to avoid attending labors in the same dress in which they attend their ordinary patients, especially the coat, as this garment must be the one most likely to be the means of conveying fomities; and at any suspicious period, when typhus or erysipelas are prevailing, to carry out the same carefulness even in the after-attendance on labor cases. I should also, after a post-mortem of any kind, or after any operation upon any case of erysipelas, or of typhus, recommend the most careful ablutions of the hands, and for the surgeon to avoid attending on a labor in any part of the dress in which such operations have been performed, not for- getting the gloves, as the hand and arm are the chief instruments of con- tact. Where, however, the disease has been unfortunately once set up in a practice, an absence from home for a fortnight or three weeks, a total change of raiment, the most careful ablutions, and a perfect avoidance of every case likely to have been the source of animal poison, should alike be adopted by the practitioner. *Part* ix., *p.* 195.

Malignant Puerperal Fever.—[Dr. G. B. Clark had two fatal cases of puerperal fever in quick succession; a post-mortem was refused in both cases, and therefore he was unable to ascertain the exact pathology of the disease; but on the occurrence of the second case, he ascertained what was supposed to be its cause. He says:]

On revolving these cases in my mind, and remembering the connection of erysipelas with this direful disease, it immediately flashed across me that I had been treating, and had then under my care, a most severe case of phlegmonous erysipelas in a sailor, who was brought into the hospital.

The disease extended from the hand to the axilla, and was treated by free incisions, aided by nitrate of silver. The man recovered from one of the most severe cases I ever witnessed. The day that I made the incisions, on that afternoon I attended Mrs. F., and I think, however painful for me to feel and relate, there can be little doubt that if no noxious matter was carried, at all events the effluvia remained, and thereby arose this malignant fever.

[Dr. Clark very prudently desisted from midwifery, and as soon as possible from all practice whatever, and took a sea voyage.]

Part xvi., *p.* 284.

Puerperal Fever.—Any fluid matter in a state of putrefaction, communicated by linen, a sponge, small particles of placenta, or by the ambient atmosphere, may induce puerperal fever. To remove such matter from the hands, wash them in a solution of chloride of lime. *Part* xxiv., *p.* 292.

Puerperal Fever.—Dr. Tyler Smith places great confidence in the chlorate of potash as a prophylactic against this fatal disease. It appears to act by liberating in the economy the oxygen and chlorine it contains. It should be given in doses from five to ten grains three times a day. The hands should be washed, and if necessary, in a solution of chloride of lime after touching any wound, purulent surface or pathological specimen; for, as Dr. Simpson remarks, the fingers may sometimes be compared to the armed points used in vaccination. Under suspicious circumstances the hands should even be washed before and after every vaginal examination. The nails of the practitioner should be kept closely cut, and some have even recommended that gloves should not be worn at all, as they have been known to become infected, and so keep up the mischief in spite of all precautions. The mucous surfaces are in the most favorable state conceivable for inoculation, and the surface of the os uteri is almost universally partly denuded of epithelium during labor. Students should not be allowed to attend labor except at certain seasons set apart for the purpose, during which time they must neither dissect, nor attend the wards of the hospital or the deadhouse. *Part* xxxv., *p.* 216.

Puerperal Fever.—In this disease Dr. Copeland says: "There is no remedy so efficacious as a decided and judicious use of spirits of turpentine." The same author also recommends camphor in doses from eight to sixteen grains; but by far the most important question is the prophylaxis of this disease. All bad or imperfect drainage must be avoided, and no medical man should attend a case of midwifery after making a P-M-examination without first washing his hands, and especially his nails, in a solution of chlorine. We must recollect that inflammation is owing to a poison, and our treatment must be directed rather to destroy or remove this poison, than to combat the inflammation. *Part* xxxvi., *p.* 232.

Secondary Affections of the Joints in Puerperal Women.—Mr. Coulson, surgeon to St. Mary's Hospital, gives the following:

Puerperal women are occasionally attacked by a severe form of disease attended by low fever, with effusion of pus into the joints, and almost always terminating in death.

The local affection occurs under two circumstances; viz., after delivery, at the full period of gestation: or after abortion in the earlier months. It is important to include the latter kind of cases, which have not been sufficiently noticed, as they throw great light on the true nature of the disease, and dispose of the theory which would attribute the secondary affections to child-bed fever.

The articular disease is merely one of the effects of pyæmia, but it receives certain modifications from the puerperal condition with which it is associated. Even in puerperal women these secondary joint affections may occur under several states which may be distinguished from each other. They are most commonly developed during the course of puerperal fever, from the third to the sixth day of the complaint. In other cases, they occur after convalescence from an attack of puerperal fever. Lastly, in some other cases they set in after parturition, without the patient having presented any symptoms of puerperal fever.

When the articular affection occurs during the course of puerperal fever, the following train of events is generally observed. For the first three or four days, the ordinary signs of puerperal fever are alone recognized; then some symptoms of phlebitis may present themselves; or these symptoms may be so slight as to be overlooked. They are soon followed by a change in the condition of the patient. Severe rigors often usher in this change; the fever increases; the countenance is anxious and sallow; the respiration becomes more hurried; there is irregular delirium; and the patient sinks.

In these cases, there are two dangerous maladies; viz., puerperal fever, and purulent infection, running their course at the same time; and it is not to be wondered at, if the general condition of the patient presents an anomalous appearance, or if it be rendered obscure by the predominance of one set of symptoms over the other.

In another set of cases, this obscurity does not exist. The patient has completely recovered from an attack of puerperal fever, or has not had any attack of that complaint; all the dangers of the puerperal state having apparently passed over. She goes on well for the first week or two; there is no fever; no abdominal pain; no apparent danger of any kind. Suddenly, a severe rigor sets in; this is followed by febrile symptoms, small, quick pulse, etc.; or the attack may commence with local symptoms, the general disturbance being scarcely perceptible. These latter cases are very remarkable, and not long ago were mistaken for rheumatism.

The disease with its local effects and constitutional symptoms, may occur after abortion in the early months. Here there are no symptoms of puerperal fever, properly so called; but there may be some slight symptoms of uterine phlebitis. These are often chronic and obscure cases; yet they proceed and terminate like the former series.

The secondary joint affections are the same under all these different circumstances. They may be either purulent or non-purulent; articular or periarticular; acute or chronic. These different conditions are found to exist in various cases; but the most common form of attack is acute, of a purulent nature, and occupies the interior of the joint. At other times, though extremely acute, the attack is non-purulent, and confined to the exterior of the joint; while in several cases, there is pus in the cavity of the joint, without any lesion of the articular tissues.

It is also worthy of remark, that in several cases some of the joints are attacked by purulent inflammation, while other joints in the same subject suffer from simple inflammation with effusion of serum.

The period at which the articular affection sets in is various. In a few cases, it has happened on the second day after delivery: in many other cases it does not appear until a few days before death, viz., from the 23d to the 25th day. Generally, however, the joints are attacked between the third and fourteenth days. The knee joint is most frequently the seat of the disease. I have found that it is attacked in one-third of the cases in which the joints have suffered; next comes the wrist joint; then the ankle, the shoulder, elbow, hip; and lastly, the smaller joints. In a few cases, the purulent effusion has been confined to the symphysis pubis; but I am inclined to think, from the history of these rare cases, that the suppuration of the pubic joint was primary, not secondary—the inflammatory action having extended from the cellular tissue of the pelvis.

The duration of the joint-disease necessarily depends on the duration of the primary affection with which it is connected as an effect. It is not often prolonged beyond a week, but it may last from one to three weeks. In chronic cases the duration may extend to three months.

I am quite unable to determine the circumstances which give rise to these differences, to explain why the effusion is purulent in some cases, serous in others; why it takes place now *in* the joint, at another time *outside* it. Moreover, the kind and seat of the effusion bear no relation to the gravity of the case, or to the intensity of the local symptoms.

The joint-affections are frequently accompanied by abscesses in the muscles of the legs and arms, preceded by pain and attended by doughy swellings. When these occur in puerperal women they should always excite attention, for they are too often the forerunner of purulent infection of the blood. The changes discovered after death are purulent effusion into the articular cavity without any alteration of tissue; frequently, signs of synovial inflammation with erosion and ulceration of the cartilages; more frequently still, purulent or serous infiltrations outside the joints, with abscesses in the neighboring muscles. In no cases have the bones been found diseased; in no case, likewise, are the lesions confined to the joints; yet in a few cases the joints and intermuscular tissue have only been affected.

The other lesions are those of purulent infection; viz., secondary deposits in the lungs, liver, etc. The brain has not been found affected, as far as I am aware. Pus is always found either in the veins or lymphatics of the uterus; or there is primary abscess in the walls of the uterus, in the cellular tissue of the pelvis, in the symphysis pubis, or elsewhere.

Practitioners are now agreed that the puerperal disease of the joints depends on blood-poisoning. The only question on which differences of opinion exists is, as to the nature of the poison. Is it pus? Is it some morbid secretion or putrid element introduced into the blood? My own opinion is that these secondary joint-affections, as well as many others, are caused by purulent poisoning of the blood.   *Part* xxxvii., *p.* 227.

Puerperal Fever.—When the fluids passing from the vagina are putrid and offensive, says Dr. T. P. Heslop, of Queen's College (which of itself, if it cause not the disease, will at any rate greatly aggravate the symptoms from absorption of the poisonous matter), inject weak solutions of hydrochloric acid at frequent intervals. A competent person must be found to do this or it will not be done effectually. *Part* xxxviii., *p.* 74.

Use of Turpentine and Opium.—The use of turpentine and opium in puerperal affections, though a treatment by no means new, does not seem to be sufficiently known or valued by the profession. The opium may be given in the form of pills, and the turpentine in that of enemata. Trousseau prescribed the opium at first in doses of 5 centigrammes during the day, gradually increasing to double the dose (centigramme =0·15432 grain); the turpentine may be administered, if given by the mouth, in the form of capsules. *Part* xxxviii., *p.* 215.

Puerperal Convulsions—Chloroform.—Two interesting cases of puerperal convulsions are related by Dr. R. T. Tracy, in which subsidence of the paroxysms and tranquil sleep followed the use of chloroform. In the first case the chloroform was given at each return of the fit, and about two minutes at each inhalation. The patient being of a very plethoric habit, ten ounces of blood were taken away prior to the administration of the chloroform. *Part* xxxviii., *p.* 227.

PUERPERAL MANIA.

Musk in Delirium of.—Pills composed of musk or assafœtida and camphor, to which may be added a few grains of calomel, and also some extract of henbane, if considered judicious, are recommended by Recamier in puerperal mania. *Part* ix., *p.* 77.

Puerperal Insanity.—The treatment generally proper for anæmia, says Dr. Mackenzie, of Paddington Dispensary for Women and Children, will be found, upon the whole, to be most appropriate for puerperal insanity. Special indications will require to be fulfilled by special means ; and slight forms of the disease will often yield to the unassisted efforts of nature. But when the attack is severe, and resists the natural efforts, as well as specific treatment, it will generally be found that this obstinacy is connected with an aggravated form of anæmia, and that in proportion as the condition of the blood is improved, will the cerebral disorder disappear. *Part* xxiv., *p.* 286.

Treatment of Puerperal Mania.—Speaking of the treatment of a case of puerperal convulsions, Dr. Mawer appends the following observations :

In the first place, it serves to confirm the imperative necessity of large and adequate depletion in the congestive variety of this formidable disease, affording at the same time ample proof of its undoubted safety and success. It also furnishes a remarkable example of the tolerance of tartar emetic—a fact long well established in reference to its use in pneumonia and some other pulmonary affections, but not that I am aware of to the same extent in cerebral disorders, as this case so strongly illustrates, a grain and a half having been taken every hour for eight consecutive hours without the least nausea resulting from it. While speaking of this valuable medicine in connection with this class of affections, it may not be out of place to add, that I have employed it with marked benefit in combination with camphor and morphia (aided by cold applications to the head, and preceded by active purgation and leeches to the temples), in two very severe cases of puerperal mania. General blood-letting being for the most part inadmissible, it is very desirable to possess a remedy so available as this proved in both the instances referred to, in controlling the excited state of the circulation, and in tranquillizing the extreme irritability of the nervous system, both which conditions are so constantly present in the more active forms of the distressing malady.   *Part* xxvii., *p.* 213.

————•••————

PULSE.

The Pulse.—[In a clinical lecture on this subject, Dr. Todd says:]

The frequency of the pulse is affected by various morbid influences, of which the following are the most potent:

The Condition of the Blood.—A poor blood is almost always associated with a rapid pulse; in animals bled to death the pulse attains an increasing frequency as the blood flows; this occurs in men who have been very largely bled, and in cases of excessive hemorrhage, whether hemoptysis, epistaxis, or hematemesis, or after surgical operations, the pulse attains great rapidity.

The Existence of a Poison in the Blood.—This tends generally to increase the frequency of the pulse, and so you find the pulse quick in the early periods of the exanthemata of typhus. The administration of alcohol to a healthy man affords a good illustration of this; as soon as he has taken a certain quantity of it, acceleration of the pulse takes place. But some poisons will produce a contrary effect, by depressing and weakening the heart's action, as you well know in the administration of digitalis, or of hydrocyanic acid. So also, some of the animal poisons, if taken in large doses, will cause depression of the heart's action and a slow pulse. We have now a case of scarlet fever, in a man named Boon, in Rose Ward, with whom the pulse was as slow as 60 before the eruption had come out fully; a state which seemed to me to indicate the use of stimulants, and under their administration the heart's action increased in force and frequency, and the patient did well.

The state of the Nervous System exercises a very remarkable influence upon the rate of frequency of the Pulse.—It is one of the features of the hysterical diathesis, that the pulse always quick, becomes accelerated under the slightest disturbance, physical or mental. Cerebral lesion sometimes causes a very depressed state of pulse; as, for example, inflammation of the brain, vomiting, pain in the head, and sluggishness of pulse, are symptoms which should always awaken the anxiety of the practitioner, as regards the state of the brain. In many instances of injury to the head, concussion, fracture with depression, the pulse becomes notably retarded until the compression of the brain has been removed. So also, in many cases of apoplexy, the pulse is sluggish, and the heart seems oppressed.

Of intermitting Pulse.—Among the most interesting modifications of pulse, which we meet with in practice, is that which arises from impairment of the rhythm of the pulse, or what is called the *intermitting pulse.*

The most common form of intermitting pulse, is that in which the phenomenon of intermission results from the prolongation of the natural period of rest in the series of changes which constitute the heart's rhythm. The heart's rhythm consists of a regular succession of first sound, second sound, rest—first sound, second sound, ·rest—and so on. Now in an intermittent pulse this rest is unnaturally long—the first sound of one beat succeeds the second of the previous beat, but after too long a pause. Sometimes the intermissions are very regular, occurring after every fourth or every third beat; sometimes perfectly irregular, at one time after every one or two beats, at another every thirty or forty.

Now what are the indications of this form of intermittent pulse? Is it indicative of organic disease? I think I may state positively that an intermittent pulse of itself affords no indications of organic disease of the heart.

Nor are we justified in pronouncing unfavorably of a patient because he has an intermittent pulse. You will meet with many persons who will tell you that they have had intermitting pulse nearly all their lives.

But undoubtedly this form of intermitting pulse denotes a derangement of the heart's action of a sympathetic nature, and almost invariably in sympathy with the state of digestion. This kind of pulse is of very common occurrence in men who work hard, neglect exercise, are irregular as to meals, and sit up late at night. It is also very common, and doubtless from the same cause, in gouty men. Intermittent pulse is not uncommouly a precursor of a paroxysm of gout. Certain ingesta are very apt in some people to cause intermission of the pulse. Tea, for example, especially green tea, is one of these; ices, more particularly cream ices, will do the same. So, also, certain medicines—as digitalis and colchicum.

I have stated that the intermittent pulse is not a necessary indication of organic disease of the heart. It is a curious fact, which is in some measure confirmatory of this remark, that of the various forms of disease to which the heart is subject, intermitting pulse is not of very frequent occurrence with any, nor is it constant to any particular form.

The intermittent pulse depends upon some interference with the healthy nutrition of the muscular system of the heart; and hence you get it so frequently in bad states of the blood—as in dyspepsia, gout, rheumatism.

You may gather, from what I have stated more than once in the preceding part of this lecture, that there is another form of intermitting pulse besides that to which I have alluded. The characteristic feature of this form is, that the intermission of the pulse does not result from the intermission of the heart's *rhythm*, but from irregularity in the *strength* of the heart's systolic contractions. The heart may never intermit, and yet the pulse may; or, in other words, the intervals between the beats of the pulse may vary considerable in duration. This form of intermitting pulse sometimes occurs alone, sometimes simultaneously with that in which the heart's rhythm is deranged. When it occurs in the progress of an acute disease, as of fever, erysipelas, etc., it must be looked upon as a sign foreboding the worst results. I apprehend that it is this form of intermitting pulse which most commonly accompanies fatty disease of the heart; and, on the whole, in all states of disease, both acute and chronic, it is that form from which we may augur least favorably for the patient.

Posture influences these two forms of intermittent pulse differently. The first form, or that which depends on a prolongation of the natural period of rest in the heart's rhythm, is diminished by the erect posture, and the heart becomes more regular in its rhythm. On the other hand, the erect posture increases the number of intermissions in the second form by embarrassing the heart's action in the way which I have already described.

[In considering the means best adapted to keep down the frequency of the pulse, we may employ either direct means acting at once upon the heart, or indirect or general means.]

Of the direct means the administration of *digitalis*, or of *opium*, is the most important. You may give digitalis as a diuretic, or with a view to obtain its specific action in reducing the frequency of the heart's action. Given with this latter view it must be administered with due regard to a correct diagosis, for while it is a very valuable remedy in one case it is a dangerous one in another. I would lay it down as a rule, that in all cases where there is regurgitative valvular disease, but especially aortic, digitalis given in doses which will depress the heart's action is a dangerous medicine; it weakens the heart, and thereby increases the embarrassment under which it already labors.

Now, opium operates upon the heart through its tranquillizing influence upon the nervous system, and so quiets the heart without weakening it, and therefore it is more generally applicable to heart affections than digitalis. The diuretic properties of digitalis may be often called into play in cases of cardiac disease; and for that purpose you may often combine it with a stimulant, as ammonia, or with some preparation of iron, so as to counteract the depressing effects. But the best combination, for a diuretic purpose, is with blue pill and squill, after a formula attributed to the late Dr. Baillie. I have seen, under the use of this combination, considerable dropsy disappear, and the heart become disembarrassed in its action in the most remarkable manner.

But then there are certain other *indirect* means of acting on the heart, as purgatives, which diminish the quantity of the blood without impoverishing it; or steel, which improves the condition of the blood already poor; rest, the recumbent position, a nutritious and moderate diet, mental quiet. It is generally from the efficacy of some of these remedies, especially the three or four last, that heart cases often experience a marked alleviation of all their symptoms on their first entering the hospital.

Part xxiii., *p.* 100.

———•◦•———

PURGATIVES.

Remarks on Drastic Purgatives.—Veratria, the alkaline principle which is supposed to give activity to colchicum, and white and black hellebore, is a powerful, and it may even be said intractable and dangerous, hydragogue-purgative. In arthritic cases, says Dr. R. Dick, attended with plethora and distinct constitutional fever, with morbid and loaded bowels, scanty and high-colored urine, and tumultuous action of the heart, veratria is indicated. Veratria, one grain; powder of acacia, two scruples and a half; sirup, a sufficient quantity.

The dose may be carried to three pills daily. This is the formula recommended by Majendie. We have seen no good effect from it in paralysis, for which some recommend it. Veratria may also be used in tincture and ointment.

Elaterium is somewhat analogous in its properties to veratrum. Its action, which is that of a hydragogue-purgative, is extremely violent. It is useful in the inflammatory anasarca of robust or young subjects ; but its use is to be deprecated in chronic dropsies, and in the cases of persons feeble or aged. I have seen it powerfully check rheumatic fever, and wonderfully relieve rheumatic metastasis to the heart. I have also seen it rapidly reduce the effusion into the cavity of the large joints, consequent on acute articular rheumatism. Some degree of its febrifuge power no doubt depends on the extreme nausea which it usually induces. From ten grains of the extract of elaterium, one grain of an alkaline principle called elateria, or elaterin, may be obtained. A tincture of this is more manageable than the extract. Elaterine, one grain ; spirits of wine, eight drachms ; nitric acid, two minims. Dose, thirty or forty drops. This dose, I may remark, will, with many persons, act drastically. Where it does not operate sufficiently, it may be repeated, in a full or half dose, after three or four hours. In suspected scirrhus of the pylorus, neither veratrum nor elaterium should be ordered, unless in very particular exigencies, and then with very particular precaution.

Croton oil is another of our drastic purgatives. In torpid states of the bowels, and when the vena portæ is in a state of congestion and distention, constituting what is called abdominal plethora, which some German writers consider a very important pathological condition, croton oil often brings sudden and marked relief. It also decidedly eases cerebral congestion and plethora, promptly dissipating the most intense and alarming headaches. Unless cautiously administered, however, it is a debilitating cathartic, and its use is not to be thought of in irritable states of the gastric or intestinal mucous membrane.

The half of the following combination will be found to be nearly corresponding in strength to a similar dose of castor oil : Croton oil, one minim ; oil of almonds, two ounces.

We may here observe that oil of turpentine has almost all the advantages, without any of the disadvantages, of croton oil, while the former possesses some good properties which the latter wants. In sluggish and flatulent states of the bowels, in tumid states of the intestinal mucous membrane, with a congested and distended condition of the rectum, oil of turpentine often gives surprising relief. Its nauseating taste and smell, and its tendency for some time after it is taken, to rise in eructations from the stomach, are its drawbacks. But this is compensated by the singularly warm and invigorating influence it has on the abdominal organs. In gouty, rheumatic, and paralytic cases, it is a most valuable means. It may be used with great benefit, in injection as well as in draught.

Part xv., *p.* 114.

Oil of Anda, a new Purgative.—[The Anda Gomesii is a Brazilian plant, belonging to the class and order Monœsia Monadelphia, N. O. Euphorbiaceæ. Its seeds are used as a cathartic by the inhabitants of the Brazils ; and the oil expressed from them has been used in North America. Mr. Ure having administered this oil in several cases, gives the following account of its effect. He says :]

It may be observed, that the average dose of oil of anda administered was 20 drops, and to secure its entrance into the stomach it was swallowed on sugar. It offered nothing unpleasant to the taste, produced none of that heat in the throat which croton oil creates, seldom occasioned nausea or griping ; it rarely operated within a period of two hours, although in

one or two instances I have known it act within half an hour after its
ingestion. *Part* xx., *p.* 290.

Best Means of Obtaining the Purgative Operation of Calomel.—[For
the purpose of obtaining the best purgative effect of calomel, Dr. Hall
recommends it to be mixed with a little table salt, and placed dry upon
the tongue ; no other purgative being combined with it, and the patient
abstaining for some time from taking water or other fluids. Dr. Hall
observes :]

This is a point of practical importance, and well worthy the attention of
the practising surgeon and physician. It is a well known fact that the inhabitants of maritime localities, and sailors, after a long voyage, in which
they have been deprived of the use of fresh provisions, and kept upon salt
meat, are more liable than others not so circumstanced to the influence of
mercurial preparations ; which arises in the opinion of Mialhe, from the
bodies of such men containing large quantities of the alkaline chlorides—
so that there is more complete conversion of calomel into corrosive sublimate than under the usual state of the body.

Children, and patients confined to a milk diet, support large doses
of calomel, because the fluids in their alimentary canals are destitute,
or contain only very small quantities of the alkaline chlorides. Patients, also, who have lived for a long time on broth, or low diet, the fluids
of whose bodies are also exhausted of chlorides, consequently bear larger
doses of calomel without the system becoming affected.

Part xxi., *p.* 151.

PYROSIS.

Ioduret of Silver.—In about one-quarter of a grain dose, three times a
day, recommended, by Dr. Patterson, in pyrosis and gastric affections.

℞ Ioduret of silver, nitrate of potassa, each ten grains. Pulverize
thoroughly and add pulv. liquorice ext., half a drachm ; white sugar,
twenty grains; mucilage of gum arabic, sufficient to mix. Divide into
forty pills. Dose, one three times a day. *Part* vi., *p.* 13.

Oxide of Silver in certain Diseases of Debility.—Sir James Eyre says,
he has found half a grain of the oxide of silver, three times a day, uniformly succeed in curing pyrosis; he administers at the same time two of
Dr. Hamilton's pills (composed of ext. colcynth, c. Ɖij. ; ext. hyosciam, Ɖj. ;
in pil. xij.) every night. He gives numerous cases illustrative of his
success. He next advances instances of similar successful results in
hematemesis and hemoptysis, but he does not exclusively confine himself
to the oxide of silver alone, but assists its administration by bleeding,
blistering, and other means.

From having found this remedy much superior to all other means employed during an active professional life of upward of thirty years, Sir
James feels fully justified in inviting a trial of the medicine. That it is a
tonic and sedative there can be no doubt, and there is also good evidence to
prove that it is a safe and efficient astringent. In the cases enumerated,
the dose never exceeded three grains a day, instead of six, as recommended
when first introduced ; and its employment where febrile action exists is
not recommended.

In addition to its value in gastrodynia, in pyrosis, in hemoptysis, in hematemesis, and in the first and second classes of menorrhagia in Dr. F. Churchill, it will be found to be productive of infinite benefit in restraining, when absolutely necessary, hemorrhage proceeding from the intestinal canal, obstinate chronic diarrhœa, colliquative perspirations, leucorrhœa, and other maladies. *Part* xi., *p.* 107.

Treatment of Pyrosis.—The mineral acids, being astringent tonics, are especially suited to relieve obstinate pyrosis in feeble individuals. Sometimes the sulphuric, sometimes the nitro-muriatic acid succeeds best; nor can the one best adapted for each particular case be always determined beforehand. If there be much debility, however, the former should be first tried, and the latter if bilious disorder be conjoined with indigestion. It is perfectly consistent practice, according to Dr. Child, to prescribe regular doses of acids and occasional doses of alkalies for the same patient, each medicine fulfilling a separate purpose. Alkalies are merely palliative, and relieve only when the irritating fluid that has been poured out is of an acid nature; on the other hand, the mineral acids strike at the root of the pyrosis, and produce a radical cure by checking the secretion of the fluid itself, in consequence of their tonic and astringent effects upon the vessels of the mucous membrane. The mineral acids, therefore, should be given, like other tonics, when the stomach is empty; while alkalies are of little use unless administered toward the end of digestion, at the moment when the acid fluids are irritating the gastric nerves. If taken with care in this manner, the one does not interfere with the action of the other. When pyrosis is obstinate, counter-irritation to the epigastrium, as by means of a blister, is often highly useful: it operates by relieving congestion of the mucous membrane, and imparting tone to the secreting vessels.

Medicines can palliate, even in the worst cases; but in order to effect a lasting cure, careful rules of diet must be enforced. In particular, fat, fried, or cured meat, pastry, nuts, cucumbers, pickles, and malt liquors, are to be eschewed. Moreover, all articles of food which, although generally wholesome and digestible, are yet found by patients to "turn to acid or water, or to ferment," as they express it, are to be avoided. Among the things in common use most apt to excite pyrosis, may be mentioned oatmeal, potatoes, fish and tea. As a general rule, a vegetable diet is more *acid-producing* than one chiefly composed of the easily digested kinds of animal foods; hence many patients remark that they are more troubled with acidity when they live on slops—farinaceous articles—than when they make use of a full meat diet. When bilious pyrosis occurs the first thing in the morning, it is often prevented by taking a little food before getting out of bed. Many patients find that exercise or constrained postures are sure to bring on an attack: hence clerks are extremely apt to suffer therefrom when closely confined to the desk. *Part* xvi., *p.* 318.

Treatment of Pyrosis.—If the disorder should seem to be caused mainly by a diet not sufficiently nutritious or consisting too much of farinaceous substances, the most effectual remedy will be a wholesome nourishing diet, containing a proper quantity of animal food *in its most digestible form.* Little permanent benefit can, indeed, be expected from medicine unless the diet is improved.

If the disorder should seem to have been induced, or to be kept up, wholly or in part, by fatigue, it is very essential that the patient should rest ; if by constipation, that this condition should be removed by purgatives, such as aloes or colocynth, that do not offend the stomach.

After these points' have been attended to, much further good may be done by medicines. Give a combination of astringent and sedative remedies, as five grains of bismuth with 1-12th of a grain of the muriate of morphia, or five grains of the compound kino powder, or an efficient dose of catechu, krameria, or logwood, with opium, two or three times a day. Astringents are useful sometimes, as half a grain of argent. nit. three times a day ; or three to five grains of nux vomica three times a day ; or quinine, or the mineral acids. If there be anæmia present, steel should be given.

The medicines of which Dr. Budd has had most experience in disorders of this class, and which are probably as efficacious as any, are bismuth, with morphia ; krameria, and logwood, with opium ; and steel.

Part xxix., *p.* 107.

Gallic Acid in Pyrosis.—Dr. Bayes says that in pyrosis, where this disease is unaccompanied by extensive ulceration, or organic malignant diseases of the stomach, or by disease of the liver, the most marked benefit will follow the use of the remedy. Gallic acid, here, not only checks the secretion with a certainty and rapidity he has never seen follow the administration of any other remedy, but it gives general tone to the stomach, increases the appetite, and (what I very little expected when I first used it) in many cases removes constipation. This I can only account for on the supposition that the relaxed atonic state of the stomach which favors pyrosis is continued throughout the alimentary canal, the constipation in these cases arising from want of power in the muscular coats of the intestines to expel the fæces. This want of tonicity is remedied by gallic acid.

Part xxxv., *p.* 94.

QUININE.

To disguise the Taste of Quinine.—Administer it in coffee.

Part xvi., *p.* 67.

New Preparation of Quinine.—Dr. Kingdon introduced a new preparation of quinine which he had lately succeeded in preparing. It is the di-arsenite—that is, it consists of one part of arsenious acid, and two of quinine ; it is a powerful medicine, and one which he has found of great benefit, especially in chronic cutaneous affections, and has no doubt it would be equally beneficial in ague, tic douloureux, and neuralgia. It possesses both the qualities of a mineral and vegetable tonic, and when the system has become habituated to either the one or the other (which we frequently find the case from long-continued use), by the administration of this medicine you will keep up the former action, while at the same time a new one is introduced into the system. He related a case which demonstrates this very satisfactorily. A young woman who had been affected with lepra six years, was admitted a patient at the Exeter Dispensary, under his care, and was ordered the liq. potassæ arsenitis, with decoct. dulcamaræ, three times a day. For a time the disease appeared to be improving, but it gradually got back to its former state, although the quantity of arsenical solution was increased to the full extent ; he then ordered one-third of a grain of di-arsenite of quinine to be taken twice a day, and the following week the eruption was much improved. It has been gradually increased to four times a day, and now she is nearly well.

Part xvi., *p.* 297.

Quinine, without its Bitterness.—To deprive quinine of its bitterness, combine ten grains of it with two grains of tannic acid. *Part* xxiii., *p.* 336.

Disguising the Taste of Quinine.—A piece of chocolate should be half masticated, and retained between the cheeks and the teeth. The quinine draught is to be rapidly swallowed; and then the mastication of the chocolate is to be completed, so that it may be swallowed also. The taste of the quinine is thus hardly perceived. *Part* xxvi., *p.* 326.

Action of Quinine.—The following are the general rules, established by M. Briquet, for giving quinine in fever: 1st. Give each hour or second hour the sixth or twelfth part of the quantity to be taken daily, and leave ten hours' interval without any quinine. 2d. Gradually increase the dose, until head symptoms, vertigo, and pain are produced. In *ague*, give the quinine so as to produce the maximum effect at the commencement of the febrile action. In *typhoid fever*, give quinine during the night, for the access comes on in the afternoon, and it requires some hours after administration before it produces its full effect. Always give it in solution: when given in the form of pills it is only one-sixth as active in three hours.

Part xxxii., *p.* 277.

Quinine.—As a prophylactic, quinine is especially valuable while in unhealthy localities. It should be given in three or four grain doses twice a day in a glass of sherry, and its use should be continued for fourteen days after leaving an unhealthy district. Its effects in tropical climates are very manifest, producing a refreshing and exhilarating effect on the system, which nothing can equal. *Part* xxxv., *p.* 17.

RECTUM.

Relaxed Rectum.—Dr. Hunt describes this as a malady of not unfrequent occurrence, and productive of much inconvenience and distress. The most prominent symptoms are obstinate constipation, a frequent desire to evacuate the bowels, a constant sensation of load in the rectum —which is not relieved by an evacuation—and the discharge, after much forcing, of mucous streaked with blood. The bladder, urethra, and other adjacent organs, often participate in the irritation. On examination, the rectum will be found preternaturally enlarged, and more or less filled with large folds of mucous membrane pressing down on the anus, which impede the evacuation of the fæces, introduction of instruments, and injection of enemata. This morbid condition of mucous membrane, the author attributes to a neglected state of the bowels, and repeated great distention of the rectum by fæces, which causes the mucous membrane, when the bowel is empty, to hang in loose folds. This disease, if neglected or mismanaged, gives rise to prolapsus ani, an irritable and painful state of the sphincter, and an intro-susception of the upper and undilated portion of the intestine, into the lower and dilated part. The treatment recommended for the simple relaxed rectum is, the avoidance of all aperient medicines, and the injection of a pint of cold water into the bowel every night previous to going to bed, the removal of the prolapsus, and the application of belladonna ointment to the irritable sphincter. In the case of intro-susception of the rectum, in addition to the use of the cold water injection, the exhibition of some mild aperient, taking care that whilst a costive and hardened state of the fæces is prevented, purging is avoided, and a course of the hyd. cum creta, with hyoscyamus or conium, or the iodide of potash and sarsaparilla.

[Dr. James Johnson disagrees with Dr. Hunt with respect to the use of mild aperients. He considers them to be essential to the successful treatment of the affection. He says:]

In cases of constipation, it is essential, to effect a cure, that the colon as well as the rectum should be acted upon. Fæces often collect above the rectum, and cannot be reached by small injections of cold water. These injections are, moreover, not so harmless as people seem to imagine; at all events, he has seen them productive of violent tormina and great pain; in some instances, producing faintness. He would, in this class of cases, administer some mild aperient, which would act on the colon, and soften the fæces in that tube—such, for instance, as the tartrate of potash or the confection of senna. These medicines produce no irritation or unavailing efforts to evacuate the rectum; on the contrary, they soften the fæces above, and soothe rather than irritate. In the second class of cases mentioned, in which there was intro-susception of the rectum, he has found Ward's paste corrugate the folds and give tone to the part. In this class of cases, when the bowels have protruded, and have not been carefully returned, it was liable to become inflamed, and be productive of great suffering.

Mr. Barnsby Cooper agreed with Dr. Johnson in reference to the expediency of applying remedies that would act on the colon in the first class of cases described by Dr. Hunt.

He recommended evacuating the bowels at night, just before retiring to bed. In diseases of the rectum, this rule was one of the greatest importance. When evacuated just before bed-time, the patient remained in the recumbent position for many hours, and the affected bowel was, during the whole of that time, in the pelvis. By this simple plan a cure was effected without the use of instruments or of medicine, both of which combined would only alleviate and not cure.

[For the support of the rectum in these cases mechanical means may be resorted to similar to those applicable in prolapsus uteri.]

In cases of constipation from relaxation, aloes in combination with sulphate of quinine was a favorite prescription of Dr. Abercrombie, and often succeeds remarkably well, especially in persons advanced in life. In cases of great dilatation, might not injections of nitrate of silver be of service, administered as recommended by Trousseau in the diarrhœa of children?

It has a great effect in producing contraction of the calibre of the vagina. In the habitual constipation which so often produces this affection, Dr. Graves, after objecting strongly to the use of mercurial purgatives, recommends the following combination:

℞ Electuarii sennæ, ʒij.; pulv. supertart. potass., ʒss.; carb. ferri, ʒij.; sirupi zingib. q. s.—Ft. electuarium.

The dose must be regulated by its effects, but in general a small teaspoonful in the middle of the day and at bed-time will be sufficient. Dr. Graves says, that the value of carbonate of iron as a tonic aperient has not been appreciated. *Part xi., p.* 160.

Irritable Ulcer of the Rectum.—Mr. B. Cooper describes this painful form of disease—painful to the patient, and sometimes not less so by its obstinacy to the practitioner. Speaking of irritable ulcer, he says: Such a condition of ulcer not unfrequently attacks the rectum, under the form of a narrow elongated fissure, running along one of the folds of the mucous membrane, near to the orifice of the anus. The edges of the fissure are free from any callosity, and it bears a strong resemblance to the cracks which frequently affect the lips. The most usual situation for the ulcer, as far as my experience goes, is at the posterior aspect of the rectum in the mesial line, although I have sometimes found it on the side of the bowel.

The symptoms of the disease are highly characteristic; a burning pain is experienced during the act of defecation, which continues for a considerable time after each evacuation. During the intervals the patient enjoys comparative ease, but still occasionally suffers from heat and lacinating pain about the anus, but nothing to be compared to the agony produced by the passage of the fæces over the ulcerated surface and through the sphincter, and which is commonly more or less in a state of spasmodic contraction. The bowels are in these cases generally constipated.

The ulcer may involve merely the edge of the verge of the anus, or extend a considerable way up the intestine, but may always be detected by passing the finger into the rectum, when the nature of the sore is readily appreciated by the extreme pain which the patient experiences directly the finger comes in contact with the fissure.

The finger on being withdrawn, will be marked with a streak of blood, and lead to the discovery of the size and position of the ulcer.

Pass the forefinger of the left hand up the rectum, and direct a straight probe-pointed bistoury along it, beyond the very extremity of the fissure ; then divide the ulcerated surface, and the fibres of the sphincter which are connected with it. In the after-treatment, advise the patient to get the habit of evacuating the bowels at bed-time, instead of in the morning.
Part xvii., p. 172.

Stricture of the Rectum.—The rectum is sometimes, Mr. Cooper observes, the seat of spasmodic stricture, resembling the stricture of the œsophagus which occurs in hysterical females. But permanent stricture is a frequent occurrence, and one of the prominent symptoms of this state is constipation, partly due to the obstruction, and partly occasioned by the avoidance of defecation by the patient, who dreads the acute pains which it occasions.

The egesta, Mr. Cooper observes, in stricture of the rectum are passed in small rounded portions, or if "figured," of very small diameter, from being forced through the contracted part; the patient usually complains of distention of the abdomen, interference with the function of respiration, and loss of appetite. With these symptoms an examination should be made per anum, at first with the finger alone, and this will probably lead to the detection of the obstruction, which is often very firm, and resists the entrance of the finger into the bowel. This excessive hardness may be produced either by scirrhus, or by a mere attack of inflammation, and therefore, the hardness alone is not to determine the judgment of the surgeon as to the disease being malignant, as that question will be best decided by the age of the patient, the length of time the disease has ex. isted, and by the nature of the pain. If, for instance, the patient be old, the pain constant, severe, and of a lancinating character, and he has great dread of exciting the muscular action necessary to the evacuation of the bowels, and if at the same time there is an appearance of what is termed malignant diathesis, the prognosis would be unfavorable. But, if the ob- struction results from simple inflammation in a youthful patient, it will be indicated by the suddenness of its appearance, by the febrile symptoms attendant upon it, and by the peculiar sensation conveyed to the finger; for although there is considerable hardness, it is not of the stony character that marks scirrhus, but gives the idea of its being a dense projection of the natural structures into the bowel, rather than an adventitious deposit. When the disease is malignant, bleeding is frequent, particularly upon examination either by the finger or instrument, and the pain lasts for a considerable time after, which is not the case with common stricture. The treatment in the non-malignant disease consists in the occasional applica- tion of leeches around the anus, the patient being kept in the recumbent posture, and I believe that enemata will be generally found better than bougies, as a mechanical means of overcoming the obstruction, unless they act, indeed, too much upon the bowels, in which case bougies must of course be employed.

The introduction of the bougie is a matter requiring considerable skill and anatomical knowledge. From want of this knowledge, indeed, unskillful practitioners often do great mischief, sometimes wounding the rectum, from which accident extravasation of fæces, peritonitis, and death, may be produced. The bougie should, therefore, only be employed by scientific surgeons. Leeches, the recumbent posture, injections, and in some cases the use of the bougies, and cupping in the loins when the pain is severe, are the means to be had recourse to in non-malignant obstruc- tion. And often, by such measures, a disease which at first appeared to be of an alarming character, is quickly removed. In malignant disease but little can be done: the adventitious matter indefinitely increases, so as at length completely to obliterate the bowel, and the patient dies from the insuperable barrier opposed to the escape of the excretions, unless an arti- ficial anus be made in the colon, or as some surgeons have recommended, a cutting gorget, or some instrument of the kind be forced through the obstruction; but this, if it afford any relief, can only do so temporarily. Scirrhus stricture generally destroys the patient, however, by the propa- gation of the malignant disease through the medium of the absorbents to some distant part: thus, perhaps, transplanting it to important vital organs, in which case the reaction on the constitutional powers is very rapid, and the patient soon sinks beneath its influence.

Part xviii., *p.* 195.

Stricture of the Rectum.—An operation for this disease was performed at St. Thomas's Hospital, as follows: The patient being placed upon her face, the stricture soon reached, the mere point of the finger getting into it, a grooved director was passed up to it, together with a bistoury. The director was next let fall out, and the knife carried through all the parts up to the coccyx. The intestine above the point of the stricture seemed quite free. The rectum was laid open, and two vessels, probably branches of the superior hemorrhoidal, spouted out pretty freely, and were tied ; the fibres of the upper and lower sphincter were also visible. The thick mucous membrane with the stricture, and the various veins and nerves were all divided. After the hemorrhage had ceased, a large plug of lint was put into the wound, and secured by a T bandage. The operation was quite successful. *Part* xxii., *p.* 216.·

Fungous Tumor of the Rectum in Children attended with Bloody Discharges.—M. Martin has already directed attention to the affection as it occurs in the adult, producing discharges which are mistaken for those from hemorrhoids. The first case occurred in a child, aged 5, about whom the author was consulted in consequence of hemorrhages which occurred during a prolapsus ani, and which arose from an excrescence that he at first mistook for hemorrhoids. Examining it more closely, he found it was a spongy vegetation, not unlike a portion of the placenta, which protruded from beyond the sphincter when the child went to stool, and was quite insensible to the touch. As the hemorrhage had been considerable, the fungus was touched with the nitrate of silver, whenever it protruded ; and, owing to its softness, four or five applications, at intervals of several hours, sufficed for its destruction. In a second case, a girl, aged 8, had become much reduced by the quantity of blood she had lost during several weeks ; and a fungous tumor, about the size of an almond, was easily removed in the same way. A third case occurred in an infant six months old, in whom efforts at stool protruded a tumor the size of a pea, which bled. The author believing it to be the germ of the fungous tumor, also treated it with caustic.

M. Leclayse believes that this affection is often mistaken for hemorrhoids ; and especially when the bleedings are said to be due to internal piles. The caustic could not be applied very high up, but as the bleeding has only occurred on the protrusion of the tumor, this has been easily reached, the application being successful even when the base of the tumor could not be attained. *Part* xxii., *p.* 218.

Irritable Ulcer of the Rectum.—Give chloroform, and divide the fissure by a longitudinal incision through the centre of the ulcer, including the sphincter muscle. The great source of mischief is now set at rest, and the ulcer heals ; but the healing process is promoted by applying a plug of lint, coated with the following application : Liq. plumb. diacet., ʒj. ; confect. rosæ, ℥j. This plug, dipped in sweet oil, is to be applied to the part. In sensitive ulcers of the rectum, and in painful affections generally, Mr. Curling uses the following ointment : Chloroformyli, ʒj. to ʒij ; zinci oxydi, ʒss. ; olivæ, ʒj ; cerat. cetacei, ʒiv. M. ft. ung. *Part* xxiv., *p.* 215.

Inflammation and Ulceration of the Rectum.—At a meeting of the Medical Society of London, Mr. Coulson said, that he saw a patient, aged thirty-four, who passed a semi-solid feculent motion once in twenty-four hours, tinged with mucus and blood, and in addition to this, within the same time, four or five evacuations consisting solely of small quantities of mucus and blood. On examining the bowel with the speculum, it was found that the mucous membrane was destroyed to the extent of two inches from the anus, and pus and blood were seen exuding from the ulcerated surface. Various local and constitutional remedies were employed with little relief except a slight diminution of the discharge. It was then suggested that the decoction of tormentilla should be tried; three ounces of this root in a

pint and a half of boiling water were boiled down to a pint, and four
ounces of the decoction were thrown up the rectum twice a day, and
retained each time a quarter of an hour. Under the use of this remedy
the pus and mucus gradually diminished, and within five weeks the ulceration had completely healed; the only medicine taken during this time was
a little castor oil, to keep the bowels loose. Mr. Coulson believed the
rectum to be occasionally the seat of inflammation, attended with muco-
purulent discharge, which, if unchecked, proceeds to the destruction of
the mucous membrane of the bowel, and to the formation of abscesses in
the neighborhood of the anus. A frequent desire to go to stool exists in
these cases; and unless this be yielded to at once, the motions come away
of their own accord, loose, and mixed with blood and mucus; at last the
patient's health gives way, and he is worn out by continued suffering.
Mr. Coulson showed a preparation taken from a patient who had died of
this complaint: the cellular tissue round the anus was hardened, the
mucous membrane of the rectum completely destroyed, and the internal
surface of this bowel presented elevated hypertrophied muscular fibres,
between which there were several openings communicating with external
abscesses, so that these in fact were the result of the disease of the interior
of the gut—the diseased action without being continuous with that within.
The ulceration of which he had been speaking, was not to be confounded
with the fissured rectum which often occurs from mechanical causes, or the
ulcerated rectum which is sometimes found in persons laboring under a
syphilitic taint. These conditions of the bowel were very painful, and the
source of great distress to the sufferer, but they easily yielded to remedies
—as the black oxide of mercury ointment (one drachm of the black oxide
to an ounce of lard) or if this failed, to a division of the surface of the
ulcers—and when left to themselves did not destroy the patient. Mr.
Coulson said it was most desirable, in all diseases of the rectum, to make
an examination of the bowel with the speculum.   *Part* xxv., *p.* 213.

Rectum— Ulceration and Excoriation of.—Keep the bowels free by
the management of diet after the confection of senna has been used.
Touch the small surface of ulceration with the point of a piece of sulphate
of copper morning and evening, and after the bowels have been opened,
apply hot water with a sponge for a few minutes, and then an ointment
consisting of hyd. c. creta and ceratum cetacei, ℥ss to ℥j.

*   *   *   *   *   *   *   *

Place the forefinger of the left hand upon the sore, and with a probe-
pointed bistoury fairly divide the ulcer longitudinally by passing through
it into the subjacent tissue. If the ulcer is extensive, or complicated with
other diseases, some addition is necessary to the treatment by simple
incision according to the complication. Sir B. Brodie and Mr. Copeland
agree in the above method of treatment.   *Part* xxvi., *p.* 187.

Irritable Rectum.—In a case of this disease, under the care of Dr.
Barlow, attended with constipation, in which repeated clysters and large
doses of castor oil had failed in giving any relief, perfect success followed
the administration of five grains of pil. saponis c. opio, given three times a
day; with ℥ij. of castor oil on alternate mornings. The opium did not in
any way interfere with the powers of digestion.   *Part* xxvi., *p.* 196.

Affections of the Rectum caused by certain conditions of the Womb.—
Mr. I. B. Brown says: Displacement forward or backward, and enlarge-

ment of the uterus, from whatever cause, whether pregnancy, hypertrophy, inflammatory engorgement, distention by fluid or by hydatids, polypi, or scirrhus, or any other disease, alike tend to injuriously affect the rectum.

As displacement may occur without enlargement of the uterus, it may operate singly in inducing rectal disease; but more often the two conditions concur, and it is then chiefly that the mischief is so considerable. The evils, too, will be greater when, with retroversion, engorgement of the body of the uterus, and with anteversion, that of its neck, go together. On the other hand, enlargement, without deviation of the womb forward or backward, may, and oftener does, act singly in provoking disease of the rectum, than either of these displacements does without it.

The conditions of the uterus under consideration act on the rectum injuriously in two ways; first, by mechanical pressure; and, second, by inducing vascular disturbance like that present in themselves. An enlarged uterus drags on its lateral ligaments, elongates them, subsides lower down in the pelvis, and so comes to press on the lower bowel, to interfere with its muscular action, and the circulation through its blood-vessels, and to irritate its mucous lining. At the same time any hyperæmic state of the uterine vessels causes an increased fullness of the hemorrhoidal, and a determination of blood to them. Thus, by reflecting on the anatomy of the parts, it will easily be understood why and how diseases of the rectum, such as hemorrhoids, prolapsus, fissure, stricture, fistula, as well as disordered functions of the bowel, as constipation, dysenteric irritation, etc., do sometimes result directly, either from the mechanical pressure of an enlarged uterus, or simply from the derangement of the hemorrhoidal circulation, resulting from uterine disease. *Part* xxx., *p.* 217.

Ulcerated Cancer of the Rectum.—For the relief of the dreadful pain caused by defecation in this disease, and which alone is a principal cause of the great exhaustion, Prof. Erichsen recommends Amussat's operation. You relieve the pain, and remove the cause which would stimulate the disease to make more rapid and extensive ravages than it otherwise would. *Part* xxxv., *p.* 106.

Rectum, Hemorrhage from.—After operations on the rectum, instead of using lint to restrain the hemorrhage, Mr. Salmon would introduce into the return a large plug of the finest jeweller's wool, and press it gently into the whole length of the wound. The wool must on no account be oiled, as it is by its loose absorbing texture, that it is so valuable. Styptics are never necessary, continued pressure is almost invariably found efficient. *Part* xxxv., *p.* 114.

———•••———

RESPIRATION.

Respiration.—The ingestion of fats and pure starch decrease respiration; sugar largely increases respiration; albumen, gelatin, milk, and all ordinary nitrogenous diet, increase it to a moderate degree only. Whilst brandy, wine, and kirchenwasser greatly decrease respiration, rum largely increases it. Ether, tea, and sugar are the most powerful respiratory excitants: ammonia, opium, morphia, tartarized antimony, kirchenwasser, and sleep, are the most powerful depressants. *Part* xxxv., *p.* 309.

Artificial Respiration—May be carried on by alternately squeezing the chest with the hands, so as to induce a forced condition of expiration, and removing the hands, when the elasticity of the parietes will restore them to a medium state and cause the entrance of air. Mr. Humphry has more than once saved life by resorting to this simple process.

Part xxxix., *p.* 95.

Artificial Respiration. Vide Art. "Drowning."

———•◦•———

RHEUMATISM.

Abstracts from the best writings on Rheumatism—Colchicum.—Mr. L. Wigan, of Brighton, confidently asserts the following mode of using this remedy to be heroic, in proportion as the case is violent and recent. Eight grains of the powdered colchicum root (preserved by being kept ground to an impalpable powder with twice or thrice its weight of white sugar), are given *every hour*, in water, or ginger, or apple tea, until vomiting, purging, or profuse perspiration take place, or at least till the stomach can bear no more. If nausea is felt after three or four doses, he stops a quarter of an hour, and gives brandy on sugar or soda water, when the medicine is again continued. The usual quantity supported is eight or ten doses; the maximum fourteen; the minimum five. After six or seven doses a slight nausea comes on; but by keeping quiet, with something in the mouth, three or four doses might be received, when perhaps the disgust becomes unconquerable. After this there is generally sound sleep, with occasional nausea on waking. The pain ceases, but the more active effects of colchicum do not take place for some hours after the last dose, and after a few hours more is succeeded by "Elysium." The inflammation of the joints subsides, and they resume their size with miraculous rapidity. The acidity of the perspiration ceases as well as the peculiar odor. As soon as a cup of souchong tea can be obtained, a sound sleep comes on, from which the patient awakes perfectly well. When enabled to do so, Mr. W. prefers giving a breakfast of bread and butter and tea only, very early in the morning, and two hours afterward to commence the colchicum. Nothing more but tea, and bread sopped in it during that day. It is well to indulge the returning appetite very sparingly on the day following, on which we may allow a small snap of devilled meat and rice, with a little curry, if desired. Afterward the patient may resume his ordinary diet as soon as his appetite indicates it. Mr. W. has never known a relapse, and strongly urges the practice. We confess to have some doubts of the safety of this plan, unless in robust subjects and in a very acute form of the disease.

Emetics, Purgatives, Peruvian Bark, etc.—Dr. Davis says that the duration of the disease, under the following plan does not exceed a week in the majority of cases: Bleeding from the arm to faintness, succeeded by an emetic of ipecacuanha and tartar emetic, and in five or six hours by a purge of calomel and jalap; after this he gives a scruple to half a drachm of powdered yellow bark, every three or four hours. This is similar to Haygarth's plan, and has the sanction of very varied experience.

Bleeding, Calomel, Opium, etc.—The late, and much-to-be-lamented Dr. Hope, after six years' experience upon 200 cases, gives decided preference to the following plan : After one, or even two full bleedings in the robust, he gave seven to ten grains of calomel, with one or two of opium, at night, a draught with fifteen to twenty minims of colchicum wine, and five grains of Dover's powder in saline mixture, three times a day. It was seldom necessary to repeat the calomel more than from two to four times, after which he continued the opium at night, with the colchicum draught and a senna laxative every morning. The patient was almost always well in a week, and able to commence his work in seven to ten days after pains had ceased. Ptyalism was avoided unless the heart was involved. In chronic cases he gave five grains of calomel, and one of opium, at night, for five or six times, with the senna and colchicum draught as before. Local depletion with some form of counter-irritation were usually employed.

Tart. Emetic, Nitre, Colchicum, etc.—In the acute stage Dr. Graves principally relies on bleeding, with large doses of tartar emetic and nitre, and in less urgent cases, particularly if complicated with bronchitis, he has derived much benefit from the following mixture :

℞ Almond emulsion, eight ounces ; vinegar of colchicum, half an ounce ; acetate of morphia, one grain ; nitrate of potash, half a drachm. Mix. Half an ounce every hour or every two hours.

If colchicum does not relieve in two or three days we must have recourse to mercury.

Peroxide of Mercury, Opium.—Dr. Pitschaft has for twenty years employed mercury, preferring the red precipitate, in doses of one-eighth to one quarter of a grain twice a day, combined with opium if the system be irritable.

Bleeding and Dover's Powder.—Dr. Christison, after premising bleeding, thinks that keeping up perspiration by frequent doses of Dover's powder for 36 to 48 hours is an admirable plan. Purging must be avoided till the sweating is over, nor is the plan so successful if commenced later than the fourth day.

Bleeding, Purging, Guaiacum, etc.—Dr. Macleod advises bleeding from twelve to thirty ounces during the first week, giving three to five grains of calomel at night, and a senna purge in the morning. Opium to the extent of two grains in the twenty-four hours is often useful, and the guaiacum is recommended as the best after-treatment. In lumbago, Dr. M. thinks well of a brisk calomel purge once or twice a week as above, and considers half a drachm to two drachms of the compound tincture of guaiacum three times a day, with a grain of opium at night, the best plan.

Tinct. Guaiacum, etc., in Lumbago.—Dr. Marryatt's principal remedy against lumbago was half an ounce of the compound tincture given at bed-time, with other means adapted to promote diaphoresis.

Diet—Hydriod. Potass—Liq. Potas.—Mr. Henry Rees says, " In all cases of acute rheumatism, the diet should be strictly regulated ; avoid rigidly, beer, wine, spirits, and animal food. Milk, beef-tea, butter, eggs, fish, etc., are all pernicious. His theory is that the disease depends on an excess of nitrogen. ,

In very urgent cases bleeding and mercury may be necessary, but he regards the hydriodate of potass as certain an antidote to the rheumatic diathesis as mercury is to that of syphilis. Its combination with liquor potassæ acts, he says, like a charm in rheumatic iritis.

Colchicum Mag. Sulph. Decoct. Bark, Soda.—Dr. Hughes never found it necessary to bleed. He gave a pill of opium and antimony at night, repeating it two or three times daily, if the pain was urgent. Calomel was only used when the inflammatory symptoms were severe. Half a drachm of the colchicum wine, with a drachm of the sulphate of mag nesia, was given three or four times a day, producing, after two or three days, copious liquid, yellow evacuations, with evident relief, when he im- mediately ordered decoction of bark with soda. In a few days the patient was well.

Emetics of Tart. Antimony.—In the report of the Worcester Infirmary it is stated " that emetics of tartarized antimony, administered at the com- mencement, have cut short the disease in acute cases."

Mixture of Nitre—Lotion Iod. Potassium.—Mr. Horne speaks very favorably of the following mixture :

℞ Nitrate of potash, half an ounce ; potassio-tartrate of antimony, two grains ; spirits of nitric ether, one ounce ; water twelve ounces. Mix. A wineglassful three times a day.

He also strongly recommends the external use of a strong solution of the hydriodate of potass when the joints are implicated—a hint worthy of trial. The same lotion he has found serviceable in neuralgic pains.

Nitrate of Potash.—Dr. Brocklesby, in 1764, first directed attention to the value of nitre in large doses, giving as much as ten drachms in the day and night. Mr. W. White, in 1774, confirmed its value, carrying the maximum dose to twelve drachms. In 1833, the same practice has been revived by Messrs. Gendrin and Solon. Sixteen cases are recorded, of which the average period of treatment was eight days. The mean quan- tity of the salt given in one day was one ounce in three quarts of water ; the total average quantity, eleven ounces. They advise commencing with two drachms and a half in a quart of fluid.

Twelve successful cases are recorded by M. Arran, where the mean dose was thirty-six grains in three pints of fluid, and the average total quantity 374 grains. The mean duration was eight days.

We suspect the above doses to be excessive, and believe M. Arran's practice the most reasonable and prudent. Such evidence is illustrative of the differences prevalent among practical men as to the necessary doses of medicine. There are enthusiastic givers as well as takers of physic.

Opium, Quinine, Warm Embrocations.—Dr. Corrigan, in a very interesting paper in the " Dublin Journal," asserts that the treatment of rheumatism by large doses of opium shortens the duration, diminishes suffering, husbands strength and lessens the tendency to complications. It is important that full and sufficient doses are employed, increasing them in amount and frequency, until the patient feels decided relief, and then continuing the same dose until the disease has steadily declined. The mean quantity given in twenty-four hours was from ten to twelve grains, but it often amounted to more than double. It does not affect the cere- bral function, and, as we have more than once observed, in some cases excites diarrhœa. The average duration of treatment was nine days. The plan is not adapted to gouty subjects. Warm embrocations, with turpen- tine, or camphorated spirits, were employed. Against the consequent stiffness he advises frictions, with half an ounce of camphorated oil and turpentine, and a drachm of sulphur. In cases with sweating, erratic pains, and quick small pulse, the combination of quinine and opium is admirable. Other practitioners have confirmed Dr. C.'s experience; and his suggestions, though not absolutely novel, possess great practical interest.

Aconite.—Dr. Busse, of Berlin, in a monograph upon the subject, advocates the value of Richter's treatment both of acute and chronic rheumatism. He gives from fifteen to sixty drops every two hours, of the following solution:

R Extract of aconite, four scruples; antimonial wine, three ounces two drachms. Mix.

It excites diaphoresis without distress, and relieves pain. The evidence in its favor is very strong.

Dr. J. B. Watkins of Philadelphia also speaks in favor of extract of aconite. It may be given in doses of one-fourth of a grain three times a day, to six grains, or even more, daily.

Mr. Curtis recommends an aconite plaster, made by evaporating four ounces of the tincture to the consistence of oil; this quantity to be spread with a brush on half a yard of adhesive plaster.

Belladonna.—Dr. Osborne ("Dublin Journal," June 1, 1840), remarks that belladonna causes an immediate cessation of the migratory pains, without benefiting those which are fixed. The dose is one-third of a grain three times a day, increased to one-half every three hours. Its effects seem limited to muscular pains.

Pills of Guaiacum, Camphor etc.—Dr. Hassack "Practice of Physic," (p. 672) considers the following pill a good diaphoretic stimulant in chronic cases:

Guaiacum, six drachms; camphor, one drachm; opium, two drachms; potassio-tartrate of antimony, one drachm. Mix. To be divided into 120 pills, two three times a day.

Alkalies, Laxatives.—Cases occur, says Dr. Watson, which are not absolutely acute or chronic. There is some fever, the joints are affected, the skin dry, thirst, the urine loaded with lithic deposits, and strongly *acid.* In this state alkalies are of great use. A drachm of the liquor potassæ daily for several days together, keeping the bowels free, has done more than any other treatment.

Rheumatic Headache—Treatment.—Against rheumatic headache Dr. Johnson has found no treatment so successful as the following: Eight grains of Dover's powder and two of calomel at bed-time on alternate nights for two or three times, followed by a third part of the following mixture the next morning, to be repeated in two hours, if necessary:

Infusion of rhubarb, three ounces; tartrate of soda, three drachms; powder of rhubarb, half a drachm; tincture of senna, half an ounce; wine of colchicum, a drachm and a half. Mix.

The same observer remarks that many of the most stubborn cases will yield to a course of blue or Plummer's pill, taken at bed-time, and followed by a warm saline colchicum draught in the morning. Flannel clothing, and an occasional warm bath, are valuable adjuvants.

Muscular Atony—Ammonia.—Dr. Paris asserts that against the muscular atony succeeding to acute disease, ammonia in large doses is the best remedy.

Treatment of an Obstinate Case.—In a very obstinate case, characterized by severe pains, relieved by heat, and unaccompanied by much swelling, oocurring in the practice of Mr. John Brady, of London, the following means proved very successful:

Compound extract of sarsaparilla, six drachms; iodine, half a grain; hydriodate of potash, half a drachm; boiling water, six ounces. Mix. A fourth part three times a day, with one of the subjoined pills.

Hydrochlorate of morphia, one grain; disulphate of quinine, nine grains; blue pill, ten grains; rhubarb pill, twelve grains. Divide into twelve pills.

Quinine.—M. Briquet has recently addressed a letter to the Academy of Medicine of Paris, stating that large doses of quinine were as successful in rheumatism as in ague. All will not coincide with M. B., and some late experience has proved that an excessive use of this agent is not without inconvenience and danger.

Sulphur.—We shall now adduce some evidence in favor of sulphur, which entitles it to the practitioner's serious attention. It is an old but very partially employed remedy, and has now almost descended from the profession to the people.

Dr. Munk states that he employed it successfully in 300 cases. It seemed more effective when combined with the carbonate of soda, in the proportion of two drachms to an ounce of sulphur. Half an ounce of the latter was the maximum quantity in twenty-four hours.

The celebrated nostrum, well known as the "Chelsea pensioner," owes its efficacy to sulphur.

Dr. Law states that in subacute rheumatism there is no one means he he has found so generally useful.

R Sulphur, one ounce; bitartrate of potash, half an ounce; powder of rhubarb, two drachms; powder of guaiacum, one drachm; powder of musk, one drachm; honey, four ounces. Mix. A dessertspoonful three times a day.

If it purge too much, a drachm of Dover's powder to be added. Dr. Graves also praises it, and substitutes the following electuary:

R Powdered bark, one drachm; powdered guaiacum, one drachm; cream of tartar, one ounce; flour of sulphur, half an ounce; powdered ginger, one drachm. To be made into an electuary with sirup. A teaspoonful three times a day.

If it purge too much, we diminish the dose; if constipation exists, we increase it. A teaspoonful of sulphur, with half the quantity of ginger, taken every morning in a glass of milk, has proved very useful. We know a lady liable to severe rheumatic pains in the scalp, who considers she can at any time cure them by a dose of sulphur at bed-time.

Professor Otto, of Copenhagen, treated four cases, three of which were chronic, with four drops every two hours of tincture made of two drachms of the carburet of sulphur in half an ounce of rectified spirits. The same quantity, rubbed up with half an ounce of olive oil, was employed as an external embrocation.

External Applications.—In chronic, obstinate affections of the joints, rubbing them with castor oil every night, and wrapping the limbs in warm flannels, is extensively employed in the East, and is said to be very successful.

The external application of colchicum has been strongly recommended, and we have ourselves found it useful in cases where the sensibility was great, the pains diffused and recurrent, and the temperature of the part raised.

, Painting the surface with tincture of iodine has been found useful. Equal parts of the compound 'camphor and soap liniments, with laudanum, is a good form of embrocation; and in case of severe local suffering, the following ointment has succeeded in allaying pain.

R Veratria, half a drachm; opium, one drachm; lard, one ounce and a half. Mix.

The endermic application of morphine is also worth remembering.

Part viii., *p.* 24.

Rheumatic Fever, General Treatment of.—Dr. R. B. Todd, in his article on the "Dietetic and Medicinal Treatment of Gout and Rheumatism," proceeds to say:

Those channels which are obviously the most favorable for the elimination of the rheumatic matter, are the skin, the bowels, and the kidneys; hence the use of sudorifics, purgatives, and diuretics is indicated. Of sudorifics, Dover's powder is among the best, and is sanctioned by the experience of many years; pure opium answers the double end of promoting diaphoresis while it procures rest and relieves pain; or the nitrate of potash may be given either in combination with opium and ipecacuanha (a nearer approach to the original formula for Dover's powder), or in solution along with minute doses of tartarized antimony. I am not in the habit of exceeding five or six grains of the nitrate of potass with one-eighth of a grain of the tartar emetic (to which, if there be nausea, a few drops of tincture of opium may be added), every four or six hours. The practice of giving very large doses of nitre, tried formerly in this country, and lately revived in France, does not appear to have any decided influence upon the mean duration of the disease. The administration of opium, however, is of great importance: it must be given in large doses, and is borne well by the patient. A good opiate should always be administered at night, and when where is much suffering, two or three doses should be given throughout the day. The irritative character of rheumatic fever is strongly in favor of this medicine.

The purgatives which seem most applicable are those which produce copious watery evacuations. The combination of sulphate and carbonate of magnesia answers very well, the addition of the alkaline earth serving to neutralize some of the free acid which is so abundantly secreted. Colchicum is useful as a purgative, and if employed in large doses, exerts a powerful action on the intestinal canal, but the employment of it is not devoid of serious objection. The tartate of potass is also a useful purgative. The best mode of promoting diuresis in this disease is to allow the patient to use simple diluents freely; to these no other limits need be put than those which his own sensations will dictate. Any more direct stimulants to the kidneys would probably excite those organs too much. The saline effervescing draughts are agreeable and cooling, and have the additional recommendation of serving for the neutralization of the free acid, in its passage through the kidneys.

The objection which has been urged against local applications to the affected joint during a paroxysm of gout, does not apply to rheumatic fever. In the latter disease the morbid element is escaping at many places, in the former at a single joint; if we disturb its attraction to this one joint in gout, it may fly to a new one, or to some internal viscus. These risks are obviously wanting in rheumatic fever, as the disease is more generalized in its effects. And experience teaches us that the greatest relief may be obtained by local bleeding in this malady.

As, however, local bleeding does not prevent a joint from being revisited by the rheumatic irritation, the employment of it in ordinary cases, and as a general practice, is not to be recommended. You may apply leeches to-day to a joint, to-morrow it will be free from pain, and the next day it may be swollen and painful again. If the pain and swelling, both or either, be great, and such as to excite apprehension for the ultimate integrity of the textures, then the application of leeches will be really useful, and should not be deferred.

When the articular affection is disposed to be chronic, and the rheumatic matter appears to linger about a joint, local bleeding may be of essential service. Its timely use, in such instances, may save the patient from a tedious convalescence, if not from a chronic rheumatism. Local bleeding, in the earlier stages of the rheumatic paroxysm, has the additional advantage of contributing to relieve the general fever in a manner not likely to injure the constitution. Warm fomentations or poultices often give considerable relief, and if agreeable to the patients, they may be used with safety. It has been proposed to foment the joints with a solution of an alkaline salt, as of soda or potass. I have seen this practice tried, but did not perceive any superiority of the alkaline fomentation over that of plain water.

I am strongly inclined to believe that counter-irritation by blisters to the affected joints will be found a very useful practice in the severer cases of rheumatic fever, even in the acute stages. It will generally, however, be advisable to precede the application of blisters by that of leeches.

Part ix., *p.* 46.

Rheumatic Diathesis.—In his article on the "Dietetic and Medicinal Treatment of Gout and Rheumatism," Dr. R. B. Todd remarks as follows:

In the Rheumatic Diathesis, if the joints suffer much, they may be best treated by local stimulation, or counter-irritation. A strongly stimulating terebinthinate liniment is often beneficial; but, on the whole, nothing is so useful in chronic rheumatic states of the joints as blisters applied in rapid succession. In some instances where there have been much pain and swelling, the application of a few leeches will almost always do good. I learn from Mr. Busk, who has had great experience in the treatment of those painful articular affections connected with gonorrhœa (gonorrhœal rheumatism), that blisters are an invaluable remedy in them, even from the first, and this accords with my own more limited experience. Doubtless in the case of rheumatic joints, blisters act in a similar way, by attracting the morbid element from the articular textures. I have lately employed pretty extensively, and with unquestionable benefit, the local application of iodine to the affected joints, for which purpose we may employ either the tincture of iodine, or a stronger compound, which is used at the King's College Hospital, and is called iodine paint, the formula of which is as follows:

℞ Iodinii, gr. lxiv; potassii iodidi, gr. xxx; alcohol, ʒj. M

The mode of application is by painting the part freely with a camel-hair pencil. More or less smarting is produced, and frequently vesication, or a herpetic eruption may come on. The painting may be repeated as

often as circumstances may demand. It is extremely useful where any effu
sion has taken place into synovial membranes or sheaths. *Part* ix., *p.* 45.

Chronic—Anodyne Pomade.—Take of Galen's cerate, 31 parts;
extract of belladonna, 8; acetate of morphia (previously dissolved), 3.
Mix well together.

This pomade is exceedingly useful in cases of muscular pains, chronic
rheumatism, etc., when rubbed on the affected parts. *Part* ix., *p.* 192.

Quinine in Articular Rheumatism.—In France, M. Briquet, M. Guérard,
and Professor Fouquier, have employed sulphate of quinine for the treatment
of acute articular rheumatism, with the most satisfactory results, the dose
varying from Əj. to ʒj. daily. Sulphate of quinine can be deprived of its
bitterness by being taken in coffee. *Part* xvi., *p.* 67.

Oil of Turpentine Externally in Rheumatism.—When the essence of
turpentine is poured over a surface, its volatilization is not attended with
any pain, or with the production of heat; but, when a compress imbued
with the oil is applied to the skin and covered with waterproof cloth, the
result is far different; violent pain follows in a quarter of an hour, and
doubtless, if the application was prolonged, vesication might ensue. It is
this revulsive action of the essence of turpentine, that M. Hervieux has
endeavored to produce, and which he has found extremely useful for the
purpose of dispelling rheumatic pain. In cases of paralysis due to disease
of the spinal cord, muscular weakness and pain were also relieved.
Part xvi., *p.* 68.

Phosphate of Ammonia.—After subduing the more inflammatory symptoms by antiphlogistic treatment, Dr. Edwards gives ten grains of phosphate of ammonia every eight hours. This medicine acts beneficially by
decomposing the uric acid or urate of soda, which is formed in excess in
gout and rheumatism. Instead of urate of soda, a very insoluble, we have
thus formed phosphate of soda, a most soluble salt. *Part* xvii., *p.* 26.

Rheumatism—Acute.—The treatment of rheumatic fever is a subject
upon which much difference of opinion exists among practitioners. Dr.
Todd insists very strongly upon the importance of curing the disease with
as little impairment of the power of the constitution as possible; and remarks that while we should aim at securing for the patient a short convalescence, we must guard equally against the danger of relapse, which the
so-called speedy cures by the heroic treatment are too apt to leave behind.

The indications are to relieve pain, to promote the action of the skin,
kidneys and bowels, to use antacids, and to give large quantities of diluent
fluids. For these purposes give a grain of opium, a grain of ipecacuanha,
and five grains of nitre, every two, three, or four hours; and a mixture
with sulphate and carbonate of magnesia. Envelop the joints in a large
quantity of cotton wool, and cover with oiled silk; changing it every
twelve or twenty-four hours. Give plenty of simple diluents, and from the
first, let the patient have a little good beef tea frequently through the day.
And when the patient begins to pass pale urine, with or without pale lithates, he will be the better for generous diet, with wine, ammonia, or quinine, even though the articular affection persists. Too much sweating,
too much purging, or too much opium, are equally unadvisable. If the
patient cannot bear opium, extract of hyoscyamus, hop or lettuce may be
substituted. If the state of the joints does not yield to the application of

cotton wool, apply a small sinapism for half an hour to redden the skin, then wash and dry the skin, and apply a blister the size of a crown-piece; the blistered surface may be allowed to heal, or may be dressed with stimulating ointment; or a succession of small blisters may be used. Watch the state of the heart from the first; and on the first indication of pericardial or endocardial affection, apply a large sinapism over the region of the heart, and when it comes off, a large blister; but *do not bleed* either locally or generally. Give calomel and opium to affect the gums; and, if needed, rub in mercurial ointment, or use it to dress the blistered surface. When delirium, resembling delirium-tremens, occurs as a complication of rheumatic cardiac affections, it is " a signal of distress," and must be responded to by an immediate alteration in the treatment. All too free evacuations, whether from the skin or bowels, must be checked; nourishment must be given frequently in small quantities; and even wine, brandy, or porter, may be administered. If the patient is wakeful, give opium. And take care that all exertion is avoided, lest fatal syncope be induced. If, however, there is coma, do not give opium, but apply sinapisms or blisters.

Part xviii., *p.* 36.

Anæmia as a consequence of Rheumatism.—Dr. O'Ferrall, of St. Vincent's Hospital, believes an anæmic condition may supervene in the course of acute rheumatism, resulting, apparently, rather from the natural course of the disease than from the remedies employed. Chalybeates should be given in this condition. *Part* xx., *p.* 34.

Acute Rheumatism.—Dr. Watson says that "the younger the patient is who suffers from acute rheumatism, the more likely will he be to suffer from rheumatic carditis."

This patient had the various symptoms of rheumatic fever. The heart's action, being examined, was found natural, with the exception of a slight systolic murmur heard over the interval between the fourth and fifth ribs, about an inch below the nipple.

The patient was ordered six drachms of lemon-juice, to be taken in sugar-water, three times daily. He was, however, in a couple of days much worse; the pains were very acute, and the joints along the arms and hands became involved; the pulse rose to 120, full; the systolic murmur was more distinct; the perspiration profuse, very acid, and the urine high-colored. Dr. Barlow, after giving a purgative draught, with wine of colchicum, prescribed a pill, composed of a quarter of a grain of tartar-emetic, half a grain of opium, and one grain of calomel, to be taken every fourth hour. These measures contributed to lessen the pains, and the patient was desired to take the pills only three times a day, with the following draught:—half a drachm of acetate of potash, and ten grains of nitre, in camphor mixture. The improvement was very great on the next day; the pills were discontinued, but the mixture persevered in. The favorable impression produced by the salts of potash increased during the next few days; all the symptoms gradually gave way, and ten days after the draughts had been first taken, and regularly continued, the patient was convalescent. He took, before being finally discharged, small doses of iodide of potassium and carbonate of potash, and left the hospital quite well about three weeks after admission. *Part* xxii., *p.* 38.

Treatment of Acute Rheumatism by Local Anæsthetics.—The application, locally, of the Dutch liquid to the joints in this disease is highly recommended. A moist compress sprinkled with the agent, is applied and renewed once in twenty-four hours, being inclosed in impervious bandages so as to prevent its evaporation. It is to be applied to each joint in succession as it becomes inflamed. The complications of rheumatism may be treated on general principles at the same time. *Part* xxiii., *p.* 54.

. *Rheumatism—Lemon-juice.*—Dr. Babington had generally ordered three ounces of lemon-juice to be taken three times a day, but he has recently ordered as much as six ounces. He states that there is no remedy with which he is acquainted to be compared in value to lemon-juice in the treatment of rheumatism. In gout and chronic rheumatism its effects are far less obvious and uniform. He believes it will be found a valuable agent in inflammatory diseases generally. *Part* xxv., *p.* 32.

Acute Rheumatism—Colchicum.—In all cases where albumen and urea are vicarious, and where coma supervenes, evidently from the accumulation of the latter principle in the blood, colchicum will prove of great value.

Part xxv., *p.* 38.

Articular Rheumatism.—In proportion as this disease approaches in its characters to gout we may expect to be successful with colchicum. Give twenty minims of the tincture of wine every six hours until some relief is obtained, or a grain of the inspissated juice or of the acetic extract of colchium every four hours. *Part* xxv., *p.* 41.

Collodion.—In gout and articular rheumatism cover the part with a layer of collodion, so as to preserve it from the atmosphere.

Part xxv., *p.* 325.

Pathology of Rheumatism and Gout.—The present theory with regard to these affections is, that they are both connected with an increase of lithic acid in the blood. In rheumatism, this is dependent on excess of the secondary, and in gout on excess of the primary, digestion. In rheumatism, however, there is considerable excretion of lactic acid by the skin (Todd), whilst in gout there is an excess of soda, which, uniting with the lithic acid, produces a compound of lithate of soda, that may be detected as such in the blood (Garrod), while sometimes it exudes into the cellular tissue of the skin, constituting tophaceous deposits. In both diseases there is an undue balance between the excess of lithic acid and the power of excretion—in rheumatism by the skin, and in gout by the kidney. This pathology serves to explain the similitudes and differences existing between the two affections. In both there is a certain constitutional state, dependent on deranged digestion, during which exciting causes occasion local effects. These exciting causes in rheumatism are bad diet, hard work, exposure to cold and wet, and its subjects generally are the poor and laboring population. In gout the causes are good diet, indolence, repletion, or indigestion, and its subjects are for the most part the rich and sedentary. The local manifestations in both are acute wandering pains, with pain and swelling—in rheumatism of the large, and in gout of the small joints, constituting the acute attack in the one, and the so-called regular attack in the other. These are combined with a tendency to various complications of the internal viscera, which are more or less dangerous to life.

The general indications of treatment are, in both diseases—1st. So to

regulate the nutritive functions as to insure a due balance between th
amount of matters entering the blood as the result of digestion, primary or
secondary, and the amount of matters discharged from the economy by the
excretory organs.   2d. To conduct the acute attack to a favorable termination, carefully watching the internal viscera and being prepared to act
with vigor should these become affected.   Hence the treatment of these
diseases resolves itself into what may be called curative and preventive,
—the first having reference to the acute attack, the second to the means
most likely to hinder its return ; the one must be carried out by remedies
which act upon the blood and execretory organs, the other by the management of diet and exercise.   *Part* xxvii., *p.* 45.

Treatment by Ash-leaves and Guaco.—Give an infusion of ash-leaves
(Fraxinus excelsior).   It possesses the advantages without the inconveniences of colchicum.   Generally, under its use, at the end of four or five
days, or sometimes sooner, the pain, redness, and swelling visibly diminish
in intensity, or even disappear.   Each dose of the powdered leaves ought
to be infused for three hours in boiling water, and before taken should be
strained through a linen cloth, and sweetened to taste.   Dr. Otterbourg
says that 32 grammes, infused in a sufficient quantity of water, may be
taken several times during the day.   There is no need to change the mode
of living.

As a tonic, guaco (Mikania guaco) is a most valuable drug after the
fever has passed off ; its effects were magical, where quinine produced
restlessness, thirst and headache.   *Part* xxvii., *p.* 249.

Rheumatism.—One of the exceptional cases in which lemon-juice is of
no avail, is that of a gonorrhœal character.   A woman, aged 30, was
admitted into Guy's hospital with rheumatism and a copious yellow discharge from the vagina.   All ordinary remedies failed to relieve, until
the purulent discharge had been removed by ʒj. doses of cubebs.
                                                       Part xxviii., *p.* 34.

Treatment of Acute Rheumatism by Acetate of Potash.—Dr. Golding
Bird seems to depend on this remedy more than any other in the treatment of acute rheumatism.   But, after all, it appears that the efficacy of
lemon-juice itself depends not so much on the acid as upon the supercitrate
of soda which it contains.   It seems that all these kinds of salts are useful
when they act powerfully on the kidney, and eliminate poisonous matter
from the system.   Thus citrate of potash, citrate of ammonia, acetate of
ammonia, nitrate of potash, as well as the acetate of potash, all act very
beneficially in rheumatism.

Dr. Bird gives half an ounce, largely diluted, in divided doses every
twenty four hours.   *Part* xxix., *p.* 43.

Chronic Periosteal.—Dr. Basham has observed that in cases of chronic
periosteal rheumatism, where the patient has been benefited by iodide of
potassium, at some antecedent period he has been salivated by mercury ;
whereas if no salivation has previously occurred, he has found the iodide
of potassium of little or no effect. ' This disease may depend upon the
impregnation of the system by mercury, or from the syphilitic virus.   If
the former, iodide of potassium is the remedy ; if the latter, alterative
doses of some mild preparation of mercury.   *Part* xxix., *p.* 45.

Occurrence of Delirium Acute Rheumatism.—When delirium occurs in acute rheumatism, says Dr. Durrant, it is of grave import. Examine the heart carefully—there is very likely to be pericarditis upon which the delirium depends. Bleed generally or locally according to circumstances, give calomel and opium, with salines and colchicum. Blister the cardiac region well, both in front and back. At the same time support the patient with broth, and even wine if necessary; always remembering that many of these apparently inflammatory diseases are asthenic and not sthenic.

Part xxx., *p.* 222.

Alkaline Treatment.—During the attendance of Dr. Swett, at the New York Hospital, all the patients admitted with acute articular rheumatism, were put under the "alkaline treatment."

The salt chosen was the tartrate of soda and potassa, a neutral salt, possessing the property of rendering the urine alkaline.

"The plan of treatment usually pursued was, if the patient presented himself with unusual excitement of the skin and pulse, to administer a mixture of sulphate of magnesia and tartarized antimony, until the skin was relaxed, and the pulse reduced to a more natural standard. The Rochelle salt was then directed, in drachm doses, every two or three hours during the day-time, till the urine was rendered alkaline, when it was gradually suspended. A lotion of carb. potassa ʒj. with opium ʒij., to the pint of water, was directed as an external application. The administration of the salt was not attended with disagreeable consequences, with the exception occasionally of some ulceration about the fauces; in no case was its action so severe upon the bowels as to require its entire suspension. The persons attacked were in full vigor of health, and the character of the disease acute in its form. The frequency of administration of the remedy was governed very much by the reaction of the urine.

On the admission of the patient, the urine was tested, and in all cases was found to be of acid reaction, and the secretion of the skin presented the usual acid odor. The treatment was generally commenced the second or third day after admission, and the urine was rendered of decided alkaline reaction in an average of five days after its commencement; the longest period it resisted the alkaline reaction having been twenty days, and the shortest two.

In one case, attended with profuse perspiration, which yielded readily to treatment, the colored shirt the patient wore entirely lost its color; and it was suggested whether the same change did not take place in the perspiration, as in the urine. The average amount of the salt administered was from five to seven ounces.

The average date of commencing improvement was seven days after commencement of treatment, coinciding, in the large majority of the cases, with the commencing alkalinity of the urine. The improvement was invariably permanent, and, after the urine was rendered alkaline, no new articulations were affected, as a general rule.

The average period of convalescence was twelve days after admission; and the whole duration of the disease, including the period previous to admission, was twenty-two days. One of the most gratifying results of the alkaline treatment was the diminished frequency of cardiac complications.

Not one patient was attacked with any heart complication during the treatment of the disease. *Part* xxxi., *p.* 43.

Treatment of Acute Rheumatism.—Lemon-juice is still relied upon extensively, but since it became known that it contained some of the salts of potash, these have been largely prescribed in the acetate, tartrate, or nitrate of potash. Give half a drachm of acetate of potash, ten grains of the nitrate of potash, and ten minims of vinum opii diluted with barley-water, two or three times a day.   *Part* xxxi., *p.* 46.

Treatment of Acute.—You must be guided entirely by the specialties of the case; there are no specifics; some preparation of iron with liquor potassæ may be given. When the liver is much deranged, calomel and rhubarb; when the urine is scanty, colchicum. As tonics, quinine and iron, alone or combined, may be given. Quassia, with an alkali, suits remarkably well. Wine is the best and most efficacious tonic in weakly habits; an opiate at bed-time is sometimes necessary. Warm fomentations are the best local applications.   *Part* xxxiii., *p.* 40.

Sulphur externally in the cure of Rheumatism.—Dr. Fuller orders the whole of the affected limb to be incased in flannel, thickly sprinkled with precipitated sulphur; a bandage is applied over this, and the whole covered with oiled silk or gutta percha, which has the effect of increasing the warmth and confining the vapor of the sulphur, and also obviating the disagreeable odor. This bandage should be constantly applied—absorption takes place, the breath, urine, cutaneous exhalations, unmistakably attest its presence. If the pain be situated where the above cannot be readily applied, substitute the compound sulphur ointment, which must be rubbed in for twenty minutes night and morning. When there is feverishness, acute pain, even when the limb is at rest, and the skin dry and inactive, no relief results from this treatment; but where there are no symptoms of active disease, and the pain is of a dull aching character, felt chiefly when the limb is in motion, and the skin acts freely, no external application proves so serviceable.   *Part* xxxv., *p.* 23.

Treatment of Gout and Rheumatism by the Silicate and Benzoate of Soda—combined with the Preparations of Aconite and Colchicum.— MM. Socquet and Bonjean have proposed, in gouty and rheumatic affections, the employment of the silicate of soda and benzoate of soda. Silicate of soda facilitates the elimination of uric acid, and its influence may be extended so far as to render the urine alkaline. This salt, moreover, by its tonic action upon the digestive functions and its diuretic properties, is said to be far superior to the carbonates of soda or potash, which are so constantly employed in the rectification of the uric acid diathesis. The benzoate of soda transforms uric acid into hippuric acid, the combinations of which are extremely soluble, while those of uric acid are hardly soluble at all. This medicine, in thus modifying the part of the acid which may have escaped the action of the silicate of soda, will thus contribute also to diminish its quantity. Colchicum will rapidly carry away, by the urinary passages, the remains of the uric acid which the blood may still contain. Aconite is used to act specially upon the painful part. *Part* xxxv., *p.* 25.

Treatment of Acute Rheumatism.—The treatment of acute rheumatism by one or other of the salts of potash has now become the established practice of the leading London physicians. Dr. Barlow has lately been trying the bicarbonate, but does not find it so effectual as the acetate which he had previously been in the habit of using. A combination of the nitrate, bitartrate, and acetate, given well diluted, is a good form of administration.

* * * * * * * * * * * *

Lemon-juice and Acetate of Potash.—If the portal system is congested, as shown by arrest of the biliary and urinary secretions, exhibit a brisk mercurial alterative and purgative, repeating this if necessary during the attack. Then prescribe lemon-juice in proportion of a teaspoonful or dessertspoonful, according to the age and size of the patient, every second hour. This of itself tends also to keep the bowels free. A little morphia, the dose being carefuly regulated, may be given at bed-time. Dr. Sandwith, of the Hull Infirmary, has recently treated ten cases with acetate of potash, with unusual success. It should be well diluted, and may be combined with lemon-juice. *Part* xxxvi., *p.* 30.

Chronic Rheumatism and Gout.—Apply thin sheets of gutta percha over the parts; this produces great local transpiration, and the pain is generally considerably relieved. *Part* xxxvi., *p.* 31.

Rheumatic Pericarditis.—Dr. Todd treats this and other forms of rheumatic inflammation on a stimulant plan throughout, not with a view of cutting short the disease, but of supporting the patient under it, and rendering convalescence more rapid. In a case lately under treatment, alkalies were given alone, till the appearance of the pericarditis, when opium in grain doses, every four hours, and eight ounces of brandy daily, were administered. Pneumonia of both lungs came on, and the brandy was ultimately increased to thirty-five ounces daily. No leeches or blisters were throughout employed. He left the hospital to all appearance quite well at the end of a month. *Part* xxxvi., *p.* 50.

Acute Rheumatism.—After having procured free evacuation by means of senna and salts, begin the administration of equal parts of vin. colch. and spt. tereb., in doses of ten drops every two or three hours. After a day or two, give in connection with these (only at different intervals, say of five hours each), tr. ferri chlor. ten drops, using as much opium as may be necessary to quiet pain. Allow a free use of coffee of average strength. If the patient's appetite remain, allow a moderate use of his usual food at the customary intervals. (Dr. Gordon.)

* * * * *

In acute articular rheumatism give large doses of iodide of potassium in conjunction with morphia. When more than one joint is affected do not use local means. (Dr. Hauschka.) *Part* xxxvii., *p.* 22.

Rheumatism, Chronic.—A case of most obstinate chronic rheumatism, for years resisting every form of treatment adopted, yielded to the use of the sulphurous vapor-bath. A bath was given every other day, the patient being well steamed for twenty minutes, and then, before leaving the bath, showered with cold salt water, to prevent a too relaxing action of the vapor. In the course of six weeks, the man stated himself to be " perfectly cured." Artificial sulphurous water may be made by adding a drachm and a half or two drachms of sulphuret of potassium to a gallon of common water. *Part* xxxviii., *p.* 22.

Rheumatism and Chorea.— Probably there is no fact in pathology better established by experience than the connection between rheumatism and chorea; the former being the cause, the disease in fact, the latter only a symptom. Always carefully examine whether there be a rheumatic history; in some cases, of all symptoms there may be only one leading to this suspicion, viz., urine highly loaded with lithates. If there be no febrile state to account for this state of urine, though not in itself actual evidence, it is in most cases highly presumptive of the existence of the rheumatic state. In one case we have seen chorea and loaded urine the only symptoms leading to the detection of acute pericarditis. (Ed. of Retrospect.)   *Part* xxxix., *p.* 72.

Hypodermic Injections.— In many cases of rheumatism, says Mr. Hunter of St. George's Hospital, great relief will be obtained by the use of narcotic injections, to relieve the pains when severe. Of course the usual constitutional treatment must be employed. In one case a man could not move his arm after acute rheumatism, on account of pain in the shoulder. The pain was removed by a single injection.   *Part* xl., *p.* 279.

RICKETS.

Rickets—Treatment of.—Mr. A. W. Close states that the softened state of the bones in this affection is owing originally to a deficiency in the supply of *the nutritive nitrogenized substances.* The affection is seldom seen during suckling, because the milk contains those elements which are exactly suited to the wants of the system. After weaning, the diet often adopted among the poor consists chiefly of potatoes, oatmeal, gruel, tea, coffee, and rice. Now *proteine* is only found in the two first in small quantities, and none in the rest. Among the middle and upper classes the diet after weaning is often sago, rice, or arrowroot, which certainly fatten the little children, but do not convey a sufficient quantity of nitrogen to the system. The diet ought to consist more of . the nitrogenized substances when there is this disposition in the system, such as beef-tea, eggs and wheat ground and made into bread without the separation of the cuticle of the grain, in which is contained the phosphate of lime, to whose absence the softened condition of the bones is usually attributed.
Part viii., *p.* 78.

Mollities Ossium.— [This disease, depending immediately upon the want of the mineral constitutents of bone, may arise either from a want of power in the organs of assimilation and absorption to take up the phosphate of lime contained in the food, or from the food itself not containing enough phosphate of lime to furnish the required supply. It is well known that when common fowls are prevented from getting lime, their eggs will be without shells, but on restoring the lime, the eggs regain their earthy covering. On the same principle Mr. Cooper proposes to treat mollities ossium. He says:]

I have on two or three occasions certainly had reason to believe that great benefit was derived from giving bone powered and mixed with bread, and at the same time draughts containing phosphoric acid, which converts phosphate of lime into a biphosphate, a more soluble salt than the phosphate, and probably much more readily assimilated. The result of this treatment was certainly such as would warrant the just expectation of facilitating the nutrition of bone.

I have *demonstratively* proved to you, I think I may say, over and over again, the advantages of applying phosphoric acid to exfoliating bone, to produce its rapid removal upon a principle precisely similar.

Part xvii., *p.* 124.

Treatment of, by Proteine.—Vide Art. " Caries."

Rickets.—In diseases arising from insufficiency of earthy phosphates in the food, give calcined bones in powder ; and when there is too rapid elimination of phosphates by the urine, combine with the calcined bones a large proportion of sugar, or add the latter to the food. The sugar will diminish the activity of the nutritive changes which take place in the tissues, and so lessen the amount of matter excreted. But "when a child at the breast is affected with this disease, owing to the poverty of the milk, the mother should take the calcined bones, but without the sugar, in order that the elimination of the phosphates through the milk may not be interfered with. (Dr. Bocker.) *Part* xxi., *p.* 147.

Observations on Rickets.—The indications are, not to cram the patients with preparations of earthy salts, for these are not deficient in the blood, but to correct disorder of the digestive system, and to invigorate the body by light nutritive diet, fresh air, cold ablutions, and the use of some medicinal tonic, such as quinine or iron. In some cases steel supports are proper. (Dr. Humphry.) *Part* xxi., *p.* 184.

Use of Tannic Acid.—Give tannic acid in doses of half a grain or a grain, night and morning, in sweetened water or any simple vehicle, and continue its use for a long time. It acts, in all probability, rather as a tonic and "histogenetic," than by arresting the excretion of lime by an astringent action on the kidney. (Dr. Alison.) *Part* xxi., *p.* 326.

Use of Phosphate and Oxalate of Lime.—In all chronic diseases which are distinguished by wasting, emaciation, ulcerations of the skin, etc. (as scrofula, especially rickets), 'a much larger quantity of phosphates is removed from the economy by the urine than ought to be in the normal state ; indeed, in some cases, to an almost incredible extent. The phosphates of lime and magnesia are held in solution in the urine by its acidity, and directly precipitated by the addition of alkalies, or when the urine becomes ammoniacal by putrescence. This precipitation is more complete by heating or boiling the urine, and by adding a solution of soda to boiling urine the whole may be precipitated ; and by always using the same solution of carbonate of soda, say, one to twelve ounces of distilled water, the degrees of turbidity may be readily recognized, and the quantity of phosphates ascertained. There is scarcely any disease in which at one time or another an increase in the quantity of phosphates does not take place ; but as the times are quite uncertain, there is necessity for almost daily examination. The increase, however, does not depend so much upon the nature of the disease as upon the individual affected. (Dr. Beneke.) *Part* xxiv., *p.* 310.

Superphosphate of Iron.—A sirup of superphosphate of iron is particularly applicable to rickety and weak children ; it is very pleasant to take. It contains five grains of iron and five of phosphate of lime to an ounce of the sirup. (Dr. Routh.) *Part* xxxvii., *p.* 242.

·SALIVATION.

Salivation by Small Doses of Mercury.—In a discussion respecting the salivation of patients by minute doses of mercury, in the Westminster Medical Society, Mr. Snow offered an ingenious explanation. He said: He did not believe that the salivation which was occasionally produced by a very small dose of mercury depended on any idiosyncrasy of constitution, which continued during the patient's life, but was the result of the presence of an excess of acid in the first passages. He had been led to this conclusion by having frequently seen patients salivated by a very small quantity of calomel or blue pill, taken at the same time with mixtures containing dilute sulphuric acid. Very lately, a man who was taking sulphuric acid freely for epistaxis, was severely salivated by two grains of calomel in a dose of cathartic pills. The acids naturally contained in the stomach were the muriatic and the acetic, and the mercury contained in a grain or two of calomel, or a few grains of the blue pill, would, of course, be sufficient to produce the most serious consequences, if changed into the bi-chloride. If the view he had suggested was correct, the means of preventing untoward effects would be to give corrosive sublimate at once, where a course of mercury was indicated, and to give it in suitable minute doses. *Part* i., *p.* 45.

Leeches—Poultices—Gargles.—Dr. Watson, in his lectures on the Treatment of Inflammation, makes the following remarks respecting the Treatment of Salivation : There are two expedients which I am confident are often of very great use in checking the violence of the salivation, and in removing the most distressing of its accompaniments. If there be much external swelling, treat the case as being, what it really is, a case of *local inflammation:* apply eight or ten leeches beneath the edges of the jaw bones, and wrap a soft poultice round the neck, into which the orifices made by the leeches may bleed ; and I can promise you that, in nine cases out of ten, you will receive the thanks ·of your patient for the great comfort this measure has afforded him. When the flow of saliva, and the soreness of the gums, form the chief part of the grievance, I have found nothing *so* generally useful as a gargle made of brandy and water ; in the proportion of one part of brandy to four or five of water. *Part* iii., *p.* 33.

Use of Tannin.—Mr. Druitt considers it the best of all local means of making the mouth comfortable in cases of severe salivation, and for all cases of relaxed sore throat attended with superabundance of mucus. It coagulates the mucus, and enables the patient to get rid of it easily. *Part* x., *p.* 139.

New Remedy for Ptyalism.—Dr. Robertson has discovered that one of the commonest plants of his district, the *Ambrosia trifida*, has more prompt remedial powers in cases of excessive ptyalism, than anything he had previously tried. The patients are described· as being generally relieved in six or eight hours of the more urgent symptoms, and completely cured in two days. The preparation employed is an infusion of the green leaves used as a gargle. Dr. Robertson suggests that the plant may also be found useful in other profluviæ, as leucorrhœa. The plant is known under the popular term of horseweed—horsemint. Dr. Robertson was induced to try it from observing that it completely cured a horse affected with slabbering. The effect is simply local. *Part* xv., *p.* 252.

Treatment of Salivation by Sulphur.—Dr. H. Smith says a good preparation in these cases is a mixture of alum and chlorinated soda; ʒij. of the former with ʒj. of the solution of the latter to ʒviij. of water; but the strength must vary according to circumstances; if there is much ulceration, a strong solution will give unnecessary pain. Oak-bark, nutgalls, and tannin are also serviceable remedies, and particularly the latter, as it is a powerful astringent. If there is inability to open the jaws, and the mouth is clogged with a viscid secretion, the lotion should be injected with a syringe, and warm water should be frequently thrown in, in the same manner to clean this away. But local measures alone will not suffice: the constitutional symptoms, which are severe and in some cases alarming, should be attended to, and we must endeavor to get the poison excreted from the system by the various depurative organs.

[Mr. Smith, after just referring to the use of tartar emetic, acetate of lead, and opium, which he thinks may sometimes be useful, observes :]

There is one remedy, however, which appears to possess considerable influence in removing salivation, and one which I think is not universally known; I mean sulphur; by referring to Mr. Colles' works I find that he recommended it several years ago. In what manner it acts we are not able exactly to tell, but it is highly probable that it enters into combination with the mineral, and forms a sulphuret, which is an inert preparation; moreover, it acts as a purgative, and also goes off by the other secretions, particularly the skin. I have had opportunities of using sulphur for ptyalism, and I have seen it used by others, and certainly, in the majority of cases, decided benefit occurred. The only objection I have noticed, is the fact that it sometimes irritates the bowels very much. I used it in a case lately, when I was obliged to suspend it for this reason. I would strenuously recommend it to those who may meet with a troublesome case of salivation. Mr. Allison has found out that chlorate of potash has a most beneficial influence over mercurial salivation, and he has tried it in numerous cases. *Part* xvi., *p.* 218.

Use of Creasote in Salivation.—Dr. Faulcon relates a case of profuse mercurial salivation, in which, after the unsuccessful employment of the usual remedies, he employed with great advantage a gargle composed of creasote ʒss., sage tea a pint,—the affection quickly yielding.
Part xx., *p.* 93.

Salivation treated by Nitrate of Silver.—Dr. Kirby applies a solution of nitrate of silver (ʒj. in an ounce), to the gums, three or four times daily with a hair-pencil. The teeth will be discolored, but the stain may be removed by a few applications of a solution of cyanide of potassium (one part of the salt to two of distilled water.) *Part* xx., *p.* 147.

Belladonna in Salivation.—A woman treated by mercury, internally and externally, for diarrhœa, was affected with profuse salivation. Dr. Erpenbeck treated this latter complaint with belladonna in divided doses, of two grains and a half, taken in emulsion every twenty-four hours. Next day the salivation had subsided, and the mouth was quite dry. On stopping the belladonna, the salivation returned, and again ceased when it was resumed. The author believes that after this fact and some similar ones, belladonna is the best treatment for salivation. *Part* xxx., *p.* 301.

Chlorate of Potass in Mercurial Salivation.—Encouraged by the success of Hunt, and others, in the employment of the chlorate of potass in the treatment of gangrenous affections of the mouth, M. Herpin has repeatedly employed it with the best effect in mercurial salivation, giving it in the dose of ʒss. to ʒj. per diem—the cure, when the case is taken early, being completed by the fourth day. He has long been accustomed to the employ. ment of this substance, as recommended by Odier, in jaundice, whether simple or complicated, with engorgement of the liver. Odier carried the daily dose as high as 150 grains.   *Part* xxxi., *p.* 235.

Mercurial Fetor and Salivation.—The best remedy for instantaneously and safely removing fetor of the breath, in the opinion of Dr. Nunn, of the Middlesex Hospital, is a strong solution of the chloride of zinc, made by mixing one drachm of Burnett's solution with seven drachms of dis. tilled water. This must be applied by the medical attendant with a soft brush to the gums, and between the teeth, the mouth being frequently washed with water. The solution acts by immediately entering into com. bination with the rotting epithelium and forming an inodorous product, which the brush removes, at the same time it powerfully constringes the enlarged vessels, and tends to restore a healthy state of the local circula. tion.   *Part* xxxv., *p.* 190.

Quinine in the Salivation of Pregnancy.—Dr. Mauthner relates that he has found sulphate of quinine, given in two grain doses, prove completely efficacious in cases in which various other means had been tried without success.   *Part* xxxvii., *p.* 233.

SARSAPARILLA.

Powder of Sarsaparilla.—[Sir Francis Smith, speaking of this medicine says :]

I have long been engaged in observing the effects of different prepara. tions of sarsaparilla, and I am persuaded that of all the forms in which it can be given, that of powder is in most instances the most valuable. The advantages which it possesses, in my opinion, may be stated as follows, viz. : 1, we can make use of it in many conditions of the stomach where a large quantity of fluid would prove inconvenient or injurious; 2, it may be taken in more certain and definite quantities; 3, its effects are, so far as I have observed, more durable. Of course certain conditions of the skin will occur, where the use of the domestic decoction will be more ser. viceable, especially if it be taken warm; and in a slimy or foul condition of the primæ viæ the infusion in lime water (recommended by Dr. O'Beirne of Dublin, not as made in the Pharmacopœia) will present special advan. tages.

Mode of Preparation and Administration of the Powder.—The mode made use of in one establishment where I have superintended its prepara. tion is as follows : A quantity of the roots of sarsaparilla, either split or not, but not cut into short portions, is either subjected to the vapor of steam for a few minutes, or if time admit, left in a damp cellar for twenty. four or thirty-six hours, and subsequently introduced for an hour into a stove or oven, moderately heated, which processes have the effect of loosening the connection between the bark and the ligneous portion, when the former may be easily stripped off, and powdered finely in a mortar, and the powder may afterward be taken simply in a spoonful of any bland fluid, or may, in cases where quinine is indicated, be united with a suitable proportion, and the flavor be covered with a little oil of cinnamon—or the powder either simply, or combined with S. of quinine, or in gouty habits, with capsicum or ginger, may be made into pills, and administered in the proportion of from two to four scruples daily.

Part ii., *p.* 68.

----•◦•----

SCALP.

Wounds of the Scalp—Contusion of the Bones.—[Severe cases of this kind, where the scalp is extensively separated and the bone denuded, sometimes run a very rapid course to a fatal termination; but whenever this does occur, it is much more owing to the contusion of the bone than the denudation. Prof. Hewett says:]

In the flat bone of the skull, with its compact tables and intervening cancellous tissue, the contusion seldom reveals itself on the surface; it is in the diploë that the blow produces its effects. Examined as to its compact tables, such a bone, externally, may be to all appearance perfectly healthy; but the contusion manifests itself in the diploë by an extravasation of blood within its cells or in breaking down of the delicate fibres of their walls. In such a condition, the bone has hidden within itself all the seeds of the future mischief, if inflammation should arise in the bone—and arise, in all probability, it will, if the diploë has been much injured; and the great tendency will be, in certain habits of the body, to produce suppurative inflammation, and suppuration in such a situation is fraught with the utmost danger.

The intimate connection of the bone to the membranes of the brain: the large and numerous venous channels in its cancellous tissue, render diffuse suppuration in the diploë not only one of the most formidable complaints the surgeon can have to deal with, but one which but too often sets at naught all his resources.

Let us look to the train of evils which may arise in the membranes of the brain, after a contusion of the bone, followed by mischief in the diploë.

For days, for weeks even, there may be no appearance whatsoever of the mischief which is smoldering. Soon recovering from the effects of the accident, if it was a slight one, the patient appears to be in perfect health. For a time, all wears a favorable aspect; but generally, within a fortnight or three weeks, the first symptoms begin to show themselves—pain in the head, feverishness, and soon an unhealthy aspect in the wound, if there be one; a spontaneous secession of the periosteum from the bone, which, if denuded, becomes dry, and may be seen gradually to lose its natural color, being first of a dead white, then of an opaque yellow, a greenish, or it may be of a brownish hue. Matters go on thus for a longer or shorter period, that is, as long as the inflammation does not spread to the inner table of the bone; but, as soon as this is reached, the dura mater becomes involved; inflamed in its turn, and it may be in a sloughy state, this membrane secedes from the bone, lymph or pus is poured out on its external surface, and as long as the inflammation is limited to the dura-mater itself, generally only that portion of the membrane corresponding exactly to the inflamed bone is diseased; but when the inflammation has once passed on to the parietal arachnoid, matter is thrown out into the cavity of this membrane, and then the visceral arachnoid, the pia mater, and the brain itself, soon present all the appearances of severe inflammatory action. The symptoms are in keeping with the progressive stages of the disease. As long as the inflammation is confined to the bone they are few, and not strongly marked; but as soon as the dura-mater is reached, then decided symptoms of the cerebral mischief soon manifest themselves; increased feverishness, repeated rigors, intense pain in the head, sickness, drowsiness, occasional wandering, coma, and sometimes paralysis.

Such cases as these strongly resemble those which, of late years, have so much occupied the attention of the profession. I allude to the diseases of the ear, where the bone is affected, and where the inflammation manifestly spreads from the bone to the membranes of the brain. In these cases the disease may lay smoldering for years. I have known it to do so for upward of twenty; and as long as the mischief is confined to the bone, the symptoms are trifling ones; but suddenly, without any apparent cause, it spreads to the dura-mater, and then follows the train of cerebral symptoms.

[Mischief so insidious in its course, and so constantly and rapidly fatal, when once fully developed, naturally led surgeons to bleed largely and repeatedly as a preventive; but we may fairly question whether we ought to bleed patients without a symptom of serious disease. We are told to do so to prevent inflammation of the dura-mater, but it is only one case in seventy where we find mischief in the dura-mater after death. As a general rule, blood ought never to be drawn without a clear indication of its necessity. In the majority of cases of severe wounds and contusions, patients recover, if kept perfectly quiet, and with an occasional saline purgative; but whenever inflammatory symptoms begin to make their appearance, then is the time to have recourse to antiphlogistic treatment, which must be more or less strict according to the nature of the case.]

Failing in our antiphlogistic remedies, have we any other means of relieving the patient? The only chance left is in the trephine. But are we to trephine all cases of blows on the head, with bare bone and symptoms of suppuration?

A close examination of cases, under such circumstances, will show that, in many instances, we really have no indications which could lead us to apply the trephine.

The dura-mater, when laid bare by the trephine, is so often found to be perfectly healthy, that its use has of late years been abandoned, although the symptoms of suppuration may have been very evident.

Part xxxiii., *p.* 234.

Scalp— Wounds of.—In spite of any treatment, erysipelas too commonly comes on about the third or fourth day; whenever such does happen, says Mr. F. C. Skey, the tonic treatment by quinine, steel and wine is the best.

Part xxxiii., *p.* 235.

———•◦•———

SCARLATINA.

Chlorine in Scarlet Fever.—[In scarlatina maligna, every practitioner is aware that frequently all his efforts are vain to check the disease. There seem to be two sources of danger—one arising from the primary impression of the contagious poison upon the body, and especially upon the nervous system, which is overwhelmed by its influence. In this case, the patient often sinks without any affection of the throat, and our chief dependence will be upon wine and bark to sustain the powers of the system till the deadly agency of the poison has exhausted itself. Another source of danger arises from the gangrenous ulceration of the throat—the system seems to be *re-inoculated* with the poisonous secretion from the throat. Wine and bark will here also be of great benefit; gargles composed of chloride of soda will be found efficacious, and if the child is too young to gargle, it may be injected into the nostrils and against the throat by means of a syringe. This will be found superior to capsicum gargles. But we think one of the most efficacious methods is that recommended so strongly by Velpeau, of blowing powdered alum up the parts by means of any tube long enough for the purpose, as two or three quills inserted into each other, so as to make one continuous tube. Dr. Watson seems to think highly of chlorine. He says:]

From several distinct and highly respectable sources, *chlorine* has been strongly pressed upon my notice, as a most valuable remedy in the severest forms of scarlet fever. I will give you the formula for its preparation.

Two drachms of the chlorate of potass are to be dissolved in two ounces of hydrochloric acid, previously diluted with two ounces of distilled water. The solution must be put immediately into a stoppered bottle, and kept in a dark place.

Two drachms of this solution, mixed with a pint of distilled water, constitute the chlorine mixture; of which a tablespoonful, or two, according to the age of the patient, may be given for a dose, frequently.

Part vi., *p.* 36.

Belladonna.—On the Protective Influence of Belladonna in Scarlet Fever, Dr. Watson says:

You are probably aware that *belladonna* is believed by many to exert a preventive and protecting influence upon the body against the contagion of scarlet fever. I know nothing, by my own experience, of the alleged conservative property of this vegetable, but in the small quantities, recommended, there can be no harm in trying it, *provided that* its employment does not lead to a neglect of other precautions. Three grains of the extract of belladonna are dissolved in an ounce of distilled water; and three drops of the solution are given twice daily to a child under twelve months old, and one drop more for every year above that age. It is affirmed that if this remedy does not prevent the disease, it will render it mild; and that if it be taken four or five days before exposure to the contagion, the resulting scarlatina never proves fatal. *Part* vi., *p.* 37.

Carbonate of Ammonia in Scarlatina.—The value of carbonate of ammonia in scarlet fever has been attested by several observers, by Dr. Picken, of Dublin, and Dr. Rieken, of Belgium; while at St. Petersburgh it is said to have been employed by the German physicians without any evident advantage. Mr. H. Freke suggests that it may act by taking the place of urea, and thus supply the natural stimulus to the renal functions; and Messrs. Herdenreich and Heim have observed, that in cases of scarlatina an ammoniacal alkali is deposited on the skin, and hence offer another explanation of its efficacy. Whatever the theory, the amount of practical evidence preponderates in favor of the administration of ammonia in scarlet fever.   *Part* xii., *p.* 27.

Treatment of Malignant Scarlatina.—Since bleeding was abandoned in the treatment of this disease, stimulants have formed the usual reme- dies. They were employed by Dr. Coley, in connection with proper local applications, at the commencement of the epidemic in Dec., 1847; but finding that he lost the first four patients in succession, and observing that the state of the fauces was identical with that which was found in the late epidemical diphtherite, he was induced to try the effects of small repeated doses of calomel, *at the very commencement of the disease.* It should be given in doses of one or two grains every four hours; and thus given does not affect the mouth. Acetate of ammonia may be given in conjuction with it; or in the latter stages, if there are hemorrhages from the mucous membrane, or petechial spots, quina with sulphuric acid may be exhibited. The best local application is a lotion with nitrate of silver, a scruple to the ounce, applied twice or thrice a day to all the parts which are ulcerated, or covered with diphtherite. If abscesses form in the glands of the neck, they are to be opened freely as soon as there is fluctuation or external redness.   *Part* xviii., *p.* 34.

Scarlatina—Some Points in the Treatment of.—The state of the throat, says Dr. West, must be carefully watched in every case of scarlet fever; and when there is much swelling of the tonsils, if the child be too young to gargle, a slightly acidulated lotion should be injected into the back of the throat, by means of a syringe, every few hours, in order to free it from the mucus which is so apt to collect there, and to be the source of much discomfort. If there be much deposit of lymph upon the tonsils, it is generally desirable to apply the strong hydrochloric acid, mixed with honey, in the proportion of about one part of the former to six of the latter, by means of a dossil of lint, or a camel's-hair pencil, two or three times in the twenty-four hours; but the strength of the application must be increased if the tonsils are ulcerated, or if any disposition to sloughing should appear. The coryza, which is so distressing and so ill-omened a symptom in cases of severe scarlatina, is best treated by throwing a small quantity of a solution of gr. j. or gr. ij., of nitrate of silver in ℥j. of distilled water up the nostrils every four or six hours. The glandular swellings are very difficult to relieve. When considerable, they do not seem to be benefited by leeches; the employment of which is also, in many cases, contra-indicated by the feeble state of the patient's powers; while they show very little disposition to suppurate, and consequently are not relieved by lancing; so that the constant application of a warm poultice is often all that can be done to afford ease to the patient. Children, in whom the local affection is severe, or in whom the disease assumes a malignant character, require all those stimulants, and that nutritious diet, which we are accustomed to give to patients in certain stages of typhus fever; though, unfortunately, the best devised means will, in many such cases, prove ineffectual. [A still more easy and efficacious application in some of these cases is a solution of crystallized nitrate of silver, (ℨss. or ℈ij. to the ℥j.) applied to the diseased parts by means of a sponge tied to the end of a bit of whale- bone, as described by Dr. Horace Green.]   *Part* xviii., *p.* 35.

Treatment of Scarlatina by Hot Water Applications.—Mr. Bulley, surgeon to Berkshire Hospital, directs to apply a thick flannel pad, wrung out of hot water till almost dry, upon the pit of the stomach and over the region of the heart, and then wrap the patient carefully in several blankets. At the same time wrap another flannel, wrung out of hot vinegar and water, round the throat. After the patient has *perspired* profusely for three or four hours, remove the flannels carefully, and give Stevens's saline powder (to an adult half a drachm) every four hours: and let him use a gargle containing ℈ij. of burnt alum, ℈ij. of Armenian bole, and ʒj. of brown sugar in ℥viij. of water. *Part xx., p.* 30.

Use of Acetic Acid in Scarlatina.—Dr. Webster, consulting physician to St. George's and St. James' Dispensary, has great faith in the use of frequent sponging with tepid vinegar and water, especially in the early stages, when the skin is hot and the pulse accelerated. This measure is very efficacious in preventing the spread of the disease. *Part xxi., p.* 350.

Yeast in the Treatment of Malignant Scarlet Fever.—Mr. Bennett states that he has found the administration of fresh yeast of the most invaluable advantage when the symptoms are of a malignant character. He says:

After ammonia, the mineral acids, chlorate of potash, etc., have failed, and the application of nitrate of silver besides, one or two table-spoonfuls of fresh yeast *frequently given* (according to the age and malignancy of the case) has, in my practice at least, been quickly efficacious as an antiseptic and stimulant. *Part xxiii., p.* 29.

Scarlatina—Delirium and Coma of.—Prof. Bennett gives the following case: A boy, aged 14, entered the clinical ward on the third day after experiencing distinct rigors. There was restless delirium, and constant moving of the head from side to side upon the pillow. He was apparently conscious when spoken to, but could not answer questions—the tongue was protruded with difficulty, dry, and of bright red color, studded with florid elevations—deglutition was much impeded—bowels open—pulse 130, weak—urine voided with difficulty, and diminished in quantity—sp. gr. 1025—not acted on by heat and nitric acid—skin hot and dry, covered with the bright red scarlatinal eruptions.— *Ordered salines and slight diuretics.* He continued in the same condition, the angina, coma, and alternating delirium, however, being more pronounced until the sixth day.

℞. Sp. æther. nit., ʒiij; pot. acet., ʒij; tr. colchici, ℥ss: aquæ, ℥iij. Ft. mist. A teaspoonful to be taken every four hours.

On the following day all coma and delirium had disappeared. He answers questions when put to him—skin cool—eruption faded—pulse 96, weak—passed 30 oz. of urine, which is turbid, with small flakes of a membraneous character floating in it. On the 8th day the quantity of urine excreted was 50 oz., and it was still more loaded with sediments which being analyzed were found to consist of urate of ammonia. Next day the urine was only slightly turbid, and on the following one, was perfectly clear. From this time the boy gradually recovered.

Commentary.—This was a very severe case of scarlatina. The angina was intense, occasionally rendering deglutition impossible. There was delirium on the third day, alternating at night with coma, which was often profound. The worst result was apprehended. It recurred to me that the head symptoms in this as in several cases of typhus, might probably depend not so much upon inflammation of the brain, as is generally sup posed, as upon absorption of, and poisoning by urea, an idea that appeared to me supported by the diminished quantity of the renal excretion, as well as its freedom from all deposit. Remembering the alleged virtues of colchicum in increasing the elimination of this excretion, I ordered it, in combination with diuretics, and the result was remarkable. For on the next day, not only had the fever diminished, but the urine was increased in amount and loaded with urates to an extent and in a form I had never previously seen. *Part* xxiv., *p.* 31.

Scarlatina.—Dr. Bennett remarks, that great watchfulness is required on the part of the practitioner, especially when the crisis is expected, that if the pulse at all falters, and prostration comes on rapidly, he may be prepared to meet it. When death does occur in a primary attack of scarlatina, it is from the same cause as in death from typhus—it is from congestion of the brain, as indicated by delirium, passing into coma, and followed by prostration of the vital powers.

All the eruptive fevers, strictly so called, invariably run a natural course, and cannot be cut short. It follows that—

The treatment of febrile eruptions has for its object conducting these cases to a favorable termination. To this end exactly the same general rules are to be followed as in continued fever, and the same indications exist for the use of salines and laxatives, cold to the head, wine and stimulants, and regulation of the diet.

Dr. Andrew Wood, physician to Heriot's Hospital, Edinburg, recommends the production of diaphoresis. He considers that the most efficient and safe method of treatment consists in acting powerfully on the skin, with a view of thereby assisting nature to eliminate the scarlatinal poison from the system. As ordinary diaphoretics frequently fail, he has recourse to the following method: Several common beer bottles, containing very hot water, are placed in long worsted stockings, or long narrow flannel bags, wrung out of water as hot as can be borne. These are to be laid alongside the patient, but not in contact with the skin. One on each side, and one between the legs, will generally be sufficient; but more may be used if deemed necessary. The patient is to lie between the blankets (the head of course being outside) during the application of the bottles, and for several hours afterward. In the course of from ten minutes to half an hour, the patient is thrown into a most profuse perspiration, when the stockings may be removed. In mild cases, the effect is easily kept up by means of draughts of cold water, and if necessary, the use of two drachm doses of sp. mindereii every two hours. In severe cases, where the pulse is very rapid—the beats running into each other—where the eruption is either absent or only partial, or of a dusky purplish hue—where the surface is cold—where there is sickness or tendency to diarrhœa—where the throat is aphthous or ulcerated, and the cervical glands swollen, then he follows up the use of the vapor-bath by four or five grain doses of carbonate of ammonia, repeated every three or four hours. Should this be vomited, then brandy may be given in doses proportionate to the age of the patients. Carbonate of ammonia he considers to act beneficially: 1st, by supporting the powers of life; 2d, by assisting the development of the eruption; and 3d, by acting on the skin and kidneys. Where the vapor bath was used early in the disease, and its use continued daily, or even twice or thrice a day, according to circumstances, he has found that the chance of severe sore throat was greatly obviated. In regard to supervening dropsy, he considers that, by the use of the vapor bath, with the other necessary precautions as to exposure, diet, etc., its recurrence is rendered much more rare. In the treatment of the dropsical cases, it was also very useful, and even might be trusted to entirely in some cases. Dr. Wood also condemns all depleting treatment, and even purgatives, during the first ten days, as not only not required, but positively dangerous, as tending to interfere with the development of the eruption. In the later stages, as well as in the dropsy, however, he thinks purgatives are often beneficial.

Part xxvi., *p.* 22.

Treatment of Coma, attending.—Dr. Murphy says that when coma exists after or during an attack of scarlatina, the electro-galvanic battery has been found successful, the same as in cases of poisoning by opium. At the same time a flexible tube may be passed into the stomach, and port wine and ether introduced. *Part* xxix., *p.* 314.

Treatment of Scarlatina Anginosa.—[Mr. P. H. Chavasse has had great experience of practice among children. The result of his treatment of scarlet fever has been so uniformly successful that he has not lost a single case for upward of seven years. He says :]

The system I adopt, in a case of scarlet fever, is to keep the bedroom cool—I may say cold—and to have a thorough ventilation through it; I, therefore, throw open the windows, be it winter or summer, and have the curtains and valances of the bed removed. If it be winter time, I allow the patient to have one blanket and a sheet; if it be summer time a sheet only to cover him. If the throat be not seriously affected, I merely order a narrow strip of flannel once around the throat. If the tonsils be much enlarged, I apply a barm and oatmeal poultice to the throat, changing it night and morning. I prescribe an acidulated infusion of roses mixture, that is to say, infusion of roses, with an excess of acid, made palatable with an additional quantity of sirup, to be taken every three or four hours. This is the only medicine I give. Where the child is old enough, I find roasted apples, mixed with raw sugar, very grateful to the patient.

Here let me pause, to advise my medical brethren always to make medicines for children pleasant. I avoid purgatives in scarlet fever. I never, on any account whatever, give a particle of opening medicine for the first ten days at least. It is my firm conviction, that the administration of purgatives in scarlet fever is a fruitful source of dropsy, disease and death. When we take into consideration the sympathy that there is between the skin and mucous membrane, I think that we should pause before giving irritating medicines. The irritation of purgatives on the mucous membrane may cause the poison of the skin disease to be driven internally to the kidneys, throat, pericardium, or brain. You may say, Do you not purge if the bowels be not opened for a week? I say emphatically, No!

Now with regard to food. If the infant be at the breast, keep him entirely to it. If he be weaned, and under two years old, give him milk and water, and cold water to drink. If he be older, give him toast and water, and plain water from the pump, as much as he chooses; let it be quite cold—the colder the better. Weak black tea, or thin gruel, may be given, but caring little if he take nothing but cold water, unless he be an infant at the breast. Avoid broths and stimulants of every kind.

Now, you must warily watch for a change of temperature of the skin. As long as the skin is hot, the above plan I steadily follow ; but the moment the skin of the patient becomes cool, which it will do probably in five or seven days, instantly close the window, and immediately put more clothes on the bed. But still do not purge.

You will find the acidulated infusion of roses most grateful to the little patient ; it will abate the fever, it will cleanse his tongue, it will clear his throat of mucus, it will, as soon as the fever is abated, give him an appetite. I believe, too, the acid treatment has some peculiar properties of neutralizing the scarlatinal poison.

When the appetite returns, you may consider the patient to be safe. The diet must now be gradually improved.

Within the last few years, I have had some fearful cases of scarlet fever ; but, relying on this plan of treatment, I have given, even in very bad cases, a favorable diagnosis. I have had cases where there have been violent headache and delirium ; where there have been immense swellings of the parotid and submaxillary glands ; where there have been enormous enlargement and ulceration of the tonsils ; where a great portion of the fluid that has been taken by the mouth has escaped down the nostrils ; where there has been a purulent discharge down the nose, which discharge has in many instances quite excoriated the skin over which it has travelled —and yet in such cases the patients have invariable recovered.

Another very important regulation is never to allow the patient to leave the house under a month in the summer, and under six weeks in winter.

Part xxxiii., *p.* 29.

Hematuria after Scarlet Fever.—In those cases where we have convulsions, coma, and death, there is no hesitation in attributing the symptoms to uræmic poisoning, any more than if the mischief were limited to renal disturbance. The congestion of the kidneys, the hematuria, which form the incipient stage of the disorder leading to this uræmia, arise undeniably from the imperfect elimination of the original virus.

According to Dr. Basham, we must endeavor to bring into activity and act upon those functions and emunctories which are not, or only in a moderate degree, implicated in the morbid disturbance, and by their agency relieve, if possible, the oppressed and impeded organs. Thus, though the surface of the body is anasarcous, we must endeavor to promote its exhaling power ; and as the intestinal mucous surface gives no indication of sharing in the morbid state of the kidneys, we must bring its secretions into activity to purge the system of the accumulated fluid, and vicariously, for a time, relieve the kidneys of their office. The intimate sympathy between the kidneys and skin, and between the latter and the bronchial mucous membrane, when the latter is the seat of inflammation, would entitle us to expect the most beneficial results by vigorously promoting the cutaneous function ; but unhappily, in these cases, the dropsical state of the surface of the skin precludes our obtaining much efficient aid in this direction. Warm baths effect oftentimes great temporary relief to the lungs ; the breathing becomes less oppressed, and the secretion from the bronchial tubes more free ; but the hot-air bath appears to be the most efficacious ; there is not that exhaustion which is induced by a succession of warm baths, and, to my observation, the amount o. relie felt by the patient is greater. To aid these external appliances, ammoniacal salines may be given internally with advantage. Active purging, however, yields the best results. It is, however, of importance to select appropriate means to obtain the greatest amount of relief, for it is not every purgative of the Pharmacopœia which answers the purpose equally well. That purgative which acts most directly as a hydragogue is the best adapted, but which, at the same time, is not followed by any disproportioned exhaustion, or by any torpid reaction. The combination of jalap and cream of tartar is most admirably suited to these ends. It acts quickly, without depressing the system, is not followed by inactivity, and induces copious watery dejections.

The appearance in the urine, revealed by the microscope, of that peculiar pigmentary condition observed in combination with albumen, indicates an advancing stage of degeneration, and if spread through both kidneys, must be quickly followed by an imperfect elimination of the chief urinary constituents; and this was evident by the singularly watery state of the urine, its specific gravity not exceeding 1.005, but containing abundance of albumen, and this latter, associated with a peculiar pigmentary matter, rendered visible after boiling by the addition of nitric acid.

It would be out of place here to enter into an investigation of the nature of the pigments that are occasionally met with in the urine, cyanurin, melanurin, etc. Experience tells me that the development of this pigmentary condition, in combination with albumen in the urine, is of the greatest import. It is always associated with the most advanced stage of renal degeneration, and in every instance in which I have seen it, it has been quickly followed by fatal results. Lehman, in his "Physiological Chemistry" (vol. ii., p. 428), says, as far as his experience goes, it is only when uræmic symptoms have manifested themselves, that this peculiarity of the urine is generally observable, and this entirely coincides with my own. We should not, then, be unprepared for the development of unfavorable symptoms whenever this peculiarity of the urine is observed. Hence the value and importance of frequent examinations of the urine in such cases.

You may learn an important point here—namely, the suddenness and abruptness with which the symptoms of uræmic poisoning oftentimes commence. In some cases, particularly in adults, the indications are progressive; but here all other things being promising, convulsions suddenly supervene; they intermit, but coma characterizes their remission, and the patient dies forty hours after the first indication of the urinous poison acting on the nervous centre. You may very properly ask, Can nothing be done in this crisis? Are there no remedies available for such a state? These cases of convulsion are not always fatal; sometimes in the intervals consciousness returns. Such cases offer a better prospect for remedial agents than when the patient remains comatose. In either state, however, an effort should be made to excite the bowels to active excretion. Enemata containing, according to the age of the patient, half a drop, or a drop, of croton oil, should be administered, and where the ability to swallow is unimpaired, you may expect some benefit from the chlorine mixture, the agency of which, according to the hypothesis of Frerichs, depends on its union with the carbonate of ammonia, into which the urea in the blood is converted, and which he considers to be the poisonous agent in these cases of fatal uræmia. *Part* xxxvi., *p.* 25

Scarlatina.—Some pathologists think that there is a most intimate connection between the materies morbi of erysipelas and that of scarlatina, as well as other acute diseases. During a late epidemic of scarlatina at Bradford, Dr. Meade being much struck with the analogy between the symptoms of this disease and erysipelas, very successfully applied the tincture of iron treatment, so useful in the latter, to the former disease, giving five to fifteen minims, according to the age of the patient, every three or four hours. He has only lost one case during the whole of last spring and winter, and almost all the cases in which he employed this treatment recovered with unusual rapidity.

    *   *   *   *   *   *   *

Scarlatina and Measles.—Mr. Witt looks upon the treatment of scarlatina and measles by ammonia as a specific. The dose given is from three to seven grains of the hydrochlorate every hour, for the first twenty-four hours, and every second hour for the next day. All acid drinks are carefully avoided. This is a matter of interest, now that the power of ammonia in retarding the coagulation of the blood has been established.

Part xxxviii., *p.* 17.

Scarlatina.—Dr. E. Bishop says that the use of tonics, either the citrate of iron, or the tincture of the sesquichloride, not varying the *plan* of treatment, even when serious complications present, will be found very successful in the treatment of scarlatina. One gratifying result is, that with few exceptions the children escape that serious and frequent sequel—anasarca.

Part xxxix., *p.* 19..

Scarlatina.—Dr. Fountain says that chlorate of potash must not be given in scarlatina, with the idea that in chlorine something like a specific has been found for the disease—if so given it will fall into disrepute. It is a very valuable remedy for meeting particular indications in the treatment of disease, by arresting the ulcerative inflammation of the fauces, and by its arterializing properties, supporting the restorative powers of nature, when aided by other appropriate treatment. It may be combined with carbonate of ammonia, with the best effects. *Part* xl., *p.* 296.

Scarlatina.—In the early stage, if attended with high fever, burning heat of skin, thirst, etc., try full doses of nitrate of potash with mucilages.

—•••—

SCIATICA.

Treatment of Sciatica and Lumbago.—[Dr. Graves justly remarks that in acute sciatica and lumbago, one of the most powerful remedies consists of morphia, calomel, and James' powder, given in the following way. Three grains of acetate of morphia, six grains of calomel, and two grains of James' powder, divided into eight portions, and one to be taken every third hour till the gums become affected. This is to be assisted by antiphlogistic measures, as blood-letting, general and local, etc., but when the case becomes chronic, and the patient must of necessity continue his occupation, if possible, he strongly recommends, from personal experience, the hydriodate of potass. He experienced, in his own person, a severe attack of this disease; against which he struggled for some time, obtaining relief. He states as follows :]

Mr. Ferguson recommended me to try hydriodate of potash, of which he was good enough to send me a drachm dissolved in a pint of decoction of sarsaparilla. I took a quarter of this daily, and may literally apply here the common phrase, that I felt each dose do me good ; in four days all traces of the lumbago were gone, and my lameness had quite ceased. I did not take more than one bottle, *i. e.* one drachm of the hydriodate, but the good effect continued after I had ceased taking it, and in less than a week I was perfectly well. Subsequent experience enables me to recommend this medicine strongly, in subacute and chronic lumbago and sciatica.

In spite of the best-directed means, sciatica is very apt to become chronic, and then spirit of turpentine, carbonate of iron, arsenic, extract of stramonium, corrosive sublimate, blue pill, and iodine internally, blisters to the loins, thigh, and calf of the leg, acupuncture, croton oil frictions, and other stimulating applications must be successively tried. On a former occasion I recommended a combination of opium, with spirit of turpentine internally, and when that fails, Dover's powder, combined with sulphate of quinine. I am sorry not to have it in my power to lay down any general principle, which would enable us to judge in what cases each of these remedies is peculiarly indicated, for experience has not confirmed any of the rules generally relied on, and therefore we must content ourselves with treating these diseases empirically. *Part* ii., *p.* 70.

Treatment of Sciatica by Irritation of the Foot.—This consists in applying an olive-shaped cautery, heated to a white heat, between the little toe of the diseased limb and the one next to it. This cautery ought to be applied to that part where the nerve bifurcates to furnish its collateral branches to the last two toes; and ought to be kept there for five or six seconds. The wound should then be dressed with simple cerate, and allowed to cicatrize. A Capuchin monk, affected with sciatica, carried with him in his travels through various towns, an instrument for this purpose. Professor Quadri has often repeated this operation at Prati, in Tuscany, with great success. These circumstances were brought to M. Caffe's memory, by reading an article on the treatment of sciatica, in which mention was made of a woman of Cassano who had a great reputation for her success in its cure. The means which she employed consisted in the application of a certain herb to the foot, which produced a sore. Various physicians, astonished at the results produced, took the trouble to find out that the remedy in question was the leaves of the *ranunculus sceleratus*, which, as every one knows, is a powerful vesicant. Dr. Fioravante has employed common blistering plaster to the same part, with the happiest results. *Part* ix., *p.* 85.

Sciatica, treated by Blisters and Morphia.—This patient was under Dr. Taylor's care in University College Hospital. It appears that in lifting a heavy weight, he had strained his back, and that a few months afterward he was suddenly seized with pain in the right hip—striking into the loins, and down the leg. On his admission he had still this pain, but there was no increased heat of skin; he was ordered to take, three times a day, two ounces of guaiacum mixture, with forty minims of am. tr. of guaiacum, and have a good diet; three days afterward he was to increase the dose of the tincture of guaiacum to one drachm three times daily; a blister to be applied to the right hip, and the blistered surface to be dressed twice a day with one grain of the hydrochlorate of morphia. Repeat the blister and morphia when necessary.

Whether sciatica be rheumatic or not in its nature, it is certain that the seat of the disease is in the sciatic nerve. In the treatment of this case, Dr. Taylor attributes the cure to the blistering and morphia. M. Valleix has published an excellent work on neuralgia. He also recommends the application of blisters, but Dr. Taylor remarks that:]

The plan of blistering advocated by M. Valleix is the application of flying blisters, as the French term them. This consists in having the blisters very small, allowing them to heal immediately, and in applying fresh ones as the seat of pain changes. This is the treatment which he has himself put in practice, and which he finds more efficacious than any other. After the application of blisters, the next best remedy in the treatment of this disease seems to be the internal administration of the oil of turpentine. Opium given internally generally has very little effect on the disease.

Part xiii., *p.* 61.

Moxas.—Dr. Thomson gives a case of sciatica which was treated with moxas. Tincture of guaiacum and aconite was prescribed and the dose increased. Aconite plaster over the seat of pain. Cupping over the part and afterward two grains calomel and one grain opium ; then a mixture of vin. colchici and tinct. aconite ; lastly, six moxas ; since which the case has done well.

The best moxas are prepared by dipping a piece of bibulous paper in a solution of diacetate of lead, drying it, and rolling it up in the form of a cylinder. It burns well and steadily, leaving an ash of yellow oxide of lead.

Part xiv., *p.* 59.

Bisulphuret of Carbon in Sciatica.—A patient, who, for five years, had suffered at times under a very painful sciatica, with commencing emaciation of the limb, loss of appetite and sleep, and against which a great variety of remedies had been employed, was at last put under alcohol of sulphur (the bisulphuret of carbon), used both internally and externally, after the method of Wutzer. At the end of five days, there was complete removal.

From the Memoir of Lampadius, it appears to have been internally employed with advantage in rheumatism, chronic gout, palsy, and cutaneous eruptions, and externally against burns: the latter use being dependent on its energetic property of producing cold. *Part* xv., *p.* 67.

Diagnosis of Sciatica from Morbus Coxarius.—[Mr. Corfe states that the following simple method enables us readily to distinguish between sciatica and inflamed or diseased hip joint, in those cases where difficulty arises.]

Place the thumb of the *right* hand firmly on the great trochanter, and the third finger on the tuberosity of the ischium ; then drive the forefinger into the space that exists midway, and a little above, these two points, and if sciatica is present, the patient will certainly wince. The fingers here describe a triangle, the apex of which, whilst it points toward the sacro-illiac symphysis, also rests upon the precise exit of the nerve from the pelvis, and the base is formed by the line from the trochanter to the ischiatic tuberosity. But in order to ascertain if disease of the hip-joint is present, reverse this triangle, and place the thumb of the *left* hand upon the great trochanter, and the third finger upon the tuber ischii, and let the forefinger be driven into the apex of that triangle, of which the two former fingers describe the base, and it will be found to be immediately over the articular surface of the hip-joint, and which will certainly cause pain if inflammation exists in it. It will be observed that the apex of this triangle looks downward toward the lesser trochanter. These directions apply to the detection of the seat of pain on the left side; but when the right hip is examined, the hands of the operator should be reversed to the above description. *Part* xviii., *p*. 104.

Sciatica Cured by Cauterizing the Ear.—[However singular it may appear, M. Malgaigne did actually apply the red-hot iron to the anterior part of the right helix in a case of sciatica, and his patient was cured forthwith. Similar success is stated to have resulted on more recent occasions at the Hospital St. Louis, and]

Dr. Lucciana of Bastia relates in the " Journal des Connaissances Médico-Chirurgicales," 1st May, 1850, a radical mode of curing sciatica, popularly practised in Corsica, and consisting in the application of a red hot iron to the ear, and exactly on its helix. The cauterization cures the sciatica instantaneously, or at least effects immediate improvement. The operation is in Corsica uniformly performed by the farrier, and the inhabitants, when affected with sciatica, lose no time in applying for his assistance. In confirmation Lucciana adduces some cases of sciatica which he had in vain attempted to cure in the hospital of Bastia by other therapeutical methods, and which yielded to the farrier's cautery, as if to a charm. *Part* xxii., *p*. 86.

Sciatica.—Sciatica, not connected with mechanical causes, as tumors, accumulation of fæces, etc., may be cured in fourteen days by rubbing along the affected nerve, from above downward, ʒss. of veratria ointment (gr. v. to ʒss.), every night at bed-time. The friction to be performed with a horse-hair glove until severe tingling is produced.

*   *   *   *   *   *   *   *

Sciatica and Neuralgia.—Some cases recorded by Dr. Belcombe were entirely cured by the insertion of a needle just at the seat of pain, to some depth, and another two inches lower in the same direction. These were kept in for two hours, and then withdrawn. In cases of *sciatic lumbago*, give acetate of potash in compound infusion of senna, the patients finding much relief from the movement of the lower bowels, and pressure being taken off the kidneys. In the *neuralgia* of the upper extremity, carbonate of iron in full doses was given. *Part* xxv., *p*. 74.

Use of Croton Oil.—[Mr. Hancock is of opinion that mechanical irritation of the nerve within the pelvis is the most frequent cause of sciatica. This may be from loaded colon or cæcum, or from tumors formed within that cavity.]

In cases where sciatica depends on local irritation of the nerve within the pelvis from accumulation of fæces in the colon or cæcum, the following pills generally produce a good effect; the patient, however, should be warned of the activity of the remedy. Croton oil, one minim; blue pill, extract of hyoscyamus, each four grains; compound extract of colocynth, eight grains; to be divided into four pills, two to be taken at night, and repeated as the case may be. *Part* xxix., *p*. 71.

SCORBUTIC AFFECTIONS.

Extract of Monesia.—Suggested in the form of pills, in scurvy. Dose, from 12 to 36 grains during the day.   *Part* ii., *p.* 77.

Tincture of Cantharides.—Mr. Irven has introduced a new remedy for the cure of this disease. He administers tincture of cantharides ; at first, in doses of from ten to twenty drops, three times a day, increasing the quantity taken in the twenty-four hours, according to circumstances, to about eighty drops. At the same time that an improvement in the general health becomes perceptible, the urine becomes clear, and is found to contain albumen, which is said to be uniformly absent from the urine of scorbutic patients.   *Part* vii., *p.* 13.

Purpura, or Land Scurvy.—Scurvy is the old name for purpura hemorrhagica, and *land* scurvy for purpura without hemorrhages : the two diseases are allied ; they are only varieties of the same disease. [It consists in a lesion of the capillary system and of the blood, which is deficient in fibrin. Dr. Laycock observes that if not checked, the disease will assume as formidable an appearance as marine scurvy ; there will be spreading ulcers, the gelatinous fungus on the skin and gums termed by sailors " bullock's liver," and finally death. He says :] The explanation of the symptoms is not difficult. The morbid condition of the blood has impaired the contractility of the vascular system. In the depending portions of the body the capillaries give way from the mere gravitation of their contents ; thus giving rise to the vibices in the legs, and in the under surfaces of the thighs. The petechiæ are really small inflamed or congested papillæ, or the mouths of sebaceous glands. The muscular pains are those of fatigue ; there is not enough fibrin in the blood for the nutrition of the muscles and the maintenance of their action.

Let the diet be varied, and consist partly of vegetables, which contain acids : rhubarb, cabbage, potatoes, sorrel, water cresses, nettle tops, lemons, oranges, etc. Give citric acid four grains every four hours ; or give nitrate of potash.   *Part* xv., *p.* 39.

Deficiency of Potash in the Blood, a Cause of.—Dr. Garrod points out many objections to the opinion that a deficiency of any of the *organic* constituents of the food produces scurvy ; and states that from minute researches into the composition of scorbutic or antiscorbutic articles of diet, and into the state of the blood in scorbutic patients, he has been led to the following conclusions :

1st. That in all scorbutic diets, *potash* exists in much smaller quantities than in those which are capable of maintaining health.   2d. That all substances proved to act as anti-scorbutics contain a large amount of *potash.* 3d. That in scurvy the blood is deficient in *potash*, and the amount of that substance thrown out by the kidneys less than that which occurs in health.   4th. That scorbutic patients will recover when *potash* is added to their food, the other constituents remaining as before, both in quantity and quality, and without the use of succulent vegetables or milk. 5th. That the theory which ascribes the cause of scurvy to a deficiency of *potash* in the food, is also capable of rationally explaining many symptoms of that disease.

If medicine is to be prescribed, give 10 or 15 grains of the phosphate, chloride, or tartrate of potash twice or three times a day either in water or with food. *Part* xvii., *p.* 23.

Treatment of Sea Scurvy.—The whole treatment of sea scurvy may be summed up in a few words. Supply the system freely with protein, by giving patients freely those vegetables in which it most abounds. Many English naval surgeons maintain that vegetable acids alone are not sufficient to cure scurvy, and that a portion of fresh animal food is necessary for a cure. *Part* xviii., *p.* 53.

Scurvy.—It would appear from experiments made on board convict ships by Dr. Bryson, R. N., that the remedial powers of citric acid and lime-juice, in scurvy, are about on a par; and that the good effects of both of them are probably increased by the addition of sugar. As a prophylactic, citric acid has not been fairly tried, but lime-juice, with sugar, is unquestionably of the greatest advantage. Nitrate of potash would appear not to possess antiscorbutic properties, and not to be adapted either for a prophylactic or a curative agent. *Part* xxi., *p.* 33.

Purpura Hemorrhagica.—Mr. Budd, physician to Bristol Infirmary, says:

Although purpura is certainly a disease connected with a dissolved and thin condition of the blood, yet it is also more than probable that weakness of the vessels themselves, from defective nutrition of their walls, has a still larger share in the result; the symmetrical distribution of the ecchymoses, proving the correctness of this supposition. On this ground, the very valuable properties of turpentine as a styptic, both applied locally and administered internally, is strongly recommended, great benefit having been produced by it, when all other measures had failed. Twenty minims of the oil may be given in emulsion every six hours. A similar testimony of the styptic properties of turpentine is quoted from the illustrious Hunter, and also from Mr. Vincent, late surgeon to St. Bartholomew's Hospital.
Part xxii., *p.* 118.

Case of Purpura Hemorrhagica treated by Turpentine.—A gentleman, aged 22, while coughing, expectorated a large quantity of dark colored blood. The respiratory sounds were natural, but the limbs were found covered with the peculiar eruption of purpura. He was an excessive smoker, and was generally from this cause in a state of salivation.

The treatment consisted in an acid mixture, and a dose of aperient pills; the bowels being sluggish. For the following three days this treatment was continued without change, except that a grain of ipecacuan was added to the pills. The hemoptysis subsided. A few days afterward, the patient suffered severe pain in the testicle, and on voiding his urine, it was mixed with a large quantity of blood. No material improvement following upon the administration of the acid mixture, aperients, and gallic acid, the treatment was changed and replaced by turpentine in the following form:

R Spiritus terebinthinæ, ʒij.; sacchari albi, pulveris acaciæ, aa. ʒij.; tinctur. lavandulæ comp., ʒj.; aquæ menthæ piper. ad ℥viij. M. Fiat mistura.

Of this he took an ounce three times a day. The turpentine has been continued with the best effects. The urine has acquired its healthy character, and the patient expresses himself as feeling quite well. In about a week the turpentine was stopped, and a few drops of the tincture of the muriate of iron, twice daily, prescribed in its place, with a compound rhubarb pill as an occasional aperient. There has been no return of the symptoms.

As to the cause of the diseased blood, Dr. Willis ascribes it to excessive smoking. He says:

I believe that the fumes of tobacco, if long inhaled, possessing as they do narcotico-irritant properties, are quite as capable of reducing the consistency of the blood as some other agents of the same character; and that the essence of purpuric symptoms is a fluid or defibrinated condition of the blood. *Part* xxix., *p.* 49.

Chlorate of Potash in Scurvy.—[Mr Corner, the resident medical officer on board the Dreadnought Hospital Ship, always relies upon the chlorate of potash in scurvy.]

Chlorate of potash has the effect of curing the spongy state of the gums in this disease much more rapidly than any other treatment. It should be combined with lime-juice. This salt appears to be curative in all inflammations of the mouth and gums whatever their cause, syphilitic and cancerous affections alone excepted. *Part* xxxvii., *p.* 29.

Purpura Hemorrhagica.—The use of the tincture of larch bark is recommended in the treatment of purpura hemorrhagica. Four cases are related in which improvement certainly seemed to date from its use. Dr. Moore remarks that the tincture is one of the most elegant forms at our disposal of prescribing a terebinthinate, either as an addition to a compatible expectorant, or other fluid mixture, or to be given *per se.* The dose is from ʒss. to ʒiij.; of the extract, from gr. j. to grs. v. The value of terebinthinates in the treatment of purpura has been long acknowledged, the difficulty of their exhibition having alone restricted their employment in many instances; whereas in the preparations of larch bark, whilst all the valuable styptic qualities of the turpentine are retained, its exhibition is not attended with disagreeable results. *Part* xxxix., *p.* 87.

—————•◆•—————

SCROFULA.

Leaves of the Walnut in Scrofula.—M. Negrier published a memoir on the use of walnut leaves in scrofula, which he regards, after numerous experiments, as one of the best antiscrofulous remedies that we possess.

M. Negrier concludes his memoir with the following directions for the preparations of walnut. The infusion is made with an ounce of the leaves in twelve ounces of boiling water; it may be sweetened with sugar or the sirup presently to be noticed. Two or three cupfuls may be given daily, or even five. The decoction is made with a handful of the leaves, boiled for fifteen minutes in a quart of water. The extract may be made in the usual manner from the dried leaves. For the sirup, eight grains of the extract are mixed with thirty-two scruples of common sirup; infants and young children may take two or three teaspoonfuls in the day; adults three drachms. The pills may be made of the extract, four grains in each; from two to four in the day. *Part* iv., *p.* 60.

Medicinal effect of Manganese in Glandular Swellings and Cutaneous

Diseases.—Dr. Krigeler, an Austrian practitioner, having remarked that many workmen who were previously affected with glandular swellings and cutaneous diseases, had by degrees got rid of those affections while employed in a bleaching factory in which oxide of manganese was used, has since employed the latter substance for the cure of such complaints with the happiest results. Its administration to children with scrofulous enlargements of the glands, in doses of one to five centigrammes (one-seventh to three quarters of a grain), has been found in a very short time to be attended by a diminution of the swellings, which have eventually disappeared altogether under the use of the medicine.

Part vii., *p.* 90.

Treatment of.—The basis of a very rational plan of treating scrofula consists in the administration of alkalies, and the continued use of highly animalized diet. Chemistry has lately shown in an interesting manner the reason of this fact, which is, that phosphates are passed in the urine of scrofulous patients to an extent many times greater than natural. The reason for the avoidance therefore of vegetable diet, which, by forming lactic acid, tends to dissolve the earthy phosphates, and the persistence in the use of alkalies, which neutralize the acid in the system, is clearly shown.

Part xii., *p.* 301.

Treatment of.—Dr. Willshire, physician to the infirmary for children, says iron is very valuable in the treatment of scrofula; to children at the breast give the vinum ferri, but for older children, nothing is better than the sesqui-oxide, from one to three teaspoonfuls daily, mixed with treacle. Quinine is also useful; but especially iodine. To the youngest children we may give a grain of iodide of potassium in distilled water, *sweetened immediately before administration*, thrice a day. If the child is above a year old, from one-tenth to one-eighth of a grain of iodine may be added; and the dose increased according to age. For external use the compound ointment, or the compound tincture of the pharmacopœia, will do; or a lotion with from gr. v. to ʒij. of iodide of potassium to an ounce of distilled water. Or when more counter-irritation is needed, paint on the skin near the affected part, a solution of a drachm of iodine and a drachm and a half of iodide of potassium to half an ounce of alcohol.

Part xvi., *p.* 60.

Scrofula.—Dr. Graves recommends cod-liver oil; enlargements of the tonsils and of the cervical glands will disappear under its use.

Part xvi., *p.* 62.

Scrofula.—In addition to the usual hygienic treatment, Mr. Bulley recommends small doses of the *purest sulphur*, which has the effect of accelerating the capillary circulation, and restoring the defective animal heat. The following formula may be used: ℞. Sulphur. purif. gr. v. ad x.; sirup simp. ʒj.; aquæ ʒvij.; bene terendo ft. haust. To be taken once or twice a day in a tumblerful of new milk. A slight chalybeate may sometimes be advantageously added. *Part* xviii., *p.* 152.

Treatment of Scrofula as it affects the External Lymphatic Glands.— Mr. Balman says, the best application for almost every kind of scrofulous sore is certainly the iodide of lead ointment; the ung. hyd. nit. oxid. is more stimulating for some very indolent and flabby sores; but the former has generally succeeded with me so well that I now seldom use any other.

The disposition to scab seems very remarkable in all these kind of sores; and however beneficial this process may be in other wounds, it very nearly always tends to impede, rather than otherwise, the healing of scrofulous ulcers, not only by preventing granulation from forming, but, by allowing the ill-conditioned materials to accumulate and fester under it, causes further destruction to the subjacent tissues. I have generally, therefore, directed a poultice to be applied until the sore becomes clean, and then endeavor to prevent their reproduction by some of the stimulating applications already alluded to. I have used a cataplasm composed of bran, linseed, and common yellow soap, with very good effect in these cases.

We have observed, that these glandular swellings are met with under a great variety of circumstances. The patient may, for example, present the fine, delicate, white skin, the tumid lip, and crimson hue of cheek, and the languid, listless, and enfeebled gait so familiar to us in persons possessing the well-marked lymphatic temperament; or all these signs of the strumous constitution may be for the most part wanting, and we have the outward characters of a sound and vigorous constitution; or there may be evidences of a previously acquired syphilitic taint sufficient to justify our pronouncing this to have been the primary *exciting* cause of the disease. A disease, therefore, occurring under so many and varied aspects must of necessity require different modes of treatment. If, for instance, the swellings appeared for the first time after an attack of primary syphilis, the iodide of potassium and sarsaparilla will be found the best remedy, all other remedies, as far as my experience goes, being perfectly useless.

I have made trial of most of the reputed antiscrofulous remedies, and must confess with very different results. The following, however, deserve some notice: mercury, barium, iodine, alkalies, cod-liver oil, etc.

The hyd. bichloride may be given in doses of from 1-16th to 1-20th of a grain dissolved in distilled water, or in the form of pill, with the ext. of sarsa. twice or thrice a day. In cachectic chlorotic, and other cases attended by a languid circulation and much general debility, barium may be used as follows: R. Baryta chlorid., gr. x.; tinct. ferri mur., 3ij. to ℥ss.; sir. aurantii, ℥ss.; aq. dest., ℥x. Mix; of this ℥ss. to ℥j. may be given two or three times a day. Cod-liver oil has little or no influence in the great majority of glandular tumors; but in some forms it is a potent remedy, as when associated with caries of the bones or phthisis. Phosphoric acid, as a medicine, is also most valuable. It may be given in the infusion of calumbo, beginning with five grains of the dilute acid of the pharmacopœia, gradually increasing it to twenty or more.

As regards the treatment of scrofulous swellings, I believe that much harm is sometimes done by the indiscriminate use of frictions with the iodine ointment and other compounds, by inducing a low form of inflammatory action in the skin and integuments, and the chance of bringing on suppuration which it is desirable in many cases, for reasons before stated, to prevent. On this account, and also from the fact that the action of all such applications is very feeble in dispersing the tumor under any circumstances, I seldom now have recourse to them.

In the absence of all signs of inflammatory action after a trial of some of the foregoing internal medicines, I prefer, as a counter-irritant, penciling the part with the solid nitrate of silver a few times, at intervals of a week or ten days. This, I think, is a milder and safer proceeding than the use of blisters, the action of which is more diffusive and irritating.

It is hardly necessary to insist upon the utmost attention being paid to a variety of circumstances regarding the general management of scrofula; such as good and wholesome food, good air, sea-bathing, exercise, and various other hygienic means, which are known to exercise the happiest effects in every form and variety of this disease. *Part* xxiv., *p.* 40.

Use of Proteine in Scrofula.—In the case of a boy, proteine, given in three-grain doses, three times a day, the dose being afterward increased to five grains, produced the most remarkable effects—iron and other tonics having been previously given without any improvement.

In another patient, aged two years, an emaciated, strumous child, with tumid abdomen and enlarged cervical glands, and numerous ill-conditioned ulcers on the loins, nates, thighs, legs, and arms, with symptoms of mesenteric disease. Dr. Taylor ordered zinc ointment, and occasionally a poultice of equal parts of linseed-meal and wheaten flour, to be applied to the ulcerated parts; and to take, proteine, two grains, soda exsiccata, one grain, three times a day, in sugar and water.

First week.—The skin has become cleaner and more healthy, and some of the ulcers have healed; several that are now open display in a very remarkable manner the appearance of softened tubercles; the child looks more lively; bowels regular; appetite better; takes beef-tea twice a day, and milk night and morning. To have mutton for dinner.

Second week.—Greatly improved in every respect; has begun to run about again, which she has been incapable of doing for the last six weeks; nearly all the ulcers have healed; abdomen smaller; has gained flesh; appetite excellent; bowels regular; sleeps well. Ordered the proteine to be continued in doses of three grains, soda exsiccata, one grain. A month afterward, the little patient was running about in excellent health and spirits. *Part* xxviii., *p.* 38.

Scrofula—Anæmia—Boils.—Dr. Christophers considers the liquor cinchonæ hydriodatus cum ferro a very valuable preparation of iodine. It may be given in doses varying from fifteen minims to two drachms. It does not produce the evil effects which arise from small doses of the other preparations of iodine. Another new preparation, the liquor cinchonæ hydriodatus, in doses varying from one to three drachms, is equally valuable in secondary syphilis when the usual treatment has failed.
Part xxxiv., *p.* 217.

———•♦•———

SEA-SICKNESS.

Sea-Sickness.—As preventives, Dr. D. F. W. Fisher recommends active exercise and a tonic regimen for some days before embarkation; and when on board, keep on deck in the breeze, make large inspirations, wear a girdle, walk quickly till perspiration or fatigue is caused, or engage in some hard work, such as helping the sailors, hard work being the surest prophylactic; and take warm and exciting drinks, as tea or coffee with a little brandy, or diaphoretic medicines, opium, saffron, or. acetate of ammonia. When the sickness has come on, nothing will do except palliatives: lie down with the head low, in a hammock or a suspended bed, and take stimulant aromatics, lemons, etc. *Part* xvii., *p.* 293.

Sea-Sickness.—We may often succeed in preventing an attack of this by creasote, and the best and most convenient form is to have it made up in lozenges, about one drop in each, one or two of which can be taken when necessary. *Part* xxxiii., *p.* 321.

Sea-Sickness.—Give from ten to twelve drops of chloroform in water, and if necessary repeat it. It is said by Dr. Landerer, of Athens, to be a "sovereign remedy." The patient soon becomes able to stand up, and gets accustomed to the movements of the vessel. *Part* xxxv., *p.* 306.

———•••———

SENSATION.

Reflex Sensations.—Dr. R. B. Todd says : The irritation of a calculus in the bladder will give rise to pain at the end of the penis, or to pains in the thighs. Irritation of the ovary will cause pain under the right or left mamma ; stimulation of the nipple, whether in male or female, gives rise to peculiar sensations referred to the genital organs ; ice suddenly introduced into the stomach will cause intense pain in either supra-orbital nerve ; acid in the stomach is apt to cause a similar pain, which may be very quickly relieved by the neutralization of the acid. Phenomena of this kind imply some closeness of connection between the nerves of the sympathazing parts in the centre, probably by means of commissural fibres connecting the respective points of implantation of the nerves with each other. *Part* xx., *p.* 51.

Sensation—Loss of, from Hysteria.—Dr. Rowland cites a case of this kind in a young woman, aged 25, which various remedies failed to relieve, who was gradually cured by the patient persevering in taking the following, in the form of a draught, three times a day. Tinct. ferri sesq., mxv. ; tinct. cantharid., miv. ; and tincture of aloes, mxx. *Part* xxix., *p.* 68.

———•••———

SILVER.

Nitrate of Silver— Use of, in Stricture of the Urethra—In Fissured or Excoriated Nipples— Skin Diseases—Affections of the Mucous Membrane of the Throat, etc.—One of the most useful remedies in medicine is the nitrate of silver; whether we regard its use externally or internally, we must look upon all improvements in its mode of application as very desirable ; the form of *nitrate* as an external application has not been improved, neither is it necessary, as its qualities in the present form are such as we require. As an *external application*, however, nitrate of silver has been greatly extended of late, and especially since some able publications on its use in different diseases. In *stricture of the urethra* it has long been used, acting, not as is commonly supposed, by destroying the stricture, but "by inducing some change in the vital actions of the part, which is followed by relaxation of the narrowed portion." In *fissured or excoriated nipples*, it is occasionally very useful, and certainly superior in many cases to the tincture of catechu, which has lately been so praised in these affections. In *porrigo*, the solid nitrate of silver, by being well rubbed on the part, .

will seldom fail in either curing the affection or considerably improving it —the cauterization should be repeated at intervals of a few days. In *psoriasis* and *impetigo*, it has also been found useful; but more especially in erysipelas, both when rubbed on the sound skin round the inflamed portion so as to separate the latter from the former, and also when rubbed all over the inflamed surface. In *affections of the mucous membrane* of the mouth and fauces, it is occasionally an invaluable application. "When the fibrinous exudation of croup commences on the surface of the tonsils and arches of the palate, its further progress may be stopped by the application of a solution composed of a scruple of nitrate of silver and an ounce of distilled water. The solid nitrate has been introduced through an aperture in the trachea and applied to ulcers on the inner surface of the larynx, in a case of phthisis laryngea with apparent benefit. (See Dr. Pereira's work on Materia Medica, p. 696.) A case of diphtherite illustrating its good effect on the mucous membrane of the throat is related in the "American Journal" of Medical Sciences, in which Dr. Gibbes applied a *saturated solution* with benefit, to an ulcer half an inch in diameter, over the left tonsil and to the fauces, by means of a small sponge, which was thrust far back into the pharynx. Every application was attended with relief, and it was repeated every two or three hours when the albuminous accumulation was present. *Part* vi., *p.* 178.

Chloride of Silver—Therapeutic Properties of.—The chloride of silver, which was formerly recommended by Poterius, as an anthelmintic and hydragogue; by Hoffmann, as an evacuant of phlegm in dropsy and melancholy; by Tachenius, as an excellent remedy combined with the sulphuret of antimony, for mania, melancholy, and epilepsy; and lastly, in modern times, by Professor Serres, for syphilis—has been employed in various cases by Dr. Perry.

He declares that he has found it preferable to the nitrate of the same metal, inasmuch as its effects are more certain, its application easier, is less disposed to decompose, and free from any disagreeable taste. The chloride of silver acts best in the form of pills; nevertheless, for young children, it can be prescribed in the form of powders, or suspended in some appropriate sirup. The use of this salt inwardly is not attended with the risk of the green or brown discoloration of the skin, as with nitrate of silver. Dr. Perry has prescribed the chloride for epilepsy; he has also given it in chronic dysentery; under its influence the number of stools and other symptoms have diminished; he has used it also in suppressed menstruation; and lastly, in the secondary form of syphilis.

Part ix., *p.* 84.

Oxide of Silver.—There are certain diseases of the mucous surfaces of the alimentary canal, bladder, uterus, vagina, etc., which often baffle our best attempts at relief, for example, pyrosis, menorrhagia, and leucorrhœa; and there are endless affections which probably depend upon some irritation in the nervous centre, either immediate or distant, which equally baffle our efforts at relief. Sir James Eyre has published a little work, in which he extols very highly the oxide of silver as a powerful tonic, sedative, and astringent, and states that in these tiresome cases it will be found very valuable. *Part* xi., *p.* 107.

Stains from Nitrate of Silver, to remove.—Moisten the spots several times with a solution of hydriodate of potash, and expose the part to the direct rays of the sun. The hydriodate converts the black stain of the nitrate into the white ioduret of silver. A trial of its use internally is also recommended in those cases where the skin has been tinted by the internal use of the nitrate.   *Part* xiv., *p.* 254.

Oxide of Silver.—Dr. Lane says that the conjunction of oxide of silver with confection of roses is injudicious, as a salt of silver is liable to be formed, though certainly the tendency of metallic oxides to be acted on by the vegetable acids (gallic, malic, or citric) varies much. The combination of essential oils with the oxide of silver is exceedingly objectionable, for the chemical union of the oxygen with the silver is not very powerful; neither is that of the hydrogen and carbon in the essential oils; the substance in question, therefore, being intimately commixed, silent or explosive composition will inevitably ensue, the oxygen and hydrogen, forming water, while the silver remains in a metallic state, or is converted into a carburet. An analogous, though more complicated action, I think, takes place where the vegetable acids are concerned. I should not recommend any druggist to dispense a prescription wherein the oxide of silver and an essential oil are conjoined, without communicating with the prescriber, if possible.

The combinations of the oxide of silver which I chiefly employ, and should recommend, are as follows: 1. With extract of gentian or chamomile. 2. With extract of hyoscyamus or conium, to which I often add a small proportion of ipecac. 3. With inspissated ox-gall. 4. With the aqueous extract of opium. 5. With compound cinnamon powder. The pills never should be rolled or kept in carbonate of magnesia.   *Part* xvi., *p.* 296.

Nitrate of Silver Stains.—Messrs. Smith have advised a process, already suggested by others, which is remarkable for its simplicity. The stained portion of linen is well saturated with a strong solution of chloride of lime. This converts the silver to a white chloride, which is then removed by ammonia, or by a solution of hyposulphate of soda. If the stain be deep in the fibre and of old standing, this process must be repeated several times before it is effectually removed.

A solution of the cyanide of potassium is also useful in the removal of these stains. The plan of converting them to iodide of silver by tincture of iodine, and washing out the iodide by hyposulphate of soda, is not always successful.   *Part* xvi., *p.* 299.

To Remedy the Fragility of Nitrate of Silver Crayons.—The brittleness of nitrate of silver is the source not only of considerable loss of the material itself, but frequently of danger to the patient, as when the fauces, œsophagus, urethra, bladder, and cavity of the uterus are being cauterized. M. Chassaignac has succeeded in remedying this evil, by having in the centre of the stick of caustic a thread of platinum wire. M. Blatin secures the same object by a wick of cotton, which is placed in the mold before the fluid nitrate is poured into it. The crayon thus prepared is rendered more solid, and, when broken, the fragments remain attached to one another.   *Part* xix., *p.* 324.

To remove Nitrate of Silver Stains.—Mr. Collins, in a number of the "Dublin Med. Press," recommends to brush over the stains on the linen, skin, nails, or teeth, with a solution of cyanide of potassium, eight or ten grains to Ʒj. of distilled water. If the stains are superficial, one or two applications will suffice; if deep, several will be required.

Part xx., *p.* 148.

Nitrate of Silver Stains.—Accident first led M. Martinenq to the observation, which he has since repeatedly confirmed, that the stains produced by nitrate of silver on linen, etc., may be readily removed by wetting the linen in a solution of *bichloride of mercury* (1 part to 31), rubbing it well, and then washing it well in cold water.

Part xx., *p.* 294.

Nitrate of Silver.—Mr. Ward recommends instead of dissolving this salt in water, to dissolve it in common nitric ether. The ether acts as a solvent of greasy matter on the skin, and from its volatility, quickly dries, enabling us to apply several coatings of the solution in a short time. The strength may vary, but about eight grains to the ounce will generally be sufficient. In erysipelas, this will be found an improvement.

Part xxxi., *p.* 236.

SINUSES.

Treatment of Chronic Sinuses by strong Nitric Acid.—Mr. Skey says, whenever inflammation, or even redness, has attended them, the application has generally failed; but the large majority of these canals are not inflammatory, but chronic.

The mode of applying the escharotic is by means of a fine glass tube of length sufficient to reach the full extent of the sinus. At one end of the tube is a small glass bulb. The air is sufficiently exhausted by the hand, when warm, to draw up sufficient acid to fill the tube, and partly so the bulb. The instrument, thus armed, is passed into the sinus, and the acid discharged, either by the hand, or by the aid of a lucifer match, while the tube is slowly withdrawn, pouring out its contents along the entire track.

Part xxxiii., *p.* 239.

SKIN.

Functions of the Skin.—1st. The skin is an external lung, an aerating mechanism spread out over the body's entire surface. Both lungs and skin abstract oxygen from the atmosphere, which they replace by carbonic acid and watery vapor. A healthy cuticle, then, must be freely permeable by elastic fluids (gases and vapors). 2d. The cuticle is very profusely perforated by minute valvular orifices, openings of the sweat-ducts; the skin is the grand drainage pipe of the body; and when, on indubitable authority, we learn that, computing 2,506 square inches as the body's superficial contents, its linear amount of drainage pipe is about twenty-eight miles—an hour's railway ride forsooth! (Wilson)—we shall arrive at something like an appreciation of the importance of keeping this pipe-age pervious.

Now, from the two just named properties, the skin is manifestly complementary or vicarious in its functions to those two vital organs, the lungs and kidneys; therefore an obstructed skin throws the whole onus of elaboration upon these latter organs, which consequently become overworked and diseased. 3d. This is not all. The skin is a decarbonizing organ; opening into the cuticle, in common with the hair follicles, are the orifices of the "fat glands," which secern an oily matter (for the skin's lubrication) from the blood; if allowed to collect, this fatty matter checks the "transpirability" of the skin, by glazing it over with a sort of natural varnish, thus throwing the whole work of decarbonization upon the liver; its fat cells become gorged, and thus arises that most grave malady "fatty liver," good enough in a pasty, that is, if there be any virtue in pâté de fois gras, but no trivial calamity to any unfortunate human possessor. Carbon is retained, moreover, in the blood, depriving the sentient lining of the arteries and left heart of their proper stimulus; and carbon thus, with saline and other impure matters circulating through the brain, deranges that organ of organs. The connection, then, between a clear head and a clear skin is closer than the unlearned might suppose. 4th. Many years back, Drs. Blackall and Osborne discovered that dirtiness was a great source of dropsy. To understand this, it must be recollected, that in an impure obstructed skin are checked two of the skin's main functions—evaporation and exhalation. (Dr. J. Coventry.)   *Part* xiv., *p.* 258.

Pathology of Skin Diseases.—According to Dr. Burgess, eruptions of constitutional origin, by long standing may sometimes assume a local character. Erysipelas and acne frequently supervene in cases of derangement of the uterine function. Strophulus is associated with the process of dentition. Urticaria, lichen urticatus, and several varieties of herpes, are often the results of a disordered condition of the digestive organs. Psoriasis and lichen agrius frequently occur during the process of gout and urinary diseases; and the hereditary nature of certain eruptions, as lepra, psoriasis, lichen, etc., is beyond all doubt. Unless we bear in mind, in our treatment of these eruptions, their intimate relation with the organic function, we are constantly liable to serious error. If, for example, we were to look upon these critical eruptions or discharges which occur at certain period of life as *local* diseases, and attempt to suppress them by topical applications, it is unnecessary to add that serious consequences would result; whereas, if they are not interfered with, they will get well as soon as the equilibrium of the system is restored. The impetiginous eczema of infants, and those eruptions which occur at the periods of puberty and the turn of life, are examples of this kind.   *Part* xix., *p.* 197.

SKIN DISEASE.

ACNE.

[Medical writers, of all ages, have found some difficulty in curing this peculiar form of eruption. Mr. Startin has been more successful; he first ascertains the exciting cause, and then applies those local and general means which increase the cutaneous circulation, viz., hot air bath, with or without sulphur; chalybeates combined with mineral acids, vegetable bitters, or iodine. He considers arsenic and mercury unnecessary, unless the state of the liver or other viscera indicate their use; he recommends a mild nutritive dietary, with such alcoholic stimulants as the stomach may require for producing healthful digestion; he considers vegetable acids, antiscorbutics, so called, and the common diet drink, worse than useless, nearly excepting even sarsaparilla.]

The external local treatment of acne is not the least important, and must be regulated entirely by the stage and condition of the disease. In its commencement, when a loaded state of the sebaceous follicles is the most prominent symptom, moderate frictions with the flesh-brush so as to keep open the pores, and the extraction, by pressure, of the larger collection of sebaceous matter (the outlet of the follicle being dilated with some pointed but not too sharp instrument), will be required; whilst a weak spirit lotion and the use of oatmeal, instead of soap, may be enjoined; as the disease advances, and the suppurating points are numerous, large and painful, the vapor douche on the face, mercurial ointment with camphor, white precipitate with camphor, or the Topique contre acne of the Hôpital St. Louis may be recommended : the latter is composed of slaked lime, ʒj.; zinc ointment, ʒj.; and camphor, Ɖj. From fifteen to thirty grains of the ioduret of sulphur to an ounce of lard, is also a useful application, as is a weak solution of bichloride of mercury in milk of bitter almonds, or thin quince-seed mucilage. The following lotion, not to be found in books, you will find occasionally very efficient: hyposulphite of soda, ʒj. to ʒij.; sulphate of alumnia, ʒj. to ʒij.; rose water, ʒviiss.; cologne water, ʒss. for a lotion, to be used by washing the part with a linen rag twice or thrice daily. Of course these proportions are not applicable in every case, but the composition is very useful in removing the unpleasant yellow stains of the cuticle as the acne declines, and it is perhaps more applicable to acne rosacea and pustulosa, than to the other varieties of the disease, as it always relieves the attendant itching.

It sometimes happens that we may have succeeded in the removal of acne, particularly acne rosacea, but that a degree of redness remains on the end of the nose, or on one or two spots on the cheeks, which, on examination, is not found to be inflammation, but a dilated state of the minute cuticular vessels; there are two ways of getting rid of this disfigurement, both of which I have constantly found successful; when the vessels are very small and numerous, not appearing to be nourished by conspicuously large trunks, the best plan is to paint them over very lightly with nitric acid, of the pharmacopœia strength, which is to be immediately blotted off with bibulous paper; by this means a blister is raised, and the cuticle detached after a few days, when it will be found that the morbid state of the capillaries has disappeared, or that they have so much contracted, that a second application at the end of a fortnight is all that is required.

The acetum cantharidis may also be used in a similar manner, though it is not so effectual. The second method has the same object in view, though the mode of its accomplishment is rather different, and it is only applicable when the red portions of the integument appear to be maintained by the influx of several larger capillary trunks—a morbid condition, which at the end of the nose, is exceedingly common. The plan I adopt in such instances is to divide each trunk in succession with the point of a fine lancet, and as the blood flows very freely, I restrain it by means of a small ring of steel or silver, which is mounted on a stem an inch or two in length, and fixed into a handle at right angles; by this means, I can, as it were, insulate the little wounded point, and arrest the hemorrhage, whilst the blood can be sponged away and the incision exposed, so that a piece of lunar caustic, the size of a grain of sand, can be introduced into it, by means of a probe with a flattened extremity, on which it has been previously made to adhere; this at once stops the bleeding, and obliterates the vessel, whilst it produces no disfigurement, beyond a temporary black spot that may be covered with court-plaster, or the blackness may be removed by wetting it with a solution of iodide of potassium; I can assure you I have cured numerous red noses by this simple procedure—which I may mention is applicable to the removal of small nævi and the congenital red marks called araneæ (from their resemblance to a red spider, with its legs outstretched).

The small mounted ring alluded to, you will find a most useful agent in arresting bleeding from leech-bites, until a grain of caustic can be accurately applied as already mentioned. I have also used it with advantage in removing cutaneous tumors of various kinds, for surrounding a troublesome bleeding artery till it could be secured; the size of the ring may be varied, but I prefer it not larger than a quarter of an inch in diameter, for general purposes; but I can imagine such a contrivance useful under a variety of circumstances requiring surgical interference, which it would be quite out of order to discuss at this moment—amongst such are deep wounds of arteries, whether the result of accident, injury, or surgical operation.

Part xiv., *p.* 240.

This disease, says Dr. Burgess, arises from so many causes, the treatment can only be successfully conducted by taking these into account. Exclusively local, or exclusively general treatment, are equally erroneous.

Part xx., *p.* 170.

Acne of the Face.—Apply a saturated solution of gutta percha in chloroform over the spots, enjoining the patient not to rub off the pellicle by washing. (Dr. R. J. Graves.)   *Part* xxvi., *p.* 287.

Acne and Boils.—These, depending on similar states of the constitution, may be treated alike. Great success has been obtained at the Hospital for Disease of the Skin, by the combination of ferruginous salts with saline aperients. In *acne simplex* and *punctata*, Mr. Startin prescribes ferri sulphat., gr. ij.; magnes. sulphat., ʒj.; ter die sumend.: an ointment of ammonio-chloride of mercury gr. x. ad ʒj.; to be applied every night. For *acne indurata*, the iodide of iron in doses of gr. iij., three times daily. For the *furunculous epidemic*, so ripe of late years, full doses of iron with saline purgatives—mist. ferri acid., ʒiij. ter die.   *Part* xxvii., *p.* 161.

Acne Rosacea.—Smear the following over the face with the finger every night; camphor, a drachm; milk of sulphur, twice as much, or the sulphur sublimatum. Afterward as much water as will render it sufficiently liquid. The camphor must be powdered by the usual addition of a little spirits of wine. (Dr. E. Wilson.)   *Part* xxxi., *p.* 195.

Use of the Acid Nitrate of Mercury in Acne.—A very minute drop of the acid is placed, by means of a finely-pointed glass brush, on the apex of any indolent tubercles, whether suppurated or otherwise. It has the effect of opening the pustule, if matter have formed, and if not, induces the disappearance of the induration. The application is followed only by a little smarting pain, and if it have been carefully made, leaves no scar. (Dr. J. Startin.)   *Part* xxxi., *p.* 240.

Treatment of Acne.—After arsenic has been given for a long time without improvement, try cod-liver oil in teaspoonful doses three times a day; it will often have a marked beneficial effect both upon the health and the disease. Lupus is equally benefited by the same treatment, but there is no cutaneous affection in which cod-liver oil has proved more effectual than in sycosis menti, or mentagra. (Dr. T. Hunt.) *Part* xxxii., *p.* 184.

Acne.—Cazenave has recently recommended ammoniacal lotions, which form with the fatty matter of the follicles a soluble soap with an ammoniacal base; the hydrochlorate or acetate of ammonia answers equally well.

Part xxxii., *p.* 187.

Treatment of the Different Forms of Acne.—In acne rosacea, and acne simplex, the acid solution of iron in half ounce doses is usually ordered, while for the tubercular form Mr. Startin places more confidence in the iodide of iron. The latter is generally given in from one to two grain doses. Malt liquors are strictly prohibited in all cases. In almost all the local use of the red lotion is directed, and any larger pustules or tubercles, which may be observed from time to time, are touched on their apices with the acid nitrate of mercury solution. In addition to these remedies the direction is mostly given to be particular in squeezing out the contents of the distended follicles as soon as they become perceptible.

The "acid solution of iron" is made by dissolving three ounces of Epsom salts, and two drachms of sulphate of iron, in half an ounce of dilute sulphuric acid, and a pint of infusion of quassia. The "red lotion" consists of two scruples of the bichloride of mercury, one of the bisulphuret, and ten minims of creasote, in a pint of water; each ounce containing two grains of the bichloride. *Part* xxxviii., *p.* 174.

ECZEMA.

Some Local Forms of Chronic Eczema.—Chronic eczema assumes different forms as it attacks different parts of the body, as the scalp, face, ears, tongue, anus, etc. Chronic eczema of the face usually is of an impetiginous character; it is generally met with in children, rarely in adults, and when it does occur in the latter, it is in consequence of extension from the scalp.

Chronic Eczema of the Face.—Mr. Erichsen mentions the case of a lady's maid, who caught cold whilst travelling outside of the carriage; her face became stiff and inflamed, and pimples with watery heads came out on the forehead and cheeks. The disease continued for three months, without interruption, in spite of treatment, when she was admitted under Mr. Erichsen's care, into the Westminster Hospital.

Mr. Erichsen commenced by ordering three drops of the liquor arsenicalis three times a day, and directed that the affected parts should be preserved day and night from the action of the atmosphere, by covering them up with lint spread well with zinc ointment.

Feb. 13.—Much better. The skin is softer, not so glazed, and the feeling of tension is less. The liquor arsenicalis was now increased to four minims for a dose, and ungent. hydrarg. precipitat. albi was substituted for the zinc ointment, it being thought that a light stimulant might be of service. Febrile symptoms arising, the arsenic was omitted for six days, when it was again resumed, and on the 25th of March, the disease was perfectly cured.

When the disease depends on irritation of the skin and mucous surfaces, it can be soonest relieved by carefully regulating the diet, avoiding all stimuli, and using one of the most efficient remedies that we possess in affections of this class—the Harrowgate waters. Where the temperament of the patient is irritable, arsenic, cantharides, etc., would decidedly aggravate the disease. Chronic eczema of the ears, which usually proceeds by extension from the scalp, is a very painful as well as obstinate affection. Mr. Erichsen observes that :

The ears, when attacked by the eczema, become exceedingly red, tense, hot, and shining ; a number of small vesicles then appear, which contain a clear transparent serum, of a reddish or pale yellow color ; when these give way, the fluid that is effused forms thin scabs or scales, which are usually cracked in all directions, and which are frequently curled up or project from the surface of the skin. If the disease continue, the pinna attains a very large size, becoming hypertrophied, and often fissured ; sometimes, indeed, the swelling goes on to such an extent as to block up the external meatus, giving rise to temporary deafness.

When it occurs in young children, it can easily be cured : it is generally in females from fifteen to twenty-five, or in women about the change of life, where it proves so obstinate. It is generally associated with irregular menstruation, or may be noticed from the fact, that it is aggravated at those periods when the uterus ought to act. Mr. E. describes a case which came under his care, a female, twenty-one years of age ; menstruation was irregular.

Both ears were found, on examination, to be affected nearly to an equal degree. They were red, glazed, much swollen, and chapped, covered with thin, flimsy, scaly incrustations, from under which a serous fluid occasionally oozes, and are very hot and tense. The integuments of the mastoid, temporal and parotidean regions are likewise involved, being inflamed and covered with thin furfuraceous laminæ.

She was ordered to apply bread-and-water poultices to the ears every night, to cover them up in rags spread with zinc ointment during the day ; to take ten grains of the pil. aloes c. myrrha every second night at bedtime, to abstain from all stimulants, and to adhere as strictly as possible to a milk diet. The ordinary means, such as mustard-and-water to the feet, etc., were likewise directed to be adopted for reëstablishing the menstrual function, and were attended with success in the course of a week. At the end of a fortnight she was much better, the ears were less tense, and not so red or swollen. She was now ordered to apply an ointment composed of equal parts of a ceratum plumbi comp. and zinc ointment, and to take five minims of tincture of cantharides, and thirty of liquor potassæ twice a day. This plan of treatment was continued until the end of April, when she was perfectly cured, the ears presenting their normal appearance, and having lost entirely their hypertrophied condition.

Eczema of the Scrotum, Penis, and Anus.—Eczema of the scrotum and of the inside of the thighs of young children is of a more active character, and is by no means so troublesome as that which occurs in more advanced life. In many cases it appears to be owing to the urine being allowed to dribble over the thin and delicate skin of these parts.

The appearance presented by chronic eczema of these parts in children is very remarkable. The scrotum and integuments covering the pubes, the inside of the thighs and penis, are of a vivid red color, inflamed and oozing; occasionally covered with soft, moist, greyish, or yellowish scabs, from under and between which a serous fluid exudes in tolerable abundance. At other times they are dry, glazed, and chapped in all directions, being merely covered here and there with thin flimsy scales. These two conditions, the moist and the dry, alternate with one another, being evideuces of the greater or less activity of the disease.

Some local forms of Chronic Eczema.—When occurring in individuals past the middle period of life, eczema attacking the scrotum usually presents the ordinary characters of that disease in its chronic furfuraceous or squamous condition. The scrotum is much wrinkled, red, dry, rough, and glazed, or covered with thin, peeling, curled, laminated, and dry furfuraceous incrustations of a whitish or greyish color, which rub off in considerable abundance, exposing cracks and fissures, from which a thin, ichorous, or bloody discharge, oozes. The itching, which is intolerable, and is more complained of than anything else, is much aggravated by any excess in diet, or when the patient is warm in bed. Every now and then, under the influence of some exciting cause, the disease assumes a more active condition, revealing its vesicular elementary character, and thus enabling it to be readily distinguished from prurigo of the region affected. Eczema involving the anus is always a most troublesome affection. It may be either an extension of the disease from the scrotum and perineum, or it may be confined exclusively to the anus and lower part of the rectum. It is occasionally seen in young children accompanied by intertrigo, or in consequence of the extension of the disease from the neighboring parts, when occurring in adults. It is characterized by occasional vesicular eruption, excoriation, fissures, and chaps, which bleed, and are excessively painful on the passage of the fæces, more particularly if these be hard or lumpy. There is always excessive pruritus; more especially, when the patient is warm in bed, or after standing for any length of time.

Eczema of the anus is more commonly a disease of individuals who have passed the middle period of life, and is not uncommonly connected with piles.

Treatment.—Cover the parts with lint, wet with lead lotion, and inclose them with oil-silk, in order to keep off the air, and to prevent urine getting upon the part. Give a small dose of hydr. c. creta at night, and a dose of castor oil in the morning: in a few days substitute zinc ointment for the lotion, and give small doses of liq. potassæ, and five grains each of calomel and magnesia, twice a day. If it be of long standing, enjoin a strict diet, abstinence from fermented liquors, salted and heating articles of food, and give 20 minims of liq. arsenici et hydrarg. iodidi twice a day, with 5 grains of Plummer's pill at bed-time, and apply a mixture of zinc ointment and the ung. plumbi acetat. to the parts by means of a piece of lint cut to the proper shape. The treatment must be persisted in for a length of time. A little extract of belladonna rubbed down with the ointment, often succeeds in allaying the irritation.

Eczema of the Scalp.—[Eczema of the scalp, however, appears to be the most commonly met with; for of all cutaneous diseases seated in this locality, as many as forty-three per cent. are cases of eczema. It is exceedingly difficult to remove: it occurs mostly in children, very rarely in adults. Mr. E. observes that,]

Chronic eczema of the scalp, although presenting considerable variety in its characters, seems to resolve itself naturally into the three following species.

1. Simple chronic eczema, which may assume either a moist or a dry form. 2. Eczema furfuracea, corresponding to the porrigo furfurosa of Willan. 3. Eczema amiantacea, which is an extreme condition of the last variety.

Simple chronic eczema of the scalp may, as has just been stated, assume either a moist or a dry form. In the moist variety of the disease there is always a very copious discharge of a thin serous fluid from a number of small openings, the remains of former vesicles, that lie closely scattered on the inflamed and tender surface of the scalp ; this discharge, which is of an acrid and irritating nature, is apt to increase the inflammation in that part of the skin over which it flows. If it be very abundant the hair looks as if it had been soaked in a thin solution of gum arabic, being matted together in locks, which have a dirty yellowish grey moist appearance, and between and under which the inflamed scalp may be seen pouring forth the discharge. As this lessens in quantity, soft yellowish-grey scabs will be formed, which gradually losing their moist appearance will be found to resemble those that characterize the dry variety of the disease. In the midst of this, acute attacks of eczema, attended by a great evolution of vesicles, by increased heat and redness of the scalp, frequently occur, adding very greatly to the severity and obstinacy of the disease ; and the distress of the patient is very often greatly increased by a chronic inflammation of the eyes and ears, which is a common complication of this form of eczema. As the discharge lessens, and the inflammatory action subsides, the moist passes, in many cases, into the dry variety of chronic eczema.

Treatment.—If occurring to a child, otherwise healthy, about the period of dentition, be careful how you check the eruption. Cut the hair, apply bread-and-water poultices, and subdue irritation by the application of rags dipped in olive oil, or smeared with zinc ointment ; or sprinkle the part with the nurse's milk. Give small doses of hydrarg. c. creta and castor oil, and lance the gums, if necessary. Fluid magnesia is often useful. If it becomes inveterate, wean the child on beef-tea, broth, and a nutritious diet, and give mild tonics, a few drops of tincture of ammon-chloride of iron, or iodide of iron, twice a day (from half a grain to two grains of the latter) ; a great part of the treatment consists in keeping the scalp so covered as to prevent the access of air.

When it becomes chronic and inactive, and presents a furfuraceous appearance, have recourse to gentle stimulants ; a lotion composed of from one to two drachms of sulphuret of potass, either alone or combined with an equal quantity of the carbonate of the same alkali, in a pint of plain, or of lime water ; wash the head with this lotion three times a day ; at the same time, every night after the last application of the lotion, apply an ointment composed of from a scruple to half a drachm of carbonate of potass to an ounce of lard, or of creasote in the same proportion, or of white precipitate ; or use the ung. hydr. nit. dil., or the sulphur ointment, or a mixture of this and tar or of creasote ointment. Do not use the oiled-silk cap ; it confines the perspiration and soddens the skin, producing a state of passive congestion which we wish to get rid of.

Chronic Eczema of the Hands.—[This generally arises from the direct application of irritating substances to the parts, as lime in bricklayers, sugar in grocers, potass or soda in washerwomen, mordants in dyers, or minute particles of steel in smiths, weelwrights, etc.]

The characters that this disease presents when attacking the hands are those assumed by chronic eczema in its worst and most inveterate forms. There is, in the first instance, an eruption of vesicles, which are most generally small and pointed, projecting but slightly above the level of the skin, and which are at first confined to a small spot, usually on one of the knuckles, or on the back of one of the fingers, whence the disease gradually creeps on until the greater portion of the back of the hand may be involved. In some rare cases, however, these vesicles are large and prominent.

[The diagnosis is of importance, particularly if there has been no local irritant, as it leads to suspicion, more especially in the better classes of society ; it may be confounded with scabies and psoriasis.]

From scabies the diagnosis is not always easy, though in the majority of cases it is not attended with any difficulty. In eczema the vesicles are usually small, agglomerated, and collected in clusters on the back of one or two knuckles, or in patches about the dorsal aspect of the hand; and occasionally we see a raw, excoriated, oozing surface, which is never met with in scabies. In scabies, on the contrary, the vesicles are generally large, more distinct, not clustered; and situated chiefly between the fingers at their roots, and not on the knuckles or back of the hand. In scabies also there is a peculiar pruritus, giving rise to an irresistible propensity in the patient to scratch himself. In eczema this is not the case, and the morbid sensation is of a smarting or burning character.

The vesicular character of the disease is a sufficient guide in diagnosis, and when it becomes chronic, and assumes a furfuraceous appearance, it is of little practical importance, as the treatment is directed by the condition of the part, and the causes of the disease. The treatment is the same as when occurring in other parts, only the hand must be kept perfectly at rest.

Treatment.—In the early stages apply water-dressing by means of oiled-silk gloves or finger stalls, and at a more advanced period, a solution of nitrate of silver (grain j. to the ounce), instead of the water-dressing ; or a solution of carbonate of soda (grain ij. to iv. to the ounce) ; or the following lotion : acid. hydrocyan., 3ss. ; zinci oxidi, 3j. ; aquæ rosæ, 3viij. ; or cover the hand with the ung. hydrarg. precip. alb., either alone or mixed with citrine ointment.

If the disease only occupy a small patch, cover it with a slice of lemon. Its spreading may be checked by applying the solid nitrate of silver around the part. Constitutional treatment must also be adopted : remove any gastric, intestinal, or uterine disturbance, and give vegetable bitters, nitric acid diluted, or small doses of bichloride of mercury ; the two latter may be given in infusion of bark. If the disease be of very long standing, give Fowler's or Donovan's solution. The hands should be kept at rest.

Part xiii., *p.* 297.

Chemical Reaction of Discharges in Eruptive Diseases.—In eczema and all eruptive diseases attended with more or less exudation, ascertain the reaction of the discharge upon test paper. If it is alkaline, apply nitric acid lotion (3ss. ad aquæ Oj.) and give small doses of the same acid, in the compound infusion of orange, internally. If the discharge has an acid reaction, adopt the reverse of the above treatment. (Dr. J. Corfe.)

Part xviii., *p.* 222.

Eczema.—Apply a lotion containing bichloride of mercury, three grains to the pint, five or six times a day.   Or, apply water as warm as it can be borne.   (M. Trousseau.)   *Part* xviii., *p.* 223.

Eczema.—In *acute* cases, says Dr. J. H. Bennett, the constitutional treatment is most important, and must depend upon the kind of constitutional affection; the disease being usually associated with either the oxalic, lithic, or phosphatic diathesis, or with a scrofulous taint.   The local treatment here is of very subordinate importance.   But in *chronic* cases, the local treatment is by far the most important, and should consist in the application of a solution of ʒij. of the subcarbonate of soda in a pint and a half of water; lint saturated with this solution being applied over the affected parts, and the whole covered with oil-silk.

*   *   *   *   *   *   *

Dr. Burgess would direct the treatment chiefly to the constitution, giving mild tonics and alteratives.   Keep the parts cleanly, and when it is thought the discharge may be safely arrested, apply mild lotions containing carbonate or bicarbonate of potash, and let the bath be frequently used.   If these remedies are not sufficient, give active purgatives if the patient is strong; or where these are not indicated, give sarsaparilla and hydriodate of potash; and employ lotions of nitrate of silver or bichloride of mercury.   If there is inflammatory tendency in the parts, apply a few leeches behind the ears.   If there is much smarting, with abundant serous exudation, give sulphuric acid internally, beginning with a small quantity, administered in barley water, and a little cold water after each dose.

*   *   *   *   *   *   *   *

Chronic of the Legs.—This disease, according to Dr. Burgess, is very difficult to manage, but is best treated by the application of the vapors of iodine and sulphur, assisted during the interim of the application by bandaging from the foot upward.   The best way to apply the vapor is the following: get a tin case or a common jar, large enough to hold the limb, and place a heated iron at the bottom of the apparatus, and a grating above it, to protect the limb.   Place one of the powders, about to be mentioned, on the heated iron, put the limb instantly into the bath, and cover the mouth over to prevent the vapor from escaping; and continue the bath fifteen or twenty minutes.   The powders consist of, sulphur, ʒiij.; hydr. sulph. rub., ϴij.; iodin. gr. x.; divided into six powders.   In a few days the proportion of iodine may be increased.

*   *   *   *   *   *   *   *

When this affection is connected with a scrofulous constitution, give col-liver oil.   *Part* xx., *p.* 168.

Acetate of Potash.—Recommended by Dr. Easton in half-drachm doses, three times a day, in eczema.   *Part* xxi., *p.* 245.

Local use of Alkalies in Treatment of Eczema.—A remedy which has been found more extensively applicable and more uniformly serviceable than any other, says Prof. Bennett, is a solution of two drachms of the sesquicarbonate of soda in a pint and a half of water; but it is necessary to place lint saturated with the solution over the affected part, and to cover the whole with oil-silk, in order to prevent evaporation.   In these cases there is an increased exudation from the skin, both of sebaceous and purulent matters; and alkalies, we know, have the property of dissolving these, and of acting as a calmative and emollient to the irritated parts. *Part* xxii., *p.* 243.

Empyreumatic Coal Oil used in Eczema.—M. Lafont-Gouzi highly extols the virtues of the oil obtained by the distillation of pit-coal in the manufacture of gas, as a remedy in certain eczematous affections, and in itch. He has used the oil in the treatment of eczema impetiginodes, of itch, of prurigo, of psoriasis, of purulent ophthalmia, of keratitis, and of otorrhœa dependent on cutaneous eruption (*otorrhées de nature dartreuse*). M. Lafont mixes eight parts of empyreumatic oil with thirty parts of axunge, and spreads the ointment over the parts affected with eczema; he asserts that it is the most active of siccatives. In cases of prurigo and of psoriasis, hé replaces the axunge with an oil of henbane containing opium (*huile de jusquiaume opiaciée*). If the disease proves obstinate, he uses the undiluted empyreumatic oil. *Part* xxiv., *p.* 257.

Eczema.—Make an ointment as follows : Oil of juniper, ℥iss.; suet, ℥ss.; lard, ℥iss. It should be applied locally to the part. *Part* xxxii., *p.* 186.

Eczema, etc.—According to Dr. Godfrey, internal remedies are most useful, ointments are injurious. The tincture of the muriate of iron given three times a day he has never known fail. The parts should be daily washed with oatmeal gruel. Occasionally a little powdered starch with oxide of zinc will aid the cure.

* * * * * * * *

Professor Malmsten, of Stockholm, has used cod-liver oil externally very successfully in intractable skin diseases. If the whole skin be affected the patient must lie in bed, all the body and bed linen being saturated with oil; an alkaline bath may be allowed once a week; but no other washing or change of clothes until the skin is restored to health.

Part xxxii., *p.* 186.

Eczema.—The value of cod-liver oil in this obstinate disease is now almost universally conceded; it should be used in conjunction with other remedies. *Part* xxxiii., *p.* 236.

Eczema Infantile.—[The great, the urgent symptom of this disease is the teasing, the intense itching, especially during the night; the child is often frantic with itching, it scratches with all its force, digging its little nails into the flesh, while the blood and ichor run down in streams.]

For elimination, says Erasmus Wilson, you may give one grain of calomel with a little white sugar to the youngest infant; when older, give it in such a dose as will produce an efficient relief to the alimentary canal; this may be repeated once, twice, or three times a week, but generally once is sufficient. *To alleviate the local distress*, apply freely night and morning the benzoated oxide of zinc ointment over the whole of the inflamed skin ; this should be allowed to remain as a permanent coating until the skin is entirely healed; it will prevent the formation of crusts by the exclusion of atmospheric air. It is very important not to disturb the ointment, but at the same time it must not be allowed to accumulate too thickly. Washing is quite unnecessary, indeed it is injurious, and must be avoided. In chronic eczema infantile, that is, pityriasis capitis, the nitric oxide and nitrate of mercury ointment of various strengths are almost specifics. For the *restoration of power* the great remedy is arsenic. As an effective, harmless tonic, it stands alone and without its peer in this vexatious disease; indeed, it is specific, it cures rapidly, perfectly and unfailingly. Two minims of Fowler's solution may be given three times a day to an infant from two months to a year old. It is very useful combined with iron as follows:

R Vini ferri, sirup. tolutan, aa. ʒss.; liq. potassæ arsenitis, m xxxij.; aquæ anethi, ʒj. M. Give one drachm three times a day after meals; if it appears to disagree it should be given less frequently or suspended. Cod-liver oil, in conjunction with arsenic, is a valuable addition.

The following formula will be found convenient:

R Olei jecoris aselli, ʒij.; vitelli ovi, j.; liq. potassæ arsenitis, m lxiv.; sirupi simplicis, ʒij.; aquæ fontan. q.s. ad ʒiv. M. ft. mist. A drachm three times a day. *Part* xxxiv., *p.* 199.

Chronic Eczema in Children.—Dr. Behrend directs, first to get the scabs or crusts separated, by means of poultices, if the spots are limited, and are not settled on the head, face, and neck, where these applications are not suitable. Before applying them, it is a good plan to moisten the surface with a solution of carb. of soda (ʒij. to ʒviii.) When the surface is large, a water dressing is to be preferred; a little sub-carbonate of pot-ash being added to the water. If situated on the head, face, or neck, paint the scabs over with a mixture of carb. of soda and cod-liver oil, re-moving the crusts carefully next morning, and moistening the surface with the alkaline lotion. This must be repeated as often as necessary, till crusts cease to be formed, and a red, inflamed, but painless surface is left. Next, we must remove this condition of the skin. One of the best means to this end, is the application of a solution of ʒj. of acetate of zinc, and the same of acetate of lead, in ʒviij. of distilled water, adding to this, at the time of using it, an equal quantity of strong chamomile infusion. The last indica-tion is to restore the activity and healthy tone of the skin, by such hygienic measures as fresh country air, free exercise, a well regulated and whole-some diet, and such local applications as weak solutions of alum and sul-phate of zinc. *Part* xxxvi., *p.* 187.

Eczema of the Face in Children.—Dr. Behrend recommends the fol-lowing application for the crusts which frequently cover the faces of children: Cod-liver oil, fifteen, and bicarbonate of soda, two parts.
Part xxxvii., *p.* 182.

Eczema—Acute.—Mr. Startin says, that the irritation of acute eczema will frequently subside most rapidly on slight ptyalism being induced. The bichloride of mercury is a good form for administration, and five or ten minims of colchicum may be given with each dose.
Part xxxviii., *p.* 174.

Eczema of the Scalp and Face in Children.—A fair-haired, blue-eyed child, aged two years, was admitted with that so common and so trouble-some form of eczema in which the whole face and scalp are involved, but the rest of the surface free. It had suffered since the age of six months, but excepting the irritation of the eruption its general health was not in-terfered with. Mr. Startin ordered as follows:

Misturæ potasii iodid. ʒj., aq. ʒv. capt. ʒj. ter die.

The surface to be washed with the yolk of egg and water, and smeared with the nitric oxide of mercury ointment. Rapid improvement ensued in this individual case; and it may be taken as a fair illustration of the treatment usually adopted. In obstinate cases the compound iodide mix-ture, which contains arsenic, is often employed.

The formulæ for the above-mentioned preparation are: of the mixture —a drachm of iodine, an ounce of liquor potassæ, and a pint of distilled water, each drachm containing half a grain of iodine. Of the liniment— olive oil, two ounces; lard, two ounces; powdered nitric oxide of mer- cury, a drachm; oil of bitter almonds, half a scruple; and glycerine, ʒj.

Part xxxviii., *p.* 174.

HERPES.

Dartres of the Perineum.—Dr. Barosh, of Lemberg, was consulted by a young man, about twenty-eight years of age, for a dartrous eruption affecting the perineum and scrotum, with which he had been afflicted from his sixteenth year, and the irritation from which was such as to cause him to be continually applying his hands there, so that he was obliged to avoid society. He had consulted the most famous physicians in Hungary, but the only thing that seemed at all to relieve him was the cold water hip- bath. When he consulted Dr. Barosch, he was exhausted by suffering, insomnia, loss of appetite, and despair; the skin was dry; the entire perineum, scrotum, and internal surface of the thigh, were covered with deep brown, hard crusts, surrounded by bleeding fissures, caused by the nails of the patient. Below these crusts the skin was hard and thickened. The fall of the crusts alternated with an acrid discharge. Kœchlin's liquor having failed, Dr. Barosch prescribed the external application of iodine as follows: Fifteen grains of iodine and two scruples of hydriodate of potass dissolved in five ounces of distilled water and one ounce of spirits of wine; make a lotion. The topical application of this solution continued for several hours, caused at first a burning sensation, which was, however, very tolerable, and was soon followed by a relief such as the patient had not experienced for two years. The use of this lotion was continued for three weeks, the patient taking baths frequently during that period, at the end of which time the cure was complete.

Part viii., *p.* 73.

Herpes Squamosus.—The cyanuret and deuto-phosphate of mercury are occasionally employed. The former is said to be preferable to the bichlo- ride, being less apt to disagree, and less readily decomposed. It is a use- ful external application in some skin affections, allaying the violent itching and irritation of what M. Alibert terms *herpes squamosus.*

Part ix., *p.* 21.

Treatment of Herpes Zostera.—The most soothing application, according to Dr. Corfe is freshly made ungt. hydr. ammonio-chlorid., smeared on the whole crop of vesicles, twice or thrice a day.   *Part* xviii., *p.* 222.

Arseniate of Iron in Herpetic and Squamous Eruptions.—Numerous facts accurately observed authorize M. Dupare in concluding that a daily dose of one-fifth of a grain of arseniate of iron, uninterruptedly repeated during the necessary time, is competent in the adult to effect the cure of an herpetic or squamous affection, however extensive or long-established.

An anti-herpetic treatment by arseniate of iron in no degree excludes the employment of topical remedies of acknowledged utility, and it is materially assisted by the internal or external use of certain non-sulphu- reted mineral waters.   *Part* xxx., *p.* 175.

IMPETIGO.

Devergie's Solution of Arsenic.—Is composed of arsenious acid, ten grains; carbonate of potash, ten grains; distilled water, six pints and a half; alcohol, fifty minims : tincture of cochineal, as much as is required to color the mixture sufficiently. Each drachm of this solution is said to be equivalent to four drops of Fowler's liquor arsenicalis. M. Devergie employs this remedy with advantage in long standing cutaneous cruptions, particularly those of a squamous and impetiginous nature. He indicates, as a constant result and symptom of cure, the appearance of dark brown spots on all parts of the skin previously diseased, which persist for some months afterward.   *Part* ix., *p.* 86.

Impetigo.—In *acute* cases, says Dr. H. Bennett, treat the particular constitutional state which may accompany the eruption ; the local treatment being unimportant. In *chronic* cases, on the other hand, be particular about the local treatment. Apply lint saturated with the solution of subcarbonate of soda (ʒij. to Oiss. of water), and cover it with oiled silk.

*   *   *   *   *   *

When this affection seems connected with the scrofulous diathesis, give cod-liver oil.   *Part* xx., *p.* 286.

Impetigo.—Apply the saturated solution of gutta percha in chloroform, by means of a camel's-hair pencil, over the patches daily.
Part xxvi., *p.* 128.

Impetigo and Eczema.—Dr. Hughes Bennett keeps the parts moist with lint saturated with a solution of half a drachm of carbonate of soda to one pint of water, covering this with oil silk. For *favus*, first remove the crusts by poulticing, then apply oil to exclude the atmosphere and prevent the growth of the parasitic fungi. These remedies should be conjoined with cod-liver oil and generous diet.   *Part* xxxiv., *p.* 197.

ICHTHYOSIS.

Ichthyosis Fortuita.—Dr. Thomson considers that in the treatment of these cases, there are three indications to be fulfilled : 1st. Augment the action of the capillaries of the skin, by giving small doses of blue pill and emetic tartar ; liquor arsenicalis ; cantharides in decoction of rumex obtusifolius, made by boiling an ounce of the sliced root of the common dock in a pint of soft water; dose ʒij. 2d. Improve the secretions generally, by generous diet, as milk, vigorous exercise in the open air, etc. 3d. Aid the action of the two former by topical means which stimulate the skin, and assist the separation of the diseased papillæ by warm baths, friction, etc.   *Part* xiv., *p.* 254.

ITCH.

Treatment of the Itch in Belgium.—The following circular was addressed to military surgeons by the Inspector-General of the Belgian army :
Each patient is to be supplied with an ounce or an ounce and a half of liquid sulphuret of lime in a small pot ; this quantity he is to rub carefully and slowly with his hands on every part that is covered with papulæ. If there be any papulæ on the back, another patient is to rub the liquid upon

that part. The operation is to be repeated three times in the twenty-four hours, so that each patient consumes three or four ounces of the sulphuret daily. A bath is to be taken every alternate day; the frictions are to be suspended on that day. Fifteen frictions (or ten days' use) are usually sufficient for the cure of the disease, if the medical officer in charge sees that the remedy is properly used. *Part* x., *p.* 97.

Treatment of Itch.—Immerse the hands of the patient in an alcoholic solution of stavesacre for half an hour together, two or three times, and the acarus scabiei will be destroyed. (Dr. Burgess.) Use a lotion made of an ounce of sulphate of copper to a pint of water: wash off the scabs before using it. It is an almost certain cure. (Mr. Lloyd.) Use a lotion of iodide of potassium in the day, and sulphur ointment at night; a cure may be expected in seven days. The lotion should be 5j. of iodide to ʒviij., or ʒxvj. of fluid. (Dr. Ward.) *Part* xiii., *p.* 307.

Treatment of Scabies.—[Mr. Corfe states that he rigorously pursues the following plan with a patient affected with itch:]

We provide him with old soiled linen and a worn out sheet; and each morning and evening he is ordered to make a good lather of yellow soap in his hands, and thus dip them wet into a basin of sifted or fine sand, and assiduously rub every part of the body on which the slightest trace of a vesicle exists. Having performed this ablution until the skin tingles smartly, he wipes himself dry, and then rubs the common ung. sulphuris firmly into the itchy parts. He is then enveloped in the winding sheet, and has a pair of old gloves on his hands, and he is left till night, when the same operation is pursued, and repeated daily until the fourth day, when he is ordered to indulge (and a great indulgence it is) in a warm bath, where he again lathers his body in plain soap and water, puts on fresh linen, and is provided with clean sheets, and the cure is from thence invariably effected. The vesicle of course is broken by the friction of the sand and soap; the acarus is exposed, and this ectozoon receives its death-blow by the inunction of the sulphur, which is oftentimes not accomplished by the mere application of sulphur ointment alone. The use of sand-soap balls is more elegant, though not more efficacious.

Part xviii., *p.* 223.

Treatment of Itch.—Use a sulpho-alkaline ointment. If there is a great abundance of pustules, and this excites too much pain, use frictions of lard and oil. Another ointment recently tried cures in three frictions, soothes the itching instantly, and does not give rise to any secondary eruption. It is composed of equal parts of fresh chamomiles, olive oil, and lard. M. Bourgignon makes an ointment by mixing 300 parts of the powder of staphysagria to 500 of lard, keeping it at a temperature of 100° C. for twenty-four hours. The frictions to be made four times a day, the cure being complete by the fourth day. *Part* xxiii., *p.* 291.

Itch—Cured in Two Hours.—In the Hospital of St. Louis, Paris, the itch is cured in two hours. The patient is first put into a warm bath, and rubbed for an hour with yellow soap. He then passes into a clean bath, where he continues to cleanse his skin for another hour. After leaving this, one of his fellow-sufferers rubs him over for half an hour with the following ointment: Axunge eight parts, flowers of sulphur two parts, and carbonate of potash one part. The patient is then examined, and sent away cured, though sometimes pretty numerous vesicles on the hands and elsewhere remain unaltered. *Part xxv., p.* 265.

Scabies, and other Parasitical Diseases of the Human Skin.—The vapor of benzoin, or benzole, which is prepared by the decomposition of benzoic acid, destroys parasites, says M. Reynal, more surely than almost any other application. It may therefore be used in pityriasis and scabies most effectually. *Part xxxi., p.* 196.

Itch— Cured in Half an Hour.—Sulphur applied in a liquid form, says Dr. E. Smith, is more readily absorbed, and consequently more certainly destructive to the insect than when used in the form of ointment. To prepare a solution, boil one part of quick lime with two parts of sublimed sulphur in two parts of water, until dissolved. The body should be previously washed with warm water, and then this solution rubbed in for half an hour. By this time the cure will be complete, and it will only be necessary to wash and use clean clothes. *Part xxxiv., p.* 195.

Treatment of Scabies by Sulphuret of Calcium.—A much more speedy and cleanly method of treating this loathsome disease than the filthy proceeding of inunction, says Dr. Kesteven, is to wash the parts affected with a solution of the sulphuret of calcium for half an hour night and morning. It is rarely that a third application is necessary, but it should be enforced to make security doubly sure. *Part xxxiv., p.* 196.

Itch.—Instead of the sulphur ointment, Dr. Fischer recommends a lotion of caustic potass, 1 part; distilled water, 12 parts. *Part xxxv., p.* 158.

Bourgignon's Treatment of Itch.--After the trial and comparison of the various modes of treatment, M. Bourgignon accords the preference to the following formula: Glycerine, 50 drachms; finely-powdered sulphur, 25 drachms; 2 yolks of eggs; and tragacanth powder, q. s.; adding essences to mask the smell. *Part xxxv., p.* 331.

Scabies.—The diagnosis of this disease is occasionally difficult; it will be much facilitated by the knowledge of the fact, that the ova of the acarus may be readily found with the microscope, attached to the roughened and undermined cuticle in the neighborhood of the vesicles.
Part xxxvi., p. 191.

Parasticides.—The following is the formula of the Hospital for Diseases of the Skin for the " compound sulphur ointment " which is in general use against scabies, favus and true ringworm, diseases which depend upon parasites, which it is necessary to kill: R Of sublimed sulphur, half a pound; of the ammonia chloride of mercury, half an ounce; and of the sulphuret of mercury, half an ounce; to these, well rubbed together, add four ounces of olive-oil, sixteen ounces of fresh lard, and twenty minims of creasote. It will be seen that we have here in combination three different drugs, each possessing great efficiency in the destruction of insect and fungus life. The object in view, that of obtaining a vigorous compound, which at the same time shall not be irritating to the skin, is, we believe, exceedingly well attained. *Part xxxvii., p.* 315.

LEPRA. •

Bark of the Ulmus Campestris (or Elm).—Dr. Sigmond thinks favorally of the use of the decoction of elm-bark, both internally and externally, in all varieties of lepra, and in other scaly affections of the skin. Four ounces of fresh elm-bark, bruised, boiled in four pints of water, form a thick decoction.

The best time to gather it is in the spring, and the most desirable parts are the smaller branches and twigs. The inner bark abounds with a mucilaginous principle (which disappears on boiling too much). Dose of the decoction, from two to four ounces, three times a day.

Dr. S. says : I have likewise found it very serviceable in tinea capitis, and more especially when it has been used as a wash externally. In those extensive papulous eruptions, known by the name of lichen, which usually terminate in scurf, the lichen simplex, which attacks the face and skin sometimes periodically, very quickly yields to the remedy ; and in the milder cases of erysipelas, when the constitution has not in any way participated, I have been in the habit of using this remedy with a success that has now enabled me to lay the result of my observations before you.

In those affections of the skin where the papulæ are in a state of high irritation, amounting to inflammation, I have uniformly found lotions or applications of mercurials, such as the unguentum hydrargyri nitratis, or ointments of lead, to be rather injurious than beneficial ; in such cases it is that I have observed so much benefit from the bark of the elm, internally taken, and externally applied, and in almost every stage of cutaneous disease. There are likewise some states of the skin in which papulous eruptions and erythematic blushes are indicative of diseased states of the internal mucous membranes, and likewise of various dyspeptic symptoms. Thus we observe where leucorrhœa exists, or where disease has been induced by dram-drinking, that redness of the skin, and disordered functions of the skin are visible ; in such instances the use of the elm-bark for some weeks, with attention to diet has been productive of the best consequences, and I have had the satisfaction of seeing some of those eruptions, which have for years baffled every attempt of the medical men, yield to a determined course of the elm-bark. It is of importance to continue it for some time, and to attend to the state of the bowels during the period in which it is taken. The state of the urine should be carefully observed ; and it will be found that, after some little time, much acid will become developed, which most probably is determined from the blood, and would have been deposited in the skin and have produced some of the disordered states which the elm-bark appears destined to avert. *Part* i., *p.* 61.

Lepra.—Dr. Ross says : The iodide of potassium has been used externally in almost all cutaneous diseases. From some experiments lately made with regard to its destructive power over the itch insect, it has been recommended for the cure of scabies. M. Schedel states, that the speediest cure of this complaint is effected by an ointment containing 3ss. to 3j. of axunge.

Dr. A. T. Thomson recommends an ointment composed of hyd. potass. 3iss., to axunge ℥iss., with tinct. opii 3j., in lepra ; this, conjoined with appropriate internal treatment, has a very good effect ; but, from a comparative trial, I think it inferior to another ointment recommended by the same author, viz.:

℞ Calomelanos, 3j. ; unguent picis, 3iv. ; unguent cetacei, 3j. M.
Part vi., *p.* 122.

Lepra, Psoriasis, Lupus, Acne, Eczema Chronica, Impetigo, Prurigo,

Lichen.—In the treatment of these and all chronic affections of the skin, which are not venereal, nor dependent on local causes, Mr. Hunt advises to first, reduce inflammatory action by depletion and antiphlogistic regimen; then administer arsenic, beginning with five minims of the liquor potassæ arsenitis thrice a day, with the meals, until the conjunctiva is inflamed ; afterward reduce the dose to four minims, keeping the eyelids slightly sore and weeping. The whole success of this treatment (which seldom or never fails in any of the above diseases), depends upon the continued and persevering use of the medicine, which is perfectly harmless, when administered with vigilance under these restrictions.

Part xiv., *p.* 247.

Lepra—Treatment of.—In obstinate cases of lepra, use fumigation with sulphur and iodine vapors.

*   *   *   *   *   *   *   *

When the functions have all been got into a healthy state, and the system is free from inflammatory action, begin with Fowler's solution of arsenic, in four or five minim doses, taken thrice a day upon a full stomach ; and, without increasing the dose, continue this plan steadily till the system is brought under the influence of the remedy. Continue the medicine for some time after the disappearance of the eruption. (Dr. Griffith.)

*   *   *   *   *   *   *   *

Let strong tar ointment (⅛ to ¼ of tar) be rubbed in gently thrice a day ; while a tepid bath is used once or twice a week. And give Fowler's solution of arsenic, beginning with five drops daily and increasing a drop every other day, until twelve or fifteen are reached. (M. Emery.)

Part xx., *p.* 174.

Syphilitic Lepra.—Dr. R. B. Todd would give five grains of blue pill night and morning, thus affecting the system slowly and gradually by a mild and unirritating preparation of the mineral. Iodide of potassium favors the mercurial influence, at the same time exercising some specific antidotal power of its own. Hyper-salivation, violent iodism, irritation of the bowels and of the skin, and peculiar nervous affections are produced when too much of these minerals is thrown into the system, with a desire to produce a rapid effect. We may withhold them for a time, renewing them again as occasion may suggest. It is sometimes much more desirable to introduce mercury also by the skin than by the stomach. Tar is also one of the safest remedies—the pix liquida. It may be given internally in capsules, or applied externally, or both. Fifteen or twenty minims may be taken three or four times a day, at the same time the patient may be tarred over the surface, and lie in tarred sheets. This is exceedingly useful, though scarcely available in private practice. *Part* xxiii., *p.* 322.

Lepra and Psoriasis—Sesquicarbonate of Ammonia in.—M. Cazenave, so well known as a very successful dermatologist, has published experiments tending to show that sesquicarbonate of ammonia may advantageously be used as a succedaneum of arsenical preparations, in lepra and psoriasis.

Give the sesquicarbonate of ammonia in the following manner : Sesquicarbonate of ammonia, ʒss. ; diaphoretic sirup, ʒvij. ; take one to three tablespoonfuls per diem. If diarrhœa, lassitude, cephalalgia, and rapid alternations of heat and cold were to occur, the remedy must be suspended.

Part xxv., *p.* 265.

Lepra Vulgaris.—Dr. J. S. Taylor directs an alkaline bath once a week, and thin oatmeal gruel instead of soup. Give half-grain doses of iodide of potassium, and three minims of Fowler's solution three times a day, and apply night and morning, an ointment composed of the nitric oxide of mercury and lard, with a few drops of creasote added.

Part xxvi., *p.* 284.

Scaly Disease of the Skin.—In these and scrofulous and cancerous diseases the galium aparine is proving very valuable. Mr. Hooper prepares an inspissated juice, a tea spoonful equalling half a pint of the decoction : 3j. of this juice may be taken three times a day. *Part* xxix., *p.* 47.

Lepra Inveterata.—In the treatment of this most obstinate affection, says Dr. Willshire, much will be gained by a proper regulation of the diet. Bread, milk, eggs, and vegetables, as potatoes, water cresses, etc., should alone be allowed, and all alcoholic drinks avoided. A warm bath twice a week is of the greatest use. The medicinal means principally of use are, arsenic, bichloride of mercury, and iodine, for which the decoction of elm bark forms a good vehicle. An ointment containing calomel and pitch is one of the best local applications. *Part* xxxix., *p.* 230.

PEMPHIGUS.

Dr. Bennett, Mr. Skey and Mr. Startin believe that arsenic is almost a specific remedy in the worst cases of this disease, as it remedies the unknown constitutional cause upon which the disease depends. It does not prevent the liability to return, but it renders the attacks less severe than the original one. *Part* xxix., *p.* 249.

PITYRIASIS.

Treatment of.—Dr. Startin recommends external applications of a soothing nature ; baths medicated with mucilage of linseed, milk, yolk of egg, etc. ; at the same time give demulcents, diuretics, etc., to increase the renal secretion. Cover the parts over with glycerine ; it remains fluid, and resists evaporation under any temperature to which the body is exposed. *Part* xiii., *p.* 306.

Pityriasis, Herpes, Eczema.—M. Cazenave uses a lotion composed of one part of alum, and sixty-two parts of water. In the slighter forms of acne, lichen, pityriasis, herpes, and even in eczema, a simple acidulated lotion. In impetigo, after the crusts have fallen off, the following application of alumina : Alum, eight grammes; infusion of Provence roses, five hundred grammes. Gowland's solution, or Bateman's mercurial emulsion, however, answer very well. M. Cazenave uses the following : Bichloride of mercury, ten centigrammes ; hydrochlorate of ammonia, ten centigrammes ; almond emulsion 250 grammes ; make a solution. In really chronic eczema he uses the following lotion : Acid nitric, twenty-five drops; acid muriatic, twenty-five drops ; distilled water, three hundred grammes. Mix by shaking. *Part* xiv., *p.* 253.

Pityriasis.—Pityriasis is closely allied to psoriasis. Dr. Wright says : Psoriasis is prone to affect the muscular parts of the body ; pityriasis chiefly shows itself upon the scalp, forehead, and face. You saw a very good case of both diseases in the person of a man named Hines, who came into the top ward of the hospital on the 28th of November last year. His arms, and hands, and legs were extensively covered with patches of psoriasis : the upper part of his face, his forehead, and scalp were completely dusted with the peculiar dandriff of pityriasis. Both, here, occurred in the same individual, and merely different in their relative intensity. The man was a brass-founder, and had lately been out of work, and indifferently fed. The disease was of five weeks' duration. He was ordered generous diet, and half-a-pint of ale daily.

R. Decoct. dulcamaræ, ʒviij.; potassæ, liq. arsenicalis, aa. ʒj.; misce fiat mist. cujus cap. coch. ampla duo ter die.

R. Pil. coloc. c., Əij.; extr. hyoscy., Əj. Misce et divide in pil. xij. quarum cap. ij. omni nocte.

This was all the general treatment the man had, and on the 23rd of December he left the hospital well. Five days less than a month, he was under medical management, and at the time of his departure there was not a trace of skin disease about him. It is probable that the medicines administered to this patient rendered him some service ; but perhaps the greater service was due to his improved mode of living.

Part xvi., *p.* 221.

Pityriasis Capitis.—Dr. Winsar recommends the following lotion : Fresh sulphuret of potash, ʒj., distilled water, ʒiij. It may be used once a day.   *Part* xxviii., *p.* 330.

Pityriasis Versicolor Curable by Local Applications.—This common disease known vulgarly as " Liver spots," and in the Nosology of Wilson as Chloasma, is one generally acknowledged to be of extreme intractability. Mr. Paget, we notice, among his out-patients at St. Bartholomew's, does not adopt any constitutional treatment whatever, but simply orders a wash of the bichloride of mercury (gr. j. ad ʒj.) He informs us that he has never known a case long resist the influence of this remedy regularly applied to the whole affected surface once in the day. At the Skin Hospital, although an arsenical course of internal medication is always prescribed at the same time, yet a mercurial lotion is also used, and may possibly be the chief curative agent. In the hands of Dr. Jenner, at the University College Hospital, the sulphuric acid has, we understand, succeeded very well. There can be little doubt but that the disease is almost invariably curable by local applications solely (parasiticides ?) In relation to this mode of cure, it is important to connect the observation of Eichstedt and others, as to the eruption depending on the presence of a cryptogamic plant. Another interesting link in the same chain of evidence has recently been made out at the Skin Hospital, namely, that it is not unfrequently contagious.   *Part* xxix., *p.* 250.

Cocoa-Nut Oil Ointments.—Use of, in Pityriasis. *Vide* Art. " Medicines."

PRURIGO.

Prurigo Senilis.—[This disease is well known to be very intractable, and is indeed set down by many authors as incurable ; hence the treatment usually recommended is merely palliative, and consists in the use of simple salt or sulphur baths, lotions containing sulphuret of potash, or corrosive sublimate, cinnabar fumigations, etc. Dr. Bellingham thinks that a good deal may be done by treatment. He says:]

Constitutional remedies appear to have little effect upon purigo ; our principal reliance therefore must be upon local measures. The local application which I have found most generally useful, both in relieving the intolerable itching, and in curing the disease, is creasote, either in form of ointment or of lotion, usually the former. The ointment may be made with from ten to twenty drops of creasote to the ounce of lard, the lotion with from twenty to thirty drops of creasote to the half-pint of water, a little spirit of wine or acetic being added in order to render it more soluble. The ointment to be useful should be well rubbed into the parts every night, and a very few applications will in general relieve the itching, prevent the development of fresh papulæ, while the old ones will gradually desquamate. If the application of the ointment is premised by the warm bath, and if the patient attends to personal cleanliness, the remedy will be more likely to prove quickly successful. *Part* xvi., *p.* 223.

Treatment of Prurigo Pudendi.—Dr. Corfe says : Prurigo, where it attacks the pudendum or scrotum, is oftentimes more effectually soothed by a lotion composed of two or four drachms of the terchloride of carbon or chloric ether, in a pint of distilled or elder-flower water, than any other application that I am acquainted with ; at the same time a warm bath administered every evening affords a calm and refeshing night's rest.
Part xviii., *p.* 222.

Treatment of Prurigo—Prurigo Pudendi (and other Species).—In those severe cases which are not benefited by our treatment, Dr. Burgess gives strychnia, beginning with one-sixth of a grain twice a day, and increasing the dose to one-fourth of a grain. Occasional doses of tincture of henbane may also be given.

Senilis.—Give phosphorus internally, in the form of phosphorated ether, having preceded it, for a day or two, by repeated doses of tincture of hyoscyamus. [The dose is not stated ; but the dose of the tinct. æther. c. phosphoro of the French, is, according to Pereira, from 5 to 10 drops.—
Part xix., *p.* 199.

Prurigo of the Genital Organs.—This affection (which often assumes the form of lichen or eczema) is well known to be very painful, distressing, and difficult to remove. M. Tournié has lately proposed calomel ointment, and a powder of camphor and starch, which topical applications he has used with much success. When the parts (genital organs, anal region, or axilla) are covered with scabs, tepid baths, and emollient applications are to be used first. When the indurated particles are removed, the affected spot is to be rubbed twice a day with the calomel ointment (one or two drachms of the calomel to one ounce of axunge), and after each application dredged with the powder (four parts of starch to one of finely powdered camphor). We mention M. Tournié's treatment as this kind of prurigo so often baffles the remedies usually employed. *Part* xxv., *p.* 247.

Colchicum in Prurigo.—Dr. Elliotson gives the case of a man, laboring under this disease in its most inveterate form, to whom half a drachm of vinum colchici was administered thrice daily. This the patient took for three weeks ; at the end of which time he was completely cured.

Colchicum would thus seem to answer well in some cases of skin diseases where the urine is of low specific gravity. *Part* xxv., *p.* 264.

Prurigo—Starch in Skin Diseases.—M. Cazenave substitutes powdered starch for poultices, especially in pruriginous affections, either simply dusted over the part, or applied after the latter has been well cleansed by an alkaline solution and thoroughly dried. The starch may be used simply, or mixed with oxide of zinc, camphor, etc. M. Cazenave treats acute eczema, acne rosacea, impetigo, and herpes, by dusting the affected regions, night and morning, with the following powder—White oxide of zinc, two drachms; powdered starch, four ounces. Very good results have been obtained in prurigo of the genital organs, the groin, or the axilla, with the following powder : White oxide of zinc, two drachms; camphor, half a drachm; powdered starch, four ounces.

Prurigo Ani et Vaginœ.—Dr. Richart recommends the following: Take equal parts of sulphate of zinc and of alum, roughly powder them, and put them into a glazed earthenware vessel; put it on a slow fire and leave it there till bubbles of air are no longer disengaged, and till the mixture acquires a stony hardness ; then powder it, and throw it by small portions at a time into boiling water. Filter, and apply to the parts with a sponge and on linen. *Part* xxx., *p.* 228.

PSORIASIS.

Psoriasis—Liquor Hydriodatis Arsenici et Hydrargyri.—[In a previous number of the "Dublin Journal," Mr. Donovan gave some account of a new chemical compound, consisting of iodine, arsenic, and mercury, and the diseases in which it would be found beneficial, namely, psoriasis, lepra, and lupus. He now presents to us the experience of some of the most eminent men in Dublin. Mr. Carmichael states that :]

I have tried the liquor hydriodatis arsenici et hydrargyri, in five or six cases of lupus, and in one case of psoriasis, with decided benefit in all.

In one case of lupus, of ten years' standing, in which great deformity had been occasioned by the disease on the features of a young lady, on whom all the usual remedies had been tried, it produced most decided benefit, and seemed to put an immediate check to the progress of the malady. She is not yet perfectly well, but sufficient advantages have ensued to promise recovery. In one of my lectures I stated the case of a man who had lost a great part of the vomer, and in whom much deformity had consequently ensued from an obstinate attack of lupus, who in the course of a few weeks so far recovered, as to be discharged from the hospital apparently well. I perceive there has been no relapse of the disease, as he was told to return to the hospital should any suspicious symptoms make their appearance.

In the case of Mr. ——, affected with psoriasis, although the disease had existed for years, most decided benefit generally followed the use of the preparation in question, so that nothing but discoloration of the skin remains where scaly spots were formerly manifested.

[Dr. Irving's case is the most interesting, not only on account of the virulence of the disease, but also because he had tried in different cases the separate ingredients of the liquor hydriodatis arsenici et hydrargyri without their having gained his confidence. In relating this case he says :]

On examination, I found his legs and arms thickly covered with large spots of psoriasis, much inflamed, and very itchy. He said they were increasing rapidly in number, and that some had made their appearance on his body and forehead during the last few days.

I directed that he should be blooded to twelve ounces, and ordered him some aperient medicine which he was to continue for a week. These means afforded him some relief; the eruption was less itchy and less inflamed. I directed him to continue the aperient medicine, and to take twelve drops of liquor potassæ three times daily.

It would be tedious to relate the entire history of this case; it is sufficient to say, that he took various remedies, Dulcamara and Plummers's pill among the number, without any benefit unless temporary relief from itching.

From the experience of many cases which I had treated without permanent benefit at the Maison de Santé, with Fowler's solution of arsenic, iodine, and mercury, separately administered, I was inclined to doubt their efficacy; I therefore determined to try the compound of these three. On the 11th of February we commenced the solution.

He took a draught containing ʒss. of liquor hydriodatis arsenici et hydrargyri three times a day from this date to the 28th of April. Twice during that period I found it necessary to stop the medicine for two or three days, and to give an opening draught, from his having complained of headache and sickness of stomach.

On the 28th of April the disease was quite cured, nothing remaining but a stained appearance of the skin.

Venereal Eruptions.—Mr. Cusack states a new and different application of the arsenico-mercurial compound, which he employed with considerable success. He found that venereal eruptions rapidly yielded to scruple or half drachm doses three times a day, that is to *one-quarter of a grain* of protoxide of mercury, and one-eighth of a grain of arsenic, or thereabouts, in the twenty-four hours. This indeed is a very small quantity of mercury to effect a rapid cure with: no one will deny that the less of it that will answer the purpose the better for the patient: and here again we perceive the effect of chemical combination, assisted no doubt by solubility. Mr. Cusack writes:

" I have unfortunately omitted to make notes of the cases in which your valuable remedy, the liquor hydriodatis arsenici et hydrargyri, was administered, and am only able to state generally, that I have used it freely in secondary venereal eruptions, both papular and scaly. I found the eruptions yield rapidly to its administration in the dose of one scruple to two, three times each day. In two instances the mouth became tender, and a slight salivation followed; but in no case have I observed any unpleasant consequences, even when taken in larger doses."　　　　*Part* ii., *p.* 50.

Uses of some of the Combinations of Iodine.—In the paper before us, by Mr. Osbrey, the effects of some of the combinations of iodine are interesting. He begins with the liquor hydriodatis arsenici et hydrargyri, in a case of inveterate psoriasis. The patient, Susan A., æt. 9, was affected with diffuse psoriasis which engaged almost her whole body, the scales on the extremities being continuous and remarkably thick. The following mixture was given:

℞ Aquæ destillat., ʒviij.; liq. hydriodat. arsen. et hydr., gtt. 80; tinct. zingiber., ʒss.

Sumat unciam misturæ omni tertia hora.

Sickness of the stomach was at first produced, which soon subsided on desisting from the medicine for a few days. In ten days the eruption began rapidly to decline upon the trunk, and the thick scales to loosen upon the extremities. The separation of the scales on the head was accelerated by applying an ointment consisting of equal parts of tar and dilute citrine ointments. " In five weeks from the commencement of the use of these remedies she improved in health, but after that period her appetite de. clined; she fell away in flesh, and her countenance became pallid. The use of the mixture was of course discontinued. All traces of the eruption had then disappeared from the surface of the trunk, and only a few patches remained on the extremities." She then went into the country, took tonic medicines, and soon recovered her health. The mixture was again com. menced, and in three weeks no trace of the disease remained.

The iodide of potassium, Fowler's solution of arsenic, mercurial altera. tives, sarsaparilla, guaiacum, and other medicines had been previously tried in vain. At the same time we think that every practitioner ought to exer. cise the greatest caution in every case where he is using the above mixture, as in the case here related we perceive that the patient's health was at first materially injured for a time. Three other cases of scaly eruptions were treated in the same way. One was affected with several thick scaly patches on the extremities for twelve months previously. These disap. peared when she had used the medicine about three weeks. The separa. tion of the scales was here also assisted by the tar and citrine ointments. Twenty-five drops of the mixture were given three times a day without producing sickness.   *Part* vi., *p.* 63.

Concrete Naphthaline in Psoriasis.—Dr. Emery, of the Hospital St. Louis, had his attention turned to the investigation of the different pro. ducts of tar as remedial agents in the treatment of skin diseases, on ac. count of the successful results he obtained from the use of tar, and because of the unpleasant odor it gave forth. Various preparations were had re. course to, the most valuable of which proved to be the concrete naphthaline which Dr. Emery tried in fourteen cases. In two cases, one of psoriasis gyrata, and the other lepra vulgaris, it failed in effecting any good; in the remaining twelve it proved more serviceable. In two of the cases, lepra vulgaris of from fifteen months to two years' duration, arsenical and iodic preparations had been previously tried; in the younger patient the arsenic at first seemed to do good, but the improvement soon ceased. An ointment prepared with two scruples of concrete naphthaline to thirty of lard was applied, causing the scales to fall off, leaving the skin of a violet color, with white circles around. A perfect cure was effected in six weeks, and although three months have passed since, there has not been any relapse. In four other cases the men were laboring under inveterate psoriasis; in one of them it had existed sixteen years, and had resisted arsenical, iodic and mercurial treatment. The tar ointment was had recourse to, and with de. cided advantage, but the man becoming impatient on account of his busi. ness, an ointment of naphthaline, twice the strength of that used in the preceding cases, was spread on compresses, and applied over the diseased parts night and morning. The man was cured in six weeks. When the ointment was applied too strong, it caused a burning heat, which was soon removed by emollient baths and poultices. The other six cases were also instances of psoriasis cured by the naphthaline ointment. Dr. Emery states that this remedy has an unpleasant odor, which passes off, and it is apt to irritate the skin and cause erysipelas if it be not carefully watched.
Part vii., *p.* 171.

Psoriasis:

If dependent on strumous diathesis, Dr. Graves uses cod-liver oil, made into an emulsion with sirup, mucilage and orange-flower water. Insert one or more issues at a distance from the part affected; and let the patient use warm baths with two gallons of *size* added to the water, or an equivalent quantity of isinglass, or calf's foot jelly.

Of the Scalp.—Use hot-air sulphur baths for fifteen or twenty minutes daily, and apply the following ointment at night: R Hydrarg. biniod., əj.; adip. ppt. ʒj.; ol. limon., gtt., v. M.

Or, give hydrarg. bichlor. gr. one-sixteenth dissolved in sp. vin. rect., 3ss., thrice a day with decoction of bark and sarza, and apply dilute citrine ointment, with a third part of ung. ceræ alb. *Part* xv., *p.* 256.

Acetate of Potash in Psoriasis.—Give acetate of potash in doses of half-a-drachm three times a day. It acts (as described by Dr. Golding Bird) by increasing the metamorphosis of tissue in the system, by which means all products of low vitality are likely to become decomposed and eliminated from the system in the urine. *Part* xxi., *p.* 245.

Use of Phosphorus.—Dr. Burgess recommends phosphorus as one of the most valuable medicinal agents we possess in those inveterate cutaneons diseases—leprosy, psoriasis, lupus—in which the skin seems to adapt itself to the morbid condition, which it retains with singular tenacity against all the usual methods of treatment.

The *phosphorus* treatment of these maladies may be either internal or external. The best method of administering the remedy internally is dissolved in oil or ether, and the phosphorated oil or ether then mixed up with powdered gum arabic and mint water. Camphorated lard is the most appropriate vehicle for applying phosphorus externally. Its energetic revulsive properties may likewise be turned to account in certain diseased conditions of the skin. Phosphorus, the iodide of arsenic, cantharides, and the biniodide of mercury, are the most powerful internal remedies for the skin diseases, we possess. *Part* xxi., *p.* 250.

Psoriasis.—" Psoriasis, so-called, lepra vulgaris, psoriasis diffusa, psoriasis gyrata, psoriasis guttata, and psoriasis inveterata, are one disease more or less chronic." The real nature of psoriasis is altogether unknown. There is no exudation, properly so called; there is considerable redness and an increased growth, or a hypertrophy of the epidermis. As there is generally a deranged state of the digestive organs, with sometimes constitutional disorder in this affection, we must correct these by suitable combinations. For the constitutional treatment, Professor Bennett advises equal parts of Fowler's solution and tincture of cantharides, in doses commencing with ten drops, gradually increased to fifteen or twenty. Most dermatologists are agreed that the best local application is the pitch ointment (ung. picis); if it causes considerable irritation it may be diluted with an equal part of lard. Some cases require only the arsenic, others the pitch ointment alone, and a third class of cases require the action of both. *Part* xxii., *p.* 244.

Treatment of Psoriasis and Lepra-Vulgaris.—According to M. Emery, the arsenical preparations, and especially Fowler's solution, are the best internal remedies. Tar takes the first place as an external application.

The combination of these is the best treatment for psoriasis. The iodide of mercury ointment is occasionally useful when judiciously applied, and next to it the iodide of sulphur. The tar ointment is made by mixing a third or a fourth of a part of tar to two or three parts of axunge. The ointment of iodide of mercury is made by mixing one part of proto-iodide of mercury with eight of axunge; and that of the iodide of sulphur by mixing from one part in thirty-two to one part in eight of lard. Besides these, dietetical and hygienic measures must be adopted. Diet mild, and not too substantial, avoiding all aliments difficult of digestion, regular exercise, frequent use of baths, and having recourse again to the treatment which had benefited them before, on the least appearance of the disease.

Part xxii., *p.* 245.

Psoriasis, Chronic.—M. Cazenave has for many years past employed carbonate of ammonia in squamous diseases of the skin. He prescribes ten parts of ammonia to two hundred and forty of simple sirup, the patient taking from six to twenty-four grains of the salt daily. *Part* xxii., *p.* 259.

Psoriasis—Dr. Graves applies a saturated solution of gutta percha in chloroform; no woollen stockings or rough garments of any kind should be allowed next the skin, lest the application should be disturbed.

Part xxvi., *p.* 288.

Psoriasis.—Dr. Crawford says the diet should be nourishing. ℞ Potass. acet., ʒij.; aquæ, ʒiij. Of this one drachm to be given in a little water three times a day. Locally, the limbs to be placed for five minutes in the morning into a tepid bath, containing one drachm of bicarbonate of soda. The scales to be gently removed with a soft flesh brush, and then the following applied : ℞ Plumbi diacet. sol., ʒj. ʒvj.; sol. mur. morph., ʒij.; a teaspoonful to be mixed with a tablespoonful of cream, and applied to the limbs. *Part* xxviii., *p.* 233.

Psoriasis Diffusa.—When in large patches over the flexures of joints, forehead, neck, chest, etc., says Dr. Bullar, give a quarter of a pint daily of the decoction of the urtica dioica (common stinging nettle), made by boiling an ounce of the leaves and stems in a quart of water, down to a pint. An extract may be made from this—dose, five grains three times a day. The same medicine is efficacious in inveterate chronic papular eruptions (lichen), and in various forms of vesicular and scaly diseases (eczema, lepra, and psoriasis), especially in cachectic states of the system.

Part xxxi., *p.* 172.

Scaly Cutaneous Diseases.—Mr. Thomas Hunt believes that if there be any medicine more safe and manageable in these cases, in careful hands, than another, it is arsenic united with chlorate of potass; but if there be any medicine more dangerous and unmanageable than another, it is the compound of arsenic, iodine, and mercury, known as Donovan's solution.

Part xxxii., *p.* 182.

Psoriasis—Syphilitic.—Iodide of potassium and sarsaparilla, says Mr. Stanley, will generally cure the disease for a time; but, as a matter of certainty and safety, 5 grains of Plummer's pill should be given night and morning, though not necessarily to touch the mouth. *Part* xxxiii., *p.* 236.

Psoriasis of the Matrices of the Nails.—In cases under the care of Dr.

Hare, at the University College Hospital, he put them upon the plan of treatment which he has found to answer very well in cases of psoriasis— viz., liq. potassæ in half-drachm doses, and liq. arsenicalis in five-minim doses, three times daily, in water. *Part* xxxvii., *p.* 308.

SYCOSIS MENTI, OR BARBER'S ITCH.

Iodide of Sulphur.—Dr. Ross says he made use of the iodide of sulphur very successfully in a bad case of sycosis menti. After soothing the irritation by extracting the hairs from the pustules, by poultices, prussic acid lotions, and warm poppy-head fomentations, an ointment of gr. xv. to the ounce was used by gentle friction morning and evening. In ten days the tuberculated indurations covering the chin were much smaller, and ultimately a complete cure was effected. *Part* vi., *p.* 123.

The Liquor Potassæ.—Given in doses of from 15 to 30 drops, three times a day—is an admirable remedy in many cases of inveterate skin diseases. According to our observations, it is far more efficacious, and perhaps, too, less injurious, than the potash in combination with iodine. The liquor potassæ may be given in milk, beer, decoction of Sarsaparilla, etc. With respect to the sulphate of iron as an external application, in sycosis, mentagra, etc., we cannot believe that it possesses any curative virtues above those of the sulphate of zinc, or of the sulphate of copper, that are in daily use. The white vitriol is our favorite, and the best way of applying it is by dipping rags of soft linen in a tepid solution of the salt, and covering these with a piece of oil-skin. If used thus, the lotion will not require renewal oftener than night and morning. In some cases, a little hydrocyanic acid may be conveniently added to the solution with advantage. (Ed. Med. Chir. Rev.) *Part* ix., *p.* 189.

Sycosis.—Sycosis, says Mr. Startin, has its site in the sebaceous follicles of the face and head, which are perforated by the hair of the beard, whiskers, eyebrows, or scalp, and unattended with any necessary derangement of the general health.

The treatment consists of plucking out the hairs with a pair of forceps, and the application of a mildly stimulating ointment composed as follows:

White precipitate of mercury, gr. xv.; strong mercurial ointment, 3j.; liquor of acetate of lead, 3ss.; recent pure palm oil, 3vj. This made a smooth, creamlike application, which suited the parts very well. To combat the general disorder, brisk acidulated saline purgatives were administered, which, when the desired effect was produced, were combined with a chalybeate.

Also daily ablutions with the yolk of an egg and water, until the cure is effected.

In one very severe case the disease had extended to the forehead, and all the hairy parts of the face, and so much hypertrophy existed in many of the diseased parts that the disfigurement was hideously great; the upper lip was quite lobulated; and a stiff yellow beard grew out of the surface, covered with fungoid-looking granulations that oozed a mucopurulent secretion. I had more leisure at that period than now falls to my share, and I spent many hours at different times in removing the hairs from this diseased mass, and in opening the tubercles when suppuration could be detected, anointing him with my own hands; in short, in carrying out the principles I have detailed. He took iron in various forms, but received the most marked benefit from the iodide internally administered, and iodide of sulphur externally, in the form of ointment (15 grains to the ounce of lard), by which conjoined means in two or three months he was perfectly freed from his disease, save that a few of the eyelashes seemed to have been permanently destroyed.

Mr. S. states, that as the implication of the hairs constitute the only difference between acne and sycosis, it becomes a rule, as conclusive as it is practically useful, that they should be extracted by a forceps from all the inflamed vari as fast as they appear; and thus the maladies will be rendered identical, and require only a similar treatment.

Fomentations of decoction of mallows or poppies, of linseed, or of warm water, in which a little sulphur and bran have been boiled (in an earthen vessel), are very serviceable, both before and after this operation, and I would recommend the sulphur-vapor douche as a most valuable accessory.

This bath can be readily applied by means of any contrivance, at the end of the steam-pipe which will exclude the nose, or as is the preferable mode, the whole face may be subjected to the sulphurous vapor, if the nose be provided with a tube for inspiration.

By paying attention to the extraction of the hairs, to the use of the scissors instead of the razor, and to washing and anointing the parts, after the manner recommended for acne in my last lecture (the use of the lancet and cauterization being also occasionally required), and the internal treatment directed as then advised, I have often succeeded in curing sycosis of twenty or thirty years' duration in as many weeks.

Part xiv., *p.* 238.

Treatment of Sycosis.—[The patient was directed to clip the beard carefully, to use no soap in washing, but to dab the face with a soft towel. Regular diet and abstinence from stimulants were enjoined; and,]

Dr. Wright ordered the following to be applied three times a day:

R Hydrarg. bichloridi, gr. ij.; acidi muriatici mij.; mist. camphoræ, ℥viij. M. ft. lotio.

Additionally he had these medicines:

℞ Inf. gentianæ, ℥viij.; liq. potassæ, liq. arsenicalis, aa. ℨj. M. ft. mist. cujus cap. coch. larg. duo ter die.

R Pil. coloc. c. ℈ij.; extr. hyoscy., ℈ij.; pil. hydrarg., gr. x. Misce et divide in pil. xiv. quarum cap. ij. omni nocte.

In less than a fortnight, we had some satisfactory evidences of improvement. The congestive and inflammatory tendency was less, as shown by the external appearance, and the patient's own remark, that he had less heat, pricking and pain in his chin, than previously. Further, there were fewer spots of suppuration, and in one or two places a little furfuraceous material had collected. You remember my dwelling upon this, as one of the best features in the manifestations of amendment, and saying that the fact of epidermal desquamation being successive of suppuration, was proof that the local inflammatory action was subsiding. Such proved to be the fact. In this case we had not a solitary drawback. The patient systematically improved from the commencement, and before two months had elapsed he was able to shave the lower part of his face without inconvenience.

[In these cases of psoriasis, pityriasis, and sycosis, alluded to by Dr. Wright, glycerine will prove a valuable application.] *Part* xvi., *p.* 222.

Treatment of Sycosis.—In regard to the treatment of this most troublesome complaint, Mr. Wilson mentions that he has found the strong citrine ointment, the iodide of sulphur ointment, and the tar ointment, to be the most useful local applications; but that it is difficult to predict in any individual case, which of these will be most serviceable, one frequently succeeding where another has failed, or even proved highly injurious. At the same time he gives Fowler's or Donovan's solution internally; but he mentions a case in which a gentleman was nearly poisoned by two drops of the former. *Part* xxiv., *p.* 258.

Mentagra or Sycosis.—Sycosis is often very troublesome and obstinate. The object of treatment is to destroy the vegetable parasite which causes or is the disease. An ointment of corrosive sublimate, one grain, and lard, two dr's, is often very useful, or the white precipitate ointment of the Pharmacopœia. An ointment composed of a scruple of iodide of sulphur to an ounce of lard is strongly recommended by Dr. Thompson. Warm fomentations and poultices are very useful. Epilation is sometimes absolutely necessary to effect a cure. The condition of the digestive organs must be attended to, and purgatives, tonics, and antacids exhibited as required. *Part* xxxvii., *p.* 179.

Treatment of Sycosis.—Dr. W. Cooke says: Poultice with linseed until the scabs are removed, and then apply constantly a lotion composed of two drachms of manganese, with potassa or permanganate of potash and a pint of water. After the ulcers are healed apply red precipitate ointment every night for several weeks. *Part* xxxvii., *p.* 182.

SYPHILITIC ERUPTIONS.

M. Cazenave considers the best remedies to be the iodides of mercury. Biett gave R hydrarg. biniod., gr. x.; pulv. glycyrrh., 3j. M. ft. pilul. lx. Dose two or three daily. But the protiodide is better; R hydr. protiodid. gr. x., pulv. glycyrrhiz. ℈ss. M. ft. pilul. lx. Begin with one, and afterward give two, three, or four, daily. In the more inveterate forms, as the tubercular, give twice the above quantity. Do not combine with opium, which neutralizes the effect. If the bowels become deranged, suspend its use for a few days.

Next in value to iodide of mercury is that of potassium, in doses of six grains daily, increased to ten, or in obstinate cases, and where the constitution is not irritable, to half a drachm in the day. Topical remedies are not of much use. To dress an ulcerated surface use hydrarg. protiod. ℈j. to an ounce of lard. *Part* xv., *p.* 242.

Syphilitic Cutaneous Eruptions.—In the treatment of these eruptions, which may come on as exanthematous affections, vesicular, papular, tubercular, pustular, and as ulcerations, Mr. Acton strongly recommends mercurial fumigations.

He does not believe the condylomata to be inoculable. As local treatment he recommends the parts to be washed with a solution of chloride of soda twice a day, the parts to be well dried, and calomel sprinkled upon them, and dry lint kept between the excoriated surfaces.

Under the head of pustulæ, he includes rupia, bullæ, and impetigo of the scalp. He finds the emplastrum ammoniaci cum mercurio an admirable local application.

In the local treatment of alopecia, Mr. Acton recommends stimulating washes, as, equal parts of rectified spirits, eau 'de cologne, and castor oil, or, if a stronger one be required, equal parts of vermy water and tinctura lyttæ, some pomade being used also.

The throat is very frequently the seat of secondary symptoms. Patches of erythema appear, which become prominent, and then pale in the centre, extending in size. They are often of a circular shape, or like the figure 8; they frequently ulcerate; their most common situation is on the tonsils, the sides of the tongue, or near the frænum; they are met with less frequently at the corner of the mouth, and on the dorsum of the tongue. Generally the patient has other secondary symptoms at the same time.

Mercurial Fumigation.—"The patient, having undressed, is seated naked on a chair in a large box, his head being the only part exposed to the air. This box is heated by a furnace, on which the bisulphuret of mercury is placed, in the proportion of three drachms for each vapor-bath. The intense heat applied soon volatilizes the mercury, which quickly fills the well-closed chamber or box with a leaden-colored vapor that condenses on the body of the patient, who is exposed to its influence for twenty minutes, during the last ten of which he perspires profusely. The box is then opened, and the surface of the body is gently wiped, so as only to remove the drops of perspiration; a gown is now thrown over the body, and towels twisted round his legs, and the patient laid on a bed, thus swaddled up, between two blankets, which are tucked carefully round him, and additional covering added. The patient is now left for half an hour, during which he perspires freely, and a glass of toast and water may be given. At the end of this time, the wet clothes should be removed, and the patient thoroughly rubbed down; after dressing he should not at once expose himself to the open air, but remain a short time in a cool room. The vapor, thus administered, may be repeated two or three times a week, for a month or five weeks, and a cure of some of the most rebellious forms of secondary symptoms may be attained. It may be readily assumed that this treatment is one that cannot be easily carried into effect in the country, as the necessary conveniences are not at hand. In these instances, the vapor-bath may be had recourse to, and the cinnabar may be placed on a metal plate over a little charcoal furnace; but, from some experiments which I have instituted, I find that the mercurial vapor is so heavy, that it will not usually rise more than a foot, and the good effects of the fumigation will be slight, as compared with those arising from the real fumigating apparatus. The body should be covered with a dark powder when the apparatus is well applied, and gold leaf will detect the presence of mercury on every part of the body. The above remarks, perhaps, explain why fumigations have fallen into disrepute, as the proper means of application are not always at hand." *Part* xxiv., *p.* 266.

Treatment of the Syphilides—Formulæ.—The following is the prescription for the mistura hydrargyri bichloridi of the Pharmacopœia of the Hospital for Diseases of the Skin: R Of the bichloride of mercury, two drachms; of strong hydrochloric acid, one drachm; of spirits of camphor, two drachms; of burnt sugar, half a drachm; of water, a gallon. The dose is from a drachm to two drachms, each drachm containing a twelfth of a grain of the bichloride. An extemporaneous biniodide of mercury is also much used, the formula for the mixture being as follows: R Of the bichloride of mercury, two drachms; of the iodide of potassium, six ounces; of the tincture of cardamoms, two ounces; and of water, a gallon. Of this, the dose, a drachm, contains a tenth of a grain of the bichloride, and two grains of the iodide. Simultaneously with the use of either of these mixtures, Mr. Startin almost always orders the "red ointment" to be rubbed into the patches of eruption, or applied to any ulcers which may exist. The formula for this "unguentum rubrum," the prime favorite of the institution, is : of the bisulphuret of mercury, half an ounce; of the nitric oxide of mercury, half an ounce; of creasote, twenty minims; and of fresh lard, sixteen ounces. *Part* xxxvii., *p.* 316.

TINEA CAPITIS OR PORRIGO.

Treatment.—Dr. Graves directs attention to the following points :

When the disease is of long standing, always insert an issue in the arm before you attempt its cure. I have seen water on the brain and other fatal consequences, from neglect of this precaution.

If this disease has clearly originated from contagion and no other evidence of derangement of the general health can be detected, we must not, from the mere presence of the cutaneous affection, infer a constitutional taint, and must avoid the common error, of making the poor children undergo a course of alterative medicines.

This affection originating in contagious matter directly applied to the skin, cannot, like some varieties of lepra and psoriasis (to which it often bears a great resemblance), be cured by internal medicines, such as mercury, arsenic, and iodine, given separately or in combination.

When it occupies the hairy scalp, the common procedure of shaving the head is injudicious, for it adds to the irritation of the skin ; and the scalp can be sufficiently exposed by cutting the hair as close as possible with a sharp scissors.

The cure must be accomplished by removing the scales as far as that can be done by diligent ablution, without using any irritating degree of friction : and when the diseased portion of the skin has been thus exposed, we must next have recourse to some application which will destroy the morbid secreting surface. Formerly this was attempted by means of an endless variety of complicated formulæ, each of which had its advocates; the list may, however, be now reduced to a few simple remedies, and in truth, with nitrate of silver, sulphate of copper, or strong tincture of iodine, every case of this disease may be cured.

I never use the solid lunar caustic, or sulphate, but prefer a solution of ten, fifteen, or twenty grains to the ounce, as the case may require. As to the application of this solution, it will not do to apply it, as is generally done, with a camel's-hair pencil, *for it must be strongly rubbed into each spot*, for which purpose a small bit of sponge, covered with fine linen, and tied to the end of a quill or slender stick, should be employed. When a large portion of the scalp is affected, it will require some perseverance to apply this lotion in an effectual manner.

An application of this nature, when effectually done, must not be re. peated oftener than once a week.

Immediately after it the whole scalp must be covered with a spermaceti dressing, and the spermaceti must be renewed at least four times daily, so as to keep the head constantly moistened with it. The head is not to be washed for three days after the application of the caustic, or of the tincture of iodine, but then it may be well but very gently washed with yellow soap and water twice a day, taking care to cover, as before, with a spermaceti dressing after each washing.

In scaly diseases of the skin, it is quite surprising how much the cure is facilitated by keeping the affected parts constantly smeared with sperma. ceti, oil, melted suet, or even candle-grease. Without this aid, the use of caustics will often disappoint the practitioner.

When the above precautions have been taken, the cure will advance rapidly, and each succeeding application of the caustic solution, or if the tincture, may be less severe. *Part ii., p.* 69.

Tinea Capitis, or Porrigo. — Dr. Davidson makes some valuable remarks on the use of *ioduret of sulphur in porrigo,* and other cutaneous affections. The following are among the cases given :

C. B., aged 10, was admitted to the Glasgow Royal Infirmary, on the 1st Feb. Scattered over the whole of the head were numerous thick greyish patches of scabs, which, when removed, left the surface underneath perfectly bare and shining, but in a day or two, numerous small pustules made their appearance, accompanied with considerable itching. The eruption appeared in the form of small pustules four years ago. In this case, the scabs were first softened by the constant application of poultices for two days; the head was then shaved. An ointment, composed of five grains of the bichloride of mercury to one ounce of axunge, was tried from the 5th of February to the 12th, without any improvement. The following was then employed :

R. Iodur. sulphur. Ðij.; axungiæ, ʒij. misce.

This ointment was applied daily to the head ; and in a few days a decided amendment was remarked.

On the 5th of March, the following report was taken.—Pustules and scales are now completely gone, but there are some bald patches on head in situation of eruption ; no itching; surface of skin pretty natural; general health good.

He was dismissed in a few days afterward.

James R., aged 12, was admitted on the 10th Feb. The whole of the head and neck was covered with thick laminated yellowish scabs, which were easily removed. Some yellowish pretty large pustules were situated behind the ears, but on the scalp they were not distinct, the hair being matted together. A fetid ichorous matter was discharged, and numerous pediculi nestled everywhere on the head. He had had the eruption for two and a half years, but the general health was pretty good.

A poultice was applied for a day, after which the following ointment was applied, even before the shaving of the head, in order to extinguish the pediculi, which it effectually did in twenty-four hours.

R. Iodur. sulphur., Ðij.; axungiæ, ʒij. Misce.

He was dismissed perfectly cured on the 29th February, or in about a fortnight after the commencement of the ointment, the skin being quite natural in appearance, without itching, and the hair growing naturally over the whole head.

D. M'I., aged 10, admitted 30th December. The whole head, particularly the forehead, was covered with a thick, dry, greyish white crust, accompanied with itching, but without discharge. The disease was of four years' duration, and was represented to be of a very inveterate kind. General health good; bowels regular; tongue clean; pulse 80.

R. Iodur. sulphur., Əij.; axungiæ, ʒj. Misce.

A fortnight after the use of the ointment, the eruption is reported to be quite gone, and the skin covering the scalp natural in appearance.

As a precautionary measure, it was continued till the 22d, when he was dismissed.

Observations.—Porrigo, in all its forms, is often a very unmanageable disease, and even when cured is very liable to return. In the treatment of porriginous affections, the following is a more particular account than what is given in the short history of the cases. The head is first well washed with soap and water, the hair is then cut as short as possible with the scissors, a poultice is applied, and continued for a day or two if necessary, to soften the crusts, which being removed as thoroughly as possible, the hair is closely shaved. In general, the ointment is not applied until the head has been shaved; but if pediculi be present, it is employed from the commencement, in order speedily to extinguish these vermin. The proportion of ioduret of sulphur employed has varied from 20 to 40 grains to one ounce of axunge.

As a general rule, the daily application of the ointment will be sufficient; but, in some cases, it is advisable to use it twice a day, in order to facilitate the cure.

Alteratives, or any particular internal treatment, have rarely been resorted to, when the general health was tolerably good. Laxatives have occasionally been prescribed, and a mild farinaceous or milk diet.

Part v., *p.* 115.

Tinea Capitis or Porrigo.—Topical Application of Iodine and its Compounds.—Dr. James J. Ross remarks as follows, regarding the topical use of tincture of iodine in cases of porrigo:

The next instance we shall bring forward of the external use of tincture of iodine is in porrigo, or, more generally speaking, ringworm of the scalp, comprising all those affections, described as tinea, porrigo, eczema, impetigo, etc. The diagnosis of these various forms, which run one into another, is often exceedingly doubtful, and, what is of more consequence, their cure is often difficult, and frequently exhausts the patience both of patient and surgeon. Hundreds of applications have been used in the treatment of ringworm, and their very number proclaims their inefficiency; while in many cases, there can be no doubt, that the cure ultimately effected, ought rather to be referred to the natural dying-out, as it were, of the disease in course of time, than to the particular remedy in use at the moment. In such circumstances, then, we are all much indebted to Dr. Graves, who has laid down certainly the most successful plan of treatment I have yet had an opportunity of trying. He recommends as a precautionary measure, that, if the disease has been of long standing, an issue should be inserted in the arm, before attempting its cure. He condemns shaving the head, for it adds to the irritation of the skin, and the scalp can be sufficiently exposed by cutting the hair as closely as possible with a sharp scissors.   The next object is to remove the concreted scales, which lie over and conceal the diseased skin : this is to be accomplished by diligent ablution, without using any irritating degree of friction.   We must next have recourse to some application, which will destroy the morbid secreting surface, or those vegetable fungi, which, according to some late observers, constitute the true pathology of the disease.   For this purpose, Dr. Graves recommends either the tincture of iodine, or a solution of lunar caustic, or blue-stone, 10, 15, or 20 grains to the ounce, as the case may require. Since reading Dr. Graves' paper, I have in several instances used the tincture of iodine, and have since been far more successful than before.   "As to the application of, this solution, or the tincture," continues Dr. G., "it will not do to apply it, as is generally done, with a camel's-hair brush, *for it must be strongly rubbed into each spot,* for which purpose a small bit of sponge, covered with fine linen, and tied to the end of a quill or slender stick, should be employed.   When a large portion of the scalp is affected, it will require some perseverance to apply the lotion, or tincture, in an effectual manner.   An application of this nature, when effectually done, must not be repeated oftener than once a week.   Immediately after it, the scalp must be covered with a spermaceti dressing, and the spermaceti must be renewed at least four times daily, so as to keep the head constantly moistened with it.   The head is not to be washed for three days after the application of the caustic, or the tincture of iodine, but then it may be well, but very gently, washed with yellow soap and water twice a day ; taking care to cover, as before, with a spermaceti dressing after each washing."   The doctor adds, "when the above precautions have been taken, the cure will advance rapidly, and each succeeding application of the caustic solution, or of the tincture, may be less severe."   I have been thus particular in transcribing Dr. Graves' directions, as there is no disease more troublesome to the practitioner, and as, from experience, I can bear testimony to the efficacy of his mode of treatment, as above explained. The surgeon, when applying the iodine or caustic, should have his hands protected by gloves.   *Part* vi., *p.* 120.

Tinea Favosa—Treatment.—The mode of treatment of this obstinate disease, employed by the *frères* Mahon, although kept secret by them, has for a long time been followed with unquestionable benefit in the Parisian hospitals.
The hair is first cut short, and the crusts then removed by emolient poultices.   The head is now frequently washed with soap and water, and the inunctions and lotions continued until the scalp is completely cleaned. When this has been effected, the second stage of the treatment commences, the object of which is to remove the hair *slowly* and *without* pain, from all the points of the scalp, occupied by the favus.   Every second day the ointment (No. 1) is applied, and its use continued according to the obstinacy of the case.   On the intervening days the hair is combed with a fine comb, to remove the loose hairs.   This mode of treatment having been continued for about a fortnight, a depilatory powder (No. 2) is sprinkled through the hair once a week ; on the following day the hair is combed, and the depilatory ointment applied as before.   At the end of a month or six weeks a more active ointment is applied every day ; and as the disease gives way the frictions are made only once a week, until the redness of

the skin has entirely disappeared. Although the formulæ of the remedies employed by the *Frères* Mahon have been kept secret, yet their composition has been very nearly ascertained by experiment and are supposed to be as follows :—

No. 1.—Slaked lime, eight scruples ; soda of commerce, twelve scruples ; lard, sixty-four scruples.

No. 2.—Wood-ashes, sixty-four parts ; pulverized charcoal, thirty-two parts.

Lotion.—Lime-water, five hundred parts ; sulphate of soda, one hundred and eighty-five parts ; alcohol, twenty-four parts ; white soap, ten parts.

Part viii., *p.* 159.

Scald Head, Ringworm of Scalp, etc.—In one of the meetings of the Westminster Medical Society, Mr. Fisher refers to the practice of treating scald head, ringworm, etc., in Brussels. This is by an ointment chiefly composed of wood soot. The common soot of the chimney is collected, placed in a quantity of water, and macerated by a gentle heat for four days ; the fluid is then strained and evaporated in an open vessel to the consistence of treacle. An equal portion of this and common lard are mixed together and applied to the part affected night and morning. The head is shaved occasionally and thoroughly washed every third day. It is supposed that the efficacy of this ointment depends upon the creasote and pyroligneous acid which it contains :

Dr. Sayer observes, that the ointment used in Brussels years ago, with so much efficacy, consisted of equal parts of charcoal, so burnt as to retain its pyroligneous acid, nitrate of potash and common brimstone, worked up with hog's lard into an unguent, and applied night and morning. The head was, moreover, washed daily with soft soap containing a great quantity of alkali, and shaved every fourth day. *Part* ix., *p.* 172.

Treatment of Porrigo.—Dr. Corrigan states that nothing is easier than to give the appearance of having cured the disease. It is merely necessary to poultice the head, or part it is on, when the scab all comes off, leaving a shining red surface, then to wash it, when it looks clean, and thus make it look as if cured. After many applications, a week, fortnight, or month, may pass over, but in all those instances where I had the opportunity of afterward observing the case, the small favi began again to show themselves, and the disease then rapidly shot up again, and spread ; indeed, so certainly was this the case, that I at last began to think the disease was incurable. To reflecting on the nature of the disease, I owe the thought of a remedy on which I place considerable reliance—it is the local application of oxymuriate of mercury, which has much power in destroying the sporula of cryptogamic plants. I have used it in the form of ointment in the proportion of five grains in very fine powder to ʒj. of ung. cetacei ; I have used it in the proportion of 10 grains to ʒj., but it sometimes gives pain in this larger proportion. A small portion of the ointment is rubbed in on the part affected every day. It has not salivated in any instance in which I have employed it. *Part* xii., *p.* 255.

Porrigo.—Mr. Startin submits the following : The first procedure I would dwell upon as most necessary to success (I speak of course from my own experience) is to avoid all unnecessary irritation ; do not use soap or apply cold lotions, or poultices, or narcotics that by their absorption may occasion fatal effects, as tobacco, etc. Do not shave the head, but use scissors, cutting the hair as close as possible, and use all applications without force or friction, following the grain of the hair, and extract with the forceps those hairs only which are loose, and can be removed without pain. The directions I am in the habit of giving are as follows: Soften the crusts, if necessary, by applying flannel wrung out of water as steaming hot as possible, without scalding or injury to the head, till the hair can be cut short with scissors, so that the root of every hair may be visible without touching the parts; wash the head with half of the yolk of a fresh egg and tepid water; dry it with a soft cloth, and anoint with an ointment adapted to the case, which in porrigo should be a sulphureous application; in impetigo the iodides of mercury or of sulphur; in pityriasis calomel, white or red precipitate of mercury; and in eczema the bisulphuret of mercury, and sometimes the black oxide of manganese; all these ingredients may be combined with creasote, with camphor, etc., as well as variously intermingled, bearing in mind that the proportions of each article must not exceed Əj. to ʒj. of lard, which is better than any oleaginous substance of which I have made trial. Of course the internal treatment must correspond to the nature of the particular affection, its stage, and the constitutional symptoms manifested. It will also be advantageous that the patient wear a light linen or silk cap, which is by no means to be rendered impervious to perspiration, but to be of a kind that can be washed daily; the lining of hats, bonnets, etc., must also be frequently cleansed and renewed. If these recommendations be attended to, I can assure you from my own experience, that a complaint which ordinarily lasts for years may be subdued in as many weeks or months.   *Part* xiv., *p.* 236.

Porrigo Scutulata (Willan)—Herpes Tonsurans (Cazenave)—(Ringworm.)—Mr. Erichsen advises to shave the head, and apply one of the stronger acids to the part. The strong acetic answers best. It may be applied by means of a piece of sponge tied to a stick, and should only be used for a few minutes. Nothing more should be done for a week or ten days, when the crust produced by the acid should be separated with a pair of scissors, and if there be any appearance of the disease remaining, the acetic acid should be applied again; but if it present a healthy appearance, let it be well washed with soap and water, and a little olive oil applied every night. When all the vegetable organisms constituting the disease have been destroyed, then use a stimulating ointment, as the ung. creasote, ʒss. to ʒj. to the ounce of lard; or apply tincture of iodine by means of a camel's-hair brush; or the ung. hyd. biniodid., diluted with six parts of the ung. picis liquid.; or a mixture of equal parts of sulphur and pitch ointment; or the carb. of potass ointment, ʒss. to ʒj. to the ounce of lard. It is often useful to alternate some of these remedies; the head should also be washed three or four times a day with a lotion of the sulphuret of potass dissolved in lime water, or with carbonate of potass dissolved in water, or with soft soap and water. Attend to the general health; if the child be of a delicate habit or scrofulous, give iron and tonics, quinine with infus. quassiæ, and a nutritious diet. All heating articles of diet are improper, also salted food; the diet should be plain, but nutritious.   *Part* xiv:, *p.* 243.

Porrigo Declavans.—According to Dr. Coley, we should not remove the hairs; but rub solution of sulphate of copper upon the bald patches for several minutes, three times a day; and give a purgative occasionally. And in *Porrigo Favosa* apply twice a-day the ung. hydr. ammon. chlorid., and give a calomel and jalap powder every three days. Treat *P. lupinosa* in the same manner. *Part* xv., *p.* 254.

Oil of Juniper in Scald Head.—The direct application of the oil of the juniperus communis has been already proved to be successful in scrofulous ophthalmia, scabies, and eczema. Dr. Sully has found besides, that it is efficacious in the most inveterate forms of scald head. His formula is, oil of juniper, one ounce and a half; axunge, two ounces; essence of aniseed, six drops. The oil may also be applied unmixed; but in either case it should be applied freely over the whole affected surface.
Part xv., *p.* 255.

Creasote in Porrigo.—Speaking of the treatment of *Porrigo Senilis,* Dr. Bellingham says: Before concluding, I may observe that the efficacy of creasote, as a local application in cutaneous disease, is not limited to cases of prurigo. In that comparatively rare, but very intractable form of disease of the scalp, the *favus confertus* of Erichsen, which is known under a great variety of names, as the porrigo scutulata, tinea annularis, scald head and ringworm of the scalp, which constitutes one of the few contagious diseases of the scalp, and is one of the few which occasions the destruction of the bulbs of the hair, and for the cure of which that most painful application, *the pitch cap*, was in former times supposed to be essential, creasote in the form of ointment and lotion will be found a most effectual remedy, provided its use is persevered in for a sufficient length of time, and attention is at the same time paid to cleanliness. On the other hand, in the vesicular and pustular diseases of the scalp, in which the eruption is usually preceded or accompanied by more or less inflammation, evidenced by the heat, redness, soreness, and discharge, creasote as a local application will be found to disagree, and will rather aggravate than relieve the disease. *Part* xvi., *p.* 223.

Ointment for Scald Head.—Norway pitch, 30 parts; turpeth mineral, 15 parts; red oxide of mercury, 15 parts; lard, 100 parts. Mix. The ointment to be applied night and morning. *Part* xvii., *p.* 196.

Favus.—By those not well accustomed to the diagnosis of skin diseases, favus has often been confounded with other eruptions of the scalp, more especially eczema and impetigo, or the combinations of these diseases known as the eczema impetiginodes; but in none of these do the yellow crusts or scales present, when examined microscopically, traces of vegetation. This furnishes the real diagnostic and pathognomonic character of the disease. There can be no doubt the disease is inoculable, and capable of being communicated by contagion. The pathology of favus is best understood by considering it essentially to be a form of anormal nutrition, with exudation of a matter analogous to, if not identical with, that of tubercle, which constitutes a soil for the germination of cryptogamic plants, the presence of which, as stated, is pathognomonic of the disease. As favus is in many cases a constitutional disease, and dependent upon the causes inducing scrofulous diseases in general, the treatment must be constitutional, and directed to remove the tendency to tubercular exudation. The internal and external exhibition of cod-liver oil with appropriate diet and exercise, has been attended by most marked advantage. As to the local treatment, Professor Bennett directs the affected scalp to be poulticed for several days, until the favus crusts are thoroughly softened and fall off, then the head to be carefully shaved, and lastly, cod-liver oil to be applied with a soft brush, night and morning, and the head covered with an oil-skin cap to prevent evaporation, and further exclude the atmospheric air.

Every now and then the accumulated and inspissated oil should be removed by gently washing it with soap and water. Whenever favus is recent, and of limited extent, it may be at once destroyed by cauterization with nitrate of silver.   *Part* xxii., *p.* 238.

Apparatus for Fumigating the Scalp, in some Chronic Diseases of that Region.—Dr. Burgess has recommended fumigation of the scalp in certain of its diseases. He thus describes the apparatus he uses for that purpose:

The vapor apparatus is extremely simple. It consists of a tin jar, about ten inches by four, with a conducting tube, on which is placed a stop-cock, for the purpose of diluting the vapor, or turning it off, and an elastic cap of vulcanized india-rubber, which fits closely to the head, so as to prevent the vapor from escaping. The great majority of diseases of the skin are constitutional, and those of the scalp are not an exception to the rule.

Favus (the *porrigo favosa* of Wilan), for example, which is one of the most unsightly, as well as the most inveterate of the eruptions of that region, may be temporarily relieved by tonics and fomentations, and the skin even made to appear clean and healthy; but the *virus* still remains, and, consequently, the "cure" will be but of short duration. In this, as in other inveterate diseases of the scalp, the application of vapor, simple or medicated, as the case may require, to the diseased scalp, will be found a very efficient remedy. Where the object is, to *alter the vitality of the parts*, it can be done more effectually by the repeated application of stimu-lating vapor (the skin being previously cleansed with any detergent wash) than by the employment of caustic lotions or ointments. Indeed, greasy applications of every kind may be advantageously dispensed with in the treatment of diseases of the scalp.

That variety of baldness, which is the result of atony, or disordered nu-trition of the hair-follicles and bulbs, will be materially benefited by the use of the vapor apparatus.   *Part* xxi., *p.* 259.

Cachexia Eczematosa in Children.—This disease is very common amongst the ill-fed and neglected children of the lower classes. There is a pale and sickly aspect, and on different parts of the scalp the hair is mat-ted together with filthy scabs of eczematous secretion, from which exudes a thin and irritating discharge. There are also weak ulcerations behind the ears, and about the angles of the mouth, and on the nares, etc.

There is no eruptive disease more easily got rid of than this, says Dr. W. S. Oke, provided the treatment be carefully carried out. The whole of the scalp having been closely clipped, and the scabs removed by poultice or fomentation, the eczematous parts are to be smeared by the ointment, 1, twice a day, and well fomented before each application. The alterative dose, 2, is to be given twice a week, and the strength supported by 3. By these means the removal of the disease will be at once accomplished.

1.—℞ Unguenti hydrarg. nit. oxidi, oz. ss. Bis die applicandum digito.

2:—℞ Hydrarg. cum cretâ, gr. iij.; pulv. rhei, gr., iv.; pulv. cinnamomi, gr. j. Misce; fiat pulvis bis hebdomadâ sumendus in theriacâ.

3.—℞ Quinæ disulphatis, gr. ij.–iij.; acidi sulphurici dil., gtt. vj.; tinct. aurantii, co. syrupi zingib. sing, dr. ij.; aquæ destillatæ, ad oz. iij. Misce capiat cochleare largum bis quotidie. *Part* xxvi., *p.* 292.

Treatment of Favus.—After removing the crusts of favus by poulticing and shaving the head, keep the surface moist with cod-liver oil, or use Dr. Jenner's lotion, composed of one part of sulphurous acid mixed with three parts of water, in the following way: Saturate lint with this lotion and apply it all over the scalp night and morning, keeping it moist by an oil-silk cap. *Part* xxix., *p.* 248.

Treatment of Favus.—From the observation of about a dozen cases of severe favus (diagnosis by the microscope in all) recently treated by Mr. Startin at the Hospital for skin diseases, we can speak with great confidence of the efficiency of the following ointment. It is the ung. sulph. comp. of the pharmacopœia of that institution:

℞ Sulph. sublimati, ℔ss.; hydrarg. ammonio-chlorid., ℨss.; hydr. sulphureti cum sulph., ℨss.; leviga simul, dein adde olivæ olei, ℥iv.; adipis recentis, ℥xvj.; creasoti, m xx. Misce.

To correct the state of general health, Mr. Startin commonly orders simultaneously a mild course of the iodide of potassium, but this, we suspect, has but a small share, if any, in the local result.

In a most disgusting disease for which as yet no real cure is known, it is much to be in possession of an almost certain means of insuring its absence. The ointment no doubt acts as a parasiticide. Before its first application it is desirable to clear away the crust as much as possible, either by fomentation or a poultice.

We may remark, that the ointment mentioned is used by Mr. Startin in the treatment of scabies, and also in that of the contagious form of porrigo. *Part* xxx., *p.* 177.

*   *

Porrigo.—The treatment now in vogue for this affection in Guy's Hospital is the iodide of lead ointment and alkaline lotions, with the internal use of the iodide of arsenic. *Part* xxxiii., *p.* 236.

URTICARIA.

In a case of this disease, says Dr. Maclagan, where the urine was of low specific gravity (1010), and was found on examination to be much deficient in urea and uric acid, colchicum was employed with complete success. The urine before taking colchicum was of a pale straw color, transparent, and left no deposit on standing.

Colchicum was then administered, and a fortnight after the urine was again examined. The *urea* was more than triple in his amount, and raised above the normal standard. The increase of *uric acid* was in a tenfold ratio, whilst the other organic constituents and water suffered a corresponding diminution, the inorganic salts remaining nearly as before. *Part* xxv., *p.* 264.

Treatment of Urticaria.—It sometimes happens, says Dr. G. Budd, that a nettle-rash resulting from defective digestion is brought on not merely by some one substance, but by several substances in common use; and it is then very difficult to detect the offending substances or to prevent the disorder by any restriction of diet to which the patient will submit.

Where it arises from defective digestion, give a dinner pill, containing three or four grains of rhubarb, and from half to one and a half grains of ipecacuanha. This remedy is a very valuable one in slowness of digestion.

It sometimes happens, especially in women, that the nettle-rash, though depending immediately on the stomach, occurs only when digestion is weakened by over-fatigue, or by anxiety or some other mental emotion, or by profuse monthly discharges, and that remedies of a different class are availing.

In some such cases, where all the means spoken of failed, the eruption was known to disappear under the use of carbonate of ammonia, alone or in conjunction with tincture of gentian.

Serpentaria is another remedy that has obtained some repute in the treat ment of this disorder. An excellent application for allaying the irritation of nettle-rash, whatever be its cause, is a lotion made by mixing ₃ss. of acetate of lead and ₃ss. of tincture of opium with ₃viij. of water.

Part xxix., *p.* 106.

Treatment of, by Quinine.—A severe case, in which the eruption had come out daily for the last six months, presented itself a few days ago. The patient was a married woman, of middle age, and of nervous tempera- ment. The following was the prescription ordered :

℞ Quin. disulph., gr. xij. ; am. sesquicarb., ₃j. ; magnes. carbon., ₃ss. ; aq. pur., ₃viij. Ft. mist. ₃ss. ter. die sumend.

The quinine in this formula is of course undissolved, and the magnesia is added in order to suspend it. To relieve the itching of the eruption, a lotion containing the dilute nitric acid was ordered to be used. With regard to the latter, it may be worth remarking, that Mr. Startin believes it quite as useful as the hydrocyanic acid for the relief of tingling, etc., while it is very much less expensive. *Part* xxx., *p.* 236.

Urticaria.—This, says Prof. Budd, is generally caused by the imperfect digestion of particular articles of food, such as crabs, muscles, pork-pie, fish, honey, mushrooms, cucumbers, almonds, and oatmeal. Our main object of treatment must therefore be to expel the offending matter as soon as possible ; this is best done by an emetic, followed by a warm quick purga- tive. If it seems rather to be referable to several articles in common use, it may be kept off by the administration of a few grains of rhubarb before dinner ; it may occur from weak digestion, attended with general debility ; in such cases the carbonate of ammonia, with the tincture of gentian, will succeed when other means fail. To allay the cutaneous irritation use a lotion composed of half a drachm of acetate of lead, half an ounce of tinc- ture of opium and half a pound of water. *Part* xxxiv., *p.* 197.

MISCELLANEOUS.

Arsenic in Chronic Scaly Eruptions.—Mr. Erichsen lays great stress upon the necessity of attending particularly to the constitution and tempe- rament of the patient before commencing the use of the medicine. It will be badly borne by individuals of a plethoric habit of body, or of a highly sanguine or sanguineo-nervous temperamant—this arises from the stimu- lating properties of the metal. In such cases, the digestive organs become so irritated, and the nervous system so excited under the use of the arsenic, that it is impossible to employ it in any such dose as can be expected to produce a beneficial effect upon the cutaneous affection. There are other circumstances which contra-indicate the use of this remedy, namely, "the complication of the cutaneous affection with other diseases," and especially with irritative or inflammatory gastric dyspepsia, accompanied with a sensation of heat and oppression at the epigastrium, increased by food, so well described by Dr. Todd. When this form of dyspepsia is present, the smallest doses of arsenic will do harm, as the usual effect of the remedy, when continued too long, is to produce these very symptoms. Besides this form of indigestion, any other local inflammatory condition of the system, or the supervention of phthisis, will contra-indicate the use of so powerfully stimulating a tonic as arsenic. Another important circumstance to attend to is the kind of disease, and the stage in which to use it. The indiscriminate use of this article in certain diseases of the skin, has no doubt frequently brought discredit upon it.

One great principle to be held in view in its use is never to administer it in the early, acute, and inflammatory stages of the affection. The solution of the arsenite of potassa (Fowler's solution), and the solution of the iodide of arsenic and mercury (Donovan's solution), are the two preparations which are most frequently prescribed in this country; and the former is by far the most popular of the two. Different authors vary a little as to the dose of Fowler's solution which ought to be given; but most of them agree that we ought not to exceed 15, or at most 18 drops in the course of the day. Mr. Erichsen, however, begins with two minims of the solution twice a-day, and increases the dose to 5, 6, or 7½ minims three times a-day, beyond which, he says, it ought not to be carried, as its good effects will be more evident from small doses continued for some time, than from larger doses which have to be sooner relinquished. Some patients, however, are so excitable, that the smallest doses are inadmissible. Another good preparation is the iodide of arsenic introduced by Dr. A. T. Thompson. The dose is the twelfth of a grain twice a day, to be increased to the sixth or fourth of a grain three times a-day, although these doses are seldom necessary. It is well to combine the extract of conium with iodide of arsenic, in order to sheath its irritating qualities, and prevent it from exciting too powerfully the mucous membrane of the stomach. By the addition of the biniodide of mercury, a compound pill may be formed, which resembles in its effects the liquor of the hydriodate of arsenic and mercury, and which has been found by Dr. A. T. Thompson very efficacious in lupus, and by Mr. Erichsen in some syphilitic eruptions, more particularly when of a squamous kind. A pill may be made containing one-twelfth of a grain of the biniodide of mercury, and two grains of the extract of conium; to be given twice a-day. The iodide of arsenic may be gradually increased to one-sixth of a grain, and the biniodide of mercury omitted at the end of a fortnight, or sooner, as it might affect the gums. The diluted biniodide of mercury ointment may in some cases, as in syphilitic psoriasis, be also applied externally at the same time. Arsenic seems to be an excitant or stimulating tonic, acting chiefly on the digestive, nervous, and integumentary systems; and when the dose has been pushed so as to irritate any one of these parts, the medicine ought to be immediately suspended, or greatly reduced in strength. The time for prescribing arsenic in a cutaneous affection requires, perhaps, as nice a discrimination as can be exercised. Mr. Erichsen points out a mode of practice which will be generally serviceable in these cases. As it is in the chronic stages that the remedy is to be used, he first ascertains whether the affection will bear the topical application of mild stimulants, such as the ointment of the white precipitate, or the nitrate of mercury diluted with equal parts of the spermaceti ointment, or a solution of the sulphuret of potassium in the proportion of about a drachm to the pint; and if any of these applications can be borne without increasing permanently the severity of the disease, the internal administration of arsenic may likewise be beneficial. In illustration of this opinion he adduces as an example that very common disease, eczema, which, when in its acute stage, in which it will bear no other topical application that the most soothing poultices and fomentations, will infallibly be greatly increased in severity by the employ-ment of arsenic, even in its most minute doses; but at a more advanced period, when it can bear topical stimulants, the same disease will be greatly benefited by the internal administration of this medicine. The diseases of the skin for which arsenic is recommended, may be of very different kinds, but they all agree in this, that they are characterized by the pre-sence of scales or scurf; and even when they do not belong to the order *squamæ* they are usually but little benefited until they arrive at that stage in which they assume a furfuraceous or scaly condition.

Part viii., *p.* 10.

Selection from the Formulary of Biett on Diseases of the Skin—Internal Remedies.—Subcarbonate of soda, half, to one drachm; barley-water, one pint. Dose, four glasses daily. Use: Lichen; prurigo; chronic diseases with itching.

Decoction of Dulcamara.—Dulcamara, half an ounce; water, a pint and a half. Boil down to two-thirds. The quantity of the remedy may be increased to one ounce, or an ounce and a half. Dose, half a glass at first; then a glass, morning and evening. Use, lepra vulgaris; chronic diseases.

Decoction of Orma.—Orma pyramidalis, four ounces; water, four pints; boil down to a half. Dose, two to four glasses a day. Use: Scaly diseases.

Sirup of fumaria, twelve ounces; sirup of viola tricolor, four ounces; bisulphate of soda, two drachms. Mix. [M. Biett often employed this mixture in cases of eczema, lichen, and several chronic diseases of the skin.] Dose, two spoonfuls a day.

Sirup of fumaria, a pint; bicarbonate of soda, three drachms. Dose, two teaspoonfuls; one before breakfast; the other at bedtime. Use: eczema; lichen; prurigo.

Pearson's Solution.—Arsenite of soda, four grains; water, four ounces. Dose, from twelve drops to a drachm or more. Use: most chronic dis-eases of the skin; eczema, impetigo, lichen; but chiefly in squamous dis-eases, lepra, psoriasis, etc.

Fowler's Solution.—Arsenious acid, and carbonate of potass, of each seventy-eight grains; distilled water a pint; alcohol, half an ounce. Use: the same as Pearson's solution. Dose, three or four drops, gradually increased to twelve or fifteen.

M. Biett's Solution.—Arsenite of ammonia, four grains; water, four ounces. Use: same as above. Dose, same as Pearson's solution.

Larrey's Sirup.—Sudorific sirup, one pint; bichloride of mercury, hydro-chlorate of ammonia, and extract of opium, of each five grains; Hoffman's liquor, half a drachm. Dose, half an ounce to two ounces. Use: syphilitic eruptions. Sirup of mezereon, two ounces; balsam of tolu, four ounces; subcarbonate of ammonia, half an ounce. Dose, a spoonful morning and evening. Use: constitutional syphilis.

Van Swieten's Liquor.—Bichloride of mercury, eighteen grains; water, twenty-nine ounces; alcohol, three ounces. Dose, a teaspoonful daily, in a glass of decoction of sarsaparilla. Each ounce contains a little more than half a grain. Use: secondary syphilis.

Powders—Pills.—sublimed sulphur, magnesia, of each half an ounce. Make eighteen packets. Dose, one daily. Use: chronic eczema; scaly diseases.

Proto-ioduret of mercury, twelve grains; extract of lettuce, two scruples. Make forty-eight pills. Dose, one to four. Use: syphilis. Or,

Proto-ioduret of mercury, half a drachm; extract of guaiacum, one drachm; extract of lettuce, two scruples; sirup of sarsaparilla, q. s. Divide into seventy-two pills. Dose, one, and then two daily. Use: syphilis.

Bichloride of Mercury.—Extract of aconite, six grains; bichloride of mercury, two grains; marshmallows powder, eight grains. Make eight pills. Dose, one to four. Use: syphilis.

Deuto-ioduret of Mercury.—Deuto-ioduret of mercury, six grains; marshmallows powder, half a drachm. Make thirty-six pills. Use: the same. Dose, two or three a day.

M. Sedillot's Pills.—Strong mercurial ointment, one drachm; soap, two scruples; mallows powder, one scruple. Make thirty-six pills. Dose, two or three daily. Use: the same.

M. Biett's Pills.—Mercurial ointment, powdered sarsaparilla, of each a drachm. Make forty-eight pills. Use: the same. Dose, one to four daily. Or,

Phosphate of mercury, half a drachm; extract of fumaria, one drachm. Make forty-eight pills. Dose, one to two a day. Use: as before.

Aconite Pills.—Extract of aconite, half a drachm; mallows powder, two scruples. Make forty-eight pills. Dose, one or two morning and evening. Use: syphilitic eruptions; nocturnal pains.

Arsenic Pills.—Arsenious acid, one grain; black pepper powdered, twelve grains; gum arabic, two grains; water. q. s. Make twelve pills. Dose, one or two a day.

Arsenite of Iron—M. Biett.—Arsenite of iron, three grains; extract of hop, one drachm; mallows powder, half a drachm; orange flower sirup, q. s. Make forty-eight pills; each contains the one-sixteenth of a grain. Dose, one daily. Use: the two preceding formulæ are chiefly used in cases of chronic eczema and lichen; in the scaly diseases, lepra, lupus, and psoriasis.

Arsenite of Soda—M. Biett.—Extract of aconite, one scruple; arsenite of soda, two grains. Make twenty-four pills. Dose, one or two daily. Use: as above.

Hydrochlorate of Iron.—Hydrochlorate of iron, twelve grains; gentian, in powder, twenty-four grains. Make twelve pills. Dose, one to four daily. Use: employed with success by M. Biett in scrofulous eruptions.

Sulphate of Iron—M. Biett.—Sulphate of iron, one scruple; powdered mallows, twelve grains; sirup, q. s. Make twelve pills. Use and dose the same.

Part ix., *p.* 73.

Use of Tar in Cutaneous Diseases.—[Mr. Wetherfield published, in 1845, an account of several intractable cases of skin disease which were cured by the use of *tar*, after arsenic and other favorite remedies had been tried in vain. As he still finds the remedy a valuable one, Mr. W. again calls the attention of the profession to the subject. He says:]

Tar was administered in these cases in capsules, each containing ten minims of simple Stockholm tar, and was first prescribed in this form by Dr. Sutro, of the German Hospital. This mode of administering the tar removes every objection on the score of taste to the use of this valuable remedy, which doubtless would still have enjoyed all the credit it obtained at the time its virtues were so much extolled in the works of Bishop Berkeley, but for its nauseous flavor in the then mode of administering, viz., tar water.

Acne.—Two obstinate cases of this disease, of several years' standing, were published in the report. The face, neck, and shoulders were much covered and disfigured by the eruption, which had withstood all kinds of treatment. One capsule was given three times a day, and continued for three months. The disease entirely disappeared.

Eczema Impetiginodes and Eczema Capillitii.—Both diseases nearly the same in character, the former attacking adults, the latter children. Two cases of the former disease, one of eight years', another one year's duration. Both cases were treated by the internal use of the capsule, and externally the ung. picis. liquid, continued between two and three months, with perfect success.

Eczema capillitii is most common in young persons, beginning on the scalp behind the ears; from thence extending to the body and limbs. Several obstinate cases, of from five to seven years' duration, have been treated with the capsules of tar and ung. picis liq. very successfully. In one case a bath of tar water was employed instead of the ung. picis, the child being but three years of age. Four ounces of tar, added to a sufficient quantity of water to cover the child's body and limbs, is the mode in which the tar bath may be made, and a very efficient remedy it is, free from the objection which might be raised against the ointment, of soiling the linen. This child took the capsules with perfect ease, and together with the warm tar bath used every other night, recovered in five weeks. Cases of this disease often run a course of five or seven years, resisting every, even the most potent remedies.

Lepra.—A case of this disease came under treatment. The patient was covered with leprous patches. He took the capsules about a month, and the disease decidedly diminished. He was unsteady in conduct, and irregular in his habits, and did not pursue the plan so as to derive all the benefit he might have done. The odor of tar was perceptible in his clothes worn next the skin.

Psoriasis Palmaris et Nasi.—In this disease, in addition to the internal use of the capsules, which should be persevered with a considerable time, the hands should be immersed in a bath of tar water every night for a quarter of an hour, then dried, and powdered with starch powder. In a case of psoriasis nasi, the cracks which form at the junction of the mucous membrane and true skin should be anointed with ung. picis liq. very slightly at bed-time, and washed off in the morning with warm water. In a case of this kind which annoyed the patient, who was a great snuff-taker, the disease was thus removed in a few days.

Prurigo Senilis.—Two cases in men, one of 85, and the other of 90 years of age. These gentlemen were subject to attacks of prurigo, attended as usual with desperate itching and irritation. Various remedies had been employed in vain ; lotions of hydrocyanic acid. hydr. bichlorid., etc., etc., The ung. picis liq. was applied freely on the legs, and over it an elastic roller, occasionally bathing the legs in bran water, to remove the deposit of tar from the skin. Fresh applications were made in this manner every second or third day. This plan soon allayed the itching. Both patients suffered repeatedly from this disease, but always found relief from this mode of treatment, and were often quite free from it for months together.

Sycosis.—A case of this disease, which had resisted a multitude of remedies, amongst others carbonate of iron in large doses, sarsaparilla and lime water, arsenic, mercury, etc., was cured by the internal use of tar in capsules, taken one morning and evening, which removed not only the mealy eruption, but pimples, which were a source of great annoyance and much pain in shaving.

Tar acts as a diuretic and diaphoretic. The odor of tar is distinctly perceptible in the urine of those who take it in capsules. The quantity is somewhat increased, and it is rendered clear and free from all deposits. A physician who took it for acne, and who had studied the analysis of urine long and carefully, told me he had found it entirely remove a deposit of phosphates to which he had been long subject. Increased perspiration, and the strong odor of tar on the linen of those who have taken it, clearly prove its action on the skin. In moderate doses it improves the digestive organs, and invigorates the general health.

Tar certainly deserves a trial in all chronic intractable and senile eruptions, where, owing to peculiar idiosyncrasy, arsenic cannot be administered.   *Part* xviii., *p.* 223.

Treatment of the more Common Forms of Skin Diseases.—According to Prof. Bennett, of Edinburgh, *Eczema* is by far the most common disease met with, both in its acute and chronic forms.

Prof. B. says : The local treatment I have found most efficacious, consists in keeping the affected part moist, with lint or linen saturated in a very weak alkaline solution, consisting of soda subcarb. 3ss. to a pint of water. For this purpose it is necessary to cover the moistened lint with oil-silk, or gutta percha sheeting, which should well overlap the lint below, so as to prevent evaporation. The usual effect is soon to remove all local irritation, and especially the itching or smarting so distressing to the patient; to keep the surface clean, and prevent the accumulation of those scabs and crusts, which in themselves often tend to keep up the disease. After a time, even the indurated parts begin to soften, the margins of the eruption lose their fiery red color, and merge into that of the healthy skin, and, finally, the whole surface assumes its normal character.

Herpes.—This disease generally runs its course in about fourteen days, and requires no treatment whatever, further than an acetate of lead lotion to allay the smarting. It is not very common.

Scabies occurs very frequently, and is cured by a host of remedies. A strong lather of common soft soap and warm water, twice a day, answers very well. The question with scabies, is not what remedy is useful, but which will cure it in the shortest period. The most extensive experience at St. Louis has shown, that the su.phur and alkaline, or Helmerinch's ointment, cures itch, on an average, in seven days. That sulphur, however, is not the active remedy, I have satisfied myself of by experiment. Soft soap, as we have seen, which contains alkali, and even simple lard, if pains be taken to keep the parts constantly covered with it, will cure the disease as soon as sulphur ointment. I have tried the Stavesacre ointment, recommended by M. Bourguignon, in only a few cases, but found it to answer very well.

Pemphigus.—This is rather a rare disease, and when chronic, coming out in successive crops, is very rebellious. Two cases which entered the infirmary last winter were cured in a few weeks by the weak alkaline wash, applied as in the case of eczema, combined with generous diet.

Impetigo.—This affection in all its forms is very common, and is best treated by the weak alkaline wash, exactly the same as in eczema. In the chronic forms which attack the chin of men, constituting one of the varieties of mentagra, the same treatment cures the most rebellious cases if the moisture be constantly preserved. For this purpose the hair must be cautiously cut short with sharp scissors, and the razor carefully avoided. If the side of the cheek covered with the whisker is attacked removal of the hair from thence also is essential to the treatment. A bag or covering accurately adapted to the part affected must be made of gutta percha sheeting, and tied on with strings. This may be covered with black silk, to allow the individual to go about and carry on his usual occupations. In this way I have frequently seen chronic impetigo of the chin, of from eight to ten years' standing, completely removed in a few weeks. But then the surface must be kept *constantly* moist, a circumstance requiring very great care and determination on the part of the patient. When it becomes necessary to shave, flour and warm water, or paste should be used, and not soap. Alkalies applied from time to time only, as in the form of wash or soap, always irritate, although, when employed continuously, they are soothing.

Ecthyma is not a common disease, and usually presents itself, as the *E. cacheticum*, requiring in addition to the alkaline wash locally, a generous diet.

Acne is a disease always requiring constitutional rather than local remedies. Although not uncommon in private, it is rare in hospital practice. Careful regulation of the diet, abstinence from wine and stimulating articles of food, watering-places, baths, etc., etc., constitute the appropriate treatment.

Rupia.—This disease I have never seen occur but in individuals who have been subjected to the influence of mercurial poisoning. Hydriodate of potassium and tonic remedies, with careful avoidance of mercury in all its forms, is the treatment I have found most successful.

Lichen and Prurigo.—In both these affections constant inunction with lard is as beneficial as constant moisture in the eczematous and impetiginous disorders. In the prurigo of aged persons, the ung. hyd. precip. alb. is a useful application, although the disease is not unfrequently so rebellious as only to admit of palliation. The chronic papular diseases often constitute the despair of the physician.   •

Psoriasis, and that modification of it known as *lepra*, are very common diseases, and are uniformly treated by me externally with pitch ointment. I have satisfied myself by careful trials, that it is the pitch applied to the part that is the beneficial agent, as I have given pitch pills, and infusion of pitch, largely internally without benefit. With the hope of obtaining a less disagreeable remedy, I have frequently tried creasote, and naphtha ointment and washes, but also without benefit. Lastly, I have caused simple lard to be rubbed in for a lengthened time, but without doing the slightest good. The oil of cade is also very useful, especially in psoriasis of the scalp. Internally, I give five drops each of Fowler's solution, and of the tr. cantharidis. It is rare that the internal treatment alone produces any effect on a case of psoriasis of any standing. If a case resists this conjoined external and internal treatment, I have always found it incurable. About a year ago I carefully treated a series of cases internally with Donovan's solution, without producing the slightest benefit.

Lupus is a constitutional disease, and must be treated by cod-liver oil, and all those remedies useful in scrofula, of which it is a local manifestation. The external treatment is surgical, consisting of the occasional application of caustics, red lotion, ointments, etc., according to the appearance of the sore.

Favus is a very common disease in Edinburgh, and is most readily removed, first, by poulticing the crusts till they fall off, and the skin presents a smooth, clean surface; secondly, by shaving the hair; and thirdly, by keeping the scalp continually covered with oil, so as to exclude the atmosphere, and prevent the growth of the parasitic fungi, which constitutes the disease. For this purpose, a gutta percha or oil silk cap must be constantly worn. A continuance of this treatment for six weeks produces a cure in young persons if combined with cod-liver oil, generous diet, and anti-scrofulous remedies internally. I have tried the lotion of sulphurous acid, recommended by Dr. Jenner, and found it successful in a few cases, but the treatment by oil is so easy, to be far preferable to it. Very chronic cases are cured with difficulty, but so long as the oil is applied the disease never returns, and mere freedom from the disgusting crusts is a great gain.

Scalp diseases must be treated according as it depends on eczema, impetigo, psoriasis, or favus, in all cases first removing the crusts with poultices, then keeping the head shaved, and lastly, applying alkaline washes, pitch ointment, or oil, according to the directions formerly given. Ringworm is a disease I have never seen in Edinburgh, and of what it consists I am ignorant. Some writers apparently consider it to be favus, and others a form of herpes. On two or three occasions I have seen a scaly disease of the scalp, in the form of a ring—that is lepra, which I have cured by pitch ointment, or oil of cade. My friend, Dr. Andrew Wood, informed me some time ago, that he banished it from the Heriot's Hospital school by condensing on the eruption the fumes of coarse brown paper, and thus causing an empyreumatic oil, or kind of tar, to fall upon the part. This has led me to suppose that it is a scaly disease, and a form of lepra or psoriasis.

So-called *syphilitic diseases* of the skin are, in my opinion, the various disorders already alluded to, modified by occurring in individuals who have suffered for periods more or less long from the poisonous action of mercury. A longer time will be required for their cure, but the same remedies locally, conjoined with hydriodate of potassium, in smaller doses, with bitter infusions, tonics, and a regulated diet, offer the best chance of success.

The great difficulty in the treatment of skin diseases generally consists in their having been mismanaged in the early stages—a circumstance I attribute to their not having, until a recent period, been much studied by clinical students. Many chronic cases of eczema are continually coming under my notice, which, in their acute forms, have been treated by citrine ointment, or other irritating applications, which invariably exasperate the disorder. I shall not easily forget the case of one gentleman, covered all over with acute eczema, who had suffered excessive torture from its having been mistaken for psoriasis, and rubbed for some time with pitch ointment. In the same way I have seen a simple herpes, which would have readily got well if left to itself, converted into an ulcerated sore, by the use of mercurial ointment. Nothing is more common than to confound chronic eczema of the scalp with the favus, although the microscope furnishes us with the most exact means of diagnosis. I need scarcely say that the correct application of the remedies I have spoken of can only be secured by an accurate discrimination, in the first instance, of the diseases to which they are applicable.

The general constitutional treatment in all these cases seldom demands aperient or lowering remedies except in young and robust individuals with febrile symptoms. In the great majority of cases, cod-liver oil, good diet, and tonics are required. In a few instances, sedatives, both locally and internally, are necessary to overcome excessive itching and irritation. These the judicious practitioner will readily understand how to apply according to circumstances. *Part* xxxi., *p.* 178.

Use of Collodion in Skin Diseases.--Mr. Wilson says: the diseases of the skin in which I have hitherto used the collodion with advantage are, chronic erythema of the face; intertrigo; chapped nipples and chapped hands; herpes labialis, preputialis, and herpes zoster; lichen agrius; lupus non exedens and exedens; acne vulgaris; and several affections of the sebiparous organs. In chronic erythema of the face, its contracting power was most usefully evinced, as it was also in lupus non exedens, and acne.

In a troublesome case of chapped hands and fingers, resulting from chronic lichen agrius, the collodion acted not merely as a protective covering, but also promoted the healing of the cracks. In chapped nipples, it was even more efficient in its protective and curative action. The gaping cracks were instantly drawn together and almost obliterated by the contracting power of the remedy, and were effectually shielded from the influence of moisture and the pressure of the gums of the infant, and all this, in consequence of the rapid evaporation of the ether, in an instant of time. In another point of view the remedy is invaluable as an application to chapped nipples—namely, as being in nowise injurious to the infant, from offering nothing which can be removed by the lips during the act of sucking, and in this particular, therefore, possessing a vast superiority over the various forms of ointments, astringent lotions, etc. As it is usually prepared, it has the consistence of sirup, and in this state is best suited for those cases in which its adhesive properties are principally needed. Where, however, it is intended to be applied to the surface of an ulcer or abrasion, or to chaps of the skin, I find it convenient to dilute it with ether, and render it almost as limpid as water. *Part* xviii., *p.* 227.

Borax in Efflorescence of the Face.—Mr. Vanoye, in these cases of red spots, or efflorescence of the face, so often seen in the young otherwise in good health, states he has found washing them several times a day with Hufeland's formula a most excellent remedy. It consists of borax two parts, orange-flower and rose-waters of each fifteen parts.

Part xxiv., *p.* 258.

Grease in Man—Inoculation of.—In a case in Guy's Hospital, three grains of quinine were ordered three times a day ; also a lotion of nitrate of silver, 3ss. to ℥j. of distilled water, applied by a sponge pushed up the nostrils ; with full diet, ten ounces of port wine, and two pints of porter daily. The solution of caustic seemed decidedly to have killed the disease. The parts around the nose, cheeks, and eyes, were much swollen, and were punctured., The streams and jets which flowed from the wounds showed the state of congestion the parts were in. *Part* xxiv., *p.* 349.

Balms for Diseases of the Skin.—Baume Chiron ou de Lausanne, employed to promote the Cicatrization of chapped Nipples and Broken Chilblains.—Take of olive oil, ten ounces ; Venice turpentine, two ounces ; yellow wax, one ounce ; alkanet root, half an ounce ; boil together, strain and add of balsam of Peru, two and a half drachms ; camphor, nine and a quarter grains ; stir constantly until cold.

Balm for Chilblains.—Take of rectified spirit of turpentine, one drachm ; sulphuric acid, fifteen grains ; olive oil, two and a half drachms ; mix. To be rubbed night and morning on unbroken chilblains.

Goulard's Balm (Oil of Saturn).—Take of essential oil of turpentine any quantity ; heat it *secundem artem ;* decant, etc. Used for dressing phagedenic ulcers, ecthyma, some chronic eczemas, and rupia.

Plenck's Mercurial Balm.—Take of mercury, one ounce ; Venice turpentine, half an ounce ; lard, three ounces ; calomel, seventeen grains and three-quarters ; elemi ointment, three ounces : mix. Used for dressing venereal ulcers. *Part* xxvii., *p.* 161.

Cutaneous Affections.—When associated with the cancerous diathesis, are best treated at the London Hospitals, by creasote made into pills with liquorice powder. *Part* xxxiii., *p.* 236.

Disuse of Soap in Skin Diseases.—Mr. Startin is very emphatic in his directions to patients suffering from cutaneous eruptions, to avoid the application of soap to the irritated part. In the general directions appended to the pharmacopœia is the following : "Avoid using soap of *any kind* to the affected part ; substitute to cleanse the skin, instead of soap, a paste or gruel made of bran, oatmeal, linseed-meal, arrowroot, or starch and warm water, or warm milk and water ; and yolk of egg and warm water to cleanse the scalp." The last named application is exceedingly useful in cases of porrigo and eczema of the scalp in children. Both of these affections are often aggravated and kept up by the persevering use of soap. *Part* xxxviii., *p.* 176.

———•••———

SLEEPLESSNESS.

Sleeplessness.—Vide Selections from Favorite Prescriptions, Article " Medicines."

Wakefulness—Hypodermic Injections.—Opium, morphia, and other sedatives, Mr. Hunter observes, will, in some cases, entirely fail in procuring sleep, or even cause a little delirium, whilst a little morphia (a third or half a grain of the acetate) injected into the cellular tissue of any part of the body, will act rapidly and effectually, procuring sleep and allaying irritation.   *Part* xxxix., *p.* 53.

---•◦•---

SMALLPOX.

Sulphur.—It would appear from the experiments of Dr. Midaveine, that sulphur possesses the same efficacy as mercury in arresting the devolopment of the small pox pustule. Dr. M. employs an ointment composed of two to two and a half drachms of flowers of sulphur to an ounce of lard, and with this rubs lightly, thrice a day, all parts of the body on which pustules exist. The nearer the pustules are to the period of their first appearance, the greater the chances of success; the papulæ then contract, become dry, and fade away. Even in confluent smallpox the patient quickly recovers his appetite, and asks for food.

Dr. Midaveine employed the sulphur ointment in sixteen cases only, and of these twelve had been vaccinated.

Gold-leaf.—Gold-leaf is used for the same purpose by the Egyptians and Arabs as related by Baron Larrey. They cover the parts with gold-leaf as soon as the eruption makes its appearance.

M. Legrand bears testimony to the efficacy of the practice, having tried it in one case, which he relates. The patient was a beautiful English girl, who had a copious eruption of confluent smallpox. On the first day of the eruption the whole of the face was covered with the gold leaves, which were made to adhere by means of gum water. The application was renewed morning and evening so long as the suppurative fever continued; and when the cure was complete, not a pit or scar was left on the face where the gold-leaf had been applied. The hands, and the rest of the body which had not been thus protected, were deeply marked with the scars of the pustules.

Almond Oil.—Barron Larrey says that he has found nearly the same beneficial results to follow from the repeated anointing of the face of the person laboring under smallpox with almond oil; a practice which recommends itself from its cheapness and the facility of its application.
                                                 Part iii., *p.* 51.

Aphorism of Practical Surgery.—It is a well-known fact that all abcesses caused by smallpox exist between the periosteum and the bone, with tumefaction of the latter, and subsequent formation of a sequestrum; but in the majority of cases, this cause produces only a swelling of the bone with denudation. It is important to distinguish these two sets of cases. (Dupytren.)   *Part* iii., *p.* 116.

Iodine a Preservative against Variola.—Dr. Schreiber states that he has found the administration of iodine useful in preventing the members of the family of a person laboring under smallpox from being infected with the same disease. The formula he used was as follows:

℞ Hydriod. potass., gr. viij.; tinct. iod., gtt. xvj.; aquæ font., ʒij. S. A. teaspoonful morning and evening.   *Part* x., *p.* 187.

Blisters in confluent Smallpox.—M. Piorry has for some time past derived great assistance from the use of blisters as a means of preventing the scarring of the face by the cicatrices of confluent smallpox. The pus, retained so long in contact with the tissues, and altered in character through the agency of the air which passes through the pustules by endosmosis, operates extensive local destruction, and proves very injurious to the system when re-absorbed. Various practitioners have proposed measures for obviating this inconvenience, as by cauterization of each pustule (impossible in the confluent disease), the opening them by scissors, needles, etc. Experience, however, shows that over such means the blister has the advantage of—1, opening at one time the whole of the pustules over which it is applied; 2, evacuating their entire contents, and preventing the consequences of the sojourn, or resorption of pus; 3, counteracting the attendant erysipelas, by diminishing the swelling: and 5, causing the scabs to fall much sooner from the face than from other parts of the body. It has an advantage over mercurial plasters in not risking the excitement of salivation, the extent of evil which results from its use being a slight ischuria. The various plasters applied as abortives in this disease, have been reproached with exerting a repellent action, and directing the morbid action upon the brain and its membranes. A blister, on the contrary, rather acts as a derivative. *Part* xv., *p.* 261.

Smallpox—To prevent Pitting from.—Professor Bennett recommends mercurial ointment thickened with starch (ung. hydrag., ʒj.; pulv. amyli., ʒij.) to the forehead and face, night and morning. The ointment forms a thick hard crust, which, as it cracks and peels off, is renewed by a fresh application. *Part* xxi., *p.* 262.

Abortive Power of Collodion on Smallpox.—A case occurred in the wards of M. Aran, at the Bon Secours, in which the good effects of collodion was proved to be as decisive in confluent smallpox as it had been found before in the more simple form. It occurred in the person of an unvaccinated young man, and the collodion was applied to all parts of the face but the lips and ears. Through this transparent covering the progress of the pustules was observed to become at once arrested, while those uncovered continued enlarging. Moreover, a part of the covering having been destroyed without being observed for some hours, the pustules thus exposed immediately began to develop themselves until again arrested by a reapplication. The ears, too, were now covered, and the progress of the pustules stopped there. In a few days the collodion peeled off, the skin looking as if after erysipelas, but no cicatrices were to be observed, though in other parts of the body they existed in abundance, the eruption having been very confluent. *Part* xxiii., *p.* 292.

Treatment of Smallpox.—After mature deliberation upon the treatment of smallpox, Mr. Pasquin arrived at the conclusion that the pitting and disfigurement of the face was dependent upon the confinement of the matter too long in the pocks, causing a slough thereby to form in the cellular tissue lying between the cuticle and the fascia of the face. This is not regenerated, hence the cuticle falls into the space where the cellular tissue is then wanting, and thus follows the pitting. To obviate this, Mr. Pasquin determined to puncture each pock previous to its arriving at perfection, and apply a common poultice. This treatment succeeded to his utmost satisfaction. As the pustules are liable to form on the tongue, fauces, pharynx, and larynx, apply a few leeches over these regions, exter-

nally, so as to diminish the circulation and to reduce the size of the pocks.
Part xxiv., *p.* 42.

Smallpox.—In a case of smallpox, under the care of Dr. George, attended by great swelling of the throat, and painful and difficult deglutition, great relief followed the application to the throat of jeweller's cotton, well sprinkled with powdered camphor.   *Part* xxvi., *p.* 290.

Smallpox—Abortive Treatment.—Professor Bennett recommends to the face the following plaster : Carbonate of zinc, three parts ; oxide of zinc, one part ; rubbed in a mortar with olive oil to a proper consistence. This may be used throughout the case, and renewed from time to time.
Part xxix., *p.* 50.

Smallpox—To prevent Pitting in.—Dr. Crawford uses a saturated solution of iodine in spirits of wine. Brush this tincture freely over the face once or twice daily, from the earliest period of the eruption, and continue it during the maturation of the pustules.   *Part* xxx., *p.* 175.

Abortion of the Variola Pustule.—Many are the remedies which have been recommended for the prevention of the pits left in the place of the pustule. Mercurial ointment has, perhaps, been most useful, though it is very objectionable. Trousseau's Elastic Collodion is much more useful and agreeable ; it is formed of collodion 30 parts, Venice turpentine 1½, and castor oil ½ part. It must be applied over the whole face three or four times a day. The result has been highly satisfactory.
In the Paris hospitals from 30 to 40 centigrammes of corrosive sublimate are added to every 30 grammes of the elastic collodion, and it is said with excellent results ; but of this mixture M. Delioux has had no experience.
Part xxxii., *p.* 188.

Prevention of Pitting in.—Dr. Stokes and Dr. Graves, of Dublin, have recommended painting the face with a solution of gutta percha in chloroform. It should be applied immediately before complete maturation. The increase of swelling after this time is moderate, and not such as to give rise to much pain, tension, or inconvenience.   *Part* xxxiii., *p.* 228.

Smallpox.—In confluent variola, as soon as the eruption is complete, the greatest benefit may be derived from a few grains of Dover's powder, given every night.   *Part* xxxiii., *p.* 308.

Smallpox—Prevention of Pitting in.—If the eruption be distinct, the solid stick of nitrate of silver should be applied to each pustule, previously moistened with a little water. If confluent, the concentrated solution of 8 scruples to an ounce of distilled water, must be applied over the whole surface. (If necessary to apply it to the scalp, the hair should be previously removed.) The application should be used on the second or third day of the eruption. Mr. Higginbottom relates a case of confluent smallpox, where no punctures were made, in which the strong solution was applied to the whole of the face and ears, the pustules were immediately arrested, and in nine days the eschar had come away from the face, without leaving pits.   *Part* xxxv., *p.* 159.

Treatment of Smallpox.—During the spring of 1858, smallpox was very prevalent in the Chatham garrison, and only one case out of thirty proved fatal under the treatment pursued by the author. The patient, under the care of Mr. Mandeville, surgeon 3d Indian Depot Battalion, was directed to take a mixture composed of 2 drachms of compound rhubarb powder, 2 drachms of tincture of hyoscyamus, and 7½ ounces of camphor mixture, in doses of two tablespoonfuls three or four times a day; but if the attendant fever was very high, there were added two ounces of the solution of acetate of ammonia to the above. This mixture was generally continued as long as the fever lasted, which was usually about the time when the pustules had fully maturated and the scabs had formed, the fever seldom extending beyond that period. It was then omitted, and bark ordered, if there had been great prostration, after a serious attack. A draught containing one drachm of tincture of hyoscyamus, in an ounce of camphor mixture, was given at night, as soon as the patient complained of any restlessness or itching, which was about the second or third day of the eruption in the confluent form; but they sometimes complained of it, on the first day, when the eruption appeared to be retarded, as if struggling to force its way through the cutis vera. This was continued every night as long as the sleeplessness from the pruritus continued, and at the same time the following liniment or ointment was laid on with a large-sized camel-hair brush three or four times a day over the face and any other part of the body of which the patient complained of being itchy—viz., half a drachm of extract of belladonna, rubbed up with half a drachm of spermaceti ointment, to which were added 3½ ounces of olive oil and 2½ drachms of chloroform. The cerate was added to give it consistence and hold the chloroform in suspension, but the bottle must, notwithstanding, be well shaken before using, as the chloroform will subside after standing for any time. *Part* xxxviii., *p.* 28.

SNAKE BITES.

Ipecacuanha in the Bites of Venomous Animals.—[A little girl was bitten by a centipede; after the usual remedies, oil, spirits, laudanum, ammonia, had been exhausted without relief to the pain.]

Mr. Collett says: I fetched a bottle of wine of ipecacuanha from the chest, and gave it to the mother to apply locally. To my surprise and delight she came out of her cabin in two minutes, to tell me it had stopped the pain instantly. I requested her to re-apply it if necessary. The pain returned once, when it again immediately and entirely relieved it. If so minute a quantity as is contained in the wine, could be attended with such good effects, I think much more might be expected from its use in the concentrated form of emetine. *Part* xvi., *p.* 331.

Snake Bite.—Dr. Bland recommends a ligature, whenever practicable, above the bite; include the bitten part between the blades of a pair of tenaculum forceps, raise it from the subjacent tissues, and cut it completely out with a scalpel; apply a cupping-glass to the wound, or use suction; give stimulants, as brandy, wine, ammonia, or oil of turpentine; bleed to relieve constriction of the chest, or pain about the heart or head; wash the head, face, and hands, occasionally in cold water; and prevent sound sleep for some time after the injury. *Part* xvii., *p.* 296.

Snake Bite.—Dr. Whitmire paints the part bitten, and the whole extent of the swelling, with three or four coats of tincture of iodine, twice daily. *Part* xx., *p.* 189.

Bite from an Adder.—Vide Art. "Bites."

Bite from a Cobra de Capello.—Give a teaspoonful of sp. ammoniæ aromaticus in a little water every five minutes. Dr. Mac Rae, when bitten by this snake, took 13 teaspoonfuls in this manner; every dose seemed to give some relief. In three hours he was out of danger.

*   *   *   *   *   *   *

D. Cole adds his testimony to the great value of ammonia administered internally in the cases of bite from this snake. He prefers the liq. ammon. fort., (P. L.) in doses of ten to twenty drops. He also states his belief that it is exceedingly dangerous to suck the poison from the wound, as, in his opinion, the deleterious principle of the poison is not neutralized by the gastric juice.

*   *   *   *   *   *   *

In twenty cases of this nature, hot brandy and water was immediately administered along with peppermint and laudanum. Not one case was lost.

*   *   *   *   *   *   *

The late M. Lisfranc spoke in the most unqualified manner of the success following the free application of ammonia to the wound, and its free administration internally.

*   *   *   *   *   *   *

Suction from the wound, or the actual cautery, or if possible, a tight ligature, combined with every means to combat torpor, ought to form the bases of the treatment.   *Part* xxvi., *p.* 334.

Bites from Serpents.—Rub the parts with the tincture of guaco, and give ʒj. doses every ten minutes. This remedy is said by Dr. Pritchard to be unerring in its efficacy.   *Part* xxvii., *p.* 250.

Arsenical Treatment of cases of Snake Bite.—Arsenic has been recently employed for the treatment of these cases, and it is singular that persons having been bitten by snakes recovered completely by this treatment, without any of the poisonous symptoms of arsenic being manifested. Mr. Ireland prescribed liquor arsenicalis, ʒij.; tinct. opii, gtt. x.; aquæ menthæ pip., ʒiss. To this quantity half an ounce of lime juice was added, and the medicine taken in an effervescent form. A grain of arsenic every half hour looks formidable treatment, but it was certainly successful in snake bite, and may be so in hydrophobia. Arsenic would seem to stimulate specially the semilunar ganglion and its tributaries, presiding over the organic life of our bodies. Its " evacuant " operation is an incident of prime importance in cases of poison. It should always be given on these occasions until the patient vomits and purges abundantly.
Part xxviii., *p.* 317.

Snake Bite.—Dr. Loundes recommends 5 grains of bicarbonate of ammonia every five minutes, and to administer an enema of mustard and water, with two drachms of tinct. of valerian, which may be repeated if returned.   Apply a mustard cataplasm over the cardiac region and then give the following: Chloroform, ʒj.; spirit, ʒij.; mist. camph., ʒiij.; M. ft. m. ʒj. every ten minutes.   *Part* xxix., *p.* 326,

Snake Bite.—A decoction or broth of the leaves near the root of the common male fern, polypodium filix mas, has been used as a secret remedy in Australia, as a specific for snake bites. Though the experiments hitherto made cannot be said to be satisfactory, it might be tried by medical men in the army, if nothing better is at hand. Probably a tincture would be more powerful. *Part* xl., *p.* 278.

Alcoholic Stimuli in Snake Bites.—Vide Art. "Bites."

SOAPS.

Medicated Soaps for the Treatment of Skin Diseases.—Sir H. Marsh recommends the following in the more chronic forms of skin disease, as chronic eczema, psoriasis, etc. :

Sulphur Soap.—Take of white Windsor soap, two ounces ; spirit of wine, colored with alkanet root, one fluid drachm. Pound the soap well in a marble mortar, so as effectually to get rid of all lumps ; add the spirit and beat into a uniform paste ; then add sublimed sulphur two drachms, otto of roses, ten drops—beat all well together.

White Precipitate Soap is made precisely as the sulphur soap, substituting ammoniated submuriate of mercury for the sulphur.

Red Precipitate Soap.—Take of white Windsor soap, two ounces ; rectified spirit of wine one fluid drachm ; pound the soap well in a marble mortar, until all lumps have disappeared ; add the spirit and beat into a uniform paste ; then add precipitated red oxide of mercury, one drachm ; otto of roses, six drops ; beat all well together.

Corrosive Sublimate Soap.—Take of white Windsor soap, two ounces ; spirit of wine, one fluid drachm ; corrosive sublimate, one scruple ; pound the soap well in a marble mortar until all lumps have disappeared ; add the corrosive sublimate, previously reduced to a fine powder, and rubbed in a separate mortar, with the spirit. Beat all into a uniform paste, adding six drops of otto of rose.

Sir H. Marsh states that the only forms of cutaneous disease that admit of the application of these soaps are those which either have passed from the acute into the chronic stage, or have not been at any period peculiarly irritable and tender ; at the same time, he has met with several cases in which the tender surfaces, at first intolerant, became subsequently inured to them ; and, after a little perseverance, the patients began to speak highly of their soothing and beneficial effects. *Part* xxii., *p.* 260.

SORES.

Sores and Wounds—Sloughing.—Dr. T. S. Fletcher advises the use of chlorine. It is a powerful antiseptic, and prevents sloughing. Make a solution of chloride of lime, two drachms of the powder to a pint of cold water. Cover the wound with pads of tow dipped in this solution, and renew them about twice a day. *Part* xxxi., *p.* 191.

Chloride of Potash in Scrofulous Sores.—M. Bouchut employs with great success, a solution of this substance (ʒj. ad ʒiij. aquæ) as a local application to external sores in scrofulous children. He has also found it highly useful in arresting the progress of ulcers supervening upon the employment of blisters, as also in ulcerated chilblains. *Part* xxxviii., *p.* 175.

SPASMODIC AFFECTIONS.

Spasmodic Affections of the Larynx—Veratria.—Dr. Bushnan has strongly recommended the ointment of veratria in the treatment of dys-menorrhœa. Dr. Bushnan supposes that dysmenorrhœa may frequently be owing to perversion of the nervous action of the lower portion of the spinal nerves, and found good effects from the external application of the oint-ment of veratria. Dr. Tunstall suggests that if the ointment of veratria has this effect on the lower portion of the spinal marrow, why may it not have a similar effect on the superior portion? and in this latter case it would be supposed to be useful in spasmodic affections of the larynx and appendages. Dr. T. accordingly tried it in the case of a schoolmistress:. she was usually seized with a sense of suffocation, the whole of the muscles employed in respiration were put into violent and convulsive action, the lower extremities became cold, the face purple, the whole surface was be-dewed with cold perspiration ; she was perfectly sensible during the whole attack; the fit usually terminated in ordinary dyspnœa, which lasted for hours, or even days. Every variety of depletion and counter-irritation had been employed; also, opiates and antispasmodics, without the least advantage. Dr. T. says :]

I therefore prescribed a scruple of veratria to one ounce of simple cerate, and directed that a small portion should be applied on each side of the cer-vical vertebræ, and rubbed well into neck, throughout its whole extent, twice a day. Although the attacks were previously rather frequent, she had not a single attack of consequence during its use. *Part* iv., *p.* 29.

Opium Smoking as a Remedial Agent.—Dr. James Johnson suggests that the Chinese mode of smoking opium may be made useful " in certain dangerous and painful maladies, where the common mode is found to be inefficient, and attended with great derangement of the digestive organs." The Chinese method induces a profound sleep and insensibility to all mental misery and corporeal pain, which cannot be induced by opium taken into the stomach, and may, therefore, at some period, be used in cases of teta-nus, hydrophobia, tic-douloureux, and violent spasms, where the com-mon mode of giving opium by the stomach so frequently fails. Dr. Johnson adds, that " the various preparations of opium might be easily smoked by means of a common pipe, and the powerful effects induced in a very short space of time without the possibility of their being rejected by the stomach, or prevented from acting energetically on the sensorium, and throughout the whole nervous system." *Part* v., *p.* 56.

Division of the Muscles of the Face when affected with Chronic Spasms. Dieffenbach performed this operation in four cases in which the disease had existed for a considerable time. The orbicularis palpebrarum was divided, also the muscles of the cheek, from the ala of the nose to the an-terior border of the masseter, and lastly, the muscles at the angle of the mouth. The result of the operation was, that the spasmodic affections were cured. *Part* v., *p.* 142.

SPERMATOCELE.

Spermatocele and Hydrocele.—[In a clinical lecture upon a case of hydrocele which had been operated upon,]

Mr. Syme stated, that he had long ceased to employ port wine for injection into the tunica vaginalis, on account of its effect proving very uncertain; and that having subsequently used a mixture of the tincture of iodine with three parts of water for this purpose, he had, during the last five years, always injected the tincture alone, and without a single case of failure or unpleasant effect, either in public or private practice. The quantity required was about a teaspoonful, or as much as filled a common sixpenny pewter syringe, which was the most convenient instrument for the operation, as the substance composing it allowed the nozzle to be readily adapted to the canula of the trocar. The fluid when injected was allowed to remain, and while producing the effect desired with absolute certainty, seemed to occasion less pain than any other agent in past or present use.

When the tumor was punctured, the fluid which issued through the tube, to the amount of a pint or more, appeared somewhat turbid, and this was attributed to its probably containing the scales of cholesterine, which are frequently met with in albuminous fluid long pent up in close cavities. The tincture of iodine, therefore, was injected as usual. But when a little of the fluid was poured from the basin, in which it had been received, into a glass vessel, in order that the gentlemen present might more readily examine it, the absence of scales, and the peculiar opalescence observed, at once suggested the idea of spermatocele, and an appeal to the microscope confirmed this suspicion, by bringing myriads of spermatozoa into view.

Had the true nature of the case been ascertained in the first instance, injection would not have appeared expedient, since spermatocele has not only resisted the means of treatment which have proved sufficient for the remedy of hydrocele, but has also shown a disposition to resent with violence even liberties of a much slighter kind.

The result of this case was, therefore, watched with interest; and when, after passing through the usual course of a simple hydrocele, under the same circumstances, the swelling quickly subsided, with complete restoration of the testicle to its healthy state, it naturally suggested another trial of the same kind. For this an occasion happened at the time to present itself, in the case of a gentleman, who had had a hydrocele tapped about twenty years ago, by Sir Astley Cooper, and afterward injected with port wine by another surgeon in London, but still suffered from it. The tumor was in every respect very similar to that just mentioned; and when punctured, was found to contain the same sort of turbid opalescent fluid. The suspicion of spermatocele was confirmed by the microscope, which detected abundance of spermatozoa; but everything went on satisfactorily after the iodine was injected, so that before the end of three weeks the testicle had very nearly regained its proper size and consistence.

The two cases just related afford encouragement to attempt the radical cure of spermatocele by the injection of tincture of iodine, although other means have been found to fail.   *Part* xxi., *p.* 236.

SPERMATORRHŒA.

Causes and Treatment of.—[A number of years ago, Mr. Phillips, at the suggestion of M. Lallemand, first applied lunar caustic to the mucous membrane of the urethra to check involuntary seminal discharges. Mr. P. says:]

Involuntary discharges are, for the most part, if not altogether, caused by irritation set up in or about the ducts connected with the testicle.

There are particular modes in which the urethral irritation is commonly excited; among these, masturbation holds a prominent place: by this practice the constant excitement of the seminal ducts ends by establishing a permanent irritation there: it may likewise happen from excess in sexual intercourse. Next to this cause we arrange gonorrhœa or gleety discharges, which, from time to time, establish chronic inflammation in the vicinity of the orifices of the ejaculatory ducts. Then follows stricture, which, by opposing an obstacle to the free passage of urine, ultimately causes the development of a morbid condition of the mucous membrane between the stricture and the bladder. The same state of these organs may result from irritation within the rectum ; that irritation may be caused by fissures of piles, or by the presence of ascarides.

The mode in which the irritation, once set up around the orifices of the ejaculatory ducts, acts, is very much the same as obtains upon the application of irritation to the mouths of other ducts ; it solicits increased action in the organ with which they communicate. Irritate the bladder, and the kidneys are stimulated to increased action ; irritate the conjunctiva, and the lachrymal secretion increases ; irritate the duodenum, and it is said bile will be supplied in increased quantity ; it is unnecessary to carry the illustration further.

In most cases the evidence of involuntary spermatic discharges is clear enough, but the time comes when the ejaculation is unaccompanied by the ordinary sensations, and the patient may then be unaware of the extent of the evil. I have again and again known cases where the spermatic fluid passed out with the urine ; others, in which the efforts at stool caused a pressure to be made upon the distended seminal vesicles, and thus their contents were squeezed out ; but the fluid may not pass until the process of buttoning up is going on, and the evil may be undiscovered. Still, unless the disorder be very advanced, in most cases the person himself is aware of it when it passes with the urine, because it almost always passes with the last drops, and can then be detected, and because a certain sensation is experienced about the neck of the bladder. But when the medical man is consulted, he calls for the recently passed urine, or requests that it may be passed in his presence, and at the bottom of the vessel he perceives small granular diaphanous particles ; and they are seen floating even before the urine cools ; if the evil be, however, very advanced, no peculiar sensation is experienced, and the granular matter may be undetected, and may assume a more uniform cloudy appearance. In cases where uncertainty remains with regard to the deposit, we may advantageously have recourse to the microscope, by means of which the little long-tailed animalcules of the spermatic fluid can readily be perceived. Under any debilitating causes, whether those causes be found in frequent spermatic discharges, disease, or old age, the fluid becomes much thinner, and the animalcules much less numerous, and they may be almost, if not altogether, wanting.

One of the general symptoms resulting from too frequent spermatic discharges, which is most distressing to the sufferer, is a state approaching to, if not at the time, actual impotency. It is not that the seminal fluid, though deteriorated, is incapable of determining fecundation, but it is that the organs are wanting in the energy necessary for projecting the fluid into the uterus; the erection of the penis, if it exist at all, being only momentary. The digestive functions become deranged; the bowels constipated; nutrition languishes; respiration is troubled; the voice fails; the heart's action is interfered with, even to such an extent as to induce the belief of actual disease in that organ, and hypochondriasis becomes complete. These things do not advance far without causing trouble in the nervous system, manifested by some perturbation of the senses, by headache, with great sense of weight or pressure, and they are accompanied by loss of memory; a timidity and apprehension which are very painful. It must be evident that as the causes of these discharges are many, the treatment must also be variable. When the irritation is in the rectum, the case will require a very different course of treatment to one proceeding from stricture of the urethra. We will therefore make such general remarks as are proper with reference to the treatment of the several varieties of the affection which we have considered. First, when the cause is masturbation or sexual excess: the causes here are voluntary, the cure must also be voluntary. Lunar caustic will be powerless, unless the patient has sufficient determination to abstain from the practice. But in many cases perfect abstinence will not suffice to put an end to the mischief; the *voluntary* discharges are got rid of, but they were persisted in so long that a permanent irritation has been set up in the verumontanum, and that irritation may, as we have already explained, excite equally injurious *involuntary* discharges: and here a remedy must be found by the surgeon. The first thing we have to do is to introduce cautiously a bougie, to pass it down toward the bladder; but before it arrives there, the patient will complain of pain which is sometimes very acute; and the point at which the bougie has then arrived is usually a little in front of the prostate. The surgeon must then carefully observe how far the penis has been extended, and a mark must be made upon the bougie to indicate the depth to which the instrument has penetrated, because that is the point upon which the lunar caustic must be applied. The depth to which we must penetrate must be marked upon the caustic instrument, which is then introduced and gently passed to the proper point, when the caustic is uncovered, and the membrane brushed over: as soon as that has been done, the caustic is again covered, and the instrument is withdrawn.

The point upon which the caustic is to be applied is, as near as practicable, about the region of the orifices of the ejaculatory ducts. It often happens, however, that the whole or several parts of the urethra are very sensitive, and it becomes difficult to know, from this circumstance, which is the most tender and irritable; but when, for example, it is found that it is seven and a half inches from the orifice of the urethra to the bladder, which is known by the urine passing along the catheter, and when it is further seen that an acute pain is felt at a little more than six inches, we may confidently cauterize the space between the sixth and seventh inches, satisfied that the orifices of the ejaculatory ducts will not escape.

In some cases the patient complains of a little heat when the caustic is applied; in others, the sensation spoken of is a coldness. I have more than once known some discomfort almost amounting to spasms at the anus, but altogether it is astonishing how rarely any complaint is made. At the next time of passing the urine, more smarting is usually experienced; it may continue through the day, but it is very bearable. In all cases it occasions a discharge, which is sometimes considerable, and at first is thin and watery, but gradually becomes thicker, and in the course of a few days ceases. In a few cases the discharge is at first streaked with blood; and in a few rare instances there may be trifling hemorrhage.

It is always necessary to guard the patient against impatience, because four or five weeks will, in some cases, pass, before the beneficial effects of the remedy become clearly evident; and this is the more necessary, because he looks with intense anxiety to the result; and sometimes it happens that a single discharge, after the application of the caustic, will dash the cup of hope from his lips, and induce the most gloomy forebodings. I may again repeat what I have said before, that I have never applied too much caustic, but I have more than once failed by using too little; and much experience is necessary to apply the proper dose. However, it is better to err on the safe side, until experience shall have given confidence in the use of the remedy. I have scarcely ever had recourse to a second application until five or six weeks have passed, and given the assurance that the first has been insufficient.

If the affection has been caused by a gonorrhœal or gleety discharge, the treatment must be the same as in the former instance.

If it has been caused by stricture, we must first restore the canal to its natural diameter; the obstacle to the passage of the urine may be removed, but the morbid condition of the posterior part of the canal, which has resulted from it, may persist; so may the specific discharges. Then the efficacy of the lunar caustic can be at once demonstrated; and a single proper and sufficient application of the remedy, with the precautions already indicated, will, in most cases, promptly cure the disease of the urethra as well as that of the spermatic organs.

If the discharge be determined by irritation of the anus, or the rectum, appropriate means must be used to cure the intestinal disorder; and it may be that when that has ceased the spermatic disorder will also cease. But it may persist, because a distinct irritation may have been determined in the urethra by the long-continued action of that of the intestinal canal; and to dissipate that, recourse must be had to the lunar caustic, under the same restrictions as have been already pointed out.

The space which M. Lallemand usually cauterizes, is from the neck of the bladder to the membranous part of the urethra; but sometimes he brushes over the internal surface of the bladder itself to a greater or less extent. He cautions us strongly against repeating the operation too soon; and advises us to wait two or three weeks before we re-apply the caustic. Many of his cases appear to have been cured by a single application. Pain and a slight discharge of blood, but never amounting to hemorrhage, seem to have followed some of his operations; but these consequences disappear at the end of from twelve to forty-eight hours. In one case they are described as lasting three weeks, but this is mentioned as a rare exception. When the emissions have been *diurnal*, M. Lallemand regards the conversion of them into *nocturnal*, and the fact of the emissions being once more accompanied with erections and with pleasurable sensations, as a sign of the favorable effects of treatment and prospect of cure.

We shall now, with great brevity, advert to other modes than cauterization, of treating involuntary seminal discharges, depending *solely* on chronic inflammation of the prostatic portion of the urethra and of the vesiculæ seminales. The daily introduction of a bougie, and the retaining it for a longer or shorter time in the urethra, may first be mentioned. This, as our own observation enables us to testify, is often useful. Leeching of and blisters to the perineum are by no means of slight efficacy, especially where the prostate is tender and enlarged. We have also prescribed tartar emetic frictions of the perineum with excellent effects. A total abandonment of masturbation, and a moderate use, or even an entire though temporary disuse of coition, are, of course, indispensable measures. One of our correspondents states that he has found opiates extremely useful. They are so in most cases, though not in all; since they sometimes seem to augment the disease. Conium is safer: and both it and opium may be used both constitutionally and as a suppository. Cold clysters are often of benefit. As regards general means, alcoholic and malt liquors must be abandoned. M. Lallemand's opinion of these is exceedingly hostile; and we believe he is right in this. The food should be nourishing, light, and unstimulant; the bowels should be of course attended to, and, as a general rule, country air and exercise prescribed. Among medicines and articles of diet, tea and coffee in excess, tobacco, camphor, nitrate of potass, aloes, must be abstained from. *Part* vii., *p.* 119.

Involuntary Seminal Discharges. — Since the publication of Mr. B. Phillips' paper on this subject, in which the application of the nitrate of silver to the prostatic portion of the urethra, as first recommended by Lallemand, is shown to be very efficacious, the subject has been taken up by other writers.

Mr. James Douglas, of Glasgow, publishes a case in which the cauterization of the urethra, though very beneficial, did not cure the affection, and for which an injection composed of one grain of opium, three grains of acetate of lead, and one ounce of mucilage, used three times a day, and doubled in strength in ten days, was remarkably efficacious.

Another paper on the same subject is published by Mr. Allnatt, in which he hesitates to believe that these discharges are always seminal. He thinks that they are often more of a mucous character, and unattended with the pleasurable sensation accompanying the emission of semen. An abundant secretion of mucus may be afforded by the prostate, the glands of Cowper, and by the internal coat of the bladder when diseased. Mr. Allnatt has before directed the attention of the profession to the effect of creasote on the mucous membrane in fluor albus, gonorrhœa, and purulent otorrhœa, and thinks that it may be useful in these mucous discharges resembling semen. In the case of otorrhœa he used an injection composed of a drachm of creasote, the same quantity of liquor potassæ, and six ounces of water; to be frequently thrown into the tube. Mr. Allnatt accidentally discovered the value of the same remedy to restrain the bleeding from piles.

Part viii., *p.* 163.

Spermatorrhœa.—In the *treatment* of this affection, M. Lallemand observes, it is more important that our attention should be directed to the present condition of the spermatic organs, than to the original cause producing this; and there can be no question that, in many cases, until this great source of irritation be removed, all the efforts of the practitioner and resolutions of the patient will be in vain. To the chapter which directs the suitable treatment, when this diseased condition arises from irritation occurring in the vicinity, we need not advert; seeing the remedies employed against ascarides, eruptions, or fissures at the margin of the anus, diseased conditions of the prepuce, stricture of the urethra, constipation, etc., are those in ordinary use.

When arising simply from debility, as it may do in persons of lymphatic temperament, and who have suffered in childhood from incontinence of urine, give tonics, as the ferruginous waters, use the local douche followed by friction, or transmit galvanic shocks through the penis and perineum; warm aromatic baths, ergot of rye, 4 to 20 grains night and morning, or small doses of copaiba or turpentine are sometimes useful. When from great nervous susceptibility of the organs, give narcotics and sedatives, as camphor in 5 or 6 grain doses, and introduce every few days a medium-sized gum catheter, and allow it to remain for an hour or more, or practice acupuncture of the perineum. When dependent upon sub-inflammatory condition of the orifices of the ducts, use tepid baths, give milk diet and light regimen, apply nitrate of silver to the parts, *sec. art.*, and let all exercise of the organs be abandoned. *Part* xvii., *p.* 181.

Spermatorrhœa and Impotence.—Let the patient sit in the hip-bath of Priessnitz for five minutes three times a day, the water being brought to the temperature of 65°. The time may be increased and the temperature lowered, until the patient sits for twenty minutes, three times a day, in water at 50°. In some cases the spine may be sponged for three or four minutes before leaving the bath. A shower-bath may be used after the first daily sitting-bath, the head being protected by a conical cap.—(REV.) *Part* xxiv., *p.* 248.

Treatment of.—Mr. Adams, surgeon to the London Hospital, recommends the application, locally, of caustic, and the internal exhibition of conium and soda in the infusion of gentian, cold-bathing, fresh air, and the almost entire abstinence from alcoholic fluids. After the secretions of the patient have been got into good order, give small doses of tinct. cantharides and the sesquichloride of iron in a bitter infusion. *Part* xxv., *p.* 216.

Spermatorrhœa.—[Mr. Milton offers the following observations on the treatment of this disease. He says:]

It consists—

1. *Of Quinine in Solution*, in the following form:

℞ Quin. disulph., gr. vj.; acid sulph. dil., ʒj.; tinct. cardam. co., ʒiij.; aq. cinnam., ʒvss. M. Sumat cochl. duo ampl. bis die.

Used in this way, one grain seems to have much more effect than larger doses with less acid.

2. *Of Local Baths of Cold Salt Water.*—I generally direct the patient to buy a pound of common salt, break a piece off as large as a walnut, and dissolve it in half a basin of water. The scrotum and perineum are then bathed with this by the aid of a sponge for five minutes every morning, and the water thrown away, so that nothing remains to excite suspicion; those patients who are under no restraint may use a hip bath of cold solution of salt water with the greatest advantage.

3. *Some Gymnastic Exercise every Day.*—The application of this

remedy must naturally be modified by the patient's position in life; but even those most restricted can take a walk early in the morning and last thing at night. When this trenches on the hours of sleep it may be regarded rather as an advantage than otherwise; the less sleep the patient has the sounder it will be; the earlier he rises the better, the erections being generally most forcible and recurring most regularly in the morning.

When the weather does not admit of out-of-door exercise, I advise reading for a fixed time, as an hour or so every night; and if the patient be restless and unsettled, reading aloud, even when he is obliged to walk to and fro to accomplish his task, will often soothe down this excitement and dispose him to sleep.

4. *Of Checking the Erections.*—It will often be remarked, that the patient has erections two or three nights successively. When these awaken him, I find it best to treat the case like one of chordee, and direct him to rise, take a teaspoonful of spirit of camphor in water. This will generally allay the priapism, and prevent its recurrence. On those nights when he expects the emissions, a dose may be taken last thing at night.

The bowels should be kept loose; and, for this purpose, five grains of blue p l may be taken occasionally, in conjunction with rhubarb. When this does not act, the sulphate of magnesia may be added to the mixture.

5. If these measures do not suffice to cure the disease, I would advise blistering. If applied on the perineum, it acts most efficiently; but, in some instances, I have seen this followed by a troublesome crop of boils; this I have never seen from a blister on the penis, where it can be applied and dressed much more easily, and where it occasions much less soreness and difficulty in walking. If the patient objects to this, it may be laid on the groin.

Those cases in which I tried steel failed. In place of acting beneficially, it seemed to heat and over-stimulate the patient, and even to dispose more to erections. In that shattered state of the frame in which the semen passes away involuntarily, and almost without an erection, it may be useful, but I am inclined to rely more on the measures I have laid down.

Some surgeons, considering this disorder, in many instances, as merely an effort of nature to throw off an accumulated secretion, recommend connection. I would neither recommend nor forbid it, unless I found it acting injuriously. In some cases the patient takes it for granted that if this be THE remedy, medicines, gymnastics, etc., can do him no good, and shaking off all restraint, gives way to the worst excesses. This plan, too, is not free from danger to the surgeon's reputation. Only very recently, a patient placed himself under my care for seminal emissions. He had suffered under them for a long time, and had consulted a surgeon, who advised him to have connection. The result was a gonorrhœa, which took two months to cure; and this mistake unsettled all his former confidence in his medical adviser.

When self-pollution or excessive connection is indulged in, I only know of one remedy, and that is, the employment of some irritative ointment to the penis, such as that of bichloride of mercury, ℨss. to ℨj.; deutiodide of mercury, Əj. to ℨj.; or of the ung. ant. pot.-tart.

The only way to break him of it, is to make the penis so sore, that he is at once awakened by the smarting as soon as he commences any attempts at friction. When once the habit is fairly broken off, he rarely recurs to it.

The despondency of spirits, the loss of appetite, flatulence, weakness, pain in the back, etc., under which many of these patients labor, are generally removed by adopting a plain diet, as weak coffee, toast, and bacon, for breakfast, an early dinner, consisting of a chop or two and bread, strictly excluding all porter, vegetables, cheese, pickles, or pastry ; as little tea as possible ; and in the evening, instead of supper, a basin of tapioca, ground barley, or arrow-root, with a biscuit.

A persevering use for a few weeks of this treatment will, I think, effect a cure even in the most inveterate cases. *Part* xxv., *p.* 241.

Lupulin (the Alkaloid of Hops) as an Anaphrodisiac.—M. Debout, of Paris, editor of the "Bulletin de Thérapeutique," has found lupulin extremely useful in chordee, priapism, traumatic orgasm, and spermatorrhœa. The lupulin should be used in powder, and triturated with lump sugar. The dose is from fifteen to thirty grains. M. Ricord and M. Puche have carried the dose from one to three drachms without any unpleasant effect.
Part xxviii., *p.* 320.

Spermatorrhœa.—According to Mr. Milton, where physical weakness is a prominent symptom, quinine has an undoubted efficacy in controlling the *night* discharges of spermatorrhœa. Spirit of camphor is the best remedy for relieving the obstinate erections which sometimes remain after gonorrhœa, a teaspoonful for a dose. Gymnastic exercise is an excellent means of controlling spermatorrhœa. The best plan is to rise at six in the morning, sponge with cold salt water, use the dumb-bells for half an hour, and follow this up with a brisk walk. For both the night and day discharges, opium is a most valuable remedy. If the costiveness is obstinate, let the patient take a pill of gentian with 1-12th of a grain of strychnia, with a tumbler of unsweetened gin and water at night, and one of cold water in the morning. If the urine scalds, and the patient complains of spasmodic pain at the neck of the bladder, and the urine be loaded with lithates, or clouded with mucus, we may give the nitro-muriatic acid with laudanum, in the decoction of pareira brava or chimaphila. In cases of extreme uneasy sensation or creeping along the vas deferens or urethra, veratria ointment, or some mild counter-irritant, are the most useful applications. The caustic holder is not to be regarded as *the remedy*, because, in truth, it is not often called for. In cases complicated with gleet, where the cautery has failed, blistering is the best remedy. A good instrument for applying the caustic is a platinum canula with stilette. After introduction, the stilette is withdrawn, and a bougie passed down prepared thus : the tip being scraped rough, it is rolled in fused caustic, and this again in melted tallow, by which means a thin film of caustic is secured.

The indigestion in this disease is best relieved by aromatic confection, with sulphate of soda and mint water. · Before resorting to the caustic bougie, the sensitiveness of the urethra must be diminished by occasional blisters and injections. In prostatic gleet, a blister repeated two or three times has cured the patient after all other treatment had failed. The same in night discharges. Quinine may be given subsequently.
Part xxix., *p.* 233.

Nocturnal Seminal Emissions treated by Digitaline.—Digitaline, of late much extolled and employed with success, according to many practitioners, in cases of nocturnal seminal losses, has yielded, in the hands of Dr. Laroche, a result which deserves to be mentioned. A young man, aged 18, presented himself some months ago to- be treated for nocturnal seminal losses. The disease had come upon him about two months previously. For twenty days, the pollutions had not omitted a single night; his strength was gone, the appetite had left him, and his sleep was troubled by unpleasant dreams. M. Laroche prescribed three granules of digitaline (equal to a grain of the powder of the plant). The night following the administration of the medicine, the pollutions intermitted for the first time. In three weeks he was cured. *Part* xxxi., *p.* 167.

Bromide of Potassium— Use of in Spermatorrhœa.— Vide Art. " Chordee."

— • ◦ • —

SPINA BIFIDA.

Spina Bifida.—Mr. Hewitt makes the following remarks regarding the treatment of spina-bifida: The dissections of the cases of spina bifida which have been published, and the preparations which are to be found in our museums, at once point out the rashness of attempting to remove these tumors either by ligature or by the knife. I do not consider this remark to be in the least invalidated by the success which is said to have attended the practice of M. Dubourg, who has published in the Gazette Médicale de Paris, 1841, a paper upon the radical cure of spina bifida. M. Dubourg operated upon three cases: in one, a ligature was applied to the tumor—the patient died two days after the operation; in the other two, which terminated successfully, the sac was removed by the knife, and · the lips of the wound were brought together by hare-lip pins and sutures. The successful termination of these two cases was, it must be confessed, very fortunate; but this success ought not, in my opinion, to lead any surgeon to adopt so rash a practice; for, laying aside the question of thus opening the theca vertebralis, there still remains the fact that, in the majority of cases, some nerves are connected with the sac, and that, when the sac corresponds to the sacrum, the chord itself is *generally* connected with the tumor. In one of M. Dubourg's cases the tumor was in the loins: in the other it was in the lower part of the cervical region. The sacs we examined after the operation, *but no nerves were connected with them.*

Several cases in which the plan of treatment adopted by Sir A. Cooper has completely succeeded, have been placed upon record by various authors; but in these cases two points of importance have not, I think, been sufficiently considered, and I would, therefore, lay down the following general rules:

1st. The tumor ought never to be punctured along the mesial line, especially in the sacral region; for it is generally at this part that the chord and its nerves are connected with the sac. The puncture is to be made at one side of the sac, and at the lowest part, so as to diminish the risk of wounding any of the nervous branches.

2d. The instrument ought to be a grooved needle, or a small trocar; for if a lancet is used there will be a greater risk of wounding some important part contained in the cavity of the tumor. *Part* x., *p.* 180.

Spina Bifida successfully treated by Ligature and Puncture.—In a case where the tumor is pedunculated, owing to the defect in the bony canal being very slight, and the neck of the tumor covered with ordinary integument, it is possible, safely and with success, to remove the projecting membranous bag by the application of ligatures. The ligature must be gradually tightened so as not completely to constrict the part for some days, and if great tension of the tumor come on, it may be relieved by puncturing with a fine needle. A case, the text of the above, is related by Dr. Wilson, of Glasgow, in which a firm cicatrix, and consequent cure, resulted. *Part* xxxviii., *p.* 144.

SPINE.

Lateral Curvature of the Spine.— Wry-neck depending on Contraction of the Sterno-Mastoid Muscle.—[The object of this paper of Mr. Syme's is to point out the kind of case in which an operation for spinal curvature may be useful, and to discourage the operations which are recommended for all other kinds of spinal distortion. We cannot always be sure whether the bones or muscles are the first cause of lateral curvature. The muscles may be so weak as to allow the spine to bend, and the bones may at the same time be so unhealthy that an undue pressure may cause a premature distortion. All the operations which have been recommended for these lateral curvatures are at least very doubtful in their efficacy, if not positively injurious, and there is only one kind of spinal distortion which it is proper to attempt to remedy by subcutaneous incisions, and that is spinal curvature depending upon wry-neck caused by contraction of the sterno-mastoid, which muscle is liable to contraction both spasmodic and permanent. Although spasmodic contraction does not generally affect the shape of the spine, the permanent contraction may do so very materially.]

Wry-neck, like club-foot, is sometimes congenital, but much more frequently, like squinting, and the *pes equinus*, occurs during childhood, in connection with some inflammatory or feverish state of the system. It depends upon a contracted state of the sterno-mastoid muscle, which has usually the feeling and appearance of a tense cord stretching from the clavicle to the ear. The head is bent toward the side affected, the face being turned to the opposite direction. Until the introduction of subcutaneous incision, the treatment of this complaint was very defective, since it consisted either in the use of mechanical support, which did little, if any good, or in cutting across the contracted muscle, together with its superjacent integuments, which was a painful and bloody operation, leaving a large sore, slow to heal, and apt to renew the evil during cicatrization. The subcutaneous process requires merely a puncture of the skin, is not attended with pain or bleeding, needs no dressing or after-treatment, and at once affords the relief desired.

There is still another condition of the complaint, of which I may mention an instance that came within my notice last summer, in the case of a boy who was brought from the country on account of lateral curvature. Observing that his head inclined to one side, I examined the sterno-mastoid, and found it, not tense and rigid as I expected, but soft and yielding. I perceived, however, that when an attempt was made to raise the head, the muscle resisted and became tense, and therefore concluded that it was the seat of the evil. Under this impression I proceeded to divide it, and succeeded in doing so, though with more difficulty than usual, from the want of tension, for which it was necessary to compensate by stretching the neck. A good effect was immediately perceptible, and the following day the patient's back was comparatively straight, which it has since, I am informed, become completely.

In concluding these remarks, it may be well to warn against mistaking for wry-neck depending upon musclar contraction, the distorted position of the head which proceeds from caries between the occiput and atlas. The latter disease, like the former, usually occurs in young persons, presents to a careless observer similar symptoms, and if confounded with it, leads to treatment not only useless, but extremely injurious. A young gentleman had for twelve months used friction and exercise under the instruction of a distinguished member of the profession, who supposed that he labored under wry-neck from the contraction of the sterno-mastoid. No benefit having been experienced, it was thought that an operation might be serviceable, and with this view I was asked to see the patient. He presented all the characters and well marked symptoms of *spondy larthrocace*, or caries at the occipito-vertebral articulation, in a stage so advanced, that there was nothing left for me but to explain the nature of the case and predict the fatal termination, which soon afterward happened.

Part vii., *p.* 143.

Treatment of Lateral Curvature of the Spine.—For many cases of this affection Mr. Stafford recommends *lateral exercise;* and for this purpose he has devised a machine, which consists of a semicircular wooden frame, resembling the platform or rocker of a hobby-horse. This frame lies on its convex surface, and the ends of a rope, which passes through two pulleys fixed in the ceiling, at a distance from each other equal to the length of the rocking frame, are attached respectively to a bar at each end of the frame. "The patient stands upon this machine, taking hold of the rope by each hand, and then rocks himself or herself backward and forward (from side to side, rather), by which both the lumbar and dorsal curve are acted on laterally." Mr. Stafford has "hardly known an instance when it (lateral exercise) has not been of the greatest service." But "lateral exercise, however, will not always recover a lateral curvature. The spine is sometimes so completely distorted and the vertebral column so entirely thrown out of the centre of gravity, that the muscles have lost their power. They are so stretched on the convex, and so contracted on the concave side of the curve, that they cannot act. In such cases lateral exercise will not alone be sufficient. More must be done—the spine itself must be elongated; and the best method of accomplishing this is by gravitation of the body. "To effect this object I have invented a machine by which the patient can be raised up from the ground by the upper part of the body, while the lower part hangs suspended. Hence the lower part, by its own gravitation, and by additional weights being hung round the hips, gradually elongates the spinal column, until it becomes nearly if not quite, for the time being, straight. In this manner the muscles on the concave side are lengthened, while those on the convex are shortened, and allowed to contract, whereby they are both put into a more favorable position to pull back and retain the vertebræ in their situation. After the machine has been used I usually recommend the lateral exercise, as the muscles and ligaments are then in the best state to be strengthened."

Part x, *p.* 161.

Spinal Irritation.—Dr. Tûrck, of Vienna, says : " If we carefully analyze the symptoms observed in well-marked cases of spinal irritation, we shall find that they·can all be elucidated on the supposition, that there is a centric change so operating as to exalt the functions of the cerebro-spinal axis. This change can scarcely be considered strictly structural, because we know that structural changes are marked by anæsthesia, or paralysis; on the other hand, we know that the circulation may be the medium through which the actual change is induced. Opium renders frogs tetanic, as strychnine acts on man and lower animals; the slightest touch of the surface in poisoning by strychnine is sufficient to excite convulsions. The poison of the rabid dog so exalts the functions of the incident excitor and reflex motor nerves of the respiratory and spinal ganglia, that a breath of air on the face will excite a convulsive gasp and general spasms. In 'spinal irritation' the change is probably in the capillary circulation : 1, of the cerebro-spinal axis ; 2, of the ganglia of the sympathetic, or ganglia of the posterior spinal nerves ; and 3, of the fibrils of the nerves themselves. This purely functional derangement of the nervous system has been termed neuræmia by Dr. Laycock, one of the recent English writers on this subject, and the class of diseases to which it gives origin, neuræmic.

" If we were to attempt an illustration of our remarks as to the diagnosis, we could not take a more apt instance than that of abdominal tenderness. Where it depends on spinal irritation, it will be found that the history of the patient presents instances of her having previously suffered from neuræmic affections. The affectible state of the cutaneous nerves of the abdomen is never observed to occur alone, the nerves of the abdominal viscera suffer also. The kidneys, for example, secrete less or more urine than natural : if less, the deficiency amounts occasionally to complete ischuria ; if more, the urine is pale and diabetic. And so there is one or other of the two opposite states of constipation and diarrhœa, but usually constipation, with spasm of the colon, giving rise to colic. In the more aggravated cases, the motor nerves of the large intestines, bladder, abdominal parietes, and lower extremities are also affected ; and tympanites, vesical paralysis, constipation, and paraplegia ensue. The tenderness experienced is not simply tenderness on pressure, but it is a *tenderness to the slightest touch,* and when there is spinal tenderness, for it is not always present in these cases, the tenderness is of the same kind. The abdominal tenderness of peritoneal or visceral inflammation differs altogether from the preceding, both in its history and concomitant symptoms. It is rarely seen in neuræmic females, except when the case is quite manifest, as for example, when there is chronic structural disease of the peritoneum or abdominal viscera, accompanied by inflammation, or when it appears in parturient females as a symptom of metritis. We believe the neuræmic state is rarely coincident with structural disease within the abdomen, or terminates in it.

" The accompanying phenomena differ widely ; in the tenderness from peritoneal inflammation it is impossible not to be struck by the peculiarly haggard expression of countenance of the patient ; in neuræmic tender-.

ness, the expression is rather that of peevishness and pain than of mortal suffering. In the latter, there is rarely or never, the grass-green vomit observed in peritonitis; the pulse, too, is fuller, rounder, and larger, nor are the knees of the patient drawn up as in peritoneal inflammation: in the latter, tenderness on pressure, and not tenderness to the touch, is the distinguishing characteristic.

" The diagnosis of all neuræmic affections, whether their seat lies in the head, thorax, or abdomen, is, mutatis mutandis, precisely similar. The previous history of the patient, and the physiological character of the symptoms themselves, will almost always enable the practitioner to decide. Inflammatory diseases of the heart, lungs, and brain, are peculiarly liable to be confounded with neuræmic affections of those organs.

" With respect to the treatment of cases of cerebro-spinal irritation, we would above all observe that it must be constitutional. They principally occur, idiopathically, in females whose parents are gouty, and of the nervous temperament, or at least who have themselves suffered from affections of the nervous system. Neuræmia of the cerebral and spinal ganglia is not unfrequently seen in females, one or other of whose parents has been insane. This we believe is extremely usual, and the fact is of importance, both in the diagnosis and treatment of the affections of all the viscera in connection with the spinal cord. While remedies suitable to the constitutional peculiarities of the case are administered, endermic medication, on the principle of incident excitor action, will be found of singular benefit ; even the metallic neurines, as arsenic, may be thus employed with safety and efficiency. We would conclude this short sketch of the treatment, by the observation that no plan whatever will be successful unless the hygienic condition of. the patient—namely, the condition as to mental occupation, sleep, diet, pure air, sufficient light, and exercise be strictly attended to."

Part xi., *p.* 13.

Rheumatic Caries of the Spine.—It is of great importance in practice to distinguish between strumous caries of the spine, and the rheumatic caries described by Sir B. Brodie, as the two diseases are quite different in their origin, progress and termination, and the treatment required is also different in each case. In the former, pain is frequently, though not invariably met with ; in the latter it is a constant symptom, whilst in paraplegia from disease of the chord alone, there is entire absence of pain. We may also be assisted in our diagnosis by the moral history of our patient, as well as by the presence of a strumous or rheumatic diathesis. But in females we meet with the most anomalous symptoms, which, if there be no rheumatic diathesis, no increase of pain on pressure, the pain shifting from one part of the spine to the other, may pretty safely be referred to hysteria.

With respect to the patholgy of the disease, Mr. Solly believes that it is local ; the mollities ossium *rubra et fragilis ;* and renders this view probable by instancing the softening of the bones of the pelvis occasionally met with, which is an entirely local disease, and from which recovery not unfrequently takes place. A medical friend of Mr. Solly's, who had suffered under this rheumatic caries, broaches the very pertinent idea that nervous exhaustion may be a cause of diminished supply of phosphatic salts to the bone, seeing that the phosphorus is an essential constituent of the brain, and, therefore, that, from the superior importance of the latter to the system, the principal portion secreted would be supplied to it in preference to the bones. On this supposition, Mr. S. would give phosphoric acid freely, for he says that, even if it does not act specifically, it is a good tonic, often agreeing better than sulphuric acid with the system. The dose he would commence with is ten minims of the dilute acid. He mentions another important fact which should be strongly impressed on the mind in the treatment of all spinal affections, namely, the necessity for absolute quiet of the mental system, on account of the close connection existent between the spinal cord and the brain.

In treating this disease as inflammatory, it is necessary to be extremely careful in our antiphlogistic measures, on account of the general depression of the vital powers attendant upon inflammation of their structure. It will scarcely ever bear active treatment, and the blood-letting should be almost invariably merely local. *Part* xi., *p.* 146.

Alkaline Urine, consequent upon Injuries of the Spine.—Dr. Snow says that the urine is alkaline, because the bladder, being paralyzed, cannot expel the whole of its contents, and a little is constantly retained. Wash the bladder out with warm water every day or two. *Part* xv., *p.* 144.

Spine—Lateral Curvature from Relaxed Ligaments.—Sir B. Brodie says that if the patient is 19 or 20, treatment is of no avail; it must be begun if possible at 13 or 14, and patiently continued. Improve the general health by country and seaside residence, open-air exercise, tonics, etc. Strengthen the muscles of the back by climbing and other exercises; for which in delicate girls friction and shampooing for an hour or two daily may be substituted. And let the patient lie down either a part or the whole of the time that she is not engaged in exercise.

In *inveterate cases*, as where one scapula is three times as far from the spinous processes as the other, it is necessary to use artificial support. The patient may walk on crutches, so high, that only the toe can be placed on the ground, or wear a machine to take the weight of the shoulders off the spine, and to make pressure on the projecting ribs. Some of the best are those made by Bigg, of Leicester Square, Laurie, of Bartholomew Close, and that known as Tavernier's lever belt.

From Rickets.—The general treatment is the same as that for rickets generally. *Instruments are worse than useless.* *Part* xv., *p.* 155.

Angular Curvature of the Spine.—Dr. Pirrie recommends the following as the most judicious plan of treatment to pursue: Any attempt to remove the curvature would be most injudicious. Anchylosis is the only favorable termination to be hoped for, and therefore the object aimed at in treatment should be to place the patient under the circumstances most likely to conduce to that result. With that view it is indispensable, first, to keep the patient in a recumbent position, so as to remove from the diseased parts the pressure of the superimposed weight, and to preserve the parts as much as possible in a state of perfect quietude in that position; and, secondly, to use all means, judicious and available in the circumstances of the case, for maintaining the general health. In some cases, local remedies are highly beneficial.

One particular advantage which results from preserving the parts at perfect rest in the horizontal position, is that the removal of the irritation caused by the superincumbent weight from the diseased parts, diminishes the danger of the formation of abscess, which is a most unpromising occurrence, and must induce the gloomiest apprehensions as to the ultimate results. One of the best means for fulfilling the above indication is to place the patient in the supine position on Earle's bed, which, beside other advantages rendering it very convenient for this part of the treatment, allows the relative position of the trunk and limbs with regard to each other to be slightly changed, without any risk of moving the diseased parts on each other. The slight change thus allowed renders the confinement to the recumbent position much less irksome than it otherwise would be. As an additional precaution for preserving the diseased parts from any movement, it is in many instances advisable to apply splints on each side of the spine. The splints in such cases must suit the shape of the parts to which they are applied.

Rest of the diseased parts, and the recumbent position, whether the body be prone or supine, are of the utmost importance from the very commencement of the disease until a cure is effected by anchylosis. When it is believed that anchylosis has taken place, and the patient is allowed to resume the erect attitude, it is a judicious precaution to employ for some time an apparatus such as that generally known by the name of the spine supporter, for removing the superincumbent weight.

[The maintenance of the general health is another important indication, but, unfortunately, some of the best means for fulfilling it are incompatible with the essential points of judicious treatment. In individuals of a scrofulous diathesis, insufficient clothing and food, or any causes acting permauently or habitually, have doubtless an influence in exciting caseous deposits in bone as well as in other textures. Hence the necessity of a generous digestible diet, pure air, and exposure to the light of the sun. As to the tonic remedies, that of iron is the most useful, but the class of medicines more immediately called for Dr. P. thinks are those which are calculated to preserve a healthy condition of the digestive organs. In cases where the disease depends upon scrofulous caries of the vertebræ, or upon softening with absorption without ulceration or caries, the surgeon should not deplete, but advise the recumbent position, quietude, and the preservation of the general health.]

In scrofulous caries, benefit will often be found to accrue from the early and very cautious employment of counter-irritation along with the treatment here alluded to. If the curve arise from inflammation of the bodies of the vertebræ, of their investing membrane, or of the intervertebral cartilages, slight local depletion by leeching or cupping at the commencement of the disease, and afterward counter-irritation, are known to be highly beneficial. The repeated application of small pieces of blister to each side of the vertebral column at the seat of the disease has been found well suited for children, and caustic issues for adults. Of the various means for producing counter-irritation, Mr. Pott gave the preference to caustic issues. It is improper to produce a great discharge, which would tend to weaken the patient, and besides, the long continuance of a profuse discharge and irritation might induce hectic fever. If abscesses form, the issues should be discontinued. Mr. Pott, whose valuable works contain many cases of disease of the spine, attended with paralysis, successfully treated by the application of counter-irritants, was the first who pointed out to the profession the results of such practice, and many have since followed it with equal success.   *Part* xv., *p.* 161.

Distortions of the Spine.—Bransby Cooper says that we should endeavor to improve the nutrition of the bones, by the use of articles of diet containing a good deal of phosphate of lime, as beef and mutton, giving at the
same time phosphoric acid, to render the salt of lime more soluble. Bottled
porter will also do good, if it do not relax the bowels. Support the
weight of the trunk by the simplest possible mechanical means, and put
into gentle action such muscles as may counteract the unnatural direction
the bones have acquired. Let such exercise in the open air be taken as
causes the least fatigue, as riding in an open carriage, or sailing on the sea.

Part xvii., *p.* 125.

Spine—Curvature of the.—Dr. Bishop says that when the spine becomes
curved from previous curvature of the legs in weak children, support
should be given by the use of leg irons, made with joints corresponding to
those of the hip, knee, and ankle. Many object to the use of leg irons,
but their objections are refuted both by sound theory and by the results
of practice.   *Part* xviii., *p.* 148.

*Functional Affection of the Spine, liable to be mistaken for Organic
Disease.*—The affection alluded to was essentially a disease of the young,
being seen most frequently between twelve and twenty years of age. Dr.
Kennedy had, however, met with it as early as nine years, and as late as
twenty-five. He had only seen it in private practice, and it was more
common amongst males than females, in the proportion of at least two to
one. It consisted in a pain in the back, combined with weakness, and
this was always referred to the lumbar region; at least he had never seen
it higher up. This pain commenced gradually, and might or might not be
attended with the feeling of weakness; and occasionally only the latter
was complained of. On examining the spine, the patient was nearly always
able to refer the suffering to a particular part; but Dr. Kennedy had seen
cases where the feeling was more diffused. It was worthy of notice, that
a rough examination of the part might be made—the spine might be
twisted, or percussion strongly used, and yet the patient would not complain. When left to their own feelings, they invariably preferred the
recumbent posture. Walking was much less irksome than sitting, and
particularly when they had no support for the back. In addition to an
ordinary chair, they would use a cushion, so that it might press on the
spine where they complained; and even when reclining at full length, they
often placed a cushion in the hollow of the back, so as to cause direct
pressure. Those whose business led them to stand or work at a desk,
seemed peculiarly liable to the affection.

On the subject of treatment, Dr. Kennedy had nothing very definite to
offer. A considerable variety of means had been used, both local and
constitutional. The former included local bleedings, dry cupping, blisters,
frictions, the cold douche, and galvanism; and the latter, aperients, tonics,
change of air, and relaxation from business. Of these two, the latter had
in his experience proved by much the most useful. He had also seen
benefit follow the application of small and repeated blisters, as also the use
of a weak stream of galvanism, applied daily, or every second day, according to circumstances. The patient, too, often got great relief from wearing a stiff belt. Still the general measures were the most important.

Part xxiv., *p.* 64.

ιaustion.—In remarking upon the beneficial effects of strych-
of impaired spinal energy, Dr. Marshall Hall says:

Such cases occur from causes of nervous exhaustion, such as excessive
study, muscular effort, sexual indulgence, etc.; and in such cases strychnia
has appeared to me the appropriate and useful remedy.

This agent acts distinctly on the spinal marrow. In excess it induces
spasmodic affection. It is therefore contra-indicated in cases of *irritation*
of this nervous centre of spasm. Its appropriate use is in spinal *exhaustion*.
It constitutes one of our best tonics, improving the general health, and
conducing to the recovery of strength and flesh.

I have given it in minute doses thrice a day, in the midst of meals, for
many months. The following is the formula which I have adopted: ℞
Strychniæ acetatis, gr. j.; acidi acetosi, ♏xx.; alcoholis, ℨij.; aquæ destillatæ,
ℨvj. M.

Of this, ten drops, containing one-fiftieth part of a grain, may be
given thrice a day; but I have generally begun with five, and gone on to
fifteen.

In two cases only have I known it to disagree. It seemed to affect the
head. In many the patient has improved in looks, as in general health and
strength, without experiencing anything but good from it.

I am giving the strychnia a cautious trial in the epilepsy attended by
pallor, thinness, and nervous exhaustion; in the paraplegia the result of
sexual excesses, and in which neither pain nor spasm has occurred; and in
the paralysis agitans.   *Part* xxvii., *p.* 58.

Spinal Curvature.—M. Piorry gives one ounce of fine filings of fresh
bones daily, either in milk, or better still, in rice milk, which entirely dis-
guises all disagreeable taste. At the same time the patient must be freely
exposed to fresh air and sunlight.   *Part* xxxv., *p.* 75.

SPLEEN.

Uses of the Spleen.—Dr. O'Beirne offers an ingenious theory respecting
the uses of the spleen, which is much the same as the one entertained by
Professor Hargrave.

He arrives at the conclusion that this viscus in the healthy state is contracted and at rest, that it contains no more blood than is poured into its
cells, after becoming venous, by its nutritious arteries; and that it performs no function but that of a *reservoir* for the relief of overloaded states
of the vena cava inferior and the whole portal system. This is easily seen
to be probable when we remember that the venæ cavæ hepaticæ enter the
vena cava inferior just as it is passing through the tendinous opening of
the diaphragm, that their mouths are large and always wide open, having
no valves and consequently admitting of reflux, and that the powers which
propel the blood of the portal system are very feeble compared with those
which propel that in the inferior cava, all which circumstances seem to
show that the venæ cavæ hepaticæ, as well as the rest of the portal system,
instead of offering resistance, are constructed not only to facilitate but to
provide for determination toward them: the blood of course would easily
find its way along the splenic vein into the spleen, and this organ would
thus act as an immense and most important reservoir to relieve venous

obstructions almost throughout the whole system, either immediately or collaterally.   *Part* vi., *p.* 54.

Engorgement of the Spleen—German Treatment of.—Dr. Schwabe has employed the following in engorgement of the liver and spleen:

℞ Belladonna root, powdered, a grain and a half; muriate of quinine, four grains; powdered rhubarb, fifteen grains; mix. Divide into ten powders. One to be taken morning, noon, and night, in any convenient vehicle.   *Part* viii., *p.* 78.

———•◆•———

SPONGE TENTS.

Improved Method of Making.—Mr. Coates says : The plan I adopt is to select a piece of the best cupped sponge, of the required form and size, and, after beating and washing it well to free it from any sand or gritty particles it may contain, to squeeze it almost to dryness in a towel. A piece of tape about ten inches long is then passed through the sponge at about one-third from its base, making a shallow groove on each side from the apertures to the base for the tape to rest in, both ends of which are tied together for the withdrawal of the tent when necessary. Having fixed one end of a piece of whipcord (say two or three yards long) to some firm object, I commence winding the other end on the sponge gradually, from apex to base, as firmly as possible. The tent is then well dried before the fire, or in an oven, previous to the removal of the cord. When it is thoroughly dry, a small hole about half an inch deep should be made in the base, with a joiner's pricker or a heated wire, for the introduction by the director. The whole surface of the tent is then slightly coated by dipping it into equal parts of melted lard and beeswax. The expansion of the tents is gradual, and never requires the aid of "tepid water injections," the moisture of the surrounding parts being quite sufficient.

No possible good can accrue from steeping the sponge in a solution of gum, which not only renders the operation most disagreeable and un-cleanly, but also prevents the close contraction by the retention of the glutinous particles in the interstices of the sponge.   *Part* xxii., *p.* 306.

———•◆•———

SPRAINS.

Application of Cold to Sprains.—Many different opinions have been entertained as to whether recent sprains should be treated by warm or cold applications. We find that Mr. Cock, of Guy's Hospital, entertains, as the result of his large experience, a very strong preference for cold. He states that the consequences of a sprain may be very much limited, both in duration and severity, by the early and efficient employment of cold. It should either be done by iced water, or by irrigation. Mr. Cock is accustomed to quote by way of illustration of the powers of cold, the certainty with which the application of ice will induce the absorption of effused blood in an ordinary ecchymosis, a power which, by the way, in certain cases of "black eye" may be turned to good account.
                                                Part xxxii., *p.* 138.

SQUILL.

Squill.—According to the "Northern Journal of Medicine," squill obviates some of the ill effects of opium. If an aperient be added besides, the good effects of opium may often be obtained when it would otherwise be inadmissible.

R Pulv. opii; pul. scillæ, aa. gr. iij.; aloes; conservæ rosæ, aa. gr. ix. Fiat mass. divid. in pil. vj. æquales. Sign, opiate pills, two at bed-time.

We have remarked very beneficial results in cases of chronic ill health with tendency to dryness of the skin, from the continued use of such combinations as the following. Besides its diaphoretic effects, it should be regarded as alterative.

R Resinæ guaiaci; extract. gentianæ, aa. 3j.; pulv. ipecacuanhæ, gr. xv. Ft. mass. divid. in pil. xxx. æquales. Sign, tonic alterative pills, two twice a day.

Or, if an aperient be required, aloes may be substituted for the gentian, and then the combination will somewhat resemble the pulv. aloes comp. of the London Pharmacopœia. *Part* x., *p.* 187.

——•♦•——

STAMMERING.

M. Colombat's Treatment.—M. Colombat has recommended a most judicious method of treatment, which if rightly pursued is always sure to effect a cure. It consists in the adoption of the following three means: 1. Giving the tongue such a position that its apex is directed upward and backward. 2. Taking in a deep breath at the commencement of each phrase, and repeating this more or less frequently. 3. Marking the time in speaking by the movements of the thumb upon the forefinger. *Part* ii., *p.* 79

Operative Treatment.—Various operations have been proposed for the cure of stuttering, which may be classed as follows:

1st. Simple transverse division of the muscular structure of the base of the tongue, performed by M. Dieffenbach by two separate methods.

2d. Transverse division, with excision of a portion of the base of the tongue, performed by the same surgeon.

3d. Mr. Lucas' method, consisting of excision of a triangular portion of the bodies of the genio-glossi muscles.

4th. A simple incision in the bodies of the genio-glossi muscles, common to MM. Amussat, Phillips, and Velpeau, though performed in a different manner by each.

5th. Division of the attachment of the tendons of the genio-glosso muscles (and occasionally of the hyo-glossi muscles also) to the lower jaw, performed, in different ways, by MM. Baudens and Bonnet.

6th. Simple division of the mucous and subjacent tissue of the floor of the mouth, occasionally found sufficient, by M. Amussat.

7th. Excision of a portion of the apex of the tongue, performed in one case by M. Velpeau.

8th. Mr. Yearsley's method of snipping off a portion of the uvula.
Part iii., *p.* 74.

Auxiliary Treatment.—Dr. Abercrombie has observed a few facts which may lead to a material improvement in the treatment of stammering : Stammerers never stammer in singing ; nor when the voice is elevated to a particular pitch, as during conversation in a crowd or in a carriage on a rough road ; on the contrary, they stammer when endeavoring to speak when the lungs have become emptied of air or nearly so. Among other indications of treatment therefore, the patient should accustom himself never to speak except with a full and continuous current of air proceeding outward from the lungs. The affection is not perceived to be owing to any defect in the organs of speech, and if he would speak in that tone of voice as if he were calling to a person at a distance, or in a tone resembling singing or chanting, he would probably find himself considerably improved : and for this purpose, Dr. Abercrombie recommends that the person should read aloud several times a day from an author whose style is somewhat declamatory. "In doing so he should be made to read in a high-pitched tone, and to stop frequently and take a full breath, so as to have the voice thrown out with a force beyond what is required for ordinary reading or ordinary conversation. With this view, it is necessary to make him stop and take a full inspiration much more frequently than would be required by any other person. In particular whenever he feels the tendency to hesitate at a word, he is to be taught to stop instantly, take a full breath, and then try it again."   *Part* vii., *p.* 78.

———•••———

STERILITY.

Carbonic Acid Gas, as a Counter-irritant.—In a discussion in the London Medical Society respecting the nature and value of counter-irritation, Dr. James Johnson alluded to carbonic acid gas, applied either as a local or a general external remedy. In the first mode of its application, the gas was admitted into the vessel from beneath, and slowly ascended until it filled the bath. The patient's body was entirely immersed, his head being protected by a covering fitting close to the upper part of the bath, admitting the head only through an aperture in its centre. When the gas was locally applied, it was conducted in tubes of various diameters, and with such variety of force as the case might require. He had tried the remedy both locally and generally ; it acted in both cases as a powerful stimulant. Its first action was the production of a momentary sensation of cold which was followed by a feeling of heat, which when the gas was applied locally, was sometimes so intense as to be scarcely tolerable. Perspiration succeeded to these phenomena. The application of carbonic acid in this manner was stated to be of great benefit in a variety of chronic diseases, in which there was no trace of inflammatory action. It was beneficial in tic-doloureux, atonic gout, and rheumatism, and similar diseases. If the reports were to be credited, it also exerted a remarkably powerful influence upon the reproductive organs. Females who for years had sighed in vain for progeny, became fertile in a very short space of time after this gas had been applied in douches to the uterus, by means of a pipe introduced into contact with that organ into the vagina. Cases in which this beneficial result had followed its use were so numerous, that the subject merited consideration.

Dr. Clutterbuck relates a case, "of great irritation and some prolapsus of the uterus" in which Dr. Rossi, of Turin, used carbonic acid gas with the greatest advantage. There was "no organic disease of the uterus, but a preternatural irritation of the genital organs altogether, and the general health was suffering from sympathy with the local disease." It was treated by the repeated local application of carbonic acid gas to the uterus, in the manner described by Dr. Johnson. The quantity of gas applied was thirty cubic inches on each occasion. Nine hundred and thirty cubic inches were applied altogether. The local disease was removed, both the irritation and the prolapsus altogether ceasing, and the health became restored. *Part* ii., *p.* 64.

Sterility—Proposed Remedy for.—Dr. Marshall Hall throws out a suggestion on the treatment of sterility, which may be tried under some circumstances. There is an extraordinary sympathy between the mammæ and the uterus, so that the functional condition of the former influences that of the latter. "This sympathy is partly nervous in its character, partly vascular. As a reflex action the uterus is made to contract after parturition, by applying the newly-born infant to the mammæ. As a vascular sympathy, uterine hemorrhage and leucorrhœa occur from undue lactation." Many cases of sterility, of course, arise from organic defect, but when the cause is of a functional and less permanent nature, it becomes a question whether or not the uterus can be stimulated so as to assume a healthy functional action in the way suggested by Dr. M. Hall, who says : My suggestion, then, is, that when the mamma is excited at the return of the catamenial period, a robust infant be repeatedly and perseveringly applied, in the hope that the secretion of milk may be excited, and that the uterine blood may be diverted from the uterus and directed into the mammary vessels, and that a change in the uterine system and a proneness to conception may be induced. I would propose that the patient should sleep, for one week before, and during each catamenial period, with an infant on her bosom. *Part* ix., *p.* 202.

Sterility.—Dr. Oldham believes that the greatest discrimination is required in the use of mechanical treatment ; both because it is not easy to distinguish cases in which there is really mechanical obstruction, from perfectly natural conditions, and also because the operations for the relief of such obstructions are not without danger. *Strictures of the os or cervix* sufficient to prevent impregnation are very rarely met with ; and the attempt at mechanical dilatation has been followed by a fatal result. The treatment of *mal-position of the uterus* supposed to be the cause of sterility, has also caused death. Lastly, *obstructions in the fallopian tubes* are probably never, when they do occur, of a kind which could be overcome by catheterism ; and as this operation will be always extremely difficult, and never without danger, its performance appears to be altogether indefensible. *Part* xx., *p.* 217.

Japanese Remedy for Sterility.—Dr. E. Williams has described a Japanese remedy for sterility. The tree is one of the order of Ternstromaceæ of Jessieu, with leaves somewhat larger than those of the congou tea, emitting an odor when bruised resembling pulegium and sabina. The mode of preparation is to take a quantity of the leaves, macerate them in as much rice spirit as will just moisten them, for six hours ; then express, and give about a teaspoonful every hour, and two or three doses will invariably bring on the menstrual secretion, which can be maintained by a dose or two daily, for any length of time. *Part* xxii., *p.* 320.

Sterility.—In those cases which cannot be accounted for by any disease, but which seem to depend on defective ovarian action, apply Professor Recamier's galvanic poultices. *Part* xxiv., *p.* 348.

Sterility from Dysmenorrhœa, etc.—When the cervix uteri is very much contracted, says Dr. I. B. Brown, introduce through the speculum a long stilette into the uterus, then over this pass the smallest sized elastic tube, and allow it to remain for a short time. Gradually pass on from this to larger tubes, until Simpson's dilators can be introduced. The best time for introducing the instrument is immediately after the cessation of the catamenia. Diseases of the rectum will also produce sterility. The rectum and uterus are both supplied by vessels and nerves from the same source, and therefore disease in the one organ must interfere with the other. When a female is suffering from bleeding hemorrhoids, during the menstrual period a diminished supply of blood is sent to the uterus, and its mucous membrane will not undergo those normal changes necessary for the reception of the impregnated ovum. The same observations apply to prolapsus ani with loss of blood at every defecation : when this is the cause, apply two or three ligatures to the prolapsed mucous membrane, and return them within the sphincter. Give opiates to keep the bowels quiet, and give good diet. After the usual operation for fissure of the rectum, you must give opium regularly and freely to relieve pain and secure perfect rest for the bowel. After a week or ten days they may be moved by injections. *Part* xxxv., *p.* 251.

STOMACH.

Atony of the Stomach.—Dr. Debreyne believes this disease is not of unfrequent occurrence, especially in women affected with leucorrhœa, chlorosis, anæmia, etc.

One important characteristic is, that the distress of the stomach is usually increased by the use of vegetable and farinaceous food, and relieved, more or less, by a generous diet of animal meat, wine, etc.

Neither opiates nor antiphlogistics are suited to such a case ; tonics alone constitute the most approved treatment, such as the use of some mild ferruginous preparation, quinine, or of some other vegetable bitter, as gentian, calumba, aloes, etc., in the form either of infusion or wine.

In a variety of *gastro-atony*, characterized by frequent returns of vomiting, from 5 to 10 grains of powdered calumba, recommended 3 or 4 times a day.

If the epigastric uneasiness should be troublesome, advised to combine with the calumba a mild opiate. *Part* i., *p.* 23.

Nitrate of Silver in Gastric Affections.—[A good case of this kind is related by Dr. Dick, in which this remedy was useful.]

A young gentleman had stomach ailments almost from infancy. The most distressing symptom, however, was eructation of an acid and burning fluid and gas from the stomach, which often commenced even during meals, and continued for hours afterward. Yet his bowels were regular, urine natural, and the functions of the skin normal, with sound sleep—and no apparent disorder or disease of any other organ in the body.

The case of this young gentleman appearing to me to betray a union of morbid secretions and morbid sensibility, I commenced the treatment with small doses of blue pill and ipecacuanha, from which no immediate benefit appeared to result. I then put him upon a month's course of nitrate of silver, with a view to allay the morbid sensibility of the mucous membrane. The effect in this, as in almost every other case in which I have tried it, was surprising and gratifying in the extreme. This patient, in common with many others who had taken this medicine, warmly expressed the great relief from irritation, flatulence, cutaneous chillness, discomfort, which it promptly procured. *Part* v., *p.* 61.

Chronic Diseases of the Stomach—Atony of the Stomach.—This kind of gastric affection, says Dr. Strange, so common among the crowded population of manufacturing towns, presents the following symptoms and physical signs : The tongue is large, flat and flabby, filling the whole width of the mouth, its surface almost uniformly pale and without scurf, presenting the appearance of boiled veal or muscular fibre which has been macerated in cold water; the face pale and flaccid, corresponding remarkably with the tongue ; the epigastrium distended, not painful, but uneasy on pressure ; the abdomen in women often pendulous and flabby, sometimes hard and tender ; the pulse is generally unaffected, or it is weak and small.

Patients affected with this form of disease complain that they have no appetite, or that they crave for things which are to them indigestible.

There is not often very acute pain in the region of the stomach or along any part of the digestive canal ; but sometimes to the sense of fullness succeeds a constriction about the lower part of the epigastrium, accompanied by eructations of gas sometimes mixed with acidity. There is flatulence, with irregularity of the bowels, a general state of costiveness being occasionally interrupted by a painful diarrhœa. A feeling of constriction, with pain extending through the back, coming on two or three hours after meals, may be owing, as is supposed by Dr. Abercrombie, to irritation created in the duodenum by the passage of insufficiently digested food into the bowel ; and I have remarked that this pain very frequently coexists with a relaxed state of the bowels and painful emotions. On the whole, however, a feeling of acute pain coming on periodically some hours after a meal is much more frequently met with in another well-marked form of gastric disorder, viz., where the tongue exhibits a degree of redness round the edges, with furred centre ; and where there is pain on pressing the epigastrium, denoting an irritable state of the mucous and muscular coats of the stomach.

With the view of reducing the irritation, if any, and of gently stimulating the stomach, I have for a length of time mainly depended upon one substance, viz., the oxide of bismuth, which has also been highly extolled by Dr. Paris and other authorities. When cases to which it is applicable are selected, I believe that not one in ten cases will occur in which much benefit will not be procured from its use. The manner in which I prescribe is as follows :

R Bismuth. trisnitrat., 3j.; morphiæ muriat., gr. ss.-j.; acaciæ mucil.,

℥ij.; sirup. zingiber.; tinct. cardam. com., aa. ℨiij.; infus. cascaill., ℥v.
M.—℥j. ter die.

This formula retains its appearance for a length of time; the mucilage
suspending the bismuth in such a manner as to give to the mixture the
consistence of cream. In pyrosis, taken at the period of attack, and in
that form of gastrodynia previously described, taken half an hour after
meals, it immediately assuages the pain and promotes digestion. In those
cases particularly where there is considerable derangement of the
duodenum, this medicine acts like a charm.

All kinds of fermented and spirituous liquors, as they debilitate as well
as stimulate, are injurious in this affection. Purgatives must not be resorted to for the relief of the costiveness which so often accompanies this
form of dyspepsia as by over-exciting they afterward debilitate the intestines. Gentle laxatives with tonics, such as small doses of aloes or colocynth
with sulphate of iron, as recommended by Dr. Abercrombie, or with sulphate of zinc, are the most beneficial.

Atonic Morbid Irritability of the Stomach.—I look upon this second
form of dyspepsia as the natural consequence of a long continuance of the
former atonic variety.

The symptoms indicating this affection differ considerably from those
characteristic of mere want of tone. The tongue is generally slightly red
at the tip or round the edges; there is a thin whitish fur all over the
centre which cannot be scraped off; a sense of heat in the throat, œsophagus, and sometimes in the stomach. The sleep is often disturbed, and
muscular efforts are weakened. The appetite is always uncertain in this
affection, following the remissions and exacerbations of the attacks. There
is a general desire for savory and solid food, although this almost invariably aggravates the symptoms. There is pain in the stomach during the
whole time the food remains there, which is sometimes relieved by vomiting
coming on from half an hour to three or four hours after a meal.
Substances in small quantities are seldom returned. In some cases there
is a sense of weight only at the stomach until about two hours after taking
food, when a sense of pain and constriction ensues, which lasts frequently
until relieved by a relaxed but unsatisfactory motion. In these cases it
has been no doubt rightly supposed that the irritable stomach pushes
onward the partially digested food into the duodenum, whence it is either
forced back by vomiting, or passes out of the bowels, after giving pain in
its whole course, in a partially relaxed and often scalding motion. This
morbid irritation of the stomach is sometimes accompanied by a degree of
pyrosis, but not by any means in a constant manner. The regurgitations
are more frequently composed of the mucus of the stomach mixed with
acidity, gas, and the aroma of the food.

When the disorder has not arrived at any very troublesome height a
similar treatment to that recommended for atony of the stomach, will be
found to answer very well. In more exaggerated cases, however, and
especially if there be much pain and heat at the epigastrium, it will be
well to begin with moderate counter-irritation, as a blister, two or three
mustard poultices, or the ung. antim. tart. All drastic purgatives, particularly mercurial ones, should be avoided, as they increase the irritation.
The oxide of bismuth, with infusion of rhubarb and magnesia, will be
found to answer the double purpose of maintaining a steady action upon
the bowels, and of correcting the acidity and heat of the stomach.

The following is a good formula :

R Bismuth trisnitrat., 3j.; magnes. carb., 3ss.; tinct. Kyoscyami, 3ij.; Infus. rhei, ʒviii. M.

One ounce of this mixture to be taken three or four times a day. After the more acute symptoms have been reduced, the mixture of bismuth with gentle stimulants and tonics, as prescribed for the atonic state, will answer well; and, finally, we may have recourse to quinine, iron, zinc, and other direct tonics.

Should there be much acidity with regurgitation some time after taking food, accompanied with a costive and unsatisfactory state of the bowels, the following pill, taken regularly after the principal meal, will be found very useful:

R Aloes in pulv. gr. iss.; ferri sulph., gr. ij.; sapon. dur., gr. vj. M.— Div. in pil. ij. simul sumend.

The soap is a great addition to the aloes and iron pill in common use, as it unites chemically with the free acid of the stomach. *Part* x., *p.* 68.

Vegetable Acids in Acidity of the Stomach.—Dr. Tracy, of Ohio, makes the following remarks on vegetable acids as correctives of acidity of the stomach: During the summer of 1841, I was myself the subject of repeated and severe attacks of catarrhal inflammation of the eyelids, which uniformly yielded to the usual treatment in the course of from three to six days. I observed that they always succeeded to irregularities of diet and regimen, or to anxiety of mind, and were accompanied by acidity of stomach. This I attempted to correct by the early and free use of soda, but in vain; it had but a very slight and temporary effect. As these attacks became more and more frequent, I observed that they were preceded by a sense of fullness and oppression in the præcordia. I had for months abstained from the use of acids, under the impression that they were not suited to my state of health; but having received no benefit from soda, I was induced to take a glass of lemonade, at the first commencement of the attack, and almost instantly I experienced very copious eructations of gas, together with much alleviation of my feelings of distress. The remedy was again and repeated, and the threatened ophthalmic attack effectually prevented. I have since resorted to my bottle of lemon sirup, whenever threatened with a recurrence of the complaint, and uniformly with complete success; all the symptoms being removed in the course of a short time. I have from the time above mentioned to the present (June, 1843), made a free use of acids, and have not experienced a single recurrence of ophthalmia, and very few, indeed, of pyrosis.

I have found vegetable acids uniformly and entirely successful in removing the disposition to attacks of acidity of stomach, in persons who, during the intervals of such attacks, were free from all such symptoms; and my impression is, that in all such cases they can be relied upon with more confidence than any other remedy. In cases of acidity, arising from pregnancy, I have found the sub-acid fruits of great service, while those that were tart could not be borne, and mineral acids were decidedly injurious, and where alkalies or absorbents were of little or no avail. *Part* x., *p.* 73.

Use of Acids in some Affections of the Stomach.—It seems to be a contradiction to cure acidity of the stomach by the administration of vegetable acids; but such seems to be the case in some peculiar and obstinate affections of this organ. Dr. Chapman, of Philadelphia, refers to the same thing in his late work on the diseases of the thoracic and abdominal viscera. He has found occasionally the most discrepant sorts of nourishment agreeing with dyspeptics. One patient was cured of his dyspepsia by drinking sour beer, another by living exclusively on raw turnips; other cases are related in which sour pie-cherries and vinegar were used. Dr. Tracy states that the vegetable acids will be successful when the alkalies have failed, and for general use he recommends lemonade or lemon-juice.

Part xi., *p.* 61.

Digestion of the Mucous Membrane by the Gastric Juice following simple Ulcer of the Stomach.—In that gastric disorder which often occurs in the advanced stages of phthisis, says Professor Budd, and is attended with increased secretion of the gastric juice, such as may produce ulceration, give liq. potassæ, fifteen drops, or bicarb. potassæ, a scruple, thrice a day, or give infusion of logwood, ℥j. thrice a day, which will also arrest diarrhœa. *Part* xvi., *p.* 149.

Simple Ulceration of the Stomach going on to Perforation.—[The symptoms of this disease, in its early stage, are not yet defined. Dr. Seymour has found, that before the fatal seizure, the patient has long felt pain after eating, unaccompanied with symptoms of acidity ; and aggravated sometimes by one kind of food, and sometimes by another, but most commonly by solid meat. As to treatment, Dr. S. observes] :

In the treatment of such cases, when there is real reason to suspect so serious a disease, soothing remedies seem to be indicated. The bowels should be carefully kept open by enemata, so as to prevent any acrid medicine coming in contact with the ulcer ; and occasional blisters to the epigastrium may be expected to be useful. Where the existence of the complaint is more clear, from the preceding pain and the subsequent vomiting of blood, a case which I have frequently seen, I know of no remedy so uniformly successful as the oil of turpentine taken internally.

Part xvi., *p.* 150.

Observations on Disorder of the Stomach.—Dr. Seymour observes, that pain dependent on excess of acid in the stomach, often becomes attended with great irritability of the heart and pulsation in the epigastrium, so that the patient is led to believe that he is suffering from disease of the heart, or aneurism of the aorta. These alarming symptoms are cured by the regular administration of antacid medicines with sedatives, or alkalies with rhubarb and calumba root. His formula is rhubarb, six grains; bicarbonate of soda, fifteen grains ; calumba powder, three grains ; compound cinnamon powder, two grains; to be taken in a glass of water, before dinner or at bed-time, and continued regularly during at least a fortnight. Pain without heartburn or vomiting, is most likely to be the result of irregular contraction of the stomach, in which case he relies on bismuth with magnesia, in the following formula—trisnitrate of bismuth, calcined magnesia, compound tragacanth powder, of each a scruple : rub together, and add water an ounce and a half; sirup half a drachm : this draught to be taken every four hours. He says bismuth is highly useful in all painful spasm arising from disorder in the intestinal canal, and states from his own knowledge that it was used with much effect at Moscow in the spasms of the Asiatic cholera in 1831.

When the pain of the stomach resists this treatment, he trusts to a grain of opium administered thrice daily; the bowels being in the meantime kept open by injections. In simple pyrosis he employs the compound powder of kino (Ph. Lond.)—namely, kino and opium with cinnamon, in doses of five grains a day, the bowels being kept free by aloes, rhubarb, or enemata. A blister over the epigastrium is sometimes useful at first. When under the idea that the liver is diseased, " calomel and purgatives are prescribed, such cases become greatly aggravated, both as to time and severity." Pyrosis is often, however, the forerunner of an incurable disease—namely, the fungoid disease of the stomach. *Part* xvi., *p.* 150.

Sarcina Ventriculi.—In a case of this disease under the care of Mr. Amyot, attended by frequent and most violent acid vomiting, after alkalies, hydrocyanic acid, creasote, nitrate of silver, and opium, had been tried, without permanent effect, ℥ss. of the concentrated essence of calumba, to the ℥viij. of water, and given every two or three hours during the attack, gave the most decided relief. *Part* xxvi., *p.* 87.

Sarcina Ventriculi.—One indication necessary to be fulfilled in the treatment of this disease is to destroy the fungus by a regular and systematic exhibition of alkalies, thereby removing the acidity so essential to its formation and development, and then to employ some remedy capable of destroying its growth. This may be done, says Dr. Hassall, by giving bicarbonate of potash and infusion of quassia, and afterward the sulphite of soda. The operation of this salt seems to be that the sulphite being decomposed in the stomach by the acids therein generated, sulphurous acid gas is liberated, the destructive effects of which upon parasitic formations like the sarcina is well known. *Part* xxvii., *p.* 83.

Sarcinæ Ventriculæ.—In a case of this disease, of many years' standing, under the care of Dr. Neale, University Col. Hospital, the following was the successful treatment: At first the diet was the same as that ordered commonly in diabetes mellitus. Three grains of sesquicarbonate of ammonia were given three times a day in one ounce of infusion of quassia, with one to two drachms of sulph. sublim., to open the bowels. Afterward the same diet was continued, but the medicine was sodæ hyposulph., ʒvj.; infus. quassiæ, ℥xij.-℥ss. ter die. The only variation made was, that precipitated sulphur was preferred to sublimed sulphur; and one ounce of cod-liver oil was given three times a day. *Part* xxviii., *p.* 109.

Sarcinæ Ventriculæ.—This disease is easily recognized, says Prof. Budd, by the vomited matter fermenting, both the foam on its surface and the sediment thrown down containing abundance of sarcinæ and torulæ. The fermentative process may be checked by giving half a minim of creasote in a pill at each meal. Common salt has the same effect. Bisulphite of soda from the liberation of sulphurous acid, has the same power. It may be given in doses of ʒss. to ʒj. in water, two or three times a day.

In chronic cases of the disorder, the drain from the coats of the stomach, and the frequent throwing up of part of its contents, causes constipation; and it is requisite to obviate this condition, since any undue accumulation in the bowels aggravates the stomach-disorder. The best aperients are probably aloetic or colocynth pills.

When the disorder is severe, and the patient reduced in flesh, opiates, timely administered, are of much service in lessening the uneasiness at the stomach, and promoting sleep.

It now and then happens, that the disorder coexists with chronic ulcer of the stomach, and that eating solid food causes *pain* in the stomach, which is different from the uneasiness that results from distention of the stomach, and pain also in the corresponding part of the back. In such cases, as in ordinary cases of simple ulcer, the diet should be of the least irritating kind.

By the various means enumerated, the disorder may be greatly mitigated, the strength of the patient kept up, and his life prolonged; which is as much as can be promised for any disorder which originates, as this usually does, in irremovable organic changes.   *Part* xxix., *p.* 108.

Epigastric Neuralgia.—[On the *slightest* pressure in the epigastric region great pain is felt in these cases—not occupying a space above the size of a five-shilling piece. The following illustrates this kind of case, which might easily be mistaken by the young practitioner. Dr. Lees proceeds:]

He says that he never experiences pain in the stomach, but that, after eating, he has been often obliged to lift his shirt from contact with the epigastrium, as the tenderness caused by even its apposition was intolerable, although it was not aggravated by increasing the pressure. The state of his general health and appetite is good; functions natural; tongue clean; bowels regular; no thirst, nausea, or vomiting. He does not suffer from flatulence, has no headache, but is very low spirited. The circulation is languid, pulse 56; heart's action feeble, but regular, and without any murmur; the abdominal muscles are in a state of constant tension, hard and rigid; there is no evidence of any tumor, nor abnormal pulsation in the epigastric region; neither pain nor tenderness in the back, nor in the course of the intercostal nerves. His easiest posture is on his left side, with the right leg drawn up. When he lies on his back with the right leg extended, the spine is arched, so that the hand can be passed freely under it, but it becomes quite flat and in contact with the bed, on the leg being flexed. The urine is of natural appearance, sp. gr., and reaction; no visible sediment, but on microscopic examination there are seen numerous very minute crystals of oxalate of lime aggregated in long masses.

He could not assign any cause for his complaint, except that he has been constantly employed in a very dusty meal-room, but he has neither suffered from cough, nor from any difficulty of respiration.

Tincture of aconite was applied over the tender part, but without any relief. Ordered:

R Infusi valerianæ, infusi cinchonæ, aa. ℥iij.

Sumat ℥j. ter in die; a small blister over the part, and to be dressed with acetate of morphia ointment, gr. j. ad ℥j.

He was allowed meat every day, and advised to walk about and amuse himself. Under this treatment he was cured.   *Part* xxx., *p.* 57.

Remedies for Stomach Disorders.—Prof. Budd remarks: Quinine, and the bitters generally, are especially grateful to persons who have injured their stomachs by hard drinking. With such persons they improve the appetite and strengthen digestion, and have a bracing effect upon the system at large.

In persons exhausted by over-work, or wherever weakness of the stomach is the result of general debility from other causes, they often do much good in the same way—*by improving the appetite* and strengthening the digestion.

They do harm in the organic diseases of the stomach; in plethoric states of the system; and generally where there is a furred tongue, or where the urine throws down a sediment of lithic acid, or of lithate of ammonia. Their most striking effect is to improve the appetite, when this has been impaired from hard drinking or from over-work, or from nervous exhaustion from other causes; and the best time for giving them is from half an hour before meals.

The different bitters have not precisely the same effect. Calumba has a sedative influence not possessed by the others, and probably on this account has had a wider reputation as a remedy for mere indigestion. Gentian and chiretta (which is of the gentian tribe, and is much employed by practitioners in India) tend to increase the secretion of the liver, or, at any rate, do not impede the secretion of the liver, which quinine and quassia seem often to do. They are, therefore, better suited to bilious persons, and to those cases of indigestion where the secretions of the liver are defective.

The different preparations of steel are especially useful in the indigestion that occurs in chlorosis, and generally where weakness of the stomach results from ánemia.

They do harm in plethoric states of the system, and generally where there is a furred tongue, or where the urine throws down a sediment of lithate of ammonia or of lithic acid.

The citrate, or ammonio-citrate is the most agreeable preparation to the taste, and generally the most grateful to the stomach. If there be any disposition to sickness or nausea, or any tendency to furring on the tongue, it may be given in conjunction with the bicarbonate of soda or potash. This makes a mixture having much the same effect as Griffith's mixture—the mistura ferri composita—and far more agreeable.

The muriated tincture of iron is more astringent than the other preparations, and may be given in conjunction with dilute muriatic acid, in the forms of indigestion suited to this latter medicine, when these exist in states of anæmia.

The sulphate of iron, like other metallic sulphates, has a tendency to cause sickness, and should not be given in cases where a disposition to sickness exists.

Steel medicines do good by improving the quality of the blood rather than by their immediate action on the coats of the stomach, and are best given at meal-times. They then are mixed with the food, and gradually absorbed with the products of digestion, and are less apt to offend the stomach and to cause headache than at other times.

Whenever steel medicines are given, it is essential that a regular action of the bowels be kept up. These medicines tend to confine the bowels and to cause evolution of sulphureted hydrogen in them: and unless this tendency be counteracted, they are apt to fur the tongue and cause headache.

The choice of purgatives is a very important matter in stomach disorders. The different purgatives exert their chief action on different portions of the intestinal canal: some excite the secretion or the peristaltic movement of one part, some of another. In disorders of the stomach and bowels, where a purgative is required, care should, therefore, be taken to select those which are least prone to irritate the injured or disordered part.

Castor oil, for example, offends the stomach, but acts very mildly on the large intestine. It should not be used in stomach disorders, or where, from any cause, a tendency to vomiting exists; but is better than any other purgative in dysentery, or during convalescence from typhoid fever, when the intestines are ulcerated, and in various other conditions where a speedy and sure purgative, and one not apt to irritate the large intestine, is required.

Senna acts chiefly on the small intestine, and, besides exciting its peristaltic action, increases the secretion from its mucous membrane. It acts, also, on the liver, increasing the secretion of bile. In conjunction with a few grains of calomel or blue-pill, it is, as every one knows, one of the best purgatives in bilious states of the system, or where an evacuant is required; but in mere disorders of the stomach it is often objectionable, from the tendency it has to cause sickness.

The best purgatives in stomach disorders are aloes and colocynth, which exert their chief action on the large intestine. These medicines may do much harm when the large intestine is ulcerated or inflamed; but in simple ulcer of the stomach, and in the most severe functional disorders of the stomach, they may generally be given without causing either pain of the stomach or sickness. In some kinds of functional disorder of the stomach, aloes seem indeed, like other bitters, to improve the appetite and strengthen digestion.

Aloes appear to act more exclusively on the large intestine, and irritate the stomach much less than colocynth, and hence, in stomach disorders are generally preferable to it.

Where, from the existence of piles, or from pregnancy, or some other condition, these medicines are objectionable, the best substitutes for them in stomach disorders are the saline purgatives, which exert their chief action on the small intestine, and have little tendency to cause pain in the stomach, or sickness. *Part* xxx., *p.* 58.

Stomach—Dilatation of, with Obstructions at the Pylorus.—A good diagnostic symptom of disease of the pylorus, says Dr. R. B. Todd, is the vomiting of sarcinæ with a peculiar yeast-like substance. Give half a drachm of sulphite of soda in an ounce and a half of water every four hours. If necessary increase the dose to a drachm. The sulphite of soda will destroy the sarcinæ, but it will not act upon a diseased pylorus. Where the disease, therefore, is simply from sarcinæ, give the sulphite, but otherwise, it is not to be depended upon. *Part* xxx., *p.* 59.

Sarcinæ Ventriculi.—Chloride of calcium, says Dr. A. Leared, is perhaps a better remedy to restrain the vomiting than hyposulphite of soda. Give the following draught: ℞ Liquoris calcii chloridi, ʒj.; aquæ ℥vij.; sumat haustum talem ter quotidie. *Part* xxxi., *p.* 92.

Gastric Affections.— *Vide* Selections from Favorite Prescriptions, Art. "Medicines."

Gastric Ulcer.—Dr. Handfield Jones thinks there are many who cannot dissever in their minds the idea of inflammation from that of ulceration, but he believes that the perforating gastric ulcer is essentially the result of a local failure of nutrition, and not in any degree *necessarily* connected with inflammation. Our chief object in treatment must be to improve the general condition of the system, by good nutritious diet, allowing five or six hours' rest between the meals; we must attend to the general mucous surface, and invigorate the organ as much as possible. For this purpose, counter-irritation, with sedatives and astringents, may be necessary at first; and, as soon as they can be borne, tonics, as acids, bitters, quinine, iron, and cod-liver oil. If there be much vomiting and pain, which the ordinary remedies fail to relieve, order strychnine, one-sixteenth of a grain; muriatic acid, one minim; water, one ounce; three times a day.

Part xxxiii., *p.* 111.

Affections of the Stomach—Excessive Secretion of Mucus and Gastric Juice.—Prof. Budd gives the following: Bismuth, combined with aromatics or alkalies, may be administered before meals with advantage. When there are fetid eructations, you may give creasote pills (containing from a quarter to half a minim) or a few grains of bisulphite of soda; or some finely powdered wood charcoal. To alleviate pain, and allay general nervous irritabiltiy, the best medicines probably are conium and belladonna, which do not confine the bowels or check the secretions as opium does.

Deficient Secretion of the Gastric Juice.—Take care that the albuminoid food be as liquid as possible; let the quantity requisite for the day's consumption be taken at frequent short intervals; and if likely to turn sour, guard it with alkalies. We often find a draught of cold water, an hour or two after meals, will remove the discomfort arising from difficult solution of meat meals; in part by replacing the gastric juice, and also by favoring the absorption of the delayed nutrimentary mass. In the way of medicines, a pill containing a grain of ipecacuanha, or capsicum, with three grains of rhubarb, may be taken before dinner. For slowness of digestion, ipecacuanha is more effectual than any of the other stimulants. When digestion is habitually slow and feeble, much lasting benefit will be derived from nitro-muriatic acid, taken half an hour before the principal meals.

Sympathetic Vomiting.—The most effectual remedies for this are, sedatives, to lessen the irritation from which it springs; alkalies, to neutralize the acids which the stomach contains; astringents, to restrain the undue and untimely secretion. The insoluble antacids, magnesia and chalk, are very suitable; bismuth has a remarkable effect in restraining undue secretion, especially when combined with magnesia or chalk. If there are any symptoms indicating inflammatory action, apply a blister to the epigastrium, and attend carefully to the diet, which should consist chiefly of milk and farinaceous food.

Pyrosis.—The classes of remedies which have been found most useful are astringents and sedatives. We might advantageously combine five grains of bismuth with a twelfth of the grain of the muriate of morphia; or five grains of the compound kino powder, or logwood, catechu, krameria, with opium, given two or three times daily before meals.

Indigestion of Drunkards.—The most efficient remedies are bitters, opium, and solid food. Gentian, quassia, and calumba, may be taken singly or combined, in the form of tincture, an hour before the principal meals; with these, small doses of opium or morphia may be advantageously combined, to tranquillize the nervous system, but in all these cases it is essential that the patient should eat as soon as possible some solid, nourishing food.

Employment of Vegetable and Mineral Tonics.—Quinine and the bitters generally do much good in persons exhausted by overwork, hard drinking, or other causes; they improve the appetite and strengthen digestion. The best time for giving them is about half an hour or an hour before meals. The different bitters have not precisely the same effect; calumba has a sedative influence not possessed by others; gentian and chiretta tend to increase the secretion of the liver; quinine and quassia seem to impede secretion. Tonics do harm in organic diseases of the stomach, in plethoric states of the system, and generally where there is a furred tongue, or when the urine throws down a sediment of the lithates. When there is any disposition to sickness or nausea, the amonio-citrate of iron, in conjunction with the bicarbonate of soda or potash, is the most pleasant preparation, and will have the same effect as Griffith's mixture. the sulphate of iron, like other metallic sulphates, has a tendency to cause sickness. Steel medicines act generally instead of locally, and are there-fore, best given at meal-times, so as to be absorbed with the food.

Part xxxiv., *p.* 71.

Ulcer of the Stomach.—If there be a constant gnawing pain at the epi-gastrium, says Dr. Brinton, apply some counter-irritant, as a blister, mus-tard poultice, etc.; if the powers are exhausted, dry cupping is the best means of mitigating it. A still more valuable remedy, in some cases of obstinate vomiting and severe pain, may be found in frequently swallow-ing small bits of pure ice. In cases of severe hemorrhage its use is almost indispensable. When severe pain is accompanied by very frequent vomiting, a very small opium pill is retained better than any other sedative. If diar-rhœa be present, the compound kino powder, combined with the trisnitrate of bismuth, is an excellent remedy. Ten or twenty grains of the trisnitrate of bismuth, with five to ten grains of the compound kino powder, has a very remarkable effect in relieving pain, vomiting, and diarrhœa. If flatu-lence be very troublesome the alkaline carbonates with bitter infusion are the best remedies. We can recommend the following combination: potass. iodid., gr. j.; potass. bicarb., gr. xv.; tinct. aurant., ʒss.; inf. calumb., ʒviiss. To be taken an hour after food. *Part* xxxiv., *p.* 76.

Syncope Senilis, arising from Gastric Irritation.—This complaint, ac-cording to Dr. Higginbottom, is common to all ages, but more particularly to infancy and old age. It is generally observed in persons above sixty, and takes place without any organic disease, although both the vascular and nervous system must be inactive and in an impaired condition.

Gastric irritation from the food remaining undigested in the stomach, appears to be the sole cause of the attack; this gives rise to syncope and convulsions which may be fatal. Vomiting at an early period is the most effectual remedy. Half a drachm of the powder of ipecacuanha, with ten or fifteen grains of bicarbonate of potash to neutralize any acidity, will produce full vomiting and raise the system to its normal condition. The nausea and ineffectual natural attempts at vomiting produce debility and exhaustion. If the first half drachm of ipecacuanha does not operate, a second dose may be given with perfect safety. In advanced age the body does not require the same amount of solid food. It has been erroneously said that "wine is the milk of old age;" the truth is that milk is the wine of old age; second childhood should be treated as directed by the late Dr. James Hamilton, of Edinburgh, "Plenty of milk, plenty of flannel, and plenty of rest." *Part* xxxiv., *p.* 99.

Treatment of Ulcer of the Stomach.—When hemorrhage from a chronic ulcer amounts to a considerable quantity, says Dr. Brinton, although it be only a symptom of the disease, yet we must direct special attention to it, and we may remark that the astringents we introduce are much more efficacious than in the case of bleeding into the lungs. If there is reason to believe that the bleeding is from a large vessel, the stomach must be kept in the state of perfect rest, the supine position must be rigidly observed, and the minimum of food that will support life, taken lest the clot which alone intervenes between life and death be disturbed.

In many cases of hematemesis, if there be no great tendency to vomiting, turpentine, or the sesquichloride of iron act admirably; but what is preferable, because it is not so apt to excite vomiting, is ten grains of gallic acid, dissolved in an ounce of distilled water by the aid of about ten minims of the dilute sulphuric acid. Among tonics, the preparations of iron claim the foremost rank. When vomiting and pain have ceased, begin with the very mildest preparations, such as the ammonio-citrate, which should always be given immediately after food. The insoluble oxide should generally be avoided. As a combination of the vegetable and mineral tonics, none is so elegant and so generally useful as a mixture of sulphate of quina and iron, kept in solution by a few drops of sulphuric or hydrochloric acid.

It is impossible to cure ulcers of the stomach by any remedies in the absence of proper regimen; drugs, although invaluable as aids to a strict diet, are powerless as substitutes for it. Milk diet, given in small quantities at frequent intervals, is the best that can be given under such circumstances; if the stomach be excessively irritable, it may be diluted with lime water. During convalescence the diet must be kept up as much as prudence will allow; ground rice with milk forms an excellent food, wheaten flour is best given as bread steeped in boiling water, and pressed through a muslin sieve while still hot (bread jelly) and boiled with milk. With respect to alcoholic stimulants we may say that it is advisable they should be studiously avoided: in cases of extreme exhaustion, where alcohol seems necessary, it must be given as an enema. But we may ask, are there no stimulants which may afford us the advantages of alcohol without its disadvantages? In such cases the peculiar stimulant effects of opium make it by far the most valuable of them all. *Part* xxxv., *p.* 55.

Cardialgia.—Dr. Tilt says, that if this does not depend upon foul secretions, requiring purgatives, give a sedative mixture before meals; an alkali after meals; three grains of blue-pill and two of extract of hyocyamus every, or every other, night; a mustard or hot linseed poultice, sprinkled with coarsely-powdered camphor, every other night. If the pains continue, prescribe a pitch, belladonna, or opium plaster: the two last may be alternated every fourth day. Often much benefit is derived from the application to the pit of the stomach of a piece of lint steeped in chloroform and covered with oil-silk. In some of the worst cases, in which the pain is agonizing, relief will sometimes be obtained by about thirty to sixty drops of aromatic spirit of ammonia, in the smallest possible quantity of water, or by the same quantity of chloroform, on a lump of white sugar.

The following liniment, recommended by Dr. Oldham, may be tried with advantage: Extract of belladonna, half a drachm; tincture of aconite (Fleming's), four drachms; for an ounce and a half of soap liniment. Dr. Shearman gives nitrate of silver and opium, with quinine and potash water, in one drachm doses; Mr. J. Frank recommends oxide of bismuth; and Hufeland writes favorably of nitrate of bismuth, in ten or twenty-grain doses. *Part xxxv., p. 58.*

Liquor Pepsinæ in Dyspepsia from Ulceration of the Stomach.—Prof. Nelson gives the following case:

Miss S. J., aged 18 or 20, was brought by her mother to me from Cheltenham, laboring under pain and fullness of the epigastrium and right side, vomiting of blood, and sometimes of purulent matter. She was excessively anæmic, her skin being nearly white, and the legs œdematous. There had been no catamenia for a considerable time, and her father, as reported, had died of cancer of the stomach. She became worse after the journey. I saw her in bed, and detected a rounded swelling to the right of the epigastrium, which I inferred might be a hepatic abscess, complicated with stomach ulceration. At this time she lay faint and helpless, vomiting everything she ate, sometimes intermixed with blood, and occasionally being composed entirely of muco-purulent matter combined with bile. She was afraid to speak above a whisper, her tongue and mouth were parched, and her legs pitted deeply under pressure; the pulse was small, frequent, and thready, about 140 per minute. Soothing poultices were applied over the swelling, large masses of hard round fecal matter were removed by injections, nitrate of silver was administered before food, and the alkalized liquor pepsinæ, with hydrocyanic acid, was given after food, at intervals of one hour. At the same time the food was entirely pultaceous or liquid, and consisted of the smallest quantities at a time, seldom more than one teaspoonful. After several fluctuations, and occasional severe attacks of purulent vomiting, she gradually began to amend. So soon as the above symptoms abated, she went through a course of quinine and steel; and, after a tedious treatment of about ten months, she recovered plumpness, color, and strength, contrary to the expectations of all her friends and acquaintances. The remedy could have little power over hepatic abscess; but I can scarcely see how, in her utterly reduced condition, she could have gone through the treatment without the support derived from the solvent action of the pepsine upon the food—oysters, arrowroot, and milk and wine, having all been previously rejected. *Part xxxv., p. 294.*

Heartburn.—In anæmic feeble persons, Dr. T. R. Chambers believes this arises generally from over-sensibility of the nerves to the natural acidity of the stomach. This is relieved by alkalies, but alkalies prevent perfect digestion by neutralizing the acidity necessary to a proper performance of the digestive function. The treatment must therefore be directed to alleviate the over-sensibility of the nerves, temporarily, by hydrocyanic acid and bismuth; permanently, by strengthening the general nervous system by quinine and iron, combined with sea-bathing, or the shower-bath. In other cases heartburn depends on too large an amount of acid being present in the stomach, resulting from chemical decomposition of the sugar in the chyme, owing to decreased vital power. The treatment here is to increase the power and vigor of the stomach. The activity of the pepsine may be much augmented by neutralizing the saliva collected in the stomach and œsophagus just before the meal, by a little hydrochloric or lactic acid; for the saliva arrests the solvent action of the gastric juice in a close proportion to its amount. The quantity of gastric juice may be further increased by supplying one of its most important constituents, water, which is best taken as cold as possible about half an hour after the meal.

Part xxxvi., *p.* 65.

Eructation and Vomiting.—When from simple relaxation of the œsophagus, Dr. Chambers gives astringents, as gallic acid combined with a little rhubarb. When from excess of air, swallowed from irregular nervous action, as in hysteria and chorea, valerian, either in infusion of the herb or combined with ammonia. When these fail, strychnine or creasote. The shower-bath is a very powerful remedy. When from the formation of foreign gases from chemical decomposition, no agent is so useful as sulphurous acid, which may be given as hyposulphite of soda; if this chance to disagree, charcoal will scarcely fail to arrest gastric fermentation. When chronic vomiting is sympathetic, *i. e.*, from some disease or condition elsewhere, as in peritonitis, pregnancy, etc., give hydrocyanic acid. When from gastric mucous flux, with copious formation of acid, give carbonate of magnesia. When the vomiting is accompanied by much local pain, as from gastric ulcer, malignant tumor, peritonitis, hernia, perforation of the gut, opium is the remedy of most value. When at the commencement of fevers and in cholera, apply chloroform on cloth to the epigastrium. Milk and lime-water, as a sole diet, will often alone stop chronic vomiting; complete rest and absence from excitement must accompany it. Chloroform does not arrest the nausea of sea-sickness, but it controls the violence of the straining. *Part* xxxvi., *p.* 70.

STRANGURY.

From Administration of Cantharides.—Dr. Seymour relies chiefly upon starch injections containing twenty or thirty drops of tinct. of opium. Cantharides should not be given to patients with *stricture of urethra.*

Dr. S. believes that cantharides should not be given to women, from its peculiar effects upon the uterine system. Camphor is recommended in some books, but is very slow in its operation. Hyoscyamus, however, increases its efficacy—especially in chronic irritation of the neck of the bladder. *Part* viii., *p.* 68.

STRICTURE.

RECTUM—ŒSOPHAGUS—URETHRA.

Of Rectum :—Dr. O'Beirne considers that it is our duty, if possible, to avoid making an opening into any part of the colon, and that in cases of stricture it might be avoided. The failure in the use of the instruments in cases of spasmodic stricture, he attributes to want of sufficient boldness in their use, and mentions a few facts to embolden practitioners, and to show the impunity with which the most obstinate constriction of the bowel in question might be overcome.

The facts were as follows : Of all the diseases in which constipation is most obstinate, tetanus is certainly the one. In some cases of this disease which had terminated fatally, he succeeded in passing the instrument to a considerable height, but only by means of long-continued, gradually increasing, and determined pressure against the point of resistance ; when first he used this force, he remembered the instrument passed rapidly upward, as if through a narrow ring, giving to his hand a sensation as if he had perforated the walls of the intestine ; accordingly he withdrew the tube, and was much pleased to see its extremity coated with fæces, and bearing no marks of blood. This circumstance had occurred to him not once, but twenty times in the treatment of those fatal cases to which he alluded. In those cases it was found, after death, that the whole of the colon was so enormously distended as to conceal the other intestines, and to equal in size the thighs of a very large man, while the uppermost part of the rectum was contracted to the diameter of the barrel of a quill, but felt much firmer. On cutting into the intestine at this point, neither the serous nor the mucous coat was found in the least thickened, neither did the muscular coat exhibit any signs of thickening other than that caused by the powerful contraction of its fibres upon themselves. It was quite evident in these cases that even this firm structure was forced at each introduction of the instrument, so as to enable the bowels to be freed. Why, then, should we be deterred from employing a sufficient degree of force in another case when the degree of resistance is infinitely less ? When the difficulty of introducing the tube is great, the application of a blister over the sacrum, extending up a little on the spinous processes of the lumbar vertebræ, would be found a considerable assistance ; and in order to effect this rapidly, if the case be very urgent, a sponge should be impacted into a tumbler, boiling water poured upon this, throwing it off repeatedly in order to produce the necessary degree of heat, and then the tumbler could be inverted over the part to be blistered. Having thus disposed of spasmodic stricture, he would now say that, in cases of the organic kind, every success might be obtained by the same means, with this difference— namely, the use of small tubes gradually increased in size. With respect to malignant stricture of the rectum, he was of opinion that this might be a legitimate case for the lumbar operation.

[Dr. Williams says that the great difficulty in the formation of an artificial anus in the lumbar colon consists in the difficulty of distinguishing the colon from the small intestine; for the signs mentioned by M. Amussat, whether taken separately or collectively, are not diagnostic, consequently there is always a risk of opening the peritoneum, and thus sacrificing the entire principle and chief advantage of the operation. M. Amussat has, however, discovered a sign which bids fair to do much toward removing the difficulty in question].

The sign rested on the fact that the small intestines sustained a motion of alternate ascent and descent corresponding to expiration and inspiration, in which the lumbar colon did not participate ; if, therefore, the exposed intestine presented this oscillation, it was small intestine—if it did not, it might be presumed to be the colon. As M. Amussat made no mention whatever of this distinctive sign in any of his publications on the subject, it was very satisfactory that it had now been made known and recorded. *Part* xi., *p.* 110.

Stricture of the Rectum and Œsophagus.—If non-malignant, these may be treated effectually with instruments, invented by Mr. Wakley; consisting of a flexible guide and four dilating tubes about ten inches in length for the rectum, and twenty for the œsophagus; the guide being also longer for the latter tube. The guide is first introduced, and over this, the directors, which fit accurately, and must be used of progressively larger size. Mr. Wakley also uses instruments for the dilatation of the os uteri, constructed on similar principles, but the dilators are shorter, and have an inverted cup-shaped rim to fit the os uteri. *Part* xxxv., *p.* 130.

Dilatation of the Urethra in Stricture.—Dr. Arnott makes use of "a tube of oiled silk lined with the thin gut of some small animal, as the cat, to make it air-tight, and attached to the extremity of a small canula, by which it is distended with the air or water from a bag or syringe at the outer end with a stopcock or valve to keep the air in when received." The canula may be of elastic gum, or of the flexible metal used to make the metallic bougies, or of silver. The instrument is easily passed, and as soon as the bag is sufficiently within the stricture as much air is to be injected as the patient can easily bear. *Part* iii., *p.* 94.

Aphorisms of Practical Surgery.—Few diseases are more difficult to cure *radically* than a very tight (très grand) stricture of the urethra. For, after the canal has been widened by the prolonged use of bougies, there is always a great tendency to a relapse of the disease. It is then that cauterization becomes useful, because we thus obtain a cicatrix *molded* upon the bougie.

There are cases of stricture, etc., in which the keeping of an instrument in the urethra, instead of being a means of cure, becomes actually an obstacle to it: Dupuytren used to cite several instances of urinary fistulæ cured by the mere withdrawal of the sound. *Part* iii., *p.* 115.

Use of Alum in the Treatment of Stricture of the Urethra.—M. Jobert regards alum as possessing many advantages in the treatment of this disease. He uses it as follows:

A bougie is selected, the finer at the extremity the narrower the stricture. By placing its extremity for a moment in a candle, it is so far softened, that on immersing the instrument in pulverized alum, it adheres to the entire heated surface; the point is then rounded off between the fingers, so as to communicate to it a suitable shape. The bougie, when thus armed, is passed into the stricture and left there for twenty minutes or an hour, according to the period of the treatment, the sensibility of the patient, etc. After a few minutes a slight smarting is felt, but no other apparent effect is perceived. On withdrawing the bougie, a few drops of whitish mucus escape, which M. Jobert considers as tending to liberate the canal of the urethra. Not unfrequently, on the day following the application, bougies of a considerable size can be passed into the bladder.

M. Jobert also uses large bougies armed with alum, in the treatment of stricture of the urethra. *Part* v., *p.* 145.

Stricture of the Male Urethra—Urinary Abscess.—Sir B. Brodie thus describes the ordinary course of the affection. The patient, he says, complains of more than usual difficulty in voiding his urine; but the difficulty

does not amount, at least in the first instance, to an absolute retention.
Perhaps he has a shivering. There is a sense of fullness in the perineum,
and some degree of deep-seated induration is perceptible in one part. This
gradually increases, and a tumor presents itself under the skin of the perineum, surrounded with more or less of œdematous effusion, especially into
the scrotum. The skin becomes inflamed, and the fluctuation of fluid is
perceptible underneath. An abscess bursts or is opened with a lancet, and
a considerable quantity of putrid pus is discharged. Here the œdema of
the neighboring part subsides. Pus continues to flow through the orifice
of the abscess, and after some time it is observed that urine flows through
it also. The discharge of pus diminishes, but the urine flows in larger
quantity; and whenever the patient makes water, part escapes through the
natural channel and part by the new opening. The abscess has evidently
a communication with the urethra, behind the stricture. If you have an
opportunity of dissecting the diseased parts while the abscess is recent, you
find it to open into the urethra by a ragged, irregular orifice. If you examine them at a later period, the orifice in the urethra is found to be
smooth, regular, and rounded at the margin; the external orifice in the
perineum is reduced to a narrow diameter, and is seen in the centre of a
button-like projection of the skin; and the abscess itself is contracted, perhaps reduced to a narrow passage, with a smooth surface, which presents
somewhat of the appearance of its being lined by a mucous membrane. We
now say that the case is one of *fistula in perinœo*. The whole of these
phenomena are easily explained. The urethra, constantly teased by the
pressure of the urine against it, ulcerates behind the stricture. If the stricture had been completely closed, as in the case of retention of urine, an
extensive extravasation of urine would have immediately taken place; but
under the existing circumstances, this does not happen, and only a moderate quantity, perhaps not more than a few drops, dribbles into the cellular
membrane, sufficient to induce inflammation and suppuration and no further local mischief. A *fistula in ano* is formed in the same manner, by ulceration of the rectum allowing the escape of a minute quantity of feculent
matter into the neighboring textures.

Sir Benjamin goes on to remark, that sometimes the abscess of the perineum is accompanied by typhoid symptoms. If the abscess is opened, the
matter that issues is putrid and urinous—if the opening is deferred the
patient may die.

"I have described," continues our author, "the simplest form of the urinary abscess. But it is often more complicated. It is not always confined
to the perineum; sometimes it makes its way forward through the upper
part of the scrotum, and presents itself on the lower part of the penis, between the scrotum and the glans. At other times it burrows in the opposite
direction, forming a large collection of matter in the nates, or it may burst
in the groin, or in the scrotum. In one case, in which I had an opportunity of examining the body after death, I found a large abscess in front of
the pubes, extending half-way toward the navel; another among the adductor muscles of the left thigh; and a third among the muscles at the upper
part of the right thigh, as far outward as the *foramen ovale* of the ischium;
the periosteum having been destroyed, and the bone itself rendered carious
to a considerable extent: and all these abscesses could be traced into an
abscess in the perineum, communicating with the urethra behind a stricture
by a small orifice. In another case—which I attended with Mr. Samuel

Cooper, there was a *fistula in perinœo*, communicating with a large abscess of the pelvis on one side of the bladder.

" I have seen a few cases in which an abscess of this kind had made its way into the rectum, forming a fistulous communication between it and the urethra. If such communication be of a large size it is a source of great distress, as feculent matter occasionally passes through it from the rectum into the urethra. If it be small, however, the absolute inconvenience is but trifling, and the patient is rendered sensible of its existence only in consequence of a small quantity of air escaping occasionally by the urethra; and this may continue, without any further symptoms supervening, for many years."

Bougie.—"The best kind of bougie," he observes, "is that in common use, made of plaster spread on linen, and rolled up. It should be smooth on the surface and neatly rounded at the extremity. The plaster bougie should be rubbed until it becomes warm, so that it may be molded by the hand, and bent into the form of the urethra. Thus bent, it is much to be preferred to the elastic bougie, which is made of elastic gum on the outside and of catgut within. The latter may, it is true, be bent into any form; but it is elastic, and however you may bend it, it always regains its straight figure; and hence it is not well constructed for being passed along the curved canal of the urethra. The bougie which is used for the purpose of examining the urethra should be of full size, that is, large enough to fill the urethra without stretching it. A small bougie may deceive you in two ways: it may pass through a stricture, and thus lead you to believe that there is no stricture, when there really is one; or it may have its point entangled in the orifice of one of the mucous follicles of the urethra, or in some accidental irregularity of the canal, and lead you into the opposite mistake of supposing that there is a stricture where none exists. If you use a bougie of the size of the urethra, you are not at all liable to the first error, and you are much less liable to the second than you would be otherwise. The bougie should be cylindrical. There is no advantage in any bougie, except a very small one, being conical. A conical bougie, becoming larger toward the point which is held in the hand, is likely to extend forcibly the orifice of the urethra, and to excite inflammation in it."

Retention from Spasmodic Stricture.—Sir Benjamin recommends the immediate and direct recourse to mechanical means.

"Begin," he says, "by taking one of the smallest gum catheters, which has been kept for a considerable time on a curved iron wire, and which retains the curved form after the wire is withdrawn. Introduce it without the wire; and as it approaches the stricture, turn the concavity of the catheter toward the pubes, elongating the penis at the same time by drawing it out as much as possible. It is not very improbable that it will pass through the stricture, and enter the bladder. The urine will then flow through it in a fine stream, and the patient will obtain immediate and complete relief.

" If you fail with the small gum catheter, try, not a plaster, but a small catgut bougie. Let this be well made; that is firmly twisted, nicely rounded at the extremity, and everywhere well polished. Observe the same rule of elongating the urethra, and it will probably enter the stricture. It is not necessary that the catgut bougie should pass on to the bladder; it is sufficient if the stricture grasps or holds it. Let it remain in the stricture until there is a violent impulse to make water. Then withdraw the

bougie, and the urine will follow it in a small stream. If the patient empties
the bladder, the object is attained; but, otherwise, re-introduce the catgut
bougie, or rather introduce another of the same size (for a catgut bougie
which has been once used is not fit to be employed a second time); and
let the patient retain this second bougie as long as he can. If the straight
catgut bougie cannot be passed, you will often succeed in effecting its introduction by bending the point of it. This contrivance enables you to
keep the point sliding against the upper surface of the urethra, avoiding
the lower part, in which the obstruction is always most perceptible, and
in which the bougie is most likely to become, as it were, entangled.

"Even where you have failed to relieve the patient by means of the catgut
bougie, you will often succeed in introducing a silver catheter, or an elastic gum catheter mounted on a firm iron stilet, into the bladder. The catheter employed on this occasion, if the stricture be of recent formation,
should be nearly of the full size of the urethra; but if the stricture has been
of long duration, it should be considerably smaller. The common silver
catheter is not so well adapted for the purpose as that which I now show
you. You will observe that it is shorter and less curved than usual, and
that it is fixed in a wooden handle, which renders the instrument more
manageable than it would be otherwise. If you use an elastic gum catheter, the iron stilet should have a flattened handle, resembling that of a common sound. You should pass it as far as the obstruction, and having ascertained where it is situated, withdraw the catheter a little, a quarter of
an inch for example, and then, as you pass it on again toward the bladder,
keep the point sliding against the upper part of the urethra, which is toward
the pubes, avoiding the lower part, which is, of course, toward the perineum. Be careful to employ no violence. If you lacerate the urethra, so
as to cause hemorrhage, you will be defeated in your object. Press the
catheter firmly, but gently and steadily, against the stricture, keeping in
your mind the anatomical position of the parts, and being careful to give
the point of the instrument a right direction. When the pressure has been
thus carefully continued for some time, the stricture will begin to relax.
It will allow the point of the catheter to enter, and, at last, to pass completely through it into the bladder. In some instances this will be accomplished in the space of one or two minutes; while in others it may be necessary to persevere for a quarter of an hour. As soon as the catheter has
reached the bladder, the patient's sufferings are at an end, as the bladder
becomes completely emptied. If you have used the elastic gum catheter,
it may be prudent to allow it to remain in the urethra and bladder for one
or two days, or even for a longer period; and this will go far toward accomplishing the cure of the stricture."

Use of Opium.—"The remedy on which you are most to rely, where
these mechanical means fail, is opium. From half a drachm to a drachm
of laudanum may be given as a clyster in two or three ounces of thin
starch. If this should not succeed, give opium by the mouth, and repeat
the dose, if necessary, every hour until the patient can make water.
According to my experience, the cases in which the stricture does not
become relaxed under the use of opium, if administered freely, are very
rare. The first effect of the opium, is to diminish the distress which the
patient experiences from the distention of the bladder. Then the impulse
to make water becomes less urgent; the paroxysms of straining are less
severe and less frequent; and after the patient has been in this state of

comparative ease for a short time, he begins to void his urine, at first in small, but afterward in larger quantities."

Warm Bath.—" It is customary in these cases to employ the warm bath. It is, indeed, sometimes useful, but you can place no dependence on it as compared with opium. It is not sufficient that your patient should sit in a hip-bath: the bath, to be at all efficient, must be complete; his whole person ought, therefore, to be immersed, and he should remain in it for half an hour, or an hour, or longer, unless he previously becomes faint. Bleeding from the arm is seldom required in cases of retention of urine from stricture; but in some instances, even where other means have failed, taking blood from the perineum by cupping gives immediate relief."

Purgatives, when induced by Spirituous Liquors.—" Purgatives require some time to produce their effect, and in most cases, at the period of your being called in, the symptoms are too urgent to admit of this delay. Where, however, a stricture is chiefly spasmodic, and the retention follows the too great use of fermented liquor or spirits, I would advise you, if you are sent for on the commencement of the attack, to prescribe a draught of infusion of senna with the tartrate of potass and tincture of jalap. As soon as this has fully operated, and the bowels are emptied, give thirty or forty drops of tincture of opium by the mouth, or order an opiate clyster to be administered, and, in all probability, the attack will subside."

" After all, there is no absolute rule as to the treatment of retention of urine from stricture. One person is relieved in one way, another in another; and you will do well in each case to bear in mind the particular mode of treatment which has proved of service, in order that you may at once resort to it, if you are called a second time to the same patient, under the same circumstances. In one instance, you will be able to pass a catgut bougie, and not a catheter; in another you will be able to pass a catheter, and not a catgut bougie. One individual is relieved by opium, another by the warm bath. A gentleman of my acquaintance, who was subject to attacks of this description for a considerable time, almost always began to make water after a pint of warm water had been thrown up as a clyster."

Sir B. Brodie relates a case of old stricture of the urethra, in which the attack of retention of urine came on periodically, and was cured like other intermittent diseases, by prescribing sulphate of quinine.

When an operation becomes indispensable, which Sir Benjamin thinks it must *rarely* be, he is of opinion that puncturing the bladder from the rectum is applicable to the greatest number of cases. But those who operate frequently must often operate unnecessarily.

Stricture in the Anterior Part of the Urethra.—Sir Benjamin observes that a *stricture at the orifice of the urethra* may be dilated by means of a common bougie, or a short metallic instrument; the size of the bougie being gradually increased, and the introduction being repeated daily or on alternate days, according to circumstances. The process of dilatation is, however, in many instances, attended with much inconvenience to the patient. In those cases, especially, in which the contraction began in early life, every introduction of the bougie causes considerable pain; at the same time that the disposition to contract is so great that the operation requires to be repeated almost daily. The consequence is that the part is kept in a constant state of inflammation, and, between the disease and the remedy, is a source of incessant annoyance to the patient. In a case of this sort, which was extremely troublesome, Sir Benjamin determined at once to divide the contracted part of the urethra. This was easily accomplished by means of a pair of knife-edged scissors, one blade with a blunt point being introduced into the urethra, and the division being made in the situation of the frænum. No hemorrhage followed the operation. A piece of lint was kept between the cut surfaces to prevent their reunion, and in about ten days they were cicatrized, being covered by what had already assumed a good deal of the appearance of a mucous membrane.

Strictures in the anterior part of the urethra, but behind the orifice, require to be mechanically dilated, by the introduction of bougies or metallic instruments. Sometimes the patient obtains relief on very easy terms, the dilatation being readily accomplished, and the use of the bougie once in three or four days being sufficient to prevent a recurrence of the contraction. At other times, however, the disposition to contract is so great, that it becomes necessary to introduce the bougie once or twice daily ; and, indeed, Sir Benjamin has known cases in which the patient was seldom able to expel his urine until the bougie had been employed.

Caustic Bougie.—Sir Benjamin conceives that the *caustic bougie* is applicable to the following cases : 1st. Those of spasmodic stricture, where two or three applications of the caustic may be sufficient to relieve all the urgent symptoms. 2dly. Some cases of old stricture, in which there is still a considerable disposition to spasm. In these last cases apply the caustic two or three times, and no oftener. It will probably relieve the contraction as far as it is spasmodic, and thus enable you to proceed more advantageously, with the use of the bougie or metallic sound. 3rdly. The caustic may be used very properly in some cases of stricture which are endowed with peculiar irritability, in which every application of the common bougie induces severe pain, or brings on spasm, preventing it entering the stricture. Two or three applications of the caustic may be sufficient to deprive the stricture of that unnatural sensibility which otherwise would have foiled your efforts to effect a cure. Yet our author seldom employs caustic for these reasons : 1st. Although the caustic often relieves spasm, it also very often induces it. It is true, that in many instances it enables a patient to make water with more facility ; but in many instances also, it brings on retention of urine. 2dly. Hemorrhage is a more frequent consequence of the use of the caustic than of the common bougie, and it sometimes takes place to a very great and to an almost dangerous extent. 3dly. Where there is a disposition to rigors, the application of caustic is almost certain to produce them ; and frequently the application of caustic induces rigors where there had been no manifest disposition to them previously. 4thly. Unless used with caution, the application of caustic may induce inflammation of the parts situated behind the stricture, terminating in the formation of abscess. *Part* vi., *p.* 92.

Stafford's Treatment of Stricture— The Lanceted Stilette.—Mr. W. Coulson arranges those cases of stricture in which the ordinary plans of treatment fail to relieve or cure under three or more classes: the first, in which there is simple stricture of the urethra, so complete, however, as sometimes to cause retention of urine ; the second, in which two, three, or more inches of the urethra, are thickened and contracted, and often complicated with fistulous openings in the perineum ; the third, in which one or more bad strictures exist in an extremely irritable urethra, which is frequently combined with an irritable state of the whole system.

Three cases are produced to elucidate the above varieties, and to show that, after every other method had failed, Mr. Stafford's mode of dividing the part with his instrument was successful. After which Mr. Coulson goes on to say:

My object in publishing these cases is to assist in removing the feeling which too generally prevails against Mr. Stafford's treatment in cases of impermeable stricture: for nearly all who have written on the complaint more or less condemn the use of his instrument. In alluding to it, Sir Benjamin Brodie says: "Mr. Stafford has invented an ingenious machine, which is intended to divide a stricture by means of a cutting instrument. If any cases occur in which this method may be useful, they are undoubtedly very few in number; and great caution must be required to avoid making false passages, which might be followed by effusion of urine and purulent deposits." These were the fears which unfortunately influenced me in rejecting for years this most valuable instrument. I say unfortunately, for I now recall to my recollection numerous cases in which I failed to afford relief for want of this or a similar instrument. I believe that there is much less danger of making a false passage with the lanceted stilette, carefully directed against an impermeable stricture, than in the use of the common catheter or sound. As to the effusion of urine and purulent deposits, how rarely do they occur, in cases where great violence has been used, and lesion of structure has taken place in the attempts to introduce instruments into the bladder. In the use of Mr. Stafford's instrument, admitting that the division is not made in the direction of the canal, it is certain to be made *anterior* to the obstruction, and consequently not likely to be attended with infiltration of urine. In lieu of Mr. Stafford's operation, Sir Benjamin Brodie proposes the following modification, which he adopted in the patient, viz.: "I then make an incision in the perineum, dilating the fistulous sinus, and laying open the membranous part of the urethra as far forward as the stricture, the exact situation of which was marked by the bougie. The bougie was then withdrawn; an instrument was then introduced in its place, consisting of a straight silver tube, closed at its extremity, except a narrow slit, through which a small lancet could be made to project, by pressing on a stilt which projected on the handle of the instrument; the round extremity of the tube being pressed against the anterior part of the left hand, introduced through the wound in the perineum and urethra to its posterior surface. The pressure of the instrument being distinctly communicated to the finger through the substance of the stricture, the lancet was protruded, and the stricture was divided. A silver catheter was then easily introduced through the urethra and divided stricture into the bladder, and allowed to remain there. The urine, of course, flowed through the catheter. At the end of two days the silver catheter was removed, and replaced by one of elastic gum. The wound in the perineum gradually healed, and the patient ultimately recovered, making water in a full stream, and being able to introduce a sound of a full size into the bladder, so as to prevent a recurrence of the contraction."

Now the following is Mr. Stafford's plan. The single lanceted stilette, or urethral perforator, is passed down to the stricture, the exact distance of which from the extremity of the urethra is first ascertained. When the point of the instrument is arrived at, and rests upon the contraction (which is known by means of its graduation), and is in an exact line with the natural course of the canal, the instrument is held and maintained in that position by the left hand, the fore-finger of which being passed through the ring on the under part of its handle, the thumb of the right hand is passed through the ring on the handle of the stilette. The stilette is then pressed gently and gradually forward, when the lancet is protruded out at its point, and is thus made to incise the stricture. The lancet must be immediately drawn back, or allowed to retire into the sheath, by the action of the spring.

In the operation which is proposed by Sir Benjamin Brodie, as a modification of Mr. Stafford's, and as a substitute for it, an external wound is made in the perineum for the purpose of preventing infiltration of urine, and next for the purpose of guiding the lancet.

I have already alluded to the little chance of infiltration of urine, and I know of no case in which it has occurred. As to guiding the lancet, I really think the instrument may be as safely guided when passed down the urethra, and held properly against the stricture, as by the finger introduced through the wound in the perinæum. The principle of the operation is Mr. Stafford's ; the modification is the opening in the perineum, which complicates the operation, inflicts additional pain, and prevents the patient, for a time at least, from following his usual avocations.

I am not wishing to urge this plan of treatment in cases where there is any passage, however small, through the stricture ; but in every case where the contraction is so great as not to admit of the introduction of an instrument, Mr. Stafford's plan, in my opinion, offers a safe, speedy, and effectual mode of cure. *Part* vi., *p.* 115.

Stricture of the Urethra.— Dr. Leroy d'Etiolles, advises when the stricture produces complete retention of urine, to endeavor to pass bougies in conjunction with bleeding, baths, etc.; try the application of tobacco smoke; should these fail, press a small catheter against the obstacle for an hour. Cut down upon the urethra posterior to the obstacle, but should a calculus be there detained, cut through the rectum. If necessary to puncture the bladder, do it through the rectum. M. Lallemand cuts down on the strictured part itself. *Part* xiii., *p.* 286.

Opium in Stricture of the Urethra.—There is a case related in the reports of the Ipswich Medical Society, of an old man with obstinate stricture, and who had passed no urine from the Saturday to the Tuesday, when it was determined to puncture the bladder. But having taken two grains of opium, and repeated the dose in an hour, the spasms relaxed and the operation was not required. *Part* xv., *p.* 229.

Instrument for Dividing Strictures.— M. Civiale has invented a new instrument for the division of indurated strictures of the urethra. The principle of the improvement consists in the division of the strictures *from behind forward*, instead of cutting in the reverse directions, as hitherto practised by surgeons. The new instrument, according to M. Civiale, has the advantage over the old method in the fact, that the extent of the incision can be precisely ascertained, and controlled by the operator, and a division of all the tissues can be performed with safety. *Part* xix., *p.* 184,

Stricture of the Urethra.—There is a form of stricture, marked by the " tightness of the contraction, the resilient disposition displayed after dilatation, and the great degree of irritation induced by attempts to effect this," in which Mr. Syme has advised the free division of the contracted part upon the director.

The best plan is to introduce a grooved director *into* the tight portion, to cut down upon it, and freely divide the stricture, and introduce a catheter into the urethra. This plan must not be confounded with that of introducing a catheter *as far* as the stricture, cutting down upon its point, and then with the knife cutting a way for the catheter to the bladder.

Part xix., *p.* 187.

B. Cooper's Treatment of.—[Mr. Cooper would substitute the name of " *irritable* " for that of " *spasmodic,*" as applied to stricture, since the latter term involves the idea of the disease being caused by muscular action : while this is not really the case, except in the membraneous and bulbous portions of the urethra.]

Irritable or Spasmodic.—Give a dose of opium with tartarized antimony, a hot bath, and warm purgative enema. These measures should always precede the employment of the catheter, and will generally be found sufficient to afford relief without resorting to its use. In obstinate cases of *mixed* stricture, cup in the perineum, give two grains of calomel and a grain of opium at night, and, during the day, small doses of the tincture of muriate of iron. At the same time employ the bougie very gently. If it produces pain and bleeding, apply caustic to the stricture to diminish its irritability and introduce into the rectum, at bedtime, a suppository containing a grain and a half of opium, and five grains of extract of henbane, mixed with soap.

Permanent.—In the first place, explore the urethra. Making the patient lie down on a sofa, introduce a bougie or silver catheter (No. 6), and press it gently, for a minute or more, against the stricture. If it should pass the stricture, do not seek to introduce it further. After the use of the bougie, let the patient keep quiet and on low diet for the rest of the day, and take a draught containing liq. potass., gtts. xx. ; tinct. opii, gtts. x. ; mist. camph. ʒiss., at bedtime, and an aperient in the morning. In about forty-eight hours, introduce the bougie again, and this time it may be passed into the bladder, and allowed to remain for ten minutes or a quarter of an hour. If No. 6 cannot be introduced, carefully try a smaller one. If no instrument can be passed, be guided as to the treatment, by the urgency of the symptoms. When there is retention of urine, and the pain complained of is very severe, put the patient in a hot bath, give a grain and a half or two grains of opium, and a purgative enema; and when the bowels are opened, introduce into the rectum a suppository, containing opium, and a quarter of a grain of belladonna. These means will generally relieve the urgent symptoms. Then proceed with the treatment, introducing a bougie gently every other day ; and while this is being done, insist on the patient living very carefully, and give such medicines as blue pill with tartarized antimony, followed by aperients. If the stricture becomes irritable, give sedatives, and apply the caustic bougie carefully. If the attempts at dilatation by the bougie fail, try the repeated injections of tepid water into the urethra. If by all these means relief is not obtained, and the patient is suffering from retention, or is threatened with ulceration of the urethra behind the stricture, the bladder must be punctured. Under very urgent circumstances we may puncture by the rectum (provided that the prostate is not enlarged); but as a general rule it is much better to cut down upon the urethra, and divide the stricture in the perineum.

The operation of *dividing the stricture in perineo* is performed with the patient in the same position as in lithotomy: an instrument is passed down to the stricture, the grooved staff being perhaps the most appropriate to the purpose. An incision is next made in the perineum, commencing at the point where the end of the instrument can be felt resting on the stricture; the groove is then to be cut into, and the knife carried down-ward with great caution, cutting the way for the point of the staff, which should be made to follow it as it gradually divides the stricture, and the staff, being pushed on, passes into the bladder. The staff should then be withdrawn, and an elastic gum catheter put in its place, and retained there for several days.

In cases of fistulous opening in the perineum being concomitant with the stricture, Mr. Cooper adopts another plan for performing this operation. He says :

Having made the incision into the perineum, instead of opening the urethra at the groove of the staff as before described, I have first opened the membranous parts of the urethra behind the stricture, and then passed a female catheter into the bladder, and drawn off the urine; thus relieving the patient of the retention, but having still to divide the stricture; this is effected by feeling within the wound for the point of the grooved staff above the stricture; and, proceeding to cut through the obstruction, carrying forward the staff as before described (first, however, having withdrawn the female catheter), the staff enters the bladder through the opening originally made for that instrument. The staff should then be withdrawn, and an elastic gum catheter inserted in its stead; this should be left in for a week, when it must be removed, and substituted by a new one. At first, some urine will escape by the wound through the perineum, as in the operation for lithotomy; but generally in the course of a week or ten days it passes entirely through the catheter. About a fortnight after it has entirely ceased to flow from the perineum, the catheter should be removed, but still for some time the patient should regularly have the water drawn off, and this, if performed with gentleness, produces much less irritation than would be excited by the constant presence of an instrument in the bladder.

When a permanent stricture occurs in the urethra anterior to the bulb, and especially in that part of the canal covered by scrotum, it is not advisable to cut down upon the stricture from without, owing to the liability to infiltration of urine if the incision be made through the scrotum, and of the difficulty of healing the wound when the opening is made anterior to it. The cure of such stricture must, therefore, be assiduously attempted by the use of bougies or caustic, or should they resist this treatment, perhaps the instrument, furnished with a cutting stilette, employed by M. Stafford, may be used; as this part of the urethra may be rendered straight, the instrument may be directed with much more certainty than when the stricture is seated in the curved portion of the canal. I should myself, however, prefer opening the urethra behind the stricture, if retention demand it, rather than to puncture the stricture itself.

Part xix., *p.* 189

Use of the Bougie in Stricture.—Mr. Solly, of St. Thomas' Hospital, says:

When the catgut bougie is used, the great secret is to handle it with the utmost delicacy, and twirl it gently between the thumb and finger when it meets with obstruction. When it is introduced it should be allowed to remain for an hour. *Part* xix., *p.* 194.

Case of Stricture attended by Profuse Discharge.—[In this case there was such profuse discharge, that gonorrhœa was suspected. The patient had previously had stricture, and as he completely negatived the idea that it was gonorrhœa, Mr. Smith suspected that he might have stricture remaining. He says:]

I requested permission to examine the urethra, and, on doing so, I discovered two irritable strictures. I told him that this was the cause of the discharge persisting, and that it was necessary for him to come to London every week to have the bougie passed. I, at the same time, desired him to refrain as much as possible from sexual connection, and from all other species of excitement.

I need not enumerate the particulars of this case, which was troublesome to treat—for the urethra was so excessively irritable that about three weeks after this, I could only introduce, with some trouble, a No. 4 bougie. In a short time, however, a good-sized instrument could be introduced, the discharge diminished, and, at the end of two months, I passed No. 12 bougie; all discharge had ceased. He had latterly used a weak solution of acetate of zinc, in order to diminish the irritability of the urethra, and hasten the cure. I advised him to return to me in another month, in order that I might ascertain if the cure was satisfactory. He visited me last week. The urethra admitted No. 12 bougie, and the discharge had never returned. *Part* xx., *p.* 159.

Strictures—Mr. Guthrie's Conclusions Respecting.—1. That a hard and elastic, or an intractable stricture is never permanently cured by dilatation, or by the application of caustic, although it may be materially relieved by the regular periodical use of a dilating instrument.

2. That the division of an old, hardened, or elastic stricture through the perineum is not usually followed by a permanent cure, although it is always attended by immediate relief. The disease being apt to return unless a solid sound or catheter is occasionally passed to prevent it.

3. That the operation of dividing the perineum and urethra in such cases is sometimes attended by severe hemorrhages, by fever, and is occasionally followed by fistulous openings, giving rise to much inconvenience.

4. That such division does, in some instances, effect a permanent cure.

5. That the division of the urethra through the external parts should never be attempted in any portion of it anterior to the bulb, such operation not being necessary; for the narrowest stricture of the pendulous or movable part may always be divided internally with much less comparative danger than by the external incision, inasmuch as the instrument can be guided through this part by the finger and thumb of the left hand of the surgeon with a certainty almost unerring.

6. That the stricture considered by all surgeons as the most important and difficult of cure—viz., at the termination of the bulbous portion of the urethra—may always be divided, when impassable, by a *straight* instru-

ment, and in general more easily than by a *curved* one; the use of which is founded on the erroneous belief that the stricture is situated in the membranous part of the urethra, instead of being, as it is, anterior to it.

7. That the division of a strictuie should, if possible, be effected by an instrument passed through it, and cutting from behind forward, rather than from before backward, although a combination of both methods will frequently be necessary to insure success.

8. That the division of a stricture by these means will not always insure a permanent cure if more than the mucous membrane is implicated, unless such parts be divided also.

9. That in cases of intractable stricture. the mucous membrane, the inner layer of involuntary muscle, and the elastic tissue external to it, should be divided when the operation is done from within, but not the outer layer of muscular fibres, which should remain as a barrier between the stream of urine and the common integuments of the external parts—an accuracy of division not always to be attained; whence, perhaps, the difficulty of effecting a permanent cure.

10. That when a permanent cure is effected in these cases, the divided elastic wall of the urethra is not re-united by a structure exactly similar to itself, but by common areolar tissue, rendering the part more dilatable under the pressure of the stream of urine; the formation of which dilatation can be aided during the progress of the cure by pressing on the divided part with the point of a solid instrument passed daily for the purpose of preventing, if possible, that contraction which always takes place during the process of cicatrization; a proceeding which cannot be advantageously adopted when the parts are divided through the perineum, lest it should encourage the formation of a fistulous opening, to which there is always a tendency.

11. That in cases of intractable stricture accompanied by one or more fistulous openings in the perineum, in *young persons,* or of middle age, the operation through the external parts, or along the urethra, may be resorted to at the pleasure of the surgeon with an equal chance of success, provided the portion of the obstruction or bank preventing the free passage of the urine be effectually divided, the *sine quâ non* of the operation.

12. That the operation within the urethra should always be preferred in *elderly* persons, particularly if somewhat stout or fat, as less likely to create severe constitutional disturbance, and if this operation should fail from any cause, it by no means interferes with the due performance of the other through the perineum, which in serious cases then becomes imperative, as the last resource capable of giving relief.

Part xxiv., *p.* 227.

Prof. Syme's Operation for Urethral Stricture.—The patient having been placed under the influence of chloroform, is " brought to the edge of his bed, and his limbs are supported by two assistants, one on each side. A grooved director, slightly curved, and small enough to pass readily through the stricture, is next introduced, and confided to one of the assistants. The surgeon sitting, or kneeling on one knee, now makes an incision in the middle line of the perineum or penis, wherever the stricture is seated. It should be an inch or an inch and a half in length, and extend through the integuments, together with the subjacent textures exterior to the urethra. The operator then taking the handle of the director in his left hand, and a small straight bistoury in his right, feels, with his fore-finger guarding the blade, for the director, and pushes the point into the groove behind, or on the bladder side of the stricture, runs the knife forward, so as to divide the whole of the thickened texture at the contracted part of the canal, and withdraws the director." A silver catheter is now allowed to remain in the bladder for forty-eight hours, after which it is to be withdrawn. After eight or ten days a moderate-sized bougie should be passed, and its introduction repeated once every week or fortnight for two months. Mr. Syme makes it an indispensable condition of his opera-tion, that the stricture should be permeable; in other words, should admit the passage of an extremely small director at least; and in order appa-rently not to limit the usefulness of his operation, he asserts that there is no truly impermeable stricture. He also condemns, in measured terms, the old operation of cutting into the perineum in search of the obstructed canal without any further guide than the point of a catheter, introduced, not through, but merely down to the contracted point. An imperfect di-vision of the contracted part—want of care to pass instruments while the urethra is healing, as all injuries of the canal are apt to occasion strictures when this precaution is neglected—and subsequent exposure to a repetition of the causes which give rise to the disease—may prevent the advantage gained from lasting so long as could be desired. The first of these cir-cumstances tending to cause relapse did not originally occur to me, but was suggested by facts falling under my observation, which led to the per-suasion that as a stricture gives the canal a sand-glass form at the part affected, it is not sufficient to cut merely the narrowest portion—the coni-cal-shaped contraction on each side of it also requiring division; so that, instead of being limited to a quarter or half, the incision should extend a whole inch through the coats of the urethra. In regard to the after-treat-ment, as wounds and bruises of the urethra are apt to induce strictures, unless a full-sized bougie be passed occasionally until the part affected recover from the injury which it has sustained, there can be no doubt that if this precaution is neglected after the operation for stricture, there must be a risk of relapse. And it is no less obvious, that however perfectly the patient may be relieved from an existing stricture, he cannot reasonably claim exemption from the production of another, if he exposes himself to the exciting causes. It will, therefore, be prudent to enjoin such a mode of life as may, as far as possible, afford protection from the influence of circumstances calculated to act in this way. With due attention to all these points, it is reasonable to expect that the obstinate forms of stricture in question may be effectually remedied by an operation of the utmost sim-plicity and most perfect safety; and that the relief will generally, if not always, prove permanent. *Part* xxvi., *p.* 199.

Traumatic Stricture of the Urethra.—Mr. Coulson asks the question, where great damage has been done to the urethra from injury, whether it would not be better to contrive some artificial outlet for the renal secre-tion, than to make repeated attempts to rectify the state of the natural canal when they are not likely to be attended by success. He thinks rather than risk repeated attacks of retention, the best plan would be to make an opening into the bladder above the pubes, or through the rectum, and by allowing the urethra perfect rest for a few days, favor its return to a normal state, and then, if after several weeks' rest, the urethra is found so mutilated as not to be amenable to the treatment by dilatation, to make such temporary opening permanent.   *Part* xxvi., *p.* 213.

New Form of Director for the remedy of Stricture by External Incisions.—In his operation by external incision, Mr. Syme has frequently found the inconvenience of not being able by ordinary instruments to thoroughly divide the contracted portion of the urethra. To this fact, Mr. Syme believes, are owing the relapses said sometimes to take place. He has had a solid director recently made, but with a long slender portion, which is grooved, and this latter part being much smaller than that usually employed, passes with more readiness completely through the stricture. The operator now cuts through the integuments above the stricture into the groove, runs the knife down until the contraction is completely divided, as is readily seen by the thicker portion of the director passing easily through the whole length of the canal.   *Part* xxviii., *p.* 215.

Stricture of the Urethra.—Dr. Dick operated in a case of stricture as follows: Making a very small opening above the stricture through the integuments into the urethra, he introduced a curved tenotome and divided the stricture from before backward. The ready passage of the sound proved that the stricture was completely divided.   *Part* xxviii., *p.* 215.

Stricture of the Urethra.—If we wish to know whether the bougie is pressing against the walls of the urethra, or has entered the stricture, we must draw it gently back; if the latter, we shall meet with some degree of resistance, as if it had been grasped by some contracted orifice. If the stricture be long and callous, the bougie may cease to advance, and in this case it should be withdrawn and a larger one introduced. Catgut bougies are going out of use; the common plaster ones are not very convenient, but they must be employed where the contracted parts are tortuous and of small calibre. Mr. Liston, however, rejected them altogether, and if the stricture was moderate, used a plated metal bougie, and if very tight, a small silver catheter. Mr. Lawrence is another high authority in favor of metallic sounds. Having been passed, the instrument should remain in the urethra a short time, and then be withdrawn, introducing it again on the third day, and if it is well borne, introducing it daily, and allowing it to remain a longer time, so as gradually to dilate the strictured part. This is a good but a tedious plan, and some surgeons prefer introducing a small instrument first, and then immediately passing in rapid succession two or three of a larger size, until the patient complains of weariness or pain. Permanent dilatation is effected by passing an instrument and allowing it to remain forty eight-hours or longer, according to the case, then this is withdrawn and a gum-elastic catheter substituted. This may be left for from two to six days; it is then withdrawn and a larger instrument passed, and so on until the dilatation is complete. For this purpose Mr. Wakley's instruments are very useful, consisting of silver and flexible tubes of graduated sizes.   *Part* xxix., *p.* 226.

Stricture of the Urethra.—Prof. Syme says: Stricture never occurs in the membranous portion of the urethra. If you divide the urethra into three portions, the prostatic, membranous, and the remaining part which is covered by the corpus spongiosum, it is in the last portion that all strictures exist. It is never necessary, therefore, to cut beyond the bulbous part of the urethra, as no strictures are beyond the bulb. If you bear these facts in mind, you need not dilate sinuses, which are sure to close when the stricture is removed. A catheter should be introduced into the bladder after the operation, and retained for 48 hours—not less, on account of the risk of extravasation of urine, and not longer, because it is unnecessary and apt to do harm.

Mr. Syme's set of bougies are exceedingly small in size. No. 1 is perhaps smaller than those made any where else. The tightest and worst strictures are *anterior to the scrotum*. A stricture in this place is felt like a small pea, somewhat elongated. This is the kind most unmanageable by dilatation, and most successfully and easily treated by division. Pass a very small director (which is here comparatively easily done, but would be very difficult at the *bulb*). Introduce the point of the knife into the groove of the director *anterior to the stricture*, and push it backward through it, while the end of the penis is held firmly. Cut *backward* in stricture anterior to the scrotum, and *forward* when the stricture is at the *bulb*. You will never meet with a tight stricture *behind the scrotum* along with an extreme contraction in *front* of it. *Part* xxxi., *p.* 159.

Stricture of the Urethra.—As a rule, Mr. Syme, in common with surgeons generally in this country, treats stricture by simple dilatation, eschewing the use of caustics and internal incisions. So firmly persuaded is he of the efficiency of the catheter, that he believes there is no stricture, however narrow, which will not admit an instrument, provided it be sufficiently small, and be employed with care and patience. He therefore believes that it is wholly unnecessary to resort to the operation of dissecting through what have been termed impermeable strictures, preferring to insinuate a catheter rather than to employ a knife in these circumstances. Hence he disapproves of that operation usually termed "the perineal section," which has been frequently resorted to in this country for the last thirty-six years. Having proceeded to employ dilatation, if he finds that the stricture rapidly reappears in spite of it, or that the process involves much constitutional disturbance, he prefers to divide freely the stricture from the perineum, upon a grooved director, performing the incisions in the median line, tying in a catheter for forty-eight hours, and subsequently passing it a few times at about weekly intervals. This proceeding, to which he gives the name of "external division," is stated by him, on the ground of an extensive experience, to be devoid of danger, and generally to be attended with a successful result, a conclusion with which our own experience of it leads us, without any hesitation, to coincide.

Part xxxii., *p.* 169.

Stricture of the Urethra.—Mr. Lawrence, surgeon to Northern Dispensary, says : The following method of applying caustic in these cases is free from the ordinary objections to the practice. Coat the end of a catgut bougie very evenly with a fine layer of caustic, by immersing it in fused nitrate of silver, to which a little water has been added. Pass a full-sized straight catheter with one terminal aperture completely *down* to the stricture, then pass the armed bougie through the catheter *into* the stricture, and by gently rotating the bougie, the whole tract of the stricture may be freely and equally cauterized. *Part* xxxii., *p.* 175.

Stricture of the Urethra.—In the employment of dilatation, says the "Lancet," the golden rule which must guide us, both in regard to the extent it may be carried at the time, and the length of interval which is to elapse between each repetition of it, is to exercise just so much pressure and dilating power as can be exerted without producing pain or uneasiness, or more than slight irritation, and not to repeat the process until any excitement produced by the previous catheterism has completely subsided. The fulfillment of these indications will conduce in the long run the most quickly and safely to a successful result. *Part* xxxiii., *p.* 194.

Maisonneuve's Method.—The method which M. Maisonneuve adopts for their radical and instantaneous cure is that by internal division. When very contracted, he commences by passing a very fine thread-like bougie into the bladder—this will require great tact and perseverance : another larger bougie is then articulated to the end of this, and pushed forward, so that the first bougie becomes coiled up in the bladder ; when this is thoroughly in the stricture it must be withdrawn, and another filiform bougie passed, to which is attached the cutting instrument of Frère Come. When this is fairly in the stricture, you must unsheathe the bistoury and withdraw the instrument, cutting through all resistance. The patient generally gets well in fourteen days. As to the possibility of relapses, nothing at present can be affirmed—it is a question to be judged of hereafter. This method of treatment has been the subject of much discussion before the Surgical Society of Paris ; the result of this shows that dilatation is still the best and safest plan, and that the cases are very few required incision. If a patient can bear with tolerable ease a moderate stricture, he had better do so than be operated on, for experience shows it is not free from danger, however practised. *Part* xxxiii., *p.* 206.

Stricture of the Urethra.—Mr. Solly, of St. Thomas' Hospital, believes that the knife ought never to be employed in any case when you can introduce the thread catgut bougie, that is, in any stricture which is pervious. When you can once introduce a bougie into the bladder you can cure that stricture without cutting. There is not one case in two hundred, of even bad strictures, where the knife need be used at all. Mechanical means must be combined with medical treatment ; if you cannot pass a bougie, give one grain of the iodide of mercury three times a day to promote absorption, and the buchu mixture to relieve irritation. To pass the bougie as far as the stricture, and allow it to remain half an hour with gentle pressure, will excite the absorbents. If you can pass a fine catgut bougie, pass over it a No. 5 elastic tube, and withdraw the bougie. As a general rule, the bougie should be passed every other day for the first week or fortnight, afterward the periods to be lengthened to once a week, then once a fortnight, but the use of the instrument must never be abandoned altogether. *Part* xxxiv., *p.* 167.

Stricture of the Urethra.—In Syme's operation for stricture, one element essential to its success has by many been entirely overlooked, and that is, the necessity of passing a full-sized bougie at intervals, gradually increasing, and for a considerable time after the cicatrization of the opening made in the urethra. In the treatment of stricture of the urethra great advantage will be gained by passing a No. 8 catheter as far as possible, and keeping its point pressing with moderate firmness against the obstruction for twelve or twenty-four hours ; systematic attempts should then be made to overcome the impediment, first, with the No. 8, and then, if necessary, others of smaller calibre. This is a powerful adjunct to the ordinary mode of treatment with the bougie, and should be employed in certain cases, which may be classified as follows: 1. Those in which the contracted portion is longer than usual. 2. Those which afford but little time for treatment. 3. Those which are likely to resist the passage of an instrument for a considerable time. 4. Those which would yield if the patient would rest, but when he cannot. *Part* xxxiv., *p.* 169.

Syme's Operation for.—Prof. Syme states that there can hardly be any serious hemorrhage in urethrotomy by external incision unless the artery of the bulb has been wounded, which may certainly be avoided by cutting in the middle line upon a grooved director. Extravasation of urine may take place if the stricture be not freely divided, or, still worse, if the stricture be undivided and the urethra be opened behind it. The urethra should be freely exposed before opening it, so that the incision of its coats may not be subcellular, which would expose the patient to the same dangers which attend internal incision. There can be no safety unless a free drain be provided for the urine through a full-sized catheter; this will require very careful management: the external extremity should be curved downward, so that the urine may fall into a vessel without wetting the bedclothes; stopcocks are productive of much danger, the person in charge gets confounded, so as not to know whether the catheter is open or shut, and if the patient makes any expulsive efforts he may do himself much injury. It will be much better to keep the catheter constantly open, so that the urine may not pass along its outer surface. The patient should remain quiet on his back, with a pillow under his knees, for forty-eight hours, no change of position being allowed. It is not desirable that the wound should heal by the first intention; if there be any tendency to this, the finger must be occasionally introduced so as to feel the instrument, or the patient will be exposed to a relapse of the disease. Strictures do not occur behind the bulb, except in cases of extreme rarity, so that incisions into the membraneous portion of the canal are unwarrantable. The danger of extravasation will be especially serious when the deep facia of the perineum has been divided; in such cases the introduction of a straight tube, as after lithotomy, will effectually prevent the risk of serious consequences.

Part xxxiv., *p.* 181.

Retention of Urine from Stricture—Syme's Operation.—When there is repeated retention of urine, says Mr. Lane, it will be necessary to open the membranous portion of the urethra behind the stricture. To do this it is necessary to hit off, with microscopic accuracy, the delicate line of the raphé, for, if we cut sidewise through the muscles, the wound will be found to gape, there will be hemorrhage and extravasation of urine. This operation is much more easy and successful than puncturing the bladder through the rectum, for, while the recent wound is healing the previous stricture will be found to give way very much, so that an instrument may readily be passed. *Part* xxxiv., *p.* 183.

Remedy of Stricture by External Incision.—Prof. Syme says, with regard to the use of external incision in the treatment of stricture, that it is not true that wounds of the urethra, like those of the skin, must heal either by adhesion or granulation, and so the old contraction be restored with greater firmness than before. It has been repeatedly shown that the most tightly contracted urethra may remain perfectly patent after division of the stricture, and in the bodies of some persons who have died several years after the operation, the canal has been found actually wider than natural, and the surface of the previously deranged mucous membrane not distinguishable from the neighboring portion. *Part* xxxvi., *p.* 173.

Source of Danger in Division of Stricture.—Out of the great number of cases operated upon by Mr. Syme, he has met with two in which during the act of micturition, acute pain in the perineum was followed by quick pulse, delirium, and death. In neither were there any signs of local mischief, but in one the kidneys were gorged with blood to an extreme degree; besides these two cases, slighter symptoms of disturbance occurred in many others. It was noticed that these symptoms were always connected with micturition after withdrawal of the catheter, therefore probably proceeding from the action of the urine upon a raw surface, produced by tearing of the imperfectly united wound in the urethra, and being of the nature of a sudden shock to the nervous system. To obviate this he introduces a short catheter by the wound in the perineum, about nine inches in length, and slightly curved in opposite directions at the extremities. By thus keeping the wound open a little longer perfect security is obtained. *Part* xxxviii., *p.* 154.

Stricture of the Urethra.— Urethrotomy.—Prof. Syme's practice is to cut from behind forward, and not backward, as is the London practice. The risk of cutting the deep perineal fascia is much lessened.
Part xxxviii., *p.* 157.

Sensitive and Contractile Stricture.—In cases of stricture so exquisitely sensitive that the passage of a catheter is followed by severe constitutional and local disturbance; also in cases in which immediately upon omission of treatment contraction begins to return, the operation of external division is most valuable. The above opinion of Mr. Bryant upon this subject is valuable, from the large amount of experience necessarily obtained at so large a hospital as Guy's. *Part* xxxviii., *p.* 158.

Stricture of the Urethra.—Syme's Operation.—Mr. Lee, surgeon to Lock Hospital, observes: It is singular that the success which has attended Mr. Syme's operation should have varied so considerably in different hands. This can be accounted for in a great measure by the kind of stricture for which the operation had been undertaken by different surgeons. An incision through the bulb is a safe proceeding, but an incision through the membranous part, involving, as it necessarily does, a division of the deep perineal fascia, is a very unsafe proceeding, and not to be undertaken except in cases of perineal fistulæ, where the parts are often so condensed by adhesive inflammation, that incisions may be made with instruments: otherwise the operation is adapted only to cases of stricture confined to the bulb of the urethra. *Part* xxxix., *p.* 207.

Internal Urethrotomy.—Mr. Thompson, of University College Hospital, considers the best instrument for ordinary use to be that designed some fifteen years ago, by Civiale, of Paris. The shaft is almost equal in size to an ordinary No. 3, the bulb to No. 5. By means of the bulb the extent of the narrowing can be accurately told. When the instrument is used, the bulb having been passed about half an inch beyond the obstruction, the cutting side must be directed downward, and directly in the middle line; the blade is made to project to the required extent, by means of an apparatus in the handle, which accurately controls it, and the instrument is firmly pressed on the floor of the urethra, and slowly and steadily drawn outward, about an inch or an inch and a half, so as fairly to divide the obstructing portion. For smaller strictures than Civiale's instrument is applicable to, Mr. T. has invented a smaller instrument on essentially the same plan. *Part* xl., *p.* 130.

STYPTIC.

Aid of Turpentine as a Styptic.—*Vide* Art. "Turpentine."

Styptic (*M. Pagliari's*).—This styptic liquor, which seems to have abundant testimony in its favor, is composed as follows: Eight ounces of tincture of benzoin, one pound of alum, and ten pounds of water, are boiled together for six hours in a glazed earthen vessel, the vaporized water being constantly replaced by hot water, so as not to interrupt the ebullition. The resinous mass is to be kept stirred round.

Part xxvi., *p.* 349.

Styptic.—*Solid Perchloride of Iron.*—The perchloride of iron is manufactured in a solid form in which state it is particularly manageable as a styptic. Another, and perhaps superior way of using it is to apply, by means of a spun-glass brush, a small quantity of the thick brown fluid, into which the solid perchloride kept in a bottle always deliquesces It is particularly useful, according to Mr. Lawrence, in such cases as excision of the tonsils, bleeding from the deeper-seated gums, etc. No inflammatory action follows the use of this drug. *Part* xl., *p.* 298.

SUPPOSITORIES.

Dr. Simpson's Morphia Suppositories.—Mr. Spencer Wells has introduced into use at the Samaritan Hospital, a form of morphia suppository, used with great advantage by Dr. Simpson of Edinburgh. Mr. Wells has found it a most convenient form of suppository after operations on the vagina, rectum, uterus or perineum of women, both in hospital and private practice, and especially so after operations made on the genito-urinary organs, as lithotrity, in cases of retention of urine, irritable stricture, etc., and after division of fistula in ano, or the removal of piles or prolapsed mucous membrane of the rectum by the écraseur. They act much more efficiently than the soap and opium in common pill use as a suppository, and are seldom or never expelled from the rectum after their introduction above the sphincter. The following is for the half grain suppository: Take of acetate of morphia, 6 grains; sugar of milk, 1 drachm; simple cerate, half a drachm, or as much as may be sufficient to make a proper consistence, and divide the mass into twelve suppositories. Then dip each suppository into the following mixture, to form a coating: Take of white wax one part, lard plaster two parts; melt together. The best way is to insert a needle into the apex of the suppository, dip it into the melted wax and lard, and immediately afterward into cold water to harden it before it loses its shape. The shape is conical, like a pastille. It is easily introduced by the finger, or more neatly by the ordinary ivory suppository syringe. Mr. Coulson has also used these suppositories lately in several lithotrity cases, and has found them of the greatest benefit in allaying the irritation which often attends the passage of the fragments of calculi through the urethra.

Part xxxv., *p.* 255.

———•••———

SUTURES.

Employment of Threads of Caoutchouc for Sutures.—Mr. Nûnnely, of Leeds, recommends the use of caoutchouc sutures.

" There are many cases where the unelastic ligature in common use is even prejudicial, and where a more elastic thread might be advantageously substituted. It produces less irritation, and holds the divided parts together with much less stretching than the common ligature, and at the same time it keeps up an equal degree of tension, ' for if the parts swell, the ligature gives way in proportion to the pressure; on the contrary, do they contract, so also does the ligature, and an equable approximation is maintained.' In hare-lip this kind of ligature might supersede the use of pins."

Part iii., *p.* 78.

Bead Suture.—Vide Art. " Palate."

Suture—New Form of.—This form of suture was used by its inventor, Mr. Spencer Wells, in an operation for the cure of vesico-vaginal fistula. It is applicable in most cases in which the quilled suture is employed, and is more easily applied. Pass a pin, armed with a shot and perforated bar, through one edge, and then through the opposite edge of the wound, then pass a second bar over the point of the pin, and then a shot, which must be pressed by forceps on to the pin, so as to fix this bar in its place, then cut the pin off close to the shot.

Part xxxv., *p.* 171.

Lead-Wire Suture.—In cases where it is desirable to place a suture to any part not easily reached, take a curved needle, and a piece of lead-wire which is very soft and flexible—the end of the needle must be so made that the wire may be screwed into it. Pass the needle through the edges of the wound, cut off the needle, and with a pair of forceps twist the two ends of the wire together, and double up the ends to prevent scratching.

Part xxxvi., *p.* 273.

Aluminium Sutures.—When union by the first intention is required, few will deny that silver sutures possess great advantages over ordinary thread or silk ones. Their great drawback is their great cost. Dr. Frodsham, surgeon to Cumberland Infirmary, says that aluminium possesses all the pliability and other properties of silver, and is only half the price. Sutures may with great advantage be made of this metal, and will be found to answer quite as well as silver.

Part xxxviii., *p.* 163.

———•••———

SYNOVITIS.

Gonorrhœal Synovitis.—Mr. B. Cooper says: Patients suffering from gonorrhœa are subject to the attacks of a peculiar form of synovitis, which so closely resembles the rheumatic affection, that it is sometimes extremely difficult to distinguish between them; and, indeed, it is only from a history of the case that a just diagnosis can be formed. It usually happens in such cases that the gonorrhœal discharge ceases simultaneously with the accession of the disease to the joint; and it is of the highest importance that the former should be reestablished as quickly as possible, the best means being the application of warm fomentations over the organs of generation. I have never known an attack of the above kind to occur unless the patient has taken copaiva, and am inclined to think that this medicine acts specifically on the synovial membranes; for I have invariably found the symptoms of inflammation greatly aggravated by its administration. Bark and alkalies, combined with opium, seem to be the most appropriate remedies, as colchicum does not afford relief. In these cases the latter circumstance constitutes a further distinction between gonorrhœal and rheumatic affections. *Part* xvii., *p.* 130.

SYPHILIS.

Inoculation as a Test—M. Ricord's Process.—In all doubtful cases, the patient is inoculated from his own sore, and if a syphilitic ulcer is produced, similar to the one from which the matter is taken, it is considered to be genuine syphilis, and treated accordingly. But instead of allowing this second sore to proceed, M. Ricord destroys the part inoculated, on the third or fourth day, before it has proceeded far enough to produce bad effects. By long experience, M. Ricord knows, even on the second or third day, what would be the effects of his inoculation, and thus destroys the part in time, as unpleasant effects might take place were the second sore to become intractable, as has occasionally happened. *Part* i., *p.* 123.

Employment of Platinum—Therapeutic Action.—The perchloride is to be regarded as an efficacious remedy in syphilis, especially of a chronic form. The chloride of platinum and sodium is more applicable to the recent forms of the disease. It is equally efficacious in rheumatic affections. Platinum must be ranked amongst the alteratives along with gold, arsenic, and iodine. It differs from mercury in producing previous excitement of the system; and it does not cause the same serious accidents which often follow the use of that drug. *Part* iii., *p.* 61.

Treatment of Chancre—Vide Preparations of Antimony and Mercury, Art. "Antimony."

Aphorism of Practical Surgery.—Syphilitic exostoses do not always disappear, although their primary cause has been entirely removed.
Part iii., *p.* 116.

Gangrenous Syphilitic Ulcers.—Nitrous acid saturated with nitrate of silver, recommended topically to arrest gangrenous inflammation and phagedenic ulceration, resulting from syphilis. *Part* v., *p.* 115.

Inoculation as a Test of Syphilis.—[Several objections have been repeatedly urged against the process of inoculating a patient to ascertain with certainty whether or not the chancre is really syphilitic. It has been urged, that by producing another sore, we increase the chance of affecting the constitution; but most surgeons now believe that one sore will produce as much mischief as two. It has been also asserted, that matter from any angry sore, introduced below the skin, is likely to cause the point to fester. This, however, is denied by Mr. Mayo. He makes the following remarks on the way in which the inoculation is to be performed :]

Before arming the lancet, the suspected sore should not have been wiped, or dressed with any chemical application, for two or three hours at least. The most convenient part for inoculation is the back of the fore-arm immediately above the wrist.

The point inoculated should be covered with a patch of sticking plaster, and not disturbed for three days.

At the expiration of that period, on examining it, either the punctured point is found to be scarcely distinguishable, having healed, and having no redness about it; or it has ulcerated, and the skin around it is inflamed, and, if the epidermis is not broken in raising the sticking plaster, there is seen a small flat vesicle containing lymph or pus, surrounded by an inflam-matory zone. Occasionally, but very rarely, the inoculated point does not become inflamed during the first three days, but on the fourth or fifth a pustule suddenly forms.

When the inoculation has taken to this extent, the evidence required is obtained. The suspected sore is certainly of syphilitic origin. And, if circumstances are not present to contra-indicate the use of mercury, a mercurial course should be immediately commenced.

In order to get rid of the artificial sore, we must freely apply the nitrate of silver, so that the texture may be destroyed to the depth of half a line, which will almost certainly destroy it, and cause the sore to heal.

Part v., *p.* 145.

Chronic Venereal Ulcers— Creasote.—In chronic venereal ulcers, Dr. R. Cormack of Edinburgh has repeatedly used creasote with advantage. It answers very well to apply it pure *once*, when there is great deficiency of action, and subsequently to employ an ointment of from four drops to thirty, to the ounce of lard. The lotion is also a very excellent form of application. In *phagedenic ulcers, ulcerated chilblains*, and sores yielding a sanious discharge, Dr. C. has often used creasote with great benefit.

In the application of creasote to ulcers and other solutions of continuity, there are several facts which the practitioner should bear in mind. *It is important to remember that water only dissolves one-eighteenth part.* If an excess of creasote be present, it will float on the surface in small globules, and can therefore very easily be removed; but if this is not done, when the lint is dipped in the lotion, these globules will adhere, and in this way a very different wash from what was intended, is placed upon the sore. In very few cases, where the raw surface is extensive, pure creasote ought to be applied to the whole of it, as severe irritation is generally the result.

Part vi., *p.* 74.

Syphilitic Sore Throat—Iodine Gargle.—Dr. James J. Ross says :

Another case in which the local use of the tincture of iodine is of signal efficacy, is that of ulcers of the tonsils and fauces—specific or non-specific. I have seen the ugliest sores in this situation put on quite a healthy ap-pearance in a few days under its use. It is highly recommended by Ricord, and certainly I do not know anything equal to it in such cases. It is best in the form of gargle; thus :

℞ Tinct. iodin., ʒj.–ij.; tinct. opii, ʒj.; aquæ, ʒvj. M. Fiat. garg. ter quaterve in die utenda.

It may be made weaker or stronger, with or without the laudanum. It requires to be well shaken when used.

The first case in which I used it, was one of irregular phagedenic ulceration near the base of the uvula, with patches of a white exudation on the back of the pharynx; the voice, respiration, and deglutition being all affected. The general aspect of the patient was cachectic, but he denied ever having had syphilis. The above gargle was ordered. An improvement was observable on the third day of its use, which went on steadily and rapidly to a perfect cure. In another bad case of syphilis, with sloughing, irregular ulcers on the velum and fauces, the local use of the same gargle (made first with ʒj. to ʒvj. and afterward increased to ʒiss), arrested the phagedenic ulceration, and reduced it to a healing sore, which soon cicatrized. Patients do not complain of the gargle being disagreeable.

Part vi., *p.* 118.

Chronic Indolent Bubo and Ulcers.—Dr. James J. Ross recommends the iodide of mercury as follows:

1. An ointment of iodid. hydrarg., ℈j. to ʒiss of lard, is extremely serviceable in various syphilitic ulcers, particularly those indolent greyish regular sores, which are seen on the arms and legs of venereal patients, and those which are left on the separation of the concreted scurvy cutaneous tubercles, which are met with on the face in bad cases. The above ointment is one of the most effectual applications for such sores that I have seen used. It is applied in the usual manner—spread on lint.

2. An ointment of this substance may be used like other preparations of iodine, with the view of causing the absorption of various tumors. Ricord uses it in this way for chronic indolent bubo. *Part* vi., *p.* 123.

Treatment of Syphilis by Tartarized Antimony.—Mr. Smee recommends the use of tartarized antimony for the cure of syphilis. Mr. Smee says that by giving *very small doses* of this medicine frequently repeated, we charge the system with it; thus irritating the capillary system, and inciting it to action throughout the whole body, causing it to throw off the antimony and with it the syphilitic poison.

He goes on to say:

As a general rule, most patients laboring under syphilis, except, indeed, if it be a sloughing phagedena, violent inflammation, or some such analogous case, no matter what form or duration, primary or secondary, p the party be otherwise robust, or at any rate, not in very ill health, will be benefited by the antimonial treatment. The medical man begins, if necessary, by ordering an aperient of colocynth, jalap, black draught, or similar purgative, and then directs the patient to take from 20 to 60 drops (30 medium) of antimonial wine, or the solution of antimony, every two or three hours regularly, and in every case where pus or a puriform discharge exists, use at the same time a lotion of chloride of soda, the strength of which should be regulated to the sensitiveness and delicacy of the part of the body affected.

Simple Sores.—In simple sores, either of the prepuce or glands, the treatment is extremely efficacious, and here had better be conjoined with a solution of chloride of soda, containing about an ounce of the latter to a pint of water, which should be applied two or three times the first day. In many cases, in twenty-four hours the character of the sore becomes changed; the surface is no longer covered with white pus, a healing edge begins to show itself, and the sores, perhaps three, four or more, are speedily healed. As soon as the character of the sore is changed, the part had better only be dabbed once or twice a day with the lotion, and at other times simply covered with a piece of dry lint; for we may be sure that here, as in all other cases, too much disturbance of a healing part only interferes with the natural healing process. Superficial sores will fre-quently, although of three weeks' or a month's standing, be healed in four or five days; but it is prudent to continue the antimony till not only the surface of the skin is not in the slightest degree raised, but even till the part affected assumes its natural color.

Indurated Sores.—The treatment of indurated sores is similar in all respects to that of superficial sores, and indeed that slight puffiness always to be seen round the most superficial sore is perhaps to be considered as a slight induration, and the dense cartilaginous hardness which occasionally presents itself is nothing but the same thing differing in degree rather than in kind , and we have the authority of some' most eminent surgeons, in confirmation of universal experience, that either produce indifferently secondary symptoms. The rapidity with which the cure is effected in these cases is proportionate to the degree of hardness. If the induration is moderate, the sore may heal, but the induration will remain ; in which case the person is by no means to be considered as cured, for the anti-mony must be continued not only till the sore is cured but till the indura-tion is removed. If the induration is very intense and hard, the sore, although healthy, will not heal till that is absorbed. In all these cases the antimony should be given very frequently at the commencement, and with the utmost regularity: for the remedy always produces the greatest effect on its first administration, and seems rather to lose its power after many days, for which reason it should be gradually increased in quantity.

Phagedenic Sores.—Phagedenic sores generally occur in poor, weakly constitutions, and require peculiar treatment on that account. The employment of antimony in these cases acts decidedly as a mild tonic ; but still, as its excreting effects seem to exceed its tonic powers, we find it advisable in these cases to conjoin the use of the remedy with that of other more potent tonics. If, indeed, the skin is cold and clammy, we should use such remedies as experience has taught us determine the blood to the surface, for a few days previous to the employment of the antimony. A grain of sulphate of quinine may be given twice or thrice a day. A grain of proto-sulphate of iron, or a grain of sulphate of zinc, may be used with great advantage for the same purpose; and the antimonial drops exhibited as before. If the patient is but slightly feeble we may begin at once with the following mixture :—

R Zinci sulphatis, gr. v.; aquæ dest., ℥ss.; vin. ant. pot. tart., ℥ss.; quaque ℥ss. vel ℈j. pro dose 2da vel tertia hora sumenda.

Proto-sulphate of iron may be substituted for the zinc with similar suc-cess. If the patient is restless or sleepless, or the nervous system much affected, the addition of about twenty or thirty minims of sirup of poppies, or a few drops of laudanum to each dose, is of much service. A little Dover's powder may be given at bed-time. Whenever iron is employed it appears to be essential that the metal should be in the state of the pro-toxide; for probably the persalts have but very little action on the system, and even that little action may be dependent upon a portion of the salt giving up one equivalent of oxygen. The nature of the salt of iron, provided it be a protosalt, does not seem to influence the result.

In all cases where the patient is feeble, he should be desired, immediately on leaving his bed in the morning, to rub his entire body with a coarse towel till the skin is red, which will further help to promote a proper flow of blood to that important organ.

Buboes.—Buboes give way to antimony perhaps more rapidly than they do to mercury, and a more favorable prognosis may be given if this treatment be adopted. It would, however, be vain to attempt the removal of an inflamed bubo containing a large quantity of pus, by any general means.

Eruptions of the Skin.—Various eruptions of the skin, the sequelæ of syphilis, as a general rule, yield favorably and rapidly to antimony.

Ulcerations of the Throat.—Ulcerations of the pharynx, uvula, and roof of the mouth, yield rapidly to this line of treatment. It is a good plan to use a gargle containing from ʒj. to ℥j. of chloride of soda to the pint of water, as that much facilitates the favorable termination of the disease. The ulceration, in these cases, rapidly loses its white layer of pus, frequently mistaken for lymph or sloughs; and as soon as a perfectly healthy surface is established the ulcer heals as rapidly as a common sore.

Ulcerations of the Mouth, etc.—Ulcerations of the corners of the mouth and tongue, and a peculiar growth of the papillæ of that organ, yield rapidly to this line of treatment.

Syphilitic affections of the testicle, rhagides digitorum, etc., yield rapidly to this plan.

Of the value of antimony in syphilitic iritis and nodes I do not happen to have had any experience. *Part* vi., *p.* 125.

Syphilitic Ulcerations of the Throat.—The inhalation of ammonia gas recommended. *Vide* Art. "Hoarseness."

Buboes.—The ferruginated pill of mercury recommended as a superior resolvent, especially with respect to buboes. *Vide* Art. "Pills."

Treatment of Chancre.—Mr. Langston Parker, of Birmingham, recommends the following mode of treating a chancre: A chancre when first presented to the notice of the surgeon, is generally in one of two states—either in that of a small pustule with its contents yet undischarged, or a minute ulcer. In whatever state it may be, our first duty is to endeavor, by the use of escharotics, to convert the specific sore into a simple one. For this purpose you will find most authors recommending either a strong solution of the nitrate of silver, or the application of this caustic in substance. When the nitrate of silver is used, if the disease be pustular, it will be necessary to open the pustule with the point of a lancet, to discharge its contents, and rub the whole surface and edges of the ulcer thus produced with the nitrate of silver, previously cut to a sharp point; if the disease be an open ulcer, it is to be treated in the same way. The nitrate of silver thus applied will sometimes have the effect of producing a simple sore, but it will more commonly give rise to considerable irritation and inflammation, while the specific character of the sore is not destroyed.

The great evil in the use of the nitrate of silver in these cases is, that it is powerful enough to irritate, but not sufficiently powerful to destroy. We want a remedy that will at once disorganize the tissue to a depth co-equal with that of the chancre. For this purpose I now employ several remedies : highly concentrated nitric acid, the acid nitrate of mercury, the acid nitrate of silver, or the potassa cum calce of the London Pharmacopœia. The second of these remedies is made by dissolving a drachm of the subnitrate of mercury in an ounce of nitric acid; the third by dissolving the same quantity of the nitrate of silver in the like quantity of acid.

When it is determined to destroy a primary venereal ulcer with any of the three first caustics, a camel's-hair pencil must be dipped in them, and the surface and edges of the sore pencilled thickly over; if the acid be sufficiently concentrated, the whole surfaces touched are at once destroyed, and converted into a yellow eschar, which, on separating, generally leaves a clean simple sore underneath. When the potassa cum calce is employed, which is the most certain of all the remedies I have mentioned, it must be made into a paste of moderate consistency, with spirits of wine, at the time it is wanted for use, and the sore and its edges covered with it. When it has been on a few seconds, a smart burning pain is felt, which continues to increase as long as the caustic is suffered to remain on, which it should be from half a minute to a minute, or even longer, according to the effects produced. After this the caustic must be all removed by means of a fine bone spatula, and the black eschar left may be covered with a poultice, a cold saturnine lotion, or fine, soft, dry lint. The pain soon subsides after the caustic has been removed. The parts touched by it are at once destroyed, and on the separation of the eschar, we have a clear grannlating sore left, which commonly heals with great rapidity, particularly if the ulcer be a recent one. A poultice is the most convenient and best application during the time the eschar is separating, if the patient can rest, which should always be urged upon him as an essential point, if it can possibly be managed. The moment the eschar begins to be detached, and a secreting surface is exposed, the poultice must be done away with, and other remedies employed. Of these, weak lotions are the best. I employ weak solutions of the nitrate of silver, acetate or sulphate of copper, alum, or zinc, or tannin in port wine, in the proportion of about two drachms of the former to six ounces of the latter.

There are certain conditions of primary venereal ulcer, which contraindicate the use of the caustic in the first instance. If an ulcer of this kind produce violent inflammation of the penis, this must be reduced by a proper general treatment before we have recourse to these remedies, which may be used after the inflammation has been subdued, if the sore be foul, and stationary, and show no disposition to heal.

Preliminary Cautions.—Whenever a patient consults you with a primary venereal ulcer, particularly if it is the first from which he has ever suffered, point out to him in as strong terms as you can the necessity of his adhering rigidly to a very abstemious diet till the ulcer assumes a granulating condition ; it is well, also, at this period, to administer repeatedly, for some few days, aperient medicine, and to insist on a total abstinence from malt liquor, wine, or spirits. If your patient, from circumstances, cannot lie by and rest altogether, press upon him the advantage of retiring early to bed, rest in bed being a most important auxiliary in the treatment of all forms of primary syphilis.   •

Mercurial Courses.—Whether it be your intention to submit your patient ultimately to mercurial treatment or not, these preliminary cautions

.should never be omitted. Many of the evils attendant on mercurial courses are to be attributed to not preparing the patient by diet, rest, and apperients, for the administration of this medicine.

If you administer mercury for the cure of a primary venereal ulcer, do not have recourse to it till your patient has been prepared to receive it by adopting, for some days, the regimen laid down, and till all inflammation produced by the action of the escharotics has subsided; you may then use it with every hope of realizing its most beneficial effects.

Mr. Parker's method of treating a *bubo* is equally judicious. When, as a consequence of a primary venereal ulcer not yet healed, or just healed, we perceive enlargement with tenderness in the groin producing stiffness when the patient walks, we may be sure that a bubo is about to form. I would not recommend you at this period to follow the old-fashioned practice of applying leeches; it is a practice generally very unsatisfactory, rendering your cure long, uncertain, and tedious; you must insist upon a strict regimen on the part of your patient, and absolute rest, if possible. You may smear the part thickly over with mercurial ointment, over this a linseed or a bread poultice, cold, and a piece of oiled silk to keep it moist, confining all by a bandage. Pressure may also be made by the emp. ammoniaci c. hydrarg. spread on thick wash leather, the plaster to be placed lengthwise parallel to the thigh, and not at right angles with it; this prevents the plaster getting displaced when the patient walks. The best means of all, however, is to paint over the enlarged gland night and morning with a strong solution of iodine in hydriodate of potass. (Iodide, one scruple; hydriodate of potass, two scruples; water, one ounce.) The effect of this is almost magical. In the intervals of the dressings pressure should be made by a pad and bandage. If the patient has not used mercury for the treatment of the primary sore, the dispersion of the bubo will be hastened by now administering it so as gently to affect the system—always presupposing that the patient is in a condition to bear mercury. Should these means not succeed (which in a majority of instances they will), and suppuration appears inevitable, hasten it by all means in your power by warm poultices and fomentations. When matter is ready to be discharged a question of very great importance suggests itself—viz., how should this be done? Many surgeons open the abscess freely with the bistoury or lancet, whilst some prefer the potassa fusa for this purpose. I would not, under ordinary circumstances, recommend either of these methods.

When a bubo is ready to puncture, I would not advise you to open it by a free incision; for, almost under every circumstance where this is practised, there is a quantity of integument in the edges, which will not unite with the granulating surface of the sore thus produced. By opening an abscess in this way the whole anterior wall of it is destroyed, and your cure must be performed by the cicatrization of a granulating surface which springs from the floor or posterior wall of the abscess. Your great object is to evacuate the matter first, then to diminish the disposition to its reformation, and lastly, to procure union of the two sides of the cavity. This may generally be done in the way I have adopted in the treatment of chronic abscesses in the Queen's Hospital.

When a bubo is ready to be opened, you should not suffer the skin to become too thin; when you practise this method, with a fine lancet make several very small punctures over the thinnest part, perhaps, six, eight, or ten; through these the matter will ooze out till the cavity of the abscess is empty. Through one of the punctures the point of a very small glass syringe may be introduced, and a very weak solution of the sulphate of. zinc injected, in the proportions of two or three grains to the half pint of water. When the abscess is quite empty, place over it a large compress of lint, and use moderately tight pressure by means of a roller. In many in. stances, if you can keep your patient quiet for twenty-four hours, you will get either partial or total adhesion of the sides of the bubo, and a speedy cure will be the result; in other instances this may not be the case, but by the daily use of the injection through one of the punctures, which should be kept open for that purpose, you will succeed in a few days, in almost every case, in effecting a cure.

I generally employ for an injection in these cases the weak solution of sulphate of zinc. I have used also a weak solution of iodine in hydriodate of potass.

Iodine, four grains; hydriodate of potass, eight grains; water, eight ounces. An injection.

The injections must be varied in strength to suit the feelings of the patient, or a gentle warmth and slight irritation should be experienced, but violent pain on no account produced. Solutions of the sulphate, or acetate of copper, alum, port wine, wine with tannin, may all be used; and if one does not succeed quickly, have recourse to another. This is the best way of treating a suppurating bubo with which I am acquainted. *Part* vii., *p.* 140.

Local Treatment of Chancres.—Dr. Strohl assures us that his local treatment of chancre is one of the most successful yet practised. It consists in cauterizing the sore if it is not much inflamed nor extensive. If it is so, he employs sulphate of copper instead, and dresses the part five or six times a-day with charpie soaked in a solution of about a grain and a half of sulphate of copper to an ounce of water. The sores will generally heal in about twelve days. At other times he uses an ointment composed of two grains of cyanuret of mercury to an ounce of axunge. This ointment is spread upon a piece of linen corresponding to the size of the sore. When this is too painful, it must be taken off for a time and replaced in a weaker form. When it has been on from four to ten hours, it is dressed with mercurial ointment, or opium cerate.   *Part* vii., *p.* 167.

Syphilitic Affections of Throat—Mercurial Cigars.—M. Paul Barnard proposed to the Acad. de la Médecine, the use of cigars impregnated with a weak solution of bichloride of mercury for persons affected with syphilitic affections of the throat and palate, as a mode of conveying mercurial fumigation. It has been proposed first to deprive the tobacco of its narcotine by frequent washings.   *Part* viii., *p.* 80.

Success of Arsenic in Syphilis.—Dr. Sicherer, of Heilbrunn, cites the following case : A lady having become affected through her husband with the virus of syphilis, had at length passed through the various stages of that disease until about to sink under final marasmus. The palate and the organs of deglutition were destroyed to such an extent that scarcely any liquid could be swallowed, and then only in a recumbent position. As a forlorn hope (for other remedies had been unsuccessfully employed), Sicherer had recourse to arsenic, ordering Fowler's solution to be taken, at first in doses of two drops, but gradually increased to thirty drops, three times a day. The remedy was continued until about two ounces of the arsenical solution had been taken, by which time a considerable portion of the impaired structures had been restored, and the faculty of deglutition regained; and after a period of ten years no relapse had been experienced.   *Part* viii., *p.* 164.

Proto-Ioduret of Mercury.—MM. Cullerier, Biett, Ricord and others employ this remedy in many forms of constitutional syphilis, especially where secondary and tertiary symptoms are combined, and in primary sores in strumous habits. Cullerier says that it is chiefly in constitutional syphilis that the proto-ioduret of mercury is administered with success. Its effects are principally evident in secondary ulcerations of the mucous membrane, cutaneous tubercles, exostoses, and chronic affections of the joints, where the other preparations of mercury have had little effect. It should always be guarded by opium, and given in half grain doses twice or thrice a day. The deuto-ioduret is more stimulating, and consequently its dose is smaller. Either of these may be employed in friction upon tumors and indolent buboes, after the removal of all acute inflammatory symptoms.

Part ix., *p.* 21.

Use of Mercury—Inunction preferred.—It is, perhaps, easier to know when we ought to administer mercury, than when we ought not. In persons of a scrofulous disposition, for example, who are disposed to phthisis, it requires the greatest discrimination: in such a case, however, we may be obliged to give it, knowing how frequently tubercles are developed in the lungs after any morbid poison has been circulating. This result may consequently follow an attack of syphilis as well as an attack of measles, scarlatina, or small pox. Sir B. Brodie prefers mercurializing a patient by *inunction*, to any other way, when the case is severe, and when the process is not inconvenient to the patient. It gripes and purges less than any other form, and is said to cure the disease a great deal better. Sir Benjamin even expresses his opinion of this method as follows: "It does not damage the constitution half so much as mercury taken by the mouth; nay, I will go so far as to say that, except in very slight cases, you really cannot depend upon any mercurial treatment effecting a certain cure, or even giving a good chance of it, by any other means than inunction. You may very often patch up the disease by giving mercury internally, but it will return again and again and you may cure it at last by a good course of mercurial ointment." In such a case, he recommends that the ointment be rubbed in at first before the fire, for three-quarters of an hour at a time, and afterward for a shorter time; the patient taking great care not to expose himself to cold. Sir Benjamin further states, that we ought not to leave off the mercury as soon as the sore has healed, but to persevere in it till the hard cicatrix has disappeared. In short, he recommends us rather to recur to the old practice of using mercury in abundance, and warns us against using it too slightly, according to some modern notions. He says: "You must not suppose that we have made an advance in all departments of surgery; on the contrary, I am sure that in some we have gone back. I am satisfied that the mercurial treatment of syphilis, as employed by the late Mr. Pearson, during a great part of his life, was as nearly perfect as possible, and it was much more successful than the less careful treatment of modern practitioners." Sir Benjamin's method of using mercury in children, is, in our opinion, very judicious, as it prevents most of the griping and purging which follow the internal use.

"Children, when born, sometimes labor under syphilis, the father or mother having been affected with it—perhaps the father and not the mother. The child at birth looks thin, and is of small size, and instead of thriving it becomes still thinner. At the end of three weeks it is covered by a nasty, scaly eruption; there is a sort of aphthæ in the mouth, and chaps about the lips and anus. I have tried different ways of treating such cases. I have given the child grey powder internally, and given mercury to the wet nurse. But mercury exhibited to a child by the mouth generally gripes and purges, seldom doing any good; and given to the wet nurse it does not answer very well, and certainly is a very cruel practice. The mode in which I have treated such cases for some years past has been this—I have spread mercurial ointment, made in the proportion of a drachm to an ounce, over a flannel roller, and bound it round the child once a day. The child kicks about, and the cuticle being thin the mercury is absorbed. It does not either gripe or purge, nor does it make the gums sore, but cures the disease. I have adopted this practice in a great many cases with the most signal success. Very few children recover in whom mercury is given internally, but I have not seen a case where this method of treatment has failed.

"Mercurial inunction may be used in certain cases in which were mercury taken internally it would do absolute harm. For example, a gentleman had a nasty phagedenic sore upon the penis; it could not be said that he was in ill health before, and therefore there was some reason to believe that the disease was spreading from the intensity of the venereal poison. He had taken calomel and opium until the gums were sore, and he was decidedly worse under it. The disease destroyed a great part of the glans, and evinced no disposition whatever to stop. It resisted all modes of treatment until he was put on a course of mercurial inunction; its progress was then arrested directly, and the sore healed with great rapidity. I have seen several instances of the same character."

Part ix., *p.* 111.

Prevention of the Contagion of Syphilis.—The problem of the means of extinguishing syphilitic contagion, appears to have been solved at the hospitals at St. Petersburg. In principle, it appears simple enough, the point to be effected being merely to prevent the absorption of muco-purulent matter, either by means of washings, which remove it directly, or by liquids, such as the chloride of lime, which have the property either of decomposing it, or of preventing otherwise its inoculation. In practice, however, it proves a matter of great difficulty, especially in the female. In St. Petersburg, the most satisfactory results are said to have followed the use of the prophylactic soap of Dr. Pfeffer. The active ingredients of this soap appear to be—in 500 grains of the substance, six grains of bichloride of mercury, four of tannin, and forty-five of chloride of lime, incorporated into a soap with soda.   *Part* ix., *p.* 180.

Treatment for Buboes.—In commenting on the process adopted by M. Regnaud of treating buboes, by first blistering, then applying a corrosive stimulant, etc., Dr. Johnson states that the plan is needlessly complicated, and that the application of the caustic potash so as to form an eschar of sufficient depth is sufficient. He further says :

Unquestionably the best method, as a general rule at least, of opening buboes is with caustic—in preference to the use of the knife—and we are therefore glad to find that Mr. Regnaud is in the habit of adopting it ; the only objection we make to his practice is as to the mode of effecting this purpose. When the abscess is once fairly open, and its surface and edges are in an unhealthy condition, few applications are so good as the tinct, benzoini comp. (Friar's Balsam), applied with lint; it is an admirable detergent to foul ulcers in general. Besides its stimulating and antiseptic properties, the balsam seems to act beneficially by totally excluding the admission of the air to the sore, in consequence of the varnished coating which it forms. When the ulcer is tolerably clean, but very tardy in healing, we have seen excellent effects from covering it daily with a layer of powdered rhubarb. As a matter of course, bark and other tonics are generally required to be administered internally at the same time.

Part x., *p.* 161.

Treatment of Secondary and Tertiary Syphilis.—M. Devergie, one of the physicians of the St. Louis Hospital, which receives a much larger number of syphilitic patients than any of the other hospitals in Paris—has met with great success in the treatment of the secondary and tertiary affections by adopting the following remedies. The patient is to drink every day about a quart of a sudorific ptisan, in which from five to twenty grains of the ioduret of potash have been dissolved, and also to take every morning, fasting, a pill composed of guiac, opium and a minute quantity of the corrosive sublimate. In the course of a week or so, a second pill is to be taken at night also. These medicines are to be persevered with for two or even three months, without intermission. A tepid bath is to be taken once a week. No wine is allowed; but milk is given freely instead. If the patient's constitution has been much damaged by irregularity or want, M. Devergie recommends the use of some ferruginous preparation, or of bark, or of both together; at the same time diminishing the dose of the sublimate, if the state of the symptoms should still require its continuance.

When, after six or seven weeks' use of these remedies, the local symptoms still exhibit an unhealthy character, the application of the crystallized acid nitrate of mercury—dissolved in water, to which a few drops of nitric acid have been added—will be found most convenient. The ointment of the proto-ioduret of mercury is also a valuable application, to promote the healing of certain ulcers. *Part* x., *p.* 172.

Treatment.—[With regard to the use of mercury, Mr. Carmichael says:]

Primary Ulcer.—1st. I do not think it necessary in the treatment of the simple primary ulcer without induration, nor for the papular eruption, and other constitutional symptoms it produces; but should the eruption linger into the fourth or fifth week after it has desquamated into scaly spots or blotches, mercury in alterative doses, either in the form of Plummer's pill or the proto-ioduret of mercury, will be of service in clearing the skin of the eruption, and in removing the pains of the joints, which are constantly present in this form of venereal. But I protest most strongly against the use of mercury at the period when the eruption first appears in its papular form, at a time that it is usually preceded and accompanied by considerable fever, like all the other exanthemata, to which class of Cullen it obviously belongs. If we should exhibit mercury prematurely during the eruptive stages of this as well as the other forms of disease, the scaly excepted, we may possibly clear the skin of the eruption, but in all probability it will return again to the great disappointment of the patient and perplexity of the medical attendant.

Iritis.—2d. For iritis I would give mercury, so as to excite its full

effect upon the system, and at the same time not neglect the usual antiphlogistic measures to remove this dangerous inflammation.

Nodes.—3d. For nodes I would exhibit mercury, and I think the
iodide of that mineral for their removal is superior to any other preparation.

Phagedemic Ulceration.—4th. For phagedenic primary ulcers I have
always found mercury most injurious.

Use of Nitric Acid.—They are most successfully treated by the application of strong nitric acid, immediately followed by a douche of cold water.
The same application is also the most efficient for phagedenic ulceration cf
the throat, which if not checked will soon extend over the velum, uvula, and
back of the pharynx, from whence it will spread upward into the nares,
and downward into the larynx. In either of which situations I need not
state the difficulty and danger of the case. Instead of the douche of cold
water, in this situation inadmissible, I employ a probang, the sponge
moistened in a solution of soda or potash will neutralize any superabundant acid applied to the ulcers.

Scaly Eruption.—During the eruption of pustules or tubercles which
cause those crusts termed rupia, I have found mercury injurious, although
its exhibition may at first flatter both patient and surgeon that the disease
is yielding to this remedy. But the natural tendency of this eruption is
also to become scaly after it has existed several weeks or months. This
scaliness is a sign that the disease is on the decline, and indicates that
mercury in alterative doses may then be employed with safety and
advantage. Should any of the constitutional ulcers on the skin spread
after the rupia crusts fall off, their progress may also be effectually checked
by the application of nitric acid to their phagedenic margins. They of
themselves first show signs of healthy reparation in their centres, which
need not therefore be meddled with. Mercury in this stage of the disease
should not be exhibited. Hydriodate of potash, sarsaparilla, country air,
and the tranquillizing effects of opium, should the patient be harassed by
extensive ulceration, are the constitutional means most to be relied upon.

Hunterian Chancre.—5th. For the true Hunterian chancre with
hardened edge and base, and for the scaly eruptions which attend it, as
well as the deep excavated ulcer of the tonsil, nodes, and other symptoms
belonging to this form of disease, mercury may be esteemed a certain and
expeditious remedy. *Part* xi., *p.* 174.

Infantile Syphilis.—[In the treatment of congenital syphilis, marked by
copper-colored blotches over various parts of the body, Dr. Bird has
found that two grains of hyd. cu. creta, continued for a fortnight or so. by
which time the eruption has usually faded very much, and then the administration of pot. iodid. gr. j. in ℥ij. sir. sarzæ, ter die, will soon effect a
cure. Dr. Bird remarks that syphilitic eruptions are exceedingly frequent
among the infants of the lower classes, and that the simple treatment just
mentioned is very effective in their cure. There are few affections among
children, the treatment of which is more satisfactory than that of syphilitic
eruptions; indeed they seem to fatten upon their medicine. If the mercury
cause diarrhœa, it is sufficient to suspend its use for a time. The diagnosis
of this disease is frequently mistaken, though of great importance, as while
it readily yields to proper treatment, it is extremely obstinate when mismanaged.]

There is seldom any real difficulty in the diagnosis of these cases when once the practitioner has learnt to recognize them. The characteristic *snuffling* will often enable him to recognize the existence of disease, even before he has confirmed his opinion by visual examination. The puckered mouth, the position of the very characteristic eruption round the lips and anus, in addition to the peculiar varnished and fissured appearance of the parts from which the scales have faded, will seldom if ever fail to convert a suspicion of the true nature of the disease into positive certainty. Condylomatous excrescences from the margin of the anus have never, in any of the cases, accompanied the earliest development of the syphilitic affection, but were always secondary, being observed in those children only whose primary affection was neglected or incompletely eradicated. When the eruption occurring on the nates and face in the first few weeks of life had been promptly treated, no condylomata appeared on the anal margin, at least so long as the children were kept in sight. But on the contrary, when the eruptions were neglected, condylomata were the almost certain results. I have not treated any case by the iodide of potassium alone, although this drug appeared to be of peculiar service after the mercury had produced a decided effect on the disease. *Part* xi., *p.* 175.

Mr. Acton employs the subjoined treatment:
Syphilitic Alopœcia.—Cut the hair close, and use warm baths; and then apply the following liniment: Equal parts of rectified spirit, eau de cologne, and castor oil; or equal parts of honey-water and tinct. cantharides. Should little red spots or blisters be produced, cease the application for a short time.

Lichen, Lepra, Psoriasis, Impetigo, etc.—Frequent warm baths, taking care to soak the head well; and cover the spots night and morning with olive oil, ℥ss. ; citrine oint., ℨj.; M. Make a liniment. Or use the following ointment: purified beef marrow, sixteen parts; sulphur ointment, sixteen parts; turpeth mineral, two to four parts; essence of lemons sufficient to scent it. (Ricord.)

Mucous Tubercles.—Use a dilute solution of chloride of sodium; dry the parts and sprinkle them over with calomel. Great cleanliness is necessary; do not use ointments.

Eczema Impetiginoides.—Cut the hair close, and apply water dressing, or lint dipped in an aqueous solution of opium; do not apply ointments. It should be a rule never to apply greasy substances to any eruption attended with oozing of fluid, since it mixes with the secretion, becomes rancid, forms a crust, the edges of which become excoriated, and what was an effect becomes a cause of irritation. Paint gummata and nodes with tinct. of iodine; it may also be applied to unhealthy tertiary ulcers.

Give internally, in secondary forms of syphilis, iodide of potassium or mercury: some prefer the former, as Dr. Williams, others the latter, as Sir B. Brodie. The following should be our guide in giving the iodide of mercury: Secondary symptoms occurring after a course of mercury, will be benefited by a course of iodide of potassium. Secondary symptoms occurring where mercury has not been used, will not yield to the iodide, but will to mercury. In order to prevent the iodide from causing pain at the pit of the stomach, or heat at the back of the throat soon after swallowing it, dissolve two drachms in three ounces of water, and let the patient take a teaspoonful of this solution night and morning in a large cup of tea, and the same quantity in half a pint of beer, or other fluid, at mid-day ; the dose to be continued and increased according to circumstances. It is of no use increasing the dose, or indeed of continuing this remedy beyond a week or ten days, if no amendment is visible. If mercury has not been given for the primary symptoms, begin with it immediately when secondary symptoms appear. Ricord gives the pure mineral, but the hydr. c. creta will answer best. If the organs of digestion be impaired, use friction ; direct the size of a horse bean of ung. hydr. to be smeared on the inside of each calf of the leg every night ; do not rub it in, as you irritate the hair bulbs by doing so, and you produce subsequent tenderness. Direct your patient to sleep in old drawers, so as to keep the bed clean. Do not use the ointment to the thighs, as is usually recommended ; it gets between the thigh and the scrotum, producing eczema ; it also dirties the patient's linen, and excites the attention of the washerwoman. Get the patient firmly under its influence before you discontinue the use of mer-cury.

Chancre.—Wash the part well with warm water, and then apply the solid nitrate of silver ; it will completely destroy the affection, if not more than of three days' standing. If it be a pustule, evacuate its contents, and the walls of the pustule are to be well cauterized. When there is a chancre of the frenum, it is more readily healed by dividing it, and caute-rizing the whole of the divided surface. To check discharge, apply a solution of pure tannin—two grs. to the ounce of water ; or sulphate of zinc solution, in private practice, as the former tells tales by staining the linen. The caustic should be reapplied as soon as the eschar is removed, or about once in twenty-four hours. If lint have been applied after the caustic, take care to soak it well before you remove it, or the eschar may be detached, and the part made to bleed. If the case be seen early, one or two burnings will suffice ; if at a more advanced period, it must be repeated at intervals of twenty-four hours—for a week or ten days, or as long as we consider any virus is secreted by the sore, which is known by the ulcers remaining stationary, and the surface being covered with a yellow pellicle ; when becoming healthy, granulations spring up and the sore heals. Caustic is not so efficacious when the chancre is situated on the frenum, orifice of the urethra, around the prepuce, or on the fourchette in the female—enjoin rest and strict attention to cleanliness, and avoid rupturing the cicatrix. *Part* xiii., *p.* 274.

Treatment of Secondary and Tertiary—Secondary form of Syphilis.—M. Ricord advises, to give the proto-iodide of mercury, and should it occasion irritation in the bowels with diarrhœa, combine it with opium. Let the diet be simple, avoiding all stimulants whether solid or fluid ; the diet, however, should not be debilitating but nutritious. Cold and damp air is very injurious ; fresh air is highly necessary.

Tertiary form of Syphilis.—The characteristic of these symptoms, is their not being transmissible hereditarily. They are manifested chiefly in the subcutaneous or submucous cellular tissue, in the fibrous, osseous, cartilaginous, muscular or nervous tissues, and organs in their locality. The remedy most to be depended upon is mercury. *Part* xiii., *p.* 280.

Repellent treatment of Buboes.—The method pursued by M. Malapert is to apply a blister the size of a crown for twenty-four hours, then raise the cuticle, and apply a pledget of lint of corresponding size, well saturated with a solution of bichloride of mercury (a scruple of the salt to one ounce of spt. vini rectif.); keep it in situ from two to four hours, and then apply cold applications for some hours; an eschar is formed, which will be thrown off, and the tumor will be dispersed. *Part* xiii., *p.* 283.

Chancre.—If seen within three days, says Mr. Acton, apply nitrate of silver freely, and secondary symptoms need not be feared, and even after this time, in nine cases out of ten, the same results will take place. There are some indications, however, against the use of caustic, and these are inflammation, or great irritation of the part; but, perhaps, the most important indication, against its use, is induration of the sore; the constitution is sure to be affected when this occurs, and mercury *must* be given.
Part xiv., *p.* 222.

Secondary Syphilis— Pains in the Long Bones, etc.—Mr. Ormerod directs us to give hydriodate of potash, five to eight, or to fifteen grains three times a day, and, if not successful in a few days, then mercury may be had recourse to. Where the secondary symptoms are scaly eruption, excavated ulcer of the tonsil, swelling of the testicle, excavated ulcer of the tongue, acute ulcers of the edges of the eyelids, iritis, purulent discharge of the meatus auditorius externus, papular eruption without fever, desquamating tubercular and pustular eruption, secondary ulcers, fissured tongue, ulceration round the nail, phagedenic ulcers of the skin, and foul sloughy ulcerations of the pharynx, they will be benefited by mercurial fumigations. *Part* xiv., *p.* 227.

Bromide of Potassium in Secondary Syphilis.—The low price of the bromide compared with that of the iodide of potassium, has induced M. Ricord to substitute that salt for the iodide in the treatment of secondary syphilitic affections. The dose of the bromide is the same as that of the iodide of potassium. It has produced the same therapeutical effects, but more slowly. *Part* xiv., *p.* 229.

Bubo.—Prof. Porter advises to open it as soon as matter can be detected, and by a very free incision, so as to prevent the lodgment of a drop of matter. *Part* xv., *p.* 236.

Treatment of Chancre.—Mr. Ormerod directs the use of the black wash to the sore, and when it is healed, and induration remains, rub on a little strong mercurial ointment, and keep constantly applied a piece of leather smeared with it.

Give in old cases small doses of hydr. c. creta, perseveringly, for a long time. If a quick action is desired give mercury by friction; but usually blue-pill is the best preparation. In phagedenic ulcers give calomel and opium so as rapidly to induce mercurial action, and when the phagedena is checked give a milder preparation. Some phagedenic sores, however, require depletion and purgatives: others wine and opium. To unhealthy and exhausted subjects give hydriodate of potash and sarsaparilla.
Part xv., *p.* 246

Secondary Syphilis—Treatment of at St. Bartholomew's Hospital— Papular Eruptions.—Treat antiphlogistically at first, then give mild mercurials, with tonics and the warm bath.

Scaly.—Give mercury, or, when slight, iodine will do.

Tubercular.—Iodine is the best remedy.

Pustular.— Give mercury cautiously, and apply yellow wash to the ulcers into which the pustules degenerate: if, however, these are large and shallow, give iodine: or if round and excavated, give opium with iodine, and nutritious diet, and apply black wash.

Ulceration of the Throat.—Give mild mercurials; or, if sloughy, iodine with wine and good diet. Use cinnabar fumigations, especially to the excavated ulcer, but with caution.

Ulceration of the Larynx, Tongue. etc.—Give mercury or iodine, or both, according to the accompanying symptoms.

Pains in the Bones.—Iodine is the best remedy; but in some cases require mercury, others incisions.

Nodes.—Give iodine; if recent and soft, apply mercurial ointment on a piece of leather.   *Part* xv., *p.* 247.

Treatment of Syphilis.—[Mr. Christophers has been in the habit of recording his experience of syphilitic cases for some years; and he has been able to observe a considerable number of cases for years after their treatment. He has come to the conclusion that syphilis, in the present day, is a disease which, even without treatment, produces few symptoms of severity; and which, itself tending to its own cure, is very amenable to rational treatment. In a case of real chancre, unless destroyed by excision or caustic before the fourth day, secondary symptoms will certainly supervene, whether the treatment have been "mercurial," or "simple:" and the severity of the secondary symptoms is in proportion, not to the number nor to the severity of the primary sores, but to their duration. If this be true, the best treatment is that by which the primary sore is most rapidly healed. Mr. Christophers says respecting treatment :]

It has been observed that some sores are very slow to heal under simple treatment, but that immediately the system is brought (though ever so slightly) under the influence of mercury, they rapidly progress toward a cure. Now here I believe the advantageous use of mercury stops; pushed beyond this, it becomes a positive evil.

I have treated cases of syphilis on a plan differing from both the mercurial and simple systems, and in every case it has succeeded well. Having first convinced myself, by the aid of inoculation (I am speaking of cases in which the sore has existed beyond the period assigned it as a local disease,) that it is a genuine chancre I have to treat, I prescribe calomel, in one or two grain doses, till the gums give the slightest evidence of its effect. This accomplished, I suspend it at once, and begin with small doses of the hydriodate of potass, with sarsaparilla; and it is a curious fact, that if the gums are made slightly sore with mercury, that action will be maintained in them by very small doses of the hydriodate, though it does not produce that effect generally, if mercury have not been given. The object in giving the mercury is speedily to heal the primary sore; the object of the iodine and sarsaparilla, to put the system in the most favorable condition to encounter the secondary affection that must (in some shape) inevitably ensue.   *Part* xvi., *p.* 213.

Comparative effects of Bromide and Iodide of Potassium in the treatment of Secondary Syphilis.—Some time ago, Dr. Egan's attention was directed to preparations of bromine as a substitute for those of iodine, which had attained a very high price. His experiments led him to the conclusion that the bromide of potassium is comparatively inert.

To detect the Adulteration of the Iodide with the Bromide of Potas-

sium.—Take of the suspected salt one drachm, dissolve in two ounces of distilled water, of sulphate of copper two drachms, dissolved in the same quantity of distilled water, mix, and put both into a clean oil flask, and boil till the vapor from the flask will not produce any effect upon a piece of paper, to whose surface a solution of starch has been applied, the fluid remaining in the flask, if impure, will immediately, on the addition of a few drops of a solution of chloride of lime, give the usual orange color of bromine which will be rendered more apparent by the addition of a little starch. Bromide of potassium is not precipitated by sulphate of copper, in which it differs from the iodide. *Part* xvi., *p.* 214.

Urethral Chancre.—When secondary symptoms appear to follow blennorrhagia, this virulent blennorrhagia as it is called, is the result of a urethral chancre; this M. Ricord has proved by observation both on the living and the dead.

During the first few days, employ the abortive treatment. The patient having passed water, M. Ricord injects into the urethra a little of a solution of nitrate of silver, fifteen grains to the ounce, from a glass syringe; the only precautions needed are to press the lips of the meatus so as to bring them in close contact with the pipe of the syringe, and to make the injection pass suddenly, so as to take the urethra by surprise. Repeat the injection at the end of two days; but if the first application does not cause pain and sero-sanguineous discharge, followed by creamy suppuration, repeat it on the same day. At the same time give copaiba and cubebs.

Part xvii., *p.* 183.

Treatment of Chancre.—M. Sisovics, chief surgeon to the general hospital of Vienna, directs at first, to use local emollients and baths; and when the syphilitic character of the ulcer is manifest, give diaphoretic drinks of decoction of sarsaparilla, or guaiacum, and then give the preparations of iodine, and use them externally in the form of local baths and fomentations. *Part* xvii., *p.* 186.

Treatment of Venereal Disease Generally.—[At the end of this course of lectures on venereal disease, published in the " Lancet," M. Ricord gives the following recapitulation of the doctrine he inculcates :]

The great class of venereal diseases comprises two very distinct orders—first, the non-virulent diseases, the type of which is blennorrhagia; the second, the virulent diseases, the type of which is chancre.

First Order.—The blennorrhagic affections do not taint the constitution, are not transmissible by hereditary, and never yield any positive results by inoculation either on the skin or mucous membranes : they are contagious in the manner of irritants, the simple catarrho-phlegmonous discharge being the most common form.

Second Order.—The *virulent* affections owe their origin to a peculiar principle, to an ulceration which can be reproduced at will, and inoculable within a certain period. The ulceration always springs up at the very spot where the virulent matter has been implanted, and its evolution takes place in a variable space of time. The virulent effect may remain strictly local, and merely give rise to consecutive phenomena, of which the most common is the suppuration of the inguinal glands; but it may penetrate into the economy, and determine in the same a set of characteristic symptoms. The general infection of the system is the result of an idiosyncrasy which does not invariably exist in every individual. The most tangible phenomenon of this infection is the specific induration of the chancre. There is no such thing as a specifically indurated chancre, without subsequent symptoms of constitutional syphilis. Once or twice in a hundred cases the induration may be ill-defined, and pass unnoticed ; but if the attention be directed to the inguinal glands (which inevitably suffer by the infection), the existence of an indurated chancre may, by their state, be inferred ; for a bubo, consecutive to such a chancre, *never* suppurates specifically. There is no constitutional syphilis without a primary local accident. When the infection has taken place, we may look for the secondary manifestations within a twelvemonth. But if a mercurial treatment be used, these manifestations may be prevented or retarded for more or less time, or perhaps forever. When no treatment, however, has intervened, there is an admirable order in the succession of the manifestations, which is denied only by those people who will not be convinced. Primary, consecutive, secondary, transitory, and tertiary accidents follow each other with the most perfect regularity. But I repeat it—a treatment breaks up the order altogether. If a mercurial course has been gone through, the secondary manifestations may, under its influence, be retarded for a variable time ; but it does not destroy the diathesis, and merely postpones the secondary symptoms. On the other hand, you will remember that the mercurial treatment does not prevent tertiary accidents, and these may even appear whilst the secondary symptoms are being kept off by mercury ; the latter may then make their appearance *after* the tertiary accidents have disappeared, and thus the order of the manifestations may be totally inverted. Constitutional syphilis can be contracted but *once*—the diathesis can never be doubled. The diathesis persists, but the manifestations are not certain or inevitable. This diathesis is not incompatible with health. Syphilitic cachexia is very rare. The non-virulent affections require no specific medication, neither do the virulent primary accidents ; mercury is used for the latter only in exceptional cases ; namely, where the chancre is indurated.

Constitutional syphilis demands a mercurial treatment ; but when the later secondary symptoms and the tertiary have come on, mercury should be abandoned, and iodide of potassium be taken up. The latter is then the medication *par excellence*. Whenever we have to treat any peculiar disorder or affection of the viscera, along with syphilis, we should never lose sight of the indications which belong to that intercurrent disease, and should even delay the specific medication, if found necessary.

[Dr. de Meric, the reporter of these lectures, subjoins the following list of formulæ used by M. Ricord at the Hospital du Midi :]

Non-Virulent Diseases.—1. *Injection for Balano-posthitis.*—Make three injections a day between the glans and prepuce with the following fluid : distilled water, three ounces ; nitrate of silver, two scruples.

2. *Abortive Treatment of Blennorrhagia.*—Make one injection only with the following liquid : distilled water, one ounce ; nitrate of silver, fifteen grains. And take every day, in three doses, the following powder : cubebs, one ounce ; alum, thirty grains.

3. *Injection for Blennorrhagia when the period for the Abortive Treatment is passed.*—Make three injections daily with the following liquid : rose water, six ounces and a half; sulphate of zinc, and acetate of lead, of each, fifteen grains.

4. *Internal Treatment of Blennorrhagia.*—Take one tablespoonful of

the following emulsion three times a day : copaiba, sirup of tolu, and sirup of poppies, of each, one ounce ; peppermint water, two ounces ; gum arabic, a sufficient quantity ; orange flower water, two drachms.

5. *Acute stage of Blennorrhagia.*—Twenty leeches to the perineum ; bath after the leeches ; refreshing drinks ; rest in bed ; low diet ; suspensory bandage. Take one of the following pills four times a day ; expressed and inspissated juice of lettuce (lactuca sativa) and camphor, of each, forty-five grains : make twenty pills.

6. *Gleet.*—Make every day three injections with the following liquid : rose water, and Roussillon wine, of each, six ounces ; alum and tannin, of each, ten grains.

7. *Subacute Epididymitis.*—Rub the testis twice a day with the following ointment: stronger mercurial ointment, and extract of belladonna, equal parts of each ; a poultice to the part after the ointment, and rest.

8. *Acute Epididymitis.*—Fifteen leeches to the perineum, and the same number in the groin corresponding to the affected epididymis ; bath after the leeches ; barley-water for common drink ; low diet, rest, and poultice.

9. *Chronic Epididymitis.*—Apply Vigo's plaster to the testes, and wear a suspensory bandage. (Simple plaster, yellow wax, pitch, ammoniacum, bdellium, olibanum, mercury, turpentine, liquid styrax, and volatile oil of lavender, are the component parts of Vigo's plaster.)

Virulent Diseases—Primary Symptoms.—10. *Abortive Treatment of Chancre.*—Within the first five days of the contagion, destroy the chancre with potassa fusa cum calce (pâte de Vienne.)

11. *Regular non-indurated Chancre.*—Frequent dressing with the aromatic wine, extreme cleanliness, occasional light cauterization with the nitrate of silver. Rest, demulcent drinks ; when there is inflammation, antiphlogistics, purgatives, and emollient applications. (N.B.—No mercury.)

12. *Phagedenic Chancre.*—Complete cauterization with the nitrate of silver, the liquid nitrate of mercury, the potassa cum calce, or the hot iron, according to circumstances. Afterward lotions with aromatic wine, three ounces ; extract of opium, three grains ; or, aromatic wine, eight ounces ; tannin, thirty grains ; or, distilled water, three ounces ; tartrate of iron and potash, four drachms ; or, in the scrofulous diathesis, distilled water, three ounces ; tincture of iodine, one drachm ; or, sulphur ointments, and sulphureous baths. Internally : tartrate of iron and potash, one ounce ; distilled water, eight ounces. One ounce three times a day.

13. *Indurated Chancre.*—Three dressings a day with the following ointment : calomel, one drachm ; axunge, one ounce. (N.B.—Mercury is used internally for the *indurated* chancre : as to the mode of administration, see secondary syphilis, No. 21, as the metal is given in the same manner in both cases.)

14. *Acute, non-Specific Adenitis, vel Inflamed Bubo.*—Twenty leeches on the tumor, emollient cataplasms, barley-water as ordinary drink, rest, broths. If fluctuation be detected, let out the purulent matter by a free incision.

15. *Abortive Treatment of the Bubo consecutive, by absorption of the Virus, to the Non-indurated Chancre.*—Deep cauterization of ten minutes' duration, with the potassa fusa cum calce, and await the fall of the eschar. (N.B.—Analogous to the early destruction of chancre.)

16. *Bubo consecutive to the Non-indurated Chancre, which inevitably Suppurates.*—Use antiphlogistics according to circumstances, and then free the purulent matter by cauterization with potassa fusa ; gradually destroy afterward, by the use of caustics, the glandular mass which lies at the bottom of the open bubo. To the poultices used after cauterization may be added an ointment, of equal parts of extract of belladonna and mercurial ointment.

17. *Horse-shoe Bubo and Gangrene.*—Horse-shoe and phagedenic ulcers in the groin, resulting from a suppurating bubo, require the dressing mentioned in No. 12. Gangrene : chloride of lime, one ounce ; distilled water, three ounces. This lotion is to be used several times a day. Or, powdered charcoal, powdered Peruvian bark, equal parts of each, to be thickly applied to the sore.

18. *Phimosis.*—Inject between the glans and prepuce the aromatic wine with opium, as mentioned in No. 12, and use emollient and sedative applications ; if gangrene be imminent, operate.

19. *Paraphimosis.*—Keep the organ raised, and surround it with cold compresses. Bland diet, refreshing drinks ; endeavor to reduce or free the constriction by an incision, according to circumstances. After the strangulation is relieved, use emollient and antiseptic applications combined with opium.

20. *Scrofulous Complications.*—Order every day the following emulsion in three equal doses : iodine, three grains ; oil of sweet almonds, one ounce ; gum arabic, a sufficiency ; almond emulsion, three ounces.

21. *Secondary Symptoms.*—Order every day three tumblers of decoction of saponaria leaves, and put into each tumbler one tablespoonful of sirop de cuisinier (N.B. Sirop de cuisinier : sarsaparilla, borage and white rose leaves, senna, aniseed, honey, and sugar ;) and take every day one of the following pills : proto-iodide of mercury, inspissated juice of lactuca sativa, of each, forty-five grains ; extract of opium, fifteen grains ; extract of hemlock, one drachm and a half. Mix, and make sixty pills.

22. *Slight Stomatitis.*—To gargle three times a day with the following liquid : decoction of lactuca sativa, five ounces ; honey, one ounce and a half ; alum, one drachm and a half.

23. *Mercurial Stomatitis.*—To gargle three times a day with the following liquid : decoction of lactuca satita, five ounces ; honey, four drachms ; hydrochloric acid, fifteen drops.

24. *Salivation.*—Order every day one drachm of flowers of sulphur incorporated with honey. As a common beverage, the nitric acid lemonade. Gargle three times a day with decoction of lactuca sativa, five ounces ; honey, four drachms ; hydrochloric acid, fifteen drops.

25. *Mucous Patches in the Mouth.*—Gargle three times a day with decoction of hemlock, six ounces and a half ; bichloride of mercury, three grains.

26. *Mucous Tubercles around the Anus (Condylomata.)*—Put twenty leeches to the perineum. Take every evening a small enema of a decoction of poppyheads, cold, and mixed with twenty drops of laudanum. As a habitual beverage, take linseed tea, sweetened with sugar and almond emulsion.

27. *Vegetations.*—Put twice a day on the vegetations the following powder : powdered savine, oxide of iron, calcined alum, of each one drachm. *Part* xviii., *p.* 205.

Treatment of Tertiary Symptoms.—[Tertiary symptoms, M. Ricord observes, will not inevitably occur in the course of syphilis, but they are very likely to do so if the treatment of the primary and secondary symptoms be not conducted with the greatest care. As soon as ever the tertiary period has set in, mercury must be abandoned, and iodide of potassium given. Nay, further, as mercury, taken in time, may prevent or retard secondary symptoms, and so may be regarded as a prophylactic against them, so may iodide of potassium be regarded as a prophylactic against tertiary symptoms; and therefore M. Ricord observes:]

To render the treatment of secondary syphilis complete and rational, it should always be followed by the exhibition of iodide of potassium. This substance is, however, not only useless, when employed against secondary symptoms and those of transition, but very often hurtful; yet, when secondaries have been of long standing, it may produce beneficial effects; it is also useful as an adjuvant of mercury, in those affections which in some degree lie between the secondary and strictly tertiary manifestations; and, finally, it is indispensable for combating the symptoms of a decided tertiary nature. In order to become well acquainted with the proper manner of administering the iodide of potassium, we should take the trouble of studying its effects, independently of its curative action. First let us see how it acts on the skin. It may produce on the cutaneous surface diverse psydracious and acnoid eruptions. The pustules are generally surrounded by a vividly red areola, and the usual seat of these eruptions is *below* the umbilical region, as the nates, thighs, etc., whereas the common acne (not to mention its other characters) is mostly situated in the upper half of the body. To these peculiarities, it may be added, that the pustules will fall in immediately the administration of the iodide is interrupted. Exanthemata, impetigo, and lichen, are very apt to be produced by the use of this salt; and what you ought especially to keep in mind is, that ecchymosis, and purpura in the inferior extremities, are sometimes caused by the action of the iodide of potassium. The effects of the latter on mucous membranes should also be carefully observed. It may cause inflammation of the conjunctiva, the sub-mucous cellular tissue lying under which gets then infiltrated and puffed up; the eyelids turn red and œdematous, and when the inflammation and effusion are not arrested, the internal parts of the eye become involved in the affection, and photophobia is the result of this state of things. The normal mucous secretion is always a little increased, but it does not take the muco-purulent character, as in the case of catarrhal ophthalmia. Coryza, of a more or less severe nature, often exists at the same time: it is preceded and accompanied by headache, and a pretty abundant mucous secretion; but this coryza never reaches the suppurative state; it never produces more than a catarrho-serous flux. These affections never give rise to any fever, and they disappear as soon as the iodide is given up. This coryza is an accident which we should not overlook, for it is of importance to avoid it when we have to treat a tertiary affection of the nasal fossæ. As for the effect of the iodide on the intestinal canal, I have to state that persons enjoying good health can bear very large doses of it; I have given as much as fifteen drachms a day. M. Puche has often given ten drachms per diem, after commencing with six; and it has been noticed that it improves the appetite of the persons who use it. With some patients a certain pleurodynic sensation, corresponding to the cardiac extremity of the stomach, is felt after its ingestion, but it never causes vomiting. The sub-mucous cellular tissue of the stomach may, by the use of this iodide, undergo the same modifications which we have noticed the conjunctiva to be subject to—a sort of hyper-secretion and intestinal ptyalism takes place, and much of the fluid which ought to have been secreted by the skin is rejected by the mouth. This liquid has a slight taste of iodine; it is not fetid in the least : the gums are not swollen, and there is no fetor in the breath, as happens in mercurial ptyalism. The same effect may be produced on the other portions of the intestinal canal; the patients are then seized with abundant serous diarrhœa. The iodine is eliminated from the system by the kidneys; half an hour after the ingestion of it, its presence may be ascertained in the urine, and it should be remembered, that the presence of iodine in the blood increases the renal secretion. I have even observed a case of polydipsia which went on as long as the iodide was used, but disappeared when the latter was discontinued, and gradually sprang up again as the use of the salt was resumed.

The effects of the iodide of potassium on the circulation are of a sedative kind; it diminishes the number of arterial pulsations and lowers their force, but they may regain their normal standard if the remedy act beneficially on the system; the same arterial energy may also reappear when the iodide causes a slight phlegmasia. This salt is somewhat antiplastic, for it has rather a tendency to liquefy the blood, and may even produce the peculiar hemorrhages of purpura. When the effect of the iodide on the nervous system is carefully watched, it is found to cause a certain excitement of the nervous centres, followed by a little uncertainty in the movements and in the intelligence.

Doses and Forms.—If the efficacy of the iodide of potassium has ever been doubted, it is because no one would venture to give it in doses sufficiently large to test it fairly. Most practitioners confined themselves to three or four grains a day—no wonder that no effects were produced. The daily dose ought to be fifteen grains to begin with; two or three days afterward, forty-five grains may be given every day in three distinct doses. If the remedy has no pathogenic effect we must be guided by the therapeutic action, so that if the curative effect be not apparent at all in three or four days, the dose should be augmented. The influence produced on the osteoscopes may very well serve as a criterion of the action of the remedy, provided these osseous pains do not arise from suppuration, and they be strictly a result of the diathesis. I have had patients in whom the removal of these pains required as much as one drachm and a half, two drachms, and even three drachms per diem.

Forms.—The iodide of potassium has been given in capsules, in solution, in sirup, etc.; rarely in the form of pill, for this salt is very deliquescent; I generally give it in sirup, and I have found bitters to be the best adjuvants—viz., sirup of gentian, of saponaria, of quassia, *de cuisinier*, of sarsaparilla, etc. One pint of sirup is to be used for one ounce of the iodide, which will give about twelve grains to the spoonful; the same quantity may also be given in the sweetened mistura acaciæ, or in the sirup of poppies, or of lactucarium. As to the diet, it ought to be of a tonic and regenerating nature—chops, steaks, wine, porter, etc. You see, therefore, that we know pretty well what ought to be the daily dose of the iodide, but we are not so well informed as regards the absolute quantity which can be given with safety; it is impossible to fix this beforehand. Neither do we know exactly how much time this medication may be continued in order to free the patient from the possibility of a relapse.

You must be careful to modify the treatment just described, according to certain peculiar manifestations. For instance, when you have to contend against syphilitic sarcocele, and the same is exempt from complications, it will be sufficient to use the general treatment.

But when there is much inflammation, you must have recourse to antiphlogistics and emollient applications; and if it were noticed that the testicle is suffering both from syphilis and struma, anti-scrofulous remedies should be added to the usual treatment of such cases. The plastic effusion will be efficiently controlled by rubbing the part with the mercurial ointment, and covering the whole with a soothing cataplasm; and much benefit will likewise be derived in these cases by the methodical compression with strips of plaster, which was spoken of when I considered epididymitis. If you have elastic tumors of the testis to treat, the best practice is to open them as soon as fluctuation is detected, and you should have recourse to sedative applications when you perceive that they are surrounded by an inflammatory areola. But when the ulceration presents no redness, nor any symptoms of irritation, a very good wash may be made with a solution of iodine in the proportion of one half or a whole drachm to 12 ounces of distilled water; and when this solution is being prepared, a certain quantity of iodide of potassium should be added, to prevent the precipitation of the iodine. If the granulations of the tertiary ulcerations are too prominent, they should be destroyed with the pâte de Vienne, or any other caustic.

When elastic tumors are not situated in the scrotum or testicle, they may be attacked by very energetic means—viz., mercurial frictions, Vigo's plaster, blisters followed by irritative dressings, as advised by Malapert, etc.; and where suppuration has occurred, the matter should be freed without delay. As for the elastic tumors situated on the mucous membrane of the nasal fossæ or mouth, they may be very beneficially acted upon by lotions containing a solution of iodine, in the proportion of two to six parts of this substance to one hundred of distilled water; in fact, the proportion of the iodine may be increased as long as no pain is produced by the application.

The muscular retraction, or plastic degeneration of the muscles, requires local applications besides the internal remedies. Topically, I use circular compression, carefully applied with strips of Vigo's plaster.

Part xviii., *p.* 206.

Proto-Sulphate of Iron in Chancre and Gonorrhœa.—[An anonymous correspondent of the "Lancet" says:]

The whole class of caustic agents, when applied to the Hunterian chancre (though the potassa fusa cum calce be used till the ulcer be "punched out," as recommended by M. Ricord) form an eschar with pus still secreting; in fact, the morbid cells have not been destroyed. The alkaloids and hydrocarbons are equally inefficacious.

If a chancre be perfectly freed from its eschar and the inclosed pus, at the bottom of the excavation may be observed minute white points or germs, secreting, slowly, the morbid virus. If, now, the proto-sulphate of iron, minutely pulverized, be dropped into this excavation, the parts will instantly assume a charred appearance, the metal is absorbed into the tissue, the morbid cells or germs will instantly cease to secrete pus, the cleared cavity will shortly granulate, and a smooth surface, without induration, will be the result of the use of the proto-sulphate of iron. The chancre is destroyed.

The proto-sulphate of iron, I have observed to be the most powerful agent for arresting decomposition in animal and vegetable substances. Inflammation and decomposition in the living tissue is likewise arrested by it.

In gonorrhœa, we have now an agent arresting the morbid cellular action in the salts which should be used in solution super-saturated.

In leucorrhœa, and in simple ulcers, the morbid action is arrested or peroxidized by this metallic salt.

Large doses of this salt have been exhibited in obstinate diarrhœa, with great benefit. *Part* xix., *p.* 186.

Creeping Bubo.—[Mr. Solly observes that there is a form of venereal affection which has not received an exact name from systematic writers, and which he designates " creeping bubo." It is that intractable sore which arises when chronic syphilitic bubo proceeds to ulceration, unstayed by mercury. Mr. Solly says:]

Its most striking feature is the manner in which it burrows under the skin, creeping onward from place to place. This creeping character has induced me, for some time past, to designate it in my clinical observations, as *creeping bubo*. It often creeps upward on the abdominal parietes, as high as the umbilicus; down the thigh, as low as the knee; round the thigh, to the anus; and over the buttock, nearly to the spinous process of the ilium.

The formidable nature of this ulcer is best seen in those cases where no mercury has been administered; for, in these, there is scarcely any attempt at the healing process. Some years ago, I had an opportunity of witnessing several cases of this kind occurring about the same time. Their extreme obstinacy astonished me. I saw every local application in the Pharmacopœia tried, but in vain. Mercury was not made use of and they continued to extend. One case sank under the disease, apparently exhausted by its depressing effects.

The appearance which creeping bubo exhibits in its *early* stage, presents some peculiarities by which it may be distinguished. The surface of creeping bubo is of a yellowish color, the discharge is thin and ichorous, the edges are everted, overlapping, corrugated, in dotted points, white, hard, and very irregular. In its early stage it is most like the strumous or scrofulous bubo, with its overlapping edges; but it differs, inasmuch as the edges of the strumous bubo are inverted, not everted, and soft, not hard and corrugated. The distinguishing marks, however, are not so easily described by the pen as by the pencil.

In this form of bubo, a mercurial treatment is almost invariably required. We must give mercury steadily, until it disagrees with the system; then abstain from it, and give tonics; and after waiting a few weeks, or even months, again return to the use of the mercurial preparations.

Part xix., *p.* 195.

Bransby B. Cooper's Treatment of Chancre—Simple.—When called to see a venereal sore, of only three or four days' duration, apply concentrated nitric acid. But if a sore has all the appearances of true chancre, begin by using constitutional treatment—giving five grains of blue pill and a quarter of a grain of opium night and morning. So long as the patient is taking mercury, apply no local remedy whatever, and then the sore will furnish, by its appearance, the best possible indication of the effect which the medicine is producing.

Irritable.—Apply nitrate of silver to the sore, and give repeated doses of opium. If when the irritability is subdued, induration remains, give mercury, as in a simple case. In some instances of irritable chancre, calomel and opium will answer as well or better than opium alone.

Phagedenic.—First evacuate the bowels, and then give repeated doses of opium, and apply soothing fomentations. If the vital powers are depressed, give bark, ammonia, and even wine ; but if there is a plethoric condition, adopt antiphlogistic measures. If the progress of the ulceration is not checked, apply concentrated nitric acid.

Gangrenous.—Keep the patient in the recumbent posture, and after evacuating the bowels, give ammonia, bark, or serpentaria, with wine or porter ; and apply black wash, nitric acid lotion, stale beer grounds, or stimulating poultices.

When the healing of chancres on the penis is interfered with by the occurrence of erections, give five or ten grains of lupulin at bedtime, and repeat it if necessary.   *Part* xxi., *p.* 269.

Diagnosis and Treatment of Bubo.—[Mr. Cooper lays especial stress upon the importance of distinguishing between a bubo arising from a virulent and one from a non-virulent disease. He says :]

Non-virulent bubo is that which attends simple gonorrhœa, and may be considered as arising from common inflammatory action, extending in the course of the absorbent vessels of the penis to the glands of the groin ; this disorder is to be treated as phlegmonous swellings in other parts of the body, either by repellents for the purpose of preventing the formation of matter, or by fomentations or poultices to produce suppuration, when that termination seems to be threatened by nature.

By repellent remedies, I mean those which have a tendency to repress the formation of matter, such as leeches and evaporating lotions ; by means of these we may succeed in preventing suppuration, but there sometimes yet remains a permanent indurated condition of the swelling, which may excite apprehension in the mind of the surgeon as to its having been produced by a specific virus, a chancre existing within the urethra. A bubo of this kind may, however, result from a mere strumous habit ; and if so, the hardness readily yields to the exhibition of iodine and iodide of potassium, and such dietetic rules as generally improve strumous constitutions ; while, on the contrary, if the hardness depends upon the action of a specific poison, a mercurial course is, in my opinion, the only safe mode of treatment.

A *virulent bubo* is marked by the same characteristic induration as a chancre itself, and the presence of this induration must inevitably give rise to the question of the virulent or non-virulent nature of the disease. The mere phlegmonous bubo has always a tendency to suppurate ; while the virulent bubo, on the contrary, seldom manifests this disposition ; and, therefore, its permanent hardness, uncombined with any symptom of suppuration, is a further proof of a virus having been the origin of a bubo.

The virulent bubo goes on to ulceration; but even this is not conclusive, for strumous ulceration not unfrequently occurs in persons of a scrofulous diathesis; therefore, as Ricord observes, there is as much difficulty in forming a diagnosis between the virulent and non-virulent bubo as between the virulent and non-virulent sore. In my own practice when the bubo puts on all the characters of a virulent or specific action, I commence at once with the cautious administration of mercury, not unfrequently combining with it small doses of iodide of potassium, abstaining at the same time from the use of any local application to the ulcerated bubo, which might tend to conceal the characteristic appearance of the sore. If the mercury be producing the desired effect, the ulcerated surface of the swelling acquires a healthy appearance, indicated by the growth of soft, red granulations, by the absence of any tendency to eversion of the edges of the sore, and by a general softness of the whole base of the tumor; indeed, the characteristics of the healing sore are as strongly marked as were the peculiarities which had before indicated its virulence. And until the induration has completely disappeared, the mercury should be perseveringly continued. *Part* xxi., *p.* 269.

Venereal Warts and Condylomata.—In long standing cases of gonorrhœa you will sometimes observe condylomatous growths about the scrotum, perineum, and verge of the anus; these, Bransby B. Cooper states, can generally be cured by an application of the yellow wash. Warts often follow also upon a gonorrhœa, in cases where the disease commences externally—that is to say, in balanitis. In the first instance they are found in points where the mucous membrane has been abraded; warty granulations spring up from these points. Whenever these warts are present with phimosis, the prepuce must be laid open immediately; this is always necessary. Sometimes these warts are very difficult to cure. When they have narrow peduncular necks, a ligature may be used to remove them; in other cases caustic should be applied to them, and savine powder may also be employed as an escharotic. Sometimes, however, neither caustic nor savine powder will remove these warty excrescences; they must then be excised, and caustic applied to the surface from which they are removed. *Part* xxi., *p.* 270.

Treatment of Secondary Constitutional Syphilis.—Surround the patient with an atmosphere of mercurial vapor, in a moist state, by the following method, recommended by Langston Parker: Place the patient on a chair, covering him with oil-cloth lined with flannel, then fumigate him with the bisulphuret of mercury, or the grey oxide, or binoxide. The patient may remain in this mercurial atmosphere for ten minutes or half an hour. Let the patient then repose in an arm chair for a short time, and let him drink a cup of warm decoction of guaiacum, sweetened with sirup of sarsaparilla. *Part* xxii., *p.* 261.

Phagedenic Chancre.—Iron is the remedy, its effects are almost magical. It is much used by M. Ricord. The following is the best mode of giving it. Potassio-tartrate of iron, one ounce; water, six ounces. Mix. Two tablespoonfuls three times a day.

* * * * * * * *

Tertiary Symptoms.—Give the iodide of potash in *large doses*, which will benefit when small ones are of no avail. *Part* xxii., *p.* 262.

Treatment of Syphilis.—[Speaking of the definition of the stages of this disease, Mr. Cooper remarks :]

If I might be allowed to express my own opinion on the subject, I would give the following definition of the three stages or forms of syphilis : Primary symptoms—the chancre or local affection; secondary syphilis—the sore throat and the various cutaneous eruptions; and tertiary—the ulcers and sores which succeed the eruptions, and which, like them, are the result of the constitutional manifestation of the disease.

The diagnosis of a primary syphilitic sore or chancre is sometimes exceedingly difficult; in fact, taking the physical characters of the ulcer alone, it is frequently impossible to distinguish it from one of a non-specific nature, frequently out of the surgeon's power to say with decision and confidence this is venereal, or that is not. There is but one true poison of syphilis, which poison produces different effects, depending on the nature of the tissue affected, and on the peculiarity of the constitution; and I believe, that all the different effects, and all the varieties of sores, depend on one and the same morbific cause, the action of which is modified by the particular state or disposition of the individual in which the symptoms are developed.

With regard to the treatment of primary symptoms we possess, happily, a remedial agent—mercury, which might be considered to have almost a specific influence over the disease, and I believe that syphilis cannot be thoroughly eradicated from the system by any other medicine, after absorption has taken place and it has become a constitutional affection. If, however, you have a patient come to you within four days after the appearance of a chancre—that is, before the syphilitic poison has had time to become absorbed, and implanted in the system, no matter if the sore be of the callous or true Hunterian description, or however ambiguous its characters, by the application of concentrated nitric acid you would effectually decompose or destroy, and render inert the specific poison.

The healing of a chancre, by the application of local means, is no proof of the constitutional subsidence of the disease. I therefore depend solely on the constitutional employment of mercury, and object to the use of black wash and similar applications, which are in themselves capable of removing the sore, and thus destroy the index which its appearance forms when its reparation is effected, only as a result of the constitutional eradication of the disease. The healing of the sore under these indications is an evidence that the system has been sufficiently mercurialized; and that its use may now be confidently abandoned. Acting under this principle and conviction, the plan I in almost all cases pursue, is to apply a simple piece of moist linen—not lint, for I have seen it (whether from the chlorine used in bleaching it, or what I do not know) excite such irritation round a chancre, as almost to produce balanitis, which all quickly subsided on the use of linen instead of lint to the sore, and administer internally gr. v. of blue pill with 1-4 gr. opium at bedtime, and v. gr. of blue pill alone in the morning; directing these pills to be made up separately, and labelled respectively "night" and "morning" pills. I tell the patient, if his bowels become constipated, to take only the morning pills both night and morning; if, on the contrary, relaxed, to take only the night pills. With this variation in treatment, according to the circumstances of the case, I continue the mercury until the sore has disappeared, and the hardness of its base subsided. I learned this treatment from my uncle, Sir Astley Cooper, and have adopted it in almost every case that has come before me during the last thirty years; and I have never yet once got into a difficulty with it, from the reappearance of the disease under secondary symptoms. Trust to mercury, but give it cautiously, give it judiciously, watching your patient during its administration, and seeing that he avoid all possible exposure to cold, and if possible keep him within doors.

Secondary symptoms are manifested in various morbid phenomena of different parts, more especially of the skin, mucous membranes, and bones. Affections of the latter, I believe, are not the result of syphilis alone, as a specific disease, but of its action, modified by the influence of mercury, which, as far as I can learn, in such cases, has always been previously administered; and I consider syphilis of itself, I will not go so far as to say incapable, but certainly not as yet proved to have the power of producing such direful morbid conditions of the osseous system.

With regard to the treatment of secondary syphilis, the iodide of potassium is the remedy held in most repute, and the one that in general produces the most immediate beneficial and successful results. But, according to my experience, iodide of potassium and iodine, although they have the power of arresting or suspending the disease *pro tem.*, are incapable of eradicating or eliminating it *in toto* from the system, and securing the individual from subsequent attacks. Sir Astley used almost invariably to prescribe the bichloride of mercury, in doses of 1-16 gr., taken in bark or sarsaparilla, two or three times a day; and I myself prefer and recommend mercury to be given. It is true, its remedial effects are not so speedy as those of iodide of potassium; but this is more than compensated for by their being of a more permanent character. Cases sometimes occur where iodide of potassium has been administered for some time, and the further continuance of its use increases instead of diminishes the symptoms it was intended to relieve. In such instances, I have sometimes seen the most marked effects accrue from small doses of arsenic, especially when combined with mercury and iodine, in the form of the liquor arsenici et hydrargyri hydriodatis, or Donovan's solution.

[It was clear in the case before them that the mercurial treatment was abandoned before the symptoms thoroughly yielded. After this he was iodized and mercurialized frequently, but with no ultimate benefit. Had he been a strong man, Mr. Cooper said he would have given him mercury and used every precaution. But being of a depraved constitution, and weak, he ordered him:]

R Iodinii, gr. ss.; potassii iodidi, ȝss.; sirupi papaveris, ȝss.; infusi gentianæ co., ȝx. Misce, ut fiat mistura, cujus sumantur cochl. ij. magna ter die, cum morphiæ acet., gr. ss. omni nocte.

I pursued this for a few weeks, and at the same time enjoined perfect rest in bed, but found little or no improvement in the sore; which, as is the character of the specific kind, healed in one part, but extended itself in another. At the same time, a number of tubercles appeared over his head and face, which are anything but a favorable indication of the condition of his system. Tubercles and blotches—the difference between the two being, that the former are elevated, but the latter even with the surface of the skin—may depend on other causes than syphilis; but, as a result of this disease, they are always unmistakable from their coppery hue, their smutty or dirty appearance, the skin in fact conveying the impression of its wanting to be washed.

Seeing that he made no progress under the influence of the medicines prescribed, I altered them, and gave him :

R Liq. hydriodatis arsenici et hydr., 3iss.; extracti sarzæ, 3j.; dec. sarzæ co., 3viij.; cochl. ij. amp. ter die sum.; pulv. opii, gr. ss. omni nocte. And since then, I must say, he has been slightly improving.

In concluding these remarks on syphilis, I may observe, that in sloughing phagedena, mercury has the effect of aggravating rather than mitigating the symptoms, and is consequently decidedly prejudicial; the remedies are the topical application of nitric acid, and the internal administration of opium. Nitric acid not only destroys the part in contact with it, but at the same time induces a more healthy action in those beneath.

Part xxiii., *p.* 203.

Prophylaxis of Syphilis.—This preservative consists of a strong alcoholic solution of soap, having an excess of alkali. Dr. Langlebert had performed several experiments by inoculating with the poison of chancres, and then employing his antidote within about five minute afterward. The effects of the virus had in every case disappeared. *Part* xxiv., *p.* 262.

Borax as an Application to Gangrenous Buboes.—Dr. Effenberger applied a solution of borax, in the proportion of from one to two drachms in a pint of water, to a large number of patients who suffered from gangrenous bubo, with great success. He had fifty cases in one year; not one had died, although there were several very severe cases, and in one the femoral vessels were laid bare. The solution was applied by means of charpie, so as to cover the edges of the sore. It was very essential that the charpie should be very frequently renewed by night and day; and to the neglect of this precaution, he attributed the failure of this practice in the hands of other surgeons. *Part* xxiii., *p.* 212.

Phagedenic Chancre.—Give iron. M. Acton trusts chiefly in the tartrate, probably any other form would do as well. If there is sloughing phagedena, give opium in large doses. Destroying the surface of the ulcer with nitric acid is useful in some cases.

* * * * * * * *

Bubo.—Give one grain doses of tartar emetic every second hour, until a marked effect is produced upon the inflammatory swelling.

Part xxiv., *p.* 268.

Mercury—Substitute for, in Syphilis.—M. Robin, of Paris, substitutes 15 grains of the bichromate of potash divided into 80 pills, with extract of gentian; one to be taken night and morning. *Part* xxv., *p.* 268.

Bubo—Opening of, by Multiple Punctures.—M. Vidal strongly recommends that venereal buboes should not be allowed to open of themselves; for when they are left to nature, the skin becomes detached and thinned, a great loss of substance ensues, a tedious recovery takes place, and an unsightly deformity is left. Opening by caustic, too, leaves disfiguring scars; and the same inconvenience results from large incisions, and cutting away, by the bistoury, portions of skin that are too much changed to unite. Still the bistoury is much more easily managed than is the caustic, and M. Vidal much prefers removing by it a portion of half dead, detached skin, or a gland which is an obstacle to reparation, to attacking such parts by caustic. By its aid the cicatrix may be rendered more regular, and cause less deformity. But cases requiring large incisions and excision are rare, especially if the bubo be early treated, and punctures are made as soon as matter is formed. The bubo should be shaved. If the abscess is recent, and suppuration not extensive, one puncture may be made at the fluctuating point. If other glands suppurate, they must be punctured in the same manner. If the collection is extensive and superficial, several punctures are required, not in the fluctuating centre, but at the circumference, by a straight bistoury passing subcutaneously to the centre; thus the skin is divided where it is adherent, intact, and possessed of its vitality. The bubo must not be pressed for two days, when it will gradually discharge itself. Sometimes the punctures close before the matter is evacuated; this may be prevented by gently pressing the abscess once a day. If they all close, it is better to allow them to do so than introduce tents, making one or two new punctures if required. By this plan not the slightest mark, or only a very slight one indeed, is left. *Part* xxv., *p.* 269.

Treatment of Syphilis.—Prof. Bennett enters into a comparison of the *simple treatment* of syphilis with the *mercurial treatment*, and gives statistics to prove the great superiority of the former plan. Prof. B. says:

The simple treatment is divided into internal or medical, and external or surgical. The first consists in the observation of certain hygienic rules, and the employment of general therapeutic means. The diet must be light and mild, meat and all stimulating viands retarding the cure; even with the lightest diet the hunger should never be quite appeased. The regimen must be the more diminished and rigid in proportion to the youth and vigor of the patient. Diluent beverages, decoctions of barley, liquorice, and linseed, alone or mixed with milk, should be taken freely, to the amount, indeed, of several pints a day. Perfect repose must be secured by confinement to bed. Constipation must be obviated by the use of emollient clysters or mild laxatives. The air should be maintained at the same temperature; this is an indispensable precaution in chronic, consecutive, and mercurial affections. Exercise is only useful in the convalescent stage. In chronic syphilis, however, it may often be carried to fatigue with advantage. Tepid baths, repeated three or four times a day, are always attended with advantage. General blood-letting is often required when the primary disease is intense, or the system excited and the patient plethoric, but should not be used indiscriminately.

In the external or surgical treatment, strict attention to cleanliness and the position of the diseased parts should never be lost sight of. Emollient decoctions or fomentations, or dressings of simple cerate, are the best applications, and the dressings should not be too frequently renewed. Leeches are generally necessary. The greatest benefit is derived from the external use of a concentrated solution of opium (in the proportion of about two drachms to one ounce of water); it soothes excessive irritability in all cases. When the suppuration is moderated and the surface of the ulcer cleansed, stimulating dressings, consisting of solutions of the sulphates of alum and copper, the nitrate of silver, and subacetate of lead, favor cicatrization.

In inveterate cases, more especially those laboring under tertiary symptoms, the iodide of potassium has been used with benefit, in doses of five grains, three times a day, conjoined with emollient applications to the affected parts.

The Mercurial Treatment consists in keeping up slight salivation, by means of the internal administration of blue-pills or some form of mercury, sometimes conjoined with mercurial frictions or fumigations, at least for the space of a month. This physiological action of the drug may be produced by administering any of its preparations continuously in small doses. If combined with opium, they act less on the bowels and more on the system generally.

It is necessary during its action, that the patient do not expose himself to cold. A certain irritability is produced, and the constant soreness of the gums, the metallic taste in the mouth, not to speak of the inconveniences of profuse salivation which occasionally occur, render this species of treatment anything but agreeable to the patient.

Part xxvi., *p.* 278.

Venereal Ulcers.—The following is the composition of Plenck's Mercurial Bahn for dressing venereal ulcers : Mercury, 1 oz. ; Venice turpentine, ½ oz. ; lard, 3 oz. ; calomel, 17¾ grains ; elemi ointment, 3 oz. Mix.

Part xxvii., *p.* 162.

Seton for Suppurating Bubo.—M. Bonnafont, chief surgeon of one of the military hospitals of Paris, has lately proposed to supersede the ordinary modes of opening buboes by the following method : A seton of a very few threads, is passed through the bubo in the direction of its long axis, and left for several days, until a kind of fistulous tract is established, The thread is then removed, and the purulent matter escapes by the small apertures, either spontaneously or by pressure. The advantages of this practice are, according to the author, the avoidance of the unsightly puckered cicatrix generally left when incisions are made, and the more rapid healing of the bubo.

* * * * * * * *

Bubo.—Dr. Clairborne applies *collodion* over a bubo when there is not much local inflammation ; the collodion is applied layer after layer, until considerable compression is produced. If there be any amount of inflammation, leeches are previously applied. *Part* xxviii., *p.* 221.

Syphilis Congenital.—Mr. Wormald, of St. Bartholomew's, says : The mildest preparations of mercury given to children are apt to run off by the bowels ; to obviate this, let a piece of flannel smeared with mercurial ointment be worn constantly over the child's belly. If the child be at the breast, mercury should be administered to the mother also.

Part xxix., *p.* 241.

Syphilis.—There is a great difference, Mr. Acton believes, between what is called the *infecting* chancre which is an *indurated* sore, and the *unindurated* sore. The former communicates constitutional syphilis, the latter does not. The infecting indurated sore ought to be treated by mercury, the *unindurated* form need not be so treated. Hence the difference of opinion amongst medical men is often founded on a misapprehension.

In treating the former, in Paris, the proto-iodide of mercury is used, but this does not answer so well in this country as mercurial friction, blue pill, or the grey powder.

Phagedenic Chancre is treated by Ricord, by first destroying the whole of the unhealthy surface with a red-hot iron, previously placing the patient under the influence of chloroform. After the sloughs have sepa rated, the surface is covered with strips of ammoniacum and mercurial plaster, and doses of tartrate of iron are given with great success, in the less obstinate cases. The most frequent variety of sore in London is the phagedenic with induration. In this the actual cautery does no good; mercury must here be given, and the system supported by bark, wine, or steel.   *Part* xxx., *p.* 172.

Bubo.—To prevent a bubo from suppurating, Dr. Thompson, at the Marylebone Infirmary employs counter irritation by means of a strong solution of nitrate of silver, three drachms to the ounce of distilled water, with twenty minims of strong nitric acid. It may be applied with a glass rod or stick, or a glass brush. The black eschar will peel off in a few days, and then it should be reapplied.   *Part* xxxi., *p.* 229.

Preservative Means Against the Syphilitic Virus.—It is stated that a *neutralizing liquid* has been discovered for this poison, composed as follows: Distilled water, ℥ixss.; perchloride of iron, citric acid, hydrochloric acid, of each ℥j. Let a drop of this fall upon the part inoculated, and allow it to remain fifteen minutes, or apply a bit of lint soaked in the fluid. If the lint be applied for an hour the antidote is complete.
                                                   Part xxxi., *p.* 236.

Plurality of Poisons in Syphilitic Diseases.—Mr. Skey, surgeon to St. Bartholomew's Hospital, believes that there are a plurality of poisons in this disease depending upon the constitution of the person affected, and not on the source of the infection. For the treatment of venereal sores, mercury, in ninety-nine cases out of one hundred, is unnecessary. We may say that there are three different kinds of venereal sores : first, the common venereal sore, where mercury is quite inadmissible ; second, the phagedenic sore, where mercury is positively injurious ; third, the true syphilitic sore, dusky, cartilaginous, indurated ; here mercury is useful, and it is the only case in which it is admissible, but it is very rare comparatively. M. Ricord, of Paris, entirely and fully coincides with these views. In the exhibition of mercury, it is a bad plan to push it where it seems to have little or no effect. It would be much better to intermit its use for a few days, and when resumed it will be far more likely to produce a beneficial impression. When pushed to salivation, it too often produces a long train of complaints, which last as long as life.   *Part* xxxiii., *p.* 239.

Tincture of Iodine in Bubo.—M. Joliclerc states, as the result of much observation, that tincture of iodine is the best application in bubo, preventing, or dissipating fluctuation, and facilitating healing if the bubo be already open. He applies it by gentle friction, so as to avoid vesication.
                                                   Part xxxiii., *p.* 242.

Common Sore or Venerola.—Mr. Skey, of St. Bartholomew's says, There are three stages through which we may trace this sore : the first is ulcerative, the pimple which comes out on the third or fourth day increases until it is about the size of a pea ; in the second stage, the sore throws up a border or elevated edge, granulations also spring up to the edge of the mound ; in the third stage, these granulations are absorbed and cicatrize. This is the ulcer of gonorrhœa inoculation, and is never followed by secondary symptoms. Mind, now, that about these sores there is no thickening, tumefaction, induration. Indurated sores, that is, with edges like cartilages, are very rare indeed. If your patient has true syphilis bubo, you feel a distinct gland inflamed under your finger. It is not like common bubo, but inflamed tissue like an abscess, running along the line of Poupart's ligament. There is no suppurative action in true bubo. None of these common complications are at all bettered by mercury. The chief and abiding principle of treatment in venerola is, to keep the parts scrupulously clean. The sore will take a certain time to heal, and you cannot stop the ulcerative process either by mercury or caustics. Above all things the parts must be kept clean, or your patient will have a "crop of sores." Simple spermaceti ointment and morphia is the nicest application. In the second stage give bark or quinine, and an extra allowance of good wine. At the end of four months you may look out for secondary symptoms, but you will never find them. In this special sore, which produces no sore throat, no eruptions, etc., mercury is never required. In fact, mercury is not more required for what are called syphilitic diseases, than for any other class of diseases. Mercury, as regards syphilis, is the greatest curse of a cure, and about the most useless thing as a remedy ever discovered. *Part* xxxiv., *p.* 211.

Obstinate Chancre.—Opium, says M. Rodet, acts most efficaciously in those cases in which mercury is of the least use, and *vice versâ.* Thus in constitutional syphilis it acts as a mere corrective, and should only be given in very small doses. When, however, the chancre manifests any tendency to phagedena, mercury should be rigidly forbidden, while opium is especially valuable in diminishing the irritability, pain, and suppuration. It is in the phagedenic serpiginous ulcers that large doses of opium act almost as a specific. It should not be given too frequently, for if the stomach be kept too constantly under its action digestion will be interfered with ; the entire daily quantity should be taken at two doses, morning and evening. Wine should also be given freely with the opium as a corrective to the stomach ; to prevent its constipating effect on the bowels, and to obviate the tendency to sleep. *Part* xxxiv., *p.* 215.

Secondary Syphilis.—[We sometimes meet with cases of secondary syphilis which resist the usual preparations of iodine. The object of this paper is to bring before the notice of the profession a new compound, which combines all the advantages to be derived from iodine, while it is devoid of its bad effects, and has proved very valuable when other combinations have failed.]

Dr. Christophers' experience of the action of this remedy is limited to cases of secondary syphilis ; but in the hands of some other surgeons, it has been found efficacious in cases of scrofula, anemia, and in the furunculoid plague.

There are two preparations: the one found so useful in treating cases of secondary syphilis) he names "liquor cinchonæ hydriodatus;" the other (that which has been found useful in treating boils, anemia, and scrofula), "liquor cinchonæ hydriodatus cum ferro." The former contains in one fluid drachm of liquor, twelve grains of cinchona flav., and one grain and a half of iodine, in the form of hydriodic acid. The latter contains, in addition to the former ingredients, one grain of protoxide of iron in each fluid drachm of the liquor. These preparations are produced by exhausting the powdered bark with an aqueous solution of hydriodic acid; then with water, and the liquor is subsequently evaporated to the above bulk.

The dose varies from one drachm to three drachms of " the liquor cinchonæ hydriodatus," and from fifteen minims to two drachms of "the liquor cinch cum hydriodatus cum ferro;" the use of the hot-air bath in order to produce profuse sweating, is a potent remedy for intractable and inveterate cases of secondary syphilis. *Part* xxxiv., *p.* 217.

Primary Syphilis—Ferruginous Treatment of.—Mr. Behrend, of Liverpool, instead of the old mercurial treatment, uses the potassio-tartrate of iron, to cure every type of primary sore: of course this does not exclude the use of caustics. He prescribes the salt in form of solution, in the proportion of one part to six of water, of which two tablespoonfuls are to be taken three times a day, and a solution of the same strength as a local application to the part. The patient must be instructed, lest he remove the lint roughly, and so destroy an incipient cicatrice or healthy granulations. In the phagedenic form, generous diet, wine, and fruit, may be allowed, but no pastry or cheese. He has not had a single case of secondary or constitutional syphilis after treatment with the potassio-tartrate of iron alone, either in hospital or private practice, except in two cases in which he combined the iron with mercurial treatment. *Part* xxxv., *p.* 171.

Secondary Syphilis.—Of the different forms of eruptions, we may mention, first, among the *rashes*, the annular form of roseola: this very soon yields to the iodide of potassium, if it be given before desquamation has' taken place, and the copper-colored stain has formed. Purpura must be treated by generous diet, iodide of potassium, and decoction of bark. Of *papular* eruptions, syphilitic lichen may be very obstinate, but it will always yield to a strong lotion of the bichloride of mercury, ten grains to the ounce. In the ulcerating form of lichen, the iodide of mercury, one grain every night, with two or three grains of the extract of conium, in the form of a pill, is the best treatment. Syphilitic prurigo yields more readily to sarsaparilla than to any other remedy. In the *scaly* forms, such as lepra and psoriasis, Donovan's solution, in doses of ten minims to half a drachm three times a day, is the most efficacious internal remedy. The best local remedies are, the bichloride of mercury lotion, and in some cases, the mercurial vapor bath, by surrounding the patient, seated on a cane-bottomed chair, with blankets, and applying a spirit-lamp to the mercurial preparation; but the simplest plan is to heat half a brick in the fire, put it in a chamber-pot beneath the chair, and throw the mercurial preparation upon it. If you use the bisulphuret of mercury, one or two drachms will be necessary; if the iodide, ten grains or a scruple; but perhaps a combination of the two is better, say ten grains of the iodide with a drachm of the bisulphuret, increasing the dose to double this quantity. At the Lock Hospital, ten grains of calomel is preferred. The patient should be kept exposed to the vapor for ten or fifteen minutes; and when the blankets are removed, he should be rubbed dry, and a wet sheet wrung out of cold water thrown over him, to diminish the sensitiveness of the skin and the relaxing effects of the vapor bath. The only *vesicular* form of disease is rupia: here mercury is most dangerous, while iodide of potassium internally, with the red precipitate ointment locally, is almost sure to cure. Among *pustular* diseases, we may mention ecthyma; this again is aggravated by mercury, but sarsaparilla often cures it. The *tubercular* eruptions are always obstinate, but the mercurial vapor bath is the best treatment. Cutaneous excrescences may be easily destroyed by strong acetic acid or the tinc. ferri mur.; but Ricord's plan of using a chloride of soda lotion for a few days, and then sprinkling the growths with calomel, is the best treatment. With respect to the syphilitic diseases of bones, it is in the hard periosteal node that the iodide of potassium, in eight grain doses, three times a day, is the specific remedy. The soft or gummy node gradually yields to repeated blistering. In chronic syphilitic diseases of the joints, the iodide of mercury is more generally useful than the iodide of potassium; these cases are very obstinate, and it may be well to alternate the remedies, at the same time giving good diet. In syphilitic angina, if not very severe, mercurial fumigation may be used, or the vapor of the grey oxide may be inhaled; but in very severe cases, the iodide of potassium internally, with the red precipitate ointment externally, acts like a charm. In the treatment of *syphilitic iritis*, commence at once with calomel and opium, say one grain of calomel with a sixth of a grain of opium every three hours, until the gums are slightly touched, but do not carry it to salivation. *Part* xxxv., *p.* 174.

Bubo.—Instead of opening these by the knife, which is the plan ordinarily employed, Mr. Turner, military surgeon at Bombay, uses caustic potass. The slough soon separates, and the result is much more satisfactory to the surgeon, as you avoid the constant opening and reopening, causing drain to the system and disgust to the patient. *Part* xxxv., *p.* 186.

Venereal Inoculation.—Prof. Porter, of Dublin, believes that secondary symptoms may be produced in the female by the seminal fluid of a man who may have had syphilis previously, and who may seem to have been perfectly cured. Thus the woman may be affected either primarily, or by a fœtus, or by the semen: were we not aware of the last mode of communication, we should be sometimes quite puzzled to account for the symptoms. *Part* xxxv., *p.* 200.

Calomel Fumigation in Syphilis.—No mode of mercurial treatment, according to Dr. Lee, removes the symptoms of syphilis so readily as fumigation; none is attended with so little mischief to the patient's constitution, and after none is a relapse so seldom experienced. Calomel is the best preparation to use for the purposes of fumigation; it is readily sublimed—is not decomposed thereby—and but a comparatively small quantity is required. It is found to answer the purpose better if combined with vapor of water; therefore, in any lamp used for this purpose, provision must be made not only for volatilizing the calomel, but a small amount of water likewise. *Part* xxxvi., *p.* 195.

Cure of Syphilis without Mercury.—Dr. Marsden believes that secondary syphilis may be treated entirely without mercury, and on the following simple plan: and not one in a hundred instances will return with constitutional symptoms. Stomachic and tonic remedies must be administered, conjoined with a good diet and the following formula, viz.:—Sulphur, one drachm; sulphuret of antimony and nitrate of potash, of each five grains; mixed into a powder, half of which must be given night and morning, and persevered in until a cure is established. *Part* xxxvi., *p.* 199.

Chancre.—Dr. Collman applies pure acetic acid by means of a glass tube, thoroughly to the part, preventing its diffusing itself around by means of charpie. On the third day a whitish eschar separates, and a clean, healthy sore is left, which will rapidly heal by common dressing. On the first and third day an active purgative is administered. *Part* xxxvi., *p.* 200.

Secondary Syphilis—Communication of.—A case is recorded by Dr. Elliotson, in which secondary syphilis was communicated from a lady's maid (having cracks in the palms of the hands and other syphilitic symptoms), to her mistress, in whom it showed itself as an eruption at the forepart of the scalp where the hair is thinnest. There had been no breach of surface to account for this. The poison had probably been communicated from the maid applying pomatums and rubbing them in with the palms of her hands.

The third or cachectic stage of syphilis does not require mercury, and yields generally to hydriodate of potass or sarsaparilla; the hydriodate is incapable of curing true syphilis in either its primary or secondary stage.

Part xxxviii., *p.* 171.

Primary Syphilis. — Dr. Thompson, of University College Hospital, says: There are two entirely distinct forms of primary sores—distinct alike in course, results, and treatment. First, the true Hunterian, or indurated chancre with hard indurated edges, feeling like a cup of cartilage imbedded in healthy tissues, and moving freely over the underlying parts; if followed by enlarged inguinal glands, these never inflame and suppurate, and the important point is, that this form is always followed by constitutional symptoms, unless destroyed before the induration appears, which happens generally in about from six to eight days. Secondly, the soft, or non-indurated chancre, with sharply-cut, even, slightly-undermined edges, much inclination to spread from the highly contagious nature of the secretion, not necessarily, though generally followed by suppurating bubo; and lastly, *there is no constitutional affection.* Both chancres should be destroyed with caustic, as early as possible, the soft to destroy its specific character, and hence its aversion to heal; the hard, for the same reason, on account of its tendency to infect the system. If induration, however, have occurred, no cauterization will avail. Thus, at the time when cauterization is of use, it cannot be determined to which variety the sore belongs. The best caustic is the Vienna paste or potassa c. calce made into small sticks. Ricord uses strong sulphuric acid made into a paste with charcoal; some astringent lotion, as a solution of tannic acid in water, should be used to restrain the abundant secretion of the soft variety, and thus prevent the spreading of the sore by infection of neighboring parts. Nothing hastens cicatrization so much as a mild form of iron given internally. Now, in this soft variety, mercury is wholly out of place and must not be employed. In the indurated variety, mercury should be commenced at once (the iodide in doses of half a grain to a grain and a half twice a day, is one of the best forms for administration), and it is undesirable to exceed very slight mercurialism; a little opium may be combined with it to prevent relaxation of the bowels, and if the stomach is irritable, inunction may be substituted.

Part xxxix., *p.* 222.

TABES MESENTERICA.

Tabes Mesenterica, and Chronic Peritonitis in Children.—Dr. West says: Chronic peritonitis, so often a fatal disease in children, differs from acute inflammation of the peritoneum, not only in its tardy progress, but in being almost invariably associated with the tuberculous cachexia.

The occasional attacks of pain in the abdomen which form a prominent symptom of this disease, may or may not be preceded by vague indications of decaying health. But, however this may be, it is not long before the appetite fails or becomes capricious, the bowels become irregular, and the motions unnatural, and thirst and feverishness set in. Occasionally the stomach is irritable, but the tongue is usually clean throughout the disease. The abdomen soon becomes large, tense, and tympanitic, and manipulation of it occasions uneasiness, or severe pain. As the disease proceeds, though pauses seem to take place in progress, the symptoms increase in severity.

The child loses flesh; the face grows pale and sallow, and anxious; the skin becomes habitually dry, and hotter than natural, and the pulse is permanently accelerated. The abdomen does not grow progressively larger, but it becomes more and more tense, although its tension varies without any evident cause, and sometimes disappears for a day or two, to return again as causelessly as it disappeared. When the tension is diminished, the abdomen yields a solid and doughy sensation, and the union between the contents of the abdomen and the abdominal walls become very perceptible. The superficial abdominal veins now become enlarged in many instances, and the skin grows rough, and looks as if it were dirty. The pain in the bowels retains the same colicky character as before, but it returns very frequently, and sometimes exceedingly severe, while the child is never free from a sense of uneasiness. The tenderness of the abdomen, however, but seldom increases in proportion to the increase of pain. The bowels are in general habitually relaxed, though the degree of the diarrhœa, as well as the severity of the abdominal pain, vary much in different cases. As the disease advances, the child becomes confined to bed, and is at length reduced to a state of extreme weakness and emaciation. Death is often hastened by the concomitant affection of the lungs; but should this not be the case, the patient may continue for many weeks in the same condition, till life is destroyed, after a day or two of increased suffering, by some renewed attack of peritoneal inflammation.

In the first stage, rely chiefly upon dietetic and hygienic means. In the second, relieve pain by the application of a large poultice, frequently renewed, to the abdomen, avoiding if possible, the application of leeches. As mild mercurials continued for a long time are of service, as soon as the abdominal tenderness is sufficiently relieved to allow of it, let the belly be rubbed twice a day with a liniment consisting of equal parts of lin. hydrarg., lin. sapon., and ol. olivæ; and give hydrarg. c. creta, with an equal quantity of Dover's powder once or twice a day. The abdomen may be advantageously supported by a well-adapted flannel bandage, with a piece of whalebone at either side. If there is diarrhœa, give a mixture with logwood and catechu. If diarrhœa is slight, or is absent, and there is much feverishness, use the tepid bath, and give small doses of liquor potassæ and ipecacuanha, with extract of dandelion, and the mercurial with Dover's powder. If a mild tonic seems likely to be borne, give a mixture with extract of dandelion, extract of sarsaparilla, and carbonate of soda; or give infusion of calumba, or liquor cinchonæ. Chalybeates will not often be borne; citrate of iron, or the ferro-citrate of quinine are the best, but must be given with great caution. Change of air, however, and especially removal to the sea-side, is the best tonic. The diet must, of course, be light and unstimulating throughout. ● *Part* xviii., *p.* 125

Oily Frictions in Mesenteric Disease.—In this paper Dr. Baur reports the great success that has attended the friction of the whole surface of the body, night and morning, with a sponge imbued with tepid oil, the patient being kept in bed, wrapped in a blanket, for two hours after. The first effect produced is abundant general sweating; the skin, losing its dry aspect, becomes supple, turgescent, and of a fresh color, a rubeloid eruption sometimes occurring. A secondary and highly benefical calming effect is produced, which is manifested in the production of tranquil sleep. As a third, there is increased secretion, especially of the kidneys and liver. It is evident that many affections may be rendered tractable by such an agent, and Dr. Baur regards it as almost possessed of specific properties in the diseases of scrofulous origin, as tabes mesenterica, or glandular tumors. He believes the frictions are powerful adjuvants in scrofulous hydrocephalus, and may even prove curative in phthisis, when steadily persevered in.

Part xxxii., *p.* 99.

Tuberculosis and Tabes Mesenterica of Infants.—Prof. Nelson, in his " Clinical Observations on the Special Application of the *Liquor Pepsinœ* in certain Diseases," says : The number of these cases that have presented themselves precludes my entering upon them individually. Let it suffice to picture them generally, and according to their broad features: to wit, the wrinkled, discontented, fretful faces of the young children, rather resembling those of old men and women in the most unhappy humor possible; the small shrunken chests; the large toad-like bellies; shrivelled extremities; and bloodless, wax-like fingers. Such patients often have voracious appetites, without any good results; the food passing off in diarrhœa, without having been digested. By means of hydrargyrum cum creta and Dover's powder, and the liquor pepsiniæ by itself after food, the changes in such children have been very extraordinary, especially when the diet has been consistent with the other treatment, and goats' or asses' milk used, along with raw egg. The same results will accompany its use amongst the pot-bellied young of the lower animals.   *Part* xxxv., *p.* 298.

Vide Art. " Marasmus."

——•••——

TANNIN.

Use of Pure Tannin—The use of tannin, or tannic acid, externally, will be found especially valuable in sore nipples, excoriations about the anus and scrotum, piles, leucorrhœa, aphthous sores in the mouth, toothache, severe salivation, and relaxed sore throat. For sore nipples, Mr. Druitt, uses it in the strength of five grains to the ounce, on lint, and the part to be covered with oil silk. For that troublesome itching about the anus and scrotum, so teasing to some people, he prefers lemon juice. In leucorrhœa, tannin will be found useful as a suppository, ten grains being mixed with a little tragacanth, and introduced up the vagina sufficiently high that during its solution and passage downward, it may be smeared over the whole surface. It is also one of the best applications for severe salivation and for relaxed sore throat, attended with an increased secretion of mucus. But Mr. Druitt, seems to think, also, that it is the best application for toothache; a piece of information which he received from Mr. Tomes. " Let the patient thoroughly wash out the mouth with a solution of carbonate of soda in warm water; let the gum around the tooth or between it and its neighbors, be scarified with a *fine* lancet; then let a little bit of cotton-wool, imbued with a solution of a scruple of tannin and five grains of mastic in two drachms of ether, be put into the cavity, and if the ache is to be cured at all, this plan will put an end to it in nine cases out of ten."

Part x., *p.* 139.

Tannin—Employment of.—Dr. Cummings states, as the result of several years' experience, that he has found tannin the most valuable of *astringents.* Thus, whenever, in dysentery, medicines of this class are indicated, it acts admirably, either given alone or combined with opium. He says, he could refer to more than a thousand cases of dysentery, diarrhœa, cholera infantum, etc., in which he has employed it, never with regret, and almost always with advantage; while other practitioners, with whom he has communicated concerning it, express similar opinions. In the sweating, or last stage of phthisis or low continued typhus, and even in the worst cases, this accompaniment of diseases of debility has been entirely or in part relieved. It is useful in almost all forms of hemorrhage, and most remarkably so in hemoptysis; and when combined with opium and ipecac, it forms a medicament very preferable to acetate of lead and other similar substances. Among other forms of hemorrhage, over which it exerts great power, is that from the bowels resulting from dysentery, and that which occurs in threatened abortion. In hemorrhoids, it is of great use as an outward wash. In epistaxis, it may be snuffed up or blown through a quill, and will almost always arrest the bleeding. No article in the whole class of astringents acts like it in severe salivation. In aphthæ and other diseases of the mouth, in which there are spongy or bleeding gums, it possesses no equal. Used as a gargle in relaxed uvula and tonsils, its efficacy is great. As an *antiseptic,* for cleaning old foul ulcers, the author has extensively used it in the form of a powder, especially when there is disposition to hemorrhage. As an astringent collyrium, it is, in his opinion, preferable to all other substances in the purulent ophthalmia of infants. He administers it internally in two-grain doses. *Part* xxiv., *p.* 350.

TEETH.

Hemorrhage from the Socket of a Tooth—Use of Plaster of Paris.—Some interesting cases of bleeding after extraction of a tooth have been related in the Journals, several of which have terminated fatally. Mr. Roberts, of Edinburgh, relates a case in which a friend of his completely succeeded in stopping the hemorrhage by filling the bleeding cavity with plaster of Paris. From the plastic nature of this substance when moistened, we may conceive how readily and completely it may be pressed into every part of the bleeding cavity, and by its rapid consolidation how it may form the most perfect plug. *Part* vi., *p.* 114.

Transplantation of a sheep's Tooth into the Socket of a Child.—Mr. R. Twiss, after having extracted the remainder of a broken front tooth from a young lady, aged twelve years, put in its place the front tooth of a yearling sheep, reeking from the jaw of the living animal, having previously shortened its root about a quarter of an inch. After the first week, during which there was little promised success (the tooth being much too small for the space, and the child not attending to directions), it became more and more firm, with every indication of its having taken root.

Mr. Twiss was led to select the sheep, on account of the extreme cleanliness of this animal, and the beauty and aptitude of the teeth for the purpose. He recommends that teeth be taken only from sheep two or three years old, as at that age they are about the size of adult human teeth, and they are more likely to grow when transplanted. The root, he observes, may be shortened or pared, if necessary, to fit its new situation. The new tooth may be kept *in situ* by waxed silk ligatures.   *Part* vi., *p.* 154.

Different Cements to stuff decayed Teeth.—1. *Ordinary Tooth Cement.* —Is generally formed of a very concentrated etherial, or alcholic solution of gum sandarac, mastic, dammar, colophony, etc., in the proportion of one-third of the solvent to two-thirds of the resins by weight. A very usual formula is: sandarac, twelve parts; mastic, six parts; amber powder, one part, to six parts of ether. This preparation is a balsam of the consistence of copaiba; it readily dries on exposure to the atmosphere, but remains for some time soft and compressible. The mass yields, with alcohol, a milk-white solution, the turbidity depending on the masticine which is precipitated.

2. *Gauger's Tooth Balsam (Balsamum Odontalgicum).*—Is chiefly in use in St. Petersburg. The recipe is as follows: Dissolve ℥ij. of picked mastic in ℥iij. of absolute alcohol. Pour the solution into a bottle capable of containing two pounds, and add of dried balsam of tolu ℥ix. Promote the solution by a gentle heat, and frequently shake the stoppered bottle. When the latter substance is dissolved, place the whole in a warm situation, to allow the undissolved particles to deposit. This balsam is viscid, and forms, when exposed to the air, a firm mass, which is neither acted upon by the saliva nor by other watery liquids. To prevent tooth-ache arising from exposure of the nerve, the decayed tooth should be well dried by means of cotton or blotting-paper, and a piece of cotton or wool imbued with the balsam is to be carefully inserted into the cavity.

3. *Vienna Tooth Cement.*—Herr V. Wirth, apothecary of Vienna, first conceived the idea of mixing with a viscid alcoholic solution of the resins powdered *asbestos*, which perfectly supplies the place of the pledget of cotton. His preparation is generally sold along with a tincture for cleansing the hollow teeth, and allaying tooth-ache. The latter tincture consists of an alcoholic solution of guaiacum and myrrh with acetic ether. Ostermaier, an apothecary at Munich, analyzed this nostrum, and has perfectly succeeded in preparing it, but we are not at liberty to publish his recipe. It will, however, be a sufficient hint to the scientific man to be reminded that powdered West Indian copal gains considerably in solubility in spirit by exposure to moderately warm air, and that pure alcohol, to which a few drops of any essential oil are added, greatly augments its solubility.

4. *Ostermaier's Tooth Cement.*—The principle of this preparation is the formation of phosphate of lime in the cavity of the hollow tooth. For this purpose anhydrous phosphoric acid must first be formed by burning phosphorus under a large basin, fifty-eight parts of pure unslacked lime in powder, are to be mixed with forty-eight parts of this flocculent anhydrous phosphoric acid, and the necessary quantity is to be pressed into the cavity of the tooth, after the tooth has been well dried; for, if the latter

proceeding be not observed, the mass will become heated, and, in expanding, fall out of its place. The application should be quickly effected, for the substance becomes quite hard and useless in the course of one or two minutes. *Part* x., *p.* 176.

Treatment of Caries of the Teeth.—Scrape out the entire of the softened carious part of the tooth, and rub its interior with a saturated solution of nitrate of silver, or with pulverized nitrate of silver barely wet. In this way the progress of caries may be effectually stopped ; and a tooth thus treated will often remain for years, though without any stuffing, and exposed to all the variations of food and drink, without giving any trouble or pain, and without any reappearance of the caries.
Part xiv., *p.* 197.

New Amalgam for stopping Teeth.—[Mr. Evans states that he has employed this amalgam successfully for a length of time. He says :]
It is composed of chemically pure tin, prepared with much care, to insure its being free from any other metallic substance, and combined with prepared cadmium, in small quantities, and mercury. In using it so much mercury should be employed as may be required to make it more or less plastic.
The cavity of the tooth being previously thoroughly freed from carious matter, can be carefully filled with paste thus formed. In the course of a few minutes it hardens into a solid, and gradually acquires a still firmer consistence and toughness, exhibiting a whitish color, or, if cut or burnished, a metallic lustre, like that of pure tin.
It retains its color perfectly, neither oxidizing on the external surface, nor on that applied to the cavity, and, of course, it does not discolor the tooth itself. It fills each crevice of the cavity, and by effectually excluding moisture and all kinds of deleterious matters, prevents the occurrence of caries, and becomes sufficiently hard to withstand the friction of mastication. To these most important advantages may be added others—*e. g.* it is easily and quickly prepared, without the trouble of beating it, as is the case with some of the amalgams hitherto used. It will not amalgamate with, or injure any gold clasps or plate bearing artificial teeth, which may be placed in contact with it ; and, in case of its removal being necessary, it can be cut out as easily as gold filling, as it forms a tough, almost ductile substance, and not a hard, brittle one, like the ordinary amalgams.
Part xix., *p.* 322.

Hemorrhage after Extraction of Teeth.—In severe cases use the actual cautery. It is best applied by means of a small rod of polished iron, furnished with a sheath ; the end of the sheath is applied to the bleeding part, and the heated iron then inserted, and passed along the sheath until it reaches the part. *Part* xx., *p.* 119.

Material for Arresting Alveolar Hemorrhage.—The difficulty that sometimes occurs in arresting hemorrhage after the extraction of teeth, especially in a person of hemorrhagic diathesis, is well known. Mr. Beardsley describes a composition which he found useful as a plug in such cases, and also for other purposes.
The proportions of the ingredients used, are, gutta percha, one ounce ; Stockholm tar, ounce and a half to two ounces ; creasote, one drachm ; shell lac, one ounce, or more, to harden it.* To be boiled together in a

small crucible, and constantly stirred or beaten, till it becomes thoroughly blended into a stiff homogeneous mass.

He has found the above composition a very ready and easy application for leech-bites, when the hemorrhage is at all troublesome. It is very adhesive when warmed, and firmly adheres all over the wounds when the part is wiped dry, and a small portion pressed on, just wetting the finger before doing so, to prevent it adhering to it also. *Part* xxi., *p.* 196.

Teeth—Loosening of the.—Use a gargle of tannic acid, three or four grains to the ounce of water. *Part* xxi., *p.* 326.

New Preparation for Stopping Teeth.—[Mr. Davenport gives the fol-· lowing recipe :]

Pour a small quantity of collodion on a plate or glazed surface; allow it to evaporate till it acquires the consistence of a thick paste, or, in more familiar language, a pill consistence ; let the cavity of the tooth be well dried, and quickly filled with the paste; in the course of a few minutes it will be hard and fit for mastication. Very slight pressure is required, and, being of a vegetable nature, somewhat analogous to the tooth itself, will resist the action of vegetable juices, and remain colorless.

[Mr. Davenport prepares his collodion in a manner different from that usually adopted. He tells us:]

The chemical manipulation is extremely disagreeable; the nitrous acid fumes are very abundant, consequently highly irritating to the respiratory organs. Great care is necessary in well washing the cotton; also, a moderate heat in drying it. The process is as under : ·

Take nitrate of potash, 4 lbs.; sulphuric acid, 8 lbs.; carded cotton wool, 8 oz.; mix the nitrate and acid in a glazed vessel, add the cotton, and constantly agitate with a glass rod for half an hour; then wash the cotton thoroughly in cold water, so that no trace of acid should be perceptible to test paper; then dry carefully, and the result will be a very soluble gun-cotton; then take 1 oz. of the cotton; rectified sulphuric ether, 16 oz. fluid ; when dissolved, add 1 oz. absolute alcohol. Allow the solution to stand twenty-four hours, and the collodion will be ready for use. *Part* xxi., *p.* 358.

Teeth—Vegetable and Animal Parasites of.—From microscopic observations made by Dr. Bowditch, he has, in a large majority of instances, found these parasites between the teeth, or at the juncture of the gums, in persons from different classes of the community, but without any disease of the mouth. He attributes their presence to a want of cleanliness; and recommends thoroughly brushing the teeth after each meal. M. Foy, a French dentist, recommends tinct. kino, tinct. catechu, aa.; a teaspoonful to be added to cold or tepid water, and used every morning.
Part xxii., *p.* 366.

Materials the best Adapted for Filling the Teeth.—Dr. Robertson says:

Pure and well-preserved gold leaf is undoubtedly the best and the most durable material which has yet been discovered for filling the teeth, and particularly so when the operation is performed in the early stages of decay, and before the slightest tenderness has been felt in the tooth. I should therefore recommend gold to be used in all cases where it is practicable, in preference to any other filling. But we have numerous cases which present themselves where gold cannot be used, and where an amalgam becomes a necessary substitute. The consideration then is, what materials are the best to form this amalgam ?

I have given much time and labor to the investigation of this subject, and after numerous experiments with the various metals, have come to the conclusion that gold, silver, platina, and tin, in their pure state, are the best ; because I have found in using them, either separately or combined, that they resist the acids of the mouth better than any of the other metals.

An amalgam of these, however, cannot be formed without mercury, but the smaller the portion the better, so that there shall be just sufficient to unite and hold in permanent combination the purer metals above specified.

The amalgams in general use, even those of the better class, which are composed of metals above mentioned, contain a great deal too much mercury; and I shall presently show that the cause for this superabundance of mercury arises from the incorrect proportioning of the metals, and the improper mode of mixing them. The method generally adopted in preparing an amalgam is to combine the mercury at once with the other metals, so that the compound may be ready for using, and when a portion is required it has to undergo a process of heating and rubbing, to bring it back from its crystallized form to a pasty state before putting it into the tooth. Instead of adopting this method, the mercury ought to be kept separate from the other metals, and only mixed with them at the time of using. This mode of mixing, with the metals rightly proportioned, will produce a harder and more durable filling, and the metals will combine with *one-third* of the mercury required in the former mode of preparing the amalgam.

Some dentists use an amalgam of palladium and mercury, which makes a firm and durable filling, but it becomes black in the tooth. A few years ago cadmium was introduced as a filling, and for a short time it promised well, and appeared to be an improvement upon former amalgams, but after a few months' trial it showed its defects, and has very properly been discarded. It neither retained its color nor its hardness, for when acted upon by the friction of the opposing teeth it soon wore away, and when not acted upon became, in parts, yellow as saffron, with the disadvantage also of having a strange tendency to produce galvanic action in the mouth. Objectionable as this compound is, it still continues to be used by a certain class of practitioners, under the title of "Parisian filling."

There are various kinds of amalgams used by the same class of individuals, which contain copper, lead, bismuth, zinc, and antimony, all of which are injurious.

The amalgam which I am about to describe contains nothing novel so far as the materials are concerned ; but it is in the proportioning of them, and by a different mode of preparing the compound, that I have been enabled, of late years, to get rid of two parts out of the three of the mercury formerly required ; and this I consider to be an important advantage.

The amalgam consists of gold, one part ; silver, three parts ; and tin, two parts ; and it is of the utmost importance that the metals should be pure, free from the smallest particle of alloy.

The mode of uniting the metals, is, first, to put the gold and silver into the crucible, and just as they are on the point of melting, add the tin, which requires less heat than the former metals. When they become melted, but not over-heated, pour them from the crucible, melt them a second time, for the purpose of having them properly mixed, and then pour them into an ingot of a shape adapted for reducing the compound into the finest powder.

The mercury is to be kept apart from the powder, and mixed with it at the moment the amalgam is to be put into the tooth. The mercury must be perfectly pure, and the quantity required will be equal in weight to the powder.

In mixing the powder with the mercury, the exact proportions of each can be ascertained to the greatest nicety, and by a very simple process, which will save time and materials, and which makes a harder compound, than by using a larger portion of mercury, and squeezing part of it out again.

A measure for the mercury may be made from a square portion of ivory, by drilling in it three holes; one may be made to contain four grains, the second eight grains and the third twelve grains. The mercury to be poured into any one of these, as more or less may be required to fill the cavity of the tooth, and by drawing the finger across, so as to bring the mercury on a level with the surface of the ivory, the portion wanted may be accurately obtained.

The measure for the powder is equally simple and convenient. It is a metal tube, with a handle attached, calculated to hold four grains, which is also got to a nicety by filling, and then drawing the finger across the mouth of the tube, so as to make level measure.

The mercury should be kept in a small bottle, with an india-rubber tube attached to its neck, and the mercury is readily passed through the tube into the measure. In this way the exact quantity of each of the metals is readily obtained.

The powder and mercury to be emptied from the measures into a glass mortar, and rubbed till they become mixed. The compound is then to be rubbed firmly with the finger in the hollow of the hand, till converted into a paste, which, before hardening, allows plenty of time for insertion into the cavity of the tooth.

I have found this compound to be far superior to the former class of amalgams. It does not, like palladium, and some of the other metals that have been used, become black in the mouth. It retains its hardness and firmness, and is not, like cadmium, liable to be worn away by friction of the teeth.

Formerly, in fixing artificial teeth upon a gold plate, it was necessary to avoid bringing the gold in contact with a tooth filled with amalgam, because a portion of the mercury united with the gold and injured it. This evil is now remedied by the compound containing so small a quantity of mercury, which is held in permanent combination with the other metals, so that not a particle of it is abstracted by the embrace of a gold clasp. With these important improvements upon former amalgams another advantage is, that it is used with much greater facility.

Part xxvi., *p.* 172.

Cauterizing the Dental Nerve.—[Dr. W. A. Roberts, before the Edinburgh Medico-Chirurgical Society, described the following method of applying the actual cautery by means of wire brought to a white heat by electricity. He says:]

After several experiments, I found that " Grove's " battery answered best, being more convenient than " Smee's;" it is much smaller, and consequently more portable and more easily kept out of sight. By this one pair of plates I can produce a more decided result than I could arrive at with six pair of " Smee's." In the porous jar I have a mixture composed of two parts of nitric, to one part of sulphuric acid. In the glass jar there is a mixture of four parts of water to one part of concentrated sulphuric acid. At the end of each of the conducting wires, you will observe a fine platina wire brought to a point. This wire is fine enough to enter the foramen of any tooth, and if required merely to cauterize the large cavity of a decayed tooth, it can be easily rolled up to act as a small ball. When the wire is to be heated, the communication is made by gently pressing upon the ivory knob while pressing down the spring; the contact is made instantaneously; by taking off the pressure, the current is broken off as quickly. I found some difficulty at first in operating, from the want of elasticity in the wires, as the thickness necessary to convey sufficient quantity of the electric fluid to heat the platina wire to a white heat, rendered them very unwieldy. This has been got over very ingeniously and satisfactorily by a plan of my son's, which consists in filling two small india-rubber tubes with quicksilver, the ends of the copper wires being inserted into the mercury at both ends, and tightly tied; by this means the communication is rendered complete, and allows of free motion. Since this was done, we find now full freedom can be obtained by having a bundle of very fine wires tied together instead of a single thick one.

The advantages, then, to be obtained by this instrument are, its easy application to the desired spot in the mouth, and that perfectly cold, instead of alarming the patient by holding a red-hot iron before his face; its being at once raised to the requisite heat, and no more than the mere point of the wire used being hot; its being at once cooled on simply removing the finger from the ivory knob; and lastly, there being no appearance of heat to alarm the patient.

When to be applied for the purpose of arresting hemorrhage, or the deadening of the dental nerve, the cavity should be first well wiped out with a piece of lint, and then the desired spot should be rapidly touched, so as not to come into contact with other parts. This can be repeated if necessary. The platina must be at least *red* hot, as it then acts instantaneously, and with little or no pain, otherwise it would cause much pain, and subsequent inflammation. I need not say, with timid persons, the inhalation of chloroform should be resorted to. I have used this form of the actual cautery with and without chloroform in many cases.

Part xxvi., *p.* 175.

Teeth—Cement for making them Insensible to Pain.—Previous to stopping teeth permanently with any metal, use a cement composed of Canada balsam and slaked lime, which is introduced into the hollow tooth like a pill. The most sensitive tooth, says Dr. I. P. Clark, of London, may, by repeating this application, be made quite insensible to the most severe operative proceedings. *Part* xxx., *p.* 137.

Some of the Effects Produced by Carious Teeth.—[The following lecture by Mr. Smith contains many interesting facts.]

On the present occasion it is my intention to describe to you some of the effects produced by carious teeth, the causes of which are occasionally overlooked by practitioners; and I am induced to do this by the occurrence of a case which came under consideration on my last admission-day.

Elizabeth H., aged 40, was sent from some distance in the country to this infirmary, Dec. 12th, 1856, to be treated for what she was told by a medical practitioner, was a cancerous tumor in the cheek. On examination, a tumor, the size of a small chestnut, was found, with an ulceration of the mucous membrane, just fitting the sharp edge of one fang of a carious molar tooth of the lower jaw, which was making its way from the gum. Being fully assured, from former experience of many cases of a similar kind, that this was the sole cause of the tumor and ulceration, I removed the tooth, and in your presence promised her it should be well in a few days. A little lotion was ordered for the mouth. She appeared again on the next out-patient day, Dec. 17th. The ulceration was healed, the tumor gone, and she was discharged cured.

Now, I tell you, that if the cause of that tumor had been overlooked, no treatment of any kind would have been of the least use; it would have continued, it would have increased, and gone on from bad to worse for months, and possibly for years, unless the tooth had been removed by the efforts of nature. I could tell you of scores of cases like the above.

Sometimes instead of the cheek, the tongue suffers from the same cause. I have detected many cases of this kind. One interesting example shall be sufficient to explain such cases to you.

More than thirty years ago, one out-patient's day, my senior colleague (Mr. Hey) informed me that a few days previously he had excised a malignant-looking tumor from the tongue of a young country-woman, who was a private patient of his; that, to his surprise, in a few days the tumor had sprouted out as large or larger than before the operation; that, as she was not in circumstances to pay consultation fees, he had requested her to be in the house-surgeon's room at twelve o'clock, in order that he might ask Mr. Chorley's opinion, along with my own, on the case. On that day Mr. Chorley did not come to the infirmary, and I went with Mr. Hey to see his patient. There was a foul, dark, fungoid tumor, which occasionally bled, and from which she suffered much pain during every attempt to speak or masticate food; it was the size of a small walnut. On examining it with the finger, I detected two broken incisors (the middle and left lateral of the lower jaw) leaning inward, and with sharp-pointed edges fitting into the centre of the tumor. I was immediately convinced that these two teeth were the cause of all the mischief, and stated that opinion to Mr. Hey, who appeared doubtful. I said that he would not be justified in applying the ligature or using any other means, without first waiting to see the effect of the removal of the two broken carious teeth. I never saw the young woman again, but I was informed by Mr. Richard Hey that the teeth were drawn, and soon afterward the tumor entirely disappeared, without any other means being resorted to.

Sometimes carious teeth produce abscesses in the cheek, neck, and throat; these burst or are opened, and form fistulous sores, which will remain unhealed for months and years unless the cause be removed, just in the same manner as you see fistulous openings in the leg in cases of necrosis, and which remain open for years until the sequestrum is removed.

A few years ago a middle-aged man asked my opinion about a fistulous sore which opened on the middle of his whisker on the right cheek. I introduced a probe, and it came in contact with the fang of the last molar tooth of the upper jaw. I persuaded him to allow me to draw it, on the promise that he should be well in a few days. I requested him to write by post on the tenth day, and let me know the result. He wrote to say the discharge ceased the day the tooth was drawn, and that it was perfectly well.

Seven or ten years ago a young woman came under my care at the infirmary with a fistulous sore in the fore part of the throat, within an inch of the sternum. It had been discharging upwards of a year. I probed it; the instrument could be passed in the direction of the molar of the lower jaw on the left side. On inquiry, she said that eighteen months before she had had a tooth drawn at the dispensary, but the fangs of the tooth were left in the jaw. Afterward an abscess formed, which descended lower and lower till it burst midway between the sternum and pomum Adami. I drew the stumps; it still discharged for a week or ten days, when it got well without any other treatment. I mention the above case to impress on your minds the possibility of the fistulous orifice being at a considerable distance from the offending tooth. The fistulous sores proceeding from carious teeth are generally in the cheek or at the angles of the jaw. On the application of the probe you will often find the instrument pass readily to the interior of the mouth; you have then only to select the proper victim for sacrifice, and you will rarely err in this respect. Where the sinus from the sore to the tooth is short, the discharge from the external sore will generally cease in a day or two after the extraction of the tooth, but where it is long, as in the above case, it may be a week or two.

As abscess in these cases always precedes the formation of a fistulous sore, it should be your endeavor to detect these cases at this particular period.

A long time ago a near relative consulted me about an abscess at the angle of the jaw, on the right side. I suspected its cause, for on pressure I could make pus appear at the edge of one of the molars. He refused to have the tooth drawn until I assured him the abscess would burst externally, and continue discharging till the tooth was removed, and that an ugly looking scrofulous cicatrix would remain for life. The tooth was drawn; the abscess discharged itself into the mouth, was soon well, and left no mark.

Now, if the cause had not been detected when it was, in ten or twelve days the abscess would have burst externally, and a fistulous sore would have been the consequence, which would have continued discharging until the teeth had been removed either by nature or art.

Whenever you extract a tooth in these cases, always examine it carefully; you will invariably find a fang deprived of its periosteum, and sometimes a little sac attached to its root, containing pus.

Sometimes, where abscess forms from a carious molar of the upper jaw, the matter, instead of making its way to the cheek, gets into the antrum.

Remove the tooth, and if this does not give sufficient outlet for the matter, perforate the antrum with a joiner's gimlet. There has been a very interesting case of this kind recorded in the journals during the present month.

A horse was condemned to the knacker's yard as being afflicted with glanders, having a foul offensive discharge of purulent matter from the nostrils, and being in the last stage of emaciation. A veterinary surgeon finding that it could not masticate its food, examined its mouth, and detecting a carious tooth in the upper jaw, extracted it The discharge ceased; the horse soon began to thrive, and got well. Here was a case in which there was as much professional credit due to the surgeon as if instead of saving a horse from the knacker's yard he had saved the life of an alderman.

Mr. Louis Oxley, the dentist, related to me a case of such interest, that I requested him to write it out for me. Here you have it in his own words :

A young woman, of rather strumous habit, complained of a dull, aching pain under the orbit. The pain lasted from three to four months, attended by a gradual elevation of the orbital surface of the maxillary. The eye above this surface became at length so affected as entirely to lose its functions. At this stage of the case the young woman, who was attended by a general practitioner, who ignored dental surgery and pathology, resorted to leeches, blisters behind the ears, and drastic purges : I need not say ineffectually. After two or three months' loss of the sight the young woman first perceived a discharge from the right nasal fossa of a thick purulent fluid. This discharge had existed for eighteen months when I first saw her, *even in spite of the aforesaid remedies !* An examination of the mouth at once revealed the cause of so much misery, and the removal of three roots in a state of periostitis was the simple means by which two most important organs regained their proper functions.

There is another case in which swelling, inflammation, and ulceration at the sides of the tongue take place, and which does not appear, as far as my experience goes, except in individuals approaching to or upward of sixty years of age; but I have seen several cases of it, and shall proceed to describe the cause. If you will examine the form of the molars of the lower jaw where they come in contact with the sides of the tongue, you will find the line from the neck to the top of the crown gives a convex outline, so that for thirty or forty years during the act of speaking or mastication, the sides of the tongue come in contact with a smooth rounded surface ; but the constant grinding of hard food, such as biscuits, etc., for two score years, where all the teeth have remained sound, wears away one-third of the upper part of the teeth, the bony part is worn away deeper by one-eighth of an inch than the enamel, leaving a sharp edge projecting into the mouth, so sharp that, by firmly pressing the finger and drawing it along the edge, you might cut it to the bone. The friction of the tongue against this sharp edge produces the effect I have described. It is only necessary to round off the edges by the use of a fine file, and the tongue will soon heal. The operation will require to be repeated in a few years.

Part xxxv., *p.* 95.

Cements for Stopping the Teeth.—M. Vagner recommends the following : A drachm of gutta percha, softened by hot water, is to be worked up with catechu powder and tannic acid, of each half a drachm, and with a drop of essential oil. For use, a morsel is to be softened over the flame of a spirit lamp, introduced while warm into the cavity of the tooth, and adapted properly. The mass becomes hardened, and even after several months exhibits no traces of decomposition. M. Pouton states that we may also obtain an excellent cement by dissolving one part of mastic in two of collodion. Having well dried out the cavity, a small ball of cotton soaked in some drops of the solution is to be introduced. It soon solidifies, and may remain *in situ*, seeming also to exert an influence on the further progress of the caries. *Part* xxxv., *p.* 99.

Application of the Electric Cautery to Dental Surgery.—The Electric Cautery is a very safe, rapid, and effectual means of destroying the exposed pulps of decayed teeth. The cavity of the tooth having been well dried out and cleaned, and the mouth protected by a soft napkin, the platinum point is introduced into the cavity of the tooth, and then heated, which is preferable to heating it before introduction. The part is distinctly illuminated, and the pulp may be destroyed almost instantaneously. In the great majority of instances there is little or no pain beyond a momentary twinge. As a rule, the tooth should not be stopped on the same day as the electric cautery has been employed, but the cavity should be filled with a combination of morphine and mastic for a day or two. If the tooth should remain tender after the use of the cautery, it is better to wait till this has entirely subsided. *Part* xxxvi., *p.* 291.

Exposed and Diseased Dental Pulp.—Mr. Underwood says: The nerve may be either removed by means of some instrument to withdraw it, as a straightened fishhook, or by destroying it entirely, or by rendering its exposed surface insensible; for the latter purpose a strong spirit solution of tannin may be applied, and the nerve becomes coated and protected by an insoluble compound formed by the albumen and tannin. As an escharotic for these purposes, nothing is better than four or five grains of recently burned quick-lime mixed with a grain of morphia; this should be taken upon a piece of wool, and placed on the pulp, and the cavity closed with wax. Next day the application may be removed, and if any tenderness remains the dressing may be applied again. A strong, saturated solution of camphor is a good anodyne application. The actual cautery may often be used with great success to instantly destroy the dental pulp.
Part xxxvi., *p.* 295.

Carious Teeth—Stopping for.—A very good and easily applied cement for stopping teeth, says M. Henriot, is soft sulphur; it is not acted on by any of the alimentary substances or dentifrices. Put some washed flowers of sulphur in a test tube, heat it over a spirit lamp to over 350° Fahr., and pour it into cold water, when it will be a spongy mass, brown, soft, and elastic. A little ball of this should be pressed into the decayed tooth.
Part xxxvii., *p.* 142.

TENDONS.

Dislocation of the Long Head of the Biceps.—Mr. Hancock, surgeon to the Charing Cross Hospital, says:

There are probably few accidents so little noticed or understood as displacement of the tendons. The subject is scarcely mentioned in any of the numerous works on dislocations, although the consequence, when unreduced, is great inconvenience to the patient, and in the case of displacement of the tendon of the long head of the biceps, which happens more frequently than any other kind, the patient is deprived in a great degree of the use of the limb.

The principal signs of this accident are pain and tenderness in front of the joint, corresponding to the bicipital groove; acute pain in the course of the biceps when it is thrown into action, the pain being referred more particularly to its two extremities; the patient is unable to raise his hand to his head, or his arm beyond an acute angle from his body; the appearance of the shoulder is somewhat altered, the head of the humerus being drawn upward, and more forward than natural, lying close beneath the acromion process, while the posterior and external part of the joint is somewhat flattened. When we consider how much in appearance these accidents resemble partial dislocations of the head of the humerus upward and forward, we can entertain but little doubt that they have frequently been mistaken for them.

In the treatment of these cases you have three principal objects in view: to overcome the action of the capsular muscles, to reduce the tendon, and to keep the tendon in its groove when you have reduced it. I am not aware of any particular symptom by which we can be guided with any certainty as to when the tendon is dislocated inward, or when outward; but, as a result of my experiments, I should imagine that it is more frequently dislocated inward than outward, the inclination of the head of the humerus, and the greater projection of the large tubercle, being unfavorable to the latter displacement. Place your patient on a low chair, and let an assistant fix his scapula by pressing upon the superior angle and costa; then separate the patient's arm from his side, as far as you can; keep his hand in the prone position, and make extension downward and outward from the wrist, until you have somewhat withdrawn the head of the bone from the acromion process. Now let an assistant sit down on the floor, underneath the injured arm, and, clasping both his hands over the deltoid muscle, draw the head and neck of the bone downward and a little backward, while you rotate the head of the bone inward and backward in the glenoid cavity, by making the patient's arm describe a circle, carrying it backward, upward, forward and inward, across the chest. Should you have reason to suppose that the tendon is displaced outward, separate the arm as far as you can from the body, and let an assistant make extension in that direction best calculated to remove the head of the humerus from the acromial process, that is, downward and outward. Unless this he done, in either form of the dislocation, the bicipital tendon remains pressed up by the head of the humerus against the acromial process, and is obviously prevented from returning into its natural position. Next place your left hand well up in the axilla, and direct your assistant, while he keeps up the extension, to rotate the arm strongly outward, and at the same time to bring it to the patient's side. Having reduced it, gently separate the arm from the patient's side; keep it steadily rotated outward, and the hand supine; place a long splint, which extends from the shoulder to the fingers, along the back of the arm and hand, and also a pad or compress in front, over the bicipital groove. Fix the whole with a roller evenly and carefully applied, and place your patient on his back in bed, where he had better remain until you consider that the parts have become sufficiently firm to prevent a recurrence of the accident.

The reason why I recommend you to separate the arm from the side after reduction, is, that by so doing you place the pectoralis major muscle upon the stretch, and consequently make its broad tendinous insertion press more closely and directly over the bicipital groove. In my experiments, the difficulty was not so great in reducing, as in keeping the tendon in its place when reduced, and certainly the plan which I am now advocating appeared to be the most efficacious.   *Part* xi., *p.* 157.

Rupture of the Tendon of the Long Head of the Biceps.—This accident, says Mr. Hancock, may be occasioned by falling upon the arm, by violent twists of the limb, without external violence referred to the part, or by the sudden and violent extension of the limb, as when we put out our arms to save ourselves in falling.   The patient experiences at the moment, a sensation of snapping in the shoulder, soon succeeded by inability to raise the hand to the head; acute pain is caused by even slight pressure in the course of the bicipital groove, or lower down, on the muscle itself; the latter becomes flabby, and the movement of the arm backward and forward produces acute suffering, mostly referred to the situation of the biceps, where it passes over the head of the humerus.

Treatment.—Your object in these cases should be to approximate the two portions of the tendon, to obtain union if possible, or otherwise to favor the attachment of the lower portion to the head of the humerus, as Mr. Stanley has pointed out.   To do this effectually, place the hand in the semi-supine position, that is, with the thumb upward, making your patient grasp the opposite shoulder; thus you effectually relax the biceps muscle, as you will at once perceive, upon recollecting that the biceps is inserted into the back of the tubercle of the radius, and that the first action of the muscle, when the hand is prone, is to render it supine before it can effect flexion of the elbow.   Now apply a roller carefully, beginning from below, carrying it up to the axilla, and fixing a compress over the course of the biceps tendon, by which means you will keep the muscle quiet and prevent spasms; and, lastly, secure the arm in this position by bandages.

Part xi., *p.* 159.

Painful Crepitation of the Tendons.—M. Velpeau gives the following account of his patient: A week since he endeavored to raise a load, having his left hand applied to his hip. He felt a violent pain in his arm, and now we may perceive a slight swelling at the lower and external part of the forearm, unaccompanied by any change of color or fluctuation. Of a regular and elongated shape, it is only painful during motion, while on applying the hand over it we may perceive a fine characteristic crepitation; and it is an example of the *painful crepitation of the tendons* which was vaguely indicated by Boyer and Desault. I first met with it in a case in the hospital of Tours, where it was suspected to be a fracture of the radius. The affection is especially observed among washerwomen, mowers, blacksmiths, locksmiths, and joiners, and when it is seated in the foot, among soldiers huntsmen, etc. Excessive friction is the condition necessary for its production. In the forearm and wrist, where it is especially met with, its recognition is very easy, the crepitation it gives rise to being quite pathognomonic, being neither like that felt in fractures, that of cartilage or emphysema: but which has been compared to the crepitation of starch or of hoar-frost—such as is produced by walking on the snow. Its seat is evidently the sheath of the tendons, and it is probably due to a slight inflammation, first causing too great dryness of the membrane, and afterward giving rise to effusion. It is generally in no-wise serious, disappearing in a few days by rest alone; but it must not be absolutely neglected, for I have seen it in some cases give rise to a fungous transformation of the sheaths; and indeed there is no reason why all the changes which occur in diseases of the joints should not take place here. If there is much pain we apply leeches and poultices, and the resolvent lotions and compression; but rest is indispensable. *Part* xvi., *p.* 330.

Tendons, Reunion of.—Mr. Adams, surgeon to the Royal Orthopedic Hospital, states that the newly-formed connective tissue, or new tendon, gradually assumes the character of the old tendon, so perfectly that no difference can be perceived; it may be formed to the extent of two inches, and it is through the agency of this that the required elongation is maintained.

*   *   *   *   *   *   *   *

Tenotomy.—To perform this operation cleanly and readily, you must use a knife with a cutting edge considerably longer than the breadth of the tendon. You must place the patient on the stomach, and let an assistant put the tendon on the stretch, by endeavoring to flex the foot, then introduce the tenotomy knife with its flat surface parallel with the tendon and close to its edge, but rather toward the posterior surface, pass it obliquely downward, keeping the point close to the tendon, and then by depressing the handle you carry it beneath the tendon; this done, turn the cutting edge toward the tendon, and divide it transversely; the division is indicated by a sudden audible snap and the yielding of the joint. In infants direct pressure of a sharp knife is often sufficient; but in adults a little cutting manipulation is required. On withdrawing the knife apply instantly a compress of lint plaster and bandage. Some surgeons recommend the tendo Achillis to be divided by passing the knife flatwise posteriorly between the tendon and the skin, and then cutting from behind forward; but the other method described is perhaps the better.

Part xxxiii., *p.* 156.

———•◦•———

TESTES.

Scrofulous Diseases of the Testis.—The following is Mr. Curling's account of the symptoms of scrofulous disease of the testis:

"The disease commences insidiously, and is insidious in its progress. The patient's attention is usually first attracted by a slight uneasiness in some part of the gland, generally the epididymis, which on examination is found to be somewhat enlarged, prominent, and hardened. Sometimes the whole organ feels slightly enlarged and indurated, though it more frequently forms a tumor with an unequal and irregular surface. The state of the testis, however, is often marked by small local effusions of fluid in the tunica vaginalis, the surfaces of this membrane being partially adherent. Very little pain is experienced in the part, and there is but slight tenderness on pressure. After the disease has lasted for some time, many months, or even a year and more, making little progress, and often remaining stationary, one of the prominences begins to increase so as to be observed externally, and to feel painful and tender; the skin over it becomes adherent, changes to a livid hue, ulcerates and bursts, giving vent to a soft caseous matter mixed with pus. This is followed by the formation of a fistulous sinus, which discharges a scanty, thin, serous pus, mixed with particles of tubercular matter and often with semen, particularly after venereal excitement. Similar changes may take place in other parts of the testis, occasioning two or more sinuses leading to the interior of the gland. These sinuses sometimes communicate, and they may continue open and discharging for a great length of time. After the deposit has all come away, if the original disease be arrested, and no more tubercular matter formed, reparative changes sometimes take place; the discharge ceases, the fistulæ close up, leaving the organ more or less diminished in size, or entirely wasted, according to the extent to which it had been disorganized by the tubercular deposit. The bursting of the abscess and escape of the tubercular matter are sometimes followed by a hernial protrusion of the testis, as after chronic inflammation of the gland."

The administration of *liquor potassæ* gradually increased to sixty or eighty drops, three times a day, in combination with *iodide* of *potassium* suggested. *Part* ix., *p.* 179.

Fungus of the Testicle.—This disease was ably treated on by Mr. Lawrence in 1808. The testicle, from a variety of causes, as a blow, or gonorrhœa, enlarges and inflames—the skin at last ulcerates, and a fungoid excrescence sprouts from the part. This growth has its origin from the glandular substance of the part, a protrusion of the tubuli seminiferi often taking place. Mr. Lawrence recommends the removal of this substance by escharotics, the ligature, or the knife. Still, as Mr. Syme says, this could not be considered as a very satisfactory operation, although a great improvement on the old one of castration, for it was plain that a portion of the gland must be sacrified in order to preserve the remainder. In order to remedy this evil, Mr. Syme proposes an improvement in the treatment. He says:

When the fungous growth is divided longitudinally, that is from the base toward the circumference, it may be seen to consist of two textures distinguished by their color and arrangement. One is brown and disposed in straight lines, radiating from the base, where they are nearly, or quite close together, toward the circumference, where they are more or less apart, according to the size of the excrescence. The other is white and glandular, lying in the spaces which are afforded by the diverging rays. The former is composed of the tubuli seminiferi, altered in situation but not in structure, while the latter is simply organizable lymph that has been effused into the interstices. The relative proportion of these textures may be seen best by making successive sections of the fungus, parallel with its base. Here the substance of the testicle appears little if at all altered, and presents a mass of uniform brownish color. But in proceeding toward the circumference, each slice shows more and more of the white interstitial substance, until it seems to be the sole constituent. In addition to these facts, which are within reach of the naked eye, Mr. John Goodsir detected in a fungus which I gave him for examination, by the microscope, that it was covered externally by a thin layer of substance possessing the characters of a granulating surface. So that the excrescence might be regarded as merely an extreme degree of exuberant granulation, or what in vulgar language is called " proud flesh."

This observation suggested to me the idea, that by the use of proper means the fungus might be made to retrace its steps, through absorption of the white substance and gradual approximation of the brown, and that

the granulating materials of the surface might thus be enabled to complete the healing process. Pressure was obviously the agent on which
reliance should be chiefly placed for producing the effect desired with this
view, and the most convenient mode of compressing the growth, seemed
to be inclosing it within its proper covering of the scrotum. There is no
loss of substance in this part, as the fungus issuing through a small ulcerated orifice, merely presses the integuments aside, so that they are found
lying in loose folds above the dense ring that encircles the neck of the
protruded mass. It must therefore be easy to obtain from this source, an
abundant supply of materials for the purpose.

Case.—Admitted on account of sores upon his legs, and a fungous excrescence from the testicle, about the size of a filbert. I cut round the
fungus, and extended the incision upward as well as downward, so as to give
it an elliptical form. The integuments were then separated on each side,
and brought over the growth, where they were retained by three stitches.
The scrotum was supported by plasters and a bandage. It appeared at
first as if union by the first intention had taken place completely; but part
of the wound suppurated, without, however, showing the slightest disposition to protrude. The patient might have been allowed to go home soon
after the operation, but was retained until the wound had fairly cicatrized.
Part xi., *p.* 122.

Fungus of the Testicle, treated by Professor Symes' Method.—Dr.
Cormack says: When in Glasgow, we saw, in the Royal Infirmary of that
city, under the care of Dr. Lawrie, a case in which this operation had been
performed with complete success. The patient, a lad, had been
kicked on the scrotum twelve months before. Suppuration, ulceration,
and protusion of the whole anterior and inferior portion of the left testicle
followed; the surface and a great part of the substance of the fungus
appearing to consist of yellow strumous deposit. On the 12th May, Mr.
Symes' operation was performed; and on the 25th, the patient was so
well as to be anxious to return home, but was prevailed on to remain a
few days longer, that the cicatrization might be more secure. Dr. Lawrie
remarked to us, that where the skin was most deficient, and with the
greatest difficulty made to cover the protrusion, *there* the cure was soonest,
and apparently most securely effected. The case was altogether a most
satisfactory testimony in favor of the new method of treating fungus of
the testicle. *Part* xii., *p.* 213.

Syphilitic Affection of the Testis.—[Syphilitic affection of the testis,
says M. Helot, may be distinguished from gonorrhœal affection by the
following circumstances:]

In the gonorrhœal epididymitis, the attack comes on suddenly with the
attendant train of inflammatory symptoms; it shows itself during the
course of gonorrhœa, or at the moment of its disappearance. On the contrary, the commencement of the syphilitic testicle is essentially chronic;
it appears, as we have above remarked, long after the primary symptoms,
constituting a consecutive affection. The gonorrhœal and syphilitic affections are thus two distinct complaints, except where the one terminates in
the other; but the course, lesions, and terminations of these two affections
show no further relation between them.

In the syphilitic affection of the testis, the organ is, even at the commencement, hypertrophied; in the gonorrhœal form, the testis, n the

contrary, commonly preserves its elasticity and its size; the epididymis is principally affected, and if, in exceptional cases, the testis itself participates in the inflammation, an inflammatory swelling follows, quite at variance with the chronic enlargement of the syphilitic complaint. In the gonorrhœal orchitis, the tumor is painful, the skin of the scrotum red, tense, and shining; the cord, when it is affected, becomes painful to the touch. In the syphilitic testicle, the enlargement is most commonly indolent from the commencement to its termination, and pressure with the hand on the testis and cord is unattended with pain. The anatomical characters of the two affections are equally opposed; thus, in the gonorrhœal affection, it is always the epididymis in which the complaint commences, and in the majority of cases, the body of the testis remains free from disease; the contrary happens in the syphilitic affection of the organ.

[Simple hydrocele can scarcely be mistaken for the syphilitic testicle; it is not, however, so easy to distinguish what has been called by Pott, Boyer, Velpeau, etc., "hematocele." M. Helot observes:]

The scrofulous affection of the testicle may, under certain circumstances, be mistaken for syphilitic affection of the testis, and the diagnosis may present great difficulties. Thus, for example, a patient having had syphilis, may be attacked with a scrofulous affection of the testis; what then are the characters drawn from tumor which may tend to clear up the case, and decide whether we have to treat one or the other affection? First of all, in the scrofulous testicle there are two varieties of swelling, one formed by the tuberculous infiltration of the whole organ, the other formed by the development of encysted tubercles, either in the epididymis or in the body of the testis. We have remarked, that in the syphilitic affection of the testis the epididymis is rarely diseased; in the scrofulous affection, on the contrary, the complaint commences usually in that organ, and extends only to the body of the testis at a subsequent period. The scrofulous testicle commences by isolated enlargements; but these nodules become chesnut-shaped, very prominent, standing out in relief, as if attached to the epididymis or testicle. We have seen, in the syphilitic affection of the testis, the cord generally remaining in a healthy condition, or if it enlarges, it does so in a gradual and uniform way, presenting no inequalities or prominences; whereas, in the scrofulous affection, particularly in the advanced stages, it is not uncommon to find the cord studded with tubercles, resembling a bead necklace. Although the course of one or the other affection is similarly chronic, nevertheless it presents differences which may be useful in forming a diagnosis. Thus the syphilitic affection of the testicle is more indolent than the scrofulous, which presents, from time to time, inflammatory accessions, characterized by a sense of tension of pain, which is augmented by the touch.* The ordinary termination, by resolution, of the syphilitic affection of the organ, opposed as it is to the suppuration of the scrofulous disease of the organ, is likewise very important in differential diagnosis.

The syphilitic is often difficult to be distinguished from the cancerous affection of the organ. How many tumors of the testis have been removed by the knife, which might have been cured had the true nature of the complaint been suspected. The rapid development in the encephalic tumor of the testis, the considerable size it will attain, its softness, which may often impose on the surgeon, leading him to believe it fluctuative; the unequal resistance it presents, the darting pains which occasionally come on, mark a striking contrast with that uniform hardness, indolent character, and moderate size of the syphilitic enlargement of the organ. The cord in the cancerous affection is often knotted, hard, and unequal, and we know how uncommon the uniform hypertrophy of the cord is in the syphilitic affection. The engorgement of the glands in the iliac fossa is observed sometimes in the cancerous affection of the testis, but never happens in the complaint we are treating of. Authors, and, among others, Sir Astley Cooper, have described, under the name of scirrhus of the testis, a variety of cancer which might be more easily confounded with syphilitic affections of the testicle, as its development is slower than in encephaloid disease, and presents, from its commencement, hard nodules; but these are hard from their formation, and become more and more so in scirrhous affections, which we do not observe in the venereal testicle. Notwithstanding the characters above given, the surgeon, amid all his doubts, has no other proof than a rational treatment to follow, in extricating himself from his uncertainty.

[The syphilitic testicle is one of the consecutive secondary symptoms of syphilis; it may be said to border on the tertiary, hence it will require the treatment applicable to these periods.]

Combine the mercurial treatment with iodide of potassium. Give three quarters of a grain of iodide of mercury in a pill every night, and one or two grains of iodide of potassium twice or thrice during the day. Continue this treatment for some time after a cure is effected. When effusion into the tunica vaginalis occurs, the fluid is generally absorbed; occasionally, however, it remains, and it is necessary to tap and inject the sac; before doing this we should endeavor to procure its absorption, by mercurial frictions on the scrotum, or the application of bego plaster with mercury. We should also try compression.   *Part xiv., p.* 229.

Treatment of Swelled Testicle by Narcotics.—Mr. Jackson relates several cases in the practice of Mr. Gay; cases of gonorrhœal orchitis, some of them very acute with febrile symptoms. The treatment consisted in low diet, a purgative dose, and the administration of tincture of henbane in the dose of one drachm three times a day. The treatment was in all speedily successful.   *Part xviii., p.* 214.

Testicle, Enlarged.—When compression is wanted, use Hutchinson's air compressor. A kind of double nightcap, made of impermeable material, such as Macintosh, or oil-silk, is folded over the testicle, and then, by means of a stop-cock and force-pump, air is forced into the bag, by which almost any degree of compression can be produced. Some forms of hydrocele may be treated in this way.   *Part xxxi., p.* 169.

Swelled Testicle.—Dissolve gutta percha in bisulphuret of carbon, and spread the substance over the part affected. (Recommended by M. Ellefson.) It immediately becomes dry and stiff, and forms a thin, tight, and adhesive covering, which loosens at the edges after three or four days, when it must be repeated.   *Part xxxii., p.* 180.

Belladonna in Orchitis.—M. de Larue recommends the following application, which, he says, promptly relieves the pain, and leads to a cure in a mean period of eight days. Lard, 60 parts; aqueous ext. of belladonna, 16 parts. It should be applied generally every two hours in considerable quantity, the parts being afterward covered with a linen compress, which is to remain unchanged.   *Part xxxvii., p.* 311.

TETANUS.

Opium Smoking—By means of the common pipe, suggested by Dr. James Johnson, as a remedial agent in tetanus, hydrophobia, tic douloureux, etc. *Part v., p.* 56.

Belladonna in Tetanus.—The value of belladonna in cases of tetanus has been repeatedly pointed out. It is surprising what large doses of the different sedatives may be given in this disease. Dr. Hutchinson, of Nottingham, publishes some cases of this description, in one of which five grains of the extract were successfully administered, and in another the dose was ultimately four grains every two hours, until the disease was completely subdued.

From the success of this treatment in tetanus, Dr. Hutchinson recommends that large doses of belladonna be given in cases of hydrophobia, so as to relieve the spasms affecting the muscles of the glottis and larynx.
Part x., p. 29.

Treatment of Tetanus—Use of Indian Hemp, Croton Oil, Opium, Emetics, etc.—In the first case recorded, Mr. Miller used the tincture of the hemp and the resinous extract. It was in a girl seven years of age, laboring under traumatic tetanus. She took three grains of the resinous extract every half hour—a full dose for an adult, under ordinary circumstances, without repetition. Narcotism was usually produced by a few doses, but only continued a short time, when the doses were recommenced.

Under ordinary circumstances, Mr. Miller doubts the efficacy of this medicine as an anodyne and hypnotic, and considers that its chief value rests in its power to subdue inordinate muscular spasm. We suspect that if the experiments of Mr. Donovan had been known to Mr. Miller at the time, he would have preferred the tincture of the resin instead of the resin itself, not only on account of its more certain effects, but also for its easier mode of administration. In a case of idiopathic tetanus in Guy's Hospital, Dr. Babington prescribed the tincture of the extract in the proportions of three grains to half a drachm of rectified spirit, to be given every half hour. The effects were variable, but upon the whole beneficial. This patient took in the space of five days 248 grains of the extract, although a single grain produced powerful effects in a healthy individual. Five doses of three grains each were given before any good effects were produced, and after that five-grain doses were administered every two hours for some time. This case shows that in cases of tetanus we must not be deterred from administering very large doses if smaller ones fail. Another authority on the use of this drug is Dr. Clendinning. He disagrees with Mr. Miller, and asserts that he has found it to be a valuable hypnotic and anodyne, both conciliating sleep and lulling pain; and another valuable quality is its power of allaying cough without the pernicious effects of opium. We protest most seriously against the baneful practice of giving opium in one form or another in bronchial affections, with the view of allaying cough. It may, indeed, allay this symptom, but it acts most prejudicially upon the mucous membrane, producing a stoppage of secretion and an increase of congestion. We hope, however, that the resinous extract of Indian hemp may afford considerable relief in a most troublesome class of bronchial disorders, in which the practitioner is incessantly called upon by his patient to give relief, which, by opium, he can only do by protracting the disease. In articular rheumatism, or severe bronchitis, we may be able, by means of hemp, to put the patient at once under the double influence of a diuretic laxative, and an anodyne antispasmodic; a saline solution, with or without colchicum, correcting the blood and secretions, unimpeded by the narcotic, whose whole influence appears to be expended on the tissues, seats of pain and irritation. Another class of cases in which we may find this medicine useful is that of low fever, by securing the enjoyment of that great restorative—tranquil sleep—without any neutralizing inconvenience. In the treatment of another case of tetanus, by Mr. Stapleton, the effect of all remedies seemed perfectly useless; and this gentleman had recourse to profound *intoxication*. Under any other circumstances we should say that this remedy was improper, but in the case alluded to it was successful. Mr. Stapleton provided himself with a mixture of alcohol and water in equal parts. He gave six ounces of this mixture at once, and four ounces more in a quarter of an hour. In twenty-five minutes the patient laid on his side and fell into a profound sleep—every muscle was in a state of quiet relaxation, and the sense of pain had vanished as if by a charm. For seventy-two hours he was kept under the influence of the remedy; when it was withdrawn the tetanic symptoms returned and were as quickly relieved, when the alcohol was again resorted to. The relief, however, was only temporary, as the patient eventually died.

[The following case of idiopathic tetanus is given by Dr. Newbigging: The patient was a baker, who, while perspiring profusely, went out to chop wood, at a time of intense cold. In the evening of the same day he complained of tetanic symptoms, which gradually increased. Dr. N. saw him first a week after the attack. The pulse was natural; bowels constipated; urine scanty. He was bled to 12 oz.; a drop of croton oil was administered, and a large blister was applied to the upper part of the spine. The bowels were opened by the oil, and he felt altogether relieved. Three days after he was again bled to 14 oz.; and a strong dose of morphia with 30 drops of tinct. cannabis ind. were given at bed-time. Three days after this, spasmodic action had commenced in the limbs; the dose of morphia was then increased, and ordered to be given four times a day, and elaterium to be used as a purgative. Next day croton oil was again had recourse to, the elaterium having proved ineffectual. Dr. Abercrombie, at the same time, recommended the use of arsenic, which was given with the morphia. He continued to improve for a week, when he was suddenly seized with great dysphagia and tremors, which were soon removed by placing him in the erect position. His medicines having been discontinued for two or three days, were renewed. About five weeks after the commencement of the attack, he expectorated a quantity of pus mixed with mucus, which expectoration continued three weeks. He had afterward thickening of the spinous process of the cervical vertebræ, and was attacked with anasarca, which was subdued by diuretics, actively administered, and in about three months he was able to return to business.]

The principal features of interest in this case of what is considered a rare disease in this country, are the gradual affection of the different muscles of the body, commencing with those of the jaw, and the successful issue of the treatment which, however varied, may be considered to have resulted from the persevering employment of croton oil and opium: for although arsenic, Indian hemp, colchicum, etc., were administered to him at different periods, I believe to none of these was so much benefit attributed by us—and he was occasionally visited by Dr. Abercrombie, Sir George Ballingal, and Dr. Duncan—as from the exhibition of opium in full doses, with the occasional use of croton oil; for, whether we consider this medicine to be endowed with any specific effect or not, as reasoning from somewhat analogous cases of nervous affections, I feel disposed to do, it certainly seemed to be followed by greater relief to the tetanic symptoms than when an ordinary purgative, such as scammony, gamboge, etc., was exhibited. I have occasionally observed benefit from the Indian hemp in allaying irritation and causing sleep, particularly when opium was contra-indicated; but I am somewhat doubtful of the value of this remedy in tetanus, and am disposed to think, that no case where opium is so decidedly indicated can be benefited by the administration of hemp, if the former powerful remedy has failed to be of service.

[It seems probable that in this case some degree of inflammation at the upper part of the spine produced the complaint, followed by formation of matter which subsequently became connected with the organs of respiration.]

A case of traumatic tetanus, which was cured by the use of emetics, is published by M. Allut. The patient was treated first by opium and musk, turpentine liniment along the spine, and leeches to the neck, but hourly grew worse. It occurred to M. Allut that he had seen the use of emetics proposed, and in despair he administered a strong dose. On returning four hours after, he found his patient decidedly better, and the urine, which had been suppressed for 24 hours, had returned. The treatment was continued for eight days, without any vomiting being produced, or more than one stool per diem, and the man made a rapid and perfect recovery. *Part* xi., *p.* 22.

Acupuncture in Protracted Lock-Jaw.—Vide Art. "Lock-Jaw."

Treatment of Tetanus.—With regard to the treatment of tetanus—opium has been given in nervous cases, as much as twenty grains every three hours. In other cases, stupor has ensued if the tetanic spasm had not relaxed. A case is recorded of a patient taking 110 bottles of port wine in forty-two days, and he was cured. Cold affusion has been said to have cured a few cases. Blood-letting is not curative, but it appears to be palliative in the acute cases. Hydrocyanic acid, mercury, digitalis, and ammonia, have been tried without effect. Dr. Elliotson gave carbonate of iron, in enormous quantities successfully. Hamilton and Abernethy have recommended purgatives, and each one recommends his own hobby. Turpentine has been considered one of the most effectual purgatives in this disease; but this, like others, cannot effect a cure. Indeed, very few of the remedies that have been tried have had any effect toward a cure. Looking rationally at the thing, says Dr. J. C. B. Williams, I should attempt to cure idiopathic tetanus on the same principles as rheumatic inflammation, using the strongest counter-irritants, liquor ammoniæ, and calomel and opium in very large doses, with colchicum, my favorite anti-rheumatic remedy. In traumatic tetanus I cannot say much about the expectation of curing this form of the disease, but there are some cases recorded of cures having been effected by Indian hemp. *Part* xii., *p.* 47.

Mitigation of the Symptoms in Fatal Cases of Tetanus.—Prof. Colles

asserts, that when cases of common tetanus are to become fatal we do not
find the paroxysms grow less frequent, but they become apparently milder,
and on the contrary, when the patient is recovering the intervals between
the paroxysms are lengthened; but the violence of the last paroxysm that
man may have may be as great as that of any of the preceding ones.
Sometimes on visiting a patient he tells you he is better—he is now able
to put two fingers between his teeth, whereas a little while ago he was
only able to put one; he *feels* himself better, his jaw can be opened more,
and his limbs are more flexible; his friends meet you with a smiling countenance, and everything is congratulation. Now, what are you to expect?
Why, that the next paroxysm the patient gets will ·carry him off—the
very next paroxysm will certainly be the fatal one.   *Part* xii., *p.* 47.

Idiopathic Tetanus.—The patient, aged thirty years, had felt for some
days unpleasant sensations, as stiffness and pain, in different parts of his
body, but on his admission to the hospital the muscles of the jaws, neck,
both extremities, back, and abdomen were in a state of rigidity; the body
was curved forward in consequence of the head and loins being drawn
backward; every two or three minutes the pain and muscular contractions
were increased, the paroxysms lasting about five or six seconds. He had
not received a wound, but had been much exposed to cold and wet. In
the treatment of this case, Dr. Watson, under the impression that the
spinal cord or its coverings were inflamed, ordered local bleeding and
counter-irritation. The pain in the loins was relieved, but there was no
alleviation of the tetanic convulsions. This led him to infer that the affection of the nervous centres was functional and not organic, consequently
care should be used, lest, by too active treatment, the patient's strength
be worn out. Do not depend so much on stimulants, but support the
strength on nutritious diet, such as animal jellies. Give opium in large
doses with hydrocyanic acid; also a well-sustained course of purgatives, as
colocynth pills with castor-oil, cupping over the spine, turpentine glysters.
A colocynth pill, with a drop of croton-oil, and occasionally an ounce of
castor-oil, and on two occasions ten grains of calomel with the aid of purgative enemata sufficed. The character of the fecal evacuations in relation
to the spasms is interesting: whilst they were natural there was no relief
of the symptoms; but when, by the use of purgatives, they became thin
and offensive, there was a very marked alleviation of the man's sufferings,
and from the stools becoming again more natural, the spasms, both permanent and convulsive, speedily gave way. This case, therefore, is one
corroborative of the opinion, that whatever else may be judged necessary
for the relief of the patient, much reliance must be placed in respect of a
cure on a decided and well-sustained course of purgatives; and this, notwithstanding the at first ordinary character of the evacuations. We all
know what a difficult thing it is, in many instances, thoroughly to unload
the bowels, and when this is at last effected, what a wonderful amelioration is produced in many convulsive diseases not very dissimilar in some
of their characters to the present. No doubt, it must be acknowledged,
that this is more likely to occur in idiopathic than traumatic tetanus, where
we have another and obvious source of irritation.   *Part* xiii.; *p.* 57.

Traumatic Tetanus—Recovery.—In the earlier stage of this case, under
care of Dr. Greenhow, calomel and opium carried to ptyalism nearly removed the symptoms: not so, however, in the more advanced stage, and

from the success which frequently results from the use of opium and tartarized antimony, a trial was made, which produced a most tranquillizing effect, causing sleep, the relief of spasms, and the general soothing of the system. Patient took half a grain of tartarized antimony, with one of opium and three of calomel, every three hours, having a double dose every night, and an enema in the morning. *Part* xiv., *p.* 54.

Electricity in Tetanus.—Try electricity. Use a *continued* current, passed *down* the nerves in the direction of their ramifications. According to Prof. Matteucci, the tendency of this *direct continued current*, when its application is sufficiently prolonged, is to *diminish the excitability* of the nerves, and thereby to produce a temporary paralysis. *Part* xvi., *p.* 100.

Traumatic Tetanus cured by the Destruction of the Cicatrix by a Red-hot Iron.—A robust youth, aged twenty-two years, was seized with trismus on the ninth day after the receipt of a wound on the temple, when it had almost healed. He experienced a painful constriction of the chest, followed by reiterated convulsions and opisthotonos. Suppression of urine, delirium, dysphagia, and unconsciousness followed.

All other means having failed to abate the severity of the disease, M. Remy, on the seventh day of the attack, determined to have recourse to the mode of treatment advised by Larrey, viz., cauterizing the cicatrix in its whole extent with an iron heated to a white heat. The symptoms immediately underwent a great improvement: the convulsive movements became less frequent, and soon ceased entirely; consciousness returned, and the urinary excretion reappeared; but the muscular rigidity continued, the slightest movement or attempt at the deglutition of fluids produced a sense of suffocation; the recumbent posture had become impossible, and the patient exclaimed against a breath of air. This condition, which lasted from four to five days, disappeared under the use of digitalis in large doses. In fifteen days more convalescence was complete.

Part xx., *p.* 62.

Tetanus—Traumatic.—Bransby B. Cooper advises, when tetanus is threatened in consequence of a punctured wound, to convert the latter into an incised wound by laying it freely open to the same depth as the original puncture; and if it is then found that a branch of nerve had been punctured or partially divided, cut it completely through. The plan of cauterizing the wound, with a view to promote suppuration, is unadvisable. Amputation is not generally advisable after tetanic symptoms have set in; there are cases, however, in which it may be resorted to, especially when the injury is so severe that the limb is not likely ever to be a useful one.

Part xx., *p.* 114.

Idiopathic Tetanus treated by Galvanism.—A case of idiopathic tetanus successfully treated by galvanism, applied in the form of shocks from an electro-magnetic apparatus, along the spine, over the masseter muscles, and in the course of the great sciatic nerves, is related by Mr. H. Hailey.

Part xxi., *p.* 91.

Case of Traumatic Tetanus treated by strong Voluntary Action of the Respiratory Muscles.—[The following case is from Cruveilhier's work on Pathological Anatomy.

The case was one of a peasant who labored under tetanus produced by the forcible separation of the thumb from the hand.].

The patient was young, and full of life and courage, and I ventured to assure him of being cured if he submitted to my orders. I placed myself before him, and instructed him to respire in a measured time, making as deep inspirations as possible. To direct him in this fatiguing exercise I beat before him the measure *à deux temps.* During an hour there was an attack of suffocation or strangulation. My place was taken by assistants, who relieved each other, and at the end of four hours the patient fell into a profound sleep. On his waking, the same system was recommenced, which was again followed by sleep. After the suspension of this treatment, there were slight exacerbations, but they speedily gave way, and he was completely cured.　　　　　　　　　　　　　　*Part* xxi., *p.* 96.

Treatment of Traumatic Tetanis.—Mr. De Ricci thinks we are justified, with the view of removing the exciting cause, in amputating the entire part, or dividing the nerves leading to it. In tetanus the energies of the brain are *minus*, and those of the spinal marrow *plus ;* therefore we must increase the first by stimulants, wine, brandy, and Indian hemp, and reduce the latter by the careful use of tobacco enemata and fomentations (fifteen grs. of tobacco to eight ounces of boiling water) every half hour, so as to keep up a state of nausea. The spine should also be well rubbed with a liniment of croton oil and turpentine. It is right to say that idiosyncrasy in some instances renders the use of tobacco extremely dangerous. The symptoms in this case, are, the countenance assuming a deadly hue and ghastly appearance, and the pulse becoming quivering and intermittent. When these occur the administration should be stopped, and stimulants immediately resorted to. These means, with paying attention to the state of the bowels by croton oil or other strong purgative, and bringing the patient under the influence of tobacco, as rapidly as possible, are the principal means upon which we have to rely.　　　*Part* xxii., *p.* 88.

Treatment of Tetanus—Traumatic.—M. Bresse, surgeon at the Military Hospital at Rennes, has cured cases by the use of frictions with the tincture of belladonna, composed of five parts of extract to eleven of alcohol, applied all over the body, more particularly over the rigid parts.
　　　　　　　　　　　　　　　　　　Part xxii., *p.* 90.

Indian Hemp in Tetanus.—In three cases of this dreadful disease the cannabis indica seemed to Prof. Miller to answer effectually. In other cases of the disease, although it failed to cure, it never failed to relieve. The dose was three grains of the extract, or thirty drops of the tincture, to be repeated every half hour, hour, or two hours, the object being to produce and maintain narcotism. There is a very marked tolerance of the remedy.　　　　　　　　　　　　　　*Part* xxiii., *p.* 287.

Traumatic Tetanus.—A case of this disease was treated locally by Mr. Eddows, and with the best success. It was traumatic, arising from injury to the ball of the thumb. The jaws became closed with slight general tetanic symptoms, a blister was applied over the back of the hand, and acetate of morphia, and afterward the tincture of aconite were applied until mxv. of the last were applied at one time. There remained a contraction of the flexors for some time, but this was removed by a splint.
　　　　　　　　　　　　　　　　　　Part xxiii., *p.* 323.

Treatment of Tetanus.—Use frictions of chloroform all over the body. Recovery was thus brought on in a case in four days.

' In a case under Mr. Cock, that gentleman pursued the tonic plan of
' treatment. Three grains of disulphate of quina were given every fourth
hour, and twelve ounces of wine allowed per day. Recovery gradually
took place.

In the Hôtel Dieu of Marseilles, a case of tetanus from wound of the
toes was arrested by large doses of disulphate of quinine, maximum forty-
five grains in one day. The cure was completed in about a fortnight.

Part xxiv., *p.* 67.

Worrara Poison as a last resort in Tetanus.—Mr. Campbell, surgeon of
the 55th regiment, India, says he thinks the Worrara poison has been
proposed justly as a last resort in tetanus, by inserting the poison in the
finger, and tying a ligature above the wound, so as to regulate its action
and effect in the system. *Part* xxiv., *p.* 336.

Tetanus and Hydrophobia.—From the experiments of Dr. Marshall
Hall, he arrives at the two following practical conclusions : 1st. That the
tetanic patient be preserved from all external excitement absolutely.
2nd. The hydrophobic patient, whilst equally preserved from excitement.
should be submitted to efficient tracheotomy. *Part* xxvii., *p.* 59.

Tetanus following Lesions of the Uterus, Abortion and Parturition.—
[From a series of twenty-four cases, Dr. Simpson proves that traumatic
tetanus does occasionally supervene as a secondary obstetrical disease. He
then enters upon the]

Nature of Puerperal Tetanus.—It will be granted, I believe, by all
pathologists that the existence of an injury or a wound upon the external
parts of the body, is by far the most common cause of tetanus. After
abortion and parturition we have the existence, upon the interior of the
uterus, of a similar state of lesion. All authorities seem now generally
agreed as to the facts (1) that the human decidua is, as was maintained in
the last century by Krummacher, the thickened and hypertrophied mucous
membrane of the uterus, (2) that the epithelial or superficial layer of it
separates from its basement or outer layer in abortion and after delivery ;
and (3) that this separation or solution of continuity of tissue, as well as
the rupture of the organic attachments of the placenta from the uterus,
leaves the interior of this organ so far in the condition of an external
wound, or with a new or raw surface for the time-being exposed. Obstetrical tetanus has, in this respect, an exciting cause essentially similar to
surgical tetanus. And perhaps the great reason why this state of lesion of
the interior of the uterus does not more frequently give rise to tetanus is,
simply this, that the uterus is itself principally, or indeed almost entirely,
supplied by nerves from the sympathetic system, while apparently, as
stated by Mr. Curling and other pathologists, tetanus is an affection far
more easily excited by lesions of parts supplied by nerves from the cerebro-
spinal system, than by lesions of parts supplied by nerves from the
sympathetic system.

Tetanus is known to follow wounds very various in their degree and
severity. " Whether (says Professor Wood) the wound is trifling or severe
seems to be of little consequence," as far as regards the supervention of
secondary tetanus. By what pathological mechanism a wound or lesion of
a part can, under any circumstances, lead on to an attack of tetanic disease,
is an inquiry regarding which we as yet possess little information ; and in

this respect, the production of obstetrical tetanus is not more obscure than the production of surgical tetanus.

The disease, when developed, essentially consists of an exalted or super-excited state of the reflex spinal system, or of some segment or portion of that system.

Treatment of Puerperal Tetanus.—In obstetrical tetanus, no kind of local treatment to the seat of the original uterine lesion could be well applied, or would probably be of any avail, if applied. And, as to *consti-tutional* means, perhaps the most important are—

1st. The greatest possible quietude and isolation of the patient from all irritation, corporeal or mental, during the course, and for some time even after the resolution of the disease.

2nd. The special avoidance of painful and generally impracticable attempts at opening the mouth in order to swallow ; but sustaining the strength of the patient, and allaying the thirst by enemata, or by fluids applied to the general surface of the body.

3rd. If there is any well-grounded hope of irritating matters lodged in the bowels, acting as an exciting or aggravating cause, to sweep out the intestinal canal at the commencement of the disease with an appropriate enema.

4th. To relax the tonic spasms of the affected muscles, and diminish the exalted reflex excitability of the spinal system by sedatives, or antispas-modies ; with the prospect of either directly subduing this morbid reflex excitability, or of warding off the immediate dangers of the disease, and allowing the case to pass on, from an acute and dangerous attack, to a sub-acute, and far more hopeful and tractable form of the malady.

Various sedatives and antispasmodics have been recommended to fulfill this last most vital and important indication in the treatment of tetanus— as belladonna, stramonium, hemlock, henbane, musk, camphor, indian hemp, hydrocyanic acid, valerian, etc. Perhaps the two drugs of this class that have hitherto been most used, and relied upon, are opium by the mouth, and tobacco by enema.

Latterly the antispasmodic action of sulphuric ether and chloroform has been repeatedly employed to allay that exalted state of the reflex nervous system, and to relax that resulting tonic contraction of the maxillary and other muscles, which constitute the essence of tetanus.

Chloroform in sufficient doses acts as a direct sedative upon the reflex nervous system, and upon exalted muscular contractility. In conse-quence of this action, it affords us one of our surest and most manageable means of allaying common convulsive attacks ; if used in tetanus its action will require to be sustained for many hours, or oftener perhaps for many days. And there is abundant proof of the safety with which its continuous action may be kept up under proper care and watching. For instance, a few months ago I saw, with Dr. Combe, a case of convulsions of the most severe and apparently hopeless kind in an infant of six weeks. The disease at once yielded, and ultimately altogether disappeared under the action of chloroform, which required to be used almost continuously for thirteen days ; as much as 100 ounces of the drug being used during the period.

Part xxix., *p.* 65.

Tetanus.—Dr. Hodges, of Somerset, recommends to apply a solution of morphia to the wound instead of giving it internally. The following is a good formula : Hydrochloride of morphia, one scruple ; tincture of hyoscyamus, two drachms; water, three ounces. Moisten a piece of lint with this solution and keep it on the wound. *Part* xxx., *p.* 39.

Tetanus.—Dr. Hobart, of the Cork Dispensary, recommends, on the first appearance of this disease, to try to remove the source of irritation, by dividing the nerves going to the part; or, if the wound be in the skin and very trifling, either make deep incisions around it or excise it altogether; but if the wound be such as would materially injure the limb independently of the tetanic complication, it is better to amputate at once. If this does not suffice, we must use some agent to render the nervous system less sensitive to the irritating cause, its effect being long kept up—such agents we have in chloroform, nicotine, and wourali. Chloroform causes congestion of the bronchial tubes, and nicotine has an extreme depressing influence on the circulation. Now wourali does not act on the heart or other involuntary muscles at all, and preference should be given to it. Artificial respiration will be necessary, if that function become seriously embarrassed. *Part* xxxvi., *p.* 40.

Traumatic Tetanus.—A case of traumatic tetanus was lately treated at St. Thomas's, with some degree of success by the administration of nicotine. At first, one-twelfth of a minim was given hourly, continued with a little brandy and water; this dose was gradually increased. The effects were found to be very transitory. It produced, at first, giddiness, profuse perspiration and nausea, together with a slower and feebler pulse, and marked alleviation of the muscular spasms. In about a quarter of an hour the pulse became fuller and stronger, the face flushed, and the tetanic symptoms as severe as ever. When given too freely, it produces faintness and sickness, even an intermittent pulse, without alleviating the symptoms. *Part* xxxviii., *p.* 46.

Tetanus.—In *acute* tetanus, Prof. Erichsen says that all drugs are utterly useless in retarding, mitigating, suspending, or arresting its progress. Division of the nerve, leading to the wound when it can be found and isolated, has been done with success, and it is better to do this pretty high up in the limb, beyond the sphere of the local irritation. The occasional inhalation of chloroform will alleviate, though it will not cure, acute tetanus. We must remember that we have an exhausting disease to deal with, and the patient will soon sink unless supported. If the case, however, assume the *subacute* or *chronic* form, calomel and opium, and even belladonna may be employed with advantage. Keep the patient quiet and support his strength. *Part* xxxix., *p.* 62.

Hypodermic Injections.—In very violent cases the injection of a third of a grain of acetate of morphia beneath the skin, says Mr. Hunter, will procure sleep and cessation of the movements for some hours. It is only a palliative, but in this manner may be used to procure the rest, the absence of which causes so much exhaustion. *Part* xxxix., *p.* 51.

Tetanus—Poisoning by Strychnia.—Wourali poison is a direct sedative to the muscular system, causing complete relaxation to the fibre. It is a direct antidote to strychnine. It does not appear to have been used in poisoning cases in the human subject, but Dr. Harley has succeeded in saving the lives of animals to which strychnine had been administered in poisonous doses. M. Vella, of Turin, has successfully used woorara in cases of tetanus at the French Military Hospital during the late war. In one case, which proved successful, two grains of woorara were dissolved in nine drachms of water, and compresses moistened with the solution were applied to the wound, the strength being gradually increased to fifteen grains in fourteen drachms of water, and the compresses renewed every third or fifth hour. This mode of treatment requires and deserves extensive trial.   *Part* xl., *p.* 42.

THROAT.

Treatment of Sore Throat, or Angina, by Alum.—*Vide* Art. "Alum."
Phagedenic Ulceration of the Throat.—Dr. J. J. Ross observes as follows on the topical use of iodine : Another case, in which the local use of the tincture of iodine is of signal efficacy, is that of ulcers of the tonsils and fauces—specific or non-specific. I have seen the ugliest sores in this situation put on quite a healthy appearance in a few days under its use. It is highly recommended by Ricord, and certainly I do not know any thing equal to it in such cases. It is best used in the form of a gargle ; thus : R Tinct. iodini, ʒj. to ʒij.; tinct. opii, ʒj.; aquæ, ʒvj. Mix. Use three or four times a day.   *Part* vi., *p.* 119.

Treatment of Malignant Sore Throat by Emetics.—In a paper " On the present state of Therapeutical Inquiry," Dr. Arnott mentions a remedy for malignant sore throat, which, like the invaluable discovery of Jenner, was found out by accident at a time when an endemic and supposed contagious species of malignant sore throat (diphtherite ?) was very prevalent at St. Helena. A sergeant's wife had four children laboring under this affection, at the same time that she was suffering from some illness for which an emetic mixture had been prescribed.]
It consisted of a strong solution of tartrate of antimony, a certain quantity of which was to be taken at intervals until vomiting should be excited. The woman, supposing that this mixture had been sent for one of her children, the last attacked with sore throat, not only administered it in the large doses intended for herself, but continued to exhibit it during the day so as to keep up a frequent and severe vomiting. I accompanied her medical attendant in his evening visit, when we found the child in a state of extreme exhaustion, but in all other respects much relieved. It rapidly recovered ; and the practice of severe and continued vomiting was adopted during my stay on the island in many subsequent cases of the same disease, with equal success. I have learned also that severe and continued vomiting was employed by the medical officers of our army in Egypt to arrest the rapidly disorganizing ophthalmia which then prevailed ; and it is manifestly applicable to other diseases of the same character, requiring the adoption of prompt and decided measures.   *Part* xi., *p.* 59.

Wound of the Throat.—[Remarking upon the difference of opinion which exists as to the treatment of cut-throat, Mr. Park relates a successful case which he lately attended. He found his patient, a woman aged 54, of melancholy temperament, lying on the floor in a state of syncope. The wound of the throat was four inches in length and gaping ; and the larynx was opened to such an extent, as to admit the point of the finger between the thyroid cartilage and the os hyoides. Mr. Park's account of the treatment is as follows :]

Having cleansed the wound, and adjusted its mangled parts, I proceeded at once to stitch it up, and to strap it closely with adhesive plaster. I applied a layer of lint and a bandage, and placed the head elevated upon the pillow, so as to keep the divided parts in juxtaposition. The pulse was so feeble, that I administered a little brandy-and-water, which revived her; and after giving the necessary instructions to the attendants, I left, and sent the following mixture: Tincture of opium, forty minims; tincture of henbane, a drachm: camphor mixture, four ounces; mix: to take a fourth part every four hours. The wound was dressed daily, the general health attended to; and it was surprising to witness how speedily the wound healed. On the first day, she could not speak at all; on the second and third, she could, but in a low, husky whisper: and on the fourth, she articulated very well. I was careful in requesting the attendants to watch and keep her perfectly quiet; and thus the case proceeded most favorably for fourteen days, when I pronounced her convalescent, and ceased to attend.

In the account of the preceding case, I trust the question, whether union by the first intention in these cases can take place, will be completely set at rest; for, notwithstanding the magnitude of the wound, there was very little suppuration, and that merely superficial; and the short space of time ere the wound had perfectly cicatrized bears out the assertion, and confirms the opinions of Sir Charles Bell and Mr. Fergusson. Of course, in all cases of this description, it will be essentially necessary for the surgeon carefully to watch the effect of closing the wound on the organs of respiration, whether the epiglottis be injured. *Part* xv., *p.* 203.

Treatment of Cut-Throat.—[Speaking of suicidal cut-throat, as discussed in Mr. Ellis's lectures on clinical surgery, the reviewer in the "Monthly Journal" says:]

Now, if (as we are led to infer from the manner in which the cases are detailed) Mr. E. advocates *immediate* closure of the wound, we consider the practice as at once dangerous and useless. Dangerous, because under any circumstances there is risk to be apprehended from swelling of the divided parts from infiltration, and this is necessarily increased by stitching the wound closely. Besides, after the active hemorrhage has been arrested, there is always more or less oozing of blood, which, if it does not escape readily by the wound, is apt to trickle down the air-passages, and may prove fatal by suffocation. Mr. Liston relates a case in his work on Practical Surgery, where the patient, except for his timely aid, would have been suffocated from the pressure caused by confined coagula, although the air-passages had not been opened into. The addition of compresses and plasters must of course add to the danger, on the interruption they cause to the breathing and circulation. And the practice is useless, because the constant separation of the deeper seated parts of the wound, caused by the slightest motion of the head, by attempts to swallow or cough, together with the passage of air and mucus between the divided surfaces, all render immediate union of such wounds impossible. Sewing up the wound, then, can only serve to render the appearance of the unfortunate patient less frightful, whilst it greatly increases his real danger. The insertion of a single point of suture near each end of the incision, in extensive transverse wounds, for the purpose of diminishing the exposed surface, is not liable, of course, to these objections. *Part* xv., *p.* 203.

Foreign Bodies in the Mucous Canals.—A portion of an ear of barley slips into the nostrils, with the stalk end foremost. The least touch' of a body so formed, in such a situation, thrusts it further inward. For one or two days it produces considerable irritation, which, however, at length subsides ; and the foreign body, coated with thick mucus, is ejected without effort. A small piece of leaf of a vegetable gets into the ventricle of the glottis ; and causes great irritation and coughing for some hours. It is soon enveloped in mucus, and comes quietly away next day.

These facts show what the surgeon should do under similar circumstances. He should not with his forceps irritate still more parts already too much irritated. He is not to allow even any effort of sneezing, in the one case, or unnecessary hawking in the other. He is to require the patient to be kept quiet, that the body may continue in one situation, so as to acquire as soon as possible the coating which facilitates the ejection.

Part xix., *p.* 157.

Treatment of Wounds of the Larynx or Trachea.—It has been a subject of much discussion, whether, in cases of free transverse division of the larynx or trachea, we ought to bring the wound together by sutures, or to leave it open. If the wound is closed by sutures there is danger of asphyxia from accumulation of blood and mucus in the tubes ; and if, on the other hand, the wound is not healed at an early period, the patient will seldom recover. Mr. Eves says :

The treatment which I should adopt in a case in which the larynx or trachea has been freely divided, would be, after all hemorrhage was perfectly stopped, and after waiting a short period to be assured on that point, to bring the parts accurately together by sutures, introduced even through the cartilages, if necessary ; then, if great difficulty of breathing should arise, so as to threaten immediate asphyxia, either from derangement of the rima glottidis, or from accumulation of fluid in the bronchial tubes and cells, I should immediately adopt the suggestion thrown out by Mr. Porter, of Dublin, and open the trachea by a longitudinal incision ; of course, this must not be thought of, except there appears an absolute necessity for such a step ; but it is satisfactory to know, that we have the means in our power of rendering that line of treatment, which is certainly the best, free from the dangers which have hitherto been apparently connected with it. I would also strongly insist upon the necessity of preventing a drop of nourishment from passing by the mouth for a few days, and the necessity of nourishing the patient by enemata. To prove the sufficiency of this mode of conveying nourishment, I would refer to a case treated in the Meath Hospital, in which Mr. Porter states, the patient was thus supported for several months, positively refusing all food by the mouth. *Part* xx., *p.* 275.

Throat—Relaxed.—Employ a gargle made with three or four grains of tannin to the ounce of water. *Part* xxi., *p.* 326.

Inflammation and ulceration of the Throat and Tongue—Nitrate of Copper.—Dr. Moore reports a case in which the uvula and soft palate, with the structures posterior to these, had been removed by the ulcerative process, extending deeply also at the base of the tongue, partially destroying the epiglottis. The mucous membrane presented an ulcerated and abraded appearance. A trace of tonsil remained ; but from pain affecting the right ear, it is natural to suppose the ulcerative process had extended along the Eustachian tube.

A variety of means having been used, the patient was eventually cured by the administration of the mistura ferri composita, with iodine, and locally, the use of a gargle of dilute hydrochloric acid and tinct. catechu. The ulcerations were touched with nitrate of copper.

Precaution in Use of Nitrate of Copper.—Dry the ulcer or part to be cauterized before applying the nitrate, and afterward smear it with oil.

Part xxv., *p.* 116.

Throat—Erysipelatous Affection of.—Dr. Todd has related several cases of this affection, which is characterized on its first approach by symptoms somewhat resembling lockjaw; in one case the patient was not able to open his mouth by the most violent effort. Then follows great difficulty of swallowing any fluids, even a little water. The best treatment seems to be, the application of the solid nitrate of silver to the fauces, and enemata of strong beef-tea, with ten grains of quinine in each, to be administered every four hours. *Part* xxvi., *p.* 77.

———•◦•———

THYROIDAL AFFECTIONS.

Biniodide of Mercury in.—Dr. Maj'sisovics, having long enjoyed a large share of practice in Vienna, where scrofulous and other diseases requiring the use of iodine are very prevalent, has had ample opportunities of administering this remedy in various forms and with variable success.

The effects of saturation with the remedy are described as the exanthema iodicum, which shows itself in dark red definite spots of various sizes, spreading over the whole body, remaining without the formation of scales, and disappearing only after a long time.

[Iodide of mercury, from the facility with which it undergoes decomposition, and its liability to produce inflammation of the stomach and bowels, is seldom used internally, but]

In the form of ointment, it is exceedingly useful in promoting absorption; the strength recommended by the author is, gr. x. to ʒij. (that of the London Pharmacopœia is, gr. xv. to ʒij.), which quantity is to be daily rubbed into the part affected. The biniodide of mercury is also but little used internally, it is, however, an excellent external application, in the strength of ʒj. to half au ounce of simple ointment, rubbed in three times a day. (The strength of the preparation in the London Pharmacopœia is, ʒj. to ʒj.)

The action of this ointment, applied as a plaster spread upon leather, is the following: In the space of half an hour, varying according to the spot where it is applied, or according to the individual constitution, burning pain comes on, which in some persons lasts two or three hours, but in very sensitive subjects even longer. In the third hour the cuticle begins to shrivel, and then rises in little vesicles filled with transparent fluid. They increase in size, and form at length a single bladder, and the fluid becomes opaque. On the second day, the raised epidermis is thicker, the quantity of fluid lessened, and upon the third day the thick and solid epidermis separates in the form of a yellowish white crust. When this has fallen off, the part underneath is seen to be already covered with new epidermis, and entirely healed, but slightly red and sensible. This is the course when the bladder is not opened; when it has been torn, the part becomes painful, and discharges pus for a long time. After three days have elapsed, the application may be made again. The patient may be allowed to walk about during the painful stage, if it be not applied upon the perineum or the lower extremities. In bronchocele its powerful effect may be mathematically shown, if the tumor is measured before the application of the plaster; for upon the falling off of the dried cuticle the size is found to have diminished sensibly. In this disease no preparation of iodine is comparable with the biniodide of mercury. It performs in one month what the other forms will scarcely do in three or four. I have treated goitres of enormous size with this medicine, and at the first application all the threatenings of suffocation or apoplexy (when they existed) ceased. Soft or so-called lymphatic tumors of the thyroid body can be entirely cured, whatever is their size. Those which are indurated, as well as endemic goitres, are harder to cure than those which are soft, and those which occur sporadically. Condylomata about the anus and perineum, or even within the rectum or vagina, are cured by this ointment; and unless they are exceedingly extensive and indurated, a single application, although very painful, combined with the internal use of iodine, has been found sufficient. *Part* xi., *p.* 176.

Bronchocele.—Mr. R. Hey, of York, says that in some cases, where surgical interference seems called for, the seton will be a legitimate and proper mode of treatment. In performing the operation, do not use a common seton needle, but get a curved trocar made, fixed in a handle, and grooved like a lithotomy staff, and having an eye behind the shoulder. Having threaded this eye with a single silk, which has a skein attached, enter the trocar at the upper part of the tumor in the median line, carry it on in a semicircular direction, so as to embrace a good deal of the tumor, and bring out the point in the median line below. Get hold of the silk thread, then withdraw the trocar, and pull the skein through. *Part* xx., *p.* 274.

Bronchocele.—A case is recorded by Dr. Terzi which was successfully treated by electro-acupuncture. The number of plates used was from sixteen to twenty, and upon the intervening discs of cloth, dipped in an acid or saline solution, a little tincture of iodine was dropped. *Part* xxi., *p.* 85.

Diseases of, and Operations on, the Thyroid Gland.—[In describing the post-mortem appearance of the gland after inflammation, Dr. Handfield Jones remarks :]

"I have more than once found the veins issuing from the gland, and passing its inferior margin, implicated in the inflammation and full of pus, or obstructed by a clot. In one case the coagulum completely obliterated all the principal venous trunks; even the lymphatic vessels, in cases of thyroiditis, often appeared inflamed, varicose, tinged with rosy lymph, or puriform matter, and with opaque parietes. The glands to which they pass are swollen, red, sanguineous, and buried in masses of plastic lymph. The ramifications of the thyroid nerves are interlaced on the surface of the injected capillary vessels."

[The medical and surgical modes of treatment of simple organic productions of the thyroid gland are next considered. Of the first we must first ascertain the cause, and, if possible, avoid or remove it. The second is to resolve the tumor. As a local application, the author prefers the protiodide of mercury. Four or five grains, with a scruple of lard, are rubbed in at each friction ; or a saturated solution of iodide of potassium in water mixed with lard may be used. From ten to twenty of these frictions will be quite sufficient to judge of the effect of the application. The absorption by the cuticle is perfect. Professor Porta generally now gives the iodide of potassium, commencing with eight grains daily, and increasing the dose to a scruple, half a drachm, or even a drachm daily. It is to be preferred to the tincture of iodine.

Extirpation of bronchocele has often been mistaken for mere enlargement of the gland or tumors upon it and external to it. Still eighteen or twenty cases are reported of it during the last century; the result in about half successful. Professor Porta has performed it four times, every time with a fatal result. The danger arises from the hemorrhage, denudation of vessels, and nerves of neck, or trachea and larynx, and diffusive suppuration; or from acute inflammation of the air apparatus; or from nervous exhaustion. The operation of extirpation of the whole, or part of the gland, should be discarded from surgical practice. Small isolated tumors may be easily and safely removed. Small accessory lobes, or isolated appendices, may increase and form tumors, the gland itself remaining normal. Professor Porta has repeatedly excised such tumors with perfect safety and success, a simple linear cicatrix remaining.]

Method of the Author.—Convinced of the difficulty and danger of isolating the thyroid gland from the part surrounding it, Professor Porta has followed a plan which he strongly recommends as safe and efficacious.

" In studying the thyroid gland, my attention has been directed to two facts which have especially interested me. First, that the arteries are inserted at the extremities of each lobe, and that their trunks run toward the superior, inferior, and external margins of the lobes; also that the large branches before penetrating the parenchyma, generally subdivide into a digitation of smaller branches. Thus, although the thyroids are *externally* four considerable arteries, *within* the tissue of the gland, they are merely branches and anastomoses of small calibre, and the embarrassment and danger of severe hemorrhage from injury to large vessels, are scarcely met with when we isolate the external portion of the tumor. In the second place, that the greater number of bronchoceles, as I have fully explained before, do not arise from degeneration of the proper glandular tissue, but from the generation of one or more non-malignant sarcomatous or encysted tumors in the midst of the parenchyma of the gland itself; that these tumors increasing, at last invade the whole space, and reduce the organ to a simple envelope or matrix, on dividing which the new products are exposed, and may be extracted with the greatest ease, injuring only small vessels, and leaving behind a fleshy sac, which, when so evacuated, falls together, and no trace of the tumor remains. . . . . The result of these observations was the following reflection : If the extirpation of the thyroid gland, and even one lobe of it, is so difficult and dangerous, would it not be better to invert the plan of operation, and evacuate the contents of the tumor, without touching its external portion, without lacerating the surrounding cellular tissue, without injuring the arterial trunks, and without dividing the principal organs of the neck ? On these grounds the new plan of operation consists in the simple incision of the external envelopes, and of the anterior surface of the tumor, at some distance from the direction of the arterial trunks; in the evacuation of the tumor by means of separation and extraction, or by excision of the cysts and nodules contained in it, without separation of the outer surface."

We are not told in how many cases the author has performed his operation, but he has selected six as illustrations, stating that in these, and in all his other cases, it succeeded perfectly in removing the tumor, and curing the patient. In only two cases did inflammatory symptoms require prompt antiphlogistic treatment. In one case a coriaceous cyst, and two sarcomatous tumors were removed from the substance of the gland. In another, the gland did not contain new products, but the enlargement was owing to simple hypertrophy. In this patient, the whole fleshy internal part of the tumor was cut away, leaving a sort of surrounding bark, about two lines in thickness. The bleeding was very slight. Cysts and sarcomatous tumors were extracted in all the other cases recorded.

The instruments for this operation are merely scalpels, blunt-hooks, dissection and torsion forceps, scissors, etc. There are three steps in the proceeding. First: division of the integuments of the neck and of the second belly of the omo-hyoid muscle, which is almost always necessary. Secondly: incision of the tumor parallel to the external incision, avoiding the branches of the thyroid arteries, or on division, at once applying the ligature or torsion, which is very easy, because the branches are mere secondary ones, running along and adhering for some distance to the surface of the tumor. Thirdly: by means of the forceps, and the back or handle of the knife, cysts or tumors are removed. When very deep and adherent, they are excised on the base. In case of simple hypertrophy, the whole internal texture of the gland may be removed. Should any arteries be injured in this last step of the operation, torsion should be employed.

Sometimes the wound heals by the first intention, but more frequently it suppurates, and cicatrizes in a few weeks. Occasionally it becomes sacculated, and requires dilatation, or becomes converted into a fistula, which does not close for a considerable time. The great object of after-treatment is to moderate inflammation which may arise, adopting active antiphlogistic measures, should its extension to the chest or head be threatened.   *Part* xxiii., *p.* 290.

Use of Iodine.—Instead of applying iodine by means of friction, in the form of ointment, to the neck in the case of goitre, M. Harmon recommends it to be tied over the part, between two layers of cotton wool in a bag. To prevent its staining the linen, a small piece of gummed silk may be placed over the bag.   *Part* xxvi., *p.* 348.

Goitre.—Dr. Mouat, of Bengal, states that upward of 60,000 cases of goitre have been treated in that country on the following plan, which generally effects a cure at once, if not, a second repetition next year suffices: Melt 3 lbs. of lard or mutton suet, strain and clean; when nearly cool, add 9 drachms of biniodide of mercury, taking care to make the powder fine by trituration in a mortar. Work in a mortar until no grains of red are apparent in the ointment, and put in pots for use, taking care always to keep both powder and ointment from the rays of light. Use as follows: About an hour after sunrise apply the ointment to the goitre with a spatula made of ivory, or thin, broad, smooth bamboo, quantity according to size of tumor—rub it well in for at least ten minutes. Let the patient then sit with his goitre held well up to the sun, and let him remain so as long as he can endure it. It is probable that about noon he will suffer severe pain from the blistering effect of the ointment, although no pustules are raised on the skin. About 2 p. m., the ointment should again be applied with a very careful and tender hand, and the patient should be dispatched to his home with orders not to touch the ointment on any account with the hand, but to allow it to be gradually absorbed, which absorption will be complete on the third day. *Part* xxxvii., *p.* 264.

TIBIA.

Nodes on the Tibia—Actual Cautery.—We are disposed to agree with Mr. Fergusson, that as a means of producing counter-irritation, the actual cautery is too much neglected; people are too much afraid of a heated iron approaching them to allow of the popular objection to this remedy being very easily overcome. The operation resembles too much that of firing horses, to become fashionable, but when properly managed, it is an equally efficient, more manageable, and less painful counter-irritation than either the caustic, potash, or the moxa. It is also of the greatest service in arresting hemorrhage. Mr. Fergusson has found it of use in some obstinate cases of nodes on the tibia. He brings a large extent of surface under the influence of the heated iron in these cases, not so as to cause a slough, but somewhat in the way which is adopted in firing horses, by which means a sudden excitement is produced over a large surface, while at the same time the skin is not destroyed, or converted into a slough. *Part* vii., *p.* 215.

TOBACCO.

Tobacco taken Moderately.—Tobacco taken moderately, says M. Raspail, is a condiment to which some people inure themselves. In whatever form it is employed, the tobacco acts evidently by property, the base of which is formed by ammonia. In fact, if we moisten common tobacco with a little ammonia, we give to it a flavor which increases its value. Pound some walnut leaves with potass in a heated mortar, and then place them in a drying stove, and you will have a powder very similar to tobacco, for the purpose of smoking, and which has even a stronger flavor, especially if a few drops of ammonia be added to it; and there is every reason to believe that common tobacco is thus adulterated to a great extent. The walnut leaves may be replaced by those of the potato, henbane, hellebore, aconite, by the grains of *elaterium* and of colocynth, etc.
Part ix., *p.* 81.

Use of Infusion of Tobacco.—The infusion of tobacco has been used with much success in many cases of prurigo. In purulent ophthalmia, also, and the scrofulous conjunctivitis of infants, it has been used with de-

cided success, and may be resorted to with confidence, when other remedies have failed. The strength of the infusion for these purposes is double
that used for enemata—viz., ʒj. to Oss. of boiling water, and shag tobacco
proves more efficacious than pig-tail. *Part* xii., *p.* 301.

Injurious Influence of Tobacco in Insanity.—[Dr. Woodward's experience is quite at variance with that of the physicians to our asylums. It
must be questioned, however, whether depriving some patients of the enjoyment of this luxury may not lead to a good deal of irritation, and thus
aggravate the disease. Dr. W. observes:]
Alcohol is not the only narcotic which thus affects the brain and nervous system. Opium produces delirium tremens, and probably insanity.
Tobacco is a powerful narcotic agent, and its use is very deleterious to
the nervous system, producing tremors, vertigo, faintness, palpitation of
the heart, and other serious diseases. That tobacco certainly produces
insanity I am not able positively to observe; but that it produces a predisposition to it I am fully confident. Its influence upon the brain and
nervous system generally, is hardly less obvious than that of alcohol, and,
if excessively used, is equally injurious. In our experience in this hospital, tobacco, in all its forms, is injurious to the insane. It increases excitement of the nervous system in many cases, deranges the stomach, and
produces vertigo, tremors, and stupor in others. *Part* xiv., *p.* 65.

Tobacco Smoking—Effects of.—From a few experiments instituted by
M. Malapert, it was found that, in the smoke of tobacco extracted by inspiration, there is 10 per cent. of nicotine. Thus a man who smokes a
cigar of the weight of seventy grains, receives in his mouth seven grains
of nicotine mixed with a little watery vapor, tar, empyreumatic oil, etc.
Although a large portion of this nicotine is rejected, both by the smoke
puffed from the mouth, and by the saliva, a portion of it is nevertheless
taken up by the vessels of the buccal and laryngeal mucous membrane, circulated with the blood, and acts upon the brain. With those unaccustomed to the use of tobacco, the nicotine, when in contact with the latter
organ, produces vertigo, nausea, headache, and somnolence; whilst habitual
smokers are merely thrown into a state of excitement, similar to that produced by moderate quantities of wine or tea.
From further investigation it was found that the drier the tobacco the
less nicotine reaches the mouth. A very dry cigar, whilst burning, yields
a very small amount of watery vapor; the smoke cools rapidly, and
allows the condensation of the nicotine before it reaches the mouth.
Hence it comes that the first half of a cigar smokes more mildly than the
second, in which a certain amount of condensed watery vapor and nicotine,
freed by the first half, are deposited. The same remark applies to smoking tobacco in pipes, and if smokers were prudent, they would never consume but half a cigar or pipe, and throw away the other. Smoking
through water, or with long tubes and small bowls, is also a precaution
which should not be neglected. *Part* xxxii., *p.* 283.

Tobacco.—The use of tobacco should be forbidden during the prevalence of an epidemic of typhoid fever; it has the effect of relaxing the
mucous membranes, and diminishing the vital force, and is very apt to produce or predispose to diarrhœa and intestinal lesion. Catechu is the best
remedy for diarrhœa arising from this cause. *Part* xxxv., *p.* 342.

TOE NAIL.

Inverted Toe Nail.—In many, though by no means in the majority of cases, the cutting the nail too short, is the primary cause of the affection. The soft parts, being no longer kept down by the projecting free edge of the nail, are forced, by the pressure of the boot or shoe in walking, against and even over the truncated end of the nail, and, as this again increases in length, it may be made to even penetrate into them—giving rise thus to inflammation, swelling, ulceration, and fungous granulations, with a degree of suffering which often renders the slightest motion of the foot unbearable.

[Many of the operations hitherto proposed are extremely painful, and while few of them afford more than temporary relief, some even tend to increase the evil. Dr. Zeis has had frequent opportunities of seeing patients operated on by Dupuytren's method of extraction of the offending portion of the nail, and he found that in every case it was ineffectual, the free edge of the nail expanding laterally, and keeping up a constant irritation. The new modes of treatment constantly met with in the medical journals are mostly mere modifications of the older plans. The most painful is that of Neret, who directs a spatula to be forced down beneath the nail to its roots, and then for the nail to be torn out. Larrey's operation differs from the former only that the third of the nail is thus treated. Baudens removes the whole of the inverted edge, together with the spongy flesh in which it is imbedded. Others advise the destruction of the nail, or a portion of it, by caustics, for which caustic potass and lime, and burnt alum have been used. Labat destroyed the root of the nail at once by the actual cautery. Donzel dissected back the skin from the root of the nail, filled the wound with charpie, and the next day with pâte caustique; removing the edge of the nail when the slough separated. Others, objecting to the destruction of any portion of the nail, propose various plans by which it may be kept from contact with the inflamed portion of the soft parts until these are completely healed. Martin recommends a triangular portion to be cut out of the middle of the nail, the base being at the free edge, and then the cut edges of the nail to be drawn together by a suture of brass-wire. This, however, from the constant growth of the nail, can only afford temporary relief. Others propose to give the nail a flatter form, by thinning the centre, and applying compresses of different kinds, whilst Bressy, after shaving the nail as thin as possible, touches it six or eight times with lunar caustic, until it shrivels up, and its edges are in consequence drawn out of the soft parts; this, however, infallibly produces entire destruction of the nail.]

Dr. Zeis considers it all-important to attend to the general health, which will usually be found more or less deranged. So soon as the nail acquires the slightest projection, he is in the habit of introducing beneath it, by means of a fine probe, a small portion of charpie, and to prevent the falling out of this, he covers the end of the toe with adhesive plaster, spread upon gold-beater's skin, which adapts itself better to the parts, and produces a less amount of pressure than when it is spread on silk or linen. The toe is then to be bathed frequently, during the day, in warm water. If the soft parts at the point of the toe, are in so swollen a condition as to interfere with the dressing just directed, or completely to cover and conceal the edge of the nail, Dr. Zeis is in the habit of removing them by the knife.

"Much more obstinate, however, are those cases in which the disease affects, at the same time, or is entirely confined to, the side of the nail. These are, especially, the cases in which the destruction of the whole, or a part of the nail, has been considered indispensable to the cure. I have, however, in such, seldom failed to secure the entire and permanent relief of the patient by rest, the frequent use of the foot-bath, and the removal, by the knife, of the fungous granulations or spongy and morbidly sensible flesh, by which the edge of the nail becomes covered. I will not, however, pretend to deny," he adds, "that cases of a very aggravated character may occur, in which the unhealthy condition of the ulceration, seated beneath the nail, will require the loosened edge of the nail to be cut away, that our applications may be applied directly to the ulcerated surface, and also to prevent the constant irritation which is kept up in it by the detached portion of the nail. It is never necessary to destroy the whole, or any part of the nail, even under such circumstances."

Part xi., *p.* 163.

Toe Nail—Ingrowing of the.—In order to heal the troublesome ulcer arising from this cause, says Dr. Newman, separate the soft parts from the nail so as to expose the whole surface of the ulcer, and sprinkle it freely with powdered charcoal, mixed with a little acetate of lead or oxide of zinc; bind a piece of lint over it, and let the patient wear a wide shoe, and keep quiet. Every day bathe the toe with tepid water, and sprinkle fresh charcoal over it, without disturbing that previously applied.

Part xxi., *p.* 260.

Onychia.—The late Mr. Colles, of Dublin, in a paper on some morbid affections of the great toe nail, divides them into three kinds: 1. The common onychia, or nail growing into the flesh, on its external edge. 2. The inner angle of the nail resting on a hard white mass of laminated horny cuticle, which may be picked out in bran-like scales, exposing a small cup-shaped cavity, without ulceration. 3. Onychia maligna depending on a morbid condition of the secreting matrix of the nail. In the first disease, only so much of the nail as is separated from the matrix, and imbedded in the fungus, is to be removed. This is done by pressing on the fungus with a spatula, raising the nail from it by a pair of strong forceps, and then by means of curved scissors passed underneath it, cutting it completely out. In the second it is to pick away the laminated scales and remove the bulbous end of the nail. In the third, the treatment is to keep the patient in bed, poultice the part for two or three days, then cleanse the ulcer thoroughly by means of a syringe and a stream of tepid water, and afterward cutting away as much of the loose nail as can be done without irritating the surrounding sensitive surface. Lastly, fumigate, night and morning, by means of a funnel, with the mercurial candle, which contains ʒj. hyd. sulph. rubrum to ʒij. of wax. After each fumigation, the toe to be enveloped in a piece of lint spread with spermaceti ointment.

Part xxvi., *p.* 328.

Onychia.—If you see this disease early, Dr. Hamilton, of Dublin, advises to poultice until you can insinuate a small shred of lint under the angle and side of the nail, by means of a small probe; you must then wet this with a solution of nitrate of silver (ʒj. ad ʒj.). Keep the lint in for forty-eight hours, and by renewing two or three times the disease will be cured. To prevent a return, caution the patient against rounding off the angles when cutting the nails, and direct him to cut them straight across.

Part xxxii., *p.* 191.

Ingrowing Toe-Nail.—The chief pain in the operation for the cure of this affection is caused by the necessity of forcing away a portion of the nail from attachments rendered excessively tender by inflammation. It is not generally known, says Dr. Long, surgeon to Liverpool Royal Infirmary, that by rubbing the nail well with nitrate of silver along the line of intended division, about two days before the operation, this tenderness is done away with, and the operation rendered nearly painless, as the caustic causes the nail to loose its attachment to the parts beneath. The best plan of doing this is to gently introduce a bit of cotton wool along the edge of the nail, thus separating it from the overgrowing granulations, and along the edge of this to apply the nitrate of silver. If the nail be very thick, it may be necessary to scrape off the blackened parts, and apply the caustic a second time. . . . . . There is no such thing as ingrowing toe-nail; it is the upgrowing of the quick through exposing the same, and taking away the natural protection and support of the nail itself. Therefore do not remove the nail, but soak the part well in hot water, and delicately remove all discharge, pass in plenty of very finely powdered burnt alum, cover all the fungus with the same, and on the next and every day do the same until no longer sensitive, then strap down the alum, first putting on the top, not under, a piece of lint. *Part* xxxvii., *p.* 176.

Ingrowing Toe-Nail.—After fomentation, Dr. Alcantara interposes beneath the nail a small piece of lint, upon which some ointment of perchloride of iron has been spread; all the surface of the excrescence, deprived of its epidermis, is covered over with this, and the dressing is renewed twice a day. At the end of four days the excrescence becomes dry and mummified, and is easily detached. The wound then assumes a regular aspect, and the cure is completed at the end of a week.

Part xxxix., *p.* 233.

—•♦•—

TONGUE.

Diseases of the Tongue.—On diseases of this organ we find very little attention has been paid by authors, except on those which are malignant. The tongue is sometimes *swollen* in dyspeptic persons, or it becomes *cracked* on the surface. These cracks or fissures are sometimes very deep, and will generally be durable. They often arise from profuse salivation at some former period of life, but, when slight, may be owing to dyspepsia. If owing to mercury, the best remedy, perhaps, is sarsaparilla, or nitric acid. We sometimes find little ulcers on the tongue, often the consequence of syphilis, and accompanied, perhaps, with little spots of syphilitic psoriasis, on the body or on the scalp. They soon disappear by means of small doses of mercury; and in one case, mentioned by Sir B. Brodie, the hyd. c. creta was given in small doses for nearly two months before a radical cure could be effected. Small doses are much to be preferred to large ones. Sir Benjamin prefers five grains of the hyd. c. creta with one or two grains of Dover's powder; and where this fails, he gives the iodide of potassium, two or three grains given twice daily, dissolved in plenty of water. If these ulcers arise from dyspepsia, which is frequently the case, one or two applications of the nitrate of silver will be sufficient to cure them. Sir Benjamin continues: "There is a disease of the tongue which I have seen every now and then, and which I am sure is very often mistaken for cancer, though it is of a different nature. It is a curable disease, although it looks like a malignant one in many respects. The first thing of which the patient complains is enlargement of the tongue, with some pain. On examination you find a tumor in one part of it, not very well defined, nor with any distinct margin. It is a softish tumor, and increases in size, and perhaps another tumor appears in a different part of the tongue, and that increases also. There may be three or four of these soft elastic tumors, with no very defined margins, in various parts of the tongue. This is the first stage of the disease.

"In the second stage there is a small formation of matter in one of these tumors—a little abscess, which breaks externally, discharging two or three drops of pus. When the abscess has burst it does not heal, but another forms in one of the other tumors. These abscesses may assume the form of ulcers, and the ulcer has a particular appearance. In the first instance it is a very narrow streak of ulceration, but on introducing a probe you find that the ulcer is the external orifice to a sort of fissure in the tongue. The probe passes in obliquely; the tongue is, as it were, undermined by the ulcer, a flap of the substance of the tongue being over it.

"The disease now becomes more painful, and at last these ulcers may spread externally. In some instances they occupy a very considerable portion of the surface of the tongue, but generally they burrow internally, and do not spread much toward the surface. This is a very distressing state of things, and a man may remain in this state for a long time. The glands of the neck do not become affected, nor does the general health suffer, except from the difficulty of swallowing food. This is one inconvenience experienced by the patient, and he also labors under a difficulty of articulation. The tongue, from its enlarged state, may become stiff, not sufficiently pliable for the purposes of speech, and the patient either speaks thick or lisps.

"In some instances the disease may be relieved by a course of sarsaparilla, with small doses of bichloride of mercury. A strong decoction of sarsaparilla, with from a quarter to half a grain of bichloride of mercury, may be taken in the course of the day. Of course, if there be anything wrong in the general health, you should endeavor to get that corrected, and attend especially to the state of the bowels and the secretion of the liver. If the secretions of the digestive organs be unhealthy, a dose of senna and salts may be given every other morning, and blue pill every other night. When the patient is brought into this state, one remedy, as I have said, is sarsaparilla with bichloride of mercury, but, according to my experience, this is not the best remedy. The remedy best adapted for these cases is a solution of arsenic. Give the patient five minims three times daily, in a draught, gradually increasing the dose to ten minims. It should be taken in full doses, so that it may begin to produce some of its poisonous effects on the system. When it begins to act as a poison, it will show itself in various ways. Sometimes there is a sense of heat, a burning pain in the rectum; sometimes griping, purging, and sickness, and nervous tremblings. A patient who is taking arsenic, especially in pretty large doses, ought to be carefully watched. At first you may see him every two or three days, and then every day : and as soon as the arsenic begins to operate as a poison, leave it off. When this effect is produced the disease of the tongue generally gets well, but at any rate leave off the arsenic, and the poisoning will not go too far ; it will do no harm. If, after a time, you find that the disease is relieved, but not entirely cured, you may try another course of arsenic. Perhaps it may take a considerable time to get the tongue quite well. Sarsaparilla, with the bichloride of mercury, may be given at one time; and at another, arsenic. You cannot give either of these remedies forever, and indeed the arsenic can only be given for a very limited period; but it is astonishing what bad tongues of this description I have seen get well under these modes of treatment, especially under the use of arsenic."

[Sir Benjamin thinks that many of these affections, which at first are not malignant, may ultimately prove so; and when they assume the malignant character, or when a disease is of a malignant nature from the first, he thinks it is the best plan to let it have its own course. As in a cancer of the breast it would be of no use to remove the small portion where malignancy first shows itself, or part of a tibia affected with fungus hæmatodes, so in cancer of the tongue the whole organ is more or less diseased from the first, and to remove the piece which first shows symptoms of malignancy, would be of little avail.]

"There is one other disease of the tongue, or rather a disease under it, which remains to be mentioned. A patient comes with a sore mouth, and you see the tongue pushed up to the soft palate. It looks as if the tongue were enlarged, but that is not the case, it is lifted up. You tell the patient to put his tongue against the incisor teeth, and on looking beneath you see a tumor. By feeling it you find fluctuation, you puncture it, and let out a quantity of transparent fluid, sometimes a teaspoonful or more. The fluid is a little glutinous, and consists of saliva. There has been an obstruction to the orifice of the submaxillary gland ; the saliva has been secreted by the gland, but could not get out by the duct, and hence it has remained till it has formed a large tumor. This is what is called ranula.

" You puncture the tumor with a lancet ; the fluid comes out, and immediately the patient is well. You see him a week afterward ; he is quite well, and there is no saliva flowing out of the orifice you have made with the lancet. But you see him a month afterward, and the tumor has reappeared, the orifice has healed, and the tumor becomes as large as ever. All you want is, to get a permanent orifice from the bag into which the duct has been converted ; but that is a very difficult matter. I have tried to effect it in various ways. I have punctured the bag, and then touched the edge with caustic potassa to prevent its healing. The patient has gone on very well so long as it did not heal, but as soon as I have left off applying the caustic the orifice has closed. I have introduced a tenaculum into the bag of the rauula, and cut away a piece sufficiently large to admit the finger ; the patient has then continued well for a longer time, because the part takes longer to heal, but contraction takes places, and the patient is bad again. I have run a seton through, and the patient has then gone on well for a considerable time. I have introduced a gold or silver ring, and kept that in as a seton. If the seton be kept in a considerable time it seems to effect a permanent cure, but even that fails, and you have to perform the operation two or three times. I know of nothing better than the use of a seton, and I believe that it is better made of metallic substance than of silk. It does not so soon ulcerate its way out, and if it remain in for a long time, the edges of the orifice through which the seton is introduced may become covered with mucous membrane. If you introduce a silk or india-rubber seton in the back of the neck, after a great length of time a sort of skin forms on the inner surface of the canal; there is a discharge of matter; and when you take away the seton the part in which it lay remains pervious. So if you keep a seton in a ranula for a very long time the opening may remain pervious. The advantage of a metallic over a silk seton is, that it does not ulcerate its way out so soon, does not get putrid in the mouth, and therefore may be kept in for a long time."

[Sometimes the tongue is affected with a tumor, which, if it occurred in the female breast, would perhaps be mistaken for scirrhus; but still it has not the character of scirrhus of the tongue—it is hard and circumscribed, and rather deeper than common scirrhus. Sir Benj. Brodie would ascertain the effects of iodine upon such a tumor, before he pronounced a decided opinion. In one case he gave eight or ten drops of the tincture of iodine three times a day, and gradually increased the dose to 20 drops. The tumor ultimately disappeared. In relating this case he cautions us against the too long continuance of iodine, without keeping our eyes on the patient. After continuing its use too long he was seized with paralysis, but on leaving off the medicine he recovered—thus showing how powerfully iodine may affect the nervous system, if used for too long a time.]   *Part* ix., *p.* 98.

Diseases of the Tongue.—[As actual disease of the tongue is often obscure, and seldom met with in private practice, attention to the following remarks taken from a lecture by Mr. Lawrence on the subject, will be of service when such do occur. Ulceration, swelling, and thickening of the mucous membrane, and hypertrophy with induration of the whole organ, are the forms most frequently met with. With the two latter ulceration is a frequent concomitant. Syphilis and cancer are the more formidable diseases, the first being by far the most frequent. Serious affections too, occasionally depend upon disorder of the digestive organs.]

Syphilitic disease of the tongue occurs most frequently in conjunction with other venereal symptoms, such as ulcerations of the fauces or mouth, and eruptions, particularly of the scaly kind. Here the nature of the malady is too obvious to be mistaken. A gentleman who had a primary syphilitic sore some weeks previously, showed me an ulcer on the right edge of the tongue, very similar to those frequently accompanying the use of mercury. The surface was raised and irregular, excoriated and partially ulcerated. There were two small superficial ulcerations of the palate, and no other symptoms. These appearances were entirely removed in three weeks under the mild use of mercury with sarsaparilla. A female, at present in the hospital, has the mucous membrane at the edge of the tongue thickened, and considerably raised, for a length of three quarters of an inch, with alteration of the epithelium, giving it a white color. It has been in this state, with considerable soreness, for three months. I lately saw a young person with thickening of the mucous membrane on both sides of the tongue, occupying nearly the whole length of the organ. It was reddened, slightly fissured, but not greatly enlarged. There was a superficial ulcer, of elongated form, on each side, about the middle of the diseased portion of the membrane. This affection, which had followed a primary sore, and was not attended with any other secondary symptom, was said to have existed in a more or less troublesome state for more than a year. I prescribed the hydrarg. c. creta, and conclude that it had the desired effect, as I have not seen the patient since. A gentleman 26 years of age consulted me on account of an affection of the tongue. There was a thickening of the mucous membrane on the middle line and at the back of the organ, constituting a flattened projection of circular form larger than a sixpence. It was redder than the rest of the mucous membrane, and had a slightly broken surface, like that of a wart. It was painful, and smarted when acids, strong liquids, or stimulating condiments were taken into the mouth. As he mentioned that he had felt some uneasiness about the throat, I inspected the fauces, and found a superficial ulcer, the size of a sixpence, on the side of the pharynx, behind the root of the tongue. I asked whether he had contracted any syphilitic complaint; he was surprised at the inquiry, but informed me that he had had a chancre several weeks previously, which had healed in ten days under the use of mercury. The tongue and throat soon became well under the use of that remedy.

Sometimes the dorsum of the tongue presents red patches, in which the mucous membrane is denuded of its epithelium, and perfectly smooth, but not ulcerated. These are sore when hot or strong things are taken into the mouth. They may last for a considerable time, particularly if they are neglected, getting better and worse. There is sometimes a combination of diseased appearances in the same case. A gentleman consulted me on July 1st. There had been a primary sore ten months ago; then an eruption, which did not last long. He had been plagued with a bad tongue for the last four or five months: it had been so swelled and painful that he ate with difficulty. The surface of the organ, in its middle portion, and over more than half its extent, the dorsum and edges being included, was smooth, the epithelium being white and opaque, as if this part had been ulcerated, and partly having a raw appearance. There were three or four small superficial ulcers with grey surfaces at the edges and tip, and small superficial ulcerations of the lips, with chaps at the angles of the mouth. In both palms there were scaly eruptions in a slight form, but not elsewhere. This patient had frequently taken the iodide of potassium in rather large doses; the tongue would get better, but the mischief would return on leaving off the remedy. I prescribed the hydrarg. c. creta, gr. iiss. three times a day. The patient did not visit me again for a week, at the end of which time severe ptyalism had been produced, with more than the usual degree of suffering. He expressed his belief, however, that the original complaint of the tongue was better. Now (August) that the mercurial affection has subsided, the tongue is quite well, though having marks on its surface of the previous disease. The beneficial influence of mercury on ulcers of the tongue, mouth, and throat, has always appeared to me to afford the most unequivocal evidence of its peculiar antisyphilitic virtues; for while the sound mucous membrane is inflamed and ulcerated by the action of the remedy, we see the contiguous venereal ulcerations altered in character and healing rapidly.

Venereal enlargement and induration of the tongue may be confounded with cancer, in which the substance of the organ is also more or less hardened. There are several and sufficient points of distinction, so that if the history be investigated, and the symptoms carefully examined, there will be no risk of mistaking the comparatively mild and manageable venereal affection for the very painful, and, I fear, inevitably fatal cancerous disease. I have always seen the latter begin on the edge of the tongue, generally at the middle or back part. It extends slowly into the substance, and may ultimately embrace the greater portion, or the whole organ. The hardness which, as in the scirrhous breast, is in the highest degree, renders the part incompressible; it is accurately circumscribed, so that we immediately feel the boundary of the disease. The hardness is less marked in syphilis, more diffused, and not confined in its origin to the margin of the tongue. Scirrhous induration does not last long, nor become considerable in extent, without the occurrence of ulceration; while syphilitic enlargement may occupy one-half, or nearly the whole organ, without breach of surface. The cancerous ulcer is deep, often with an ash-colored or partially disorganized and bleeding surface. Sometimes profuse and alarming hemorrhage occurs. The margin is hard, raised, and everted, or ragged and excavated. The induration is considerable in proportion to the ulceration, especially at the commencement. The secretion from the sore is thin and offensive. The induration, in syphilitic ulcerations, is comparatively inconsiderable; the surface is of better character, and the ulcer seldom penetrates deeply. Cancer of the tongue is a hardened mass, which becomes ulcerated; syphilitic disease is an ulceration of which the base and edge are sometimes thickened, moderately indurated, and raised. The pain of cancerous ulceration is most severe, and so much aggravated by motion of the organ, that articulation, mastication, and swallowing, are attended with the greatest suffering. The aid of opium is absolutely neecessary to procure temporary ease. The uneasiness in syphilitic cases is comparatively inconsiderable. The absorbent glands soon become enlarged and indurated in cancer of the tongue, while they seldom suffer in syphilitic ulceration; if they do, it is simple enlargement. *Part* xii., *p.* 188.

Morbid States of the Tongue.—Dr. Wright says: As a rule the tongue is a very faithful indicator of the condition of the alimentary organs; but its evidences are not unexceptionable. A furred tongue, for instance, is a common indication of dyspepsia, but it is not a constant one. You sometimes meet with irritable, nervous subjects, whose tongues are habitually furred, yet without any signs or symptoms whatever of gastric derangement. Others, again, will have clean tongues, and of natural redness, whilst they are suffering from severe stomach disorder. I called your attention to a case of this sort the other morning, in the person of a female, the subject of very severe pyrosis. During the three weeks that she has been under my care, the tongue has never lost its cleanliness or good color. I once had a dispensary patient affected with scirrhus of the pylorus, of which he died, yet up to the time of his death the tongue was scarcely ever furred or dry. Various circumstances exert a remarkable influence upon this organ. Some people, otherwise healthy, get a furred, clammy tongue if their stomachs are empty a little longer than usual; others have their tongues furred always when their stomachs are full; the coating continues only during digestion, and passes off as this function ceases. Mental and moral emotions affect the condition of the tongue in a singular manner. It may happen, that in dyspepsia, the disorder the brain suffers, sympathetically with the stomach, has as much share as this organ itself in giving the tongue its characteristic coating. Certain it is, as I have said, that the feelings of the mind will, in a very few minutes, render a clean tongue a foul one. Among the profoundly studious, among those terrified by sudden apprehensions, or shocked by the sudden advent of ill news ; among the hypochondriacal, hysterical, gloomy, and desponding, you will find many examples of the mind's influence, in this particular, upon the body.

A few days ago, in calling upon a patient, one of the first things I did was to look at his tongue. I found it, as usual, very pale, flabby, and moist, but without any coating After having made other necessary inquiries, I was informed by my patient that his heart, which has long been disturbed by mental emotion, the other night_beat with unusual vehemence and irregularity. On my asking if he could account for it, he told me that he had just then received the distressing intelligence that an uncle, from whom he expected a competency, had not left him with a shilling! This pitiable tale, told with much earnestness and visible feeling, occupied little more than twenty minutes; at the end of that time I again looked at his tongue, *and'found it coated with a thick white fur!*

I mention these things, thus generally, to you, not only as items in pathology with which you ought to be made familiar, but also suggestive of a discreet rule of practice, viz., to let the examination of a patient's tongue be *one of your first duties at his bed-side.*

Besides moral and mental states, there are certain physical ones, of which the tongue is an occasional, though not an invariable evidence. Our hospital opportunities have lately given me the occasion of showing you these pathognomonic facts somewhat strikingly. I have dwelt with particularity upon them at the bed-side, and have no doubt that they are still fresh in you remembrance. You have seen in several varieties the dark, dry tongue of typhoid fever; the glassy, bright red tongue, with its elevated papillæ, in sub-acute gastro-enteritis; the brown furred tongue of dyspepsia, with bilious derangement; the pale, flabby, furred, sodden, tongue of chlorosis, habitual drunkenness, debility of the gastric apparatus, etc.; the pale or patched, trembling tongue of the hypochondriac, the dissipated, the excessively weakened, from whatever cause; the dry, contracted, dusky-red tongue of gastric irritation, etc.

A morbid state of the tongue not only indicates (with rare exceptions) the condition of the gastric apparatus, and of the system in general, but an improvement of its appearance denotes, also, that the patient is advancing toward recovery. This change sometimes occurs with singular suddenness, and the patient as suddenly gets well. You remember the girl Scandret, in the middle ward, whom we had some difficulty of relieving of fever that had supervened upon dyspepsia. Her tongue was broad, flabby, indented at the edges, very trembling, and completely covered with dense white fur. She complained of a feeling of hollowness or sinking of the epigastrium, with frequent darting pains there, and occasional fits of nausea; her food always lay like a load in her stomach, and oppressed it with flatulence. She was ordered the twelfth of a grain of strychnine, three times a day. She had only taken five doses up to the time of our next visit, and you remembered how altered she then was. Her tongue had no indentation on it : scarcely any fur; its trembling was almost imperceptible, and its size diminished. She had no gastric pain or flatulence after the first dose of strychnine. In four days afterward she left the hospital, apparently quite well. I told you that the appearance of her tongue, and her expressed symptoms, indicated that her stomach was suffering from *irritability, the result of local nervous debility :* the manner in which she improved under the strychnine confirms me in that opinion.

There was another case to which I called your particular attention, a short time back, in the person of a girl. When convalescent from fever, she one day begged to be allowed some beef for dinner. Her tongue was very furred, but there was nothing else to prohibit the gratification of her appetite; and she asked so imploringly that I ordered her some roast beef, at the same time remarking to you that it was not improbable her anticipated meal would clean her tongue. The next day confirmed what I had said ; we found her with neither fur nor fetor in her mouth, and she required no more medicine during the few remaining days that she was in the hospital. It is not always safe to gratify the inclination of patients' appetites, for they are sometimes disposed to crave for very strange things. Inclination and appetite have frequently a great share in promoting good digestion. I have known oysters, lobsters, pork, pastry, and such like allowed almost *ad libitum,* for once, to patients, not only with impunity but with advantage. I mention these as curiosities of experience, not as examples for imitation.

Part xv., *p.* 106.

*Tongue—Inflammatory and other Affections of.—*Dr. Fleming says, that sudden and alarming swelling sometimes takes place in the tongue, which seems to be merely an unaccountable and active hyperæmia, readily yielding before inflammation has had time to be lighted up, by incision, by leeching copiously, both locally and under the chin. Another affection is " an inflammation, circumscribed or diffused, originating in the loose cellular tissue between the genio-hyo-glossi muscles," the treatment for which is antiphlogistic, but if it does not readily yield, Dr. Fleming recommends a free incision to be made under the chin in the median line, through the integuments and fascia, and through the raphé of those muscles, delaying the advancement of the suppurating process. Dr. Fleming says, the best treatment for the abraded surface of the tongue, sometimes met with, and for a peculiar kind of ulcer, which is accompanied by a small tumor about the size of a pea, and which he states may occur without the slightest suspicion of a syphilitic taint, is the iodide of iron, with hemlock, and the local application of the nitrate of copper. Dr. Fleming thinks it a tuberculous disease, and says it is by no means uncommonly met with. The nitrate of copper, he says, is almost invaluable also as an application to the small excoriated ulcers, of a semi-phagedenic character, occurring in the genitals of both male and female. It is very deliquescent, and can be applied only in its liquid state. The surface of the ulcer should be well dried previously, and afterward covered with oil.   *Part* xxii., *p.* 367.

*Tongue—Tumors of.—*For the removal of these tumors, the surgeon has choice of three methods. Amputation by the knife gets rid of the mass at once ; strangulation by means of ligature prevents any loss of blood ; and excision performed carefully by a wire heated by galvanism accomplishes both these objects at the same time.   *Part* xxvi., *p.* 340.

*Percyanide of Mercury in Syphilitic Ulceration of the Tongue.—*Mr. Wormald, at St. Bartholomew's Hospital, has recently been employing a saturated solution of the bicyanide of mercury, as an application to syphilitic ulcerations, abrasions, etc., on the tongue. Without speaking very enthusiastically respecting it, he states that he has obtained more satisfactory results from it than from any remedy he had previously employed. The solution is painted over the affected part, care of course being taken that the patient do not swallow any quantity of it. The extremely intractable nature of this form of syphilis is matter of general remark.

Part xxxii., *p.* 181.

Tongue, Deep Fissures of.—Dr. Fleming, surgeon, Richmond Hospital, Dublin, uses locally the nitrate of copper to the ulcerated surfaces, and gives chlorate of potash in from five to fifteen grain doses, with bark and sarsaparilla. The nitrate of copper is almost invaluable in this class of ulcers, and it will be found equally valuable in small excavated semi-phagedenic ulcers which occur on the genitals. It is a very deliquescent salt, and can only be applied in the liquid state, by means of a small piece of cedar. *Part* xxxiii., *p.* 178.

Glycerine and Borax in Cracked Tongue.—Dr. Brinton advises to apply a lotion composed of two scruples of borax, one ounce of glycerine, and four ounces of water; at the same time give the iodide of potassium and bark. *Part* xxxv., *p.* 59.

———•◦•———

TONSILS.

Pulvis Aluminis et Capsici.—℞ Alum, three parts; concentrated tincture of capsicum, one part. Mix and dry.

Dr. Turnbull has found a very small quantity of this powder applied to the tonsils, more efficacious, in some cases, than an alum and capsicum gargle. *Part* v., *p.* 84.

Chronic Enlargement of Tonsils—Iodide of Zinc.—Dr. J. Ross says: The first notice I saw of the medical use of this compound was in the review of Dr. Cogswill's essay on iodine in "Johnson's Journal" (Jan. 1839, p. 118). It is there stated, "During the two last years we have been in the habit of employing a strong solution of the iodide of zinc, as an application to the tonsillary glands, when affected with chronic enlargement, and we can recommend it to our readers as the best local remedy we know for that most obstinate complaint." To this statement I fully subscribe. In those cases of hypertrophied tonsils where I have used it, the diminution in their size was most marked and speedily produced. In two patients in whom these glands were so much enlarged as almost to fill up the isthmus of the fauces, and interfere materially with deglutition, they were quickly reduced to nearly their natural size, and gave no further inconvenience. A solution may be made of 10, 15, or 30 grains to the ounce of water, and applied to the tonsils daily, by a piece of sponge tied to a quill or thin piece of wood. After using this for some time, I employ the substance itself, undiluted; a little of it is exposed to the air till it deliquesces, and then applied in this state to the tonsil, by means of a camel's-hair brush. This is a much more effectual plan than Dr. Cusack's mode of applying the nit. argenti point by point; indeed, it is superior to every local application I know of being used in such cases, always, of course, excepting the knife. *Part* vi., *p.* 124.

Chronic Congestion of the Tonsils.—Dr. Becker has found extract of green walnut shells of great efficacy in congestion of the tonsils. The

mode in which he uses it is in the form of a solution of the extract of one
part to fifteen of distilled water, to be applied externally with a brush.
Part xi., *p.* 59.

Excision of the Tonsils—Follicular Disease of.—Extirpate (as also the
uvula) if much hypertrophied and indurated, and apply strong solution of
nitrate of silver. (Dr. H. Green.)

*   *   *   *   *   *   *   *

Hypertrophy and induration of the tonsils occur frequently in young
persons and children, independent of follicular disease of the throat. In
some instances, the affection appears to be congenital, or is hereditary; in
others, it is the result of repeated attacks of chronic inflammation of the
tonsillary glands. When the hypertrophy is accompanied by induration,
whether this condition coexists with follicular disease, or is the effect of
chronic tonsilitis, excision of the enlarged gland is almost the only method
of treatment by which permanent and effectual relief can be obtained.
This fact ought to be better understood by the profession than it seems to
be, for the practice of painting these morbid growths with the tincture of
iodine, or of cauterizing them with the solid nitrate, is still continued, and
patients are daily being subjected to this still annoying and useless practice,
often month after month, with the apparent expectation on the part of
their attendants that enlarged and indurated tonsils may be discussed by
these applications.—(Rev.)   *Part* xvi., *p.* 126.

Tonsils—Chronic Enlargement of.—Apply nitrate of silver, either the
solid caustic, or a solution gradually increased from three grains to two
drachms to the ounce of water; paint the tonsils twice or thrice at one sitting, and then let the mouth be well washed with water. Dr. Naudin
makes the application every two or three weeks.   *Part* xvii., *p.* 94.

Evils attending Excision of the Tonsils.—With respect to enlargement
of the tonsils affecting the permeability of the Eustachian tube, Mr. Harvey said that he considered it to exist much less frequently than had been
supposed; and in cases where this occlusion did exist, it was not from
the enlarged tonsils pressing upon the mouth of the tube, but from thickening, the result of inflammation of the lining membrane.

Excision of the tonsils was not, therefore, expedient; indeed, in many
cases which he had examined, that proceeding had been attended with
enlargement of the follicles of the pharynx, continued heat and thirst, constant desire for deglutition, disturbance of the general health, and impairment of the voice. Enlarged tonsils were more frequently found in
females than males; and when enlarged in childhood, generally assumed
their natural size at puberty. They appeared to the author to have some
intimate sympathy with the sexual organization. The treatment of enlargement of the tonsils consisted of small doses of the bichloride of mercury
and colchicum; the latter, with guaiacum, was most efficacious.
Part xix., *p.* 160.

Tonsils—Enlarged.—Do not remove them by the knife in children, as
the operation is troublesome, and sometimes serious; and, besides, they
often diminish in size spontaneously after puberty. When the patient is
old enough to exercise self-control, the operation is safe enough. •
Part xxi., *p.* 25.

Tonsil—Enlarged.—The excision of enlarged tonsils is recommended, as performed by M. Lisfranc, of Paris, by grasping the tonsil with the forceps, pulling it inward from the side of the fauces, or merely held steady in its natural position, and then passing a straight narrow blunt-pointed bistoury, the blade being sheathed except rather more than an inch from the point, through its base. It may be done with perfect safety, with immediate relief, and with little hemorrhage succeeding.

Mr. Harvey recommends the bichloride of mercury, in small and divided doses, with tincture of rhubarb and of bark, to be taken at bedtime; also the tincture of colchicum, to be taken internally, and applied externally with lin. saponis. When the scrofulous character predominates, he uses the cod-liver oil. Of all the remedies advised to be used in the chronic state, Mr. Harvey thinks colchicum is the best. He was led to this con-clusion from investigating the history of this affection, and the contents of the tonsils, resembling very much those concretions found in the joints of gouty and rheumatic patients. *Part* xxii., *p.* 215.

Angina Tonsillaris.—Dr. Flange states that the employment of the zincum aceticum in this disease, and especially in thirty cases occurring during an epidemic of scarlatina, where it was exhibited in very different degrees of the affection, has been followed by almost immediate relief. He prescribes from ℈j. to ʒj. in from ʒvj. to ʒviij. of water, giving a table-spoonful in some mucilage every two hours, in severe cases, and frequently gargling the throat also with the same. *Part* xxii., *p.* 365.

TOOTHACHE.

Oil of Ergot.—Suggested to relieve the pain; applied on a small piece of cotton, within the cavity of the tooth. *Part* ii., *p.* 42.

Oil of Valerian.—Suggested in cases of pain arising from carious teeth, unaccompanied by inflammation of the fang. *Part* ii., *p.* 56.

Creasote, generally gives relief from pain; applied directly within the cavity, but is thought to hasten the destruction of the teeth.
Part vi., *p.* 73.

Gregorian Paste.—Currie powder, made into a paste with brandy, is an excellent remedy for toothache, and forms the celebrated Gregorian paste.

Augustura Bark.—When purely nervous, fifteen grains of Augustura bark every four hours has often cured it in a few hours.

Odontalgic Pill.—Dr. Handel, of Mentz, strongly recommends the following:

R Opium, half a drachm; extract of hyoscyamus, camphor, of each six grains; oil of hyoscyamus, one drachm; cajeput oil, tincture of lytta, of each eight minims. Mix. Insert a little into the tooth as a pill, or on lint.
Part viii., *p.* 29.

Aqua, or Liquor Ammoniæ.—Recommended in odontalgia, in doses of 20 to 40 drops, thoroughly blended with a cupful of thick gruel, and taken whenever the paroxysm of pain supervenes. *Part* ix., *p.* 33.

Chloride of Zinc in Toothache.—According to Dr. Stanelli, the chlo-ride of zinc, liquefied by exposure to the air possesses the property of calming dental pains. His mode of application is most simple. By means of a small hair pencil, a small quantity of it is applied to the cavity of the painful tooth, and in the space of a few minutes it appeases the most acute sufferings, without causing any irritation. Before proceeding to the application, it is indispensable carefully to surround the tooth with cotton wadding, and, when the chloride has been applied, to well fill the cavity with this same cotton. The mouth is finally washed with a little warm water. The author affirms that he has obtained uniform success from this means in more than fifty cases, and that he has never observed the progress of the caries rendered more active by it. *Part* ix., *p.* 178.

Use of Pure Tannin.—Prof. Druitt considers tannin the best remedy for toothache :

"It will often be found that the gum around a carious tooth is in a spongy, flabby condition ; a little piece of it, perhaps, growing into the cavity. The ache, too, is often quite as much in the gum as in the tooth itself. But, be this as it may, when the tooth aches, let the patient wash out the mouth thoroughly with a solution of carbonate of soda in warm water ; let the gum around the tooth, or between it and its neighbors, be scarified with a *fine* lancet ; then let a little bit of cotton wool, imbued with a solution of a scruple of tannin, and five grains of mastic, in two drachms of ether, be put into the cavity, and if the ache is to be cured at all, this plan will put an end to it in nine cases out of ten. I think that practitioners are to blame in not paying more attention to the cure of toothache ; I am convinced that in most cases it is as curable as a colic or a pleurisy ; the chief point being to open the bowels, and put the secretions of the mouth in a healthy state, and to apply some gentle astringent and defensative to the diseased tooth till it is capable of being stopped by some metallic substance. I say emphatically a *fine* lancet, because the coarse, round, blunted tools that are generally sold under the name of gum-lancets, only bruise the gum, and cause horrible pain. The lancet which I use is sickle-shaped, cutting on both edges, and finely ground ; and if guarded with the middle finger of the right hand, it may be used in the case of the most unruly children without any possible ill result."   *Part* x., *p.* 139.

New Remedy for Toothache.—Sulphuric ether, saturated in the cold with camphor, and then a few drops of liq. ammoniæ added. It acts as a cautery. M. Cottereau, who has employed it for four years, says it is always attended with success. The rapid evaporation of the ether causes a slight deposit of camphor in the dental cavity, and this protects the nerve from the air. The ammonia cauterizes.   *Part* xiv., *p.* 324.

Toothache—Morphine Locally to the Gum.—Three hours after the last meal in the evening, rub a quarter of a grain of muriate of morphia gently upon the gum, for about three minutes ; then incline the head to the affected side, and keep in that position for ten minutes, taking care neither to spit out nor swallow the saliva. Repeat it in two hours if relief is not obtained, except there is headache or sleepiness.   *Part* xvi., *p.* 89.

Carvacrol, a New Remedy for Toothache.—Carvacrol, according to Professor Schweitzer, is formed by the action of potassa, iodine, or hydrated phosphoric acid, upon oleum carui, ol. thymi : and according to Claus, by the action of iodine upon camphor.

Carvacrol is an oily liquid, very similar to creasote, with a very unpleasant smell and strong taste. Applied on a piece of cotton to a decayed and painful tooth, it gives immediate relief.

[The following has also been used with success:]

A mixture of two parts of liquid ammonia of commerce with one of some simple tincture is recommended as a remedy for toothache, so often uncontrollable. A piece of lint is dipped into this mixture, and then introduced into the carious tooth, when the nerve is immediately cauterized, and pain stopped. It is stated to be eminently successful, and in some cases is supposed to act by neutralizing an acid product in the decaying tooth. *Part* xvii., *p.* 58.

Toothache.—Having dissolved some gum copal in chloroform, clean out the hole, moisten a little cotton with the solution, and introduce it into the decayed part. *Part* xviii., *p.* 105.

Toothache.—Dissolve a little gum mastic in chloroform, so as to thicken the fluid, and then apply it to the tooth on a little cotton wool.
Part xix., *p.* 67.

Toothache.—Apply a minute portion of arsenic, not exceeding the twentieth part of a grain, in combination with creasote and muriate of morphia, on a little cotton wool, to the sensitive portion of the tooth, and retain it *in situ* for twenty-four hours, by softened wax. Then clear away the dead dentine, lay open the pulp cavity, and remove the pulp; if the operation gives any pain, desist from it, and renew the arsenical application until the following day. When the pulp and carious dentine have been removed, plug the tooth in the usual way. If there is a discharge from the pulp cavity, after subduing the tenderness by the arsenical application, and before proceeding to plug the tooth, get the condition of the pulp cavity which gives rise to this secretion, relieved by the daily injection of a solution of alum or of nitrate of silver. In the still more advanced stages of toothache, hardly anything but extraction will do good.
Part xix., *p.* 323.

Toothache.—Let the mouth be first cleansed with warm water containing a little carbonate of soda; then remove any foreign body from the cavity, dry it, and drop into it from a point, collodion in which morphia has been dissolved, fill the cavity with asbestos, and saturate this with collodion; lastly, place over it a pledget of bibulous paper. By occasionally renewing this application, a more durable stopping with gold may at last be effected. *Part* xix., *p.* 324.

Toothache.—Apply a bit of cotton saturated with a drop or two of strong tincture of capsicum (capsic. bacc., ℨiv.; sp. vin. rect., ℥xij).
Part xxi., *p.* 262.

Toothache.—The most intense toothache connected with decayed teeth, is relieved in a moment by the magic touch of the membrana tympani with a blunt probe. Agonizing neuralgia of the face is relieved in the same way. These effects are supposed to be obtained by the influence of the chorda tympani nerve. *Part* xxiv., *p.* 336.

Emetics in Toothache.—Sometimes this is owing to the stomach, and is not relieved by any remedy, not even by the extraction of the tooth. In this case try an emetic of ipecacuanha. *Part* xxx., *p.* 137.

Toothache.—A few drops of chloroform on a bit of cotton, applied to the commencement of the meatus auditorius, often gives great relief. The chloroform must not be dropped directly into the ear.   *Part* xxxv., *p.* 32.

Toothache.—For the last thirty years, Mr. Hearder, of Plymouth, has been in the habit of using galvanism for the relief of toothache ; those cases yield most easily in which the pain originates in the tooth itself. A metal disc covered with moistened cloth and connected with the positive pole, is placed on the back of the neck, a similar disc connected with the negative pole being placed either on the tooth itself or gum ; the degree of power necessary is very feeble. Most cases are relieved permanently, many for a considerable period, and very few not at all. Of course, in cases of abscess at the root of the tooth, the symptoms, as might be expected, are aggravated.   *Part* xxxviii., *p.* 253.

———•••———

TOURNIQUET.

Proper Mode of Applying the Tourniquet.—When you first put on the tourniquet, says Prof. Liston, no pressure must be made on the vessels ; the surgeon must be ready to make his incision before it is screwed up ; for if you allow it to remain on a minute or two, the whole limb is gorged with blood. If you are desirous that the patient should not lose blood, it is of the utmost moment to attend to this point. Put on the tourniquet ; you may even allow the surgeon to transfix the limb with his knife ; the instant the principal vessel is about to be divided, screw it up quickly, and again, as soon as the larger arteries are secured, take it off. If you go on screwing it up, look at the end of the vessels, then unscrew it ; if you see something bleeding, try to catch the vessels, and then screw again ; there is an immense quantity of blood lost, the veins pour it out as fast as the arteries, you do not know what you are tying, and you are almost certain to tie a great many vessels unnecessarily.   *Part* xi., *p.* 185.

Arch-Tourniquet.—[Dr. Oke, of Southampton, has caused to be constructed an arch-tourniquet on a somewhat novel plan.]

It consists of an arch, a pad, and screw. The flanks of the arch are perforated with holes for the action of the external screw, which is worked by a short handle, as in the common tourniquet. The pad is of the ordinary size, flat on one side and convex on the other. Upon its flat surface there is a smooth cavity for the reception and working of the point of the screw. Mode of application : Let the arch embrace the limb, so that one of the perforations of the flank may be exactly opposite the cavity on the flat side of the pad, previously applied over the trunk of the artery to be compressed. Then fit the external into the internal screw, and work it upon the pad till sufficient pressure be made to stop the circulation of the artery.   *Part* ix., *p.* 174.

Military Tourniquet.—This consists of an ordinary straight stay busk, of sufficient length to embrace the largest limb, and by a series of notches at both extremities, may be so reduced as to fit the smallest. The limb being surrounded by this, all that remains is to direct the pressure upon the artery, by means of a screw. The pads are made of box-wood, and the busk is covered with a sheathing of india-rubber, so as not to absorb moisture.   *Part* xxxv., *p.* 87.

Vide Mr. Guthrie's remarks on, Art. " Amputation."

———•◦•———

TRACHEA.

Removal of Foreign Bodies from the Trachea.—The case of Mr. Brunel, in whose windpipe a half-sovereign was accidentally lodged, has given rise to one or two practical suggestions which on future occasions will be found valuable. Although the symptoms in such case may not be immediately dangerous, disease of the lungs would very probably take place sooner or later, and, therefore, it would be always wise to take the necessary steps for the removal of such a foreign body without loss of time. The opening of the trachea in Mr. Brunel's case answered one important end, viz., it enabled the patient to be inverted without giving rise to violent symptoms of suffocation, which took place on this change of position before this orifice was made. From this circumstance Sir B. Brodie comes to the conclusion that in all similar cases where it is necessary to invert the body for the sake of dislodging a foreign substance from the lower part of the windpipe, or its bifurcations, tracheotomy ought always to be previously performed. This will always act like a safety-valve to prevent suffocation, and will also enable the practitioner to manipulate with the forceps or any other instrument that he may wish to use. At the same time it will be seen from the experience of Mr. Erichsen that such an opening in the trachea does not materially diminish the irritability and contractility of the glottis ; and for this reason he has suggested an instrument which will answer the double purpose of intercepting any foreign body which might fall downward toward the larynx during the inverted position of the body, and of a scoop, so as to extract the substance when it is caught in its net. " It consists of a pair of cross-action forceps, the blades of which terminate in branches 2¼ inches in length, and slightly bowed at the extremities ; within the bowed part is inserted a piece of delicate but strong net ; the forceps open to the extent of three quarters of an inch, which will be sufficient to obstruct all passage through the windpipe in the ordinary situations for tracheotomy." When the patient is inverted it is evident that any foreign body would be very likely to fall into this net, and might then be removed at once, or by a pair of common forceps.   *Part* viii., *p.* 124.

Cases of Spontaneous Expulsion of Foreign Bodies from the Air-Passages.—A case of spontaneous expulsion and subsequent recovery is given by Mr. Plant, in the Dublin Hospital Reports. A piece of wood had been passed into the trachea, and at first had lodged in the right bronchus. At the end of four weeks, during which time the boy had suffered much from troublesome cough, it was thrown up from the bronchus into the trachea, where it could be detected moving up and down. As there appeared to be no particular danger, Mr. Plant, trusting that, as it had been thrown up from its first situation, it might also be ejected from the trachea, deferred operating. At the end of the fifth week it was so, and the boy recovered. Another case of this nature is given by Stalpart Vander Wiel. A small piece of bone passed into the trachea of a girl while she was engaged in supping bouillon. The symptoms were constant cough, fever, and ultimately hemoptysis, with purulent expectoration. At the end of four months the bone was coughed up, and the girl recovered. Mr. Howship relates a case in which a nail had passed into the trachea of a man aged 65. The accident occurred on the 15th of August: severe pulmonary symptoms followed, and the man was given up by the faculty, but the nail was discharged on the 12th November, the patient recovered, and was alive twelve years afterward, though subject to frequent pulmonary affections. In a case given by Dr. Lettesom, the covering of a button remained in the air-passages for eight months, when it was coughed up, and the pulmonary symptoms subsided. The admission of an ear of grass into the air-passages appears not to be an uncommon accident, and almost invariably gives rise to very distressing symptoms. Dr. Donaldson, of Ayr, relates one of this description, in which the grass remained in the right bronchus for seven weeks, giving rise to intense bronchitis; it was then expectorated, and the patient recovered.

Part xii., *p.* 186.

Case in which the Larynx of a Goose was Impacted in the Trachea of a Child.—The children in Dr. Burow's vicinity are very fond of blowing through the larynx of a recently-killed goose, in order to produce some imitation of the sound emitted by this animal. When given to them for that purpose, it has usually ten or twelve rings of the trachea connected with it.

A boy, aged 12, while so engaged (Nov. 1, 1848), was seized with a cough, and swallowed the instrument; a sense of suffocation immediately ensued, which was, after a while, replaced by great dyspnœa. Dr. Burow found him laboring under this eighteen hours after, his face swollen, of a bluish-red color, and covered with perspiration. At every inspiration, the muscles of the neck contracted spasmodically, and a clear whistling sound was heard; and at each inspiration, a hoarse sound, not very unlike that of a goose, was emitted. As, on passing the finger down to the *rima glottidis,* it was found closed, Dr. Burow felt convinced (improbable as, from the relative size of the two bodies, it seemed) that the larynx of the goose had passed through it. Tracheotomy was at once performed; but owing to the homogeneousness of structures of the foreign body and of the part it was in contact with, the greatest difficulty existed in distinguishing it by the forceps. Moreover, so sensitive was the mucous membrane, that the instant an instrument touched it, violent efforts at vomiting were produced, and the entire larynx was drawn up behind the root of the tongue. At last, after repeated attempts, Dr. Burow having fixed the larynx in the neck by his forefinger, so that it could no longer be drawn up on these occasions, he contrived to remove the entire larynx of the animal. The child was quite well by the ninth day.   *Part* xxi., *p.* 203.

Improved Mode of Applying Nitrate of Silver to the Interior of the Larynx and Trachea.—To apply nitrate of silver to the trachea, use an instrument having a small grindstone, five or six inches in diameter, which, being caused to be rapidly revolved by means of a pulley and strap, and the salt being placed upon it, a fine dust is thrown from it, which, by the mouth being opened and the breath drawn in, is placed in direct-contact with the diseased surface of the trachea or larynx.

Part xxii., *p.* 150.

TRACHEOTOMY.

Tracheotomy.—[The larynx occasionally requires to be opened during the existence of ulceration on some of its upper portions. When this has been accomplished, Mr. Liston recommends that the surgeon should touch the parts with a solution of nitrate of silver, by means of a piece of sponge at the end of a bent probe, carried upward through the wound in the throat. It may happen that it is not necessary to open the trachea, but only to make an orifice in the crico-thyroid membrane.]

In cases where there is obstruction at the rima glottidis, as where swelling has followed a scald of the glottis, the high operation might answer, and in cases where a foreign body, not of large size, is lodged in the ventricle of the larynx, an opening in the crico-thyroid membrane might suffice, and it is much simpler than tracheotomy. It can be done at once with any pointed instrument that comes readiest to hand, as a penknife, and without any great incision. You feel for the space between the cricoid and thyroid cartilages, and there make a longitudinal incision, right into the tube. This might be resorted to where a person is suffering from the lodgment of a foreign body in the œsophagus, and in such cases it has been done successfully too. A patient may labor under serious and alarming obstruction of breathing in consequence of some large body pressing on the back of the trachea, and you may have nothing at hand to displace or extract it, but you may save the patient, in the meantime, by performing laryngotomy, and allowing him to breathe until you can examine what the foreign body is, and take proper means for its removal. In the majority of cases the operation of tracheotomy is to be preferred, as for the extraction of loose foreign bodies, or of those lodged in the lower part of the canal. In all diseases of the larynx and glottis you will also act more wisely by opening the windpipe. You thus get a large opening, and in a part of the canal which you are certain is quite pervious and clear; you thus insure the free breathing of the patient.

This operation, as I said before, is one not attended with great difficulty or danger. The wound can be made down upon the windpipe without involving any vessel of importance. There are sometimes arterial branches running across the windpipe; but this is very rare.

There is no muscular substance to divide; but there are a few veins, lying over the windpipe and the thyroid body, to be avoided. The wound heals immediately; everything is in favor of it, and it is, therefore, very different from a wound across the windpipe.

If you make an opening to extract a foreign body, and succeed, the wound will heal as far as you wish it to do; you must, in fact, try to keep it open for some time; you must not dream of sewing it up, because blood, even in a small quantity, might insinuate itself into the windpipe, or become infiltrated in the cellular tissue, or collect in the cavity of the wound, and cause injurious or fatal pressure: you put a bit of lint betwixt its edges, and cover the surface of the wound with a pledget dipped in cold water, which is to be frequently renewed. After the incision has been made six or eight hours, you may then bring it together, or apply some strips of plaster: it will generally heal with great rapidity. You find m cases where a foreign body has been lodged in the wound for many days or for many weeks, or even months, that, upon its withdrawal, the parts contract so much that, in twenty-four hours, if it were necessary to introduce an instrument again, you will find it very difficult to accomplish.

There is no difficulty in getting down to the windpipe in an adult patient, if he is at all steady and willing, as most patients who have suffered from difficulty of breathing are, to submit to the operation. You place the patient on a chair (this is better than the recumbent position), turn his head back, and have an assistant to support it. You make an incision from the top of the sternum upward, toward the cricoid cartilage, fully an inch in length, through the skin and the subjacent tissue. You expose, at once, the sternohyoid muscles, and cut between them, push the veins out of their place downward, clear the windpipe upward, by pushing the isthmus of the thyroid body out of the way, if it is there, and then you are quite prepared to cut into the passage. You desire the patient to swallow his saliva, and, taking advantage of the windpipe being pulled downward, you push the knife into it at once, with the back toward the top of the sternum, and, by a little sawing motion, divide three or four of the rings. There is generally no difficulty in doing this, and no bleeding; but if any vessel be wounded you may tie it, or wait a little before you open the windpipe. If you operate for the extraction of a foreign body, the probability is that it will slip out of itself at once; by the relief of the respiration, and the cessation of struggling and exertion on the part of the patient, the bleeding, principally venous, will cease immediately. If there is any arterial bleeding, you will take care to arrest it; you then dress the wound, and allow it to come together in due time. If you operate for an obstruction at the top of the windpipe, you must keep the opening in the tube pervious; and for this purpose you introduce a properly-formed canula. Veterinary surgeons do not hesitate to cut a large square hole in the trachea, and some surgeons, practising on the human body, have proposed to cut out an oval piece of the rings and their connecting membrane; but that is, at least, quite unnecessary, and, indeed, it may be hurtful, by leading to an after contraction of the windpipe.

In children you may sometimes find difficulty in performing the operation. The neck is short, and often very fat. The space in which you cut is very limited; the windpipe also is exceedingly small, and in all cases where the operation is required, the breathing is embarrassed, and the parts are in constant motion. You must have the patient well secured; you cut down upon the fore part of the neck, right in the median line, expose the sternohyoid muscles, separate the connecting cellular tissue, and clear the trachea. You cannot make a young subject elevate the windpipe well or certainly, by swallowing his saliva; you must therefore stretch and fix the tube before cutting into it; you do this by putting a sharp hook in it. You then pull the larynx upward, push in your knife, and make a sufficient opening.

In some individuals, when the operation is performed for disease at the rima glottidis, the canula may soon be removed safely, and the wound permitted to heal; but sometimes it must be worn for several weeks.

The same precautions are to be observed here as in wounds after the patient has attempted suicide; the wound must have a covering of loose texture to prevent cold air getting into the passages.

Part xi., *p.* 171.

Tracheotomy.—When the operation of tracheotomy is to be performed, says Professor Colles, you will find things in a different condition from what you might suppose from performing it on the dead subject. It is all very well to say, throw the head back, and give yourself room, but you cannot put your patient into the position you would wish, on account of the difficulty of breathing; it is so great that he cannot bear such a position an instant, and that in which you find him is generally a bad one, for he is leaning forward; and you must put up with the inconvenience.

Part xii., *p.* 186.

Tracheotomy in Acute Diseases of the Larynx or Trachea.—M. Trousseau has recorded the results of his experience in 121 cases of croup, in which tracheotomy was performed. He advocates the rather early performance of the operation.

If you cannot avoid the thyroid veins, cut straight through them; the hemorrhage ceases on the introduction of the canula. If the case be not very urgent, keep the edges of the wound apart by some instrument, for a short time before introducing the canula, in order to allow of false membranes being expelled. You may expedite this by dropping water into the bronchi, and sponging the trachea. If the canula become obstructed, remove it immediately and empty it, and when the canula is withdrawn introduce the dilator. After the fourth or fifth day, diminish the size of the canula, and by the thirtieth day, it may be dispensed with. Drop into the air-passages, fifteen or twenty drops of a solution of nitrate of silver (gr. v. to ʒj.), and cleanse the trachea with a sponge dipped in the same solution. *Part* xiii., *p.* 237.

Tracheotomy.—Dr. Marshall Hall observes as follows: In every case the first thing to be done is to make an incision of appropriate length through the integuments merely. All the other tissues down to the trachea are to be *pushed aside* without further incision, which may be done without the slightest hemorrhage. For this purpose either an eye-probe may be used, or the double-acting forceps closed. Either of these being introduced, and gently moved in different directions, the trachea is at length laid bare, and this part is *kept exposed* by applying and expanding the forceps.

At this moment, either an incision may be made into the trachea, by means of a minute scalpel, such as is used in operations on the eye, and this incision may be kept open, by means of the double-acting forceps, whilst a silver tube is introduced; or the tenaculum canula may be applied, and a portion of the trachea removed, and the tube may be inserted, or not, according to the views of the operator. *Part* xix., *p.* 151.

Indication for the Performance of Tracheotomy.—Dr. G. H. Rees says: Do not operate for croup or laryngitis in children if the ribs are motionless during inspiration, as this indicates that effusion has taken place into the pulmonary tissues. If the lungs were free, the ribs would be pressed inward or backward by the external atmospheric pressure, when attempts were made at inspiration while there was some serious obstruction to the air-passages.

If the altered movement be considerable, the lungs are yet free, and incision may afford relief. *Part* xx., *p.* 83.

Tracheotomy.—[If there is a necessity for enlarging the wound in the tracheotomy to introduce the canula, the knife should be carried upward, and not below. The reason of this, says Prof. Fergusson, is, that]

There is always much less danger in carrying your incisions upward, in this operation, than in cutting at the lower part of the wound; for, if you happen to get very low down, you might come in contact with important blood-vessels; the arteria innominata, in some cases, rises very high, and that might be wounded; but more especially might the vena innominata be in the way. At the upper part of the wound you may cut without much fear; it is true, there is the isthmus of the thyroid body in the way; but this does not matter much, so that you keep exactly in the median line. You must not misunderstand me, and fancy that I would wish you to cut through the isthmus. You ought, if possible, in opening the trachea, to get below this process on all occasions; but it is not easy or judicious to do so in many instances. In the case under notice, the neck was very short, and I was obliged to divide the isthmus of the thyroid body. It is most important to recollect these two points in performing the operation of tracheotomy : in the first place, not to use your knife freely at the lower part of the wound; and to take especial care not to deviate from the middle line.   *Part* xxv., *p.* 197.

Tracheotomy.—Dr. Gerson, of Hamburg, has invented an instrument which is similar to a three branched speculum in principle, for the purpose of opening the trachea without risk of hemorrhage.
                                                         Part xxvi., *p.* 336.

Tracheotomy.—Recommended by Dr. Marshall Hall, in cases of hydrophobia.   *Part* xxvii., *p.* 59.

Impromptu Tracheotomy.—If you are called suddenly to a case requiring tracheotomy, without proper instruments, take a pair of pointed scissors, and, the integuments having been divided with a lancet or sharp penknife, pierce the trachea with the scissors, and separate the blades. You may then insert the handle of a teaspoon and turn it one quarter or half way round.   *Part* xxx., *p.* 132.

Tracheotomy.—When the trachea has to be opened to *extract a foreign body*, don't be satisfied with making a mere slit, but make a sufficiently large valve-like aperture, larger than the size of the body which has passed.
                                                         Part xxx., *p.* 133.

Dr. Marshall Hall's Tracheotomy Scissors.—To facilitate this operation both in epilepsy, hydrophobia, and other cases, Dr. H. invented a pair of scissors, made so as first to divide the skin over the trachea, and then being pushed into the tube and the blade *opened*, as large an aperture may be made as required. An instrument called a cage is then introduced so as to keep the orifice open.   *Part* xxx., *p.* 271.

Tracheotomy.—Before opening the windpipe, always introduce a hook into one side, so as to keep the part steady. The opening is then made much more easily, and the orifice kept open and prominent for the introduction of the canula.   *Part* xxxi., *p.* 226.

Tracheotomy.—Mr. T. S. Wells, of Samaritan hospital, recommends to fix the trachea by passing a tenaculum, grooved on its convex surface, beneath the lower edge of the cricoid cartilage; by this the trachea must be drawn upward and forward; then pass a knife along the groove, and divide three or four of the tracheal rings: nothing can be easier, simpler, or safer, if the hook be used to fix the trachea. *Part* xxxv., *p.* 93.

Tracheotomy.—[We must admit that tracheotomy is a heroic remedy, and only appropriate to Herculean forms of disease. But Dr. Marshall Hall says:]

I am persuaded that life may be saved, where imminently threatened, by a simple pair of pointed scissors. The integument, being taken up horizontally by the thumb and finger of the left hand, should be divided longitudinally by the scissors; these should then be promptly forced into the trachea, to the proper depth, and opened horizontally to the just extent; the scissors must be then turned, being kept in their place, and opened in the direction longitudinally; the operator has thus made, in a little more than a moment of time, an opening through which the patient may breathe until further appliances can be obtained.

The scissors would be better if they were notchéd on the external edge, so as to prevent them passing too deeply. The opening made must be kept patent: a tracheotome made of silver wire, capable of being introduced readily and expanding within the edges of the opening, is undoubtedly the best of any. *Part* xxxv., *p.* 94.

Foreign Bodies in the Air Passages.—Tracheotomy.—An ingenious and advantageous plan of operating in these cases, is to lift up a piece of the trachea like a flap, with a common tenaculum, after the tube has been laid bare, and then, having allowed the foreign body to be expelled, to drop the flap down again into its original position. *Part* xxxvi., *p.* 170.

Foreign Bodies in the Trachea—Tracheotomy.—In performing tracheotomy for a foreign body in the air tube, says Mr. J. Adams, if the offending substance does not escape at the time of operation, or cannot be discovered, the tracheal tube is not adapted to maintain the patency of the opening made, as a foreign body could not readily escape through it. A strong metallic wire speculum, something like those used in operations on the eye, as invented by M. Luer, of Paris, could be easily modified so as to maintain the patency of the opening, and at the same time allow of the exit of any offending body. If such an instrument were used in case of croup, any false membrane making its appearance at the opening could be extracted. The complete arrest of all hemorrhage would be necessary before an opening was made into the trachea, as the passage of blood into that tube would not be prevented by the speculum. *Part* xxxviii., *p.* 147.

Foreign Bodies in the Trachea.—Tracheotomy.—The opening required, says Mr. F. C. Skey, is large, in fact, sometimes as large as it can be made, if in a child of four or five years of age. There is no increase of danger or difficulty in making a large opening instead of a small one. It is little or no use employing forceps of any kind for the purpose of extracting the offending body, it is preferable to await the return of cough, which in the act of expiration, will inevitably carry the foreign body with the current of air through the larger and nearer orifice, in preference to the smaller and more remote one. *Part* lx., *p.* 275.

TRANSFUSION.

Transfusion of Blood.—Dr. Prichard mentions the case of a gentleman who had been reduced to an exhausted and exsanguineous state by a long continued draining of the system through the kidneys.

"His early complaints had been of dyspeptic symptoms. These were followed by emaciation and loss of strength. His actual state was that of extreme inanition ; his pulse was feeble, jerking, very compressible, the calibre of the artery apparently not filled ; he had palpitation of the heart, increased by the slightest exertion, while any effort brought on an approach to syncope. No disease was discoverable by the sounds of the heart or respiratory organs, though some suspicion was entertained of slight dilatation. "The state of the urine alone threw some light on the nature of the disease. It had long deposited a very copious sediment, of a whitish color, slightly tinged with purple, which was redissolved by dilution, with the addition of an alkali. It appeared to consist of lithates, with some chyle; it was thought probable by the medical gentleman who had previously attended the patient, and by myself at our first meeting, that an exhausted and exsanguineous state, brought on by a long continued draining of the system, constituted the principal disease, or at least that which first required attention. Under these circumstances, it was determined to try a restorative and repletive plan. A nourishing diet was ordered, with malt liquor and some other stimulants. His stomach would receive but little, and at length rejected food. His exhaustion increased to that degree that immediate fatal syncope was threatened. We determined, the patient being obviously *in extremis*, to try the effect of transfusion, and as patients under cholera had borne the injection of large quantities of fluid, there seemed to be no danger in injecting a considerable quantity of blood. Sixteen ounces were taken from the veins of a hale young man, a· servant of the patient, and were injected most skillfully by Mr. Clark. The patient was immediately revived and roused. On the following day he appeared much stronger, but complained of some sense of fullness about his head, and a few drops of blood escaped several times from the nostrils. This subsided; his appetite became good, and he ate plentiful meals of meat, and drank porter, etc. He gradually recovered his strength. The urine improved under the use of alkalies with lime-water, and these were nearly all the remedies used except a few bottles of an effervescing solution of citrate of iron. After two or three months he left his chamber, and then his house, and is now travelling on commercial business." *Part* viii., *p.* 78.

Case of Transfusion.—[Mr. Brown relates a case of transfusion which he performed in November, 1837. His patient, who had been subject to epilepsy, was suddenly attacked, during labor, with most alarming prostration. The child's head was opened and delivery speedily effected, but she did not rally ; the lochial discharge was not more than usual. Stimulants were given, and friction along the spine made use of, with other means likely to restore her, but without effect. Mr. Brown then recommended transfusion, although he very much doubted its efficacy. He describes the operation and its effects as follows :]

Maw's instrument was the one employed ; the central cup, designed to hold the blood, was surrounded by hot water, intentionally made two degrees above the temperature of the fluid. I took from the woman about

℥iv., which were received in the prepared vessel, and in the quickest manner I could, while my assistant was engaged in receiving the blood into the apparatus, I punctured the right basilic vein of the patient, and most readily (after sending a stream of blood through the instrument, to expel the atmospheric air which it contained) passed the extremity of the tube into the vein. The piston was slowly worked : after its second movement the patient expressed that she could feel the tranfused blood " go along her arm into the heart, and quite warm it." Before I had injected the remainder of the blood, she gradually improved both in color and in warmth, and avowed her delight that I was no longer of a " green color, but quite right." Her subsequent recovery took place without any untoward symptoms. *Part* xiii., *p.* 341.

Operation of Transfusion of Blood.—Dr. Routh has collected together all the recorded cases in which transfusion was performed, and from these data has come to conclusions very favorable to the performance of the operation. According to him it should be employed—

Firstly. In all cases of collapse induced by hemorrhage, whether primary or secondary.

Secondly. In that state of extreme exhaustion from dyspepsia, where collapse is imminent, it might be advantageously employed. There are many cases in which dyspepsia has persisted for a long time, and perhaps been neglected, and where, notwithstanding, no organic disease can be detected ; in which no food can be retained on the stomach, and the remedies employed are powerless. Here the patient will sink from inanition, if something is not done. In these cases it is highly probable, that were the operation more frequently resorted to, life might often be saved. Dr. Blundell kept a dog alive three weeks, by consecutively transfusing the blood of another dog in his veins.

Thirdly. In some cases of stricture of œsophagus, where no food can be taken, to give the patient time to rally, so as to admit the introduction of bougies subsequently.

Fourthly. In the collapse which follows long-continued fevers, more especially those of a typhoid character, produced frequently by supervening diarrhœa, or by the crisis of the disorder. It is exceedingly probable, transfusion here might be most advantageous.

Fifthly. In the collapse, or great exhaustion following diarrhœa, dysentery, and cholera.

As a rule, the quantity transfused should not be less than 6 oz., nor more than 16 oz.

The operation may be executed in three ways : 1. By receiving the blood in a vessel, and allowing it to enter the body by gravitation. 2. By interposing a tube between the blood-vessels of the emittent and recipient persons, and trusting to the force of the circulation for the transmission. Both these methods have given place to the third or injecting process, which is effected by the stop-cock stomach pump ; but, instead of the tube through which the pump would be filled, there is a funnel-shaped basin to receive the blood. Much nicety is required in its make.

" So little is the theory of transfusion understood by instrument makers in general, that instruments are made and sold for the purpose that are wholly inapplicable. The basin should be cased like a plate, that it might contain hot water. The piston should fit accurately, and at the same time work freely. I think that an interruption by some elastic material in the tube that is to convey the blood, is advisable, for then the pipe that is inserted into the vein is less likely to be disturbed by any motions which may arise in the working of the syringe or movements of the patient. At least three persons are required for the safe and efficient performance of the operation, and their attention should be wholly given to it. Supposing everything ready, the instrument quite clean, air-tight, and thoroughly warmed, the basin filled with hot water, a vein in the patient's arm should be punctured, and the finger applied to the orifice till the tube is ready to be inserted. It is quite unnecessary to dissect out a vein, and place a probe under it before making the puncture, as has been recommended. A vein in the arm from which the blood is to be taken, is next to be opened by a fine cut, and the stream directed into the centre of the basin, the arm being held close to it. When sufficient has entered, the syringe should be filled, and the piston pushed in a little till blood flows at the end of the pipe, which is then to be introduced into the vein. The injector now works the syringe till the desired quantity has been thrown in. There should be no cessation to the stream of blood entering the basin till the operation is ended, so that after each occasion of the syringe being filled, there may be at least an ounce of blood at the bottom of the basin, or else air would probably be sucked in. The accident to guard against is the transmission of air. The greater facility with which this is likely to occur when transfusion is performed through the jugular vein, points out the impropriety of selecting this vein for the operation. It would be worse than useless to attempt to transfuse unless an expert bleeder be procured. Much of the success of the operation depends on the dispatch, as well as the steady and uninterrupted course that is pursued ; for, with the disadvantage of the blood travelling over dead surfaces, very little exposure of it to air must be apt to destroy vitality. *Part* xx., *p.* 130.

---•◆•---

TUBERCLES.

M. Lombard's Conclusions regarding Tubercles.—1. Tubercle is a secreted substance, deposited under the form of yellowish opaque grains. It grows by superposition. 2. There are two species of tubercles, the simple and the multiple ; the latter forms by the aggregation of several simple tubercles. It contains organized parts within. 3. Granulations are a form of chronic pneumonia; they do not pass into tubercles. 4. The softening of a tubercle depends on the action of the surrounding living parts. 5. Simple tubercle never softens from the centre to the circumference. 6. The multiple tubercle often softens from the centre to the circumference. 7. The most frequent seat of tubercle is the cellular tissue. Tubercle is sometimes to be seen in the lymphatic vessels. Tubercle does not occur on the free surface of mucous membrane so long as it is entire. 8. Tubercles are often hereditary. 9. The lymphatic and sanguineo-nervous temperaments are predisposed to tubercles. 10. Infants and females are most subject to tubercular diseases. 11. Inflammation is an exciting cause of tubercles. 12. The same is to be said of passive congestions, of over-activity or deficient activity of an organ, and probably also of the alterations of the fluids. 13. No certain sign of the rise of tubercles is known. 14. The hectic fever which occurs in tubercular diseases results from the act of elimination. 15. To prevent the tendency to tubercles, we must counteract the influence of hereditary disposition, of temperament, of age, of sex. 16. In persons with predisposition to tubercles, inflammations should be guarded against with the greatest care, or arrested as promptly as possible. 17. The same rules apply to passive congestions. 18. The absorption of tubercles is very probable. 19. To obtain the cure of tuberculous ulcerations we must prevent the formation of new tubercles, and confine the work of elimination within certain limits. 20. Tubercles may remain long in the organs in a latent state; to obtain this result we must seek to arrest the process of elimination by antiphlogistic means, and above all by revulsives. *Part* xi., *p.* 52.

TUMORS.

Erectile Tumor Cured by Vaccination.—A child thirteen months old (not vaccinated), had a small erectile tumor over the left eyebrow. M. Pigeaux inserted nine points of vaccine matter over its whole surface. The vaccine eruption was confluent on the tumor, but followed its usual course; on the 25th day the scabs fell off, and nine-tenths of the tumor had disappeared. The surface of the tumor was now powdered with alum, and the scab was removed every four or five days, to permit a fresh application of the powder. At the end of three weeks the whole of the erectile tissue was destroyed; the bottom of the wound threw up healthy granulations, and in seven weeks it was completely healed. For the success of an operation of this kind, it is necessary that the points of insertion be sufficiently numerous to produce a confluent pock; and should any portion of erectile tissue remain after the removal of the scabs, it must be destroyed by some caustic like the powdered alum. *Part* vii., *p.* 168.

Mode of Taking out a Fatty or Steatomatous Tumor from the Breast.—On this subject Sir B. Brodie says: We know of no internal medicine, nor of any local application that will disperse these tumors, and the only thing to be done is to remove them by the knife. This may be done when the tumor is quite small. I do not, however, generally recommend the operation at this period; first, because the tumor may never increase, and as long as it is small it is of no consequence; and secondly, because the operation is really more easy when the tumor has attained a certain size. Still, it is better not to let the tumor go to any *very* large size; and for this reason, lest the pressure of the skin should cause it to contract adhesions to the neighboring parts. Where such adhesions have taken place the operation is rendered difficult, and you cannot be certain that you do not leave some small portion of it, which may be the nucleus of a future growth. As soon, then, as the tumor becomes large enough to be troublesome from its bulk, you may dissect it out; and this is a simple operation if you know how to do it, and very difficult otherwise. Make a free incision of the skin, not upon the tumor, but into it, cutting fairly into its substance. Do not spare the incision through the skin, but let it extend from one end to the other. Then lay aside your knife, and you will find that with the fingers you can easily separate the cyst that contains the adipose matter from the neighboring textures, pulling out one lobe after another, till at last the tumor remains attached only at one corner, that is, at the point at which the vessels run in and out. You have no bleeding in any other part of the operation, but in this last part of it you will generally find one or two arteries which you must secure by ligature. When the tumor is situated under a muscle, the operation is to be performed in the same way, with this exception, that besides laying open the skin, you must freely divide the muscle, cutting across the fibres.

[Sir Benjamin gives a curious case, which illustrates the value of liquor potassæ in some of these fatty deposits. It is as follows:]

A man came to this hospital some seventeen or eighteen years ago, with a very odd appearance—an enormous double chin, hanging nearly down to the sternum, and an immense swelling at the back part of the neck—two great tumors as big as oranges sticking out, one behind each ear. The patient stated that these tumors had begun to form three or four years before, and had been gradually increasing in size. They gave him no pain, but they made him miserable, and in fact had ruined him. The poor fellow was a gentleman's servant, and having such a strange, grotesque appearance, nobody would hire him. I gave him half a drachm of liquor potassæ three times a day, and gradually increased the dose to a drachm. This was taken in small beer. About a month after he began to take it, the tumors were sensibly diminished in size. He went on taking the alkali a considerable time, and the tumors continued decreasing. It was just then that iodine began to have a sort of reputation, much beyond what it deserved, for the cure of morbid growths, and I gave him the tincture of iodine. It was curious that while he took the tincture of iodine he lost flesh generally, but the tumors began to grow again. Finding this to be the case, I left off the iodine, and gave him the liquor potassæ a second time. He took an immense quantity altogether, and left the hospital very much improved, being directed to continue to take the medicine for some time longer, off and on. I had lost sight of him for some time, when I happened to be requested to visit a patient in Mortimer street. I did not observe the servant that opened the door, but as I came down he stopped me in the hall, and said that he wished to thank me for what I had done for him. To my surprise it was this very man. He had gone on taking the caustic alkali for a considerable time, and you may suppose how much he was improved by his being able to get a situation as foot-man. There were some remains still of the tumors, but nothing that any one would have observed. _Part_ ix., _p._ 117.

Sanguineous Tumors on the Heads of Newborn Infants.—[Mr. Adams has met with several cases of a rare form of infantile pathology, which is scarcely mentioned by British authors. All obstetric practitioners are acquainted with the caput succedaneum, as it is usually termed—a soft tumor formed by effusion of the serum of the blood at the presenting part of the child's head, and which, though usually requiring none but the simplest treatment, sometimes, though rarely, inflames and gives rise to abscess. There is, however, another class of tumors found under the same circumstances, which, on account of their rarity, have either attracted little attention, or have been mistaken for a totally different pathological state. For our knowledge of these we are indebted entirely to French and German writers. They applied various names to these tumors, for which Naegele has substituted *Cephalhæmatomata.*]

Cephalhæmatomata may exist in three forms, viz., under the aponeurosis, under the pericranium, and under the bone.. The *first* kind, viz., that wherein the blood is effused under the aponeurosis formed by the expansion of the occipito-frontalis muscle, is generally considered to be of a simply contusive character, as evidenced by its mode of production as well as by its external and internal anatomical characters. This is the simplest, but at the same time the rarest form of the cephalhæmatoma. In general it disappears rapidly, and requires only mild discutient treatment. The *third* variety in the above list, the *subcranial* cephalhæmatoma, which has its seat between the dura mater and the bone, has been but rarely observed, and very little of a satisfactory nature is known regarding it. The symptoms are those of cerebral compression, but it is impossible to diagnose its existence during life, and it can only be guessed at when it coexists with an external cephalhæmatoma, which, according to M. Baron, frequently happens. The *second* variety, or that in which the tumor exists beneath the periosteum, although much more frequent than either of the two preceding, is on the whole a rare affection. I place it last, because it is to it I mainly wish to direct attention, as being the most interesting in a practical point of view.

Mr. Adams then relates two of the best marked cases of the second variety. He was sent for to examine the head of a healthy male child, which he had delivered eight days before; the presentation was in the second position of natural labor, and the duration of labor six hours, of which the first stage occupied five. The mother and friends were alarmed at what they called "a hole in the child's skull." There was a soft fluctuating tumor over the left parietal protuberance, which felt as if circumscribed by a ridge of bone that seemed to mark the boundary of an opening into the skull. But, on more careful examination, the bone could be felt in the centre of the apparent hole, which, together with the absence of pulsation, etc., satisfied him that it was a case of cephalhæmatoma. Evaporating lotions and slight pressure with a bandage were accordingly used, and in three weeks the tumor had entirely disappeared.

Another case of exactly the same nature occurred in the practice of Dr. Menzies, which was left to the efforts of nature, and recovered without any treatment. The presence of a bony ridge, circumscribing the tumor, which gives the impression of an opening in the cranium, is the most striking peculiarity, and of the greatest practical importance. The bone within the circle can generally be felt uninjured on pressing the finger firmly from the edge to the centre. The time the tumor takes to become fully developed varies from a few hours to as many days, and it seldom disappears entirely within four or five weeks. Various are the opinions as to its causes, some holding that it is a consequence of severe labor or the use of instruments, while others say that when it occurs it is almost always after very easy labors.

But the most important researches on this point have been made by M. Valleix. He considers that cephalhæmatomata do not exist before the occurrence of labor, and that they are the consequence of force or pressure employed upon the child's head during delivery. For a right understanding of his views it is necessary to advert to the anatomy of the parietal bones in the infant. At birth the pericranium adheres but slightly to the bone, with the exception of a few lines at the sutures and fontanelles, and consequently a slight force is sufficient to strip it off. In doing so, numerous vessels are seen to enter the fissures of the bone. The bone itself ossifies from one point in the centre, *i. e.*, the parietal protuberance, and bony radii shoot from the centre to the circumference. These radii are best seen on a dried preparation. Haller noticed, that on compressing the head of an infant even slightly, after removing the pericranium, he saw springing from between these radiated fibres innumerable drops of blood, which, collecting together, formed a thin layer over the bone. M. P. Dubois, after corroborating Haller's experiment, suggested that the fact furnished a probable explanation of the formation of the bloody tumors of the head. M. Valleix, after numerous observations, confirms the theory of Dubois, and concludes that if pressure, and above all, if circular pressure, is made upon a point of the cranium, blood will spring from the surface of the bone, and by its upward pressure strip off the pericranium, which is easily detached; that as the liquid blood accumulates under this membrane, new outlets will be opened up for the escape of more blood, and thus at length a tumor will arise. Assuming this as a settled point, he considers that the pressure of the child's head against the mouth of the uterus causes, according to the degree of pressure, either the simple sero-sanguineous tumor, an ecchymosis, or a sub-pericranial cephalhæmatoma.

The contents of the tumor may vary in quantity from a scruple to nearly eight ounces. Dr. W. Campbell, in one case which he punctured, obtained a large teaspoonful, and in another half a teaspoonful of slimy sanguineous matter.

There are but few diseased appearances occurring on the heads of newborn infants likely to confuse the diagnosis; and it requires little more than a knowledge of the existence of such affections, and of their distinguishing characters to prevent our falling into error. A favorable prognosis may in general be given. If, however, the cephalhæmatoma be of great size, or remain undiminished for several weeks, the bone is apt to become affected, when, from the excessive discharge, and the constitutional disturbance attendant upon the extension of the disease to the brain, death will almost inevitably result.

Regarding the treatment of cephalhæmatoma there needs not much be said. In many cases—I might almost say in most cases—no treatment is required, or at least the treatment adopted may be of the simplest description, and used principally with the view of preventing the parents or friends from becoming anxious. When the tumor is small, causing no uneasiness, and not threatening to inflame, there may be used a simple evaporating lotion, such as a solution of muriate of ammonia with alcohol, and this treatment may be conjoined with slight pressure. But when the tumor is large, and does not diminish at the end of a fortnight or three weeks, these means are likely to fail, and it may be necessary to adopt more active measures to procure absorption or evacuation of its contents.

[Dr. Zorer, of the Foundling Hospital of Vienna, employs cold applications of calomel when cerebral congestion is supposed to exist, and almost invariably opens the tumor, a most injudicious practice when hastily adopted.]

Lowenhardt recommends puncture with a trocar, and strapping; and to this plan I am inclined to give preference, using, however, the ordinary knife for subcutaneous puncture instead of the trocar. Where the contents of the tumor are fluid, it will be equally efficacious, and the wound will be more readily disposed to heal by the first intention. The wound must afterward be treated on the ordinary principles, and the simpler the dressing the better. In making the incision, care must be taken to avoid the arterial vessels; for, in a case operated on by M. Valleix, death followed the division of a small branch, and Smellie records a similar unfortunate case which happened in the hands of one of his pupils.

Part xi., *p.* 207.

Encysted Tumors—Cure for Encysted Tumors, or Wens of the Head, or other Parts of the Body, without Cutting them Out.—First make a longitudinal cut along the scalp. This is performed with little loss of blood. Next, press out the contents of the cyst, and apply freely, alcohol in the cavity, with a camel's-hair brush. Then place in the cavity, also, from two to six grains of nitrate of silver, and bring the edges together with strappings, when inflammation takes place. Should it inflame too much, apply cold water dressings, and give a few doses of active purgative medicine. This plan, says Dr. Harvey, has ever been found to complete the cure in a few days. *Part* xi., *p.* 156.

Pulsating Tumors of Bone.—[Mr. Stanley remarks that there are three distinct sources of pulsation in the tumors of bone: 1. The proximity of the tumor to a large artery; 2. The development of blood-vessels and blood-cells, constituting a sort of erectile tissue within the tumor; 3. The enlargement of the arteries of the bone in which the tumor has arisen. Of these, the first is by far the most common. The tumor generally consists of soft, fibrous, and dense osseous tissue. Such cases have frequently been mistaken for aneurism, and the principal artery supplying the part has in consequence been tied. On the subject of pulsation in the tumors of the bone dependent on the development of blood-vessels and blood-cells, forming a sort of erectile tissue within the tumor, Mr. Stanley remarks, that assuming these cells to be continuous with the surrounding arteries, the rush of blood into this structure might give to the whole mass a pulsation resembling that of aneurism. Several cases of the third variety are referred to. The density and resistance of the investments of the tumor are specially noticed by the author as appearing to have a material influence in causing pulsation in them, for it may be doubted whether any of these tumors would pulsate without the resistance derived from the bone or its coverings.]

After some observations tending to show the little value to be attached to the presence of bellows-sound in the diagnosis between aneurism and the pulsating tumor of bone, Mr. S. proceeds to relate the case of pulsating tumor of the ilium which occurred in St. Bartholomew's Hospital, in which a ligature was placed around the common iliac artery. The patient, a man, aged 42, had on the inner side of the right upper arm, a tumor about the size of a small orange, very loosely connected with the surrounding structures, free from pain, and without pulsation. This tumor was first observed about ten years ago, and during the last three years it had ceased to grow. The pulsating tumor of the pelvis had its chief attachment to the left ilium, and projected from both surfaces of the bone. It reached downward to Poupart's ligament, and to the extent of about three inches into the abdomen. It felt moderately firm, and a little below the crista, near the anterior superior spine, a small movable piece of bone was discovered apparently involved in the tumor. Everywhere within reach of the fingers the tumor pulsated, not with a thrill of vibration, but with the

deep heavy beat of aneurism. By the ear resting against the abdominal
parietes, a bellows-sound was plainly recognized. After a minute description of the local features and constitutional phenomena of the disease, the
author observes, that in deciding on the nature and treatment of the case,
the following points were involved—was this pulsating tumor an aneurism?
and if so, from what artery had it arisen; or was it one of the pulsating
tumors of bone? He then states the argument which, in consultation, led
to a preponderance of opinion in favor of this tumor being an aneurism.
In the uncertainty respecting the origin of the supposed aneurism from the
external or internal iliac artery, the decision would obviously be that the
common iliac should be tied, and the man having decidedly expressed his
feeling in favor of submitting to the operation, the author considered it his
duty to undertake it.

The case proceeded favorably to the middle of the second day, when
symptoms of peritonitis ensued, and he sunk on the morning of the third
day from the operation. On examining the body, the effects of peritonitis
were observed in the deeper parts and left side of the abdomen. In the
wall of the left ventricle of the heart there was a medullary tumor about
the size of a filbert. Medullary matter was found in the bronchial glands,
and a few deposits of the same kind in the lungs. A minute description
is given of the tumor in the pelvis, which was connected with the ilium,
and composed of a spongy tissue with cells and convoluted vessels distributed through it. The tumor in the arm, which had all the marks of
an innocent structure, was found to the surprise of the author, identical
in structure with the tumor in the pelvis.

Notwithstanding its density, says M. Roux, the osseous structure may
become the seat of a transformation similar to that which, in the soft
parts, constitutes sanguineous (erectile) tumors. The capillary vessels,
more especially those which depend on the arterial system, become extraordinarily developed. Perhaps when they are thus amplified, the network
which they form naturally may assume a different arrangement; perhaps
the capillaries are differently interlaced, anastomosed. However this may
be, as these capillaries become dilated and filled with blood, the bone
softens, swells, and probably there is destruction of the proper fibres of the
thin lamellæ which constitute its substance. At last, the disease progresses to such an extent that the external lamellæ of the bone, even those
formed by the compact tissue, are reduced to a kind of thin, flexible envelope, through which the pulsations of the tumor may be felt, and which
rupturing divides into little fragments, or disappears entirely. This state
of the osseous substance may be compared to aneurism; it is indeed, an
aneurismal state of the capillary system of the bone. The flat bones,
which have a well-marked diploic structure, such as those of the skull and
pelvis, and the spongy portion of the long bones, are the most liable to the
disease. The immediate cause is nearly always a blow. As is the case in
the soft tissues, sanguineous fungus tumors of the bone are not always be-
nignant; they may be endowed with a force of expansion and a rapidity
of growth, which alone would render them extremely formidable, and present, on anatomical inspection, the most heterogeneous structure; or the
cancerous element may manifestly be superadded. When this is the case,
these tumors approximate very closely to the degenerescences of the osseous structure, known under the name of spina ventosa or osteosarcoma.
These latter appear to be merely different forms of cancer of bone, a dis-

ease which has been but imperfectly described hitherto, and which it will, perhaps, be ever impossible to delineate with precision, so great are the anomalies which it is susceptible of presenting. These tumors are so rare, that M. Roux has only seen a few well-marked cases during his long surgical career. The only methods of treatment which can be adopted with any chance of success are—the ablation of the tumor along with the part of the bone which is diseased : the amputation of the entire part or organ affected ; and lastly, the ligature of the principal artery of the diseased region.

M. Lallemand, of Montpellier, describes a sensation of crackling to be perceptible to the finger when pressure is made upon the tumor. This is due to the breaking down of minute osseous septa which exist in the substance of the morbid mass. The noise produced has been compared to the " crumpling " of parchment. The above phenomenon also presented inself in a case treated by M. Roux. *Part* xi., *p.* 180.

Adipose Tumor in the Spermatic Cord—Unique Case.—The patient, 43 years of age, in the autumn of 1842, discovered an enlargement in the left side of the scrotum. This was at first supposed to be hernial, but by careful examination with an exploratory needle, the disease was considered to be confined to the spermatic cord. As the tumor increased in size, Mr. Edwards was consulted.

He considered the tumor to be irreducible epiplocele, but advised the patient to consult Mr. Lawrence. By him endeavors were made, but without success, to reduce the supposed hernia, and a suspensory bandage was directed to be worn. In the spring of 1844 slight enlargement had taken place, and a change in form was perceptible. No effect resulted from the administration of iodine, which was used both internally and externally. At midsummer, 1844, there was a manifest increase in size, though slight, and the tumor had assumed a lobulated form. The lobules were very hard, not unlike scirrhus, and insensible. In April, 1845, the tumor had enlarged to the size of a melon; the left testicle lay in front, and both spermatic cords could be felt in a sound condition. Mr. Travers was now consulted, and he convinced himself that the mass was unconnected with either abdomen or testicle, and advised operation. Sir B. Brodie and Mr. Lawrence, on examination with a candle, were convinced that it was not hernia, and agreed in recommending excision of the tumor.

Mr. Lawrence thus describes the symptoms : " Upon first view it would be pronounced a scrotal rupture. It was a pyriform enlargement occupying the whole left side of the scrotum, extending to the abdominal ring. The integuments and cellular tissue were perfectly natural. But a circumstance was immediately perceived at variance with the supposition of a rupture; the left testicle lay on the front of the swelling; it was loose and movable on the mass ; the cord could be traced a little above it, and was then lost in the tumor. When firmly grasped, the mass was found to be of an unequal consistence ; portions were solid and firm, but the greater part was soft, so that I examined it with a candle, supposing it might contain fluid ; there was no transmission of light. Judging from the mere manual examination, it might have been a large scrotal rupture, with various contents, principally omentum ; or it might have been a tumor not of uniform consistence. It had the doughy feel belonging to omental rupture ; and the omentum, when long out of the abdomen, becomes some-times much enlarged by the deposit of fat in its texture, especially in corpulent persons, but this gentleman was thin. Although the swelling was continued upward, careful examination showed that it had no con-nection with the cavity of the abdomen ; the cord could be felt free above, close to the abdomen. The conclusion was obvious ; the swelling could not be a rupture, but I could not make up my mind as to its real com-position. Although the nature of the disease was doubtful, there were no evidences of dangerous character, nothing to contra-indicate the operation of removal, which had become urgently necessary from the great bulk of the tumor, and its rapid rate of increase during the last few months."

Mr. Lawrence, assisted by Mr. Travers, removed the diseased mass. The first step was an incision into the swelling. Two elliptical incisions were now made, including a considerable portion of the skin of the scrotum. An attempt was made to save the testicle, but the different constituents of the spermatic cord were so entangled with the substance of the tumor, that after some loss of time, the entire contents of the left scrotal sac were turned out. Mr. Lawrence thus describes the tumor after excision : " This mass, measuring about eight inches in length, by six in width, was taken from the scrotum. It presents the ordinary appearance of adipose swelling, the component masses of fat being larger, and the surface being partly lobulated. On a superficial view of its exterior, and of the cut surface after it had been divided, it might have been taken for a mass of beef suet. Swellings of the scrotum, in the great majority of instances, are ruptures or morbid conditions of the testis, its coats, or the spermatic cord. Diseases of the cellular structure, excepting inflammations and effusions of blood, serum, pus, or urine, are very uncommon. I do not remember to have met with a tumor in this situation ; and the fatty growths so common in the adipose tissue, are what we should have least expected in a part which naturally does not contain a particle of fat. I have never seen in the scrotum, the cellular tumor which is sometimes met with in the external organs of the female." The ligatures came away kindly, and in three weeks the patient walked about his house. He now walks from Islington to the city without inconvenience. *Part* xii., *p.* 225.

Removal of Tumors by a Flap Operation.—[Every practical surgeon must have noticed the facility with which a tumor loosely connected with the parts on which it rests can be raised, and also that this facility is diminished when the skin is dissected off it. By the ordinary mode of incising, the operation becomes converted into a digging ; this is proposed to be remedied by using a flap. The mode in which Mr. Chippendale operated in a case of this sort, is best described in his own words, as follows :]

Raising the tumor as far as I could from the body with one hand, I passed a long narrow knife under the skin near the border of it, in the direction of its long diameter ; having cut through the connections at its base, and the edge of the knife having arrived at the opposite border, it was turned toward the surface of the body, and the skin severed. The whole was now turned out, and the tumor dissected from the flap thus formed, with the greatest facility. The few vessels which bled had liga-tures applied, which in a quarter of an hour, were again removed ; the flap was laid down on the wound with two points of suture in the long side, and the edges secured with adhesive plaster; the whole was healed in a few days, leaving a scar representing three sides of a rectangular parallelogram as thus [.

The skin when thus divided, so soon shrinks, that it can seldom be necessary to take any portion of it away; but should a case occur where such a proceeding became necessary, a portion could be taken from the free border of the flap, so as to make it fit the exposed surface, as parts are brought to coincide in autoplastic operations. *Part* xii., *p.* 251.

Pulsating Tumors of Bone.—[These tumors so nearly resemble aneurisms that they are liable to be mistaken, even by the most eminent surgeons; they have, indeed, been named osseous aneurisms. M. Dupuytren regards them as accidental development of erectile tissue, generally implicated with the cancérous element. He has recorded many of these cases. Mr. Teale observes:]

A case of pulsating tumor of the ilium, supposed to be aneurism, recently occurred at St. Bartholomew's Hospital. Mr. Stanley describes the tumor as pulsating throughout its whole extent; not with a thrill or vibration, but with a deep heavy beat of aneurism; and a bellows sound was distinctly audible. A ligature was applied to the common iliac artery. The patient died on the third day, from peritonitis. The tumor on dissection, was found to be composed of a spongy tissue, with cells and convoluted vessels distributed through it. In the wall of the left ventricle there was a medullary tumor, of the size of a filbert. After relating the case to the Medico-Chirurgical Society, Mr. Stanley alluded to several others, in which tumors originating in the bones had been mistaken for aneurism. Two such had occurred at St. Bartholomew's Hospital: one was an encephaloid tumor of the humerus: the other a morbid growth, consisting of a soft fibrous and dense osseous structure, originating in the femur, and supposed to be popliteal aneurism. Mr. Stanley also referred to a case of great interest, which had occurred to Mr. Guthrie. In this instance, a medullary tumor, situated in the gluteal region, presented so decidedly the characters of aneurism, that it was regarded as such by Sir Astley Cooper and other surgeons, and accordingly Mr. Guthrie applied a ligature to the common iliac artery. *Part* xiii., *p.* 235.

Treatment of Pendulous Tumors.—[These tumors after remaining stationary for years, often become the seat of morbid action: hence the general rule of practice is to remove them when first presented. The chief point of importance in their removal is a consideration of the proper part of the pedicle at which the division is to be effected. Dr. O'Ferrall observes :]

If the section be made too near the bulb, an unsightly projection will remain after the operation; if it be done too near the other extremity of the pedicle, the integument, on retracting, will leave a wound, and consequently a scar, much larger than could have been anticipated. Allowance, then, must be made for the elongation of the pedicle by the weight of the bulb, and for the contraction of the stalk, which always follows its division —the same process which renders it unnecessary to tie the neck of a uterine polypus close to the mucous surface from which it has grown. The best mode of proceeding is, to poise the tumor on the hand, and allow the surrounding skin to retract and recover its pristine position, and then to make the section of the pedicle a little below its origin. Should the nutritious artery be large enough to deserve attention, the jet of blood may be prevented by previously including the neck of the tumor in a provisional ligature, and, when the section is accomplished, tying the divided artery. The provisional ligature may then be removed altogether. A slight touch of the nitrate of silver, just sufficient to produce a delicate white coating, will not only shorten the duration of the subsequent smarting, but lessen the probability of any reaction, especially of an unhealthy kind. Simple water dressing will then complete the local treatment.

In operating on the adipose pendulous tumor, the extent of interference with the pedicle will be regulated by the presence or absence of fatty matter in its substance. If the growth extend through the neck into the subcutaneous cellular membrane beyond it, such an incision must be made as will allow of its complete extraction. In such a case, the small cavity then left should be filled with lint dipped in olive oil, and the integument brought gently over it, to prevent an unnecessarily large cicatrix. The lint is withdrawn when suppuration is established, and the integuments brought together by adhesive plaster.

The proceeding in the case of pendulous nævus is somewhat different, and must be adapted to the peculiar circumstances of the case. It is not usual for the pedicle, in such instances, to be entirely free from all traces of erectile tissue. Should the pedicle be implicated, or should the vessels of the cellular or dermoid tissues beyond it be hypertrophied, a simple section would be inadequate to the cure; hemorrhage of a troublesome nature would be the immediate result, and reproduction of the disease the more remote consequence of such an imperfect procedure. The diseased part must be included in an elliptical incision, and thus freely and completely removed. It may happen that the erectile formation may extend irregularly, for a considerable distance, beyond the origin of the pedicle. In such cases, the amputation of the pedicle alone would entail the consequences already alluded to, while the excision of the whole of the morbid structure might be forbidden by its extent, or by the importance of the parts in which it is found. The following is the mode I would recommend under such circumstances, and when the removal of the pendulous tumor is desired on account of the inconvenience it occasions. The tumor being held horizontally and on the stretch, the point of the style or nail cautery, described by Dr. Wilmot, should be passed through the cervix in several places, so as to insure the obliteration of the vessels contained in that place. The whole cervix may be traversed by these punctures at one or several successful operations, according to its breadth. When the vascular character of the cervix is thus changed, its section may be performed, without risk of hemorrhage.

When a pendulous tumor is known, or suspected to be malignant, great care must be taken to remove the entire of the morbid parts. If the heterologous structure be confined to the bulb of the tumor, and the pedicle or surrounding skin be healthy, there can be no reason for doing more than simple section of the former; but the section should not, for obvious reasons, be made too near the bulb. But should the neck of the tumor be thickened, hardened, or irregular, a free elliptical incision should be made in the integument beyond it, and all suspicious parts satisfactorily removed.

Part xvi., *p.* 313.

Tumors of the Neck connected with Blood-vessels.—[Some years ago Mr.

Liston punctured a tumor in the neck, from which considerable hemorrhage occurred, and which the operator then supposed to be an abscess in communication with an artery. Professor Syme has published the account of a similar case in which he tied the artery, but after death the tumor was found not to communicate. Mr. Syme says:]

About a month ago a young man called upon me to get my opinion of a swelling in his neck. It was seated on the right side, and occupied the upper triangular space. It was of an oval form, quite circumscribed, and obviously consisted of a bag containing fluid. Upon more particular examination, I found a distinct pulsation of the kind which I had been accustomed to regard as characteristic of aneurism, being an expansive impulse, not limited to a portion of the tumor, but felt equally at every accessible point, even from the mouth, and more especially in a lateral direction. The patient stated that the swelling had commenced about nine months ago—and had progressively enlarged without any cause that had been ascertained. He also stated, that when he worked hard, or walked fast, the tumor increased in size, and had a strong beating in it. I felt satisfied that there was an aneurism of the carotid artery, but expressed no opinion at the time, and desired the patient to call again for further examination. When he did so, I varied the process by placing him in different positions —by trying the effect of pressure on the tumor and artery—and by listening to the sounds of the tumor. There was no distinct aneurismal " bruit," but a very strong loud pulsation, that implied the action of the heart upon an extensive surface. Finding my impression thus confirmed, I informed the patient of my apprehension ; but before giving a decided opinion, requested that he would call once more. He did so a few days afterward, and I then felt fully warranted in informing him that an operation would be requisite for his relief. Next day he placed himself in my hands for this purpose. After he had been confined to bed for a few days, I tied the artery below the crossing of the omo-hyoideus, as the tumor prevented this from being done higher up. The textures of the neck were more than usually adherent, and the vessel was not exposed to view with nearly the same facility as upon the former occasions which have required me to perform the operation. I nevertheless succeeded without any tearing, or undue disturbance of the parts, in passing and tying the ligature, so as to relieve me from the slightest apprehension of any bad consequences. The tumor immediately sustained a very distinct diminution of bulk, which was remarked not only by the gentlemen present, but by the patient. He went on most favorably after the operation until the fifth day, when hemorrhage took place from the wound, and notwithstanding every effort to effect prevention, recurred from time to time until the evening of the twelfth day, until it proved fatal.

The parts concerned were examined next day in the presence of Drs. Scott, Duncan, Mackenzie, Peddie, Brown, Gillespie, and Ballingall.

We found a tumor, extending from the ear to the extremity of the omo-hyoideus, and completely occupying the upper triangular space of the neck. At the lower part it seemed to terminate in the sheath of the vessels, which looked like a prolongation of it downward, but was found to be merely enveloped by the bag, which I dissected out entire from the coats of the vessels to which it had intimately adhered. The cyst, when opened, was found to possess a tough consistence, and to contain a fluid

like thin gruel. At the posterior part, when viewed internally, it displayed a sacculated or honeycomb-looking structure.

[Another case has been reported in which a large abscess in the neck
(treated by a quack) had not been opened, but allowed to go on till it
burst by several openings. When the discharge had gone on for about a
month, alarming and repeated hemorrhages took place from the openings.
After death,]

The blood-vessels were injected, and it was found that ulceration had
occurred in the subclavian artery, as it lies upon the first rib. The rib
was in a carious state, as well as the bodies of the contiguous vertebræ.
The situation of the ulcerated opening in the artery was toward the
bone, and occupied about one-fourth of the calibre of the vessel; the
opening was of oval shape, and well defined. There was no enlargement
of the capacity of the vessel at the point.   *Part* xvii., *p.* 141.

Treatment of Erectile Tumors.—M. Behrend, of Berlin, treats these
tumors by the application of the concentrated acetic acid, followed by
lint dipped in distilled vinegar. Under this treatment the tissue becomes
pale and hard, diminishes in bulk, and is at length completely thrown off.
He also, in some cases, enjoins the repeated division of the dilated vessels,
by puncturing them with a needle with double-cutting edges.
Part xviii., *p.* 230.

Tumors—Encysted.—In cases of small sebaceous tumors, instead of dissecting out the cyst, puncture the tumor, squeeze out the contents, and
apply nitrate of silver all over the internal surface of the cyst. The most
convenient way of applying the nitrate, is, to have a probe coated with it.
Part xix., *p.* 271.

Neuroma, or Tumor of Nerve.—No measure is successful except that
of excision. The tumor may either be dissected out of the mass of nerve-
fibres among which it has grown, or it may be cut away together with the
piece of nerve to which it is attached. The latter measure is generally
quite safe and practicable. Lastly, amputation may be resorted to [if the
disease is situated in an extremity], when other means fail, and the symptoms are urgent.   *Part* xx., *p.* 59.

Extirpation of Erectile Tumors by the Cautery.—Dr. Douglas Maclagan makes the following remarks : "These erectile tumors, which consist
essentially of a congeries of enlarged blood-vessels, are commonly treated
by ligature; but this causes a good deal of suffering, and often much constitutional irritation, before the strangulated mass finally separates. The
method of applying the cautery is to pass a large red-hot surgical needle,
which may be readily heated by a gas-flame, once or twice through the
base of the tumor; and the object is to cause effusion of lymph, and thus
to alter the structure of the tumor, and to arrest its growth.
Part xxiii., *p.* 154.

Fibrous Tumors.—[According to Dr. G. M. Humphrey, with the exception of the fatty, the fibrous are perhaps the most common of the simple
growths. They resemble the natural fibrous tissue as found in areolar
membrane, in ligaments, tendons, etc. Their miscroscopical examination
is also distinctive. In some instances, the fibres are disposed more or less
concentrically. These tumors generally do not attain to a very large size.
In other instances, the component fibres interlace in a complicated irregu-

lar manner. These kinds may attain to a very large size; they are commouly round. In a third, but more rare class, the tumor consists of an aggregation of small nodules, or masses closely compressed together, having an uneven, knotty outline, and looks like a conglomorate gland.]

When you examine fibrous tumors with the naked eye you may observe that many or most of them consist of two structures, viz., dense opaque fibres, or bands, coursing about and interlacing in the midst of a more clear, hyaline, softer substance; the latter being contained in the meshes formed by the interweaving of the former, much in the same way that the fatty is related to the fibrous element of an adipose tumor. The actual difference between these two components of fibrous tumors seems to depend upon the larger quantity of fluid—serous or aqueous fluid—which exists in the softer substance; and the proportion which this substance bears to the rest of the mass varies exceedingly. In some instances it is scarcely perceptible, the tumor appearing to consist almost entirely of the tough, opaque, fibrous element; in others the latter structure forms but an insignicant part, or may not even be distinguished at all in the soft, succulent, cellular mass of which the tumor consists. When a tumor of this latter kind is opened, and the fluid allowed to drain away, the mass shrinks, and soon loses a half or two-thirds of its weight. Now and then the fluid is contained in distinct cysts with smooth walls, lying in the interstices between the interlacing fibres; thus constituting one of the forms of "sero-cystic sarcoma," and consist of a thickened condition of the cellular tissue excited, perhaps, by chronic inflammation, or some long-continued irritation, or they may take place without any obvious cause.

Fibrous tumors vary so much in the compactness of their structure, and the mode of arrangement of their fibres, that in the classifications of tumors made by Abernethy and succeeding pathologists, the several members of this class were arranged in separate divisions. The name "cellular sarcoma," or "vascular sarcoma," was given to those in which the structure was soft and succulent, resembling the common cellular tissue, the chief bulk and weight of the mass being dependent on the larger quantity of fluid contained in the spaces between its solid elements. Tumors of this kind grow, as we might expect from their structure, more quickly than the other varieties of the class; they are found generally in parts where the cellular tissue is naturally lax and abundant—in the scrotum for instance, and in the labia pudendi, occasionally in the ovary, or in the cellular tissue surrounding the lower part of the uterus and the vagina. They are generally invested with a thin capsule, which separates them from the surrounding parts; their connections are loose, and though they may attain very large size, they are easily dissected out. The capsule is not, however, always present: on the contrary, the tumor may be blended with the surrounding cellular tissue, so that it is not easy to define its limits very clearly. Those enormous tumors of the scrotum which are occasionally met with in this country, and are more common in warm climates, appear to be of this nature.

The testicles and penis are commonly buried in these masses. Sometimes the skin is affected in a similar manner, becoming greatly thickened and tuberculated, so as to present the usual appearance and characters of elephantiasis. When an incision is made into a scrotum thus diseased, a large quantity of serous fluid drains away, and the size of the mass soon diminishes. I have occasionally met with ill-defined tumors under the skin of the face and in other parts of the body, which I could account for only on the supposition that they depended upon a hypertrophic condition of a small portion of the subcutaneous cellular tissue. You will perceive that there is a near relation between tumors of this kind and that thickened condition of the areolar and fibrous tissues which occurs in warts, polypus, pterygium, and the like; indeed, we cannot draw any clear line of distinction between them.

Another species of fibrous tumors has been called the "mammary sarcoma," from the resemblance of the tumors to udder; their fibres being interwoven so as to form a toughish, doughy, pale mass, intermediate in consistence between the cellular sarcoma and the tumors next to be described. The specimens of mammary sarcoma are generally found in the neighborhood of the breast; they have been know to attain a very large size, and are usually capsulated.

The third species of fibrous tumors, which is by far the most common, and in which the characters of the class are most strongly marked, was not distinguished by Mr. Abernethy with a particular name. These tumors are remarkable for their great hardness, and on this account are very often described under the name "scirrhus," a word which has been so indiscriminately used in former times as to have retained hardly any definite meaning at all, but which is now by all accurate pathologists applied exclusively to one of the varieties of cancer; they are more frequently found in the uterus than in any other part of the body, and were described by Dr. Baillie under the name of the "fleshy tubercle of the uterus;" the term "fibrocalcareous" has also been applied to them, because of their liability to undergo calcareous degeneration, a peculiarity which I believe is not shared by either of the other varieties of fibrous tumors.

In each of these species there is a general correspondence to be remarked between the characters of the tumors and those of the tissues in which they grow. Thus the soft, succulent, "cellular" tumors are found in the loose cellular tissue of the scrotum; the "mammary" tumors are found in or near the breast; and the last variety, the "fibrous" tumors—strictly so-called—are found in the uterus, among tendinous structures, in the periosteum, and in the dura mater.

The characters of these three species of fibrous tumors are so far distinct that I have thought it worth while to direct your attention to them; at the same time you should know that the intervals between them are filled up by intermediate gradations, just as it is in natural structures with regard to the areolar and fibrous tissues. Here, for instance, is a round tumor growing in the tough cellular tissue which forms the soft, strong padding at the extremity of a finger: it is scarcely hard enough to belong properly to the third species just mentioned, yet it is too firm to be classed with either of the other two; and you will find many specimens not strictly included in either of these species, but serving to connect them more closely together.

A fibrous polypus consists of a fibrous tumor, which, projecting into the interior of the uterus, has become pedunculated. It corresponds in structure with the fibrous tumors growing in other parts of the uterus, though I think its structure is not generally quite so dense. It is covered by the mucous membrane of the uterus reflected over it, together perhaps with a thin layer of uterine tissue; these converging at the upper part of

the polypus, pass from it to the uterus, and constitute the pedicle, which
is generally narrowest at the middle, expanding below over the polypus,
and again expanding above where it is connected with the uterus. The
pedicle thus consists entirely of stretched uterine structure, forming, in
reality, no part of the polypus, which explains the fact of its not being
necessary to remove the entire pedicle in order to prevent a return of the
disease after operation. The mucous membrane covering the polypus is
sometimes very vascular, so as to bleed profusely when it is lacerated or
superficially ulcerated. This was the case with a patient lately in the
hospital, who had been greatly reduced by repeated hemorrhages and
continual oozing of blood fiom the vagina; on examination I found a
fibrous polypus presenting at the os uteri, and the lower end of the tumor
rough from superficial ulceration. The os was sufficiently dilated to permit
the introduction of the finger and Gooch's canula, with the assistance of
which the tumor was tied at its upper end, and the patient quickly recovered.
  When the tumor is situated near the exterior of the uterus it projects
into the abdominal cavity, carrying before it the peritoneum, together
perhaps with a thin layer of uterine tissue. In process of time the tumor,
gradually projecting more and more, may become pedunculated; as in this
instance, where a large fibrous tumor hangs from the left cornu of the uterus
by a pedicle thinner than one's little finger. Under such circumstances
the tumor is likely to contract adhesions to the adjacent viscera, and in
some instances it has been known to be quite detached from the parent
organ and transplanted as it were to a new soil. When this has taken
place, I believe the tumor always ceases to grow and becomes calcified.
  In like manner, when the tumor is situated near the internal surface of
the uterus it projects into the cavity of the organ, carrying before it the
mucous membrane, with perhaps a thin layer of uterine tissue. As it
increases it projects more and more into the uterine cavity, where the
resistance is least, its basis of attachment to the uterus gradually narrows
and at last forms a mere pedicle. In this manner is formed the *fibrous*
polypus which differs from the *mucous* and *uterine* varieties of polypus
described on a former occasion, inasmuch as it is the result of a fibrous
tumor forcing its way into the cavity of the uterus.
  Under ordinary circumstances fibrous tumors occur in considerable
numbers in the same uterus; in some of these specimens there are five, six,
or even more, indeed they are rarely single, except when they project into
the cavity of the uterus, and distend its walls; there is then commonly
only one tumor. This exception is a matter of some practical importance,
inasmuch as it gives us greater confidence that we may be able to effect a
permanent cure by our operations upon polypi, and that the patient will
not be troubled with relapses from the presence of other tumors. I do
not mean to say that such is invariably the case, for you will every now
and then meet with an instance of fibrous polypus, associated with fibrous
tumors in other parts of the uterus, and such a coincidence may be
adduced as an argument in favor of the view which regards the polypus
to be of the same nature with the tumors, but it is certainly not the
general rule.
  In the greater number of cases the fibrous tumor in the uterus consists,
as I have said, of a firm globular mass growing from one centre without
any peripheral processes or lobes; this, however, is not their constant
character. Sometimes there are several nuclei, forming distinct masses,

closely packed together. Here is a specimen of an uneven, granulated, or finely lobulated tumor in the fundus of the uterus, which appears to consist of a number of separate masses less closely packed; it looks something like a salivary gland, but is of firmer structure.

Again, fibrous tumors are generally distinct from the surrounding uterine substance, and separated from it in their whole circumference by a well-marked capsule. Exceptional cases, however, do occur, in which the line of demarcation between the tumor and the uterine tissue is less marked.

In this specimen the tumor consists of a thickened, coarse, hypertrophied state of one side of the fundus uteri. Rarely is the os uteri the seat of fibrous tumor at all, but when it is so the tumor, so far as I have been able to ascertain by the examination of specimens in different museums, consists of an enlargement of one or both lips of the os uteri, the posterior lip being most frequently affected. The tumor thus formed partakes of the usual characters of fibrous tumors, except in the continuity of its structure with the uterine tissue; it may attain to a very large size, filling the vagina, or even projecting externally.

All the changes to which fibrous tumors are liable may be observed in those affecting the uterus. They are: calcareous degeneration, softening, and the various effects of inflammation.

Calcareous degeneration commences with the appearance in the substance of the tumor of one or more small grains of hard, straw-colored substance, consisting of carbonate, with some phosphate of lime. They are generally near the centre of the mass at first, and gradually extend toward the circumference; they increase at the expense of the fibrous structure, and are evidently the result of a transformation of it—a conversion of the fibrous into earthy matter. In course of time the earthy grains enlarge and coalesce, forming very hard, branching, knotty masses, like coral, of straw-color. They are closely connected with the remaining substance of the tumor; indeed they are continuous with it, so that they cannot be cleaned without great difficulty, or the help of maceration. Such masses may attain to considerable size, involving the greater part of the tumor, but they generally contain enough of the fibrous structure in their interstices to disclose their real nature. In a few instances the calcareous degeneration has commenced upon the surface of the tumor, and I have seen one case in which it had converted the outermost layers of the tumor into a hard shell, inclosing the central part like a kernel. It may take place in the tumors which project into the peritoneal cavity, or in those which hang polypose into the uterus; but I have not met with an instance in which it affected a tumor formed by the hypertrophy of an appreciable portion of the uterus, such as those originating in the os uteri just mentioned. Neither have I known it to occur in the cellular tumors, in the mammary sarcoma, or in any of the softer varieties of fibrous tumors.

Softening appears to take place in two ways: first, as a chronic process, affecting some circumscribed portion of the tumor, which is usually at or near the centre. The change is observed to commence with a slight discoloration—a yellowish or dark tinge—which is followed by a loosening or incipient disintegration of the structure; at the same time a line of demarcation is formed round the altered portion, which becomes separated like a sequestrum from the surrounding mass. Both the detached portion and the cavity are at first rough and shreddy on their opposed surfaces; the former undergoes still further disintegration and solution, becoming broken up into a number of small fragments, which float about in a dark, dirty, turbid fluid, and which may, ultimately, quite disappear.

The process of destruction may go on in the adjacent portion of the tumor, enlarging the central cavity, till the whole is reduced to a fluid or semifluid mass, walled in by the cellular capsule of the tumor, which now stands in the relation of a cyst-wall to the disorganized contents. Uterine tumors, which have undergone this change in a greater or less degree, have more than once been mistaken for ovarian cysts, and tapped accordingly. There is a specimen in the museum of the College of Surgeons, with a history appended, to the effect that an encysted tumor formed in the uterus, and the patient was twice tapped and the cyst emptied, the disease having been supposed to be ovarian dropsy during life; it was, probably, a case of the kind I am now describing, if we may judge from the appearance of the sac, and from the knowledge that cysts are very rarely produced in the walls of the uterus. In some instances the softening process is completed at one spot without extending to the circumference; the ragged processes hanging into the interior of the cavity are removed, the latter acquires a smooth lining, and looks like a simple cyst lying in the substance of the tumor. You must not mistake for cavities thus formed, the vacancies occasioned by enucleation of portions of the tumor after death. It is necessary to give you this hint, because I have known such an error to have been made.

The second mode in which softening takes place is more rapid and more diffused; the whole or greater portion of the tumor being affected at once. The change commences with the infiltration into the mass of a serous fluid, whereby its texture is loosened, and its components separated; at the same time the tissue of the tumor is softened, and interstitial absorption is set up in it. As the result of these processes combined, the tumor is soon broken up into detached fragments, and reduced to a diffluent pulp, or it may be, completely liquefied. It may even burst into the cavity of the uterus or the abdomen, and its contents be discharged. These changes are probably occasioned by some altered state of nutrition analogous to inflammation; they may be induced by an accidental cause, an injury, or pregnancy, and purulent fluids are sometimes found mixed up with the softened substance of the tumor. Nevertheless, they are not necessarily attended with any constitutional disturbance at all corresponding with the extensive destruction which is in progress.

Suppuration has been now and then known to take place in a fibrous tumor, and ulceration sometimes extends into it after penetrating its coverings, as in the case of polypus. Here is a specimen of large fibrous tumor of the uterus, projecting into the peritoneal cavity, and covered with a coating of cancer, which was diffused over nearly the whole interior of the abdomen. At one part you may see that the cancerous disease has penetrated the tumor, and destroyed its substance for about an inch. Dr. Lever, in his work on disease of the uterus, relates a case where melanosis was deposited in the structure of a fibrous tumor.

We cannot say that these tumors are attended with any particular train of symptoms, they have hardly any nervous link connecting them with the rest of the body. The drain upon the vascular system, occasioned by them is scarcely appreciable, neither do they return to it any noxious element, or communicate an evil influence in any other way. The symptoms to which they do give rise are almost entirely dependent on their effects upon the neighboring organs and tissues, and therefore vary with their position. Thus, if they be placed near the lining membrane of the uterus, they occasion the several symptoms of chronic inflammation of that membrane, such as uneasiness, discharges of mucus or blood, with, perhaps, the pains of forced uterine contractions, sensations of weight, bearing down, etc. When situated more in the middle of the uterine wall, or nearer to its external surface, they may exist for a long time, and attain considerable size, without giving any indication of their presence. In some cases, by their pressure upon the rectum or bladder, they occasion an irritable disordered state of these organs, or difficulty in voiding the urine and fæces. These and other symptoms of the like kind are rather casual results of the tumor's relation to certain external parts, than of any intrinsic quality of its own.

The fibrous tumors of the uterus become the subject of treatment only when they grow from the os uteri, or when they project into the cavity of the uterus and the vagina, assuming the polypose form. In either case they may be removed by ligature, or if their pedicles be narrow, may be excised, as recommended and extensively practised by Dupuytren. In a few cases an incision has been carried through the coverings of a fibrous tumor, projecting into the cavity of the uterus or vagina, but not become polypose, and attempts have been made to turn the mass out of its bed by dissection, and by tearing the fine filaments which unite it to its capsule. This proceeding, though successful in a few instances, is for obvious reasons, seldom to be attempted. The application of iodine externally, and its internal administration, has been recommended with the view of promoting the absorption of these tumors, and is said to have been attended with success. I have seen it tried in a few instances, but the result has not been encouraging.

Fibrous tumors affecting the bones are usually found upon those of a spongy nature, upon the ends of the long bones, the phalanges, pelvis, and lower jaw. So far as I have seen, they are confined to the *exterior* of the bones, growing from the periosteum, and creeping along the surface of the bone in such a manner as to prove almost to a certainty that they originate in some morbid condition of the periosteal fibres. The bones underneath these tumors may suffer absorption, in consequence of the pressure produced, but do not seem to be affected in any other way. They appear upon the maxillary bones more frequently than upon any other part of the skeleton. On the lower jaw they spread along the ramus, encircling it beneath and on the sides; so that the bone is almost concealed by the tumor. In some instances they form within the substance of the jaw, probably from periosteum lining the sockets of the teeth, and as they increase the walls of the bone become spread out over them. They grow up around the teeth, and where they project into the mouth, may be soft and fungous. In the upper jaw they form now and then in the antrum, and gradually distend the walls of the cavity; more frequently they commence on the outside, and grow along the surface of the bone, projecting into the mouth, nose, orbit, and toward the cheek, so that the natural outline of the maxilla can scarcely be recognized.

In some instances these fibrous tumors of the jaws have exhibited a semi-cartilaginous structure; and now and then fibres, or plates of bone, are formed in various parts of them. The progress of the disease is well illustrated by the series of tumors of the jaws in the College of Surgeons, from the museum of the late Mr. Liston. These preparations furnish ample proof, if proof were needed, of the skill of that illustrious operator; they show also how necessary it is to bear in mind the mode of growth of these periosteal fibrous tumors of the jaw; because from their disposition to creep along the surface of the bones, they are liable to return after removal, unless the immediately adjacent as well as the affected part be excised. The histories attached to the specimens teach us that very large fibrous tumors, both of the upper and lower jaw, together with the bones on which they grow, may be removed successfully.

Nearly allied to these tumors of the periosteum, and forming a close connecting link in pathology between them and the common warts and polypi, are the tumors of the gum called " epulis." They are of two kinds; one consisting of a red granulated or nodulated growth springing from the sockets of the teeth, originating apparently in a morbid condition of the membrane lining the sockets, and caused in many instances by a diseased state of the teeth. Such a growth requires to be extirpated, and it is not enough simply to slice off the tumor, for it is deeply rooted and will most likely reappear unless the alveolus from which it springs, be removed with it, which may easily be done by cutting a notch in the jaw with the bone forceps or a small saw. The second kind of epulis is exemplified by this specimen of tumor of the gum on the outside of the upper jaw; it is a red, soft, pulpy growth, as large as a walnut, in appearance resembling swollen gum; indeed it consists evidently of a growth of the gum. It is slightly lobulated on the surface, and tolerably defined at the circumference, where it is continuous with the surrounding gum. The patient was a healthy young woman, and the disease had been observed to follow the extraction of a tooth six months before she came to the hospital. The tumor was closely connected with the bone, so I removed the portion of the maxilla on which it rested, including the sockets of the canine and first molar teeth. Seven years have now elapsed since the operation was performed, and the patient is still quite well. The tumor was very vascular, bled frequently and might have been mistaken for a malignant affection.

Fibrous tumors are not uncommonly found in nerves. In some cases they form distinct round masses within the neurilemma. In others they appear to consist of an increase of that fibro-cellular tissue which unites the nervous filaments together. These tumors are in some cases attended with a good deal of pain, felt in the course of the nerves and easily excited by pressure, a slight blow, or a quick movement. Excision is the only remedy, and it must in each case be uncertain how far it will be possible to effect that without injuring the structure of the nerve. Not long ago I removed from within the sheath of the medium nerve near the wrist, from a woman aged forty-eight, this spherical tumor; it is as large as an orange, presents a semi-opaque glistening appearance, not unlike brawn, with more opaque yellow spots interspersed here and there. It resembled some of the varieties of encephaloid disease so closely that I should have been apprehensive as to the result had it not been gradually forming many years, during which time the woman enjoyed good health. It was attended with a good deal of pain and a shrivelled state of the fore and middle fingers. Some filaments of the nerve were removed with the tumor, never-theless, the patient recovered completely, regaining the use of the hand; the fingers were also in course of time restored to their natural condition.

It has already been intimated that fibrous tumors occur in several other parts of the body besides the uterus, the periosteum, and the nerves. Here is one as large as a walnut and of spherical shape, growing from the inside of the dura mater, and causing an indentation in the surface of the brain. Sometimes they form in the substance of the testicle, the prostate gland, the ovary, and even the walls of the alimentary canal. Very rarely are they to be met with in any other of the internal organs.

One point more requires to be specially mentioned in relation to these growths; viz., their occasional liability to return after they have been to all appearance completely extirpated. Where this has taken place the tumor has, I believe, generally grown quickly in the first instance, has been composed of several detached portions, of which one or more may have been left behind in the first operation, or has consisted in a thickened morbid condition of the tissue in which the growth occurs, affecting a considerable area and probably not having such definite limits as these growths usually present. To the latter circumstance I have already directed your attention in speaking of fibrous tumors of the periosteum, and have said that the same feature is to be observed in some of the adipose tumors, more particularly those under the skin.   *Part* xxiii., *p.* 236.

Diagnosis of Tumors in the Neck.—[This always presents great difculties when the tumors are of large size, only slightly painful and fluctuate indistinctly. If a complete and accurate history of the case cannot be obtained, more than a general diagnosis may be impossible ; but when the precise position of the tumor at its commencement can be made out, when its relations to the larynx and trachea, and its mobility in regard to them and the surrounding parts when it was of small size, can be ascertained, together with the rapidity and manner of its growth, Dr. Redfern thinks there will be little difficulty in arriving at a satisfactory conclusion.]

A *tumor* developed in the substance of *the thyroid body* presents itself in the front of the neck, is usually larger on one side than the other, is firmly connected with the larynx and trachea, moves freely with the larynx in deglutition, and when it is displaced laterally by manipulation. The other features vary with the nature of the tumor.

In ordinary bronchocele (hypertrophy) the swelling is soft, projecting, elastic; without fluctuation, pain or tenderness on pressure; it occurs usually in early life, in the female sex, and in particular districts of country ; it is simple in its nature throughout, and presents no tendency to degeneration or change of structure; it in no way interferes with respiration or deglutition, nor does it affect the patient's health or comfort until it becomes of very large size, when difficulty of respiration and deglutition, with frequent headaches, occasion the greatest distress, and may end with the death of the sufferer.

In cystic disease of the thyroid the nature of the tumor becomes manifest, sooner or later by the presence of fluctuation in one or more cysts, by a glairy, serous, or sero-sanguineous fluid escaping readily along a grooved needle when introduced, the fluid containing no cellular formations when examined microscopically, or having such a structure as is consistent with the idea of the existence of cancer—by the formation of the tumor taking place at or after the middle of life—by its slow and painless growth, and by the slight inconvenience it occasions as long as its size is not very great.

In *cancerous disease of the thyroid* (usually scirrhus) the tumor appears between forty-five and sixty-five years of age, is of great and uniform density, and generally painful; it is developed rapidly, and may attain a large size in the course of a few months; it accompanies the larynx in its movements, but shortly limits their extent by attaching the organ to the surrounding parts; it occasions great difficulty of deglutition and respiration from an early period; hoarseness, cough, and spasmodic action of the muscles of the larynx and pharynx come on and increase in their intensity—the distress and anxiety of the patient, his sallow complexion and emaciation, marking him out as the subject of a steadily advancing and destructive malady.

In *medullary cancer of the thyroid* the surface of the tumor may be even and tense, or indistinct fluctuation may be perceived, the other characters depending on the steady infiltration of the surrounding textures, distinguishing the disease from other tumors of the same part.

Enchondromatous tumors are to be recognized by their great density, the slowness of their growth, and the absence of any signs of the extension of the affection to the surrounding parts, and of general evidence of the existence of malignant disease.

The diagnosis of *tumors of the neck not connected with the thyroid body*, is to be established by reference to the general characters which distinguish them in other situations, every particular of their history and mode of growth being carefully ascertained as essential points, and sufficient care being exercised lest the presence of a quantity of coagulable fluid, in the interior of a cancerous tumor, lead to the belief that it is of a cystic character. *Part* xxiii., *p.* 279.

Tumors, Encysted.—Evacuate the contents by making a small oblique opening on the cyst. Inject then an alcoholic solution of iodine, closing the aperture with diachylon or charpie. As soon as the inflammation has subsided, the cyst becomes detached, and may be extracted by means of the forceps. Usually, however, M. Borelli has found that two or three injections are necessary to promote a complete separation. *Part* xxiii., *p.* 295.

The Cold Douche in Promoting Absorption.—Dr. Sloan submitted to its action, cases of an encysted tumor—a goitre and a scirrhous mamma—and in all there has been decided improvement. The water with which he has practised is supplied to the town from a basin 100 feet above the lowest street. He applies it by means of the gutta percha tubing fixed to one of the pipes, allowing the stream to strike the object at from six inches to two feet from the end of the tube; at all events, before the column of water is broken. A pressure of less even than forty feet of water produces excellent effects. The application should be continued until a decided sense of pain is induced, or for something less than five minutes. *Part* xxiii., *p.* 306.

Sanguineous Pelvic Tumor in Females.—M. Nelaton calls attention to a peculiar form of tumor, hitherto much neglected by authors. These tumors are usually preceded by some general symptoms, as *malaise*, disturbed menstruation, pains in the hypogastrium, and a feeling as if a heavy body were about to escape from the vagina. The abdomen is sometimes enlarged, and a hard, very painful tumor is felt by the patients in the hypogastric region; in other cases they are not aware of its existence, and, when it is pointed out to them, they cannot say how long they have had it. On examination, the abdomen is found to be inflated, tense, convex, and painful. The decubitus is dorsal, with the thighs flexed on the pelvis. By palpation in the hypogastrium, a tumor is felt in the cavity of the pelvis (*petit bassin*). This is sometimes confined within its inner border, and sometimes extends as high as the umbilicus; it is commonly inclined toward the right iliac fossa. The tumor is small, rounded, without knotty projections, and becomes gradually lost in the pelvic cavity; it is scarcely movable, and is of pretty firm consistence, sometimes presenting fluctuation. On vaginal examination, there is found, between the uterus, a tumor, advancing toward the orifice of the vulva in proportion to its size. It is smooth, rounded, and fluctuating, varying from the size of a large goose-egg to that of a thumb, without pulsation or expansive movement; it may narrow the vaginal canal so as only to permit of the passage of the index finger. The uterus may be raised by the tumor, so that its body is felt above the pubes; and its neck may be so much elevated, that the forefinger can only with great difficulty reach it.

The treatment of these tumors consists in evacuating the liquid which they contain. M. Nélaton proposes to employ a large trocar, and then a simple lithotome to enlarge the opening. The patient is placed on her back, on a tolerably high bed, with her legs and thighs bent, as in the position for lithotomy. By introducing a speculum into the vagina, the tumor is discovered toward its base, at the posterior wall. The point where fluctuation is most apparent having been discovered, a long trocar is introduced, with a canula sufficiently long to allow the escape of the matter, which is liquid, black, and viscid, like treacle. The incision ought generally to be three *centimètres* in extent; it should be made in the axis of the vagina, so as to avoid wounding the uterine arteries. It should also be carefully ascertained that there are no arteries on that part of the wall in which the incision is made. The incision should be neither too wide nor too deep, so that the rectum may be avoided. When some days after the operation, the liquid which escapes has become purulent and fœtid, disinfectant injections should be employed. The strength of the patient should at the same time be supported by quinine and other tonics. The walls of the tumor should also be explored with a scoop (*curette*), so as to remove any adherent clots, which may be in a state of commencing putrefaction.   *Part* xxiv., *p.* 297.

Calcification of Fibrous Tumor of the Uterus.—Mr. I. B. Brown exhibited a specimen of fibrous tumor, which had been transformed by calcification into a solid, heavy body, weighing eight ounces. It was situated at the fundus of the uterus. The sides of the uterus were not adherent to this body, but were distended so as to form a sort of close-fitting bag to the tumor; the neck of the uterus was drawn up and lost in the body, and the os was elongated and thin. This interesting specimen was found in a patient aged seventy.

The calcareous crust of this tumor consists of semi-transparent plates, overlaying each other, having a glassy fracture; these dissolved in dilute muriatic acid allowed an abundant escape of carbonic acid, leaving a residue of an imperfect fibrous basic substance.   *Part* xxv., *p.* 292.

Fibrous Tumor of the Womb removed by Incision and Enucleation.— Mr. Teale recently removed a large fibrous growth from the interior of the uterus. The tumor had protruded through the mouth of the womb and filled the vagina. It was so large that the fingers could not be passed above it to determine its mode of attachment. The treatment adopted in this case, which Mr. Teale also recommends in similar ones, is, to pull down the tumor beyond the external parts, if necessary, by midwifery forceps or other means, and partially or completely invert the womb. The operator can then ascertain whether the tumor be pedunculated or imbedded in the wall of the womb. Should the latter mode of attachment be found, he recommends the investing membrane of the tumor, a little below its attachment, to be carefully cut through in a transverse direction, by long curved probe-pointed scissors, to such an extent as to allow of the tips of two or three fingers to be insinuated between the investing membrane and the tumor, and the process of enucleation to be completed by detaching the upper part of the tumor from the wall of the uterus, after which the remaining attachment of the investing membrane may be divided by the scissors, and the tumor removed. If the uterus should remain inverted, it must be immediately replaced by gentle but firm pressure, which may generally be done without difficulty, as the os uteri has been so long subject to distention that it will offer but little resistance. *Part* xxviii., *p.* 289.

Nerves—Excision of Tumors of (*Neuroma*).—When a tumor pressing upon, or in any way implicating a nerve, has to be excised or dissected out, make a clean incision of the nerve either above or below the tumor before the operation, as this will not only considerably lessen the pain, but also the subsequent inflammation. The consequent paralysis lasts only a short time, as the divided nervous extremities soon reunite. *Part* xxx., *p.* 309.

Tumors of the Upper Jaw.—It is a common opinion that these tumors originate within the antrum of Highmore. Mr. Hancock does not agree with this opinion. Mr. Ormerod, of St. Bartholomew's, has taken pains to classify these tumors, which he does as follows:

1. Epulis.
2. Cystic tumors, consisting of the walls of the bone expanded on or into a sac, with more or less of solid growth; the walls in some parts being quite membranous and transparent, and the sac filled with glairy fluid, or a firm substance contained in cells, or accompanied with a granular fatty substance, partitioned by fibro-cellular substance; also consisting of a single bony cyst lined by a membrane, with a second canine tooth adherent to it, and having its cavity filled by a glairy fluid.
3. Cartilaginous and osseous tumors from the upper jaw-bones, as round tumors growing on their outer surface here and there, but chiefly as a mass growing from their inner surface, so as to fill up the maxillary sinuses, the septum nasi and spongy bones being also affected. The thickening is dense, hard, and ivory-like.
4. Fibrous tumors from the upper and lower jaw-bones, consisting of white or pale yellow, firm, and nearly homogeneous, with or without specks of bone, or of dense, more or less fibrous, or even obscurely fibrous, substance, containing at times one or more small cavities filled with. pus, with a glairy fluid, or with blood; growing on a healthy bone and periosteum, or from the alveolar and outer surface of the bone, or originating in the cancelli, and being accompanied with a perfectly healthy condition, with absorption or consolidation of the surrounding bone.
5. Medullary tumors from the upper or lower jaw, consisting of round

lobed, or nodulated masses, with a smooth membraneous covering, or with
a rough fungous or ulcerated shreddy surface; invested by a thick capsule, by a dense periosteum, or by partial thin laminæ of bone; composed
of round lobes, connected together by cellular tissue, or formed of an
almost homogeneous mass; made up of a structure of a soft medullary,
brain-like, spleen-like, or firm fatty nature, with cells and bony spiculæ,
sometimes commencing in the neighboring glands, and extending to the
jaws secondarily.

In addition to these, Mr. Stanley enumerates fatty and erectile tumors of
the jaw; whilst Mr. Paget adds what he terms myeloid tumors of the
part; but whilst the examples he quotes resemble so much, on the one
hand, the fibrous, on the other medullary tumors, their true character,
whether innocent or malignant, is so very doubtful, that I should hesitate
in admitting them as a distinct class.

I have never met with a fatty growth so invading the upper jaw as to
require the removal of any portion of that bone, and therefore I do not
presume to offer any opinion upon that form of disease.

Mr. Stanley states that the erectile tumor is a very rare form of disease;
but that it occurred to M. Gensoul in one of his successful cases. The
tumor was soft and vascular, and quicksilver, impelled into the morbid
structure, readily pervaded it throughout. I have not seen a similar case,
nor have I been able to meet with any recorded elsewhere. It is occasionally very difficult to form a correct opinion of the exact point of origin of
a fibrous tumor of the upper jaw. It will sometimes commence by a contracted pedicle, enlarge, and spread out, and not only fill the antrum, but
extend into the nares; by its peculiar and irregular appearance giving rise
to the supposition of its being a polypus of the nostril, and leading to
abortive attempts for its removal by the polypus forceps. Mr. Stanley,
although not mentioning the disease, has the following observations bearing upon this point: "A tumor gradually increasing within the antrum
may occasion yielding of the walls equally in all directions; but in some cases,
disease extends chiefly in one direction, and causes difficulty of diagnosis.
In a case I saw, a morbid growth originating in the antrum had extended
only in the direction of the nostril, and portions had been extracted by
polypus forceps."

[Osseous tumors are the most frequently met with amongst the non-malignant growths of the upper jaw. Mr. Hancock has two specimens of this
disease:]

The first case is that of a young man, aged 22, a farmer, residing in Lincolnshire, who was sent up to me on the 1st October, 1848, by Mr. Young,
of Gosberton, whose patient he was. This case was a striking example of
what has been affirmed elsewhere, that "osseous growths are in some instances combined with hypertrophy of the surrounding bones, producing
general enlargement." The whole of the bones on the right side of the
head and face were very much enlarged and thickened, the bone at the
fronto-malar suture presenting a surface of more than a square inch, and
this, I believe, is the usual origin of the tumors in question. I believe that
they should not be regarded as originating within the antrum, or from
causes connected with the teeth, but from excessive development or hypertrophy of the bone itself, which, in its growth, extends in various directions, invading the antrum of Highmore, and in some instances entirely
obliterating that cavity. M. Paget, in his Lectures on Surgical Pathology,

in allusion to these tumors, says : "More commonly, it is almost limited to the antrum ;" but he singularly disproves his assertion, and confirms my views, by his illustrative example. He says : "In this case, it may exist with little deformity. In the museum of St. Bartholomew's Hospital is a specimen, in which both the antra appear nearly filled by the thickening and in-growing of their walls; only small cavities remain at their centres. The new bone is hard, heavy, and nearly solid, yet it is porous or finely cancellous, and is neither so compact nor so smooth on its cut surface as that of 'ivory exostosis.' The same disease is manifest in a less degree upon the outer surfaces of the maxillary bones, and on the septum and side walls of the nose."

I have operated upon three cases of this form of disease. One of these I have just related, and in the other two the antrum remained; in one of these there was general hypertrophy of the bone, causing great disfigurement, and necessitating its entire removal. The swelling did not arise from, and was not confined within, the cavity, but was, in truth, a portion of the general thickening and enlargement of the bone. I have a preparation, which was taken from a child of six years of age, upon whom I operated in April, 1852, and is a well-marked example of the fallacy of Mr. Stanley's position, that "morbid growths mostly arise from either of the lateral parts, not from the front of the jaw—a fact which might be explained by the consideration that irritation more frequently originates in a molar than in an incisor tooth," as does the following case :

A child was admitted, under my care, into the Charing Cross Hospital, in August, 1852, with tumor of the left upper maxilla. It appears that in December, 1851, she fell and bruised her face. Soon afterward a tumor was observed on the left side, just below the orbit. This was unattended with pain, but it gradually increased in size until, at the time of admission, it was about the size of a walnut. Upon careful examination, I found the hard palate and gums perfectly healthy; the tumor was smooth and solid. Upon carrying my finger behind the soft palate, I could not detect anything wrong in that situation; but as I otherwise could not detect the extent of the mischief, or what was the extent of operation required, I introduced a small exploring trocar into the tumor, and felt it enter a solid mass, which prevented my giving the instrument any lateral motion. I next perforated the upper jaw above the alveolar process corresponding to the molar tooth, and found the instrument enter a cavity, in which I could freely move its point, and from which I decided the case was hypertrophy of the anterior portion of the maxillary bone, and I acted accordingly, confining the operation to the simple removal of the part affected, without interfering either with the floor of the orbit or the roof of the mouth.

The last form of abnormal growth is the encephaloid or medullary sarcoma ; and it is here that a correct idea of the origin of these growths becomes of so much importance. I have throughout this paper been at great pains to disprove the opinion so universally maintained, and so decidedly advocated by Mr. Stanley, that morbid growths commonly originated within the antrum, not only because I felt, from what I had observed, that such opinion was wrong, or rather open to very many exceptions, but because the statement, backed by such an authority, gives rise to the supposition that medullary sarcoma usually commences within the antrum ; and that, if attacked sufficiently early, it may be eradicated by operation. At the risk of appearing tedious, I feel that the importance of the subject fully justifies my again quoting Mr. Stanley. He says: "But even with the help of the most careful examination, whenever the disease fills the antrum and nostril, it will be uncertain whether or not it extends pos. teriorly beyond the front surface of the pterygoid processes of the sphe. noid bone. Whilst Mr. Liston has observed: 'If anything is to be done, it ought to be undertaken with a thorough determination to go beyond the limits of the morbid growth, to remove the cavity which holds it, and thus get quit, if possible, of all the tissues implicated, or which may have become disposed to assume a similar action.' I know from experience, that this step, if adopted in time, may prove successful." It may appear pre. sumption in me to differ from such authorities as these, and men of such experience, but my own experience leads me to an opposite conclusion.

I entirely differ from the opinion that medullary sarcoma commences in the antrum of Highmore, and extends backward to the pterygoid pro. cesses; but, on the contrary, from what I have observed, I firmly believe that the disease commences in the cancellated structure of the body of the sphenoid bone and bones at the base of the cranium; and that, however early we may perform the operation, we never succeed in eradicating the mischief, which is sure to return at a longer or shorter period, according to circumstances.

I have performed, and assisted at many operations for the removal of the upper maxilla for this disease; and where the mischief, as far as external examination and the introduction of the finger behind the soft palate went, appeared to hold out every reasonable prospect of its complete removal, but in no one instance was this satisfactorily accomplished, and in no one instance did the disease fail to reappear, whilst post-mortem examination demonstrated its growth from the body of the sphenoid bone, the basilar process of the occipital bone, etc. This disease will sometimes extend into the orbit, in some instances causing the eyeball to protrude, in others presenting us a firm tumor on one side of the eyeball. But it should be borne in mind that, notwithstanding the absence of external swelling of the cheek, these growths rarely, if ever, originate in the orbit, or are confined to that cavity, but that the swelling in the orbit is almost invariably an extension of the disease in that direction, its origin being in the cancellated structure of the bones at the base of the cranium, and that it mostly, at the same time, invades the spheno-maxillary fossa and antrum of Highmore, so that it can never be entirely removed by dissection from the orbit.

I have a lady at present under my care, who consulted me for protrusion of the left eyeball, with apparent commencing chemosis of the conjunctiva and indistinctness of vision. The protrusion is not very great; but pressing the base of the eyelids near the margins of the orbit, gives the sensation of an elastic body between the orbit and the eyeball. There is no swelling of the cheek; but, upon examining the mouth, I find the gum is beginning to separate from the molar teeth, and the dental margin to become everted, whilst separation is also commencing between the hard palate and its covering, the bone appearing softer than natural when pressed upon. Carrying my finger behind the soft palate into the spheno-maxillary fossa, I can distinctly feel an irregular growth in that situation.

This case shows the impropriety of operating upon orbital growths of this description, the tumor in that situation being commonly but a local manifestation of disease extending into the upper jaw and elsewhere, where the knife cannot penetrate. In some instances the tumor will be more isolated or partial, and equally, if not more malignant, if we may judge from the rapidity of its growth. It will not present the same elasticity to the touch, feeling more like an enchondroma, and when cut into, it has very much the appearance of a fibrous growth.

A woman brought her child, aged two years, to me at the Ophthalmic Hospital with a conical tumor of the orbit, at the inner and upper part; it was very firm to the touch, and the mother said it caused the child great uneasiness. She had perceived the swelling about a month before. I entertained some doubts as to the nature or the swelling, and expressed them to the mother, at the same time telling her that I could not recommend any operation. At this time the disease was apparently confined to the orbit, as by careful examination I could not detect any manifestations elsewhere. She pressed me to do something, and therefore I endeavored to remove it, and found it to consist of dense fibrous structure, invested by yellow, firm substance; it penetrated so deeply, however, that I could not get the whole away, and the swelling rapidly reappeared, the disease seeming to be lighted up with fearful intensity. The child lived two months afterward, but had become a most frightful object. The tumor protruded from the orbit, extending upward toward the forehead, outward, invading the temple, and downward through the upper maxilla and mouth to the neck.

These cases justify the opinion that fungoid or medullary growths of the orbit rarely exist as independent disease, but that they almost always coexist with the same disease in the antrum and spheno-maxillary fossa; at all events I do not recollect an instance where this was not the case, and I have seen many of them.

Having endeavored to point out the inadvisability of performing operations in cases of medullary sarcoma of the upper jaw, I will now advert to some of the most prominent means of diagnosis between this disease and other abnormal growths of that part. The diagnosis between fibrous tumors and medullary sarcoma is very obscure; some idea may be obtained from puncturing the tumor, and from the degree of resistance to the lateral motions of the instrument presented in the former disease, as well as from the absence of spiculæ of bone discernible in some forms of the latter; but the principal diagnostic signs which we posses are, the condition of the teeth, gums, and bones of the part. It is true that the bones, in certain conditions of health—as in the case to which I have alluded—may, from pressure, become carious, or even destroyed by necrosis; but they are never converted into that soft degeneration so characteristic of medullary sarcoma, or the malignant disease. Pressure on the hard palate is met with firm, hard resistance; whereas in medullary sarcoma—in all cases where the tumor projects from the cheek, and in very many of those wherein the disease manifests itself in the orbit—the palate upon the affected side is elastic to pressure, usually more congested than natural, whilst the gums are congested and thickened, the dental margin is thickened and everted from the teeth, which become irregular, loosened, and projecting. When seen for the first time, this condition of the gums and teeth may be mistaken for abscess or disease connected with the teeth, with which, however, it has nothing to do, and from which it may be distinguished by the comparative slight pain which accompanies it, by its gradual progress, by the absence of inflammatory swelling of the cheek, and by the character of the enlargement of the gums.

In this affection the gums are spongy and elastic, and, when pressed upon, are found, in a great degree, to have lost the support of the alveolar process, which becomes softened by the disease : whereas in inflammation and abscess resulting from disease of the teeth, or alveolar sockets, of a simple character, the pain is very great, the swelling of the cheek is evidently of an inflammatory character, whilst the enlargement of the gums is smooth and firm, and the firm resistance of bone beneath may almost always be detected. In medullary sarcoma this state of the gums should be regarded as the result, not the cause, of the disease ; and for the reasons which I have already given in the early part of the paper, the teeth, though loose and comparatively useless to the patient, had better not be meddled with.

Bony tumors, though more easily distinguished from medullary sarcoma than fibrous growths, may, upon superficial examination, create doubts in the minds even of well-informed surgeons. As I was going down into the operating-theatre, to remove the upper jaw from a child aged six years, a surgeon of some standing, who had examined the child in the ward, said, "Surely, Mr. Hancock, you will not meddle with that; it is malignant." He was misled by a certain degree of elasticity presented at one point of the tumor, and which I have observed in all the cases which have fallen under my observation. They have not been of that form denominated ivory exostosis, but have all presented a certain degree of yielding to the touch; but they have this marked distinction from the medullary sarcoma : in this latter disease the surface of the tumor is uneven and elastic, but the elasticity is superficial; whereas in osseous tumors the elasticity is deeper seated, and the yielding or elastic substance is evidently covered by a thin shell, which recedes when pressed upon, but appears to recover itself when the finger is removed. We have not the crepitation in these cases as in osseous cysts, but the elasticity is covered by a thin, smooth investment, and is not so immediately upon the surface as in osteo or medullary sarcoma. Puncturing these tumors with an exploring needle, or what I prefer, a small trocar, will also assist us in our diagnosis. In medullary sarcoma, the instrument appears to enter a soft mass, and with but little force a considerable degree of lateral motion may be given to the instrument; but not so in osseous tumors. Here, though it may be introduced with difficulty, still it will appear to be clung to by the structure into which it penetrates, and lateral motion cannot be obtained except with that degree of violence which we should be unwilling to employ ; and, again, as in fibrous growths, the condition of the gums and teeth will pretty surely mark the non-existence of malignant disease. The teeth will, in many instances, be perfectly sound ; and though, in others, the patient may have lost some of those organs, the gums may have healed, and will not show any of that spongy appearance, or tendency to eversion, so characteristic of the malignant disease. I never saw a tumor of the upper jaw of a malignant character unaccompanied by mischief about the palate and gums; but an osseous tumor may have attained great size, and cause considerable deformity, without projecting into the mouth, or complicating the palate or gums at all; and this is an additional reason for employing an exploring needle or trocar, this instrument, in some cases, affording us the only means of ascertaining the extent of operation to be performed—

whether the whole, or a portion only, of the upper maxilla is to be removed. Mr. Fergusson has laid down that rapidity of growth is a diagnostic sign of malignant tumor; this, however, is not entirely to be depended upon, as the growth of bony tumors will sometimes be extremely rapid, as in one case wherein the tumor attained a great size in less than five months.   *Part* xxxi., *p.* 136.

Tumors of the Jaws.—[In a clinical lecture on this subject, Mr. Syme makes the following important general remarks which will apply to tumors affecting both upper and lower jaw.]

There are some anatomical differences between them, which lead to pathological differences. In the upper jaw, the hollow of the maxillary antrum exposes to a condition which cannot exist in the lower jaw—viz., inflammation and suppuration of the cavity. The antrum also serves as a receptacle for polypus growths, which, however, are mere intruders from the nasal cavity, and not diseases of the jaw itself. In both jaws the bone is apt to die from the effects of inflammation. In the upper no reproduction of bone takes place after removal of the exfoliation; in the lower the bone is denser, and the periosteum more capable of reproduction, and there is no instance in the body of a more complete restoration of bone. I have repeatedly seen almost the whole lower jaw, including the condyle, thrown off as an exfoliation, yet complete reproduction has taken place. These are all the differences which it is necessary for me to notice now. There has been a notion prevalent, that tumors of the upper jaw originate in the antrum. This is erroneous; their origin is in all cases similar to tumors of the lower jaw.

Tumors of the jaws are chiefly of five different kinds—three solid and two fluid. Of the solid, you have one growing from the surface, and two in the interior of the bone. The one on the surface is denominated "epulis," or "epulotic tumor;" it appears on the gum, and increases in size without limit to its growth, and at last becomes inconvenient from its bulk; it is also liable to bleed, and may become as serious, in this respect, as if it were malignant. Epulis grows from the surface of the bone, and requires for its remedy the removal of the part to which it is attached. The knife never cures the disease completely, and it is always requisite to take away more or less of the alveolar process, in order to do which you must extract one or more teeth.

The other two forms of solid tumor originate in the osseous substance, and are divided into simple or local, and malignant, or those where there is some constitutional derangement connected with the local condition, which produces a tendency to a return of the disease after its removal. The first kind are generally of firm consistence, and slow growth, and accompanied by a healthy state of the constitution; the second are of soft consistence, and rapid growth, and the patient's constitution commonly unhealthy. But these kinds pass, by various degrees, insensibly into each other. The slower the growth, the firmer the consistence, and the more healthy the constitution, the greater will be the probability that the disease is entirely local, and that the removal of the tumor will be followed by a permanent cure. But tumors of the most rapid growth and softest consistence have sometimes been taken away, without any return of the disease; and hence the general rule is, that if such tumors are distinctly limited to the jaw, they should be removed. You must bear in mind, however, that a malignant growth is apt to extend its roots beyond the bone from which it originated, in this respect remarkably differing from the simple, local, or fibro-cartilaginous growths, to which your attention was lately directed. The other day, a lady, said to be laboring under polypus of the nose, consulted me. I found, however, that the soft mass which showed itself in the nostril was really a tumor proceeding from the superior maxillary bone; and further, a swelling at the inner canthus, showed that the disease was not limited to that bone, but extended up to the ethmoid, and probably to the base of the skull. I therefore advised her against any interference; but had the disease appeared limited to the superior maxilla, I should have recommended excision of the bone. I could mention several cases, where the removal of soft tumors of the jaws of rapid growth has been followed by permanent recovery.

The fluid tumors of the jaws are of two sorts, being collections either of serous or purulent fluid; the serous or cystic are not unfrequently mistaken for solid tumors; they grow in the substance of the bone, and are generally at some parts of their extent as hard and as unyielding as bone, so that if their examination be limited to these parts, the tumors will be supposed to be solid. Even so accomplished a surgeon as M. Gensoul, of Lyons, had once made his incision and exposed a tumor of the jaw, when all at once the knife entered a cavity, from which serous fluid escaped. I have myself met such cases, and seen them in the practice of others. It is therefore necessary to examine a tumor of the jaw over its whole surface; then, if it be cystic, you will be almost sure to find some yielding point where the bone gives way like pasteboard, and is perhaps felt to crackle under the finger.

These cysts frequently exist independently of any other morbid condition, but sometimes, and especially in the upper jaw, they are connected with displaced teeth, one of the permanent set having taken a wrong direction, so that, when the cyst is opened, the tooth is found lying in its interior: I have, in this theatre, more than once found such a state of things present. Whether this be the case or not the treatment is the same—viz., to open the cavity freely and stuff it with lint. The prognosis is, however, more favorable if a tooth be found in the cyst; it is then almost certain that the cavity will contract and heal. This may occur in other cases, but it has also been noticed that cysts, after being opened, are not unfrequently followed by the formation of a solid tumor. I could mention to you cases where I have opened cysts containing nothing but serum, in the place of which solid tumors have afterward been formed. It is also possible that the cysts may be complex, and so extensive as to require removal. A patient left the hospital only a few weeks since who applied to me five years ago on account of a large cystic tumor of the lower jaw, which I opened, and gave exit to a large quantity of albuminous fluid, and stuffed the cavity with lint. The swelling afterward contracted to a considerable extent, but never entirely disappeared, and she returned two years later with the tumor as large as when I first saw her, and affecting the jaw more extensively. I again opened and stuffed it, and the tumor again contracted to a certain extent. It, however, again increased, and I repeated the process for the third time, but with the same result, the patient returning last autumn with the tumor larger than ever, and extending now from the symphysis to the coronoid process. I removed half the jaw by disarticulation, and on examination we found that the cyst, instead of being simple, was complex, consisting of four chief cavities, the walls of which were studded with smaller cysts of various sizes. It was clear that in this case nothing short of excision of the portion of the bone affected could have produced a cure.

Tumors depending on purulent collections are not at all uncommon. They are almost invariably in connection with the stump of a tooth. A portion of a stump may remain after the extraction of a tooth and be forgotten, and the tumor may be supposed by the surgeon to be solid. Generally, however, the parietes, like those of serous collections, will be found to yield at one place, and you find an additional guide to your diagnosis in the presence of the diseased tooth. I lately saw a tumor of the lower jaw, which was removed under the supposition that it was solid throughout; but on being sawn through, it proved to be an abscess, the osseous wall of which had undergone immense thickening, except at one small point in immediate connection with a diseased tooth, which had never caused any pain. In that case, it may be doubted whether it would have been possible to afford relief otherwise, even if the real nature of the disease could have been made out, from the difficulty of affording a free outlet for the discharge. *Part xxxi., p.* 140.

Fibrous Tumor of the Womb.—Give the liq. calcis chlor. from 30 to 50 minims, twice a day for months, or give the Kreuznach-water (artificially prepared by Mr. Hooper) ʒj. three times a day in warm water, at the same time using an injection for the vagina of ʒij. to the ʒj. of water. Dr. Preiger, however, chiefly depends on baths and fomentations composed of the Kreuznach-water, and some extraordinary effects have no doubt been produced by him, as we have seen. *Part xxxi., p.* 212.

Iodine in Fibrous Tumors in the Uterus.—Dr. West almost invariably orders for those of his patients at St. Bartholomew's who are the subjects of fibrous tumors of the uterus, a long course of one or other of the preparations of iodine. The following is the prescription which was ordered for a middle aged woman, who applied with that disease.

Potassii iodidi, gr. j.; sirup ferri iodidi, mxx.; aquæ carui, ʒss. Ter die sumend. *Part xxxi., p.* 311.

Atheromatous Tumors of the Scalp.—[These consist essentially of a diseased sebaceous follicle, lined inside by tessellated epithelium, and combining a cheesy-looking matter; if they contain a darkish-colored matter, it is a sign of disintegration, not unfrequently followed by ulceration, which may readily be mistaken for a malignant growth. Mr. Erichson says:]

The mode of removal of these tumors before ulcerating is very simple. A single incision is made across the wen or cyst, and then, with a strong drag of a forceps, a sort of evulsion is practised, the entire growth coming out like an almond from its husk or shell. They are found also under the eyelids, and are made worse by any practice but one—namely passing a small probe through them on the conjunctival surface, and stirring up the contents with the probe dipped in nitric acid. *Part xxxii., p.* 196.

Vascular Tumors.—Elastic ligatures are much superior to inelastic ones in the removal of vascular tumors, etc. To apply it the elastic thread must be stretched to its full extent, and tied in a single knot; it must then be slipped over the tumor and tied, by a double knot. Strangulation follows, and the tumor falls off in a few days. *Part xxxv., p.* 93.

Sebaceous Tumors.—Pass through the centre of the tumor a needle carrying a thread, and tie the same as a seton; the tumor will inflame, pus will form and be evacuated through the apertures. The thread may be removed in a fortnight. This treatment is only applicable to those tumors which are more or less in a fluid state. The size of the thread must depend upon the size of the tumor. (M. Marchand.) *Part* xxxv., *p.* 170.

Uterine Fibroid Tumor—Enucleation of.—In making the opening through the uterine wall, the French and American surgeons prefer the use of the knife. In a case of Dr. Simpson's, caustic potash was applied an inch behind the os uteri. Our own opinion is decidedly in favor of the knife, and to make the opening through the uterine structures from within the uterine cavity, rather than from the vagina. Then comes the question, ought we to enucleate at once by instruments, or wait for the expulsive action of the uterus? Before we can answer this, we ought to be able to say whether the organ is, in such cases, always in a condition to exert it. Is it hypertrophied? This is by no means invariable. Hence how hopeless it would be in certain cases to wait for any expulsive uterine action, for the uterus may be actually atrophied, although this is very rare. We may generally expect hypertrophy if the fibroid growths project into the cavity of the uterus and irritate the mucous membrane; or if the tumor be vascular; also if it be developed during or shortly after the period of conceptivity. On the other hand, we should expect atrophy if the tumor occurred during the period of decrepitude. If the uterus be hypertrophied, will it always exert its expulsive action? In all the cases recorded it has not failed to occur, so that after making an artificial os, the cellular attachments of the tumor must be separated and expulsion waited for. If the pains do not come on, the operation of separation must be repeated, the uterus will be sure in time to expel the exposed and partially separated tumor. Ought the tumor to be enucleated at once, or the uterus be allowed to expel it, either partially or entirely? In favor of the latter method we may say that it bears a more close relation to the natural process of effecting the same object; there is less risk of hemorrhage, and lastly, the cavity left is much smaller, and the uterus is more likely to contract on it. In the removal of these tumors, we should recommend, 1. That the incision through the uterine walls be made sufficiently large. 2. That the separation of the cellular attachments be as extensive as possible. 3. That the cyst of the tumor me not cut into. 4. That ergot be given. 5. That the hand be introduced as soon as the dilatation of the os will admit to remove the tumor. (Dr. Grimsdale.) *Part* xxxv., *p.* 234.

" *Phantom Tumors* " *of the Abdomen.*—Dr. Greenhow relates the following among other remarkable cases:

Mrs. ——, aged forty-four, having borne a family, had suffered for several years from menorrhagia, alternating with profuse leucorrhœa. She had also suffered from a variety of other ailments referable to spinal irritation, itself due, I do not doubt, to the disarrangement of the uterine system. I was consulted by her, somewhat more than three years ago, for a tumor in the left hypochondrium, the appearance of which had been long preceded by occasional attacks of pain in that situation, of such intensity as to make her writhe about in bed, and for the relief of which opiates, even in large doses, were of little avail. This pain was of paroxysmal character, often coming on very suddenly, and sometimes without apparent cause, although more frequently as a consequence of over-exertion. It sometimes lasted for many days without intermission, but with variable intensity. The employment of counter-irritation to the spine, and of tonic treatment calculated to improve the general health and lessen the uterine flux, were of essential service; and when, at a subsequent period, I sought for the tumor, it was not discoverable. After an interval of many months I was again consulted for the tumor, which, sure enough, had very evidently returned, and is described in my notes of the case as " an ovoid movable tumor, free from tenderness, and apparently floating loose in the left hypochondriac region; it is difficult to estimate its size, but it appears to be somewhat reniform, and at least twice the natural size of a kidney." It is further added that the patient was in all other respects in good health; that no fullness, tenderness, or pain existed in the posterior lumbar region, and that the urine was normal. Notwithstanding that I believed the tumor to be of the same character with those already related, I thought it desirable that the patient should have the benefit of a second opinion, particularly as I had been unable to find it on a previous occasion. An eminent physician who was called to my assistance, devoted much pains to its elucidation, but without arriving at any more satisfactory conclusion as to its nature than myself. We agreed that it could not be ovarian, from its position; that it was too movable for an enlarged kidney, which was also discountenanced by the absence of any unusual fullness, resistance, or tenderness posteriorly; and that it had not the character, neither had the patient the aspect, of malignant disease. Although in great doubt on the subject, we treated it on the supposition that it might eventually prove a hydatid growth. Some time afterward other symptoms of spinal irritation manifested themselves; and although I had never seen an avowed case of Dr. Addison's " phantom tumors," I began to suspect that this would prove an example of them, as it subsequently did. The patient very shortly after the consultation, went from under my immediate observation, although she continued to act under my instructions. In the course of a few weeks she wrote me word that the tumor had dispersed; and a few months ago, being again in town, she afforded me several opportunities of satisfying myself that the tumor really was gone. *Part* xxxv., *p.* 247.

Arterial Tumors — Aneurisms.—Mr. Cusack, of Steevens' Hospital, Dublin, applies compression by means of conical weights, which, suspended to a frame arching over the limb, may be exactly applied to the artery; five and a half to seven and a half or eight pounds, are generally required to arrest the pulse of the femoral artery completely. At first the circulation must only be partially arrested, and the weight must be applied every alternate hour. After the lapse of six or eight days the weight may be increased till the circulation is completely arrested, the pressure not being continued, however, more than an hour and a half at a time. This mode of applying pressure appears the best hitherto suggested, as it approaches the nearest to manual pressure. It is easily applied, and has proved very satisfactory in its results. *Part* xl., *p.* 307.

TURPENTINE.

To Prevent Nausea, from Administration of Turpentine.—It is stated that turpentine when made into an electuary with mucilage, honey, and a little magnesia, may be given without exciting the disgust and nausea, so frequently caused as ordinarily prescribed.   *Part* xii., *p.* 301.

Oil of Turpentine as a Styptic and Astringent.—As an *astringent*, in doses varying from 20 minims to a drachm, according to the urgency of the symptoms, and repeated every three or four hours, turpentine is one of the most efficacious remedies which we possess. The best vehicle for its administration, in the first place, is water, flavored with sirup of orange, or any other agreeable aromatic. It may afterward be advantageously com-bined with any other therapeutic agents, which the special nature of the case may require : thus, in epistaxis depending upon the rupture of one or more small vessels, and where much arterial blood has been lost, muriated tincture of iron will form a valuable adjunct. In hematemesis and other sanguineous discharges from the bowels, it may be united with compound infusion of roses, sulphate of magnesia, iced-water, and solutions of tannic or gallic acid. In some forms of hemoptysis, it may usefully be added to infusions of matico ; in hematuria, to the decoctions of uva ursi, chima-phila, pyrola, etc. ; or to tincture of the sesquichloride of iron. In purpura hemorrhagica, the decoctions or infusions of the barks form with it an excellent adjuvant. In hemoptysis, it has speedily and effectually arrested the hemorrhage ; and is a much safer remedy than lead.

Dr. Smith states that in his experience, there is no single medicine in the materia medica, that can be compared with it as a *styptic*, either as to cer-tainty of action, or to the safety of its effects. It is compatible alike with acids and alkalies.   *Part* xxi., *p.* 116.

Baths containing Oil of Turpentine.—[Dr. Smith recommends the em-ployment of alkaline camphene or turpentine baths, in chronic rheumatism, lumbago, sciatica, gout, and other affections. He says :]

I have employed camphene in the form of a bath, mixed with common soda ; or two pounds of the latter with from a quarter of a pint to half a pint of camphene, and half an ounce of oil of rosemary, will form an excel-lent bath. In delicate skinned patients, females and children, ʒij. of camphene will be sufficient. I may remark, *in limine*, that the alkaline camphene bath possesses virtues peculiarly its own. In the coldest day in winter, as I have verified in more than one instance, it may be employed with the most perfect safety. Whilst the individual is in the bath, he experiences, to my knowledge, no disagreeable annoyance from the disen-gaged vapor ; on the contrary, if we except the taste of the turpentine, which for some time remains in the mouth, a sense of calmness and tran-quillity very often follows a previously disturbed, irregular, or excited con-dition of the respiratory or sanguiferous systems. After five minutes recumbency in the bath, the pulse is found to become fuller, softer, and slower ; I have seen it fall from 100 to 80. The respiration also becomes freer, deeper, and less labored. On coming out of the bath, the whole skin has a peculiar velvety, soft, and agreeable feeling ; the breath is strongly tainted with the terebinthinaceous odor. If it have not been too hot, a pleasurable tingling warmth is experienced throughout the whole cutaneous surface; and this, with the preceding symptoms, may continue twenty-four hours. One great advantage of this bath will be found in the circumstance that it may be employed at a heat from 10° to 15° below the temperature of the ordinary warm one, without including that sensation of chill to which some delicate constitutions are so peculiarly obnoxious; ten or fifteen minutes is the length of time a patient ought to remain in a bath of this description. In the first instance, it is well for patients to commence with a smaller quantity of the turpentine and soda, say a pound of the latter, with two or three ounces of the former, and gradually increase its strength on each repetition of the bath, to the first mentioned proportions. This bath may be taken every second or third day, according to the urgency of the symptoms and the nature of the affection for which it is prescribed.

Part xxi., *p.* 355.

———•♦•———

ULCERS.

Baynton's Method of Treating Ulcers.—[Mr. Joseph Bell, brings forward cases to show, the efficacy of this mode of treatment, which he justly supposes has fallen too much into disuse. There is no doubt that the practice is excellent; but the troublesome attention which it constantly requires must always be an impediment to its general and continued use, especially amongst the classes of poor people in whom the most troublesome cases occur. Mr. Bell says:]

To explain at any length the method of this celebrated surgeon, may seem to some superfluous. It is, however, my decided conviction that the majority of practitioners are either ignorant of it, or do not put it into practice.

Baynton's system consists of three parts: First, straps of adhesive plaster, from two to three inches broad, and of sufficient length to surround the limb, and to overlap a few inches. These straps are to be applied by placing the centre of the strap exactly opposite the ulcer, over which the free ends are to be crossed, pulling them as tight as the feelings of the patient will permit. The first strap is to be placed a little below the lower margin of the sore; the second is to overlap it a little; the third to overlap the second a little; and so on till the ulcer is completely covered; a soft piece of cloth is then to be placed over the ulcer; but I frequently dispense with this. Secondly, a bandage is to be applied, from the extremity of the limb to the articulation above the sore. Thirdly, this bandage is to be kept constantly wet with cold water. The dressing to be changed every day, or every second day, according to the quantity of discharge and irritability of the ulcer. Such then is the Bayntonian system, which when properly applied, is competent to cure, speedily and effectually, the irritable or inflamed, and the varicose, as well as the indolent or callous ulcer; proper attention, of course, being paid to the improvement of the general health—a *sine qua non* in every plan of treatment.

Part iii., *p.* 105.

Ulceration of upper part of Rectum and Sigmoid Flexure—Case of—Cured by Lime Moxa.—Dr. Osborne of Dublin relates the case of a female who labored under the symptoms of ulceration of the upper part of the rectum and sigmoid flexure, for above a year, and had constantly most severe pain in those parts on passing her motions, which were accompanied by discharges of purulent and sanious matter. On being examined, the rectum and lower part of the colon were free from contractions, and the fecal masses which occasionally passed, although productive of great suffering, yet showed that the passage was not considerably narrowed ; a lime moxa, which extended to about the size of a crown, was applied over the sigmoid flexure, and was immediately followed by a diminution of pain and an almost complete cessation of the discharge ; and before the ulcer produced by the moxa had filled up by granulations, all the symptoms of the internal ulceration had entirely disappeared. *Part v., p.* 129.

Treatment of Old Ulcers by the use of Corrosive Sublimate and Tincture of Iodine.—E. B., aged 43, was admitted into hospital with a large, foul, and painful ulcer on the lower part of the left leg ; extending from the instep nearly six inches upward, across the whole front of the limb. Several useless attempts being made to effect a cure, Mr. Furgusson put her on a course of mercury, in the following way. "Twelve grains of the bichloride of mercury were made up into 240 pills ; two of these were taken for a dose immediately after dinner, the first day, four on the third, six on the fifth, and so on ; increasing the dose by two every second day, until the patient should take thirty pills at a time. After this, if necessary, the dose was to be gradually diminished every second day by two pills, until the number decreased to two. The patient proceeded till she took eighteen pills for a dose, which affected the system, and she then desisted taking any more. Meantime, Mr. Partridge had recommended the sore to be lightly touched with a strong tincture of iodine, which had an excellent effect ; and it was supposed, by the combination of the two remedies, a most obstinate case was cured. *Part v., p.* 144.

Outward Applications to Ulcers—Chemically considered.—On examining the composition of the more common medicinal applications to indolent ulcers, it would appear that, 1st, their energy on the animal tissue, and their caustic properties, are in direct ratio to the rapidity with which they part with their oxygen ; and 2d, the bases of those compounds which experience has taught us to prefer, are, when deprived of their oxygen, perfectly inert, and their affinity for oxygen is comparatively slight. Three qualifications, therefore, appear necessary to constitute a good outward application to an indolent ulcer. 1st. A substance containing a large proportion of oxygen, or of an electro-negative body. 2d. A compound that will part with its oxygen to the animal organism moderately slow. 3d. A compound whose elements, when its oxygen is abstracted, possesses no chemical or solvent powers on the tissues, nor poisonous effects on the body generally.

Guided by these views, Mr. Sankey is led to recommend the employment of various compounds to indolent ulcers, such as the iodate of the protoxide of mercury in the strength of ℈ss. to ℨss. to the ounce of lard ; the iodide of starch ; the oxide of silver ; pectic acid applied as a poultice ; the iodate of peroxide of mercury ; the preparations of periodic acid, the bromates ; succonates ; the precipitate formed by tr. opii on Goulard water ; mucic acid ; alloxan ; hydrated peroxide of iron, etc. In angry and inflammatory ulcers, on the other hand, which are attended with increase of circulation, and consequently, with excessive supply of oxygen, the oxygenated compounds would be prejudicial. Cold lotions or poultices, for chemical reasons, would be indicated ; or, if ointments are used, those only containing a preponderance of electro-positive elements, as ung. cetacei, creasote, etc.; perhaps, also, the application of turpentine, or the non-oxygenated essential oils, as the ol. limon. *Part* vii., *p.* 168.

Simple Ulcers of the Cervix Uteri—Cauterization of.—M. Lisfranc, greatly vaunts the mode of treating ulcers of the neck of the uterus, by the application of escharotics. That which he prefers greatly to all others, is the solution of mercury in an excess of nitric acid. The speculum uteri, he says, is indispensable. The escharotic is never to be applied otherwise than very lightly; nor with a view to destroy the ulcerated or altered surfaces, but to modify their vital state—to produce a *new action* in the parts. A soft brush, or dossil of lint, is the proper tool for making the application, and the speculum is immediately afterward to be filled with tepid or cold water—the abraded surfaces are to be washed clear of all remains of the caustic, which is only felt as peculiarly painful, when it is suffered to come in contact with the sides of the vagina. *Part* viii., *p.* 155.

Phagedenic Ulcer of the Septum Nasi—Chloride of Zinc.—Dr. Zwerina gives the following case: A woman, aged 30, who had suffered from severe pain and enlargement of the right tibia, which was judged to be syphilitic in its nature, was at the same time affected with an ulcerous disease of the nose, which by and by perforated the septum, and threatened to destroy the whole member. The disease of the leg was arrested under the use of mercurial inunction, that of the nose resisted all the topical applications that were made to it—sublimate, arsenic, red precipitate, sulphuric acid, nitric acid, etc., until the chloride of zinc was called into requisition. One grain and a half of the salt was dissolved in one ounce of distilled water, and the scabs being removed, the sore was pencilled over several times a day with the solution. At the end of a fortnight, a healthy granulating surface was found underneath the thick crust which now covered the sore, and this being removed from time to time, and the solution re-applied, at the end of five weeks, the cicatrix was perfect, and the patient well. *Part* viii., *p.* 155.

Use of Turpentine.—Mr. Hancock recommends turpentine in those ulcers which are prevented healing by deficient action, where the ulcer is sluggish, surface-smooth, without granulation, or of a greenish foul appearance; discharge serous, edges rounded, smooth, and callous, and the surrounding skin is pink or blue. It should not be exhibited where the patient is plethoric, the ulcer inflammatory, and the pulse full and frequent, or where it produces nausea, or other unpleasant symptoms; in the last case substitute cajeput oil, three drops three times a day, or give capsules, each containing twenty to twenty-five drops of the turpentine. Continue the use of the turpentine until good healthy granulations appear, with the secretion of good pus. *Part* xiv., *p.* 321.

The treatment of Ulcers.—With respect to ulcers with exuberant granulations, Bransby Cooper says:

In such cases pressure is indicated, which is best effected by the application of bandages; but, should such means not succeed, escharotics may be required to keep down the tendency to hypertrophy. Sulphate of copper I consider the best application for this purpose. Nitrate of silver, which is very frequently employed, tends, in my opinion, rather to increase their growth; for, although when first applied, it removes them, yet they appear to return with increased vigor after its escharotic influence has ceased.

[Indolent ulcers will generally require both constitutional treatment, and stimulating applications to the sore. Mr. Cooper says:]

Bark and acids are indicated, having taken care first that the bowels are freely opened and the secretions generally natural. Stimulants should be applied to the ulcer, either the ung. nitrici oxidi, or the ung. zinei; or, should lotions be preferred—and, indeed in some cases they seem more suitable than greasy applications—nitric acid lotion, or zinc or lead in solution, may be substituted; but at the same time, the patient should be kept during a large portion of the day in a recumbent posture, and much benefit is sometimes derived from the elevation of the affected limb. Porter and generous diet will also expedite the cure, by exciting the reparative process. The pressure and support of a bandage is occasionally useful, but in languid or indolent ulcers its utility is doubtful; for I have frequently observed that a tendency to slough follows its application, as if the granulations were too tender to sustain the slightest pressure.

When these ulcers prove very stubborn, and resist all the constitutional and topical remedies, I have lately witnessed the best results from stimulating their surface by subjecting it to a stream of negative electricity.

At a convenient distance from the indolent ulcer (not less than five or six inches) a portion of the cuticle is raised from the cutis by the application of a piece of emplast. lyttæ of the size of a half-crown. The cuticle is detached by a pair of scissors, and on the exposed cutis a piece of zinc foil is placed, of the same size as the denuded spot. A plate of silver foil is laid on the original ulcer, and the two plates connected by means of a thin copper wire. The size of the silver plate is immaterial. Both zinc and silver are now covered with pieces of moistened lint and oil-skin, and the apparatus, as recommended by Dr. Bird, is complete. In a few hours the surface beneath the zinc becomes white, and a slough begins to form, which in a short time is thrown off, leaving a healthy ulcer behind. In the meanwhile a great change has taken place in the original ulcer; it has thrown aside its indolence; the granulations are sprouting and contracting; new skin is forming at the margin, and the whole surface looks healthy and animated. *Part* xvi., *p.* 228.

Callous Ulcers of the Leg.—Prof. Syme's method of treating these tiresome cases was to apply a large blister over the sore and neighboring swelled part of the limb, which has the effect of speedily dispersing the subcutaneous induration and thickening, so as to relax the integuments, and thus remove the obstacle opposed to healing action. In the course of a short time, seldom exceeding a few days after the blister has been applied, the surface of the ulcer, however deep it may have been, is found to be on a level with that of the surrounding skin; not, of course, through any process of reproduction or filling up, but merely from the removal of interstitial effusion, allowing the integuments to descend from the position to which they had been elevated, as may be readily ascertained by measuring the circumference of the limb, before and after it has undergone the effect of blistering. But, along with this change of form, the ulcer in other respects no less speedily requires the characters of a healing sore, assuming a florid color, affording a moderate discharge of purulent matter, and presenting a granulating surface with surrounding margin of cicatrising pellicle. No subsequent treatment beyond the attention requisite for insuring quiet and cleanliness is needed, and recovery is completed, not only more quickly, but with much less tendency to relapse, than when accomplished by other means.

With regard to the varicose ulcer, the author states that his opinion is not in favor of aiming at what is called the "radical cure," by obstruction of the vein or veins concerned. He has frequently practised the method of Velpeau, who accomplishes the object of obliteration by passing a pin through the skin under the vessel, and then tying a thread lightly round the included part; and has never met with any bad consequences from doing so: but he is nearly satisfied, from what has fallen within his own observation, that the operation is barren of good effects in permanently remedying the tendency to ulceration. The *black wash* has long seemed to him the best application for promoting cicatrization of the ulcer. If the sore comes under treatment in an inflamed or irritated state, poultices should be employed in the first instance; and if the depressed surface and thick edges denote a complication of the callous condition, blistering will be proper instead of such relaxing means. *Part* xvii., *p.* 188.

Phagedenic Ulcers.—[Phagedenic ulcers may occur in other cases than syphilitic ones. The disease is very rapid in its progress, and is attended with severe pain preventing sleep, headache, fever, furred tongue, and tenderness of epigastrium.]

"In the local treatment," Professor Cooper says, "bleeding can rarely be resorted to with advantage; venesection exposes the patient to the risks of hemorrhage, on account of the natural tendency of this disease; and leech-bites assume a morbid action, as is just what we see in hospital gangrene. Mr. Welbank found an application of strong nitric acid to the surface an excellent means of arresting the ravages of gangrenous phagedena. His mode of applying it was, after protecting the surrounding skin with a thick coating of cerate, to dip lint in the acid and apply it to the part, the surface of which was thus converted into a firm and dry mass. Simple dressings were afterward employed, and an evaporating lotion. In France a solution of chloride of sodium, consisting of one part of the concentrated solution in eight of water, is employed, either mixed in a poultice or used with lint. The dressings most used are bread or carrot poultices, a watery solution of hyoscyamus, the liq. opii sed., with a pledget or poultice over the lint. From a consideration of the predisposing cause you will infer the propriety of attending to diet and regimen; when great debility exists, you are to employ bark, quinine, and wine, with a light nourishing diet. In St. Thomas's Hospital it is customary to allow a mutton chop with eggs and milk." *Part* xvii., *p.* 195.

Treatment of, by Proteine.— *Vide.* Art. "Caries."

Treatment of Specific Ulcers—Strumous.—A weak solution of iodine, or the black wash, are useful stimuli to strumous ulcers. If there is a mass of strumous matter forming beneath the skin, paint it over with tincture of iodine, or solid nitrate of silver.

Phagedenic.—In cases of phagedenic ulcer with extensively undermined edges, in which, if an escharotic were used, a large quantity of skin would have to be destroyed, take small strips of lint thoroughly saturated with black wash, and thrust them with a probe to the very bottom of the sore, so as to bring the black powder into contact with its entire surface. Afterward apply strapping, *sec. art.*

A suitable course of medicine and generous diet are accessories in the treatment which must not be omitted.

Menstrual.—Mr. Critchett next proceeds to speak of the *menstrual* ulcer. He says:

There are two or three modifications of this disease met with in practice; thus you have a class of cases, in which, the uterine function being entirely suspended, the system finds relief in a constant discharge from the surface of a sore, which discharge is altered in quality and increased in quantity at the usual monthly period. In other cases the uterine function is performed, but the sore becomes inflamed and painful, and increases its amount of discharge at that period; thus giving evident signs of sympathy and co-öperation with the uterus. There is, again, a peculiar and very formidable class of sores, which occur either at the period when, in the natural course of things, the menstrual function is about to cease; or where, from some organic change in the menstrual organs, this discharge no longer takes place.

The first form of this disease to which I have alluded, and which may be distinguished as "the true menstrual ulcer," occurs generally in young females, soon after the age of puberty. It is often, in the first instance, of a strumous character; or it may have arisen from some external injury. The uterne function not being very fully and regularly established, by degrees it ceases, and its place is supplied by the ulcer.

I have invariably found that the breaking out of the sore has preceded the suspension of the menstrual discharge, or has been first formed prior to that period of life when the function of the uterus commences. I note this especially, because it is an important element in the consideration of the treatment of these cases. The appearance of the ulcer is characteristic of its nature: it is generally rather large, its edges are ragged, its surface is irritable, dark-colored, and exhibits specks of blood; the surrounding parts are of a deep red-color, but not much swollen; the discharge is thin, and often mixed with blood; the pain and soreness are generally distressing and much aggravated at the period when the uterine function is due. When this vicarious discharge is fully established, the disease becomes most intractable. I have met with cases that have existed above three years, having resisted all the ordinary methods of treatment adopted on these occasions.

If we consult surgical authorities on this subject, we invariably find the matter rather briefly dismissed, somewhat in the following way: "Restore the healthy functions of the uterus, and then the ulcer will heal." This sounds very rational and very proper, and no doubt answers exceedingly well when it can be accomplished; but, according to my experience, it is always difficult, and very frequently impossible.

I contend that it is scientifically more correct, and practically far more efficacious, to adopt a method the very converse of the one I have above stated—viz., "Heal the ulcer, and the uterine function will speedily be restored to health and regularity."

I commence, then, at once to attack the ulcer. Some stimulus is often useful in allaying the irritation; a solution of the nitrate of silver is generally the best. I then apply strapping rather tightly; for I find in all those cases in which I have, as it were, to compel a cure in spite of the rebellion of the constitution, rather tight and very accurately applied support is necessary.

As the discharge is copious, it should be applied frequently, either alternate days, or every day. The wound will soon take on a healthy action, and begin to heal, and you will naturally suppose the cure is at hand; but as the monthly period approaches, in spite of all your efforts, the aspect of the sore changes, the discharge again becomes thin and copious, and much of the improvement that has taken place during the previous month is lost. You must not be discouraged by this, but must start again, and each month you will find you gain more than you had previously lost, until, at last, you succeed in entirely closing the wound, and then you are safe; the ulcer being healed, the uterus spontaneously resumes its healthy and regular function—at least, such has been my experience. But even suppose such a result should not invariably occur, you have then a simple case of amenorrhœa to deal with, which is surely far more easily controlled when uncomplicated with a vicarious discharge from an ulcer in the leg.

When sores occur about the time of the cessation of the catamenia, take care, before healing them, to get a freely-discharging issue made.

Part xix., *p.* 200.

Treatment of Indolent Ulcers.—Mr. Chapman's plan is as follows: Dress the sore with a compress of lint dipped in cold water, and folded once, twice, or three times, according to the amount of compression deemed necessary; or, if the ulcer is very deep, cover it first with soft sponge torn up into very small shreds, and soaked in water, and over this apply the wetted lint in a single layer; then take three or more moistened strips of linen or calico, about two and a half inches wide, and apply them round the leg in the same manner as Baynton's strapping. Cover the whole by a calico bandage, placing compresses of lint about the malleoli, so as to insure the bandage being evenly applied. Soak the bandage with cold water, and envelop the limb in oiled silk, reopening this from time to time, to renew the cold affusion. At first the ulcer may require dressing every day, but after a time, an interval of three, four, or even five days, may elapse between the dressings. *Part* xix., *p.* 203.

Use of Chloride of Zinc.—Dr. Brookes states that the chloride of zinc exerts a good effect in stubborn ulcers, especially with callous, hard, everted edges, and will rapidly set up a healthier action when other remedial means have failed; the surface will speedily granulate and heal.

Take two parts of chloride of zinc, and three parts of gypsum; mix them, and spread the powder over the surface of the sore, protecting the edges of the healthy skin with vinegar. In about a quarter of an hour apply a poultice. *Part* xix., *p.* 205.

Foul and Flabby Ulcers.—Bi-sulphate of iron and alumina, is recommended as an excellent application. *Vide* Art, "Iron."

Chronic—Use of Collodion.—Apply collodion, in the following manner: Dry the ulcer with bibulous paper; wash it over with ether, by means of a soft brush; again dry with the paper; then apply the collodion with a brush in a circular manner, so as to cover the edges of the ulcer to a greater or less extent, as may be deemed necessary, and varnish over so much of the ulcer itself as to leave a small central opening for the escape of discharges. Any stimulus judged to be favorable to cicatrization may be applied in the dry form before beginning to paint with the collodion.

Part xix., *p.* 318.

Chronic Ulcers—Treatment.—Dr. T. H. Burgess recommends, to em ploy fumigation in the following way. R Sulphuris, ʒiij.; hydr. sulph. rubr. ϴij.; iodinii, gr. x. M. Ft. pulv. sex. Put one of these powders upon a heated iron at the bottom of a large jar or tin case, the iron being covered by a grating. Immediately put the limb into the jar, and close it up to prevent the escape of vapor; and continue the bath for fifteen or twenty minutes. In a few days the proportion of iodine may be increased.

Part xx., p. 168.

Treatment of Ulcers by means of Opium.—Mr. Skey says: Mr. P., placed himself under my charge, with a large chronic ulcer on the calf of the right leg. Its margin was irregular and jagged, and was elevated to at least one-third of an inch above the base of the ulcer, which base was pale and bloodless. This wound was about the size of a man's extended hand, including the fingers, or even larger. It had existed for, I think, seventeen years. All remedies had failed, and the cure had long been abandoned as hopeless. I gave Mr. P. half a grain of opium night and morning. In three days he himself noticed the singular red color of the entire margin of the ulcer, which in a week extended over the base. I rolled and strapped the limb; the entire sore consequent on its depressed surface being placed beyond the influence of the pressure. Within two months that sore was reduced *to the size of half a crown*, and the *only remedy employed was half a grain of opium night and morning*, which, by the by, had a very beneficial influence on his health. *Part xx., p.* 177.

Treatment of the "Warty Ulcers of Marjolin," by means of the Chloride of Zinc.—[Dr. Fearnside proceeds to describe the case which fell under his care. His patient was a large unwieldy man; having the aspect of a man accustomed to indulge in malt liquor. About nine years previously he had sustained a severe injury in the front of his right leg. Inflammation and a swelling ensued, the size of a pullet's egg, which underwent little change for some years. But 10 or 12 months prior to his coming under Dr. Fearnside, pain was felt in the tumor, which acquired a dark red color, the skin covering it being indurated and uneven, and the discharge thin, fetid, and often bloody. Dr. Fearnside continues:]

When I first saw him, the morbid growth presented the following characters: From the centre of the front of the right leg, occupying a space of about three inches in diameter, there sprung a dark grey substance, which projected at least two-thirds of an inch above the surrounding skin. Its surface had a granular appearance—at first view not unlike the head of a cauliflower; on closer examination, it was seen that this was occasioned by the prominent extremities of coarse fibres which arose from the base of the ulcer, and were collected into masses, separated from each other by deep fissures. The margin of the sore was thickened, elevated, and possessed little or no connection with the fibrous structure above described: the surrounding integument had undergone considerable warty induration and discoloration. A thin ichorous discharge proceeded from the part; the pain experienced was not violent; there was no enlargement of the popliteal or inguinal glands. He complained of being weakened by repeated loss of blood, but his health was otherwise good. He had been previously under the care of one or two medical men, and had been advised to submit to amputation of the leg, on the supposition that the disease was fungus hematodes. The case was considered a favorable one for the employment of the chloride of zinc.

On its first application, the remedy was mixed with flour. (Canquoin's formula.) But little pain was occasioned by it, and the resulting slough was not deep. When it was next employed, it was blended with pure sulphate of lime, as proposed by Mr. Ure. The whole of the morbid growth was covered to the depth of a third of an inch with a paste composed of one part of chloride of zinc and two parts of sulphate of lime. The application gave rise to severe pain, which was only partially under the control of opium. At the expiration of four days an extensive and deep slough was produced, which separated in the course of the ensuing week or ten days. The greater part of the sore was then covered with healthy-looking granulations; but to get rid of two or three small masses of whitish semi-cartilaginous substance, as well as to overcome the indurated condition of the margin of the ulcer, it was requisite again to have recourse to the caustic paste. The subsequent progress of the case was, upon the whole, highly satisfactory. No hemorrhage ensued after the first complete application of the chloride of zinc. In the course of a month small florid granulations had arisen to the level of the adjoining surface, and cicatrization commenced. *Part* xxii., *p.* 249.

Treatment of Varicose Ulcer at St. Thomas's Hospital.—After all other measures have failed in the treatment of this affection, in cases at St. Thomas's Hospital, perfect success has followed the application of a caustic issue, by rubbing potassa fusa along the chief vein between the ulcer and the heart. *Part* xxii., *p.* 256.

Ulcers external to the Anal Aperture.—Mr. Hilton directs these to be treated by the recumbent position to relieve the hemorrhoidal veins, keeping the bowels open by castor oil, which acts on the entire course of the intestinal canal, and lubricates the hard exterior of the fecal mass as it passes through the rectum; and by applying the following ointment: ungent. opii, ʒj.; ung. hydrarg. fort., ʒiij., to be applied two or three times a day. *Part* xxiii., *p.* 176.

Cicatrization of an Ulcer promoted by the Electric Moxa.—[The attention of Mr. Cooper was formerly directed to this process for the promotion of the cicatrization of obstinate ulcers, by Dr. Hull, of the United States. Instead, however, of employing the galvanic battery which is cumbersome, he used one introduced by Dr. Golding Bird, merely using two plates, one of silver and the other of zinc, connected by a copper wire. The case in which the apparatus was used, was an ulcer originally produced from a gun-shot wound situated on the inner side of the right foot and below the ankle. The charge of shot passed obliquely through the soft part of the right instep, and injured the navicular bone. During the treatment several small pieces of bone came away, as often as two or three times a week. The wound never, however, completely healed, and previous to the application of the electric moxa, it was the size of the hand.]

Carrot poultices were first used, and leeches were from time to time applied round the sore. Warm water dressing was subsequently employed, and the patient took sarsaparilla, but this treatment continued for about six weeks, proved unavailing as regarded the cicatrization of the ulcer.

At this period Mr. Cooper ordered the electric moxa to be applied; this was done in the following manner: a small oval piece of blistering plaster, about the size of a crown piece, was placed six inches above the sore. On the following day, a blister having formed, the cuticle was removed, and a plate of zinc, previously cut so as accurately to fit the vesicated surface, was applied on the same. A silver plate was then placed on the original sore, and the two metallic agents connected with a copper wire. This simple apparatus was secured on the limb by means of a few narrow strips of adhesive plaster, the whole being covered with wet lint, and a loose bandage, which latter was kept constantly moist.

On the next day the silver plate was raised for the purpose of examining the sore, and a most decided improvement was observed, the granulations looking more healthy and active. On the second day, however (the moxa having remained in contact with the limb for forty-eight hours) there was pain and considerable redness over the whole leg, with enlargement of the inguinal glands. The moxa was therefore removed, the stimulating effects having evidently caused inflammation of the absorbents; yet the original sore had a more healthy appearance, and was evidently decreasing in size. On the fifth day the inflammatory symptoms had considerably subsided and the sore was improving fast. On the ninth all pain and redness in the leg had disappeared, and a slough separated from the blistered surface to which the zinc plate had been applied. The original ulcer was found much decreased in size, being now no larger than a crown piece; the granulations assumed a healthy appearance; they rose to the level of the margins, and were covered and protected toward the centre of the sore by a whitish layer of healthy pus. The borders were becoming flattened and regular, and the gradual extension of the cuticle could be distinguished within them.

The cicatrizing process went on uninterruptedly. About four months after admission, the ulcer was quite healed up, and the patient left the hospital in good health. He was, however, recommended not to bear the whole weight of his body upon the leg for some time to come, and allow the soft parts about the ankle to gain tone before he used them freely.

Part xxiii., *p.* 293.

Phagedenic Ulceration.—Sarah H——, aged 6, a strumous child of low powers, living in an unhealthy neighborhood, was admitted as an out-patient on July 18th, with acute phagedenic ulceration of the side of the tongue, gums, and lips; it was of one week's duration, and was now spreading rapidly.

Caustic was freely applied. Ten grains of chlorate of potash in water to be given three times a day; and the sore to be sponged frequently in the course of the day with a solution of nitrate of silver (three grains to the ounce.) In a few days the phagedenic action was checked; and at the end of a fortnight, healthy granulations were seen fast repairing the breach. Bark and soda were now substituted. On August 8th, the child was perfectly cured.

Phagedenic Ulceration of Labia and Bend of Thigh—Recovery.— Jane J——, aged 20 months, a stout, healthy-looking child, brought up by hand, had been ailing one week, was brought to the surgery with extensive, spreading, superficial ulceration of both labia and bend of the thigh on the right side, almost running into gangrene. This was accompanied with great œdema, and excessive pain and difficulty in micturition.

Ordered stale beer grounds poultice; nutritious diet; and ten grains of chlorate of potash in barley-water three times a day.

This treatment was pursued with speedy success, subduing the phage-denie tendency, and causing a healthy action to be set up in the ulcerating surface. In a few days, a simple bread cataplasm was substituted; and at the end of three weeks the child was quite cured.

The above cases fully prove the value of nitrate of silver in solution and stale-beer grounds as applications in phagedenic action; at the same time the effects of chlorate of potash must not be forgotten as an important agent in checking acute ulcerative spreading. *Part* xxiv., *p.* 220.

Granulating Surfaces.—To protect raw granulating surfaces from the atmosphere, lay a thick semifluid aqueous solution of gum tragacanth on the raw surface; if it is imperfect in any part repair such by another layer. This application, says Professor Miller, produces no irritation, and being translucent permits a complete surveillance. *Vide* " Collodion."
Part xxiii., *p.* 288.

Obstinate Ulcers—Tincture of Cantharides.—Mr. Tait gives the following mixture, which has been recommended as being of great utility in these affections: Tinct. of cantharides, 12 drops; iodide of potassium, ʒss.; compound tincture of cinchona bark, ʒj.; water, seven ounces. Mix. ʒj. ter die; and apply the following lotion: Tincture of cantharides, twelve minims; diluted nitric acid, twenty drops; compound tincture of cinchona, two drachms; water, one ounce. The tincture of cantharides is of great utility in indolent ulceration, dependent either upon atony of the engaged parts, or system generally. It is useful—1st. Where the granulations are exuberant, but pale, weak, and flabby. 2d. Where there is deficiency, or total absence of granulations, the ulcers being deep and scooped out, with raised and indurated edges. 3d. Where the granulations are not defective, but cicatrizing irregularly, sometimes in the centre, at other times on one side, the lymph which is thrown out and organized on one day being absorbed the next. *Part* xxiii., *p.* 325.

Chronic and Secondary—Use of Phosphate of Lime.—In chronic ulcers, resulting from scrofulous diathesis, Dr. Reneke recommends the use of phosphate of lime, in doses of from eight to twenty grains per diem. It should be ordered to be taken with the breakfast, dinner, and supper, so as to be thoroughly mixed with the food. These cases are accompanied always by a want of the proper cell growth, which the phosphate is said to increase in a remarkable manner. The phosphate, nevertheless, cannot be said really to cure the scrofulous dyscrasia, but we shall certainly promote the cure in the most efficient manner by its administration.

In persons who have suffered from secondary ulcers, ulcers of the bones, etc., and who have become exceedingly weak and emaciated, give (along with the preparations of mercury, of which the iodine may be preferred) the phosphate of lime in doses of fifteen to twenty grains during the day.
Part xxiv., *p.* 303.

Ulcers.—Mr. Holt, of Westminster Hospital, recommends to exclude the atmospheric air by the following treatment, after the inflammation has subsided. From a piece of adhesive plaster somewhat larger than the sore, a portion, just the size of the sore itself, is cut out; the plaster is then applied to the part, and painted with collodion. Oiled silk is now placed over the ulcer, and made to adhere to the plaster by means of the collodion, by which process the air is completely excluded from the ulcerative surface. The whole is then secured by strips of adhesive plaster placed crosswise, and by a roller running from the toes to above the knee. *Part* xxv., *p.* 266.

Treatment of Ulcers of the Leg.—The facilitation of the flow of blood toward the heart is the great object to be attained in treating ulcers of the leg. Many methods have been proposed whereby to effect this. That employed in the Middlesex Hospital, is the most easy and rational; the limb being raised high above the level of the body on an inclined plane. By such a plan ulcers commonly heal rapidly.

The out-patients of the London Hospital are treated as recommended by Mr. Critchett, by strapping the whole leg from the toe to the knee with inch-wide strips of plaster, and applying a bandage as tight as can be borne. The plaster should be made of unirritating material, and spread on unglazed calico. In the London Hospital the emp. plumbi is used. At St. Bartholomew's, Mr. Wormald directs the application of a folded compress of lint over the trunk of the internal saphena, immediately below the knee, to be fixed with considerable tightness, by means of a broad strip of sticking-plaster. The same object is gained yet more effectually by Mr. Startin's elastic spiral bandage, as used at the Hospital for Diseases of the Skin. These ulcers are essentially of an inflammatory character, and the blistering the edges by some blistering fluid (Bulleyn's is the best) is often followed by remarkable benefit. At the Hospital for Diseases of the Skin the patient is put under a continued course of iodide of potassium, or biniodide of mercury, and the following ointment is applied to the ulcer: Hyd. bisulphuret, hydrarg. nitric. oxyd. aa. $\mathfrak{z}$ss.; creasote, mxx.; adipis recentis, $\mathfrak{z}$xvi. Misce.

* ' * * * * * * *

In an obstinate case of this disease, Mr. Gay, finding the skin immediately in the neighborhood of the ulcer very tense, and unable to yield further to the contracting power of the scar, divided that part of the skin where the tension existed in the greatest degree. Three weeks after, the ulcer was quite closed. Mr. Gay observed that it was only by altering the direction of the traction, and transferring it to more healthy and movable parts, that any advantage can be expected from measures similar to the above. *Part* xxvii., *p.* 159.

Cancroid.—Dr. Roe, of Westminster Hospital, recommends from one eighth to one-fourth of a grain of ammonio-sulphate of copper three times a day. It may be continued for many months. *Part* xxvii., *p.* 248.

Ulcers—Indolent and Callous.—Instead of employing the expensive and troublesome plan of strips of adhesive plaster, Professor Syme recommends to apply a large blister. This quickly relieves the hard swelling of the limb, and allows speedy healing and sound cicatrization without further trouble.

* * * * * * * * *

Varicose.—Professor Syme recommends to apply simply the common black-wash lotion. Under this plan they generally readily heal.
Part xxvii., *p.* 352.

Venereal Ulcers.—Instead of the violent treatment which has been commonly employed for this kind of ulcer—such as rubbing over the surface · with caustic potass, and pushing it into the several sinuosities—Prof. Syme recommends to apply a blister over the sore, and administer small doses

of iodide of potassium to the extent of two grains twice or thrice a
day. *Part* xxvii., *p.* 353.

Treatment of Indolent Ulcers by Incisions.—The principle in Mr. Gay's
method of treating ulcers which have resisted all other modes, is to relieve
the tension of the skin or other tissues, by making incisions at right angles
with the line of tension ; or where the tension is at the edge of the sore,
to supply new skin altogether by a species of plastic operation.

Mr. Chapman proposes a modification of Mr. Gay's new operation,
where the edges of the ulcer are adherent to the tissues beneath ; this is,
to glide a double-edged bistoury under the tense margins of the sore, so
as to set them free, and allow of their edges being brought as near into
contact as possible across the suppurating surface. *Part* xxviii. *p.* 240.

Treatment of Callous Ulcer by Excision of the Margin.—Mr. Hain-
worth thus describes the disease : The apparently sunken, nearly circular
or oval ulcer, varying in diameter from one-third of an inch to three, four,
or five inches, having a level, pale-red, glassy surface, void of granulations,
excreting a thin, scanty, unirritating fluid, with a hard, precipitous, white
or dusky edge, surrounded by integument, thickened and indurated by
infiltration of lymph and serum, even now occupies too many a bed in our
great hospitals, and too frequently exhausts the patience of sufferer and
surgeon, dresser and nurse.

From this description it will be seen, that those ulcers are purposely
excluded from consideration which are either inflamed or irritable—which
depend simply on a varicose state of the veins—which are complicated
with diseased bone, or with any special local or constitutional cause.

The primary obstacle to the successful treatment of this ulcer is the presence of a compact and effete solid ring of cuticle. This must be excised
by carefully shaving off the accumulated cuticle without wounding the
cutis. *Part* xxix., *p.* 242.

New Mode of Treating Ulcers from Irritation of the Nails.—[Mr. Ure
related the following case of a young woman, aged 23, who was under his
care at St. Mary's Hospital.]

Four months before admission, the great toe of the right foot became
uneasy and swollen, the patient having pared the nail the day preceding.
Ere long, a painful and irritable sore made its appearance by the side of
the nail, which discharged from time to time a quantity of thick, bloody,
and sometimes black-looking matter.

As the sore was rather in an inflamed state on her admission, poultices
were applied. On the third day, when all surrounding inflammation
seemed to have subsided, Mr. Ure prescribed the use of a salve composed
of one grain of finely levigated arsenious acid, incorporated with an ounce
of spermaceti ointment. He was led to try this remedy by the suggestion
of Mr. Copeland, who deemed it almost a specific in ulcers of this nature.
This was steadily employed for about ten days, without producing any
marked change on the sore. Mr. Ure then ordered, instead, the continuous application of a hot saturated solution of alum. This induced rapid
absorption of the thickened parts, and prompt cicatrization of the ulcerated
surface, so that the patient was enabled to leave the hospital, cured, in the
course of three days. Mr. Ure observed that, while alum is soluble in five
parts of water at 60° Fahr., it is soluble in little more than its own weight

of water at the boiling temperature. A hot saturated solution is, consequently, more energetic in its action than a cold one. *Part* xxix. *p.* 247.

*Extensive Phagedenic Ulceration, Successfully Treated by the Actual
Cautery.*—[This patient, 25 years of age, ten days after exposure to contagion, observed a small pimple near the frenum on the penis. Caustic was
liberally applied, apparently with success. At the end of a fortnight,
swelling in the groin came on, an abscess formed, which burst spontaneously. The sore on the penis was nearly healed. Subsequently the opening in the groin extended rapidly, and he soon labored under all the symptoms of irritative fever.]

Where the chancre had existed there was a slight depression, some discoloration, but no hardness of the base; it had been cicatrized for two or
three weeks. In the groin was a foul ulcer of the size of the palm of the
hand; its surface presented a yellowish dark aspect; the edges of the
wound were ragged, uneven, and undermined, secreting a thin, fetid,
sanguineous discharge; an areola of a livid tint surrounded the wound for
a considerable extent. Ordered to be confined to bed, to live on broths,
jellies, and farinaceous food. The compound decoction of sarsaparilla with
nitric acid, twelve grains of Dover's powder, at bed time. To the ulcer,
the nitrate of silver, an opiate lotion, and poultice of linseed-meal. To
give the symptoms and treatment of this protracted case *in extenso* would
be tedious. Suffice it to say he took the compound decoction and extract
of sarsaparilla, the mineral acids, quinine, opium, and various preparations
of iodine; to the wound were applied the strong nitric acid, muriate of
antimony, the balsam of Peru, different kinds of lotions, ointments, and
poultices. The edges of the ulcer were cut away by means of curved
scissors; a moderate allowance of stimulants and a suitable regimen enjoined; still, however, the phagedena continued progressing, so that when
all treatment to stay its progression had failed, it was determined to apply
the actual cautery. It was done at once; and the parts covered with lint,
spread with cerate composed of two parts of resin cerate, and one of oil
of turpentine; forty drops of tincture of opium were given to procure
sleep. The recovery of the patient thereafter was truly remarkable.

Part xxix. *p.* 247.

Cancerous Ulcers.—Mr. Weeden Cooke recommends a carrot poultice
to be applied to cancerous sores when offensive. It should be changed
every few hours. Mr. Chatterley says that wood soot (not powdered
charcoal) answers very well for the same purpose. The wood soot should
be sprinkled from an ordinary tin pepper box, on the outside of the other
dressings used. It may be obtained from chimneys of fire-places in which
wood and nothing else is burned, or from the ovens of ham and bacon
curers. *Part* xxix., *p.* 321.

Treatment of Phagedena.—For a considerable period past, a mild form
of hospital phagedena has been prevalent in the various London insti-
tutions.

It has generally attacked superficial wounds, whether those resulting
from accidents or operations, and, in a few instances, even stumps have
been affected with it. The treatment which has certainly been found of
most general benefit has been the application of pure nitric acid. In a
case under the care of Mr. Coulson, a man in good health, admitted on
account of a laceration on the dorsum of the right foot, had the wound

so severely affected by phagedena, that amputation was seriously proposed. The nitric acid was freely applied, by soaking a piece of lint, and then pressing it into the sore; it was allowed to remain seven hours, and completely achieved its intention. The gangrene ceased to spread, the sore took on healthy action, and rapidly cicatrized. Neither in this nor in any one of several other cases in which the dorsum of the foot was the affected part did any sloughing of the tendons follow the use of the acid. It appears to be in cases of simple phagedena that the local use of nitric acid is most to be depended upon, since those of syphilitic origin not unfrequently resist its influence. A case of the latter character, occurring in a young and seemingly healthy woman, was lately under the care of Mr. Stanley, in St. Bartholomew's Hospital, and, in spite of all measures, ultimately terminated in death. Nitric acid had more than once been freely applied, and opium, cinchona, chlorate of potash, etc., had been fairly tried. In the Middlesex Hospital, the favorite treatment for phagedena is by opium pushed freely until its effects become apparent. Some very successful cases are accredited to this plan. It is observed, that there seems scarcely any limit to the quantity which may be borne, and that, generally, before any narcotic effects become apparent, the sore takes on a healthy action. Now and then the acid succeeds admirably in syphilitic cases; as a rule, however, they seem more amenable to constitutional than local measures.

The most convenient mode of applying nitric acid is by means of a glass brush; in the absence of which, however, a glass rod succeeds very well.
Part xxx., *p.* 177.

Ulcer of the Leg in Elderly People.—According to Mr. Skey, of St Bartholomew's, opium has a wonderful effect as a stimulant in these cases. Give good diet, and a common opium and soap pill at bedtime. Assist by strapping and bandaging if necessary. The soap and opium pill may be given, once, twice, or three times a day if necessary, and if other symptoms do not forbid its exhibition. Sometimes the soap and opium purges; in this case leave off the soap, and give half a grain of extract of opium night and morning, or once a day; increase to one grain if necessary. Opium gives energy to the capillary system of arteries, promotes warmth, and thus secures an equable balance of the circulation.—*Vide* Art. "Opium." *Part* xxxi., *p.* 192.

Use of Acid Nitrate of Mercury—For Sloughing Ulcers.—The practice of treating unhealthy ulcerations wherever situated, by means of caustics, is much pursued at this hospital, and with excellent results. The pain attending the application of nitric acid has been much overrated by the profession generally.

Its powers in case of phagedena are now widely recognized. The pain spontaneously caused by an unhealthy sore during a single night is probably much more than that produced by an application of caustic. In most cases of sloughing or unhealthy ulcers, Mr. Startin employs either the solution of the acid nitrate or the arsenical paste. The rapidity with which the surface granulates afterward is often surprising.
Part xxxi., *p.* 240.

Spender's Chalk Ointment in Ulcers of the Leg.—The following formula has been very successfully used in chronic non-specific cases of this kind: R Cretæ prep., ℔iv.; adipis suilli, ℔j.; olei olivæ, ℥iij.

Having heated the oil and lard, add gradually the chalk, finely pow.
dered.

The ointment and a bandage being once applied, it is left until the
cicatrix forms and becomes firm. *Part* xxxii., *p.* 196.

Phagedenic Ulceration.—When situated upon an extremity, and the
sore can be well exposed, Mr. Cock, of Guy's Hospital, advises to try con.
stant irrigation. You must have a reservoir above the bed filled with lukewarm water, to which a little chloride of lime or soda has been added as a
preventative of smell. Then by means of an elastic tube a stream must be
kept continually flowing over the sore. By this means all particles of discharge, etc., are washed away as soon as formed, and a speedy arrest of
morbid action is secured; of course this is based on a supposition that
phagedenic action is a process of local contagion, the *materies morbi* by
which the ulcer spreads being its own pus. *Part* xxxiii., *p.* 233.

Astringent Lotion for Ulcers.—A lotion, consisting of half a drachm of
the tincture of catechu, to a pint of the decoction of oak bark, is a favorite
one at the Aldersgate-street Dispensary, as an application to foul and
indolent ulcers on the leg. Mr. Savory, the surgeon to that institution,
finds it superior in efficiency to most other astringents. It is applied freely,
a piece of lint being well soaked in it and laid over the sore.
Part xxxiii., *p.* 238.

Cancerous Ulcers.—From a trial of a great variety of applications, the
following lotion seems to answer perhaps the best: ℞ Plumbi acet., Ɵij. ad
ʒj.; creasoti mxl. ad ʒj.; aq. fluvial., ʒxij. M. Ft. lot.

The acetate of lead and the creasote form a uniform mixture, and there
is no separation of the latter ingredient. A piece of lint soaked in the
lotion, and applied to the ulcer twice or three times a day, is Mr. Valen-
tine's mode of applying it. The whole is covered by an oiled silk.
Part xxxiii., *p.* 239.

Ulcers—Spreading and Sloughing.—Mr. Stanley, of Lock Hospital, says
that the best of all the usual remedies for such affections is the external
application of the "Friar's Balsam," (tict. benzoin co.)
Part xxxiii., *p.* 237.

Treatment of Ulcerated Legs.—The most important point, in the
opinion of Dr. Thos. Westlake is to get rid of the superincumbent column
of blood which impedes the circulation; this is best done by means of a
flannel bandage, from seven to eight yards long and three inches wide,
applied very carefully, so as to give complete and uniform support to the
affected limb. In indolent ulcers the compound tincture of iodine is the
most safe and efficient stimulant. In irritable ulcers, the application of
the following lotion—iodide of potassium, one scruple; hydrocyanic acid
(Scheele's) half a drachm; camphor mixture, one oz.—applied for four or
five minutes with lint well saturated acts like a charm. The following
ointment may be afterward employed; spermaceti ointment, half an
ounce; iodine, five grains; extract of belladonna, one drachm.
Part xxxiv., *p.* 197.

Ulcers of the Leg.—Dr. J. K. Spender says: we must endeavor to
preserve the purulent secretion which nature has provided as a protective
covering; if this be deficient, the best ointment as a substitute will be one
composed of two parts of lard and three of chalk mixed when heated and

fluid; this must be applied spread on linen and over this a flannel or calico bandage. If the ulcer be extensive and the discharge great, it should be dressed every day, but generally ulcerated legs are disguised much too frequently; all interference should be postponed as long as possible. One great advantage of the chalk ointment is, that it neutralizes the acrid secretion, and allows the dressing to remain much longer than otherwise, without interfering with the healing process. When removing the dressing, be careful that you do not take away the ointment which may adhere to the ulcer, or you will very much hinder its healing.

General principles of treatment often require some modification in practice. The instances in which the chalky incrustation and compression has answered best are superficial ulcerations, however extensive the surface, and whether dependent on varix or not. Deep and callous ulcers require a special treatment, which is best fulfilled by the addition of a stimulant to the chalk ointment, and the best is, the nitric oxide of mercury; ointments of tar and chalk, and iodine and chalk, are found to subdue many forms of irritable ulceration. Dr. Hughes Bennett and others confirm the value of tar in all dermal affections of a psoriasical character. The use of bandaging is of equal importance, to afford a support to the veins. Poultices are generally injurious, and cannot be condemned in too emphatic terms; they relax and weaken the structures and granulations, which rather require tonics and support. The application of a poultice is nothing less than a mischievous interference with the natural healing process. Lotions of every kind are equally prejudicial. The constant application of cold water is exceedingly injurious. To keep patients in bed is a useful element in the treatment of varicose ulcers of the leg, but compression answers every object to be gained by the assumption of the recumbent position; and whenever compression is resorted to, exercise confers the direct and positive benefit of assisting and sustaining those processes necessary for restoration, it sets up an additional energy in the process of reparation by its direct effects as a stimulus. Of the various measures which have been proposed for the treatment of varicose ulcers of the leg, we may notice Mr. Syme's proposal for blistering the edges of the callous ulcer. Mr. Holt has proposed the exclusion of atmospheric air by the application of plaster, oiled silk, and collodion. M. Denonvilliers has recently brought glycerine into notice as a clean and useful application to ulcers. Dr. Neumann is an advocate for the application of charcoal. Mr. Gay maintains that the edge of the ulcer is not free to contract, being bound down to the tissues beneath, and therefore recommends an incision to be made through the healthy skin and superficial facia, within a short distance of the edge of the ulcer, in a direction parallel to the direction of the axis of the limb. Mr. Chapman adopts a modification of this, but considers the cases very rare where it would be required. To Mr. Hainsworth is due the credit of reviving the ancient practice of excising the margin of the callous ulcer. The late Dr. Golding Bird and Mr. Spencer Wells have explained and illustrated the application of the electric moxa. Mr. Skey advocates the use of opium upon principles which are unquestionably authentic and sound. *Part* xxxiv., *p.* 202.

Ulcers of the Leg.—If the ulcers are *gangrenous*, they may readily be made healthy by applying a powder made of equal parts of fine charcoal and chalk, and over this a poultice, or dry lint and bandage. If *very pain-*

ful and irritable, apply a dossil of lint dipped in chloric ether, and over this the bandage. If sanious, or fungoid, apply freely the nitrate of silver, or sulphate of copper. If sluggish, they must be roused into action, by applying the nitric oxide of mercury ointment. If the edges are hard and cartilaginous, draw the edges tightly together by straps of plaster, and apply a flannel bandage as tightly as possible, to awaken the absorbents into activity. For simple sores, the simple ointment is best, with a bandage as tightly applied as it can be borne. If much matter is discharged, they should be dressed daily, and in all troublesome cases a flannel bandage is absolutely indispensable; it will be found to be very much superior to the usual calico bandage, if properly applied. (Dr. Hunt.)

Part xxxv., *p.* 166.

Ulcers— Old Callous.—Dr. Watson, surgeon to the Royal Infirmary, Glasgow, says: If an ointment consisting of anhydrous sulphate of zinc, mixed with glycerine, spread upon bits of lint the size of the ulcers, be applied to them, and allowed to remain a few hours, most acute pain will be caused, and the ulcer will be corroded; but when the slough separates, the granulations will rapidly spring up to a level with the surrounding parts, and in most cases will soon become skinned over. The sulphate of zinc is as suitable, but not superior to the chloride for this purpose.

Part xxxvi., *p.* 259.

Powdered Chlorate of Potash as an Application to Ulcers, etc.—Mr. Hutchinson, of the Metropolitan Free Hospital, says that finely powdered chlorate of potash is an excellent application to cachectic ulcers; it seems to speedily induce cicatrization, and is very convenient of use; it is of great use in cracked nipples and open buboes; it should be dusted into the sac with the finger, and it may also be prescribed internally at the same time. *Part* xxxvii., *p.* 175.

Ulcers of the Leg.—At the Hospital for Skin Diseases, the patient is always directed to bandage the limb, though no very particular attention is paid to this part of the treatment. Internally the mistura hyd. com. is mostly ordered, and to the sore itself the unguentum rubrum is applied. If the ulcer is sloughy or very unhealthy looking, the acid nitrate of mercury is applied as a caustic previous to the use of the ointment. Confinement is not insisted on. From the rapid healing which often ensues, probably the mercurial induction, both internal and local, has usually a considerable share in the cure. *Part* xxxviii., *p.* 173.

Caustic Lint.—Nitrate of silver is never applied to sores, except in the solid state or in solution. In the former case its action is often too severe; in the latter it is sometimes too transient. M. Riboli has conceived the idea of dissolving nitrate of silver in a small quantity of water, soaking pledgets of lint in the solution, and drying them. This caustic lint, applied to ill-conditioned ulcers, produces a more permanent effect than the remedy in a liquid state; and as the author proposes different degrees of concentration for the solution the activity of the treatment may be varied, according to the nature of the case, and the more or less advanced stage of the affection. *Part* xxxix., *p.* 232.

UMBILICAL CORD.

Advantages of retaining Undivided for a Short Time after Birth.—In all cases where the infant is born weakly or in a state of asphyxia, M. Baudelocque recommends not to cut the umbilical cord for some time at least after birth. He relates that since he has followed the opinions of Smellie, Levret, Chaussier, etc., on this subject, he has not lost a single case, although when born the child might be in a state of pretty complete asphyxia or apoplexy. He states that, though a child be born in an apoplectic or asphyxiated state, the circulation still continues through the umbilical vein, even though the umbilical arteries should have ceased to beat, and that premature section of the umbilical cord takes away one of the chief aids to its revival. *Part iv., p.* 135.

Treatment of Hemorrhage from the Navel of New-born Children.—Ordinary remedies are insufficient to arrest the bleeding. Kolophonian, alum, the various styptic fluids, turpentine, ice, amadou, compression, etc., have been employed in vain. Cauterization has been several times tried, both with the nitrate of silver and the actual cautery. In fact, the use of the ligature appears to be the only means worth dependence upon as capable of restraining the bleeding, and the mode of its application *en masse*, as advised by Dubois, is to be preferred. But in the best manuals and treatises we find no advice given as to the method of securing immediately the umbilical arteries, and, so far as we know, it has never been accomplished, from the many difficulties attendant upon its performance. It has, therefore, been proposed to secure all the three vessels together, by pulling the navel-knot forward, and passing around it a ligature with the help of hare-lip pins. At first sight this operation seems to have much in its favor, though experience does not confirm it. Nevertheless, up to the present time, it has been of most service.—ROGER, *in Journ. f. Kinderh.*

Part xxix., *p.* 311.

UMBILICUS.

Treatment of Urinary Discharge from the Umbilicus, in Infants.—B. Cooper says that, in infancy it is not uncommon for a urinary discharge to take place from the umbilicus, in consequence of the open state of the urachus; in such a case you should first ascertain that there is no obstruction to the passage of the urine through its natural canal, and if that should be the case, as frequently happens from congenital phymosis, the cause of the obstruction should be removed, and then, upon gentle pressure being applied to the umbilicus, the urachus generally closes, although there have been instances in which the defect was never remedied.

Part xviii., *p.* 203.

Hemorrhage from the Umbilicus after Separation of the Funis.—When a disposition to this hemorrhage is known or suspected, says Mr. Ray, apply collodion after the separation of the funis, and before the usual compress is applied; and examine the part every day. When the bleeding actually occurs, it is necessary to adopt mechanical means to check it *without the least delay.* For this purpose, first pinch up the umbilicus between the finger and thumb, in the manner recommended for leech-bites; and if this is successful, fill the depression of the umbilicus with cotton wool, and coat it over with collodion, or apply plaster of Paris mixed up with water. If these means do not control it, make an eschar with a probe, director, or skewer, heated to whiteness, and afterward coat with collodion. Lastly, if other means fail, tie the vessel, first introducing a fine probe into it, to act as a guide for the incision. Ligature is not recommended except as a last resource, because in these cases there seems to be a hemorrhagic diathesis, and, consequently, it is undesirable to make incisions.

Part xix., *p.* 256.

----•◦•----

URETHRA.

Inflammation of Mucous Membrane of Urethra—New Mode of Introducing the Catheter.—Dr. Patterson, of Rathkeale Infirmary, gives the following case: The patient labored under most distressing inflammation of the mucous membrane of the urethra, and his bladder was greatly distended with urine, which he could only pass in drops and in extreme agony; there was a most unbearable desire to empty the bladder, occasioned, in a great measure, it may be presumed, by that organ's partaking of the inflammatory action. The morbid sensibility of the urethra was such as that no instrument of any kind could be introduced, and the patient's impatience could not wait the abatement of the inflammation, under the employment of the most active means. In this case I attached an injecting apparatus to a curved elastic catheter, and, having inserted the extremity of the tube a little way within the orifice of the urethra, I, in the gentlest manner, injected, or rather insinuated a little warm decoction of linseed, just so as to moderately distend the urethra; I then gradually urged the catheter onward, and succeeded in getting it into the bladder, with little or no pain or inconvenience to the patient.

Part iii., *p.* 97.

Mechanical Injury of.—Obstructions of the urethra may arise from *mechanical injury* to various parts of the urethra, as, from the violent pressure of some circular body, as a ring round the penis, or a blow upon the urethra as it passes under the pubes where the mucous membrane is especially liable to suffer from such a cause. Sir B. Brodie gives the following directions with regard to the treatment:

"In all cases," he says, "in which there is reason to believe that the urethra has been divided or lacerated in consequence of an injury inflicted on the perinæum, it is the duty of the surgeon not only to look at the great and immediate danger, but to guard against future ill consequences; and much may be done at this period toward preventing a most serious inconvenience, which would be relieved with difficulty afterward. If there be a penetrating wound, in which the urethra is probably implicated, an elastic gum catheter should be introduced with the least possible delay, and allowed to remain in the urethra and bladder until the healing of the wound is far advanced, or, at all events, until it is ascertained that the urethra has not suffered; the catheter being, however, occasionally removed for a limited time, if it seems to act as a source of irritation.

In cases of contusion of the perinæum, when the effusion of blood in the perinæum and scrotum, and more especially the discharge of blood from the urethra, or any other circumstances, lead to the suspicion that the urethra has been lacerated, the same treatment should be had recourse to, the gum catheter should be introduced as soon as possible, and allowed to remain for at least some days after the occurrence of the accident. The extravasation of blood does not in itself justify the making an incision in the perinæum ; and indeed, according to my experience, there can be no worse practice than that of making an incision in a case of simple ecchymosis, either in this or in any other situation. But where such extravasation exists, there is always reason to apprehend that there may be further mischief; the progress of the case, therefore, should be carefully watched, and, on the first appearance of any symptoms which might be supposed to indicate that urine had escaped into the cellular membrane, or that suppuration had begun to take place, a staff should be introduced into the urethra instead of the gum catheter, and a free incision should be made from the perinæum into it, the gum catheter being replaced afterward.

But it may be that these measures of precaution have not been adopted in the first instance, and that you are not consulted until after the lapse of a considerable time, when the wound or laceration of the urethra is already healed, leaving the urethra contracted in the situation of the cicatrix. Here you may, perhaps, succeed in gradually dilating the urethra, as where there is an ordinary stricture. But in a case which I have already mentioned, I have stated that "this was not accomplished without a great deal of local and constitutional disturbance;" and so it has been in all cases of this kind which have fallen under my observation. Nor will the occurrence of such difficulties be a matter of surprise to any one who bears in mind that here the object is to dilate, not a genuine stricture, but a cicatrix, of the urethra, and who has not observed how the cicatrix of an old sore leg inflames and cracks when the subjacent muscles begin to increase in bulk from exercise, or how the endeavor to extend forcibly the contraction after an extensive burn produces the same result. It may be that these difficulties are insuperable under the method of treatment by simple dilatation ; and under these circumstances, a small staff having been introduced into the bladder, the cicatrix of the urethra should be divided by an incision from the perinæum, a gum catheter being introduced afterward, and allowed to remain until the wound is healed over it. But even then much remains to be accomplished. The cicatrix has still a greater disposition to contract than an ordinary stricture; the bougie or catheter must be had recourse to almost daily, and the patient must be contented if he can persevere in the use of instruments of a moderate diameter, as the urethra will invariably resent the attempt to keep it dilated by those of large dimensions."

The condition of the patient is improvable, where the injury of the urethra is limited. But where there has been actual loss of some portion of the canal, the patient must either be content to void the whole of his urine by the perinæum, or submit to an operation for establishing a communication between the anterior and posterior portions of the urethra. This operation is best explained by a case.

"A young man, in making a leap on horseback, received a violent blow on the perinæum from the pummel of the saddle. The immediate consequence of the injury was hemorrhage from the urethra, and this was followed by extravasation of urine and sloughing of the perinæum to a considerable extent. A catheter was at first introduced into the bladder, but it was afterward removed. The sloughs having separated, the sore in the perinæum gradually closed, a small fistulous opening only being left immediately behind the scrotum, through which the whole of the urine was discharged. He was in this state seven months after the occurrence of the accident, when he arrived in London, and Mr. Baker advised him to have my opinion on the case.

On introducing an instrument into the urethra, I found an obstruction of the canal immediately below the pubes. Several ineffectual attempts having been made to penetrate the obstruction in the usual manner by bougies and sounds of various sizes, I had recourse to the following operation: The patient having been placed in the same position as in lithotomy, a staff was introduced into the urethra, and held by Mr. Hilles, who, with Mr. Baker, assisted me in the operation, with the extremity of it resting against the obstruction. I then made an incision in the perinæum, extending backward from the part in which the staff was to be felt, in the direction of the prostate gland. It was now evident that not less than three-quarters of an inch of the urethra was deficient below the pubes, the place of it being occupied by a rigid cicatrix. This having been divided longitudinally by the point of the scalpel, I was enabled, though not without some difficulty, to pass the staff from the part at which the extremity of it rested, into the sound portion of the urethra toward the bladder, and then into the bladder itself. The staff was then withdrawn, and an elastic gum catheter having been substituted for it, the latter was allowed to remain in the urethra and bladder. On the ninth day after the operation, there being some degree of irritation at the neck of the bladder, the catheter was removed, being reintroduced, however after two days more. From this time it was removed at intervals, which were sometimes longer, sometimes shorter, according to circumstances. The wound in the perinæum gradually healed, and in less than ten weeks from the time of the operation was reduced to the diameter of a small pea. The patient was now able to introduce a silver catheter of the size of his urethra into the bladder without difficulty, and he repeated this operation so as to draw off his urine three or four times daily. When he voided his urine without the catheter, by placing the point of his finger on the opening in the perinæum, he was enabled to discharge the whole in a sufficient stream by the urethra. . *Part* vi., *p.* 101.

Importance of Discriminating Diseases of the Urethra.—(M. Civiale mentions two mistakes which are often made in the treatment of diseases of the urethra.) One consists in regarding as a poisonous discharge produced by gonorrhœa, that which is innocuous, and caused by irritation merely in the passage; such, for instance, as the presence of a stricture; the former being a virulent poison capable of reproducing *ad infinitum*, while the latter is perfectly harmless.

Want of due discrimination in this case not unfrequently inflicts an irreparable injury on the patient. For example; when a stricture, attended with a discharge from the passage, is observed soon after an attack of gonorrhœa, the patient naturally considers that he is suffering from the gonorrhœa, which had not been properly cured; and should the person who has the treatment of the case entertain the same opinion, the result will be that the patient will continue taking copaiba, cubebs, etc., off and on for months, perhaps years, to the great injury of his stomach and system in general, while the stricture all the time is gradually getting worse. There is a curious point in reference to the effect of copaiba on this kind of discharge, and it is this—the discharge is always relieved, but never removed by copaiba, unless in conjunction with the use of bougies. This fact again tends materially to perpetuate the erroneous treatment, as the inference at once suggests itself, that copaiba, etc., will cure this discharge if persevered in, inasmuch as it always exerts a marked influence on it. But however good the argument, the practice is bad, for it will never cure such a discharge. The practitioner very commonly remains in ignorance of his error, by reason of the patient becoming dissatisfied with his treatment, on feeling no permanent benefit from it, and therefore, soliciting the assistance of various others for the relief of what he and they regard as an incurable clap.

Occasionally, the discharge caused by the irritation of a stricture is attended with many of the symptoms of a regular gonorrhœa; but when it is generally known that it is so, there will be experienced but little difficulty in practice, in distinguishing these discharges, which differ so materially in their effects on the system.

The other mistake refers also to the presence of a stricture. It is the received opinion, being so laid down in all works on surgery, that the stream of urine through the urethra bears an exact ratio to its calibre. It would be so, were the urethra a dead body; but being endowed with vitality which is acted upon by muscles—whether in its substance or not is immaterial—the result is, that a person afflicted with a permanent stricture may pass his urine in a good stream, because when he feels a desire to evacuate, his urethra, obedient to his will, opens out, so to speak, at its strictured part, and discharges a larger-sized stream than would have passed through it, had it been an inanimate body.

In practice this consideration is of high importance, for if a person afflicted with a permanent stricture passes his water in a fair stream, a surgeon in this particular, misled by his teachers, will pronounce the case not to be stricture, to the great injury of his patient. Indeed, no error that can be made in surgery is attended with more serious results than this, because the case, from being misunderstood, gradually gets worse, in spite of all treatment, bougies not being introduced, until some exciting cause having supervened, irritation comes on in the passage; no urine whatever can be passed; and the patient's life will be in extreme danger, should he not then be efficiently treated.   *Part* xix., *p.* 185.

Vascular Tumors at the Orifice of the Urethra.—Mr. Norman, Surgeon to the Marylebone General Dispensary, directs to remove them by excision or by the ligature, the latter being preferable in consequence of the serious hemorrhage which sometimes attends excision: in either case apply a powerful caustic afterward to prevent the growth being reproduced. For very small tumors it will be sufficient to use the actual cautery, or caustics, such as potash, nitric acid, and pernitrate of mercury: nitrate of silver is less efficient and much more painful.   *Part* xx., *p.* 162.

Vascularity of the Lining Membrane of the Female Urethra.—Under the name of " Vascular Tumor of the Orifice of the Meatus Urinarius," says Dr. Gream, of Queen Charlotte's Lying-in-Hospital, this affection was first described by Sir Charles Clarke, in his valuable work on the " Diseases of Women."

I have ventured to refer to this affection under another name, because my own experience, confirmed by that of others, tends to show that it does not always appear as a tumor, but that it may be present under other forms, accompanied by the same general as well as local symptoms.

Dr. Ashwell has correctly described the disease, but he speaks of it more especially as a tumor, and states that it is rarely seen after the cessation of the menses. I am led to think that he is mistaken in this respect, for I have witnessed the disease as often in elderly women as in the young.

It may be present as a simple vascularity of the lining membrane of the urethra, without any elevation whatever, extending some little distance toward the bladder; the membrane itself being highly florid in color, and extremely tender when touched, or during the passage of the urine. This is the usual character of the disease, when it is confined within the canal; but Sir Charles Clarke relates the case of a patient in St. Bartbolomew's Hospital, in whose urethra there was a tumor of a scarlet color, nearly filling up the canal. The occurrence of a tumor, however, within the urethra is unusual.

The second form in which the disease appears, is that of a flattened vascular spot, with but slight elevation, surrounding the orifice of the urethra, highly florid in color, and exquisitely tender when touched; it is so little elevated that it can scarcely be called a tumor. The redness extends from it into the canal for some little distance, but the membrane within, although florid in appearance, is quite smooth on its surface; whereas the external spot of vascularity is slightly granulated, because it is not modified by pressure from the sides of the urethra.

In the third stage, the disease consists of a distinct tumor, granulated, and attached, sometimes by a broad base, sometimes by a narrow one, and, in some instances, even by a slender pedicle, to the side of the urethra, or just externally to it; and, in almost all cases, some dilated vessels will be seen extending from its base to within the urethral canal.

When there is an actual prominent tumor, the local pain and the constitutional symptoms are greatly increased in severity. In some cases, the peculiar scarlet color of the part has attracted the notice of the patient; but in many instances, particularly when the vascularity is within the urethra, not only has the actual seat of the disease escaped her observation, but it has also been overlooked by her medical attendant, who has referred to the uterus as the diseased organ, has stated that its cervix was inflamed or ulcerated, and caustic has sometimes for weeks, or months, been applied, without affording the least advantage to the patient.

This vascular disease is not at all to be considered as similar to an affection situated in the same parts, having its origin in a varicose state of the veins.

In the vascular disease in question, the blood contained in the vessels is arterial, while in the venous enlargement it is dark colored, and the distended veins have the same appearance which veins have in other parts of the body when in a varicose condition. Attention is first called to the vascular disease, by an uneasy sensation at the lower part of the body, and pain passing down the thighs; and pain when urine is voided, or when the part is touched; slight bleeding also occurs occasionally, owing to the rupture of some dilated vessel, whose covering is always much attenuated. There may be frequent desire to pass urine; and walking causes great suffering; while accompanying these symptoms, there is always copious mucous discharge, which is excessive when the disease appears in the form of a tumor. Owing to which, as well as to the constant uneasiness and frequent·acute suffering, the patient becomes emaciated and weak, and it is surprising to find so many and such severe symptoms arising from a disease whose extent is confined within such limited bounds ; but there is clear evidence that it does produce them in the fact that, immediately upon the destinc-tion of the vascular spot, or even on its partial removal, a comparative freedom from the symptoms is at once enjoyed.

The only mode of cure is the destruction of the entire congeries of vessels ; and if the smallest part of it is left, the disease will most certainly return.

Having several times been called upon to treat cases which had been before apparently cured (by myself and others) it occurred to me that the application of strong nitric acid, in the manner adopted by Mr. Henry Lee for the destruction of hemorrhoids (and which proves so successful,) would be equally applicable to the vascularity of the female urethra.

But there is a difficulty in exposing the part sufficiently, and in prevent-ing the sides of the vagina from collapsing too soon after the application of nitric acid; and this is overcome by the use of a speculum, invented, I believe, by Mr. Hilton, for the removal of hemorrhoidal excrescences. A portion of the side of the speculum, extending nearly to its internal extremity, can be removed after its introduction into the vagina, and if this part of it is just under the pubes, the spot of vascularity will project into the tube; but should only the lining membrane of the urethra be vascular, it will be readily exposed by pressing the speculum firmly toward the pubes against the surrounding part; and the acid can be applied while the pressure is kept up.

A small rod of glass, or a piece of hard wood in the form of the stick of a camel's hair pencil, is the best thing with which to apply the acid; and this should be held to the part for about a minute, care being taken that each enlarged portion of the vessels is completely destroyed, and in about three or four minutes the pain attending it ceases, and the speculum can be removed. It will be better to examine the part in about four days from the time of the application of the acid, and it often will be found healed with no trace of the complaint left. More frequently it presents an unhealed sore, but an absence of the disease. If, however, there be any vessel remaining having the peculiar scarlet color, it should be again touched with the nitric acid, otherwise the symptoms will rapidly return.

Part xxv., *p.* 297.

Impermeable Urethra.—In cases of complete obstruction from wounds, Prof. Syme would introduce an instrument like the common lithotomy staff, but grooved on the concave side, through the fistulous opening of the perinæum into the bladder, then pass the guide director employed for the division of strictures by external incision, down to the seat of obstruction, and thrust it through the opposing structures (in the course which it ought to take were the canal free) forward into the bladder ; the obstruction may then be divided in the same way as in the usual operation for stricture. It must be remembered that this is not the remedy for stricture, but for obliteration of the canal. *Part* xxxv., *p.* 125.

Dilatation of the Female Urethra.—There are various means of dilating the female urethra, as sponge-tents and metallic dilators ; but these cause

great pain, and, worst of all, are very liable to be followed by permanent incontinence. Weiss' dilator, though simple and easily applied, drags the urethra into a sort of triangle, the pressure falling entirely upon three points.
What is wanted is a uniform pressure, and one capable of dilating quickly,
as being less liable to be followed by incontinence. This desideratum is
supplied by *fluid pressure*. The apparatus, used by Mr. Wells, surgeon to
Samaritan hospital, is an elastic tube, having at one end a syringe and at the
other a female catheter, the latter having a piece of India-rubber tubing
closely fitting over it. The syringe must be furnished with a stop-cock.
The catheter being introduced, the India-rubber tubing may be gradually
distended with water by means of the syringe. The whole process will
not occupy more than ten minutes, and, besides, the other advantages
possessed by it, will not be accompanied by much pain.

Part xxxviii., *p.* 223.

Urethral Caruncles.—If these florid painful growths be removed by the
knife alone, even if the piece of mucous membrane upon which they are
seated be also removed, a permanent cure is seldom effected. The use of
caustics is not attended with better results. The actual cautery alone, says
Prof. Simpson, will destroy these growths effectually. An iron of proper size and shape, adequately heated, may be employed, or the requisite
degree of heat may be applied through the galvano-caustic wire. The
latter method is especially useful when the caruncles extend up the urethra
higher than the orifice, because you can introduce and apply the wire,
before heating it by the transmission of the galvanic current. Apply immediately afterward cold water and cloths soaked in it; and subsequently
treat the ulcerated surface, after the slough separates, with very frequent
applications of black wash, zink lotion, or other surgical applications.
Though this is the best mode of treating these growths, yet even this is not
absolutely a certain method of cure, as cases now and then occur in which
the growth will return in spite of all. Round the larger projecting tumor
a number of small painful red spots of mucous membrane generally exist,
and the removal of these is essential to the radical cure. The best local
application to relieve the irritation and pain is an ointment made up of two
drachms of the dilute hydrocyanic acid of the pharmacopœia to an ounce
of lard. A bit of this ointment, about the size of a pea, applied to the
part three or four times a day, often relieves the pain more effectually than
any quantity of opium administered internally, or than any other form
of local anodyne.

Part xl., *p.* 209.

———◦•◦———

URINE.

Retention of Urine—Case Relieved by the action of Cold.—The operation of cold as an excitor of the expulsor fibres of the bladder, has been
most interestingly illustrated by Dr. Currie, in his "Medical Reports."
"My friend, Dr. Ford, has mentioned to me the case of Mr. C——, of Bristol, who was instantly relieved of an obstinate stricture of the bladder,
of thirty hours duration (during all which time not a drop of water had
been passed), by placing his feet on a marble slab, and dashing cold water
over the thighs and legs. The effect was instantaneous; the urine burst
from him in a full stream, and the stricture was permanently removed.

The common remedies, particularly opium and bleeding, had been tried in vain." Facts of this kind have been noticed by several other observers.

Part viii., *p.* 47.

Urine as a means of Establishing the Diagnosis and Treatment of Diseases.—Dr. F. Simon gives the following valuable communication: Among the earlier investigators who paid attention to the urine, though very partially, I may mention Brandt, Kunkel, Boyle, and Bellini; Boerhaave, however, attempted an analysis of the urine, which, considering the time, was extremely good. Scheele's discovery of uric acid, and Cruikshanks' of urea, contributed essentially to a more correct knowledge of this secretion. The latter surgeon had already examined the urine in several diseases, especially in diabetes and dropsies. At the commencement of the present century it was chiefly Berzelius and Prout who made the urine the subject of extended inquiries; Berzelius demonstrated the existence of lactic acid, which, by the earlier chemists had been considered to be acetic acid; the analysis communicated by Berzelius, in 1809, of the composition of the urine, has been till within the last few years the only correct examination of the same; Prout has continued his inquiries up to the latest period. Of the more recent works on the constitution of the urine, those by Leeanu are the most prominent; within the last years, Becquerel, Lehmann, and Simon, have employed themselves with examinations of the urine in the healthy and morbid state. Several constituents of the urine, both in the state of health and disease, are very accurately known, as uric acid, urea, lactic acid, the salts and the sugar of the urine; of others, probably not less important, we have a very imperfect knowledge, as of extractive and coloring matters. Regarding the quantitative composition of the urine, which is rather changeable, numerous investigations have been made by the above-named chemists. Leeann also investigated the varieties which may be shown in healthy urine, according to age and sex.

The quantity of urine passed in the twenty-four hours, and its color, are frequently of importance. A diminished quantity of the urine passed in twenty-four hours, is under circumstances a sign particularly of acute diseases; an excessive increase of the urine, if permanent, is oftentimes indicative of serious diseases. A dark-colored, flaming, or fiery red urine commonly indicates an inflammatory affection; a dark brown red is generally observed in typhus. But the urine may also be colored blood-red or brown-red by bile-pigment, which is easily detected by its reaction with nitric acid; the latter constantly indicates an affection of the liver; a blood-red urine commonly contains blood; there is then for the most part found in it a sediment of blood-corpuscles, which are recognized with the microscope; but should a little blood be contained in the urine and this in a state of solution, it may be discovered by adding nitric acid, which occasions a precipitation of coagulated albumen colored red by hematine. This bloody urine indicates a bleeding in the kidneys, bladder, or, in the case of women, of the uterus. Blood flowing from the urethra comes in drops. If the blood is discharged in masses after clear urine, it comes from the bladder, and in that case it often stops up the passage from the bladder by coagulation; if the blood is distributed through the urine, partly dissolved, and not in very large quantity, it comes from the kidneys; if it be dark, and mixed with mucus and pus, it owes its origin to an ulcer. The presence of stone-colic shows that the blood has been poured out during the descent of a renal calculus.

Blue urine has been observed, though not frequently; in the majority of cases it probably owes its origin to the use of certain medicines; black urine has likewise been observed; the connection, however, is not yet known between the coloring matter and the morbid process; greenish urine indicates, according to Prout, an oxalic acid diathesis; sediments of oxalate of lime form, or mulberry calculi pass away; a urine, which is pale-colored, and has a bias to green, frequently indicates the presence of albumen, which is readily detected by heating to boiling or by nitric acid. In this case the urine is not perfectly clear, but slightly opalescent; its quantity may be increased, diminished, or natural. The oxalic acid diathesis of the urine indicates, according to Prout, functional disturbances in the chylo-poietic system; albuminuria ordinarily indicates dropsy and an affection of the kidneys. The reaction of the urine is important for the physician. Natural urine, it is well known, has an acid reaction; the quantity of free acids in the urine and the intensity of the reaction may increase to an extraordinary degree in diseases, more particularly in rheumatism, gout, in disturbances of the digestive organs, and in certain stages of typhus; to judge correctly of the intensity of the acid reaction, reference must be had to the quantity of the urine; the greater or less acid reaction is known by the effect of the urine on litmus paper of a weak blue color, which becomes colored so much the more rapidly and the more deeply reddened, the greater the acid contents of the urine are. Urine with a neutral reaction commonly forms the transition from the acid to the alkaline reaction, and *vice versa*. The alkaline reaction of the urine is of great importance to the physician; it commonly depends on carbonate of ammonia, the presence of which is recognized by the odor, and the white cloud, which a glass rod develops when moistened with an acid salt and brought near to it. The urine also may have an alkaline reaction through its containing carbonate of soda, which salt finds its way into the urine by the long-continued use of carbonate or bicarbonate of soda with vegetable acids. The urine, alkaline by carbonate of ammonia, is but seldom evacuated in this state from the bladder; during its discharge it is commonly neutral, and becomes alkaline only in a shorter or longer time after; badly-cleaned vessels may moreover contribute much to this, a circumstance which ought to be taken into account. Urine which already on voiding it has an ammoniacal reaction, and has also a very bad smell, indicates always a serious affection of the nervous system, and especially of the spinal cord. In certain unfavorable stages of tabes dorsalis, phthisis of the spinal cord, paralysis of the lower extremities and of the bladder, the voiding ammoniacal urine is ever an unfavorable sign; in other affections of the nervous system, also, as in typhus, ammoniacal urine is observed, which, however, assumes this reaction in the majority of cases not till after it has stood for some time. In typhus the reaction of the urine may be of importance for the prognosis when the urine, after it was observed to have an acid reaction through one, two, or three periods of seven days, is finally found to be neutral, and then to have an ammoniacal odor and reaction; when this reaction lasts for several days, probably during one entire period of seven days, and then again passes into the acid, this seems in most cases to indicate a favorable termination to the disease. The urine having an ammoniacal reaction in typhus has usually a dirty, turbid, yellow-brown or red-brown appearance, and forms sediments which disappear in a great measure on the addition of free acids; also in catarrhus vesicæ, or in phthisis vesicæ, the urine becomes ammoniacal in a very short time after being voided ; the large quantity of vesical mucus or pus indicates this affection ; finally, the formation of urinary concretions, consisting of earthy phosphates, is in part occasioned by the neutral or alkaline reaction of the urine ; the urine voided in this urinary affection, is not so dark as the urine in typhus, and commonly forms sediments of phosphate of lime, and of ammonio-magnesian phosphate. If the vesical calculus exercise an irritating influence on the parietes of the bladder, a great quantity of vesical mucus is commonly mixed with the urine.

The specific gravity of the urine, though by itself it possesses no great diagnostic value, as it depends on the variable quantity of water in the urine, may, however, claim the attention of the physician under certain circumstances ; the clearer and the more like water the urine appears, the less is its specific gravity ; the deeper and darker-colored, the higher the specific gravity. This general law may admit of an exception in one case, namely, in diabetes mellitus.; in this disease a urine is voided either normal or pale, seldom deeply-colored, the high specific gravity of which (1020–1060) is in contradiction to the color ; this high specific gravity imperatively requires a more strict examination of the urine. More than all other signs, the correct examination of the sediments is of importance to the physician. Healthy urine forms only after long standing a light, sinking cloud of vesical mucus ; every other separation in the urine is of a pathological nature. The urinary sediment consists either of organic formations, as mucous corpuscles, purulent corpuscles, blood, etc., or of heavy, insoluble salts or acids, or lastly, of an admixture of both ; the microscope will throw light on this.

The sediment consists of organic formations. If the urine has not a blood-red color, the sediment is white, grey, dirty-yellow, and with the microscope can be seen mucus, or pus-corpuscles ; here the sediment is constantly mucus, if the urine contain no albumen ; it is probably pus, if the sediment is deposited rapidly after the urine is voided, and the urine contains albumen. It is not necessary now to state of what importance it is to discover and appreciate mucus and pus in the urine ; in catarrhus vesicæ the mucous sediment frequently assumes a very glutinous quality ; this, however, happens only when the urine begins to become ammoniacal, which, in urine containing mucus, often occurs in a very short time, as we have already mentioned ; the same may be said of pus, and it is good in this case to test the presence of albumen not by boiling heat, but by nitric acid. If the sediment is blood, the blood-corpuscles are then seen with the microscope ; the urine standing over this is also of a blood-red color. Of the import of blood in the urine I have no remark to make. If the urine contain albumen, and there exist at the bottom a mucous sediment, it is of great importance to examine this with the microscope. We may find therein, as I have observed, peculiar long prominences, partly filled, partly transparent, and round spheres, twice or thrice as large as mucus corpuscles, filled with dark, granular contents, which beyond a doubt have their origin in the kidneys, and denote a morbid state of this organ. These peculiar forms I have frequently, and at different times, found in the urine of a person laboring under morbus Brightii.

The sediments which are not of an organic nature, may in like manner be easily recognized with the microscope and some few reagents ; they are either crystalline or amorphous, present themselves either in acid, neutral or alkaline urine, and are readily distinguished ; in acid urine sediments of uric acid present themselves, urate of ammonia, urate of soda, oxalate of lime, cystin. The greatest number of sediments which present themselves in acid urine consist of urate of ammonia ; less frequent are those consisting of uric acid, still rarer are those consisting of oxalate of lime, and the most uncommon of all are those consisting of cystin. Sediments consisting of earthy phosphates do not occur in urine having a strong acid reaction. Every sediment occurring in acid urine from yellow to brown, from red to purple-red, appearing under the microscope as an amorphous precipitate, or as large and small globules aggregated together, which is dissolved entirely or almost entirely on warming the urine, is urate of ammonia ; to this belong accordingly all the so-called critical separations in the urine ; the species of separation of the urate of ammonia is very various, and it appears sometimes as mere turbidness, without forming any sediment whatever, sometimes it lies at the bottom of the vessel as colored mucus or pus, at other times heavy, like an earthy precipitate. In the case of those diseases, which in the course of their development admit a termination by a critical separation in the urine, the kind of separation is of importance. The heavier the sediment lies at the bottom, and the clearer the urine is that stands over it, the more decided is the crisis allowed to be ; whilst the lighter the sediment floats, and the less disposition there is to a perfect deposition, the more imperfect is Nature's effort to break down the disease by a crisis. The various colorings of the sediment are characteristic of some diseases ; in acute rheumatism of the joints, in intermittent fevers, the critical sediment is observed to be colored red up to a brown red ; in acute diseases of the liver the sediment is rose-red ; in typhus it has a dirty-red color ; in some diseases the appearance of the sediment appears to be of no constant critical import, as, for example, in typhus.

A sediment in the acid urine, which is not dissolved on heating the urine, and which appears crystalline when observed either by the unarmed eye, or with the microscope, and is colored yellow up to vermilion-red, is uric acid. It ordinarily appears in the form of rhombic plates, and in the majority of cases mixed with urates of ammonia, where it then forms the undermost and dark-colored layer of the sediment. That the deposit of uric acid is of critical import, is scarcely to be doubted ; in gout and in cases of renal calculi, where the deposits consist of uric acid, uric acid or the discharge of gravel form the most perfect crisis ; in many other diseases we still want the necessary observations concerning the critical value of uric acid secretions. The sediment of oxalate of lime presents itself more rarely than those before mentioned ; it usually forms a white precipitate ; observed with the microscope, it appears in the form of small octahedra, or of little spheres arranged one by the other ; it is not soluble in acetic acid, but readily in hydrochloric acid ; when sulphuric acid is poured on it, it disappears, and after some time long lancet-formed plates of sulphate of lime are seen.

Respecting the diagnostic value of the oxalate of lime in the sediment, sufficient observations are still wanting ; it is probable that it is connected with serious disturbances in the chylopoietic system ; that we should be attentive to the possible formation of stone of oxalate of lime, where the sediment shows itself frequently and permanently in the urine, is of importance ; however, the physician, in order to judge of the phenomena more correctly, must also have reference to the diet, as oxalic acid may be conveyed into the body by various sorts of food.

The occurrence of cystin in the urinary sediment is very rare. It is easily recognized by its remarkable form; it forms faint yellow-colored hexahedral plates. According to Prout, the appearance of cystin in the urine is a very unfavorable sign, it indicates the formation of cystin calculi. In neutral urine, or that with an alkaline reaction, besides the sediments already mentioned, precipitates of earthy phosphates present themselves; they are readily known by this; that they disappear on acidifying the urine with acetic acid or acid salts; the phosphate of magnesia, commonly combined with ammonia, is distinguished by its crystalline form; it appears in colorless prisms obliquely tinctured, very frequently in the form of a roof; the calcareous phosphate appears almost always as an amorphous precipitate; as the earthy phosphates are constantly present in the normal urine, their precipitation is commonly to be looked on as a consequence of the formation of ammonia, the free acids by which the earthy phosphates were previously dissolved being neutralized by this alkali; in some cases, on the contrary, the appearance of earthy phosphates in the sediment is of diagnostic value. In affections of the spinal cord the phosphate of magnesia, more especially, appears to be secreted in great quantity; in affections of the mucous membrane of the bladder, the phosphate of lime appears in large quantity; in three cases of inflammations of the respiratory organs, at the time when resolution of the disease set in, I have seen the previously acid urine become neutral, and have observed, as a precipitate, the secretion of a considerable quantity of already formed crystals of ammonio-magnesian phosphate, perceptible to the naked eye, at the same time that in two of these cases the clear urine held so large a quantity of urate of ammonia in solution, that precipitates of uric acid were instantly produced by every acid. When calculi of the bladder are present, which consist of earthy phosphates, the urine frequently contains sediments of earthy phosphates, with which a greater or smaller quantity of mucus is mixed. In scarlatina the urine is observed to be turbid at the time of the desquamation, often also before the occurrence of the same on the outer cuticle; when it is observed with the microscope, an extraordinarily great quantity of the epithelium of the vesical mucous membrane is seen in it. It is, therefore, to be admitted, that the desquamation goes on also on the mucous membrane of the bladder; and if, as frequently appears to be the case, the scaling off takes place earlier on the mucous membrane of the bladder than on the external skin, one may determine the commencement of the scaling off by examining the urine.

The knowledge of the chemical composition of the urine is of very great value for diagnosis and prognosis; especially as far as concerns the presence of matters which are not found in the normal state of the urine; albumen is readily discovered in the urine by heat or by the addition of nitric acid; if the urine is acid, heat is preferred; if alkaline, nitric acid. The presence of albumen in the urine is always of great import, and the correct estimation of the same as a means of diagnosis not altogether easy; cases are known in which albumen was observed in the urine of healthy individuals, or set in in consequence of disturbance occurring in the digestive organs; in the great majority of cases, albuminuria is the attendant of dropsical phenomena, or the forerunner of them, the urine is then commonly clear, evinces a tendency to green, and contains much albumen; but there are cases of dropsy known, which set in altogether without albuminuria. That the presence of albumen in the urine does not infer the presence of Bright's degeneration of the kidneys, has been sufficiently proved; where degeneration of these organs is suspected, great attention must be directed to the mucous sediment of the urine. In violent inflammations, as well as in typhus, small quantities of albumen are sometimes found in the urine; the urine is then generally very dark, and has an acid reaction ; according to Becquerel, this appearance of albumen in cases of inflammation appears to be connected with a congested state of the kidney, and as this, unless the disease is itself an inflammation of the kidneys, seems to occur only in very violent and intense inflammations, the appearance of albumen in the urine accompanying inflammation might be a sign of the intensity of the inflammation. In consequence of inflammatory exanthems, especially in the desquamatory stage of scarlatina, albumen sometimes is observed to exist in the dark-colored urine, and sometimes, though more seldom, blood. It is, therefore, a matter of importance for the physician carefully to examine the case, as this heterogeneous mixture is not unfrequently the forerunner of dropsy; however, dropsy has been observed after scarlatina without albumen in the urine, and albumen in the urine without dropsy following thereon. At the commencement of diabetes mellitus, albuminuria is no rare phenomenon, and of great importance to the physician. The occurrence of albumen in this case is not constant, but alternating, it appears, before a trace of sugar can be observed, and when the sugar begins to form, it sometimes ceases again, and passing off, it gives way to the albuminuria.

To demonstrate the presence of sugar in the urine is the principal means of satisfying oneself of the existence of diabetes mellitus. If the quantity of sugar is considerable, it is easily discovered in the alcoholic extract of the urine after evaporation; if only traces of sugar are present, the sulphate of copper is used to demonstrate its presence, as we shall see at another time. Gall pigment in the urine is constantly a sign of the liver being affected; we have already stated that this can be discovered by the addition of nitric acid ; but to infer the presence of gall pigment from the color of the urine is sometimes fallacious.　　　*Part* viii., *p.* 49.

Changes produced in Urine by Disease.—Dr. Shearman gives the following :

Excessive indulgence in animal food, with too little bodily exercise, dyspepsia, and want of perspiration, are always attended by increase in the quantity of uric acid and urates. Uric acid is frequently produced in great quantity in the bladder, by the hydrochloric acid formed in the stomach from disease of that organ ; which, being absorbed into the blood, and secreted by the kidneys, forms hydrochlorate of ammonia, and deposits the uric acid. In fever, and in all diseases accompanied by rapid emaciation, the urine is of a high specific gravity, a dark brown-red color from excess of urea, uric acid, urate of ammonia, and sometimes blood and purpurine. The lateritious sediment, is urate of ammonia. And in extreme cases of acute rheumatism and hypertrophy of the heart, very large quantities of uric acid and urate of ammonia are commonly found. In all acute diseases attended by great emaciation, inflammation, or disorganization, with unhealthy digestive organs, as long as the kidneys remain healthy, uric acid is secreted in abundance ; but if the kidneys become diseased, as in morbus Brightii, diabetes, etc., then the secretion from the kidneys is perverted ; part of the nitrogen remaining in the circulation, and the carbon, hydrogen, and oxygen, assuming the forms of albumen, sugar, hippuric and oxalic acids, etc. In diabetes mellitus, when starch, sugar, etc., do not undergo the changes required to be converted into carbon or fat the starch is converted into grape-sugar by oxygen, and the sugar is excreted by the kidneys. In gout and rheumatism, urate of soda is found both in the urine and deposited in the joints and sheaths of the tendons. When pressure on the renal veins exists to such an extent as to prevent the return of blood to the cavæ, as from a tumor, pregnancy, or diseased viscera, the elements of the blood are often poured out by the kidneys ; and on examination, we find albumen, blood-discs, and the coloring matter of the blood (hematosine). And in granular diseases of the kidneys, and anasarca after acute disease of the skin—as scarlatina and extensive burns—albumen in large quantities is detected, but when the kidneys and skin regain their natural functions, uric acid and urea are again secreted in the place of albumen. In all diseases of an anæmic or chlorotic nature, attended by languid circulation and extreme debility, independent of acute disease, deficiency of urea and uric acid is found, and no deposit takes place unless there is a very small secretion of urine. In hysteria there is a large flow of limpid urine, of low specific gravity, and of a green color. In chlorosis, the urine is also of a low specific gravity, and green ; and this green color is owing to the mixture of cystine with hemaphacin. When the functions of the skin are impaired only, an excess of urea and urate of ammonia is always the result ; and if, in this case, profuse perspiration occurs, the fluid goes off by that process instead of the kidneys, the specific gravity of the urine becomes increased, and deposits frequently take place in the bladder in consequence, forming calculi, owing to deficiency of fluid ; but, if the skin is imperspirative, then the kidneys carry off the extra quantity of water, and the urine becomes lighter ; but the animal acid (lactic or butyric), which ought to go off by the skin, is secreted by the kidneys, and combining with the ammonia or soda of the urates, produces uric acid. When the functions of the liver are deranged, carbon is eliminated with hydrogen and cholesterine from the kidneys, which gives the peculiar color to the urine in all cases of jaundice. In organic mischief in the liver and spleen, or great congestion of the vena portæ, the urine is very red, purple, or copper-colored, owing to purpurine and urate of ammonia ; but when bile is circulating in the system from disease of the gall-ducts, etc., the urine is very brown, and easily shows the bile by the proper tests. In contracted, hobnail, or cirrhosed liver, the extent of the disease may generally be measured by the quantity of purpurine in the urine ; and usually in ascites from diseased liver we find purpurine ; but in ascites from peritoneal disease we find none. The purpurine appears to proceed from the altered condition in the portal circulation. When the liver and lungs are both so diseased as to prevent the proper quantity of carbon being carried off by their functions, hippuric acid is sure to be found in the urine.

In cases where organic mischief exists in the kidneys, the urine is frequently semi-solid when cold, and of a dark color, like a mass of black currant jelly. And when hemorrhage from some part of the urinary organs takes place, the urine is red, and shows quantities of blood-discs under the microscope. In fungus hematodes of the kidney, the urine looks like infusion of roses while warm, and like red currant jelly when cold, taking the form of the vessel. During the progress of pneumonia, less carbon will be eliminated from the lungs, and therefore more will be in the urine and

liver; consequently hippuric acid is often found. And in confined situations, where animals are obliged to breathe impure air, the globules of the
blood are not sufficiently supplied with oxygen, carbon cannot be con.
verted into carbonic acid in the lungs, and life could not go on unless the
kidneys secreted more nitrogen and carbon in the forms of urate of ammo.
nia and hippuric acid. In hepatitis, the carbon is not converted into bile ;
and, as long as the other secretions are going on properly, the carbon which
ought to form the bile is converted into fat and oil, and is found in the
blood and urine. We often meet with melancholy, highly nervous, emaciated
patients, simulating diabetes mellitus, but even more depressed in spiiits,
who merely complain of great debility and exhaustion, with some little
pain in the back or loins, for which we find it very difficult to prescribe
effectually. Dr. G. Bird has clearly shown that most of these cases are
owing to imperfect assimilation in digestion, converting the urea of the
nitrogenous part of the food into that state which is secreted by the kid.
neys as oxalic acid and ammonia instead of sugar, which, combining with
the lime of the phosphates, produces the oxalate of lime diathesis; and it
is to the derangement of the stomach, duodenum, and liver, that we must
look for success in the treatment of these cases.

Alkaline Urine.—When, from any cause, as the consequence of wear
and tear in old age, excess of study, or great excitement of the brain, an
injury to the spine, or stone in the bladder, the kidneys or bladder are
deprived of their natural supply of nervous power, the elements of urea
combine with the elements of water, and are converted into carbonate of
ammonia, which, by irritating the mucous membrane, and neutralizing the
solvent phosphoric acid, throws down the triple phosphates, and phosphate
and carbonate of lime, and renders ·the urine alkaline. Thus we find in
almost all cases of long-continued calculi in the bladder—let the calculus be
composed of what it may—that the urine is strongly alkaline, ammoniacal,
and deposits phosphate of lime, which sticks to the bottom of the vessel
like birdlime. The fusible calculus is composed of ammonio-phosphate of
magnesia and phosphate of lime. In persons who are confined to very
sedentary habits, with great mental exertion, for a length of time, and then
obliged to use violent muscular exercise for a few days, as clergymen with
small livings, lawyers, and schoolmasters, alkaline urine, with abundance
of earthy phosphates, is usually the consequence; and this unnatural secretion brings on a degree of debility not easily accounted for in any other
manner. In irritative dyspepsia in gouty habits, the urine often contains
the phosphates in abundance ; and whenever the triple phosphates, with
alkaline urine, are deposited for a length of time together, both in the
night and morning urine, accompanied by emaciation, there will always be
found organic disease, either in the digestive organs, kidneys, or bladder,
if not in the spine. Dr. Golding Bird gives the following rule respecting
the phosphates, which will be found very useful in practice : That where
the presence of phosphates is only found in the evening urine, organic disease is rarely the cause of it; but where they are found equally in the morning and evening urine, you may be sure organic disease exists. In bad cases
of typhus fever, the urine is frequently ammoniacal toward the close of
the disease, the nervous system of the kidneys being too depressed to
secrete urea, and its elements being converted into carbonate of ammonia,
just as they would be in common chemical decomposition out of the body.
During retention of urine fron diseased prostate gland, stricture of the

urethra, or where a catheter is obliged to be worn, the urine is always alkaline, owing to irritation in the mucous membrane.

It is easy, after a few trials, to discover, in a few minutes, the contents of almost any ordinary specimen of urine; and, without this knowledge, it is quite impossible to become acquainted with the changes which are constantly occurring in the urinary organs. For instance, you are called to a patient complaining of excruciating and deep-seated pain in the abdomen, shooting down the thigh, which resists the usual soothing mode of treatment. Examine the urine, and you may there find blood, pus, oxalate of lime, uric acid, or phosphates. This at once explains the nature of the malady, and you can confidently tell your patient that he has a small calculus of a certain description in the ureter, and your treatment is no longer empirical. Or you may be consulted by a person with various anomalous symptoms of a cachectic nature, which you would find it impossible to give a name to unless you examine the urine chemically, when you discover either albumen, sugar, or oxalate of lime excreted; and this at once explains the case. A patient consults you, much reduced in strength, depressed in spirits, and emaciated, his appetite being good, and digestive organs healthy, as far as you can discover, there being no evident cause for such a state. Take the specific gravity and quantity of the urine. If it is high, without deposit, and the quantity not great, add nitric acid to it in a watch-glass, and you will most likely discover a large quantity of urea, sufficient at once to account for the symptoms; or if the quantity of urine be large, you may discover sugar. During the course of febrile and inflammatory diseases, urate of ammonia is generally deposited. But if the symptoms increase, instead of diminish, under this deposit, examine it, and perhaps you may find the deposit to consist of phosphates and purpurine, and the urine alkaline. This will at once warn you to be watchful of your patient, and cautious in your prognosis. Suppose you have a surgical operation to perform on a patient apparently out of health, but with no decided disease. If, on examining the urine, you find albumen, oxalate of lime; or the ammonio-phosphates of magnesia in abundance, you may feel assured the person is in an unfit state to bear any operation; and by waiting, and attending to his general health, you will feel more confidence in the successful event of such an operation. *Part* xii., *p.* 96.

Test for Sugar in Urine.—Lowig recommends the following: Evaporate the urine to the consistency of sirup; treat with alcohol; then to the solution add an alcoholic solution of potash; if sugar be present, a white precipitate is formed, consisting of a compound of sugar and potash; wash this with alcohol, and dissolve in water; thus a saccharine solution is formed, which may be examined in any way, and if required, the amount of sugar determined quantitatively. *Part* xii., *p.* 117.

Alkaline Urine.—Use strychnia when the affection follows injury or lesion of the spine, as recommended by Dr. Golding Bird.
Part xiv., *p.* 97.

Influence of the Rhubarb Plant in producing Oxalate of Lime in Urine.—[The oxalate of lime in urine, can only be considered diagnostic of disease, when the oxalic acid is known to have been generated within the economy, and not introduced from without, for, says Liebig, the analysis of urine, when made without respect to the inorganic salts, acids, and bases of the aliment, teaches nothing. Are there any kinds of food which may be the means of impregnating the urine with oxalate of lime? Dr. Wilson says:]

The young stalks of the rhubarb plant, which of late years have come into such general use in this country for tarts in the spring, and sorrel, of which our neighbors, the French, consume a good deal in salads, and in other ways, both contain oxalic acid; and hard water contains lime. Dyspeptic persons who drink such water, and eat such articles of food, and are thus daily introducing, without suspecting it, the constituent ingredients of the mulberry calculus, are very likely indeed to incur the pain and the exceeding peril of a renal concretion of that kind. You must see, therefore, the great importance of detecting the oxalic diathesis, and of forbidding, to those who have it, all such viands as contain the oxalic acid, and of recommending them to use pure water, even distilled water for drinking. *Part* xiv. *p.* 108.

To Render the Urine acid.—Dr. Bird states, that, the benzoic is the only acid, the exhibition of which will render the urine acid.

Part xv., *p.* 143.

Alkaline Urine.—Wash the bladder out every day or two with warm water; the urine is rendered alkaline by retention of a few drops in the bladder. But Dr. Snow considers it important to distinguish those cases in which the urine is *secreted* alkaline. *Part* xv., *p.* 144.

Incontinence of Urine in Children.—[In the incontinence of urine occurring during sleep, in children, and unconnected with organic disease, Dr. Chambers advises the following treatment.]

Let the patient abstain from drinks for three hours before bed-time; empty the bladder on going to bed, and awaken in three hours to make water again. Blister the sacrum occasionally, to prevent sleeping on the back, and to stimulate the bladder; use cold shower bath or douche, and give ten drops each of tinct. cantharid. and tinc. ferri mur. thrice a day. Sometimes cauterize the orifice of the urethra, that the passage of urine may excite pain. *Part* xv., *p.* 145.

Incontinence of Urine in Young Persons.—M. Gerdy advises to give strychnine, gr. ¼ to gr. ½ daily, and small enemata of quinæ sulph.; or give ext. belladon. gr. iij. daily. Continue the remedies for some time after it is apparently cured.

When the urine is catarrhal, inject into the bladder a solution of nitrate of silver; give ergot of rye and camphor, aa. gr. x. daily, and rub the perineum and pelvis with camphor ointment. Or give strychnine or quinine, or four grains of cantharides powder daily. *Part* xv., *p.* 146.

Benzoic Acid in Incontinence of Urine.—Dr. Fraene recommends giving six grains, night and morning, increasing the dose to twelve grains. He succeeded in curing a case with this after three weeks of unavailing treatment with other means. *Part* xv., *p.* 146.

Retention of Urine from Spasmodic Stricture.—Dr. Lanyon recommends tinc. secale cornutum; half a drachm infused in three ounces of boiling water, and strained when cold; one ounce to be given every six hours; or two scruples of ergot of rye may be given twice a day, an hour or two before the bladder is distended. *Part* xv. *p.* 147.

Retention of Urine treated by Galvanism.—Mr. Donovan gives the case of a lady who, after delivery, could not evacuate her bladder. The catheter had to be used thrice a day, and Drs. Radford and Goodwin employed all the usual remedies for a fortnight, when it was decided to try galvanism; the first application was successful. *Part* xv., *p.* 234.

Dry Cupping in Retention of Urine.—M. Vandenbroeck, principal physician at Mons, informs the Society of Medicine at Anvers, that for more than twenty years he has replaced the use of the catheter in both sexes by the application of large cupping glasses to the superior and internal part of the thigh. In nine cases out of every twelve, the emission of urine, he says, was made at the end of some seconds. He does not assert that this has any effect in mechanical retention of urine. *Part* xvii., *p.* 181.

Ergot of Rye in Retention of.—In retention of urine from paralysis of the bladder, cerebral or otherwise, Dr. Allier, of Marcigny, recommends small and repeated doses of ergot, up to seventy-five grains a day, to be continued in decreasing doses, for eight or ten days after the cure.
Part xviii., *p.* 143.

Suppression of Urine.—Dr. J. C. Hall advises to give a drop of croton oil, with a full dose of calomel and colocynth; follow this by a draught containing sulphate of magnesia, cream of tartar, and infusion of senna; and then give a large stimulating clyster; so that the bowels may be freely purged. Then cup over the loins, or bleed, if the state of the pulse admits; and give warm baths. Afterward apply a blister to the loins, and give full doses of powdered cantharides,—a remedy, which, however inapplicable theoretically, has been followed by the best results.
Part xx., *p.* 100.

Uric Acid Diathesis.—Mr. B. B. Cooper would order low diet and vegetable food; employ the warm bath, and give carbonate of soda or potash, or liquor potassæ, taking care not to give them till three or four hours after a meal, otherwise they may interfere with digestion. Some vegetable acids may be given, but everything liable to generate acid in the stomach must be scrupulously avoided. *Part* xx., *p.* 149.

Use of Test Paper.—H. Bence Jones believes that the reaction of test paper on urine made at any one hour of the day should never determine the use of acid or alkaline medicines. The different deposits which take place in the urine are far better tests of the state of the urine, and of the necessity for these remedies. If you are guided by the reaction of test paper, the total quantity of urine made in twenty-four hours must be examined. *Part* xxi., *p.* 161.

Relation of the Specific Gravity of the Urine to its Solid Contents.—
Tables have been constructed professing to tell how much solid matter is contained in urine of any specific gravity. It is said, that by taking the specific gravity and referring to the table, the quantity of solid matter may be immediately determined.

From experiments, Dr. H. B. Jones has come to the conclusion that the quantity of solid contents cannot be determined by taking the specific gravity. *Part* xxi., *p.* 162.

Detection of Oxalate of Lime in the Urine.—Dr. H. B. Jones says: Oxalate of lime is so frequently found in the urine of those who are in a good state of health, that I do not consider it as indicating any disease, but only a disorder of no serious importance. It scarcely indicates a more serious derangement of the general health than a deposit of urate of ammonia does. It may occasionally be found in the urine of all who lead sedentary lives, taking insufficient air and exercise, and more food than is requisite for the daily wants of the system. I have found it in the urine of those who are free from every complaint. Even in the urine of healthy children it may very frequently be seen. I have met with it in every kind and stage of disease. In the fracture wards of St. George's Hospital, I have very frequently found it. The most severe case I ever saw, was an artist, aged thirty, dying of an abdominal aneurism. In cases of indigestion, especially where flatulence occurs; in cases where no indigestion ever was felt; in skin diseases; in cases where the skin never was affected; in cases of acute rheumatism, of acute gout, of fever; in sciatica in a gentleman, seventy-four years old, with spermatorrhœa; and in the diseases of women and children, octohedral crystals occur. So frequently is oxalate of lime mixed with urate of ammonia in sediments and calculi, that I have returned to the conclusion which Dr. Prout originally published in the second edition of his work. After giving some details of twelve cases of oxalic calculus, he says, "We are authorized to draw the following conclusions: 6th. That from the dissection of calculi formerly mentioned, it appears that the oxalate of lime diathesis is preceded and followed by the lithic acid diathesis—a circumstance which seems to be peculiar to these two forms of deposit, and when taken in conjunction with the other circumstances already related, appears to show that they are of the same general nature, or, in other words, that the oxalic acid merely takes the place, as it were, of the lithic acid, and by combining with the lime naturally existing in the urine, forms the concretion in question. 7th. (Dr Prout continues:) The diathesis being of a similar nature, the principles of treatment adapted for counteracting the original tendency to it must be also similar." And, as a medicine, muriatic acid was used to change the diathesis from the oxalate of lime to the lithic acid.

I find that the two deposits together may be met with daily on careful examination, by the microscope, of the urine in different cases of disease; Thus at one hour we may find oxalate of lime alone; at another, oxalate of lime with urate of ammonia; and at a third examination, oxalate of lime and phosphate of lime, or phosphate of lime only; the variations in the acidity of the urine being the chief cause of the difference in the deposit.

It requires no skill and no preparation of the urine to find the oxalate of lime. The urine should be left to stand for twenty-four hours in a bottle, or tall glass; the upper part of the fluid should be poured off, and the last few drops remaining in the glass or bottle should be examined. A magnifying power of 320 times is generally sufficient, but the crystals are sometimes so small, that twice this power is necessary to determine the form. Generally oxalate of lime octahedra are thus found without the least difficulty, sometimes in large single crystals, very frequently in aggregations of small octahedra, forming microscopic calculi. Dr. Golding Bird was the first observer who stated that these crystals, which had for some time previously been observed in urine, were oxalate of lime. The chemical proof is difficult, if not impossible, to obtain, for the octahedral crystals are rarely present in sufficient quantity to admit of perfect examination.

Part xxi., *p.* 163.

ı *Test for Sugar in Liquids.*—Chlorine, M. E. Maumené, (of Rheims,) observes, contrary to the assertion of Liebig, acts on sugar at a temperature of 212° Fah., and even in the cold, after a long period. A brown substance, partly soluble in water, is produced by its dehydrating power. The chlorides *e. g.* chloride of tin, bichloride of mercury, chloride of antimony, by their affinity for water, possess this property in a still greater degree.

A strip of any kind of tissue that is not acted upon by chloride of tin— *e. g.* white merino—is to be saturated with a strong solution of this salt, and then dried. Thus prepared, the tissue forms a convenient test of the presence of sugar in any liquid. A few drops of a very dilute saccharine fluid placed on the merino, and exposed to a temperature of from 260° to 300° Fah., will immediately produce a dark brown or black spot.

By the help of this test the presence of sugar in the urine can be readily detected. Ten drops of diabetic urine, the author stated, diffused in half a pint of water, would in this way yield a brownish black spot. Ordinary urine, urea, and uric acid, produce no results of this kind.

Part xxi., *p.* 168.

Incontinence of Urine in Children.—Examine the urine; and if, as will usually be found, it contains lithic acid, Mr. Simon recommends the following treatment: Give hydr. c. creta, or some mercurial, till the tongue is clean, and the intestinal secretions are healthy (for they will generally be found disordered). Then give a little quinine twice a day, before breakfast and before dinner; and give daily, a single large dose of bicarbonate of potash in copious solution, five hours after dinner. Let the quantity and quality of the diet be also carefully regulated. If these measures are adopted, blistering, etc., will seldom be called for. *Part* xxi., *p.* 242.

Retention of Urine.—When the bladder cannot be evacuated by the catheter, after leeching, aperients, warm baths, and opium, are we to puncture the urethra behind the strictured portion (Sir A. Cooper,)—or make a free opening in the perineum over the strictured part (Liston,)— or perforate the bladder through the rectum? Mr. Gay, of the Royal Free Hospital, advocates the latter, and states that he has never met with one unfavorable result from the practice. *Part* xxii., *p.* 232.

Retention of.—Mr. Tatum, of St. George's Hospital, reports a case in which retention of urine had taken place from stricture. All means of passing the catheter both before and after the warm bath, and after the most patient and cautious manipulation in trying to accomplish this object had failed, and it was only after a large dose of laudanum had been twice given, and the warm bath repeated with a soothing enema, that the catheter could be introduced. The symptoms again coming on after some time, the same means were again repeated, but it was not before a purgative draught had been given, eight leeches applied to the perineum, and the opium and warm bath again resorted to, that the stricture yielded so as to allow the instrument to be passed, and the bladder to be emptied.

Part xxii., *p.* 234.

Hints in Treating Urinary Affections.—[Dr. Bird concludes his work on the above subject by the three following rules.]

1. Whenever it is desirable to impregnate the urine with a salt, or to excite diuresis by a saline combination, it must be exhibited in solution, so

diluted as to contain less than 5 per cent. of the remedy, or not more than 25 grains in an ordinary draught. The absorption of the drug into the capillaries will be insured by a copious draught of water, or any diluent, immediately after each dose.

2. When the urine contains purpurine, or presents other evidence of portal obstruction, the diuretics or other remedies employed should be preceded or accompanied by the administration of mild mercurials—taraxicum, hydrochlorate of ammonia, or other cholitic remedies. By these means, or by local depletion, especially by leeches to the anus, the portal vessels will be unloaded, and a free passage obtained to the general circulation.

3. In cases of valvular disease, or other obstructions existing in the heart and large vessels, it is next to useless to endeavor to excite diuretic action, or appeal to the kidneys by remedies intended to be excreted by them. The best diuretic will, in such cases, be found in whatever tends to diminish the congested state of the vascular system, and to moderate the action of the heart; as digitalis, colchicum, and other sedatives, with mild mercurials. *Part* xxiv., *p.* 155.

Conditions of the Urine as Indicative of the State of Disease.—[The following valuable remarks on the state of the urine are made by Dr. Dick, in considering the subject of dyspepsia.]

Urine which immediately on being voided gives out a sensible smell of ammonia, generally indicates that the vital powers have suffered declension; that disease has become chronic; that the patient is past middle life, or is prematurely aged, etc.

In arthritic and rheumatic cases, the mineral and vegetable acids are carefully to be shunned. Among the latter the oxalic is the most objectionable; next, the malic; then, the tartaric, citric, and acetic. There can be little doubt that these acids act injuriously by their astringent effect on the cutaneous and mucous surfaces, by their thus interfering with their own elimination and that of the uric and lactic acids; thereby loading the blood with acidulous principles; whence follows that peculiar irritative condition of the nerves, constituting local affections, such as sciatica, lumbago, gout, or the systemic disturbance of rheumatic fever. It is amazing how difficult it is to rid the blood of this acidulous diathesis (if the expression may be used) when once it has been formed. The excernents seem to find it a peculiarly hard task to eliminate acids. Years of rigid attention to the dietetic ingesta are necessary. Hence the rarity of radical cures of gout and rheumatism. *Part* xxiv., *p.* 160.

Phosphatic Diathesis.—Dr. Beneke found the phosphates to be present in the urine in very different and nearly all sorts of diseases, varying on different days in one case, and always remaining of nearly the same amount in others; proving that it is not the disease itself which causes the excretion of phosphates, but that there must necessarily exist some other cause in the economy to account for the excretion alluded to. In all cases of rapid emaciation there was a large excretion of the phosphates, and sores of blisters in these cases scarcely healed at all, or not until long after. We may provide persons in this condition with the largest quantities of albumen and fat, but we shall never produce thereby a remarkable increase of tissues or complexion—that is to say, of formation of cells, if we do not diminish at once the excretion of phosphates by the urine. A hypernormal excretion of earthy phosphates by the urine is independent of the nature of the disease. When we observe such an excretion, we find a corresponding deficiency of formation of cells, emaciation, and loss of strength; but this deficiency is not always exclusively caused by a hypernormal loss of phosphates, it is often only the result of fever or suppuration, or of any other loss of material necessary for the regeneration of tissues and organs. It is to be observed we shall never be able to judge of the quantity of the earthy phosphates present in an ounce of urine, unless we examine the whole quantity which is passed during the twenty-four hours. Although albumen and fat are present, the phosphate of lime increases the produce of cells, and in this manner we may promote the cure of diseases showing a deficiency of formation of cells, especially in scrofula. On the other hand, in all wasting diseases, a hypernormal quantity of phosphates is always excreted, especially in those cases where the phosphate of lime proves most beneficial. This quantity, from Dr. Beneke's investigations, is not increased by the administration of the phosphate of lime, but on the contrary, by its use the quantity in the urine often decreases considerably. *Part* xxiv., *p*. 312.

Urine—Deficiency of Urea in.—In all cases where the renal secretion is deficient in urea and uric acid, these existing in the blood, Dr. Maclagan, of Edinburgh, recommends colchicum. *Part* xxv., *p*. 38.

Causes of Albuminous Urine.—In the normal state the albumen is burnt in the blood, and the nitrogenized residue of this combustion, viz., urea and uric acid, is eliminated by the urine. The combustion is, however, not so complete as not to allow some little albumen to escape with the renal secretion; but this albumen, besides being very small in amount, is somewhat different from the ordinary kind. M. Robin thinks that if during a sufficiently long time the albumen underwent in the circulation a much smaller amount in the combustion than is habitually the case, it might pass unaltered into the urine, instead of being thrown off in the form of urea and uric acid.

The urine becomes albuminous in croup, in complete ascites, and in cases of capillary bronchitis, with emphysema, accompanied by much dyspnœa; in pulmonary phthisis, especially when complicated by pneumonia and marked with difficult breathing; in gestation, when sufficiently advanced to occasion a habitual congestion of the kidneys, owing to an impeded abdominal circulation; and in such states of the system in which a very incomplete respiration causes a marked diminution of combustion. The urine is also albuminous in cyanosis, of whichever nature it may be; in affections of the heart when they exist in such degree as to keep the patients in a state of semi-asphyxia; and, of course, in such cases where an obstacle to the circulation of the blood, or of malformation of the heart, prevents the hematosis from being as rapid as under ordinary circumstances. The urine is likewise albuminous in idiopathic or traumatic lesions of the nervous centres, which cause a lowering of temperature, and thereby a marked decrease of combustion; in diabetes, a disease where very often a lesion of the nervous centre seems to be the origo mali; where the great abundance of sugar in the blood seems to be an obstacle to the combustion of albumen; and where finally the natural heat is lowered by one or two degrees with patients who are severely affected. The urine is albuminous in that kind of nervous exhaustion which characterizes the state of frame called lumbago, which exhaustion must be connected with a great diminution of calorification, and slow combustion. The urine is likewise albuminous in consequence of severe exposure to cold of a large surface of the body.

Finally, Bright's disease, where the urine is always albuminous and anæmic, is especially attributed to many of the causes which have been above enumerated as capable of exciting the passage of albumen into the urine.

When the activity of the combustion which takes place in the blood is too feeble to burn the whole of the albumen which, in the normal state, should be consumed in a given time, the general vitality is diminished, and thus more or less albumen is allowed to pass unaltered into the urine, viz., just so much organic matter as escapes the transformation into urea or uric acid. The proportion of urea contained in albuminous urine should therefore be smaller than it is found in normal urine, and such is found to be the case in the following diseases, the only ones, according to the author, in which experiments have been made, viz.: pulmonary phthisis, diseases of cerebro-spinal axis, extensive and acute bronchitis with intense dyspnœa, and Bright's disease. *Part* xxv., *p.* 134.

Urœmia, or Urœmic Intoxication.—According to Frerichs, a train of symptoms frequently arises in Bright's disease, due to the contamination of the blood with the excrementitious constituents of the urine. There are two forms of uræmia, acute and chronic. Early in Bright's disease, patients often complain of headache or of a confused sensation in the head; their eyes grow dull and expressionless; they are forgetful and indifferent; and slow and inactive in their movements. If the urinary secretion becomes more abundant, these symptoms diminish, or they may disappear entirely. In other cases they increase in intensity, the drowziness passes into stupor; at first, the patient may be aroused by loud calling and speaking, and then he gives rational answers; subsequently, the coma is complete, and the respiration becomes stertorous. Delirium is an infrequent symptom; when it does occur, the patient will repeat over and over again the same word or sentence. Convulsions frequently precede death.

The acute form of uræmia commences suddenly, and manifests itself in the three following ways: by depression of the functions of the brain, by irritation of the spinal cord, and by both sets of symptoms conjoined. In the first form, the patients sink suddenly into a state of deep stupor, out of which they are very soon unable to be aroused. The face is mostly pale, and the pupils immovable; in other cases there is circumscribed redness of the cheeks, the conjunctivæ are then injected, and the pupils small. The pulse ranges between 60 and 90; on the occurrence of coma, it usually increases in size and hardness. The respiration is sometimes stertorous, the character of the stertor differing, as Dr. Addison pointed out, from that in cerebral hemorrhage.—In the second form, convulsions occur suddenly, similar in character to those seen in eclampsia and epilepsy. The whole muscular system is usually affected. Consciousness is undestroyed.—In the third form, coma and convulsions are conjoined.

These acute forms of uræmia are usually the result of sudden suppression of urine, particularly in Bright's disease, from scarlet and typhus fevers.

Acute uræmia may be readily confounded with cerebral hemorrhage, hysterical convulsions, reflex spasms of various kinds, narcotic poisoning, typhus fever, etc.

Closely allied to the foregoing disorders of the nervous system, as consequences of uræmia, are certain affections of the senses. The most striking of these is loss of vision; *Amaurosis urœmica.*—Like coma and convulsions, this local nervous affection may be slowly developed, or it may manifest itself in a few days or even hours. The patient complains of a sensation, as though a mist lay before his eyes, which from time to time becomes denser. The only change perceptible to the physician is some sluggishness of the pupil. Landouzy affirms that amaurosis is one of the most constant symptoms of Bright's disease.

The sense of hearing is affected by Bright's disease about as frequently as that of vision.

During the convulsions, the pulse, on account of the disturbance of the respiratory movements, is accelerated, and at the same time it is often irregular; in the intervals between the attacks of convulsions, it resumes its normal rate and regularity.

A febrile disturbance (*febris urinosa*) closely resembling typhus fever in its general characters, is sometimes produced by uræmia.

The cessation of the symptoms of uræmia is usually accompanied by a profuse secretion of urine.

Vomiting is one of the most constant and early symptoms of uræmia. The vomited fluid is generally alkaline, and contains carbonate of ammonia; when acid, the presence of ammonia in the egesta is proved by the addition of liquor potassæ. Frerichs says, " I have frequently sought for undestroyed urea in the vomited matters, but always in vain." Further, in uræmia produced by extirpation of the kidneys, and injection of urea into the blood, Frerichs always found a large quantity of carbonate of ammonia in the vomited matters, but not a trace of urea.

It is doubtful in what relation the diarrhœa, which occurs in Bright's disease, stands to the uræmia.

The older physicians frequently asserted, that in cases of suppression of urine, the breath and perspiration had a fetid urinous-odor. Many modern observers have denied this. Frerichs says, that whatever difference of opinion there may be as to the existence of this odor, it is a fact, that when the symptoms of uræmic intoxication, coma, convulsions, etc., commence, carbonate of ammonia is mixed in considerable quantity with the expired breath, and that the quantity of the ammonia is in proportion to the intensity of the uræmic phenomena.

" I have," he writes, " repeatedly demonstrated the ammonia contained in the expired air of sick men, and of animals into whose veins urea was injected after extirpation of the kidneys; reddened litmus paper quickly turned blue in the air issuing from the mouth and nostrils; a rod moistened with hydrochloric acid produced, when held in the same air, a more or less thick cloud. Animals into the veins of which urea was injected, continued quiet and awake so long as the expired air was free from ammonia, but as soon as a rod dipped in hydrochloric acid produced a white cloud when held in the expired air, the disorders of the nervous system characteristic of uræmic poisoning manifested themselves."

Frerichs' own observations have not enabled him to say anything definite as to the state of the sweat in uræmic intoxication.

After death from uræmia, no lesion of structure of the central organs of the nervous system can be detected. The membranes of the brain and spinal cord are normal; the quantity of fluid in the ventricles rarely exceeds an ounce—i. e., is within the range of health. In four cases of amaurosis uræmica mentioned by Landouzy, in one recorded by Bright, and in one observed by Frerichs, the optic nerves and the visual apparatus appeared normal. The stomach, also, even when during life it has been the seat of severe symptoms, is usually found after death unchanged in texture. So the intestinal mucous membrane may be normal in appearance, when during life there has been profuse diarrhœa. The kidneys exhibit the lesions characteristic of one of the three stages of Bright's disease. The blood is sometimes firmly, at others imperfectly coagulated; Frerichs thinks that in all the cases of uræmia he has seen occurring spontaneously or produced artificially, it has exhibited a peculiar shade of violet. Christison, Jaksch, and Hamernjk, have observed cases in which the blood had an ammoniacal odor similar to that of decaying urine. Chemical analysis proves, Frerichs affirms, that the blood, in every case in which the symptoms of uræmia are present, contains carbonate of ammonia, and also, usually, traces of undestroyed urea. The quantity of carbonate of ammonia varies greatly.

The above are, according to Frerichs' researches, the most important facts known concerning uræmia.

The cause of the symptoms of uræmia has been generally sought in the retention of the constituents of the urine in the blood.

The following is Frerichs' own theory of uræmia. The symptoms of uræmic intoxication, he says, arise in consequence of the urea accumulated in the blood being converted, by the agency of a suitable ferment, into carbonate of ammonia, while yet within the vessels. For the supervention, then, he adds, of uræmic intoxication, two agents are necessary— 1st, an accumulation of urea in the blood; 2ndly, the presence of a ferment by the agency of which the decomposition of the urea may be effected.

If the urea, after collecting in quantity in the blood, be suddenly decomposed, then the symptoms are those of apoplexy; if its decomposition is effected more gradually, then the symptoms resemble those of typhus terminating in coma and convulsions.

With the causes which occasion the development of the ferment, we are, Frerichs says, but imperfectly acquainted. In the acute blood-disease— e. g., typhus, scarlet fever, and cholera—this agent is rarely absent. Slight febrile disturbance, as from exposure to cold, or trifling local inflammation, seems in some cases to give the impulse necessary for the destruction of the urea. In cases of Bright's disease which arises during pregnancy, the ferment is usually developed.

The presence of the ferment is manifested only by its effects. Frerichs offers no other proof of its existence.

In order to demonstrate its truth, it must, he says, be proved—

1st. That in every case of uræmic intoxication, a resolution of urea into carbonate of ammonia takes place.

2nd. That the symptoms characteristic of uræmia can be produced by the introduction of carbonate of ammonia into the blood.

Two series of experiments are described by Frerichs, as offering the required proof.

"In the first series of experiments, a solution of from thirty to forty-six grains of urea was injected into the veins of animals, the kidneys of which had been previously removed. They remained for some hours perfectly free from convulsions. . . . In from 1¼ to 8 hours they became restless, vomited acid chyme, or a slimy yellow alkaline mass, according to the state of fullness of the stomach at the commencement of the experiment. At the same time that ammonia was perceptible in the expired air, convulsions supervened, which occasionally ceased and returned again, and gradually passed into stupor with stertorous breathing. In some cases, convulsions were absent, and then sopor and coma were the first symptoms. After death, which took place from 2½ to 10 hours from the time of the injection of the urea, ammonia in large quantity was found in the blood; the contents of the stomach emitted, in most cases, a strongly ammoniacal (urinous) odor, and contained much carbonate of ammonia; in one case only was it somewhat acid, and even then it contained ammonia. This basis was detected in the bile and other secretions. The stomach was usually injected, and of a dusky-red color. The brain and its membranes were normal in appearance; and the quantity of fluid in the ventricles was not increased.

"In the second series of experiments, a solution of carbonate of ammonia was injected into the veins of animals. Convulsions, often very violent in character, instantly ensued, and stupor quickly supervened. The respiration was difficult, the expired breath was loaded with ammonia, and vomiting of bilious matters occurred. The stupor lasted for some hours, and ammonia was expired during the whole time. Gradually, however, the latter disappeared, and then by degrees, the animals recovered their senses. When more carbonate of ammonia was injected, while the animal lay in a state of stupor, the convulsions and vomiting recurred, and the urine and the stools passed away involuntarily; after the lapse of five or six hours the ammonia again disappeared from the blood, and the animal again became lively."

Although death by uræmia is the natural termination, so to say, of Bright's disease, yet the fatal result is sometimes caused by other lesions —e. g., by inflammation of serous or parenchymatous structures, by sinking from vomiting, diarrhœa, dropsy, tubercular suppuration, asphyxia, etc.

The diagnosis of uræmia from *apoplexia cerebri*, typhus, gastritis, convulsions of various kinds, and narcotic poisoning, is to be made by a careful examination of the quantity and quality of the urinary secretion, the presence of ammonia in the expired air, and the symptoms of disease derived from the organ the functions of which are disordered; thus uræmic coma is distinguished from that dependent upon hemorrhage into the brain, by the absence of paralysis of the voluntary muscles, the more frequent and softer pulse, and the more rapid breathing. The character of the stertor, too, differs in the two. The early occurrence of delirium and coma, and the absence of the eruption and of enlargement of the spleen, aid in diagnosing uræmia from typhus fever. At the same time it must be borne in mind that an eruption closely resembling the mulberry rash of typhus is sometimes present in the uræmia which follows cholera.

In the treatment of *uræmic intoxication*, the first object to be attained is the restoration of the urinary secretion. Mild diuretics are the best remedies for the accomplishment of the desired end. Should these fail, then hydragogues are to be employed. Little hope can be entertained of diureties acting, in the advanced stage of degeneration of the kidney. The second object is to prevent the injurious influence of the carbonate of ammonia developed in the blood on the nervous centres. When convulsions have commenced, this indication requires our first attention. Hydrochloric and the vegetable acids, Frerichs says, are the remedies which naturally suggest themselves; they pass into the blood, and are excreted again, either in their primitive or an altered form, with the urine. At the same time the patient may be washed with vinegar, and enemata containing acetic acid administered. If marked symptoms of cerebral congestion are present, purgatives and bloodletting may be required.

Vomiting, consequent on irritation of the kidneys, is to be relieved only by treating the local affection; that from chronic dyspepsia, consequent on the abuse of spirituous liquors, or disease of the heart, by bitters, narcoties, and antacids. Uræmic vomiting is most obstinate. Christison recommends creasote. Narcotics, Frerichs says, are of no service.

Diarrhœa, when it occurs during the latter stages of the disease, is very obstinate. Frerichs has generally found relief follow the use of liq. ferri muriatis.

In *bronchial catarrh*, expectoration is to be favored, if deficient, by senega, ammoniacum, etc.; if in excess, it is to be restrained by tannic acid, acetate of lead, muriate of iron, and other astringents. Alum is sometimes extremely useful.

When the disease is the consequence of pregnancy, it is a question in some cases whether premature labor should not be induced.

Part xxv., *p.* 135.

Test for Sugar.—Dr. H. B. Jones gives the following: Test a portion of urine with a solution of sulphate copper and liq. potassæ; a blue solution is first produced, heat it, and the blue color becomes slightly yellow on the surface, and rapidly changes into that of a reddish yellow precipitate, which is the mixture of the color of the urine and the color of the sub-oxide of copper. With this test, independent of sugar, a large quantity of animal matter or of urea will produce a blue color, but when heated the reduction of the copper does not take place near so rapidly.—A salt of another metal may be used instead of the copper, as silver with a drop of ammonia. The sugar takes the oxygen from the silver, and it is deposited in a beautiful metallic form on the glass.—Another easy test is allowing a drop of diabetic urine to dry on the glass, and examining it by the microscope, when remarkable tufts of stellated crystals will be seen.

Part xxv., *p.* 155.

New Test for Sugar.—It is stated by Professor Böttcher, that the least quantity of sugar in urine, or any other fluid, may be detected by adding a little carbonate of soda and a small quantity of magisterium bismuthi, and boiling briskly; when the liquid cools, the bismuth, if sugar be present, is reduced, and forms a black powder. *Part* xxv., *p.* 160.

Mode of Testing for Glucose or Diabetic Sugar.—The only tests on which Lehmann places any reliance are Trommer's, the fermentation test and the development of the torula, and the application of Biot and Soleil's polarizing apparatus. The following is the best method of applying Trommer's test to an animal fluid suspected of containing sugar:

The fluid to be examined is treated with caustic potash and filtered if necessary—that is to say, if there be too great a precipitate; an excess of caustic potash is productive of no harm, as it should be present in more than sufficient quantity to decompose the sulphate of copper; the latter, which must be added gradually, and in a diluted state, usually gives rise to a precipitate, which disappears when the fluid is stirred; as the quantity of the oxide of copper which is soluble is proportional to the quantity of sugar which is present, very little sulphate of copper must be added at a time, if we suspect that only a little sugar is present in the fluid. On allowing the azure solution thus obtained to stand for some time, there is usually formed a more pure red or yellow powder than the precipitate, which is at once thrown down on boiling the fluid. Moreover, very prolonged heating is improper, for there are several substances which by prolonged boiling separate suboxide of copper from alkaline solutions of oxide of copper; amongst them we may especially name the albuminous substances, which with oxide of copper and potash yield very beautiful azure-blue, or somewhat violet solutions, and by very prolonged boiling, separate a little suboxide of copper, although without the aid of heat they have not this property.

If a specimen of urine contain very little sugar, or if we are searching for sugar in some other fluid, it is advisable to extract the solid residue with alcohol, to dissolve the alcoholic extract in water, and to apply the potash and sulphate of copper to this solution. By proceeding in this manner, we usually obtain the reaction in its most distinct manner. If, however, we are seeking for very small quantities of sugar, as, for instance, in chyle, blood, or in the egg, we must neutralize the aqueous fluid, previously to its evaporation, with dilute acetic acid, in consequence of the solubility of albuminate of soda or of casein in alcohol, thus preventing any albuminous body from remaining in solution. If the reaction do not properly manifest itself in the alcoholic extract thus obtained, or if we would carry the investigation further, we must precipitate the sugar from the alcoholic solution by an alcoholic solution of potash, dissolve the compound of sugar and potash in water, and now apply the sulphate of copper: if only a trace of sugar be present, we obtain a most distinct and beautiful reaction. *Part* xxv., *p.* 160.

Operation for Retention of Urine occasioned by Inveterate Stricture.— Mr. Simon advocates a modified perineal operation in certain cases. He opens the urethra by puncturing a very small incision immediately in front of the prostate gland. He then runs a short, elastic catheter along this wound into the bladder. He then leaves the stricture untouched for ten days more or less, during which the urine flows through the perineal catheter; at the end of that time, the stricture is sufficiently relaxed to begin its dilatation with a middle-sized instrument. *Part* xxv., *p.* 222.

Retention of—Puncture of Bladder through the Rectum.—Pass the index-finger of the left hand into the rectum until the prostate gland is felt; the finger must be pushed, if possible, behind this part; seek now for fluctuation, which, however, is not always easy to find. The anterior part of the bladder having been pressed upon, and the posterior part of the prostate gland recognized, glide the instrument along the palmar surface of the left index-finger until it is in contact with the distended bladder resting upon the rectum—take out the director—introduce the trocar—and push it upward and forward one or two inches into the bladder. The greatest care should be taken that the prostate gland be not transfixed; it might be a fatal mistake.

After puncturing the bladder through the rectum, the patient should be kept in bed at least three weeks after the sinuses are securely cicatrized, as from its weak and feeble organization, the newly formed cicatrix is liable to give way.

In this case, stricture of the urethra had been the root of the evil. This had been followed by abscess, fistula in perineo, and retention of urine;

for the relief of the last of which the bladder had been punctured through
the rectum. Mr. Hilton believes the operation is free from danger if carefully performed; there is very little risk of hemorrhage; the operation is
by no means of a protracted kind; it does not tax the patient's strength;
is not exhausting, and entails no drain upon the system. As the lower
part of the bladder is punctured, the accumulation of mucus, urine, pus, or
other secretions, is not allowed, the viscus being completely emptied; you
prevent the urine finding its way into the urethra, and give an opportunity
to the false passages of healing, and the natural urethra of recovering
itself. The seat of the stricture is kept in a state of rest; no local excitation is used, and all irritation, muscular contraction, or spasm is forestalled.
There is, on the other hand, no chance of the bladder contracting away
from the instrument; it *contracts toward it.*　　　　　　*Part* xxvi., *p.* 216.

*Retention of Urine—Puncturing the Bladder through the Symphysis
Pubis.*—Dr. Brander recommends puncturing the bladder through the
symphysis pubis. He performed the operation first on the dead subject,
and then carefully dissected the parts and found that in all respects it had
been a successful one. The operation has now been performed several
times with complete success. He employs a flattened trocar.
　　　　　　　　　　　　　　　　　　　　　　　　Part xxvi., *p.* 251.

Presence of Pus in the Urine.—Dr. R. B. Todd says that when the
urine contains pus it is muddy from the first; hence the difference between
this and urine containing lithate of ammonia, the latter only becoming
muddy after a certain time. Phosphatic urine is also muddy when passed,
but in this case it is much paler; and after standing some time there is a
deposit as in the case of pus, but in phosphatic urine it is white instead of
being yellow, and flocculent and light instead of being thick and heavy.
A little acid renders phosphatic urine clear, while if pus be present it
increases the turbidity. In cases of phosphatic deposits also the urine is
generally alkaline; in purulent, the urine is generally slightly acid. The
pus is also rendered glairy and stringy by liq. potassæ. Again, if the
urine be rendered acid by applying heat, the pus coagulates. Lastly,
examined by the microscope, it consists of two essential parts, liq. puris
and pus globules, which are characteristic.　　　　*Part* xxvii., *p.* 89.

*Fetid, Phosphatic, Mucous Urine—Prolapsus of the Anterior Wall of
the Vagina an Occasional Cause of.*—Dr. Bird remarks that middle-
aged females sometimes suffer great distress from symptoms similar to
those occasioned by enlarged prostate in the male; that is to say, there is
great irritability of the bladder, the urine when passed being fetid, ropy,
and containing much mucus. He endeavored to trace these symptoms to
a similar cause, namely, a prevention of the complete emptying of the
bladder, and the retention of a portion of urine, so as to produce in it
decomposition. Such a cause, he considers a prolapsion of the anterior
wall of the vagina. He says: Almost the first case in which I recognized
the condition to which I am alluding, occurred in the person of a stout,
tolerably healthy-looking woman.

She complained of great sense of distress in the lower part of the abdomen, with weight and bearing down. Walking was painful to her, and
she was almost constantly tortured with a desire to empty the bladder.
The urine was very offensive, and contained a large quantity of dense,

ropy mucus, mixed with phosphates. Suspecting the possible presence of a calculus, I introduced a catheter, but little urine escaped, and no concretion could be felt. But on examining the vagina, a large pink looking sac depended from its anterior wall, and almost separated the labia. She was, indeed, suffering from prolapsus of the bladder into a pouch formed in the anterior vaginal wall. By keeping the bladder emptied by the daily use of the catheter, the urine soon recovered its healthy appearance, and the mucus decreased considerably. The decomposition of the secretion in this vesical pouch had evolved ammonia, which had irritated the bladder, and caused a copious secretion of mucus, loaded with the earthy salts, from its lining membrane. I sent the patient to my brother, Dr. Frederick Bird, as I believed no permanent cure could be obtained while the prolapsus existed. He applied the actual cautery to the anterior wall of the vagina, and the result was most satisfactory. After the slough came away, sufficient contraction occurred to prevent the formation of the vesical pouch, and the patient remained free from the ailment which had so long distressed her.

In another case the condition of the patient was relieved by introducing an injection of infusion of galls three times a day into the vagina, wearing an abdominal support with a perineal pad, and the administration of quina and iron with dilute phosphoric acid.   *Part* xxvii., *p.* 193.

Characters of Urine Depositing Oxalate of Lime.—The principal characters which have been noticed as belonging to urine containing oxalates, are the following: (1) A density somewhat higher than natural, indicating an excessive elimination of urea, or of the indeterminate extractive matters of the urine. In the series of cases recorded by Dr. Golding Bird, one-half of the specimens ranged from 1015 to 1025. Some were as low as 1009; some as high as 1030. In the cases recorded by Dr. J. W. Begbie (Monthly Journal, March 1848,) the average density was 1028 ; the extremes being from below 1015 to above 1030, and in one case 1040. Dr. Prout states, in general terms, that the urine in such cases is of moderate density. (2.) A color, according to Dr. Prout, pale citron yellow, or greenish; according to Golding Bird, amber, never greenish; according to Dr. Begbie, amber, darker than in health. (3.) An odor generally natural, rarely aromatic, like mignonette (Golding Bird) ; on the other hand, aromatic, occasionally approaching to that of the sweet-brier, noticed in urine containing the cystic oxide (J. W. Begbie). (4.) A reaction almost always more or less acid, frequently powerfully so.   *Part* xxix., *p.* 137.

Oxaluria.—The terms oxaluria and oxalic acid diathesis are now well understood to mean that morbid state of the digestive and assimilative functions in which oxalic acid is eliminated by the kidney in combination with urine. It is by no means an uncommon complaint. The prevailing forms of the crystals are the octahedral and the dumb-bell. It is at present believed that the former consists of the *oxalate*, and the latter of the *oxalurate*, of lime ; and this is likely, because therapeutic agents do not act alike in both cases. In a case of this disease under the care of Dr. Gray, of Glasgow, marked by the presence of dumb-bell crystals, after other remedies had failed, one grain of nitrate of silver was given every six hours. In two days it was diminished to half a grain, and ℨj. of the acidulated tincture of calumba was given night and morning. It should be observed, that where oxalate of lime appears in octahedral crystals, the nitromuriatic acid with a vegetable tonic will generally effect a cure. If the dumb-bell form appears, nitrate of silver is very useful. Where both kinds of crystals are present, these medicines should be given alternately.   *Part* xxix., *p.* 142.

Morbid Condition of the Urine connected with Chronic Disease.— Indigestion.—When alkalescent from *fixed alkali*, says Dr. H. B. Jones, it is from the stomach. Take more air and exercise, with mild nutritious food. Give vegetable acids, as lemon-juice or citric acid, but not tartaric. Seventeen grains of dry citric acid are about equal to half an ounce of lemon-juice, and one lemon generally gives one ounce of juice. Twelve ounces of lemon-juice, equal to 408 grains of citric acid, may be given in one day if necessary.

When alkalescent from *volatile alkali*, it arises from affection of the mucous membrane of the bladder. In this case buchu, pareira brava, turpentine, cubebs, copaiba are used. Buchu is given when pus is present; pareira brava when there is ropy mucus. Buchu is good when the urine is acid, pareira when it is alkaline; in short, when you want a stimulant give buchu; when you want a demulcent give pareira brava; when you want an astringent give uva ursi.   *Part* xxix., *p.* 145.

Sulphuric Acid, versus Urine.—Mr. J. E. Huxley has pointed out that, in the wards of insane establishments which are wet and dirty, no scrubbing or scalding will effect more than a temporary improvement, as the floor becomes a reservoir for the perpetual exhalation of the volatile ammonia. But if dilute sulphuric acid be poured over such floors, in the proportion of one ounce of acid to twenty-four of water, and allowed to remain twenty-four hours, a white film (sulphate of ammonia) will form, which may be removed by washing, and will leave the room sweet. The principle is that of converting a volatile into a fixed salt that may easily be got rid of.
                                                              Part xxxi., *p.* 232.

Test for Sugar.—Dr. Garrod considers that sugar in very small quantities may be detected by treating the fluid with trisacetate of lead, filtering, removing the lead with bicarbonate of soda or potash, and again filtering, by which means a colorless urine is produced, giving, on the addition of a few drops of concentrated solution of potash and heat, a *bright orange* color.   *Part* xxxi., *p.* 277.

Retention of Urine.—Dr. H. Thompson insists upon the principle, that when perineal abscess is found co-existing with retention of urine, it is very rarely necessary to have recourse to any severer measures than the opening of the abscess, and the passing of the catheter; and, further, that the sooner the necessary opening is made, the less likely is the patient to become the subject of extravasation at the time, or to suffer from urinary fistula afterward.   *Part* xxxii., *p.,* 169.

Urine, Extravasation of, from Injury to the Perineum.—Dr. Fletcher says we may have extravasation of urine from a rupture of the urethra without any swelling in the perineum, and in all such cases, where there are all the general symptoms of extravasation and you have reason to fear escape of urine, you must make a free and deep opening into the perineum, exactly in the medial line.   *Part* xxxii., *p.* 179.

Purulent Urine from Chronic Pyeletis.—Dr. Basham of Westminster Hospital says the value of the information to be derived by examining the chemical and microscopic character of the urine depends much on the care and accuracy with which these chemical and microscopic facts are applied to the condition and symptoms of the patient. The special characters of these deposits, if correctly interpreted, become highly significant and instructive, great aids to diagnosis, and the eventual basis of treatment. The cause and nature of a dropsical condition of the system are at once recognized, when in albuminous urine there are found epithelial, fibrinous, or waxy casts of a tubular character, glandular epithelial cells loaded with fat, or blood discs with amorphous fibrin, stained with hematin. The pathology of dropsy with such concomitants differs materially from that in which the urine is free from such deposits. But, on the other hand, cases occur in which there is no dropsy—no anasarcous state, yet the urine contains albumen, to which is added the presence of pus corpuscles, minute membranous coagula entangling clots of blood, blood discs in abundance, and shreds of amorphous fibrin. If, in such cases, there is great irritability of the urinary organs, frequent micturition with pain referred to the neck of the bladder, perineum, or penis, a suspicion at once exists of disease of the renal organs very different in character from that which we predicate on the first example. It is, however, only by a cautious comparison of the symptoms experienced by the patient with these morbid products in the urine that a correct and satisfactory diagnosis can be obtained. The presence of pus corpuscles in the urine is not, alone, sufficient to induce suspicion of renal disease. In gonorrhœa, or other inflammatory affections of the urethra, in catarrh of the bladder, or gouty inflammation of this viscus, pus would be present in the urine. In stricture, in chronic gleet, membranous *debris*, often entangling minute clots of blood, may be, and often are, present, and yet no suspicion of renal disease from any such appearances would be warranted. It is therefore by a careful comparison of the sedimentitious matters in the urine with the general symptoms of the patient, that we are enabled to arrive at a correct and intelligible diagnosis.

The symptoms most characteristic of pyeletis or inflammation of the pelvis of the kidney, are, rigors, with lumbar pains, sometimes dull and continuous, sometimes pungent and darting; often extending and becoming fixed at the crest of the ilium, or prolonged to the outside of the thigh, with numbness in the direction of the external crural nerve. Occasionally there is retraction of the testicle of the same side; there is frequent micturition, and great irritability of the urinary organs. The patient complains of pain in the perineum, or in the neck of the bladder, or feels a darting pungent sensation along the urethra, fixing itself in the glans penis till temporarily relieved by passing urine; the quantity passed rarely exceeds one or two ounces, and the urgency for passing this small quantity recurs at very short intervals of time. The pain in the bladder, perineum, or penis, is always relieved by micturition, and there is no difficulty or obstacle to the free passage of the urine.

The urine when first passed is cloudy, or even milky, but when set at rest, separating into two portions, an upper, clear, natural-colored fluid, not ropy, but containing albumen; a lower and distinct sediment of a yellowish color, consisting of pus corpuscles, amongst which oftentimes may be seen minute fibrinous shreds or membranous flocculi, with small coagula of blood attached. Earthy amorphous matter is also present in some cases. Hematuria, sufficient to cause discoloration of the urine, may or may not have occurred ; yet, in most cases, although the urine is not discolored, scattered blood discs may be detected by the microscope.

If the disease be of a certain duration, there may be fullness and enlargement of the kidney of the affected side ; for if a concretion becomes permanently fixed in the pelvis of a kidney, a partial obstruction of the ureter follows, and the usual conditions of an encysted and sacculated kidney have commenced. If, on the other hand, the calculus descends into the bladder, a train of symptoms sufficiently characteristic follows, which clearly indicate its descent into that cavity.

But we have to interpret from these symptoms the part of the urinary apparatus which is the seat of the disease, for these conditions, in some respects, are common to many different disorders ; yet if they be carefully analyzed, and a just comparison established between the one and other, we shall ultimately arrive at a correct diagnosis of the disease. Turbid and troubled urine, with painful and frequent micturition, may occur in stricture, gleet, or gonorrhœa ; but, in the two latter, the character of the pain during the passage of the urine, and the appearance of discharge at the orifice of the urethra, not to say the stains on the linen of the patient, would make the case sufficiently clear. In stricture, in addition to a turbid urine, when gleet is present, there may be membranous shreds, and even minute coagula, such as have been noticed in the urine of the patient under consideration. But, in such a case, the pain and distress are felt during micturition, not before ; the urine passes with difficulty, or in drops, or in a diminished stream, and an exploration of the urethra proves the impediment to the free excretion of the urine. In calculus of the bladder, similar conditions of the urine might exist, and much pain be experienced in the bladder, perineum, and penis ; but the pain in such cases is most aggravated after micturition ; as the bladder fills the pain diminishes ; just the reverse happens in the painful and irritable bladder of renal disease. Moreover, an exploration of the bladder establishes the presence of a stone. In the case before us, the patient refers the commencement of the pain to the region of the kidney, and describes the pain as if descending thence in the direction of the bladder, and becoming pungent and stabbing in the perineum, and occasionally extending itself to the extremity of the glans penis. These distressing sensations are always relieved by micturition, and there is a temporary lull till the urine collects again, even in small quantity. This fact is of much importance in the diagnosis of renal disease, and taken in conjunction with the history of the case, with the albumen and amount of the purulent sediment in the urine, and the peculiar character of the lumbar and regional pain, constitutes very fair evidence of inflammatory action of the pelvis of the kidney.

In cases of inflammation of the bladder, cystitis or catarrh of the bladder, and limited to that cavity, the character and quality of the urine differ much from what is excreted in renal disease. The urine is contaminated by the inflammatory exudation from the vesical mucous membrane ; pus cells, and the so-called exudation corpuscles, are present in abundance ; but the pus corpuscles do not subside as a distinct and well-defined precipitate, they are entangled in a ropy magma, in which numerous crystals of the triple phosphate are visible ; this viscidity and these crystals being rapidly developed by the agency of the alkaline urine always voided in inflammation of the bladder. This character of the urine will suffice to distinguish vesical from renal inflammation.

The ready separation of a turbid or milky urine into two parts, a clear supernatant portion containing albumen, derived from the liquor purus, and a sedimentary portion of pus corpuscles distinctly precipitated, voided by a patient who suffered from severe regional pain either in the kidney or bladder, perineum or penis; and if, in the first-named position, aggravated by pressure or motion, or when, in the latter parts, relieved temporarily by micturition, and in whose urine gravel, or blood, or both, had been previously, or at some antecedent period, present, to such a collection of symptoms there should be little hesitation in referring them to a chronic inflammation of the pelvis of the kidney.

In the treatment of these cases our chief reliance must be placed on the palliative agency of opium. If it be a case of calculous pyeletis—that is, chronic inflammation of the pelvis of the kidney arising from the irritation of the calculus impacted therein—it is quite obvious that so long as the irritating agent remains, so long will the symptoms of chronic inflammation continue. We have no remedies that can either dissolve or remove such a concretion, and the progress of the case must ultimately depend on the form and composition of the calculus, some of which escape into the bladder, with symptoms characteristic of their descent through the ureter; and, if their diameter be but small, may be excreted through the urethra; this is more likely to happen in the female. These are the most favorable terminations to renal calculus. In other cases the calculus having escaped the kidney, lodges in the bladder, and gives rise to the usual symptoms, relief from which can only be obtained by the assistance of a skillful surgeon. But in by far the more numerous cases of calculous pyeletis, the concretion grows by the apposition of fresh matter, becomes impacted in the head of the ureter, does not completely occlude the outlet, but becomes branched and irregular in shape by the constant deposit of phosphatic matter derived from the action of alkaline purulent fluid on the urine, still secreted by the intact part of the kidney; the fluid retained in the pelvis of the kidney is constantly exerting a dilating influence, and in the progress of the case a renal tumor is felt, distinctly fluctuating, and if the history and symptoms of such a case be carefully collated, the diagnosis is not difficult. It must be clear that medicinal remedies can exert no curative influence in such a case. To palliate and relieve must be the limit of our aid.

In the case which has formed the subject of these remarks, you have seen that perfect quietude, the warm-bath, cupping on the loins in the early period, and opiates, were the agents through which partial relief was obtained. The buchu, the sesquichloride of iron, and the nitro-muriatic acid, although severally administered, cannot be said to have done anything for the relief of the patient. *Part* xxxiii., *p.* 123.

Oxalate of Lime Deposit.—When examining urine, microscopically, which contains oxalate of lime, it is possible that the crystals may be obscured by opaque urates. When such is the case, says the editor of the "Medical Times and Gazette," they must first be dissolved out by liquor potassæ, or they may very much deceive you, by leading you to suppose that there is very little oxalate of lime, when it is present in great abundance. *Part* xxxiii., *p.* 127.

Tests for Sugar.—*Kledzinsky's* fluid, composed of potash, glycerine, and saturated solution of sulphate of copper, when added to diabetic urine and boiled, turns it of an opaque amber color; with non-saccharine urine, there is a white flocculent deposit. *Maumene's Test* is made by soaking white merino, or any woollen fabric, in a solution of bichloride of tin, and drying in a water bath: when dipped in suspected urine and carefully dried, the cloth becomes of a darkish brown or almost black color.

Part xxxiii., *p.* 128.

Liebig's Method for the Rapid Detection of Sugar.—Dissolve a small quantity of ox-gall in the suspected fluid in a test tube; then add rapidly an equal quantity of strong sulphuric acid. If sugar is present, a beautiful purpurine is immediately produced.   *Part* xxxiii., *p.* 129.

New Test for Sugar in Urine.—Krause advocates the use of the test-fluid, originally proposed by Luton, containing the bichromate of potash in solution. He proposes that the fluid should be made thus: Dissolve ʒj. of bichromate of potash in ʒij. of aq. destill., with the addition of ʒij. of concentrated sulphuric acid. When glucose urine is treated with an equal bulk of this fluid, the reddish-yellow color changes, in a short time (*instantly* by the application of heat), into a beautiful bluish-green color, more or less dark, according to the degree of concentration, and carbonic and formic acids escape during effervescence. A dirty brownish-red color (with occasionally a tinge of green) results if no sugar be present. Whilst Krause deprecates neglect of the well-known tests proposed by Trommer and others, he considers this one as more certain and less difficult than any other.   *Part* xxxv., *p.* 64.

Sugar in the Urine—Tests for.—Dr. Garrod, of University College, says: Moore's test, or that by boiling the urine, to which an equal bulk of liquor potassæ has previously been added, may be much increased in delicacy by first adding a drop or two of the potash solution to insure slight alkalinity, and then some good bone black or animal charcoal. This mixture must now be filtered, and we thus obtain a liquid perfectly color-less, and on adding a further excess of liq. potassæ, and boiling, the yellow or orange color is much more readily observed than in the urine before preparation. Should no change of color take place, we may safely conclude that no sugar exists, or, at any rate, such traces as may safely be disregarded.   *Part* xxxv., *p.* 301.

Retention of Urine.—If a catheter cannot be passed, Mr. Forster, of Guy's Hospital, would place the patient under the influence of chloroform; if the stricture be spasmodic, it will be at once relaxed, and even if a permanent one, will often be relaxed so far as to admit of the passage of an instrument.   *Part* xxxvi., *p.* 182.

Constituents of the Urine and their Sources.—The following, by Dr. A. H. Hassall, of Royal Free Hospital, are the sources from which the different constituents which come under the name of *Essential Constituents of the Urine* are derived:

Urea is a nitrogenous compound, derived from the disintegration of some of the nitrogenized tissues, according to Dr. Prout, the *gelatinous* tissue of the body. The principal part of the *nitrogen* of the disintegrated tissues is eliminated from the system through this compound.

Creatine and *Creatining* are also nitrogenous bodies, derived, as appears from the researches of Liebig, from the disintegration of the *muscular* tissue.

Uric acid, according to Dr. Prout, results from the disintegration of the *albuminous* tissues. But it is probable that uric acid is in some cases in part derived from elements of food rich in nitrogen, imperfectly assimilated, and the same, perhaps, is also true in some cases with urea.

The *coloring matter* of the urine, which is a non-nitrogenous substance, and extremely rich in *carbon,* is supposed to be modified hematin, set free on the decay and breaking down of the blood corpuscles, and to be the vehicle by which much of the excess of carbon contained in the system is eliminated.

The *sulphuric acid* is formed in part by the oxydation of the sulphur contained in the proximate nitrogenized animal principles, as well as in taurine.

The *phosphoric acid* present in the urine proceeds in part from the oxydation of the phosphorus which forms one of the constituents of the nervous tissue, and especially of the brain.

The *silica* is set free by the disintegration of the osseous tissues.

Lastly, the *ammonia* of the urine is in part derived from the decomposition of the urea.

On the other hand, the constituents termed *Non-essential,* as all the chlorine of the chlorides, and great part of the sulphuric, phosphoric, and silicic acids, are derived from the articles of drink and food consumed, together with the several bases, excepting part of the *ammonia,* as lime, *magnesia, potash,* and *soda,* with which the chlorides, sulphates, and phosphates, are in combination. Part, however, of these salts are, during assimilation, received into, and imbibed by the different tissues, and become set free again on their disintegration.

The presence in the urine of either of the essential constituents in increased or diminished amount, signifies the extent of the decay and disintegration of the particular tissues from which they are derived.

Part xxxvii., *p.* 90.

Discrimination of certain Organized and Disorganized Matters and Principles in the Urine.—Dr. A. H. Hassal gives the following: *Discrimination of Epithelium.*—Occasionally, deposits appear in the urine bearing considerable resemblance to mucus or pus, and which it is impossible to distinguish by the eye alone, but which, when examined under the microscope, are found to consist almost entirely of epithelium. These deposits occur especially in the urine of women, the epithelial scales being derived, for the most part, from the vagina. More rarely, however, the deposit consists of the epithelium of either the renal tubules or bladder. Each of these three varieties of epithelium possesses well-marked structural peculiarities, by which it may be distinguished, either as they occur separately or when mixed together.

Discrimination of Pus.—A deposit of pus in urine is distinguished from one of mucus, first, by its appearance; it is more opaque and cream-like, and forms a more decided and equal sediment, and when the urine is shaken, it becomes equally diffused throughout, without any ropy or tenacious shreddy substance being visible.

If, however, the urine be very alkaline, the appearance presented by the purulent deposit is very different; it becomes acted upon by the alkalies of the urine, and is then converted into a semi-transparent, tenacious substance, very closely resembling mucus, from which, by the eye alone, there is no means of distinguishing it. This change of appearance is often observed in urines which contain pus, and which have been kept for some days; the deposit, from being soft and opaque, gradually becomes transparent and ropy. The appearances presented to the naked eye by a deposit of pus in fresh urine are often quite decisive.

The outward characters of the deposit having been carefully observed, a portion of the urine, after filtration, is to be boiled in a test-tube; if this prove albuminous, there will be stronger reason for regarding the deposit as one of pus, for, with a mucous deposit, as already stated, the urine is scarcely ever albuminous.

When we come to examine a deposit of pus with a microscope, we find that the granular corpuscles are much more numerous than in mucus; that they are more readily acted upon by dilute acetic acid; and that a large number of nuclei are disclosed in them; also, that there is an absence of the fibrous shreds as well as of epithelial scales.

Thus, by the several characters, external and microscopical, now enumerated, pus and mucus may in general be easily and satisfactorily distinguished when in a separate state; when, however, these deposits are mixed together, the distinction is much more difficult, and in some cases quite impossible.

When pus has been acted upon by the alkalies of the urine, and converted into a substance resembling mucus, the distinction between the two may still, in general, be effected by means of the microscope; for in this case, while there will be an absence of epithelial scales, the pus corpuscles will be found to be considerably larger than they are under ordinary circumstances.

Another difference between mucus and pus is that the latter contains a rather larger proportion of fatty matter; this is seen under the microscope in the form of small, shining droplets or spherules, either free or contained in the granular corpuscles, or the fatty matter may be extracted by means of ether. The quantity of fatty matter in mucus is very small, and frequently it is almost entirely absent. When, therefore, fatty matter is left, on the evaporation of the etherial solution of a suspected deposit of pus, there is further reason for considering that the deposit really consists of that substance.

We have noticed that pus acted upon by alkaline urine becomes converted into a ropy substance, similar to mucus; this conversion is more marked, and is almost immediately effected, by the addition to the deposit of a solution of either ammonia or potash.

Urine containing pus, is most commonly either neutral or slightly acid, and becomes alkaline only slowly, while mucous urine, on the contrary even if acid when first passed, very quickly becomes alkaline and ammoniacal.

The liquid portion of pus, liquor puris, differs essentially from that of mucus, and holds in solution the following substances: albumen, a peculiar compound, pyin, or tritoxide of protein, which is soluble in water and precipitated by acetic acid, fat, and salts. The salts consist for the most part of chloride of sodium, with small quantities of phosphate, sulphate, and carbonate of soda, chlorides of potassium and calcium, earthy phosphates, and traces of iron, thus showing a resemblance in composition to the serum of blood.

Deposits of triple phosphate, especially when the crystals are small, are very apt to be mistaken for pus—an error which is at once rectified by the employment of the microscope.

Discrimination of Albumen.—The detection of albumen in urine is very simple. A small quantity of the urine is to be heated until it boils, in a test-tube, over the flame of a spirit-lamp. As soon as the temperature of the liquid becomes raised to over 170° Fahr., the albumen will become coagulated; and if the test-tube be set aside for a time, it will become deposited, when it may be collected, dried, and weighed. The precipitated albumen is soluble in solution of potash, but insoluble in nitric acid.

There are certain sources of failure and fallacy attending the detection of albumen in the urine:

Thus, if earthy phosphates be present in excess, they will become precipitated as soon as the urine is boiled; this precipitate resembles somewhat, and might be mistaken for, albumen, from which it is, however, distinguished by its solubility in nitric acid.

Again, it has been noticed, that, when urates are in great excess in the urine, a white precipitate of uric acid is occasioned on the addition of nitric acid, which might also be mistaken for albumen.

Dr. Owen Rees remarks, " I have observed this in cases of typhus fever of low type, and also in several cases of smallpox. This precipitate is distinguished from albumen by the fact that the addition of hydrochloric acid to a second portion of the urine will occasion a precipitate equally with the nitric acid, if it be owing to uric acid, but no precipitate will ensue if albumen be present."

A precipitate likewise occurs when nitric acid is added to the urine of a patient who has taken either copaiba or cubebs, and which, at first, closely resembles albumen. This precipitate arises from the deposition of the resinous matter contained in the above-named medicines. It is distinguished from albumen by its not subsiding as distinct deposit, and by its producing a permanent opacity of the urine.

Another method of distinguishing albumen in such cases is by acidulating the urine with acetic acid, and then adding a solution of ferrocyanuret of potassium. If albumen be present, it is thus immediately thrown down; whereas in the other case, if acetic acid produce a slight turbidity, this will not be increased by the addition of the ferrocyanuret of potassium. Lastly, no precipitate is occasioned by boiling, and the urine of persons taking copaiba or cubebs evolves, when first passed, the strong odor of those drugs.

But it sometimes happens that albumen is present, and yet is not precipitated on boiling; this happens whenever the urine is alkaline, the albumen being kept in solution by the alkali. In this case it is necessary first to acidify the urine with nitric acid, and then to boil. But nitric acid in excess precipitates albumen from the urine as well as heat. It is, therefore, best in most cases, to test both with nitric acid and heat, and it is always proper to ascertain whether the precipitate which appears on boiling is soluble in excess of nitric acid or not.

In employing nitric acid, the reagent should be added in excess, as it sometimes happens that the albumen first thrown down is redissolved; but when an excess of the acid is used, the albumen is thrown down permanently, and is not redissolved.

Dr. Bence Jones has stated, that he has found a few drops of a mixture of one part of nitric to three of hydrochloric acid much more decided in its effects, and much more delicate in its indications, than pure nitric acid. This is explained in the evolution of chlorine gas by the extraction of the hydrogen of the hydrochloric acid, one of the most delicate precipitants of the protein compounds being thus set free. But this test, like the ferro-cyanide of potassium test, has the property of precipitating other protein compounds besides albumen, as mucus, etc.

The quantity of albumen in urine varies greatly, from a mere trace to some grains to the ounce; and according to the quantity present, so varies the appearance of the urine on the application of heat. If the quantity be very considerable, the urine will become almost white, and nearly solid; whereas, if it be very small, the deposit may be so trifling as altogether to escape detection, until the test-tube be set aside for some hours so as to allow of the subsidence of the deposit. In this way the presence of a very minute quantity of albumen will be detected. When but little more than a trace of albumen exists in the urine, it is best to take a very large test-tube, and to boil some five or six drachms of the urine.

Albumen is also precipitated by dilute hydrochloric acid, ferrocyanide of potassium, bichloride of mercury, alcohol, creasote, tannin, and many other substances. It is not precipitated, however, by phosphoric and acetic acids, which exert a solvent action upon it, nor by strong hydrochloric acid, with which, when warmed, it forms a purple-colored solution.

A remarkable substance allied to albumen has been detected in urine, by Dr. Bence Jones, in case of rickets. It differed from albumen by not being precipitated by either heat or nitric acid; but on boiling the urine, and allowing it to cool, a precipitate fell which redissolved on the application of heat. Alcohol added to the urine readily coagulated this substance.

Determination of Chyle.—Urine containing chyle is usually more milky and opalescent than when it contains only oil. In chylous urine ex-amined microscopically and chemically, all the usual elements of chyle will ordinarily be detected, as oil, albumen, and granular organic corpuscles, resembling the white corpuscles of the blood. The albumen is to be de-tected after filtration of the urine by coagulation in the ordinary manner. The oil may, or may not, be visible under the microscope in the form of droplets; but if present it may always be obtained by agitation with ether; lastly, the granular corpuscles are distinguished from the flat globules by their size, granular texture, and by the action of acetic acid and ether upon them; by the first reagent, nuclei are disclosed in the corpuscles, while in ether they are insoluble, and thus distinguished from the fatty globules, for some of which they might be readily mistaken.

The milky appearance presented by chylous urine is occasioned partly by the oily matter and the granular corpuscles present, and partly by pre-cipitated albuminous, or more probably fibrinous matter. Chylous urine when first passed, and while still warm, does not usually present the same degree of opacity and milkiness which it acquires when it becomes cold. This depends on the solidification both of the fatty and fibrinous matters present. If the quantity of chyle present be very considerable, the urine will sometimes acquire a gelatinous or semi-solid consistence, owing to the coagulation of the fibrinous element.

In some of the cases of chylous urine which fell under the observation of Dr. Prout, the albumen did not coagulate on the application of heat, but it did when nitric acid was added, and hence he was led to consider that this albumen was in an imperfect state.

The proportion of fat present in chylous urine may be so great that it may interfere with the gelatinization of the spontaneously-coagulable albumen or fibrin, but as soon as the fat has been removed by means of ether, the solidification will in some cases, take place.

Determination of Fatty or Oily Matter.—Urine containing fatty or oily matter is usually, but not always, more or less turbid, and if the fat occur in connection with chylous matter, it will not only be turbid, but it will possess a whitish and milky appearance more or less marked. Usually when a drop of such urine, especially if it has been allowed to stand at rest for some time, and it be taken from the surface, is examined under the microscope, droplets or spherules of oil will be seen, which are readily distinguished by their strongly refractive properties, as well as by their solubility in ether.

Should the presence of fat be suspected, and no globules of oil be visible under the microscope, a portion of the urine should be agitated with ether, which will dissolve out any oily or fatty matter which may be present, and which may be obtained in a separate state on the evaporation of the ethereal solution.

That the substance thus contained consists really of fat is known by its greasy appearance, its insolubility in cold water, by its breaking up into droplets when agitated with hot water, and its solubility in ether.

It is not very often that a urine is met with containing only fat, for when this is present, it is usually derived from chyle, some of the constituents of which are generally present in the urine with it.

But minute quantities of fat may be present in urine, independent of chyle, as in certain forms of Bright's disease, and also without occasioning the slightest turbidity. In this case, the fatty matter is found in the cells and renal casts thrown off, and which have become deposited from the urine after it has stood for some hours.

The microscope affords the only means by which the presence of oily matter in connection with the renal cells and tubules can be ascertained.

In the Mauritius, fatty urine is epidemic, and it accompanies a peculiar form of irritative fever.

A peculiar kind of fatty matter, to which its discoverer, Dr. Florian Heller (Heller's Arch., 1844 and 1845), gave the name of *uro stealith*, has been detected in one instance in the urine. The patient, a weaver, twenty-four years of age, labored under all the symptoms of calculus, and passed some small concretions, which, on examination, were found to be composed of the peculiar fatty matter in question. These concretions possessed the following characters: When fresh, they were soft, becoming when dry, hard, yellow, wax-like, brittle, and amorphous, and presenting by transmitted light a greenish-yellow color. On the application of heat, they puffed up, inflamed, emitted a peculiar pungent odor, between that of shellac and benzoin, and left a voluminous ash. In hot water they softened, but did not dissolve; they were readily soluble in ether; the residue, on the evaporation of the ethereal solution, assumed a violet color. On the application of a gentle heat, nitric acid dissolved them with a slight effervescence, forming a colorless substance.

Determination of Fibrin.—Fibrin is distinguished from albumen by its undergoing solidification when effused from the blood-vessels. It usually occurs in the urine in connection with blood, but not always so. Sometimes it exudes from the blood-vessels of the kidneys, and solidifies in the renal tubules, in the form of casts. In other, but very rare cases, the effused fibrin does not solidify until after the urine has been voided.

When the fibrin solidifies in the kidneys, the casts are usually met with in the urine. Whenever, then, these casts are observed under the microscope, or the urine becomes at all gelatinous on cooling, and this whether it contain blood or not, fibrin is present.

Now, almost constantly, albumen is voided at the same time with the fibrin; whenever, therefore, the latter is present in the urine, the former is almost sure to be found.

There is a form of deposit of frequent occurrence in the urine, and which, since it bears much resemblance to a renal cast, may here be noticed. It consists of long threads of very variable diameter but which are all more or less striated, showing that they are made up of fibrillæ of fibrin. They are met with in abundance in urines depositing oxalate of lime; also in those containing excess of earthy phosphates and mucus, or which contain semen; besides, wherever irritation of the bladder from any cause exists, and as an evidence of which irritation they are to be regarded. They are found alike in the urine of men and women.

Determination of Keistein.—Another substance of great interest, met with in the urine of pregnant women, and with the characters of which it is necessary to become acquainted, is that known by the names of keistein and gravidine.

After the urine of a pregnant woman has been exposed to the air in a cylindrical glass vessel for two or three days (and never later than the sixth day), a fatty looking pellicle forms upon the surface, which at the end of two or three days, when the urine is becoming alkaline, gradually breaks up, and falls to the bottom as a sediment, frequently evolving at this stage a powerful odor of cheese.

This scum or pellicle, viewed under the microscope, is seen to be constituted of three distinct elements, and to consist of a granular base in which are imbedded well-defined crystals of the ammonio-magnesian phosphate, and droplets of oil. The only essential and distinctive constituent of keistein is therefore the granular matrix. This is not acted upon by acetic acid, but is dissolved by ammonia, and this it is that evolves during decomposition the cheesy odor above referred to. When this scum is collected in any quantity, it presents a greasy and opaque appearance, resembling spermaceti, arising partly from the large quantity of triple phosphate present.

The triple phosphate may be dissolved out by means of acetic acid, and the oil by ether; the cheese-like substance being left behind.

The scum of keistein is distinguished from the ordinary phosphatic crust or scum, not only by the presence of oil and the casein or cheesy substance, but also by its not remaining on the surface beyond three or four days from its complete formation.

The urines on which keistein is formed rarely become turbid on boiling, or throw down any deposit on the addition of nitric or acetic acid, showing the absence of albumen but not necessarily that of casein, since this would not be precipitated by acetic acid unless it were present in large amount.

Determination of Blood.—When blood is contained in urine in amount at all considerable, its presence is sufficiently indicated by the eye alone. The urine will be observed to possess a reddish color, and if it be set aside for some time, a reddish or rust-colored precipitate will subside, the presence of which is so peculiar that it cannot be confounded with any other colored deposits which occur in the urine, as uric acid and the urates.

Moreover, if the quantity of blood be very considerable, the urine will become more or less gelatinous, and if a portion of it be boiled, it will be found to abound in albumen.

When the quantity of blood is very minute, the microscope affords the only ready and certain means of determining its presence. By this instrument, if the urine be fresh, the presence of the red and white corpuscles of the blood will be revealed in any sediment from urine which has been allowed to remain at rest a sufficient time. If the hemorrhage proceed from the kidneys, casts, containing blood corpuscles, are sometimes met with.

Determination of Bile.—When bile is contained in urine in considerable quantity, its presence is sufficiently indicated by the color of the urine; this is especially the case in jaundice, in which the urine usually possesses a dark-yellowish green or brown color, which is exceedingly characteristic.

When the quantity of biliary matter in the urine is less, the tint of the urine is only deepened and rendered of a brown or reddish hue. When this is the case, it becomes necessary to seek for the presence of bile, for which there are several tests.

One of these is Pettenkofer's test, which consists of sulphuric acid, free from sulphurous acid, and sugar. It is used as follows:

To a small quantity of the urine, in a test-tube, about two-thirds of the bulk of sulphuric acid is to be added, drop by drop, so that the temperature of the mixture may not be raised above 144° Fahr., at which the color characteristic of bile is destroyed.

To this mixture a grain or two of sugar or sirup is to be added, the whole shaken, and then allowed to stand at rest a few minutes. Should bile be present, the liquid will have assumed a more or less intense red color with a tinge of violet. This remarkable development of color is not due to any change effected in the coloring matter of the bile, since it takes place equally when the above reagents are added to a solution of decolorized bile.

Should the suspected urine contain albumen, this should be first removed by coagulation and filtration, because with albumen and sulphuric acid and sugar a nearly similar color is developed.

If the quantity of bile present be very small, the urine should be evaporated to dryness on a water-bath before the test is tried, and the bile dissolved out either by means of a little water or alcohol.

Another test for bile is that commonly known as Heller's test, which is thus employed:

A little white of egg is added to a small quantity of the suspected urine, and after the mixture has been well shaken, a few drops of nitric acid; this causes the precipitation of the albumen, in combination with some of the coloring matter of the bile, the precipitated albumen thereby assuming a dull-green or bluish color.

When the quantity of bile is very small, the urine should be evaporated as before, and the albumen added to the aqueous solution.

A third test for bile in urine depends upon the action of nitric acid upon the brown coloring matter of the bile, called biliphœin. Two or three drops of nitric acid are to be allowed to fall upon a little of the urine spread out in a thin layer on a white surface. When bile is present in amount at all considerable, the mixture assumes a variety of changing and evanescent tints, green, violet, yellow, and pink, the latter color usually predominating. As in the case of the previously described tests, should the quantity of bile present be very small, the urine must be evaporated before the nitric acid is added.

According to the late Dr. Golding Bird, it occasionally happens that bile exists in urine in a modified, and, perhaps, oxydized state, in which it does not exhibit, with the tests above noticed, the characteristic reactions, the urine becoming merely imperfectly reddened. Ammonia, Dr. Bird states, then becomes a valuable test, it immediately producing a deep red color. There are certain fallacies attending the ammonia test, arising chiefly from the presence of vegetable coloring matters in the urine, as those of rhubarb and senna, and on which ammonia acts in a nearly similar manner.

Lastly, there is the microscopic test, which has already been described, for bile when present in urine in small quantities.

Detection of Seminal Fluid.—In some cases a mucus-like deposit occurs in urine, which, on examination with the microscope, turns out to be semen; this is shown by the presence of the well-known seminal animalcules and corpuscles. The animalcules are nearly always dead, owing, perhaps, partly to the length of time which usually elapses before the urine is examined, and partly to the injurious action exerted upon them by the urine itself. Spermatic animalcules are occasionally seen in urine in small number where there is no visible deposit.

Mixed up with the spermatozoa, octahedral crystals of oxalate of lime are frequently noticed. Some observers have gone so far as to state that whenever these crystals occur in urine, spermatic fluid is always present, a statement which is certainly erroneous. *Part* xxxvii., *p.* 91.

Mode of detecting Sugar in the Urine.—Dr. A. Becquerel, physician at the Hospital of La Pitié, in a series of lectures, pointed out the following facts: "First, that nearly all urines become discolored, impart a green color to, and even precipitate the cupro-potass solution of Barreswill, or that of Frommerz, if heated with these reagents. Second, that a great number of these same urines become brown, in like manner, on the addition of caustic potass, however pure that may be."

He strongly insisted on the erroneous conclusions to which the reaction afforded by these tests might lead, and showed that nothing is more easy than to avoid this source of error, and that there is at our disposal a much more sure, expeditious, and certain method of detecting the presence of sugar in the urine than is usually employed.

"We take a certain determinate quantity of urine, say 60 grs.; this we treat with a small quantity of solid and crystallized acetate of lead, say 4 grs.; on heating this mixture, there is immediately formed a copious precipitate of a dirty white color; the liquor is then to be filtered, and the solution treated by sulphate of soda in excess. If, for example, we have added four grs. of acetate of lead, we add eight grs. of sulphate of soda. This being done, the mixture is again heated, and sulphate of lead is deposited; we then filter once more, and there is afforded a clear transparent liquid, which contains the sugar, when there is any, and some unimportant salts. The liquid thus obtained is neither acted on by the cupro-potass reagents, nor browned by the caustic potass, *unless* sugar is present. These two re-agents are in this way perfectly reliable, very accurate, and afford no results when no sugar is contained.

" Should the urine under examination contain albumen, it is immediately coagulated by the acetate of lead at the same time as other organic matters, and gives no further trouble.

" Thus, in all cases where it is desired to ascertain the existence of sugar in the urine, whether along with albumen or not, we possess two excellent reagents in the cupro-potass solution, and in the caustic potass itself; only we require, in the first place, to treat the urine with the acetate of lead and the sulphate of soda, by which means we get rid of all such matters as decompose or discolor the cupro-potass or caustic potass tests." *Part* xxxvii., *p.*104.

--- ◦ ◦ ◦ ---

UTERINE HEMORRHAGE.

Oil of Ergot of Rye.—Diffused through water, recommended by Dr. Samuel Wright to be injected into the uterus in *severe cases of flooding.*
Part ii., *p.* 42.

Modes of Arresting Uterine Hemorrhage.—[Dr. W. Tyler Smith treats this subject under several heads. He speaks first of]

The Different Modes of exciting Reflex Contraction of the Uterus in Uterine Hemorrhage.—Reflex contractions may be excited by stimuli applied to certain organs at a distance from the uterus; by stimuli applied to certain other organs and surfaces in the vicinity of the uterus; and lastly, by stimuli applied to the uterus itself.

[Under the first division Dr. Smith mentions as excitors of contraction, the *mammary nerves* (called into exercise when the child is put to the breast,) the *pneumogastric* (when food, hot or cold drinks, or emetics are taken into the stomach,) and the *abdominal intercostal nerves.* Respecting the latter, he says:]

The cutaneous nerves of the abdominal parietes are excitors of the uterus in an extraordinary degree. The sudden impression of cold or heat upon the abdominal surface will almost always excite the most energetic contraction of the uterus affected with inertia, and from which hemorrhage is taking place. We may contract the relaxed and diffuse uterus to a firm ball, by douching the abdomen with cold water from a height; or by plashing a towel, taken out of cold water, upon the naked abdomen ; or by suddenly placing the hand, taken out of iced water, upon the umbilicus. If the surface of the abdomen should be cold, the sudden impression of heat produces a similar contraction.

About the true mode of action of irritation of the mammary and pneumogastric, and the abdominal intercostal nerves, there can be no doubt whatever. These nerves are too remote from the uterus, in their peripheral extremities, to admit of any other explanation save that of the reflex function.

[Under the second division, or organs and surfaces in the vicinity of the uterus, Dr. Smith refers to irritation of the *vulval, vaginal, vesical,* and *rectal* nerves, induced by the application of cold to those parts. He says :]

This group of organs, it will be observed, is in the immediate vicinity of the organ from which the blood flows, and they are in great measure supplied by nerves having the same origin as the uterine nerves. But what I wish to insist upon is this, that all the actions I have been describing are *reflex* in their nature. Physiology repudiates the idea of uterine contractions, excited by means of continuity or contiguity of the organs excited with the organ which contracts. The peripheries of the nerves of the bladder, rectum, vulva, and vagina, receive the impression, and the incident nerves, the spinal centre, and the motor nerves of the uterus distributed to its muscular structure, are all concerned in the muscular contraction which ensues. Though the organs excited are near the uterus, which contracts, the route of the nervous action is precisely the same as it was in the case of the stimuli applied to the mammary or the pneumogastric nerve.

I now come to the consideration of the contraction of the uterus, and the arrest of hemorrhage by irritation of the uterus itself, through the medium of stimuli applied to

The Uterine Nerves.—The power we possess over the uterus by this means is very great indeed, and the modes by which we can exert it are very various. We may excite the nerves of the external surface of the uterus, the nerves of the internal surface, or the nerves of the os uteri. When we produce uterine contractions by irritating the uterus through the abdominal surface, we act on the first series of nerves; when we inject cold water into the uterine cavity, we act on the second, and when we irritate the os uteri by digitation, we act on the third. These measures are of great importance in our attempts to rouse the uterus itself to action. We may excite the organ by introducing ice into the cavity, by injecting cold water into the cavity, or by injecting stimulating solutions.

Besides digital irritation of the uterus through the abdominal parietes, there is another external mode of inducing uterine reflex action, in the use of the abdominal bandage. The compression of the uterus thus occasioned, increases uterine action, or evokes it when it has disappeared; it is certainly one of the best means we have of preventing that inertia of the uterus after delivery which so strongly tends to hemorrhage.

The introduction of the hand into the uterus, or the irritation of the os uteri by the fingers, or the whole hand, excites the uterus very powerfully. Besides the mere introduction of the hand, irritation of the internal surface of the organ by the tips of the fingers is sometimes practised.

The different modes of exciting direct or centric Spinal Contractions of the Uterus, in Uterine Hemorrhage.—If we administer a dose of the ergot of rye to a patient suffering from hemorrhage, we observe in many cases that uterine contraction will follow. I have no doubt that the true channel through which the ergot acts is the blood, and the organ it reaches and affects, through this channel, is the spinal centre. We may illustrate its *modus operandi* by referring to the action of emetic substances on the stomach. There are certain substances which, when taken into the stomach, immediately excite all the motor actions of vomiting. This happens, for instance, when sulphate of zinc comes into contact with the mucous membrane of the stomach. Sulphate of zinc, then, appears to excite the actions of vomiting in a reflex form. But again, in the case of the stomach, there are other medicines—the potassio-tartrate of antimony, for instance, which acts as an emetic only after it has been taken into the circulation, and which acts more promptly when injected into the blood itself. I believe the action of this medicine to be perfectly analogous to the action of the ergot of rye; that the one acts upon the medulla oblongata and the motor nerves of vomiting; the other, upon the lower medulla spinalis, and the motor nerves of uterine action. The ergot, therefore, is a remedy of centric utero-spinal action.

Ipecacuanha is another medicine which is sometimes given in uterine hemorrhage. This medicine, by its emetic action, excites contraction of the abdominal muscles, and compression of the uterus, which in turn may re-excite some amount of uterine reflex action, but over and beyond this it appears to have a special action upon the uterus, increasing its contractile power beyond what we could imagine to occur from the merely secondary effects of vomiting. Ipecacuanha, then, appears to influence both the medulla oblongata and the lower medulla spinalis.

Opium is also, in hemorrhage, a remedy of direct spinal action. In moderate loss of blood it undoubtedly promotes uterine contraction, and arrests the flow of blood. Opium is an excitant of spinal action of the direct kind, and thus it is that its administration is beneficial in hemorrhage, with uterine inertia, and injurious in puerperal convulsion, of the active kind. As a minor remedy of the same spinal relations as the foregoing, the biborate of soda may be mentioned. It may be said, briefly, that all stimulants taken into the stomach and received into the blood have a centric spinal action in hemorrhage from the uterus. But one of the most important agencies of a centric kind, and one different in its nature from the foregoing, consists in the influence of emotion. Where sensibility is present, the influence of emotion comes in aid of the reflex action. It is only the hopeful and confident emotions which excite muscular contraction. The depressing passions paralyze the uterus as well as other muscles, and they are, in truth, not unimportant as causes of hemorrhage.

[Dr. Smith next speaks of "the different modes of exciting uterine action by stimulating the muscular irritability of the organ," as distinguished from the excitement of muscular action through the nerves. He mentions three methods by which this is performed: the application of cold, mechanical irritation with the hand, and the use of galvanism. With regard to the latter, he says:]

In patients perfectly paraplegic, with entire loss of reflex uterine power, the uterus has been excited to contractions sufficient to expel the foetus by means of galvanism. Dr. Radford, of Manchester, applied this power to the arrest of uterine hemorrhage. One pole of a galvanic trough being placed within the os uteri, and the other applied over the fundus, it has been found, that, on making and breaking the galvanic circle, powerful uterine contractions occur.

The Different Modes of arresting Uterine Hemorrhage mechanically.—There are various modes of compressing the uterus mechanically, which are resorted to in cases of hemorrhage. One mode is that of grasping the uterus through the abdominal parietes, and holding the organ so firmly as to prevent the further effusion of blood, while other means are being applied to insure the permanent contraction of the organ. Another mode sometimes followed is that of introducing one hand into the uterus, and then exerting pressure with the other hand externally, so as to compress the bleeding portion of the organ between the two hands. A third mode of mechanical arrest, and one which is exceedingly useful, consists in the abdominal bandage, made to embrace the pelvis tightly, and having several towels or napkins folded into a conical shape placed underneath.

Compression of the aorta, so as to cut off the supply of blood to the uterus, and prevent arterial hemorrhage, has been insisted on by Baron Dubois, M. Chailly, and others. Several years ago, I pointed out that the directions given by obstetricians were wrong, and that we should make pressure upon the inferior cava instead of the aorta. The great hemorrhages, those which kill, are from the veins, and not from the arteries, and further, not from the veins which are returning blood from the uterus, but from the vena cava and the heart itself. When the uterine veins are open, there is a great column of blood between the uterus and the right auricle, to the sudden escape of which there is no let or hindrance except uterine contraction. The compression of the great vessels is, however, at best palliative, not curative, but it may give time for the application of other remedies.

The various forms of plugging the vagina and the uterus are a distinct class of obstetric remedies in hemorrhage. Mechanical plugging is extremely useful in hemorrhage in many forms of abortion, in certain hemorrhages during delivery, and in cases of placenta prævia. The sponge or linen plug is useful in moderate floodings of the impregnated, and also of the unimpregnated uterus. This form of plug, when it fills the whole of the vagina, acts by preventing the escape of blood externally; this favors the coagulation of the blood effused behind the plug, and though the plug itself does not reach to the bleeding surface, the coagulated blood is converted into a secondary plug, which acts directly upon the mouths of the bleeding vessels. But beside the common form of tampon, we often convert the fœtus itself into a plug, having precisely the same mechanical action. Thus when, in hemorrhage before delivery, we rupture the membranes, beside the other results, the body and limbs of the fœtus come into direct contact with hemorrhagic tissue. So in placenta previa, when the presentation is allowed to remain, but the placenta is torn away, the fœtal head becomes in effect a tampon to the os and cervix uteri of the most powerful kind. Again, when turning is performed in these cases, the feet are brought down, and engaged in the os uteri as a plug. These instances only differ from the plug of sponge or linen in their being more effective, and in being applied from within instead of from without. After delivery, no form of plugging can be of much service.

The arrest of Uterine Hemorrhage by Astringents and Refrigerants.—These remedies, consisting of the acetate of lead, the mineral acids, alum given internally, and used in the form of injection, the sustained application of local cold, etc., are useful in all hemorrhages which do not proceed from patulous vessels sufficiently large to require the contraction of the muscular organ in order to close them, or when the uterus is so far undeveloped as to render its muscular contraction impossible. Such are hemorrhages occurring in the course of uterine disease, or in menorrhagia; uterine floodings in the early months of pregnancy, and the profuse lochial discharges which sometimes occur a few days after delivery, when the uterus has become perfectly contracted.   *Part* xix., *p.* 237.

Principle of Treatment by Cold in Uterine Hemorrhage.—Dr. Gooch mentions the case of a lady that he attended, in whom, both before and at the time of labor, the force of the circulation was very great; " she was flushed and had a quick pulse." After delivery, she had a most violent flooding; and Gooch remarks that, " after the violence of the hemorrhage was over, although the abdomen was covered with pounded ice, it returned again and again, slightly in degree, yet sufficiently, in the debilitated state of the patient, to produce alarming occurrences of faintness; the uterus, too, which had become firm and distinct, became so soft, it could no longer be felt. Finding the ice so inefficient, I swept it off, and taking a ewer of cold water, I let its contents fall from a height of several feet upon the belly; the effect was instantaneous; the uterus, which, the moment before had been so soft and indistinct as not to be felt within the abdomen, became small and hard, the bleeding stopped, and the faintness ceased—a striking proof of this important principle, that cold applied with a shock is a more powerful means of producing contraction of the uterus than a greater degree of cold without the shock." *Part* xix., *p.* 246.

Accidental Hemorrhage.—Prof. Murphy, of London University College, says: *The treatment* must be prompt and decisive. Accidental hemorrhage usually occurs in the first stage of labor, when the membranes are unbroken, and the liquor amnii prevents the uterus contracting about the body of the child. In order, therefore, to control flooding, the uterus should be made to contract as much as possible, and coagulation promoted in the spongy structure of the placenta; both objects are accomplished by rupturing the membranes, because the uterus contracts on the body of the child, and the placenta being compressed between both, the blood is prevented escaping so freely from its uterine surface. This effect may be rendered more perfect by using means to increase the tonic contraction of the uterus, which rupturing the membranes alone will not always accomplish. Therefore, ergot of rye, or the electric current, may be used; a drachm of the former infused in a wine-glass of water, may be given alone, or, what is better, in combination with opium. Thirty or forty minims of tincture of opium may be added to the infusion, and in proportion as exhaustion increases, larger doses of opium may be repeated. When you wish the aid of the electric current, the electro-magnetic apparatus should be employed, and currents passed either transversely or in the longitudinal axis of the uterus; rods, holding sponges moistened in a saline solution, are connected by wires to the apparatus, and may be applied to any part of the abdomen; a sponge may be introduced within the vagina, and connected in the same manner with the battery; by these means currents may be made to pass in any direction. The only objection to this mode of exciting the uterus is the delay which might arise in preparing the instrument.

Turning was formerly a universal practice in cases of accidental hemorrhage. It is now very rarely resorted to, and Dr. Murphy thinks it will very seldom be found necessary. *Stimulants* must be given even largely, and if all means fail, transfusion may be cautiously resorted to.

Part xix., *p.* 248.

Post-partum Hemorrhage.—Post-partum hemorrhage may occur either before or after the expulsion of the placenta. In the former case, its causes are three, inertia of the uterus, irregular contractions of the uterine fibres, and morbid adhesion of the placenta. Professor Murphy observes:

Inertia of the uterus is equally the cause and the effect of hemorrhage. You should be careful to recognize true inertia as soon as it presents itself; you may do so before any hemorrhage takes place, even when the child is being expelled. The fundus of the uterus has not its usual firm

VOL. II.—51

feel under the hand ; it seems spongy or like dough, and is larger than it ought to be, because it very seldom contracts to its full extent. After the delivery of the child, when the uterus generally remains contracted, it will not do so. You may have followed the contracting uterus with the hand, moderately compressing it, and in a short time you find that it has eluded your grasp, and cannot be felt. Strong frictions over the lower part of the abdomen may again excite its action ; but it is only for a moment— again it is lost. While this want of tone may be observed in the uterus, a corresponding amount of constitutional irritation may be noticed in the patient. The pulse is increased in frequency, and assumes the jerking hemorrhagic character ; the patient is watchful and restless ; complains of sinking, and does not experience that relief from the termination of her sufferings that is usual after delivery. All these symptoms may precede any hemorrhage, and should be most carefully watched ; they are the monitors of what is approaching. Hemorrhage generally begins with a slight draining from the vulva, just sufficient to soil the napkins that are applied, but in a short time, if no means for prevention are used, the stream rapidly increases to a torrent, deluging the bed, and forming a pool on the floor beneath. If the attendant is not on his guard, this may be the first notice of danger, because the patient is sometimes too much exhausted to give any intimation of her condition ; she lies on her side in a listless, dosy state ; syncope may follow, and hemorrhage for a moment cease, but it soon returns with the pulse, a violent gush of blood places the patient at once "in extremis;" a more prolonged syncope returns, from which she may never recover. Sometimes a fit of convulsions precedes dissolution.

The treatment of such cases must be direct : 1st. To restore the tonic contractile power of the uterus. 2d. To remove the placenta. 3d. To prevent, as far as possible, any subsequent relaxation of the uterus.

In order to accomplish the first object, you must endeavor, by every means in your power, to support the general circulation, which every symptom points out to you is struggling to maintain itself.

If there be great exhaustion, the patient should be given a drachm of tinct. of opium in brandy ; this may be repeated in more moderate doses, until the pulse becomes steady. If the stomach be very irritable, and reject this, it will sometimes bear broth when taken cold, and morphia may be substituted for tincture of opium. Smellie used to give potable soups, dissolved in water. The patient should be kept in a perfectly horizontal position. The arms and legs should be wrapped in hot flannels, the curtains drawn back, the window raised, and a free circulation of air secured in the apartment. Locally, every means must be employed to retard the force of the circulation in the uterus. The most convenient mode, I think, is to have a bucket containing flannels, over which may be thrown lumps of ice, and a sufficient quantity of water poured over the whole. These flannels may be wrung out, and applied from time to time to the hips and vulva. At the same time that these means are being carried into effect, the strongest pressure should be maintained on the fundus uteri, to prevent its relaxation. The success of your treatment becomes evident when you feel the fundus first become distinct, and then more firm, under the hand. In many cases the pressure is sufficient to cause the expulsion of the afterbirth, but if not, it becomes your duty, in this favorable opportunity,

2dly. To remove the placenta.—For this purpose, let one hand still compress the fundus, or assign this duty to an assistant, clearly explaining what is to be done, and then pass the hand into the vagina to the os uteri; sometimes, by drawing down the band again slowly, the back of it being pressed strongly against the posterior wall of the vagina and the perineum, the uterus is excited to contract and expel the placenta into the vagina, from whence it may be removed.

If not, draw down the funis to its full extent, as far as it will go, and let the hand in the vagina, guided by it, press forward into the uterus. The fingers formed into a cone will readily dilate the os uteri sufficiently to admit the hand; and here, again, it sometimes happens that the act of dilatation will excite a sufficient contraction to expel the placenta; if not, you must proceed; but, as a precaution, it would be well to give the patient a full dose of opium previous to entering the cavity of the uterus; when the placenta is reached, do not at once seize it in order to draw it down, rather seek to pass the hand above it, toward the surface of the cavity of the uterus. This portion of the uterus is now placed between the introduced hand and that which compresses it externally through the abdomen; by increasing this pressure, the irritation very seldom fails in causing the uterus to contract; the moment this is observed, let the hand be slowly withdrawn, having the whole placenta within it, and let a strong pressure be made on the fundus uteri externally. Thus, the placenta may be safely withdrawn, and if the uterus be properly secured, no further hemorrhage will take place. Our next object is, therefore, to do this, and

3dly. *To prevent, as far as possible, any subsequent relaxation.*—It is necessary to press very firmly with both hands on the fundus, and to continue this pressure for some time; if fatigued, an assistant may continue it; but you must be particularly careful that he understands your object. In order to insure this effect, by the continuance of the pressure, the abdomen must be very carefully bandaged.

Hemorrhage after the separation of the placenta may depend upon inertia of the uterus, an over-excited circulation in a plethoric patient, or upon mismanagement. The last is by far the most frequent cause; the patient may be too soon disturbed after her delivery, for the purpose of changing the dress or bed-clothes, or her friends may keep her in a constant state of excitement by their kind, but too officious, congratulations. The result is flooding. Again, if she escape these dangers immediately after delivery, your patient may be allowed perhaps on the third or fourth day to get out of bed; the circulation is again excited in the uterus, still very large and easily distended, and hemorrhage is the consequence. You are not even safe on the tenth or fourteenth day. One of the most alarming hemorrhages I ever had to treat occurred on the tenth day after delivery.

Part xix., *p.* 254.

Method of plugging the Vagina with a Caoutchouc Bladder.—M. Diday, having a case of *metrorrhagia*, in which the patient had become reduced to almost the lowest point of exhaustion, resolved to avail himself of one of Dr. Gariel's ingenious applications of vulcanized caoutchouc. The apparatus consists of a small bladder of caoutchouc, to which is attached a long tube. Rolled up so as not to exceed the little finger in size, it was passed as deeply into the vagina as possible, and kept there by the end of the finger; it was then inflated through the tube, until the small body, which had been introduced almost imperceptibly, acquired a volume constituting a sphere of about 33 centimetres in diameter. The air **was** retained by tying the tube. No means of retaining it *in situ* were required, and the hemorrhage entirely ceasing, it was removed sixty-four hours after, as easily as introduced, by allowing the air to escape through the tube. *Part* xxi., *p.* 202.

Uterine Hemorrhage.—In a most dangerous case of this nature, Dr. Sweeting gave five grains of acetate of lead every hour for forty-eight hours. As the hemorrhage returned on the suspension of the medicine, the same dose was given every four hours, and continued for a fortnight with complete recovery; the patient having taken in sixteen consecutive days 576 grains. *Part* xxiv., *p.* 114.

Indian Hemp.—Dr. Christison considers Indian hemp exceedingly valuable in restraining uterine hemorrhage. The tincture of the hemp is the most efficacious preparation; it may be given in doses of five to fifteen or twenty minims, three times a day in water. *Part* xxiv., *p.* 321.

Post-partum Hemorrhage.—Dr. Thos. Elliott recommends the following plan of treatment with a view of inducing uterine contraction, it being, in his experience, an " unfailing remedy."

Inject into the rectum 4 oz. of turpentine, 4 oz. of cold water, and a handful of common salt, forcibly retaining this by pressure from a folded napkin, until violent tenesmus is induced; this will invariably be attended with contraction of the womb. Turpentine is used because it is a powerful stimulant and restorative to the whole system, and, moreover, possesses considerable anti-hemorrhagic properties. *Part* xxxvii., *p.* 205.

Opium in Uterine Hemorrhage.—Dr. Gabb, of Bewdley, states that opium has a very different effect in large and in moderate doses on the uterus. In large doses it relaxes and favors hemorrhage; in small or moderate doses, as 25 minims, it stimulates and causes contraction. It is especially applicable in cases of deficient power from exhaustion or fatigue, being here, perhaps, the best remedy which can be employed.

Utility of Galvanism in accidental Hemorrhage.—Dr. Stafford, of Birmingham Lying-in Hospital, recommends, if you have a case of accidental hemorrhage during labor, and the os be pretty well dilated, to apply galvanism to the abdomen, which will probably soon bring on uterine contractions, and the head of the child will descend low enough to admit of the forceps being applied. This is especially valuable, as in these cases ergot of rye often entirely fails to induce contraction.

Part xxxvii., *p.* 208.

Post-partum Hemorrhage.—Dr. W. Thomas, F. R. C. S., says: In these alarming and dangerous cases, where the countenance is blanched and the pulse imperceptible, do not, as is too often taught, hesitate to give stimulants freely; their revivifying influence once seen can hardly be forgotten. The great thing to stop the hemorrhage is to empty the uterus; introduce the hand at once and remove the placenta, keeping up the pressure externally with the other hand; this should always be done half an hour after delivery, if the placenta be not then expelled.

Part xxxviii., *p.* 210

Hemorrhage from Carcinoma Uteri.—In cauliflower excrescence of the uterus, says Prof. Simpson, the hemorrhage is occasionally most violent and alarming. Simply plugging the vagina does not suffice to check ιt, and the use of some powerful styptic means becomes necessary. Of these the simplest and surest is the perchloride of iron dissolved in glycerine. It may be applied by a sponge or piece of lint. Tannin also is very useful; it may be applied in the form of a medicated pessary; it rapidly coagulates the effused blood, and thus prevents the further flow.

Part xl., *p.* 234.

—•••—

UTERUS.

Diagnosis of Diseases of the Uterus—Simpson's Uterine Sound.—To assist in the diagnosis of diseases of the womb and its appendages, Dr. Simpson has been in the habit of using a metallic *uterine sound* or *bougie*, of nearly the size and shape of a small male catheter, which is to be introduced into the womb and manipulated in the way which we will describe.

In diseases of these parts, we have only been able hitherto to extend our physical examination to the neck and lower portion of the body. If the womb were very large, we might, perhaps, feel the fundus through the walls of the abdomen, but from its mobility and low situation, this would be of little service; in short, we are constantly in doubt when examining any tumor in this region, whether it be an enlargement of the whole mass of the womb or a distention of its cavity, or a morbid growth; and, if the latter, whether the growth be seated in the womb itself, or in one of the ovaries or other neighboring parts.

It is particularly useful when we want to ascertain the state of the fundus, body, and cavity of the womb, and also when any particular solid tumor or fluid cyst is connected with that organ. It is provided, like the common male sound, with a flat handle, and terminates in a rounded knob or bulb. Its stem is thicker at its upper part, and tapers gradually from the knob to the handle. By being thin next the handle, it allows of more extensive movement in the mouth and neck of the womb, and its increased thickness at the other end gives it strength. The stem is about nine inches long, and graduated so as to enable us to measure the depth of the parts. In introducing this bougie, the patient may be placed on her back or left side, and having felt the os uteri, the practitioner can easily glide the instrument into the womb, the internal surface of which, when in a healthy state, is not more sensible than that of the vagina, so that when any severe pain is felt, it may be considered as indicative of some morbid condition. When the instrument is in the womb, the practitioner can give that organ sufficient resistance for its exploration by the fingers, and he can alter its position as he pleases. He can thus fix the fundus, and even move it about, so as to enable him, with his other hand on the abdomen, to examine its external surface and walls, and to ascertain what connections any other tumor may have with it. The great mobility of the uterus is well known. Its position is changed by many of the movements of the bladder and rectum; it may be drawn down by instruments till the cervix reach the external parts; and therefore the uterine sound will enable us to move it about in rather a startling manner. The instrument being metallic, can be bent to any shape, so that when we want to bring the fundus uteri more immediately under our fingers in our hypogastric examinations, the extremity should be bent upon its stem at as nearly a right angle as the conformation of the genital canals admit, and, after being introduced, its handle should be well retracted toward the perineum. By this proceeding, the body and fundus of the womb will be more easily and fully turned forward.

This mode of examination will also be particularly valuable in the early stages of ovarian tumors. The ovary lies behind the womb, so that if the sound shows the tumor to lie on the *anterior* surface of the uterus, or, in other words, if the uterine cavity runs up the posterior surface of the morbid mass, the disease may be considered as certainly not ovarian. This remark will only apply to those cases in which the tumor is still not so large as to have passed out of the pelvic cavity and become abdominal.

Part viii., *p.* 106.

Excision of the Os Uteri.—[Excision of the os uteri was, on account of the marvellous cures said to have been frequently performed by it, in cases of cancer of the uterus, very slow in establishing itself as a legitimate practice in this country. Cancer of the uterus is in reality of very rare occurrence, and removal of the diseased part presents even less chance of recovery than of any other part in which this disease may exist. Cauliflower excrescence, as Dr. Clarke named it, is, however, very much more common than was formerly supposed, and it has been ascertained that the removal of this by the knife or scissors, is an operation perfectly safe and effectual. Dr. Clarke, when he wrote, had little to offer as regards treatment.]

Professor Syme says: A great step in advance has been made through the establishment of the important fact—for which we are chiefly indebted to the surgeons of France—that excision of the os uteri, executed either by knives or scissors, is an operation perfectly safe and effectual when employed for the removal of growths not possessing a malignant disposition. In performing the operation, it is always desirable, and, in general, easily practicable, to draw the tumor fairly into view, so that the excision may be effected without taking away either more or less than what is requisite, and without injuring the neighboring parts. The most convenient instrument for this purpose is that which Dupuytren employed—the hooked forceps of Muzeux, who invented it for facilitating the removal of enlarged tonsils—or " vulsellum," as it has been improperly named by some writers.

By means of the double-hooked extremities of this instrument deeply inserted into the morbid growth toward its base, where the texture is of firmest consistence, the tumor may usually be induced by steady traction of moderate force, to descend and present itself to view, when a bistoury or curved scissors may be used without any difficulty or danger. The assistance of a speculum should be taken to insert the forceps, and if it seems necessary, in order to obtain complete command over the excrescence, additional instruments of the same kind are to be fixed into different parts of its substance. If the tumor cannot be made to protrude without resorting to an unsafe degree of violence, it may at all events be brought down in this way, so as to be within reach of the fingers, which will then form a safe guide for the scissors. The hemorrhage is seldom more than very trivial, and when at all considerable, may be suppressed by filling the vagina with lint. In a case which happened fourteen years ago, and was, I believe, the first of the kind subjected to operation in Edinburgh, I visited the patient about an hour after cutting off the excrescence, and to my no small alarm, found the blood dropping from her bed upon the floor. As there had been frequent and profuse hemorrhage from the disease, I considered it necessary to use the most efficient means for preventing any further flow, and therefore pulled the bleeding surface into view, transfixed its base with a needle, conveying a double ligature, and tied both the threads firmly. Recovery was accomplished without any untoward symptom.

In removing polypus of the uterus, evulsion, excision and ligature have been employed, and each of these modes of operation may be rendered the most eligible by peculiar circumstances of particular cases. But, in general, the combination of tying and cutting certainly seems to be the best plan of proceeding. It has the recommendation of facility, efficiency, and safety. It accurately determines the limit of destruction, prevents the possibility of hemorrhage, and relieves the patient from the fetor, and other unpleasant consequences, which attend the slow separation effected by ligature. Finally, it has the testimony of experience in its favor.

Part xii., *p.* 286.

Uterus—Diseases of.—Dr. Kennedy, of the Dublin Lying-in Hospital, directs, in first examinations, to use the *four-bladed speculum*. If the os is not readily caught, ascertain carefully its position with the finger, pass the instrument well up, and if, on withdrawing the plug, the os is not seen, withdraw the speculum slowly, expanding it at the same time.

When making applications in the os or the vagina, use Ferguson's glass speculum.

Congestion.—Apply three to six leeches *directly* to the uterus, or scarify, injecting warm water through the speculum for some time after. Repeat this several times, and then make a caustic issue over the pelvis or sacrum. Inject cold or tepid water into the vagina thrice a day; also mild astringent lotions. Give alteratives—Pullna water, sarza, iodine, pil. plum. and taraxacum. Be cautious about using tonics. If the menses are interrupted, use the hip-bath, and apply a few leeches to the uterus, at the period.

Chronic Catarrh.—Dilate the os internum by gutta percha bougies, and apply nitrate of silver by a porte-caustique, or nitrate of mercury by a camel-hair brush with a graduated handle introduced through a gum tube. After cauterizing three or four times, at intervals of eight or ten days, use, every three or four days, lotions of nitrate of silver or copper, ten grains to the ounce, and afterward milder lotions with lead or zinc. Apply leeches ; use counter-irritation by sinapisms, tartar-emetic ointment, or an issue ; and give cubebs, or mild tonics and alteratives.

Inflammation.—Use general and local depletion, antiphlogistic regimen, mercury and counter-irritation, the warm bath and soothing injections, and perfect quiet.

Ulceration—Mild.—If it is not easily detected, brush over with a ten grain solution of nitrate of silver, which will mark its outline ; then use, for ten days, a lotion with plumb. acet. gr. j. ad aq. dest. 3j. In applying lotions, lay the shoulders lower than the hips, and inject a continuous stream, for some minutes, by a " gum-elastic siphon."

Granular.—Get rid of or relieve the inflammation by depletion, etc., then apply caustic, at intervals of seven or ten days, three or four times, using in the interim mild astringent or emollient lotions, according to the symptoms.

Cock's Comb Ulcer.—Apply caustic more freely, using the nitrate of mercury, so as to form a slough.

Bleeding Ulcer.—Lay a piece of lint carefully round the margin of the ulcers, then apply caustic *freely;* apply it also to the interior of the uterus, if the lining membrane is diseased, taking care to have the caustic melted into a porte-caustique, to prevent its breaking ; afterward wash out the vagina with a stream of water. Continue the application at intervals, till the muco-purulent discharge ceases, and the mucous membrane ceases to bleed on being touched.

If aphtha appear when an ulcer is nearly healed, apply a stream of borax or weak nitrate of silver lotion.   *Part* xv., *p.* 283.

Ulceration of the Cervix Uteri in Virgins.—Dr. Henry Bennet has found that inflammatory affections of the os and cervix uteri do occur in the virgin, and that, too, not very unfrequently ; being a cause of those cases of severe dysmenorrhœa, and leucorrhœa, which so inveterately resist treatment.

[Dr. Bennet remarks that from what we know of the diseases of mucous membranes generally, we cannot suppose that a mere increase of secretion from the mucous membranes of the female genitals, should produce that excessive debility and anæmia which we frequently see accompanying it ; but we can readily understand that the assimilating processes should be affected by ulcerative inflammation in an organ with such extensive sympathetic affections as the uterus. Very marked general debility (in the absence of any decided cachexia) should lead us to suspect lesion of the cervix or os uteri—in this case, palliatives, as rest, injections, etc., may be tried ; but if they fail, or the case do not admit of delay, we must at once resort to a digital examination. Dr. Bennet observes, that,]

A satisfactorily digital examination of the uterus may be nearly always made in a virgin, without injury to the hymen, especially when the vagina and external genital organs have been relaxed by long continued congestion and inflammation. The hymen is nearly always sufficiently dilatable to admit the index, introduced slowly and with proper care. Generally speaking, the os and cervix are reached with ease, the cervix not being retroverted, as it is when inflamed in most married females ; and when once the finger has reached the os nearly all doubts may be solved. If the cervix is free from disease, it is soft, and the os is closed ; if it is inflamed and ulcerated, the cervix is enlarged, swollen, and the os is more or less open and fungous. This open and soft state of the os may also exist from mere inflammation of the cavity of the cervix.

If possible, we must introduce the speculum without dividing the hymen. The existence of the disease once ascertained, it is to be treated secundum artem.   *Part* xvi., *p.* 278.

Varicose Ulcer of the Os and Cervix Uteri.—Dr. Whitehead, of Manchester and Salford Lying-in Hospital, treats such cases as follows : Bleed from the arm, and cup, or apply leeches ; confine the patient strictly to the recumbent posture, and give three to five grains of calomel, with hyoscyamus or opium, followed by a saline aperient. Apply to the ulcer at first a strong solution of nitrate of silver, and afterward the solid caustic, and if there is much discharge of blood, apply strong solution of sulphate of zinc with vin. opii and tincture of matico. (Or gallic or tannic acid, in the form of solution or ointment.)   *Part* xvii., *p.* 259.

Preternatural Elongation of the Cervix Uteri.—Dr. Coley, of Pimlico Dispensary, says that at first, when consisting chiefly in passive congestion, it may be relieved by rest in the horizontal position, and the introduction of a soft sponge to support the parts, and the internal use of iodide of iron, or of mercury. But if permanent hypertrophy remains, excise the part; the operation is perfectly safe and easy, in the absence of specific disease.

Part xvii., *p.* 260.

Retroflexion of the Uterus.—In recent cases, replace the organ by the uterine sound, and let the woman lie for a length of time on the side or face: at the same time prevent accumulation in the rectum or bladder, and restore the tone of the parts by astringent injections. In more chronic cases, besides the above means, such treatment must be adopted as will relieve other co-existing disease, as congestion or chronic inflammation of the uterus or ovaries; and after the uterus has been restored to its position, it must be retained there by wearing one of Dr. Simpson's wire pessaries.—(Drs. Simpson, Beattie and Hensley.)

Dr. Braithwaite considers the best plan of proceeding, in the introduction of the sound or uterine pessary for retroflexion, is to place the female on her knees and elbows, with her face on a pillow. Then placing the forefinger of the left hand upon the os uteri, the point of the sound is very easily passed into the cervix, and by gently depressing the handle, as with the male catheter, the sound passes to the fundus uteri. *Part* xvii., *p.* 265.

Treatment of Ulceration of the Os and Cervix Uteri with Collodion.—Dr. Mitchell adopts the following method : The patient being placed upon her left side, and the speculum introduced, the ulcerated surface is to be wiped dry with a succession of pieces of soft lint until the adherent mucus is removed.; a camel's-hair pencil dipped in the solution is then to be rapidly applied to the ulcerated surface, and allowed to dry, which will occupy a couple of minutes—a second, third, and fourth coating, if necessary, can thus be applied ; the first coating is followed by a slight burning sensation caused by the ether, followed by a sensation of coldness from its evaporation. The application requires to be renewed at the end of forty-eight hours, as the secretion collects underneath the varnish, and detaches it. In cases of simple abrasion, three dressings have proved successful : in more obstinate cases, and where large granulations have been present, I have used nitrate of silver, acid nitrate of mercury, and potassa fusa first, and then applied a varnish of the gun cotton over the eschar, and have succeeded in curing extensive ulcers of the cock's-comb variety in half the time I have been able to succeed without the solution.

In cases of vaginitis without ulceration, I have found the painting of the walls of the vagina with the solution most beneficial. The difficulty, however, is to dry it well, which requires time and trouble, but in my mind, the result amply repays both, the friction of the surfaces is prevented, and the amount of suffering, pain and inflammation consequently much diminished. *Part* xviii., *p.* 270.

Uterus—Hypertrophy and Induration of the.—Dr. Oldham advises to reduce the size of the uterus by the application of four or six leeches to the upper and back part of the vagina once or twice a week. Blister the sacrum or inguinal region, when these parts are the seat of continuous pain ; or rub them well with a liniment composed of tinct. aconit. (Fleming) ʒiv.; ext. belladon. ʒss.; lin. sapon. co. ʒiss.; M. Internally give the solution of bichloride of mercury, in doses of one or two drachms twice in the day, combined with vegetable tonics, or chalybeates, and occasionally, if the bowels are torpid, with a little tinct. rhei. Let the colon and the rectum be cleared out daily by a tepid or cold milk-and-water injection; long continued exercise or standing to be avoided; and sexual intercourse abandoned or nearly so. The application of potassa fusa, and other escharotics, to the uterus, is much to be deprecated unless there be fungoid granulations about the os and cervix. But with a view of strengthening the structures below the uterus, cold hip baths may be used, and astringent injections efficiently given, such as decoction of oak bark or tormentilla, solution of sulphate of zinc, etc., or vaginal suppositories, made of ten or twelve grains of tannin mixed up with honey. A mechanical support should be afforded by means of a perineal pad, attached to a firm, elastic, abdominal belt. *Part* xviii., *p.* 293.

Uterine Catarrh.—Prof. Strohl, of Strasbourg, recommends the use of injections of liq. plumbi acetatis, or of a solution of ʒj. of iodide of iron in ʒxij. of distilled water. Inject the fluid very slowly, through a caoutchouc tube introduced about three lines into the os uteri, and of such diameter as not completely to fill the orifice of the uterus. *Part* xix., *p.* 270.

Ulceration of Os Uteri.—The best way to apply Vienna paste to the os uteri, for the purpose of changing the morbid action which gives rise to congestion of that part, says Dr. Mitchell, is to use a glass rod, expanded at the end into a circular disc. The paste is spread upon this disc, and the rod introduced through the speculum, and pressed against the part we wish to act upon. *Part* xix., *p.* 270.

Inversio Uteri.—When the organ is not affected with malignant disease, and no other special contra-indication exists, and the patient's health is suffering, Dr. Higgins believes that extirpation of the womb is a proper proceeding. In performing the operation, tie a flat tape, half-an-inch wide, round the inverted vagina, as high up as possible. This, when tightened, acts as a tourniquet, without injuriously pressing on the parts—it allows sutures to be easily inserted—and, if retained on for some time after the operation, it keeps the parts closely in apposition, and prevents dragging upon the sutures. *Part* xx., *p.* 223.

Climacteric Disease in Women.—Dr. W. Tyler Smith directs to remove any obvious cause of uterine irritation, by appropriate treatment. Use moderate depletion from the uterus, by incisions made into the os, or, still better, by the application of three or four leeches to the os. And use cold hip-baths, or cold injections into the vagina or rectum. If there are any dysmenorrheal symptoms, use injections with decoction of poppies and laudanum, into the rectum and vagina; if there is menorrhagia, let alum baths (ʒxvj. of alum to each gallon of water, at temp. 98°) be used in the intervals between the periods. Keep the bowels lax, but avoid drastics, and especially aloes; and promote the alvine, renal, hepatic, and cutaneous secretions. Let the diet be light and nutritious, with very little wine and no malt liquor or spirits. Let the clothing be warm, and in winter let flannel jackets and drawers be worn. And for the severe symptoms of nervous irritation, give moderate doses of sulphuric ether and valerian. Sulphuric ether is at this period a more decided sedative upon the female constitution, than either morphia, opium, or hyoscyamus. *Part* xx., *p.* 232.

Cauliflower Excrescence of the Os Uteri.—According to Dr. Watson of Glasgow, as this disease is, in all probability, not of a malignant nature, we may hope by its removal to effect a permanent cure. It is necessary, however, that the removal should be complete; and the safest and most efficacious mode of accomplishing this end is by free excision of the affected lip, or, if necessary, of the entire neck of the uterus. *Part* xx., *p.* 242.

Rupture of the Uterus.—Dr. J. C. W. Lever recommends full doses of opium at intervals during several days. A case so treated has recovered, though the rupture was so extensive that the hand could be passed into the cavity of the abdomen. *Part* xxi., *p.* 305.

Erectile Engorgement of the Cervix Uteri.—Dr. Tilt gives the following case: A few months since I was consulted by a lady, aged twenty-five, who had menstruated for the first time at the age of fourteen years, and who did so regularly till she married, three years ago. Since then she had suffered from dysmenorrhœa, and latterly from backache and leucorrhœa. After adopting the usually employed method of treatment by injections and tonics for three weeks, I made an examination, and found the vagina hotter and more irritable than usual; and on applying the speenlum, its field was filled by a well circumscribed substance of a bright red color, and yielding to pressure. On enlarging the aperture of the speenlum (Coxeter's), it was easy to see that the whole mass was formed by a swollen lip of the os uteri, which on being carefully dilated, did not present any erosion or ulceration, either on its external portion or in its cavity. The internal mucous membrane was redder than usual, and there was an increased flow of the normal glutinous secretion. I scarified the swollen surface, and ordered tepid injections, mild purgatives, and repose. A few days after the tumor was smaller, more livid, less painful, less tense on pressure, and I whitened it by rapidly passing the nitrate of silver over its surface. I ordered injections with cold solution of alum. I repeated the application of the nitrate of silver every five days for a month; and finding that the swelling did but slowly decrease, I applied iodide of iron to it every four days with a large camel-hair pencil, and in three weeks the swelling disappeared. The patient was under treatment for three months; and never during repeated speculum examinations could I find any other lesion of the neck of the womb, except an increased intensity of color.

Sometimes both lips are swollen, but generally only one is so. Out of twenty well-marked cases of this description which I have observed, in two the swelling was general; in eight the posterior lip was swollen; and in ten the interior. Most of my twenty patients were of a lymphatico-sanguine temperament; they were all married, and in five the complaint came on within the six months which followed marriage. In almost all the cases intercourse was painful.

I never employ potassa fusa in this form of uterine disease; I principally make use of nitrate of silver, and I have with advantage alternated its use with that of the solid sulphate of copper, or a strong solution of diacetate of lead, or of the iodide of iron. *Part* xxii., *p.* 278.

Uterine Neuralgia.—M. Valleix has pointed out a class of cases in which the cervix uteri, usually insensible, becomes the seat of the most acute suffering of a neuralgic nature, and has pointed out the diagnostic distinctions between these and cases of painful inflammatory congestion of that organ.

In all the cases which have come under M. Valleix's notice, the affection has been accompanied by pain following the course of the lumbo-abdominal nerves. He therefore regards the neuralgia of the cervix as part of

the more extensive lumbo-abdominal neuralgia. This feature is of importance in reference to the diagnosis of neuralgic from other pains of the
cervix uteri.

The subjects of this neuralgic affection present all the characters of
sufferers from chronic uterine congestion, with which disease the former is
almost always confounded. The pain is much augmented at the menstrual
period-producing dysmenorrhœa. The vaginal discharge which occurs in
these cases is analogous to the increased secretion from the mucous membrane of the eyelids in certain affections of the trifacial nerve They are
both functional disturbances originating in disordered nervous influence.

Careful exploration is of the first importance to its detection. The neck
of the uterus will be found tender to the touch, often so to a great degree,
the tenderness being most acute at the sides of the cervix, while the anterior and posterior surfaces are free. The cervix is of its ordinary form
and size.

On examining the abdomen and loins, a neuralgic pain will be detected
in the hypogastrium a little beyond the middle line on one side, most frequently the left only. Along the course of the first pair of lumbar nerves
will be discovered other points, more or less acutely painful, and more or
less isolated. The painful point always corresponds with the seat of pain
in the uterus.

The chief diagnostic features are, the degree and isolation of the tenderness, the intermittent character of the pain, and the occurrence of the neuralgia of the abdomen and loins.

Apply blisters to the hypogastric region, cauterization of the cervix,
narcotic injections, with absolute rest and general treatment.
Part xxii., *p.* 307.

Purulent Discharges from the Uterus.—Dr. Lloyd uses an injection of
a solution of chloride of zinc, gr. j. to the ʒj. every eight hours.
Part xxiii., *p.* 210.

Inversion of the Uterus.—Drs. Denman, Burns, and Merriman advise
the uterus with the attached placenta to be returned ; but the latter mentions an instance in which he first detached the placenta, and the patient
did well.   *Part* xxiv., *p.* 278.

Carcinoma Uteri.—To relieve the excruciating pain, apply the vapor
of chloroform to the os uteri by means of Dr. Hardy's "anæsthetic
douche."

The apparatus for applying it consists of a small metallic chamber ; to
one end of this a gum-elastic bottle is attached, to the other, a pipe furnished with a valve. On the end of the chamber there is also a second
valve to admit atmospheric air for the working of the instrument. In
order to charge it with chloroform it is necessary to unscrew the stopper
in the side of the chamber, within which a piece of sponge is placed for
holding the fluid.

The quantity poured in should not be more than the sponge will absorb,
otherwise, instead of vapor, fluid chloroform will be thrown against the
affected part. When charged, the vapor may be conveyed to the part requiring its application by any convenient pipe, if closely fitted to the one
on the instrument, pressure being made on the elastic bag to produce
expulsion of the vapor.   *Part* xxix., *p.* 279.

Uterine Catarrh and Internal Metritis.—It may be stated with a great degree of confidence, that the general opinion of medical men with regard to the seat of leucorrhœal discharges, is, that they depend upon organic lesions of the os uteri and its vicinity. In these cases the treatment is effective and satisfactory. But in some cases the lesions may be in the mucous membrane lining the womb, and it is in these cases especially that there is the greatest uncertainty, both as regards the diagnosis and treatment.

A sound symptom to judge by in this disease, is, that lateral pressure all down to the neck of the womb gives considerable pain. Dr. E. J. Tilt recommends the application of the tincture of iodine to the inside and outside of the neck of the womb in such case. The second application may take place ten days after the first, and then repeat it every four or five days, if necessary, for three months. The uterine mucus should be first cleared away. The best injection in such case is ʒj. of the acetate of lead and one pint of decoction of poppy heads. As a remedy, five to ten grains of ergot of rye, given three or four times, proved as useful as any.

Part xxix., p. 285.

Intra-Uterine Speculum.—For the exploration of the cervix uteri and using various applications, an ingenious speculum is used by M. Jobert; a very small instrument with a long handle—sufficiently small to be passed up the common vaginal speculum. *Part xxx., p. 203.*

Uterine Affections.—*Vide* Selections from Favorite Prescriptions, Art. " Medicine."

Inflammation of the Os and Cervix Uteri.—[Besides arising from general unhealthy conditions of the system, it may be induced by causes of a mere local nature, as exposure, violent horse exercise, improper irritation of the part, but especially by the too frequent application of caustic to the os uteri, with such short intervals that the eschar produced by one application could not have healed before the next was made, and this continued for such a length of time as to produce the most serious mischief, both local and constitutional. Dr. Rigby says:]

This form of inflammation of the os and cervix presents features which distinguish it from the ordinary species I have been describing. It would, perhaps, be correct to call it a highly irritable condition of the uterus (which not only involves the ovaries, but frequently implicates the spinal cord to a serious extent), were it not for the actual alteration of structure and permanent injury of the part which has suffered more immediately from the treatment.

The patient complains of constant pain in the uterine region, but generally more behind the symphysis pubis than is usually the case in ordinary inflammation of the cervix, extending from hip to hip, and in aggravated cases darting up the spine with neuralgic severity. It is increased by standing or by any exercise whatever. Sitting down upon a hard seat, or the passage down the rectum of solid fæces, produces great suffering, inasmuch as when once the pain is brought on, it will continue severely for some time after. The moment she assumes the erect posture she has a sensation of weight, bearing down, and burning heat in the pelvis, which are quickly followed by the pain itself.

The catamenial periods usually follow each other too quickly; are almost always very profuse, and invariably attended with great suffering.

If the ovaries are involved, the symptoms of ovarian dysmenorrhœa will also be present. She has a constant ichorous watery discharge, which is sometimes very profuse. The bowels are unhealthy; the urine thick; the tongue pale, dry, and rough, with red papillæ; the face sallow and wan; the spirits depressed; the pulse feeble and very irritable; and she has lost strength and flesh.

On examination, per vaginam, this canal is found soaked in the thin, watery discharge already mentioned. On gently touching the os and cer-vix uteri with the finger, the patient feels as if the parts were raw, from the aggravated sensibility which now exists in them; firmer pressure with the finger brings on the neuralgic pain already described. The os uteri is usually swollen, uneven, and knobby—it is frequently dragged forward, or to one side, without any corresponding displacement of the organ itself. Whether this alteration of shape is owing to cicatrization in the part itself and surrounding vagina; or whether it depends on different portions being affected with different degrees of induration, it is not easy to deter-mine; at any rate, the cervix usually has a strong degree of hardness, and the uterus above it feels large, hard, and very tender to the touch.

Seen through the speculum, the os uteri does not present the dark red tinge, more or less mottled with patches of a brighter color, as in cases of ordinary inflammation, but has a pale ashy hue, much injected with vessels, just as is occasionally seen in the irritable throat and tonsils of an unhealthy person who has been suffering from repeated attacks of quinsy.

The discharge is evidently uterine, and is constantly oozing from the os uteri in considerable quantities. If the uterine sound be passed, it gene-rally penetrates half an inch, or even a whole inch, beyond the usual dis-tance, showing that the uterine cavity is enlarged; and intense pain is produced the instant it touches the internal surface of the uterus, indicat-ing great irritability of that organ, and probably inflammation of its lining membrane.

The treatment of this affection will necessarily differ a good deal from the ordinary forms of inflammation of the os and cervix; the indications, it is true, will to a certain extent be the same, but the local as well as the general condition of the patient is very different. The inflammation of the os and cervix in these cases is seldom of such a nature as to require the application of leeches to the part itself, and the extreme irritation which they not unfrequently produce contra-indicates any local applications but those of a soothing character; while the enfeebled state of the patient's health renders any depletion very questionable.

The general treatment is by no means so simple or so easy as in the other case. The health has been so much deranged by the long-continued effects of severe uterine irritation, and the strength so broken down by frequent attacks of menorrhagia, and profuse leucorrhœa during the in-tervals, that it is difficult to adopt any distinct line of treatment at first starting, beyond the attempt to regulate the liver and bowels, by the mild-est remedies, and soothe the irritable system by gentle sedatives.

A course of taraxacum, with decoct. sarsæ comp. and liq. calcis, is valu-able in the early stages of treatment, as it obviates the necessity of mercu-rial alteratives, which are usually contra-indicated by the mucous irritation of the intestinal canal. It is of great importance to allay this condition as quickly as possible, not only because we thereby remove a fruitful source of uterine irritation, but because it also enables us to employ remedies which we could not otherwise do. When this has been arrested, we may generally pass at once to the use of mineral acids and tonics, and, if necessary, these will pave the way to a course of cod-liver oil. If the season of the year permit, a residence for some months at the sea-side will be most desirable. The patient should use sea-water in her morning ablutions, and if her health be sufficiently improved, and the weather warm enough, she may bathe in the sea with advantage.

The local treatment, as I have before stated, must be essentially of a soothing character. Liq. plumbi diacet. in decoct. papaveris forms one of the best injections where there is any amount of heat, swelling, or discharge ; in other cases, the plain poppy decoction appears to be the only local application which will give relief. As it is desirable she should retain injections of this sort for fifteen or twenty minutes, she ought to lie upon her back, with her heels drawn up to the nates, and thus give the vagina such a direction that the injection will remain in it as long as she preserves this position. The suppositories of diacetate of lead and extract of conium are also very valuable in these cases, and by being in a more concentrated form, and capable of being retained much longer, produce a much greater effect. The warm hip-bath is very useful, and with some patients appears to be the only thing which gives relief. If, however, the weather be mild, the sooner she can gradually come to the use of cold water the better ; and she may always be looked upon as having made good progress, when, during her residence at the sea-side, she is able to bear cold sponging with sea-water, and bathing in the open sea. For those who are able to enjoy these advantages, the salt towel which I have before recommended will be an excellent adjunct to the cold sponging. But it will be needless to enter into further details ; they will vary more or less with every patient, or with the same patient at different times, and will be naturally suggested by the peculiar features, etc., of each case. The indications of treatment are to allay irritation and restore tone, but the treatment itself must necessarily be modified by the circumstances of each particular case.

Part xxxiii., *p.* 248.

Uterine Neuralgia.—This is often conjoined with uterine deviations, says Dr. Tilt, and may be alleviated or removed by sedative injections into the bowels—say from fifteen to thirty minims of Battley's solution, with a drachm of tincture of henbane in a teacupful of warm milk. No remedy is so valuable in neuralgia as heat (cauterization with a red-hot iron), but as this is so very objectionable, apply to the most painful part a hammer previously plunged in boiling water. *Part* xxxiv., *p.* 239.

Carbonic Acid as a Local Anæsthetic in Uterine Disease.—Prof. Simpson has used carbonic acid gas applied as a local anæsthetic very successfully in neuralgia of the uterus and vagina, and in various morbid states of the pelvic organs, accompanied with pain and spasm. It may be very conveniently generated in a common wine bottle, by mixing six drachms of crystallized tartaric acid with a solution of eight drachms of bicarbonate of soda, in six or seven ounces of water. A long flexible caoutchouc tube tightly fixed to the cork, conducts the gas from the bottle into the vagina

Part xxxiv., *p.* 251

Uterus—Cancer of.—Dr. West remarked at St. Bartholomew's that hemorrhage is an almost constant symptom of commencing cancer of the os uteri, quite as valuable as hemoptysis is in respect to tubercle in the lungs.

It is peculiarly valuable when the subject of the affection has previously ceased to menstruate.   *Part* xxxv., *p.* 254.

Uterus and Bladder—Reciprocal Sympathies between.—Dr. Montgomery communicates as follows: in the human female, there is an intimate reciprocal sympathy between the uterus and bladder, and other parts of the urinary apparatus; so that, under a variety of circumstances, when the former organ is the seat of any anomalous action, or brought into a state of exalted sensibility, whether from natural or morbid causes, the latter is not only liable, but very apt to sympathize, and suffer correspondingly.

This is constantly exemplified in the increased urinary irritation so often accompanying ordinary healthy menstruation, and still more remarkably, when the latter function happens to be painfully performed. Again, in early pregnancy, the same thing is observed; and the remark is trite, that morbid actions in the uterus, whether benign or otherwise, often have the earliest announcement of their invasion in symptoms of disturbance first noticed in the functions of the bladder.

Thus, congestion or slight ulceration of the cervix uteri, and still more strikingly, malignant affections of that part, frequently excite, in the first instance, in the patient's mind, only apprehensions of gravel, or some vesical disease, for which alone she is induced to seek advice; but woe betide us, in this and many other circumstances, if we let ourselves be beguiled into the belief that because a particular organ or locality is affected with certain anomalous symptoms, it is therefore the seat of some disease, of which these symptoms are to be taken as indications; and so prescribe. Could we, for instance, expect to cure the itching of the nose and angle of the eye which accompanies the presence of intestinal worms, by applications to the Schneiderian, or conjunctival membrane?

Mrs. C. had, for a long time, intense, intolerable, distracting itching of the perineum and anus, which really rendered her life miserable, and for which she had consulted many, and used a multiplicity of remedies: many of them, no doubt, very appropriate for *pruritus*, but *not for her*. When she came under my care, I also, at first adopted the wrong course; I prescribed *for the symptom, and not for its cause*. But fortunately, after seeing her a few times, something led me to suspect the existence of intestinal worms. I gave her a dose of the Kousso, which caused the expulsion of some very large lumbrici, and all her troubles were forthwith at an end.

Mrs. M. consulted me for pruritus of the pudendum, from which she suffered to such a degree, and it was accompanied with other symptoms of so distressing a kind, that she declared she loathed herself, and felt her life an intolerable burden to her. She had used gallons of lotions, and all sorts of ointments, without the slightest relief. Examination showed an intense congestion of the cervix uteri; this was made the object of treatment, and on its removal, the pruritus and all its miserable concomitants totally ceased.

I have already called the consent between the uterus and bladder a reciprocal sympathy, because it equally acts in the reverse direction, irritations of the bladder being frequently found to influence and disturb the functions of the uterus—a fact which should not be forgotten in practice, and especially in the treatment of the disease of pregnancy, when the administration of the more irritating diuretics should be avoided, lest they should excite contraction of the fibres of the uterus, and so induce premature expulsion of its contents.

And again, we must remember that vesical disturbances may produce a group of symptoms so closely resembling those arising from disease of the uterus, as to be mistaken for them. .

Several years ago, the wife of a general officer, at that time holding the highest military command in this country, began to complain of distressing symptoms, having all the characters of those produced by uterine disease. Such was her own conviction, and on her consulting an accoucheur, he pronounced the affection to be cancer uteri, and could only promise palliation. But she had many friends, and some of them urged upon her the necessity of having another opinion; to this she at last consented, and the gentleman called in pronounced the case to be one of stone in the bladder; the stone was extracted, and the lady passed at once from a state of pain and misery to one of comfort and happiness.

A few years since, a patient came to consult me, stating that, to gratify her friends, she had come to town for my advice, although quite aware she could not be cured. She also handed me a written statement of her case, which set forth that she had had seven labors of terrible severity, owing to contracted pelvis, always requiring instrumental delivery; that for some months she had exhibited unequivocal symptoms of the existence of cancer uteri; and I confess, that from this account, and the woman's own description of her symptoms, I thought there was little room to doubt as to the nature of her malady.

However, I instituted a careful examination; on doing so, I could discover no disease of the uterus, but the neck of the bladder was distended and felt very hard. I passed a sound into it, which at once struck against a stone of considerable size. Mr. Fleming now saw the case with me, the stone was removed, and the woman soon returned home well, and continued so. *Part* xxxvii., *p.* 229.

Uterine Excitement.—Bromide of potassium has a decidedly sedative effect upon the generative system. Dr. Simpson recommends its use in spurious pregnancy. Some time since, Dr. Locock advocated its use in cases of epilepsy in females apparently having a monthly return.

Part xl., *p.* 181.

UVULA.

Vide Arts. "Palate"—"Throat"—"Chronic Phthisis."

VACCINATION.

Vaccine Crusts, the most Effectual Packages for Vaccine Virus.—[The following is from Dr. Epps' Medical Director of the Royal Jennerian and London Vaccine Institution, who states:]

The indurated pock, the scab or crust of the vaccine pock, contains the dried matter in its cells, which, being broken down, and moistened with the wetted point of the lancet, has been found effective in hot climates, when attempts to preserve the vaccine ichor in other forms have failed. The crusts or scabs we have been able to collect in this country, we learn by letters from the East and West Indies, have withstoood the heat of their vertical sun, and spread protection through the plantations and the surrounding districts.

N.B.—These crusts, when levigated and moistened, and worked into a fine pulp, have been used by many practitioners in tropical climates with the most signal success.   *Part* iii., *p.* 54.

Dr. Gregory's Lecture on.—The surgery of vaccination, simple as it may appear, has been a fruitful theme of controversy. Differences of opinion have existed with respect to the selection of lymph, the mode of making the incisions, and the number of incisions necessary to insure a full effect. Each of these points merits attention.

Dr. Gregory observes, that one of the earliest and most important disputes which chequered the career of vaccination (inasmuch as it led to the secession of Jenner, in 1807, from the original Jennerian Institution) had reference to the mode of taking the lymph. Dr. Walker adopted the plan of detaching the epidermis from the vesicle, and vaccination with the lymph (or fluid) which exuded from the abraded floor of the vesicle. Jenner objected strongly to this, and employed only the superficial lymph. Dr. Walker persevered in his plan; and it is but fair to confess that his vaccinations have stood the test of time fully as well as those conducted according to the Jennerian method.

The proper time at which lymph may be taken so as to obtain it in the most efficient state for propagating the disease, has also been a subject of discussion. Some have objected to the employment of very early lymph, others have scruples in taking lymph after the first appearance of areola, and all parties have concurred in condemning the use of lymph taken on, or after the tenth day. The facts bearing on this question are as follows: The younger the lymph is, the greater is its intensity. The lymph of a fifth-day vesicle, when it can be obtained, never fails. It is, however, equally powerful up to the eighth day, at which time also it is most abundant. After the formation of areola, the true specific matter of cowpox becomes mixed with variable proportions of serum, the result of common inflammation, and diluted lymph is always less efficacious than the concentrated virus. After the tenth day the lymph becomes mucilaginous, and scarcely fluid, in which state it is not at all to be depended on. Out of a dozen incisions made with such viscid lymph, not more than one will prove effective. The scabs of cowpox, ground to powder, and moistened with lukewarm water to the consistence of mucilage, will sometimes reproduce the disease in all its purity—a satisfactory proof that the alteration which the lymph undergoes in its progress to maturity is not of a specific kind, liable to influence the result of the subsequent vaccination, but simply dilution.

Cowpox matter differs in intensity according to the source from which it has been obtained. Very pure lymph, of great intensity, will often prove efficacious when taken from the arm on the ninth and even on the tenth days. Experience teaches that all vesicles are not equally fitted to produce the disease in purity; but it requires a practised eye to detect these minutiæ. Irritable sores are often produced by draining the vesicle too much. Infantile lymph is more to be depended upon than the lymph obtained from adults. The matter of primary vaccinations is more energetic than that of secondary vaccinations. These statements may serve as a guide in the selection of lymph wherewith to vaccinate. The number of incisions which it is requisite to make in order to produce a full constitutional effect, has been always a disputed point. At an early period of vaccination one vesicle was held to be sufficient. Then three, four, or six, were recommended. In Germany, great importance is attached to the raising of numerous vesicles, it being a received doctrine in that country that, unless some decided constitutional effect be produced, little reliance can be placed on the process as a security in after-life. Common sense dictates that the greater the number of vesicles, the greater will be the local inflammation, and, on this theory, the greater the probability of constitutional sympathy. Some of the German inoculators have been in the habit of raising from twenty to thirty vesicles in each subject. In forming a just judgment on this matter, the nature and quality of the lymph must always be taken into account. Lymph recently derived from the cow possesses so much intensity, and fixes itself with so much more of a poisonous character upon the skin of the arm than lymph long humanized or habituated to the human constitution, that a single incision made with it is equivalent to six or eight made with lymph of minor energy.

Dr. Gregory recommends, that with lymph of ordinary intensity five vesicles should be raised, and that these should be at such distances from each other as not to become confluent in their advance to maturation. Vaccine lymph should always be used in a fluid state, and direct from the arm, wherever practicable, for it is a very delicate secretion, and very slight changes in it are capable of materially altering its qualities. Lymph which has been retained fluid for four or five days, is very apt to occasion that irritable vesicle described as the most frequent of all the anomalous appearances.

When lymph fresh from the arm cannot be obtained, other means must be had recourse to. Vaccine virus may be preserved fluid and effective for two or three days in small bottles, with projecting ground stoppers, fitted to retain the matter. It may be preserved for a like time in small capillary tubes having a central bulb. This is the mode usually adopted in France for the transmission of vaccine lymph to the Provinces, and which proves very effectual; but if we attempt in this manner to transmit lymph to the East or West Indies, we fail utterly. Most surgeons have seen what are called ivory points. These, when well armed and carefully dried, are very effective. They will retain their activity in this climate for many months, and they are found to be the most certain mode of sending lymph to our colonies. Some practitioners prefer glasses to points, but they are less certain. The employment of scabs for the propagation of cow pox was first recommended in 1802. It is a very excellent mode of transmitting vaccine matter to distant countries, but some nicety is required in operating with scabs, which experience alone can teach.

Part viii., *p.* 204.

Value of Vaccination and Re-Vaccination.—[M. Serres presented to the Academy of Sciences, in the name of the committee appointed to decide on the merits of a number of treatises on this subject, a report, from which the following is taken :]

Vaccination preserves the human species from variola, but its preservative power is not absolute. Variola itself, either spontaneous, or produced by inoculation, does not preserve absolutely from future attacks, therefore it is not extraordinary that vaccination should not. Thus Mead mentions having seen three variolous eruptions take place successively on the same woman ; the son of Forestus was twice attacked with variola, and Dehaen states that one of his patients was attacked six times by variola with impunity, but died of a seventh invasion of the disease. Although, however, vaccination is sometimes powerless to preserve us from variola, it always diminishes the gravity of the malady. This property, which Jenner and his first successors did not even suspect, is thoroughly proved by the various facts which have been recently accumulated. In one of the most terrible epidemics of variola that has taken place in Europe since the discovery of vaccination—that of Marseilles, in 1828—more than ten thousand persons were attacked. Of these, two thousand only had been vaccinated, and of that number forty-five only died, whereas, one thousand five hundred of the eight thousand who had not been vaccinated, were carried off by the pestilence. Vaccine matter evidently loses part of its efficacy in passing from arm to arm ; it is therefore desirable to renew it as often as possible. A remarkable fact mentioned by one of the competitors, supplies us with a means of renewing it, as it were, at will. A cow was vaccinated with matter taken from a child. Not only did the pustules rise, but they were communicated to other cows, so that cow pox was observed nearly in its natural state. The pustules were identical in both cases. The propriety of re-vaccination is now fully established. In Germany, the various governments have been induced to pay great attention to re-vaccination, owing to the circumstance of epidemics of variola having latterly manifested themselves with a severity to which we had become quite unaccustomed, since the introduction of vaccination. Re-vaccination has, consequently, been resorted to on a very extended scale, and has had the effect of arresting the epidemics. Thus, in Wurtemburg, forty-two thousand persons who have been re-vaccinated, have only presented eight cases of varioloid, whereas, one-third of the cases of variola have latterly occurred on persons who have been vaccinated. It is principally between the ages of fourteen and thirty-five that vaccinated persons are exposed to be attacked by variola. When there is an epidemic, the danger commences earlier, and children of nine years of age may be seized. Prudence, therefore, requires that, under ordinary circumstances, re-vaccination should be performed at the age of fourteen or fifteen, and four years earlier if within the radius of an epidemic of variola. *Part* xii., *p.* 126.

Instrument for Vaccinating.—[Dr. Weir introduced to the Edinburgh Obstetrical Society a new instrument for vaccinating.]

It consists of a small handle of ivory, with four needle-points projecting from one extremity, and a small curved knife for collecting and separating the vaccine matter at the other. The skin is opened by a crucial scratch with the needle-points, which are held vertically, and are lightly applied, so as merely to remove the cuticle. The advantages of this instrument over the lancet are, that the operation is done more speedily, and that it opposes a larger surface for the absorption of the lymph, which is less liable to be washed away by too great an effusion of blood.

Soak a piece of sugar with the lymph, pound it when dry, and keep it in a well-closed bottle. Apply this powder by sprinkling it on the exposed surface with a hair-pencil. *Part* xvi., *p.* 230.

Vaccination.—Dr. W. S. Oke directs to make at least six punctures, each produced by carrying the point of a lancet, held flat to the arm, obliquely downward through the cuticle into the surface of the cutis. If possible, use fresh lymph; and never take lymph from a vesicle after the eighth day. Let the instrument used to apply the lymph remain inserted a few seconds, and then be wiped upon the orifice of the puncture. Lastly, if the development of the vesicle is not satisfactory, or if there is only one vesicle, use Bryce's test to try the efficacy of the vaccination. It consists in inserting fresh lymph on the evening of the fifth, or morning of the sixth day; then, if the second vesicle progresses rapidly, and overtake the first, it will show that the vaccination has been successful. *Part* xxi., *p.* 36.

VAGINA.

Adhesions and Strictures in the Vagina during Pregnancy and Labor.—Adhesions and strictures of the vagina may, no doubt, frequently exist in the virgin subject, as well as in one who has been previously impregnated and undergone parturition. When it occurs in the latter subject, it will generally be the result of pressure or injury during labor. The walls of the vagina may become glued together either at one point or throughout the whole surface, or bridles of lymph may be found in different parts. The formation of these cicatrices somewhat resembles the same process from burns.

"The most usual complication is a falciform band encroaching on the area of the vagina, or one or more rings of cartilaginous hardness either traversing its whole circumference, or only contracting a segment of it; and with these there is too frequently found a vesical fistula." If the constriction is slight, it will not be necessary for the practitioner to interfere much during labor.

The relaxation of the parts will almost invariably be sufficiently accomplished by the judicious use of tartar emetic, given in nauseating doses. In most instances, this practice will entirely supersede the use of the lancet. Cases of the greatest rigidity, almost resembling a "cylinder of iron" round the finger, have been relaxed by this medicine in less than six hours. Sometimes, however, a perfect occlusion exists, and in this case, we must have recourse to an operation, which must at all times be dangerous on account of the proximity of the bladder on one side, and the rectum on the other.

"The best instrument," says Dr. Doherty, "which we can employ, is a straight bistoury, covered throughout with sticking plaster, except over a small portion of its extent. It can be safely introduced by carrying its flat surface along the finger, passed into the vagina. In making our incisions we should never allow them to go beyond the sixteenth of an inch in depth at once, and we should frequently withdraw the knife and make a careful examination of the progress we have made. A pair of flat wooden spatulas, introduced one on either side, will, by keeping the parts asunder, facilitate the operation. It will also be found a useful precaution to pass the finger of the left hand up the rectum, in order that we may judge how far our incisions may be carried without endangering that intestine; and it is a matter of prudence to avoid as much as possible, cutting toward the bladder, lest, from its close proximity and intimate connection with the vagina, we open into its cavity. Having thus, step by step, and with the utmost circumspection, separated the adhesions as far as we think prudent,

we should wait until the opening has had an opportunity of dilating under
the pressure of the presenting part, when if the head be still prevented
from descending, we may endeavor, in the same cautious manner, to enlarge
the canal a little more."

[The next question is, how long are we to wait before operating, when
only a severe constriction exists, and when the child's head must of
necessity tear through the parts, if those parts are not artificially liberated.
We must remember that in all severe constrictions of the vagina, its
parietes are not the only parts implicated. The neighboring viscera will
frequently be too adherent, and therefore any laceration of the vagina will
also lacerate those viscera; hence the necessity of timely interference with
the knife or other instrument, when we feel convinced that the head will
not pass without this. The constriction should, therefore, be nicked in two
or three places, the incisions never exceeding the sixteenth part of an inch
in depth, and being directed laterally or backward rather than forward,
and the finger of the left hand at the same time being kept in the rectum
as a guide. Dr. Rigby recommends that this should be done during a
pain, when the patient will probably be unconscious of the act; but the
correctness of this practice is certainly questionable, as few patients can
be sufficiently quiet on such an occasion for the surgeon to be particular
in the depth and extent of his incisions; and moreover the incisions might
be very suddenly enlarged if made during a pain. On all these occasions
we are not warranted in resorting to an operation, till we feel convinced
that relaxation of the parts has been carried to the utmost, and that any
further delay might produce laceration.]   *Part* v., *p.* 148.

Vagina and Urethra—Disease of.—The value of the speculum is incal-
culable in all cases where there is reason to suspect disease of the neck of
the uterus.

Local Treatment.—In vulvular inflammation, Dr. Mitchell, of Dublin,
recommends the hip-bath and poppy fomentations. For the itching, nitrate
of silver ʒj., aq. dest. ʒj., applied three or four times a-day; or tincture of
matico. Both may be applied either with a camel-hair pencil or with a
stick, to which a piece of sponge is tied. Lotions of the soluble salts of
lead, zinc, mercury, narcotic preparations, borax, hydrocyanic acid, bread
crumb soaked with liquor plumbi diacet., gelatine and bran baths.

General Treatment.—Mild saline purgatives, rest, sea-bathing, alterative
doses of mercury, as Plummer's pill, gr. v. nocte maneque. Brandishe's
alkaline solution, twenty drops in an ounce of any bitter infusion; balsam
copaiba. For pain in the back apply cautery to the sacrum.
                                                        Part xiv., *p.* 306.

Vaginitis.—Dr. Mitchell recommends to paint the walls of the vagina
with several coats of collodion, taking care to allow the first coat to dry
well (which requires two or three minutes at least) before the second is
applied.   *Part* xviii., *p.* 270.

Vagina—Plugging the.—The vagina may be easily and efficiently
plugged by means of a little bladder of caoutchouc, of suitable form,
introduced in a collapsed state, as recommended by M. Diday, and then
inflated by means of a long tube attached to it.   *Part* xxi., *p.* 302.

*Vaginal Cystocele, or Prolapsus of the Anterior Wall of the Vagina
and Bladder—Operation for its cure.*—[The case was so aggravated that

with the least exertion the anterior wall of the vagina became so prolapsed
that a tumor was produced by it of the size of a man's fist, producing
several ulcerated patches from the friction of the parts. All means of
relief which had been suggested, having done no good, Dr. I. B. Brown,
of London, determined to try to effect this by means of operation.]

The patient having been prepared for the operation, by emptying the
bowels, was placed under the influence of chloroform, and then put in
position for lithotomy, each leg being held by an assistant and well bent
back on the abdomen, a third assistant holding up the tumor with Jobert's
bent speculum, and pressing it under the pubes in its natural position. A
piece of mucous membrane, about one inch and a quarter long, and three
quarters of an inch broad, was dissected off longitudinally, just within the
lips of the vagina. The upper edge of the denuded part being on a level
with the meatus urinarius, the edges were drawn together by three interrupted sutures, this being repeated on the other side of the vagina. The
next stage of the operation consisted in dissecting off the mucous membrane laterally and posteriorly in the shape of a horse-shoe, the upper edge
of the shoe commencing half an inch below the lateral points of denudation,
taking care to remove all the mucous membrane up to the edge of the
vagina, where the skin joins it. Two deep sutures of twine were then
introduced about an inch from the margin of the left side of the vagina,
and brought out at the inner edge of the denuded surfaces of one side,
and introduced at the inner edge of the other denuded side, and brought
out an inch from the margin of the right side of the vagina, thus bringing
the two denuded surfaces together and keeping them so, by means of
quills, as in the operation for ruptured perineum. The edges of this new
perineum were then brought together by interrupted sutures, and the
patient placed in bed on a water-cushion. Two grains of opium given
directly, and one grain every six hours; simple water-dressing applied to
the parts; beef-tea and wine for diet. A bent metallic catheter was
introduced in the bladder, to which was attached an elastic bag to catch
the urine; by this means the bladder was constantly kept empty. This
patient progressed satisfactorily from day to day, without a single unfavorable symptom. It is scarcely possible to imagine a more satisfactory
result from any operative procedure. The benefits from this operation for
vaginal cystocele will be equally, if not more, applicable to vaginal recto-
cele, as well as to prolapsus of the entire vagina, and also, with some
slight modifications as to denudation of the mucous membrane, to prolapsus uteri. *Part* xxviii., *p.* 279.

Vaginitis.—M. Demarquay has found a composition, consisting of
eighty parts of glycerine and twenty of tannin, of great service. Copious
injections of warm water should be previously used, and the part freed
from mucus, etc., by lint; then a plug should be introduced, saturated with
this composition, and allowed to remain to the next day.
Part xxxiv., *p.* 254.

Vaginitis, with Superficial Inflammation of the Cervix Uteri.—M.
Foucher introduces every morning, with the assistance of the speculum,
a good-sized pledget of cotton wool, well smeared over with tannin ointment, into the vagina, bringing the pledget in contact with the cervix.
By means of a thread attached to it, this may be withdrawn by the
patient, either in the evening or next morning, and the parts having been

well washed out with cold water or weak alum water, a fresh pledget may be introduced. By a little practice, patients soon learn to apply the cotton wool for themselves.   *Part* xl., *p.* 214

———•◆•———

VAGITUS UTERINUS.

Case of—Its Medico-Legal bearing.—Cases of vagitus uterinus are by no means common, and many alleged instances of this kind, reported in medico-legal works, are unworthy of credit. Any authentic or well-observed case is, therefore, acceptable. The following has been communicated to Dr. A. S. Taylor, by Dr. Crothers, who says: I was called upon to attend Mrs. W., in labor of her sixth child; her former labors had been quick. On my arrival I found her suffering from very strong pains; and on examination the membranes were tense, and protruding through the os uteri.

The labor not progressing as rapidly I expected, I ruptured the membranes, found the face presenting, and apparently arrested at the brim. I endeavored to move it into a more favorable position, when happening to introduce a finger into the child's mouth, I was very much surprised to hear a *distinct cry*, which was repeated two or three times, and so loud as to alarm the mother and attendants. The former was quite frightened, so that I had a good deal of trouble to compose her. I do not now remember if the child cried afterward, without the fingers being introduced; but several times it did so, and so audibly that I think the lungs must have been pretty well filled with air. I was obliged to complete the delivery by the forceps. The child is now a fine healthy boy.

Remarks.—The possibility of a child in utero, having its lungs so filled with air, as to be able to utter an audible cry, has been doubted. The above case, with a few others of a similar kind, reported in medical periodicals, removes all doubt on the subject.

In all the authentic instances that have been hitherto published, the uterine cry has been heard only where the face has presented, and the accoucheur has by any accident introduced his fingers into the mouth of the child. The air thus finds a passage to the lungs.

The only case in legal medicine on which the production of a uterine cry has any bearing, is in the application of the lung-tests in cases of infanticide. The air found in the lungs of a child may have been received into them before birth. Thus the fact that these organs floated on water, either entire, or when divided into small portions, would not furnish conclusive evidence, that the child had been born alive. It would merely prove the establishment of respiration, and not the fact of birth. The uterine cry has less interest, in a practical view, than vaginal respiration during the passage of the head; because in a case of unassisted labor, it is not easy to perceive how it could possibly occur; and if an accoucheur were present, then the case would not be likely to come before a medical practitioner as one of infanticide.   *Part* xxii., *p.* 315,

VARICOCELE.

Radical cure of Varicocele by Invagination and Shortening of the Scrotum.—The mode of operating here recommended by Dr. Lekman, is very similar to that which has been adopted successfully for the radical cure of hernia. A portion of the relaxed and elongated scrotum is to be pushed up on the forefinger of the left hand, and *invaginated* into the part above it, till the finger reaches the external abdominal ring. Holding the parts in this position, a broad curved needle, with a double thread passed through an eye near its point, is to be carried along the left finger, through the bottom of the inverted portion of the scrotum, and to be made to penetrate it and the integuments immediately over the external ring. The thread is then to be removed from the eye, and the needle drawn back and again carried through the inverted portion of the scrotum and the integuments at a distance of about half an inch from the parts previously penetrated. The threads passed through the two apertures being now drawn, the invaginated portion of scrotum may be pulled up to any desired height; in general, it must be drawn very nearly to the external ring; for in the subsequent progress of the cure, the relaxation of the parts is so great that the folds and wrinkles thus produced are almost entirely obliterated. The threads then having been drawn must be knotted, and the parts thus tied up must be left for eight or nine days, under a soothing and cooling regimen, by which time adhesion will have taken place between them at the cut edges, and, by the excoriation which the discharge produces between the opposed surfaces of the inverted portion of the scrotum and that into which it is pushed. *Part* iii., *p.* 108.

Treatment of Varicocele.—[This disease, which consists in a dilatation of the veins of the chord, is treated in various ways by different surgeons, and very much according to the peculiar treatment of varix, which each surgeon adopts. Cumano employed the ligature and extirpation at the same time; Mr. Warren excised or tied the varicose veins of the scrotum; M. Moulinie combined excision with ligature; Delpech divided the scrotum, exposed the cord, and tied or incised the veins; in some cases, he passed a small bit of sponge under the dilated veins and fixed it with strips of sticking plaster—it is said he cured six out of seven patients in this way. Bell has tied the spermatic arteries for this affection. Within the last ten years several new methods of treating this disease have been tried, all based on the results obtained from M. Velpeau's experiments on the acupuncture of vessels. This eminent surgeon adopts the following method:]

The patient is placed on his back, the scrotum shaved, and the vas deferens held aside. I then seize the scrotum from behind, and with the thumb and index finger of the other hand I bring the mass of varicose veins forward toward the integuments, and fix them in a fold of skin; an assistant holds one end of this fold, while I support the other. I then pass a needle under the veins, in the way described for varix, and bring a ligature round it; a second needle is passed within about an inch of the first one. You must avoid inserting the needles too low or too high, and separating them too far from each other. If the lower needle, for example, be placed too low down, you may wound the tunica vaginalis; if the superior needle be inserted too high up, you will have difficulty in separating the veins of the cord; finally, if the needles are placed too close to each other, the two wounds may unite and form one. The needles being placed, the ligatures are wound circularly round them, in the same way as for varix of the lower extremities. When the eschars are detached, the needles are withdrawn from the tenth to the twentieth day. Unless the inflammation which supervenes be severe, the patients are not confined, and a cure takes place in about a month. I have never seen phlebitis occur after this operation; in two cases, however, where the inferior needle was inserted too low down, inflammation of the tunica vaginalis came on. The whole of my patients, then, were cured in a short time; and, of those whom I have since met, not one has suffered a relapse. *Part* v., *p.* 136.

Varicocele treated by the Needles and the Twisted Suture.—It seems pretty well understood that all cases of varicocele do not require operative interference, proper and well-regulated support generally affording sufficient relief where the affection is not of a severe description. The distended veins of the cord, however, may cause such painful dragging and disturbance of the general health, as to call for some remedial means. M. Boyer advises an incision to be made over the external ring, to lay open the fibrous sheath of the spermatic cord, and to tie everything contained in it but the vas deferens and the artery. Though hazardous, the author prefers this method to the ligature as advised by M. Ricord, cauterization, or to the rolling up of the varicose plexus, as advocated by M. Vidal. In one case, Mr. Fergusson passed three needles under the scrotal veins, and twisted strong silk round them, as in the hare-lip operation. After a few days the needles were removed, which were very nearly out, and in five days afterward the sores were rapidly healing, and the patient was soon discharged cured. *Part* xxiv., *p.* 242.

Treatment of Varicocele by Gutta Percha dissolved in Chloroform.— Dr. Carey says: After having used gutta percha considerably for other purposes, a knowledge of its properties forcibly suggested it in solution, as admirably fitted to fulfill the desired objects sought in the treatment of varicocele. In order to apply it, the patient is placed upon his back, and by means of cold, the scrotum is corrugated until it is drawn firmly over the root of the penis, compressing the testes firmly in the upper portion of the inguinal pouches; then, by means of a camel-hair pencil, after the hair has been removed, apply the solution freely over the site of the scrotum, allowing it to extend on all sides some distance by a thin attachment; but over the scrotum proper lay on a succession of coats, until a thickness of a line uniform throughout is obtained, which will be sufficiently strong to form an artificial pouch of the nature and character desired. This thickness will be so yielding and pliable as not to afford the wearer any considerable inconvenience. Soon after the solution is applied to this sensitive part, the patient will complain bitterly of the burning sensation experienced, depending upon the presence of the chloroform; but this temporary inconvenience will soon pass off. The constitutional indications, if there be any, must not, of course, be neglected.
Part xxv., *p.* 245.

VARICOSE VEINS.

Varicose Veins cured by the Formation of Small Eschars.—Mr. Skey, of St. Bartholomew's Hospital, treats these cases by forming small eschars a little larger than the diameter of a split pea, the number being regulated by the extent and complication of the disease. This is effected by applying a small portion of the caustic paste through an opening made in three or four thicknesses of adhesive plaster. A piece of plaster may be laid, then, over each quantity, and may be removed in from twenty minutes to half an hour. Rest in the horizontal position is desirable, but not essential. The healing of the ulcers, which are sometimes slow and tedious, should be pushed by bark, wine, good diet, and stimulants, if necessary.

Part xxiii., *p.* 151.

Varicose Veins and Ulcers.—These obstinate and disagreeable affections, have lately been treated by the application of a convoluted spiral strap of vulcanized india-rubber, instead of the ordinary uniform elastic apparatus used. If there are ulcers along with the varicose veins,—first wet with a solution of glycerine. 3ss. to 3viiss. medicated with a little nitric acid, a little common blotting paper, and apply it over the wound, and over this a pledget of lint or linen wet with the same solution. These may be secured by a turn or two of the calico roller, and over this is placed the convoluted spiral bandage. Mr. Startin, the author of this mode of treatment, states that great success has resulted from its employ-ment.

Part xxiii., *p.* 276.

Treatment of Varicose Veins by Needles and Sutures.—It is an established rule in surgery that as long as varicose veins of the lower extremity, or varicocele, do not create much inconvenience, this abnormal state of vessels should not be interfered with ; but when the dilated veins become very troublesome, or threaten to give way, it is urgent that relief should be afforded.

Mr. Fergusson has operated with much success on various patients with the needles, and sutures, in cases of varicose veins of the lower extremity; and as some surgeons are rather timid on this subject, we mention the following case : The patient, twenty-six years of age, a servant, has always enjoyed good health, but having had much standing work in her situation, and many pairs of stairs to ascend in the day, has lately found the veins of her leg enlarging considerably. When admitted the pain and inconvenience had much increased, the left saphena vein being large, tense, and tortuous.

Mr. Fergusson transfixed the vein with needles, and applied the twisted suture, as in hare-lip cases; the patient was enjoined perfect rest ; some pain and tenderness arose in the vein ; this was, however, soon subdued by fomentations, and the patient was discharged in a few weeks with complete obliteration of the vessel.

Part xxv., *p.* 194.

Varicose Veins—On the Obliteration of.—Mr. Henry Lee operates upon these cases in the following manner : He first introduces a needle under the vein to be obliterated, and leaves it there for a few days. 2nd, after that time, when the blood on either side of the needle has become coagulated, the operation is completed by dividing the vein by a subcutaneous incision. The vein must be blocked up before incision is performed, and then we know that no abnormal product, as pus, can pass into the current of the circulation from the division of the coats. Hence the blood must

be kept at rest for a certain time in the vein. By this plan we are assured
that the coagulum so formed consists of blood alone, and no other vitiated
fluid.   *Part* xxvii., *p.* 124.

Varicose Veins cured by Injection of the Perchloride of Iron.—In a case
of large varicosity of the saphena vein, under the care of M. Follin, injection
of the perchloride of iron produced coagulation and effected a cure.
                                                 Part xxix., *p.* 208.

Varicose Veins.—Compressing the vessel at various points, by passing
a hare-lip pin beneath, and applying the twisted suture, is insufficient to
cut off all channels of communication, excepting it excites subacute inflammation throughout the veins in the neighborhood, and this end is far more
safely attained by the application of caustic issues, which Mr. Skey has
shown to be superior to any other mode of treatment at present known.
The caustic recommended is composed of three parts of quicklime and
two of caustic potash, made into a paste with spirits of wine. In applying it, cut a small hole about the size of a split-pea, or a fourpenny-piece,
in adhesive plaster, put this exactly over the part, then apply the paste ;
in from ten to twenty minutes the pain will have ceased, and the paste
must be removed. The issues must not be applied too closely one to
another, for they approximate afterward by the contraction of the skin.
                                                 Part xxxv., *p.* 91.

Varicose Veins treated by Needles and Subcutaneous Section.—Mr.
Erichsen's practice is to pass pins under these veins, generally in three
places, for which purpose the vein must be lifted up, and the pins passed
well under them, so as to avoid puncturing them ; over each of these a
figure of 8 suture must be applied. In about three or four days, he withdraws the pins, and divides the veins subcutaneously. In no instance have
any bad effects followed this plan of treatment.   *Part* xxxv., *p.* 91.

Varicose Veins—Ligature of in Pregnancy.—It has been shown by
the results of a case of Mr. Erichsen's at University College Hospital, that
even during pregnancy (should such a procedure be necessary from dangerous hemorrhage) varicose veins may be safely ligatured. Mr. Erichsen's
method, it will be recollected, consists of placing pins under the veins,
and tying them over a piece of gum elastic bougie.   *Part* xxxvi., *p.* 169.

Varicose Veins.—A case presented to Prof. Erichsen, at University
College Hospital, where a mass of enlarged veins, the size of half an
orange, was situated in the popliteal space. A pin was passed under the
upper extremity of the tumor, and tied in the usual way, and the parts
below were injected with a solution of the perchloride of iron, by means
of a small French syringe, the piston of which works with a regulating
screw, and the point of which is made sharp, and intended to penetrate
the integuments. The intention of this operation is to coagulate the blood
in the large vessels, and thus cause their obliteration. *Part* xxxix., *p.* 162.

Varicose Veins and Ulcers.—For some time past the following method
has been followed at the Great Northern Hospital by Mr. Price, in the
treatment of varicose veins of the legs, whether associated with ulceration
or not. The leg is firmly incased in a bandage which is saturated with a
mixture of starch and glue; a uniform support is thus afforded to the
swollen vessels. This bandage, when well applied, can be worn for weeks
or months ; but the rapid subsidence of the swelling of the leg, in some

instances, may require a recasing of the limb at an earlier period. This plan of treatment, in many cases, has proved as effectual as obliteration of the vessels by the twisted suture, and it moreover possesses the advantage of being available in almost every instance of varicose enlargement of the superficial veins of the extremities. When there is also ulceration, a *window* must be cut somewhat larger than the circumference of the sore or sores, to admit of the treatment of the sore without disturbing the case.

Part xxxix., *p.* 232.

VEINS.

Treatment Required after the Spontaneous Introduction of Air into the Veins.—[The possibility of the introduction of air into the veins during surgical operations is now generally acknowledged, as well as the situation in which only it can happen, accurately pointed out. Mr. Erichsen in this interesting paper confines his remarks to the *spontaneous.* introduction of air into the system, that is to say, when it is not purposely injected into the heart, but when it gains admittance into that organ either in consequence of one of the large veins in its vicinity being opened at a point where the flux and reflux of blood are naturally observed, or, during operations, under such circumstances, whether of disease of the coats of the vessel, of traction in the removal of tumors, or of contraction of surrounding muscles, that it forms an unyielding, uncollapsing tube, into which the air is apt to be sucked in to supply the vacuum, which the action of inspiration has a tendency to occasion within the thorax.

Mr. Erichsen, before giving his own views of the cause of death in these cases, sums up those of previous writers on the subject, which he arranges in four classes, viz.: 1st. That death ensues from over-distention of the right cavities of the heart. Of this opinion are Nysten, Dupuytren, Cormack, Amussat, and Bouillaud (partly.) 2d. That death ensues from the irritation occasioned by the passage of the air through the vessels of the brain.—Bichat. 3d. That the heart's action is arrested in consequence of the deleterious influence of the carbonic acid which is eliminated from the venous blood.—Marshall de Calvi. 4th. That the circulation is arrested in the lungs, either, as Piedagnel and Leroy have supposed, in consequence of these organs becoming emphysematous, or, as Bouillaud and Mercier (partly) think from obstruction of their capillaries, or, as the reviewer in Dr. Forbes' Journal is of opinion, in consequence of the respiratory changes being interfered with.

Mr. Erichsen states his own opinion to be: 1st. That the primary arrest of the circulation that takes place in the capillaries of the lungs, or in the terminal branches of the pulmonary artery, in consequence of inability in the right ventricle to overcome the mechanical obstacle presented by air-bubbles in the vessels of those organs. 2d. That respiration and animal life cease in consequence of a deficient supply of arterial blood to the central organs of the nervous system. Mr. Erichsen then proceeds to that part of the subject which is the most interesting to the practitioner, namely, the plan of treatment to be adopted.]

And first of all, as most important, let us take into consideration the best way of preventing the occurrence of the accident in question. Before doing so, however, it may be better, in order to understand the principles on which we should act, to give a brief summary of those circumstances that

are peculiarly apt to occasion the introduction of air into the circulating
system during operations. Now it is well known that what is called by
the French writers the " canalisation " of a vein, or its conversion into a
rigid uncollapsing tube, is the condition of all others which is most favorable to the introduction of the air into it. Indeed, except in those situations in which there is a natural movement of flux and reflux of the
blood in the veins, this accident cannot occur unless these vessels be canalized, or, in other words, prevented from collapsing. This canalization of
the vessel may be occasioned in a variety of ways. Either the cut vein
may be surrounded by indurated cellular tissue, which will not allow it
to retract upon itself, but keeps it open like the hepatic veins; or the
coats of the vessel may have acquired, as a consequence of inflammation
or hypertrophy, such a degree of thickness as to prevent their falling together when divided. Again, the principal veins at the root of the neck
have, as Bérard has pointed out, such intimate connections with the neighboring aponeurotic structures that they are constantly kept in a state of
tension, so that their sides are held apart when they are cut across. The
contractions of the platysma and other muscles of the neck may likewise,
as Mr. Shaw has shown, have a similar effect. In removing a tumor also
that is situated about the neck, the traction exerted upon its pedicle may,
if this contain a vein, cause it to become temporarily canalized.

The introduction of air into a vein will be favored by the vessel being
divided in the angle of a wound, the vein being, when the flaps that form
that angle are lifted up, rendered openmouthed and gaping.

[In looking over all those cases in which the wounded vein is particu-
larized, Mr. Erichsen found that the wounded vessels were always in
one or other of the abovementioned conditions] and consequently, what
the surgeon should peculiarly guard against in the removal of tumors
about the neck and shoulders, viz., incomplete division of the veins and employment of forcible traction on the diseased mass at the moment of using
the scalpel.

If this be necessary, the chest should, for reasons that will immediately
be pointed out, be tightly compressed, that no deep inspirations may be
made at the moment that the knife is being used, or before a divided or
wounded vein can be effectually secured.

But although it be necessary for the spontaneous introduction of air
into the circulating system, that the vein be either canalized in one or
other of the ways that has just been mentioned, or else that it be opened
where the venous pulse exists, yet it is only during the act of inspiration
that air can gain admittance into the vessel; and it is the more ready to
do this the deeper the inspiratory efforts are. If a vein be opened at the
root of a dog's neck, it will be found that it is only during inspiration that
air rushes in; that none gains admittance during expiration, and but
little, if any, when the inspirations are shallow, as when the chest is
forcibly compressed by the hands; and that the rapidity of the spontaneous introduction of air is, _cœteris paribus_ in proportion to the depth
of the inspirations.

This depends upon the tendency that there is to the formation of a
vacuum within the thorax, more particulary in the pericardium, during inspiration; at which time the blood is carried with increased velocity
along the veins in the neighborhood of the heart; and when expiration
takes place a temporary retardation occurs. This is particularly evident

during excited respiration. Now, during operations the state of the breathing is such as to dispose the patient peculiarly to the entrance of air into the veins. When a patient is under the knife, the respirations are generally shallow and restrained, the breath being held, whilst every now and then there is a deep gasping inspiration, at which moment, if a vein be opened in which the pulse is perceptible, or that is canalized, air must necessarily be sucked in; and, as has already been said, in quantity and force proportioned to the depth of the inspiration. This, then, being the case, the mode of guarding against the introduction of air into the veins is obvious. The chest and abdomen should be so tightly bandaged with broad flannel rollers or laced napkins, as to prevent the deep gasping inspirations, and to keep the breathing as shallow as possible, consistently with the comfort of the patient.

The surgeon must be careful not to remove the compression until the operation be completed and the wound dressed, for if this precaution be not attended to, as the patient will most probably, on the bandage being loosened, make a deep inspiration, air may be sucked in at the very moment that all appeared safe.

It has been fully proved from the experiments of Nysten, Cormack, and Amussat, as well as from recorded cases of recovery in man, that it is necessary that a certain quantity of air be introduced before death can take place, in confirmation of the observations made long since by Nysten, that a few bubbles of air would not occasion death. Magendie states, that he has several times, whilst injecting medicinal saline solutions into the veins of patients, seen air introduced without any bad consequences ensuing. In order, then, that the accident prove fatal, it is necessary that a certain quantity of air be introduced into the venous system. This quantity it is impossible to determine accurately, for obvious reasons.

What, then, are the measures that a surgeon should adopt in order to prevent the occurrence of a fatal termination in those cases in which air has accidentally been introduced into the veins during an operation? Beyond a doubt, the first thing to be done is to prevent the further ingress of air, by compressing the wounded vein with the finger, and, if practicable, securing it by ligature. At all events, compression with the finger should never be omitted, as it has been shown by Nysten, Amussat, Magendie and others, that it is only when the air that is introduced exceeds a certain quantity that death ensues. All further entry of air having thus been prevented, our next object should be to keep up a due supply of blood to the brain and nervous centres, and thus maintain the integrity of their actions. The most efficient means of accomplishing this would probably be the plan recommended by Mercier, who, as it has already been stated, believing that death ensues in these cases, as in prolonged syncope, from a deficient supply of blood to the brain, recommends us to employ compression of the aorta and axillary arteries, so as to divert the whole of the blood that may be circulating in the arterial system to the encephalon. This appears to me to be a very valuable piece of advice, and to be the most effectual way of carrying out the first indication, that of keeping up a due supply of blood to the brain and nervous centres. The patient should, at the same time that the compression is being exercised on his axillary arteries and aorta, or, if it be preferred, as more convenient and easier than the last, on his femorals, be placed in a recumbent position, as in ordinary fainting, so as to facilitate the afflux of blood to the head. The compression of the axillary and femoral arteries may readily be made by the fingers of two of those assistants that are present at every operation.

For the fulfillment of the second indication, that of maintaining the action of the heart until the obstruction in the capillaries of the lungs can be overcome or removed, artificial respiration should be resorted to, as the most effectual means of keeping up the action of that organ. Thus Sir B. Brodie states that he has seen, in a dog that was beheaded, and whose cervical vessels were tied, the contractions of the heart maintained by artificial respiration for two hours and a half, at which time there were thirty-two pulsations in a minute, and from my own observations, I can state that, by the same means, this organ may easily be kept in action in an animal that has been pithed for an hour and a half. For the purpose of keeping up artificial respiration, the Humane Society's bellows, if they be at hand, might be used, or, if they cannot readily be procured, a split-sheet might advantageously be employed. Before inflating the lungs, it will be necessary to remove everything that can compress the chest or interfere in any way with the free exercise of the respiratory movements. Friction with the hand over the præcordial region, and the stimulus of ammonia to the nostrils may at the same time be resorted to.

The third indication—that of overcoming the obstruction in the pulmonic capillaries, would probably be best fulfilled by the means adapted for the accomplishment of the second, viz., artificial inflation of the lungs. That the action of respiration if kept up sufficiently long, would enable the capillaries of the lungs to get rid of the air contained in them, appears to be the case, for I have several times observed that, if a certain quantity of air be spontaneously introduced into the jugular vein of a dog, and artificial respiration be then established and maintained for half or three quarters of an hour, but a very small quantity indeed, if any, will be found, on killing the animal, in the cavities of the heart, or in the branches of the pulmonary vessels.

If by these means we should succeed in warding off an immediately fatal termination to the accidental introduction of air into the veins, we must watch carefully for the supervention of pneumonia or bronchitis, which disease Nysten has shown to be very apt to occur in those animals that recover the immediate effects of the accident. That the same danger exists in man is evident by the two cases that have occurred to MM. Roux and Malgaigne respectively. In Roux's case the patient lived seven days after the accident, at the expiration of which period he died of pneumonia; whilst Malgaigne's patient died on the fourth day of bronchitis. In recapitulation, then, the following are the principal points that it has been endeavored to establish in this paper:

1st. That the primary arrest of the circulation takes place in the capillaries of the lungs, or in the terminal branches of the pulmonary artery, in consequence of inability in the right ventricle to overcome the mechanical obstacle presented by air-bubles in these vessels.

2d. That respiration and animal life ceases in consequence of a deficient supply of arterial blood to the central organs of the nervous system.

3d. That as air enters the veins in quantity, in force, and in rapidity, proportioned to the depth of the inspirations, the best mode of preventing the occurrence of the accident, or, at all events, of lessening its probable fatality, would be in all operations about the dangerous region—the root of the neck and summit of the thorax—to bandage the chest tightly with broad flannel rollers or laced napkins, so as to prevent deep gasping inspirations, and to keep the breathing as shallow as possible, consistently with the comfort of the patient.

4th. If the air have already gained admission, prevent its further entry by compressing, or, if possible, ligaturing the wounded vein by which it entered.

5th. Keep up a due supply of blood to the brain and central organs of the nervous system, by placing the patient in a recumbent position, and by compressing his axillary and femoral arteries.

6th. Maintain the action of the heart, by artificial respiration and friction on the precordial region, until the obstruction in the capillaries can be overcome or removed.

7th. Remove, if possible, the obstructions in the capillaries of the lungs by artificial respiration.

8th. If the patient survive the immediate effects of the accident, guard against the supervention of pneumonia or bronchitis.   *Part* ix., *p.* 149.

VENTILATION.

Importance of Ventilation.—According to Mr. Squire, the usual argand gas-burner consumes above five cubic feet of gas per hour, producing rather more than five cubic feet of carbonic acid, and nearly half a pint of water. Shops using thirty of these lights, therefore, in an evening of four hours, produce upward of nine gallons of water, holding in solution the noxious products of the gas. An argand lamp, burning in a room twelve feet high and twelve feet square, containing 1728 cubic inches of air, with closed doors and windows, produces sufficient carbonic acid, in rather more than three hours, to exceed one per cent, which is considered unfit for respiration, and when it amounts to ten per cent, it is fatal to life. A man makes, on an average, twenty respirations per minute, and at each respiration inhales sixteen cubic inches of air; of these 320 cubic inches inhaled, thirty-two cubic inches of oxygen are consumed, and twenty-five cubic inches of carbonic acid produced.   *Part* xi., *p.* 108.

VERMIFUGES.

Observations on Vermifuge Medicines.—Dr. Cazin, of Boulogne-sur-Mer, states that he has frequently employed the common *spigelia* or *wormgrass.* He administers it in the form of decoction, prepared by boiling two drachms of the herb in a quart of water to one-half. The decoction is then expressed, strained, and flavored with a little lemon juice and a sufficient quantity of sugar. The dose for an adult is two wine-glassfuls, followed by a wine-glassful every six hours until the desired effect is produced. To children and delicate persons a smaller quantity is to be given.

Wormwood (absinthium) is an excellent indigenous anthelmintic : it is also a powerful tonic and stimulant, the use of which, continued after the expulsion of the worms, prevents their reproduction. M. Cazin often uses

VOL. II.—53.

a wine prepared by digesting an ounce of wormwood, with an equal quantity of garlic, in a bottle of white wine, of which he gives from one to three ounces every morning. This wine is well adapted for poor lymphatic subjects, wasted by wretchedness, and suffering from the influence of a marshy soil. The absinthium maritimum is likewise a very good anthelmintic. M. Cazin gives it to the extent of one or two drachms boiled in four or five ounces of water, with the addition of some white sugar, or of any anthelmintic sirup. This is a quite popular remedy in the maritime districts, and almost always succeeds with children affected with worms.

Assafœtida possesses acknowledged anthelmintic properties, and is suitable for cases of sympathetic nervous affections produced by the existence of worms. It thus, like valerian, fulfills a two-fold indication. In a case of nervous affection, which M. Cazin believed to be idiopathic, the administration of assafœtida both determined the disease and revealed its true cause, by effecting the expulsion of a number of lumbrici. This result has, in three cases of chorea and in two of epilepsy, enabled him to recognize that sympathetic irritation, depending on the presence of intestinal worms, was the sole cause of disease in these instances. Under ordinary circumstances, M. Cazin frequently combines assafœtida with calomel in pills. This combination, of all those that he has employed, succeeds best in expelling lumbrici. He has also combined it with black oxide of iron, particularly in anæmic patients. Assafœtida may be given in powder, in doses of from four grains to half a drachm.

The essential oil of *turpentine* is not merely useful in cases of tænia, but is also decidedly efficacious in expelling the lumbrici. M. Cazin has sometimes, in cases of lumbrici and ascarides, administered with advantage turpentine enemata, prepared by suspending, by means of yolk of egg, from one drachm to half an ounce of the oil in decoction of tansy, absinthium, worm-seed (semen-contra), or Corsican moss.

Common salt is very destructive to worms; it is given alone in large doses dissolved in water; it should be taken on an empty stomach. M. Cazin also frequently administers it in the form of enema, with brown sugar, linseed or poppy oil, and a sufficient quantity of water. With children it almost always succeeds.

Like all tonics, *iron* has the advantage of destroying worms, at the same time that, by imparting tone to the intestines, it prevents their reproduction. From six to eight grains of iron filings, mixed with an equal quantity of rhubarb, and taken two or three times a day, have often been sufficient to expel the worms contained in the intestines.

M. Cazin succeeded in rapidly curing a boy nine years of age, emaciated and pale, whose sleep was disturbed, and who was suffering from spasmodic movements similar to those which characterize chorea, by the exhibition of pills of sulphate of iron, combined, according to Puller's formula, with aloes, senna, etc., under which treatment he voided twenty-three lumbrici in four days. He has also used with remarkable success Bosen's mixture, containing extract of black hellebore and sulphate of iron. But what he chiefly gives to children, as well as to adults, is the sirup of citrate of iron (four parts of citrate to sixty of simple sirup, and one of essence of lemon,) in doses of from two drachms to half an ounce to children, and from half an ounce to two ounces to adults.

M. Cazin remarks that *calomel*, so efficacious as an anthelmintic, ought never to be combined with an alkaline chloride, as the formation of corrosive sublimate would probably ensue from their admixture. In like manner, the combination of calomel with cherry-laurel water, or emulsion of bitter almonds, would give rise to the development of two formidable poisons, corrosive sublimate and cyanide of mercury.

The effects of the *male fern, tin, pomegranate bark, hellebore,* etc., require merely to be noticed ; and the properties of the pomegranate root bark are so well known that they need not be dwelt upon. M. Cazin has remarked nothing particular respecting other anthelmintics. He merely says that *cod-liver oil* has succeeded with him in the cases of two females, one of whom passed twelve lumbrici the same day that she had taken in the morning three table-spoonfuls at intervals of an hour.

But whatever be the medicine selected, we must not, like routine practitioners, be content when the worms are killed and dislodged, with this merely palliative cure. A very important indication remains to be fulfilled, viz. to prevent their reproduction. This object is attained, according to M. Cazin, by the adoption of a tonic and stimulant regimen, which must be long continued, and, above all, by the employment of bitter and chalybeate preparations. He has found the ferruginous chocolate to be sufficient, in the case of children, to prevent the relapses which are for many years very apt to occur. Wine taken while fasting has succeeded with the poor inhabitants of the marshes, accustomed to live only on vegetables and milk ; and he has also remarked its efficacy as a preventive of worm affections in other instances. *Part* xxi., *p.* 154.

VOMITING.

Creasote and Acetate of Lead in Vomiting.—Dr. Cormack, of Edinburgh, states that creasote, in medicinal doses, is almost immediately sedative and calming ; but these effects are of short duration ; *so that it is a drug which requires to be given in often repeated small doses.*

Creasote is one of the best medicines which we possess for stopping vomiting. In the vomiting of pregnancy, an affection so distressing to the patient, it seldom fails. If the sickness come on regularly after rising in the morning, Dr. C. prescribes two or three drops to be taken five or ten minutes before getting out of bed. This generally proves effectual; but if it does not, the patient ought to be directed to repeat the dose in two hours. In more troublesome cases, when the sickness occurs at intervals during the day, one or two drops should be given every two, three or four hours.

[In a case communicated by Professor Simpson, the creasote failed to relieve the distressing sickness, while doses of *acetate of lead* proved successful. In the sickness and vomiting following a drinking debauch, creasote is sometimes very useful. In such a case a single dose of four drops was found to relieve speedily. In sea sickness it will often be found efficacious ; but " it is worthy of notice as a general remark that creasote, though excellent in allaying vomiting, *often excites it when it does not exist.*"]

In *vomiting connected with hysteria*, creasote proves a very valuable remedy, and so far as Dr. C.'s experience goes, he is inclined to think, that Dr. Elliotson and others, who have recommended it very strongly in this class of cases, have not done so without sufficient cause. In at least ten cases of this kind, Dr. C. has tried it in doses varying from two to eight drops, and in all excepting one, it proved an admirable medicine, not only relieving the vomiting, but also apparently, in most instances, calming the nervous excitability. In the case in which it apparently did no good, the dose could not be increased beyond six drops thrice a day, on account of the vertigo which it occasioned. The patient was ultimately much benefited by sponging with cold water, and taking four grains of the saccharine carbonate of iron three times a day.   *Part* vi., *p.* 72.

Atonic Vomiting.—Dr. Debregue gives the following : In the vomiting that may be considered to be nervous or spasmodic in its nature—*i e.*, when it is not connected either with inflammation or any bilious disturbance of the stomach—he recommends very highly the use of columba powder : it possesses, he says, a sort of specific virtue in such cases nearly as great as bark does in agues. He gives it in doses of from 15 to 20 grains in two or three spoonfuls of red (French) wine, before meals The addition of a few grains of magnesia, or of a minute dose of opium, may be necessary, if much acidity or gastralgia be present; and, should the patient be feeble and anæmic, the subcarbonate of iron may be very advantageously combined with it. Opium is freely used by Dr. D. in various abdominal affections, after the state of the intestinal secretions has been ascertained to be tolerably healthy.   *Part* x., *p.* 27.

Vomiting of Pregnancy—Strychnia—Recommended in minute doses, by Dr. Golding Bird.   *Part* xiv., *p.* 98.

Observations on Vomiting.—For sympathetic vomiting occurring especially in females, Dr. Seymour, of St. George's Hospital, uses the following formula: Carbonate of ammonia, a scruple ; water, an ounce and a half; sirup, a drachm ; fresh lemon juice half an ounce ; draught to be taken every 4 hours. The following draught, according to our author, answers the same purpose : Sulphate of magnesia, a scruple ; carbonate of magnesia, 10 grains ; mint-water, 10 drachms ; laudanum, 3 to 6 minims ; this draught to be taken every four hours. The same means, he says, often afford relief for considerable periods of time, even when the vomiting is symptomatic of much more serious disease or injuries. In symptomatic vomiting, a blister or mustard poultices often put an end to the morbid sympathy. From half a grain to a grain of opium, made into the smallest size, and as fresh as can be procured, is often successful where all has failed. He has seen equal parts of milk and lime-water succeed where everything else had been tried in vain. In hysterical vomiting, he gives his testimony to the value of creasote, the dose being one or two minims thrice daily. Among other means of checking vomiting, he mentions the successful use of savory meat —the jelly of meat taken in very small quantity regularly thrice a day. Against the vomiting of phthisis he recommends four grains of the extract of conium, to be taken twice or thrice a day, followed by this draught : Lime-water, one ounce ; cinnamon-water, half-an-ounce ; sirup. a drachm. Our author affirms that vomiting occurring almost always after cough in phthisis at an early period, marks a severe and rapid form of it ; and at a late period that large collections of matter are locked up in the lungs. In the vomiting attending what was formerly termed the iliac passion in a young woman, after the case had become hopeless, he succeeded by administering two grains of calomel, made up with a grain of the soft and recent extract of opium; and when the endeavor to vomit returned, by forcing the patient to swallow half a bottle of soda-water in a state of effervescence; "the expansibility of the gas, and the downward impression in swallowing, had the desired effect." Such cases as this, marked by feculent vomiting, he regards as the idiopathic iliac passion, being plainly unconnected either with hernia or intus-susception.

[In the vomiting of Asiatic cholera, one of the best remedies consisted of a scruple of Epsom salts, with five grains of magnesia, and two or three minims of laudanum in a tablespoonful of water every three or four hours, or oftener.] *Part* xvi., *p.* 151.

Vomiting during Pregnancy.—According to Dr. Churchill, if all other means fail in its relief, premature labor must be induced.

Part xvii., *p.* 208.

Vomiting.—In obstinate vomiting, try Sir James Murray's new salt, "the bisulphate of iron and alumina," given in doses of five or ten grains, every two or three hours. *Part* xix., *p.* 312.

Use of Sub-nitrate of Bismuth.—Vomiting may depend upon a simple gastric neurosis, and then M. Monneret thinks the bismuth can be very usefully employed. It is also useful in the vomiting of pregnancy, and that accompanying dysmenorrhœa; but its efficacy is less certain than in affections of the gastro-intestinal tube, and is never so great as when diarrhœa, colic, and flatus are present. From whatever cause pain manifests itself during digestion, we may relieve it by mixing the sub-nitrate freely with the articles of food. *Part* xx.. *p.* 92.

Vomiting—Sympathetic.—Dr. Selkirk advises iodide of potassium in combination with infusion of quassia; a wineglassful of the infusion with three or four grains of the iodide three times a day. *Part* xxi., *p.* 152.

Vomiting—Obstinate.—In a case treated by Dr. Heath of Newcastle-on-Tyne, where all the usual remedies had been tried in vain, a small quantity of chloroform was inhaled to quiet the stomach, but not to produce insensibility. Half a grain of morphia was then given and the inhalation renewed. The patient was kept fully under its influence for a few minutes, and when consciousness returned he was free from all feeling of sickness. The inhalation was kept up slightly for an hour and a quarter. He had no return of the sickness for twenty-four hours. A slight return was checked afterward in the same way. *Part* xxviii., *p.* 310.

Treatment of Vomiting.—Dr. Lees, of Meath Hospital, says: If vomiting be caused by some structural disease of stomach, as ulcer, scirrhus, etc., give a drop of creasote, or five or ten drops of medicinal naphtha, or a combination of bismuth with gallic acid and opium, as recommended by Dr. Turnbull. If caused by a morbid state of the blood, as in scarlatina, erysipelas, cholera, etc., our treatment must be chiefly directed to eliminate the "materies morbi" from the system by means of the skin and bowels. Vomiting may be from a mechanical cause, as from the violence of an habitual cough, or a stooping occupation. If vomiting be from a sympathetic cause, as disease in the womb or brain, or calculus in the gall duct, kidney, or ureter, we must endeavor to remove this, the origin of the vomiting. Thus it has been necessary in some cases to produce abortion, the life of the patient having been in danger from the long continuance of this distressing symptom. If caused by the passage of a calculus, either from the gall-bladder or kidney, large doses of opium are required, the first dose combined with aloes and carbonate of soda. In some cases chloroform may be given with good effect. For the cure of nervous vomiting, that is, vomiting induced by some modification of innervation of the stomach, unconnected with any change of structure, a proper regulation of the mind is essential. A slight but continuous action must be kept up by some mild aperient medicine. In some cases, effervescing draughts, with prussic acid or laudanum, will succeed; and in hysterical cases, assafœtida, valerian, and creasote will be found useful. When the patients are anæmic, give iron with bitter tonics. External counter-irritation is often of much use. The diet must be very simple and easily digestible.   *Part* xxxvi., *p.* 275.

Vomiting of Pregnancy— Oxalate of Cerium.—Prof. Simpson states that cerium has a peculiar sedative and tonic action on the stomach, resembling in some degree the action of the salts of silver and bismuth. It is of all remedies the most generally useful in cases of obstinate vomiting from pregnancy. It does not invariably nor certainly act thus in these cases, but it is more certain than any of the remedies previously in use. The oxalate is the salt most readily procured. It may be given in doses of one or two grains three times a day, or oftener. *Part* xl., *p.* 185.

Curdled Vomitings of Children.— Vide " Marasmus."

———•◦•———

VULVA.

· *Inflammation of the Mucous Follicles of the Vulva.*—M. Robert believes this affection frequently accompanies blenorrhagia, or occurs in women liable to inflammatory affections in these parts, from pregnancy, abortion, etc. The chief seat of the inflammation is in those two large mucous follicles at the entrance of the vagina. Its cure consists in introducing one of Anel's stylets into the follicle, and then laying its cavity open by means of a pair of probe-pointed scissors, and cauterzing its internal surface with nitrate of silver.   *Part* v., *p.* 143.

Treatment of Pruritus Vulvæ.—Having been a great many times consulted for the relief of pruritus vulvæ, and most frequently in pregnant women, says Dr. Meigs, I have rarely had occasion to order anything more than the following formula, viz.: ℞ Sodæ borat., ℥ss.; morphiæ sulphat., gr. vj.; aq. rosa destillat., ℥viij. M. F. sec. art. mist. I direct the person to apply it thrice a day to the affected parts by means of a bit of sponge, or a piece of linen, taking the precaution first to wash the surfaces with tepid water and soap, and to dry them before applying the lotion. I can confidently recommend the prescription as suitable in most cases of this most annoying malady.   *Part* xii., *p.* 297.

Follicular Disease of the Vulva.—Mr. Oldham has met with several cases of a form of disease attacking the follicles which are freely scattered over the mucous membrane of the vulva. It is a painful affection, very difficult of cure, and is attended with leucorrhœal discharge. In its treatment arg. nit. and nitric acid are of no use. Hydrocyanic acid lotion is serviceable, or an ointment made of two drachms of prussic acid and a scruple of diacetate of lead, with two ounces of cocoanut oil. The parts are to be first washed with infusion of roses, and the ointment applied two or three times a day on lint.

Or try a lotion of lime-water with opium ; or make a poultice of bread, saturated with decoction of conium leaves, to a pint of which add two drachms of the liq. plumbi diacet.

When irritation is excessive, prescribe vapor-baths, either simple or medicated with sulphur. Attend to general health, order a nutritious but unstimulating diet ; avoid wine and porter ; give milk with lime water ; keep the patient at rest ; forbid sexual intercourse. There should be change of air. Give the vegetable tonics, as cascarilla, columba, cinchona, sarsaparilla, etc. ; keep the bowels open with small doses of magnes. sulph. in infusion of cascarilla or chamomile. When the symptoms are decidedly abating, give a mild mercurial course with sarsaparilla. *Part* xiv., *p.* 307.

Vulva—Prurigo of the.—Prof. Simpson recommends in severe cases of prurigo of the vulva, vagina, or cervix uteri, to brush the affected parts over with hydrocyanic acid, the strength of that of the Edinburgh Pharmacopœia. *Part* xxi., *p.* 289.

Blenorrhagia of the Vulva.—Mr. Acton would enforce cleanliness. A soothing plan should be first employed, and separation of the surfaces attempted ; then lotions of nitrate of silver, ℨj. to ℨij. of distilled water, with the addition of warm baths. If the inflammation has gained the deeper structures, leeches may be employed in addition, to the groins ; and if abscess should form, it must be opened immediately, though we should pause when the inflammation occurs round an already-formed cyst.

Part xxiv., *p.* 345.

Prurigo of the Vulva.—Prof. Simpson believes this may be relieved, and generally cured by the assiduous and persevering application of a solution of borax, five or ten grains to the ounce of water, or in a little infusion of tobacco. An ointment of the iodide of lead, or of bismuth and morphia, is very useful. Chloroform, applied locally in the form of vapor, is one of the most certain means which can be employed. These remedies should be alternated. In the more obstinate cases astringents will be found of much use : alum, or aluminated iron, or tannin. Of course the general health of the patient must be attended to. Arsenic, aqua potassa, and other alterative medicines of that class may be required.

Part xl., *p.* 214.

WARTS.

Treatment of Venereal Warts.—If they are pedunculated, Bransby B. Cooper recommends the ligature ; in other cases, caustic or powdered savine. If these means are insufficient, excise the warts with the knife, and apply caustic to the cut surfaces. When there is phimosis with warts, the prepuce must always be laid open immediately. *Vide* "Condylomata." *Part* xxi., *p.* 270.

Warty Excrescences.—Mr. T. W. Nunn, acting on the principle of Dr. Arnott, of using congelation as an anæsthetic agent, has recently applied little wedged-shaped pieces of ice to the necks of large warty growths depending from the labia minora, till they became blanched and cold ; and he then removed a great many of them with a single stroke of the knife, without causing the patient any but very slight pain. *Part* xxii., *p.* 314.

Non-Specific Affections.—These, which consist of *warts, vegetations, herpes preputialis, eczema, and excoriations,* may be treated with strong acetic acid. Mr. Acton recommends the powder of oxide of zinc in the more simple forms, and in the obstinate a powder composed of equal parts of ærugo and pulvis sabinæ. *Part* xxiv., *p.* 346.

Unexpected Effects of the Employment of Carbonate of Magnesia in Case of Warts.—In the case of a girl affected with gastralgia, whose hands were covered with warts, Dr. Lambert gave carbonate of magnesia. Two months after, though the stomach affection was unaltered, the warts had disappeared. In another case, the same dose, a teaspoonful night and morning, produced a similar effect in five weeks. *Part* xxvii., *p.* 161.

WATER.

Artificial Harrogate Water.—Where the genuine Harrogate water cannot well be procured, the following will be found a good substitute:

ARTIFICIAL HARROGATE WATER.

R Sulphatis potassæ cum sulphure, ʒj.; potassæ bitartratis, ʒss.; magnes. Sulphat., ʒvj.; aquæ destillat. ℔ij.

Solve.—Capiat dimidium p. r. n

The above is sufficient for a quart, and ought to be taken early in the morning before breakfast, and be followed by a walk, to produce the desired aperient effect. *Part* v., *p.* 85.

Waters of Vichy and Carlsbad.—Dr. Cahill considers the waters of Vichy and Carlsbad very valuable in gout, rheumatism, gravel, and affections of the liver and spleen, owing to their strong alkaline character, which is principally due to the large quantity of bicarbonate of soda which they contain; they are very mild and gentle in their operation, and not like the waters of Homburg, Weisbaden, and Kissengen, which contain chloride of sodium, and are severely purgative. *Part* xxxiii., *p.* 295.

Kreuznach Waters.—Dr. Prieger thinks there is no reason to believe that these waters, whether employed on the spot, or elsewhere, have any power in removing undoubted fibrous tumors of the womb, although we may speak with the greatest confidence of their efficacy in diminishing general hypertrophies of the uterus, not having an isolated form, or independent growth. *Part* xxxv, *p.* 308.

WHEY.

Different Kinds of Whey.—The following is a translation of the directions given in the "Pharmacopœia Borussica" of 1829, for the preparation of five different kinds of whey:

1. *Serum lactis dulce, Sweet Whey.*—Take an ounce of the dried stomach of a calf, infuse with six fluid ounces of cold water for ten or twelve hours, add an ounce of this liquor to nine pounds of fresh cow's milk, warm gently, and after coagulation is effected, decant and strain the liquid.

2. *Serum lactis dulcificatum, Sweetened Whey.*—Take three pounds of

cow's milk, boil, and at the commencement of ebullition add one drachm of bitartrate of potash ; when a coagulation is effected, and the whole has become cool, strain, and boil with a sufficient quantity of white of egg beaten up into a froth, until the albumen is coagulated ; strain, and add as much prepared chalk (or shells) as is required to neutralize the acid, and filter.

3. *Serum lactis acidum, Sour Whey.*—The former without addition of the chalk.

4. *Serum lactis aluminatum, Alum Whey.*—5. *Serum lactis tamarindinatum, Tamarind Whey.*—In these respectively a drachm of crude powdered alum, or one ounce of the pulp of tamarinds, is employed instead of the bitartrate of potash.   *Part* xxviii., *p.* 321.

WHITLOW OR FELON.

Use of Potassa Fusa.—Whitlow, paronychia, or felon, may be removed, according to Dr. Barnes, of St. Louis, U. S., in the early stages, and in the later stages may be much relieved, by applying potassa fusa. Slightly moisten the end of a stick of this caustic, and rub it over the surface of the diseased and adjacent parts for a few seconds, until the patient complains of much pain. If this pain or burning sensation lasts for a few minutes, the application has been sufficient; if it subsides more quickly, reapply the caustic for a short time. Be very careful not to destroy the skin.   *Part* xvi., *p.* 326.

Whitlow—Deep-seated.—Dr. Hamilton, of Richmond Hospital, Dublin, gives the case of a man forty years old, who was seized with a deep-seated whitlow. Deep incisions were made in the front of the first phalanx, out of which matter gushed, to the man's great relief. Incisions were afterward made in the palm and dorsum of the hand, but still the finger was obliged to be removed at the metacarpal articulation.

The symptoms are usually as follows : The affected finger becomes painful, the pain increasing to the greatest degree, so as to prevent sleep, and often to cause the patient to spend the night walking about his room in torture. This will be at first accompanied by little swelling, and little redness, more especially in front, although the greatest suffering is complained of there. The finger will be kept bent, any attempt to straighten it increasing the pain, as does also pressure over the affected part. By keeping the finger flexed, the skin in front is relaxed as well as the tendon, relieving the painful tension, and the pressure of the tendon on the inside of the inflamed sheath. The back of the finger next becomes red, swollen, and shining, pitting on pressure. You might be misled by this, and think it was the place to make your incisions in search of matter, but it will be found that pressure on this part can be borne, whereas in front, where Boyer says this whitlow always occurs, it cannot ; and when the finger is attempted to be straightened, the suffering is at once referred to the front. After the third or fourth day, this part will be found swollen and prominent, particularly on a side view, but no fluctuation is discernible. If no treatment is adopted, the disease will often proceed from the finger to the palm, which becomes red, swollen, and tender, the back of the hand particularly

so, of a deep shining red, pitting on pressure, and fluctuation is soon apparent either over the knuckle of the affected finger, or in the web between
the fingers. In the palm of the hand we often observe that the matter,
after having made its way out through a small opening in the skin, does
not pierce through the cuticle, which in the laboring classes is excessively
thick, but separates it extensively, and you have a considerable collection
of pus only covered by cuticle, before you come to real abscess; as the
palm becomes engaged, other fingers get flexed, and cannot bear extension, and the pain shoots up the arm to the shoulder; in a woman, I knew
it extend to the breast of the affected side. In most instances the inflammation with suppuration stops at the finger and palm, particularly when
treatment has been resorted to; but if not, it may go up the front of the
wrist to the forearm, in which case the patient recovers after weeks of
suffering, worn out by sleepless nights and profuse suppuration, with bent,
emaciated fingers, and a stiff wrist, and a nearly useless hand. Should'
the disease not extend so high, or not be so violent, it may end with a
stiff, bent finger. I should say when there has been suppuration the finger
is invariably stiff, and usually bent, from adhesion of the integuments to
the sheath of the tendons, and of the tendons to the inside of the sheath,
while in the state of flexion. If the inflammation is very intense, the
tendons die, and protrude through the natural or artificial opening that
has let out the matter, and throw off greyish white sloughs; where a
portion of the flexor profundus is totally destroyed, the finger may be
quite straight, being kept so by the extensor tendon. Such is the case in
the man now in the house, who came to the hospital after having suffered
from whitlow six weeks. I took away a dead portion of the flexor tendon,
one and-a-half inch long, from the sheath. I am going to remove his
finger, as he presents a further step in the disease, viz., the periosteum is
stripped from the bone of the first phalanx by effusion of pus, and the bone
is killed.

The death of the bone is most common in the last phalanx, particularly
of the thumb. In such a case you will find, though the matter has been
let out by a free opening, the disease lingers, the part continues red and
swollen, the opening discharges abundance of thin matter, they are large
flabby granulations around it, and if you feel the end of the finger, there
is a pseudo-fluctuating feel, as if it was extensively undermined; a probe
passed in removes every doubt, by grating against the rough bone. It is
best not to wait till it separates of itself, but enlarge the opening, and seizing the dead bone with a forceps, divide any ligamentous connections at
the joint, while they are on the stretch. The parts soon heal, the finger
shortened, bent forward, and clubbed at the end, the nail irregular, but
still a useful finger.

The fever, in deep-seated whitlow, often runs high, and I have known
delirium at night, but I never met with a fatal termination, except in one
case, a man who crushed his thumb while intoxicated; deep-seated
paronychia followed, inflammation of the veins up the arm, and death.

On looking over the notes of many cases, I find the most frequent seat
of deep-seated whitlows to be the middle finger, next the ring, and then
the index finger, all before the thumb. This agrees with Boyer's experience; it differs from what we perceive in the superficial paronychia, in
which the index finger and the thumb are so much the oftenest affected,
and at their extremities. The part of the finger in the deep-seated parony-

chia most commonly engaged is the sheath of the flexor tendon over the first phalanx; this sheath is not only the longest, but the strongest, and most complete. A few cases, when suppuration was threatened, subside and terminate by resolution. The majority run rapidly into suppuration, which is more or less extensive, according to the intensity of the inflammation. Such is an outline of the symptoms and pathology of deep-seated whitlow. You see that it is an inflammation of the inside of the sheath of the tendons, that nature makes vain efforts to get out the matter confined in the strong fibrous envelope; you have witnessed the disastrous effects of the unrelieved diseased action, the periosteum, the tendon, the bone, all at last engaged, and the finger, or even the hand, permanently injured or even lost. You will at once naturally arrive at the conclusion, that a free incision into the sheath, early performed, is the only treatment. Yet how is it that so many come to the hospital, where this has never been done, and all the destructive consequences allowed without an incision ever having been made?

I believe it arises from timidity, a fear of wounding blood-vessels, particularly when the disease approaches the palm; there the palmar arch becomes a kind of bugbear. Some years ago, I made careful dissections of the hand, with a view of furnishing myself with precise rules for making incisions in deep-seated whitlows. Permit me to call your attention to a few practical conclusions I arrived at:

"There are two principal wrinkles or lines running across the palm of the hand; one, nearly transverse, corresponds to the joints between the metacarpal bones and first phalanges, and is situated about an inch behind the first transverse lines on the fingers. The second begins from the first, at the articulation of the index phalanx with its corresponding metacarpal bone, and goes in an oblique direction across the palm toward the pisiform bone at the inside of the wrist; *it answers pretty nearly to the course of the ulnar or superficial or palmar arch.* These two lines, which are very regular, will be found to serve as excellent guides in making our incisions in paronychia with confidence.

" On the fingers there are three bundles of transverse lines; the two from the tip correspond to the articulations, that next the palm does not correspond to any joint, but is situated about the centre of the first phalanx end of the sheath of the flexor tendon.

"The palmar fascia goes about as far as the transverse palmar line before it sends off its four processes which go between the fingers, and are attached to the sides along with the tendinous insertions of the extensor muscles and the lumbricales.

" The web between the fingers contains the digital artery from the palmar arch and its division, and is filled up with loose cellular tissue, allowing matter easily to go from the palm to the back of the hand. As the superficial palmar arch, the only one likely to be wounded, corresponds to the oblique line which is behind the transverse line, the distance increasing as it approaches the inside of the wrist, you can, in all the fingers, *safely* make your incision as far as the transverse line; nay, in all fingers but the middle, you can cut beyond this as far as the centre of the hand, and in the index finger even further. But it is worse than useless ever to carry your incision from the finger further than the transverse line, so as to endanger the arterial arch at all, as after going so far it is quite sufficient to pass a director under the palmar fascia, which alone confines the matter, if it has gone into the hand. On the director, you could, if desirable, cut out through the fascia, and even the annular ligament. Whereas, if you cut down without a director to the palm, through all the parts to the bone (which in the palm is unnecessary, as there is nothing below the palmar fascia or annular ligament to confine matter), you could scarcely avoid wounding the arteries or large nerves. In the same way in the fingers after the sheaths of the tendons are divided, nothing remains to confine matter. These sheaths extend from the tip of the fingers to the transverse palmar line or metacarpal phalangeal articulation; they are thick and strong between the joints, thin opposite to them; you should avoid over the joints, and confine your incisions to the strong part of the sheaths between them, cutting to the bone if you choose, or what is generally enough, down to the tendon, taking care to open the sheath well, and always keeping in the centre to avoid the digital arteries running along the sides of the fingers. In the thumb it is particularly necessary to observe this last rule, as otherwise, after cutting beyond the first joints, you would be very likely to wound the superficialis volæ.

"Bearing these facts in mind, you will have no hesitation in making sufficiently free and deep incisions. I repeat, take care that your cut is long enough to open the sheath freely; a mere deep puncture through it may let out matter, and give ease for the time; but not allowing free vent, will cause the pus to seek another outlet, and much mischief ensue."

In spite of free incisions the diseased action is not always stopped. In such cases, though there is at first much relief, the unpleasant sensations return; the next night the patient will be kept awake by deep-seated, throbbing pain, and you may be sure that the matter is working its way out in some other direction, and is not getting free exit, and you will probably discover some swollen, tender spot, to repeat the incision. If the disease presents itself in a more advanced and aggravated form, not only engaging the finger, but extending to the palm, back of the hand, or even the wrist, which last is very rare, you will have to follow the matter, regulating your incisions by the rules I have mentioned. Some authors have made a separate division of paronychia, which they name paronychia periostei, from supposing the disease in this form to commence in the periosteum covering some part of the phalanges, with suppuration between the periosteum and bone, death of the bone, etc. I regard the affection of the periosteum rather as a secondary effect of the deep-seated paronychia, whose seat we have seen to be the sheaths of the tendons, but when neglected, to engage finally all the tissues, the periosteum among the rest, and the bone. When the first or second phalanges are stripped of periosteum, and dead, it is best to remove the whole finger at the metacarpal articulation.

If it is the last phalanx, it can be removed alone, and as I have already said, a useful finger will remain after the opening is healed.

Part xxxi., *p.* 183.

--- •◆• ---

WORMS.

Tape-worm—Treatment of.—In 206 cases of tape-worm, Dr. Wawruch found the following treatment the most efficacious: As a preparatory step, all the patients took a laxative decoction with sal ammoniac, for three, four, or five days, and ate nothing but weak soup, thrice a-day. In 8 cases the worm was expelled by the mere effect of continued abstinence. The anthelmintic remedies employed were castor oil and the powdered root of the male fern. From one to two tablespoonfuls of the oil were given as a dose, alternately with one or two drachms of the powder twice or thrice a day.

Enemata of oil and milk were frequently thrown up, to attract the worm toward the large intestine, and it was observed, that the effect of the drastic was always most sure when given a certain time after the last dose of fern, than at once. The drastic purge employed was composed of equal parts of calomel, gamboge, and sugar, two to eight grains of each for a dose. In many cases a single dose brought the worm away, but in others three to six doses were required. The period at which the worm was discharged was very various. The tænia is not exclusively a *solitary* worm, for in nine cases there were two worms, of different ages and development; in two cases, three worms. In one very remarkable case, four worms were discharged, and this patient still suffers from the complaint.

Generally speaking, the patient may expect to be entirely free from his disease, if he pass ten or twelve weeks without discharging any remnants of the worm. *Part* iv., *p.* 26.

Tape-worm—Mode of giving Turpentine.—Dr. Bellingham does not think it necessary to administer this remedy in the large doses which were formerly given. He states that it will be equally effectual if the system be kept for some time under its influence by giving it in moderate doses, two or three times in the twenty-four hours, occasionally exhibiting a larger dose; and if no cathartic effect follows, he combines it or follows it up with castor oil. *Part* vi., *p.* 74.

Oleum Santonicæ, or Chenopodii as an Anthelmintic.—[Dr. Monsarret made use of this medicine when some obstinate cases, supposed to be owing to intestinal worms, came under his notice. He began with four to eight or ten drops on lump sugar or milk to a child, and so on in proportion. He says:]

Its effects surprise me, not having had much previous faith. In almost every case, I could observe innumerable quantities of lumbrici were discharged. In adult cases I have used it to the extent of half a drachm, or more, for several days, with success; then, as a precaution, prescribing the following draught:

R Ol. ricini, 3vj.; ol. terebinth., 3ij.; spts. lavand., 3j.; ess. m. pip., gtt. xx. M. Ft. haust. *Part* ix., *p.* 73.

Santonine—A Tasteless Worm Medicine.—This is now recommended on good authority as a remedy for worms, especially lumbricales, in this form. Take

Santonine, one drachm; sugar, five ounces; gum tragacanth, half a drachm. Make into 144 lozenges; of these a child may take from five to ten daily, or santonine may be given in powder with sugar.

Part x. *p.*, 184.

Lumbricoides—Pulmonary Disease arising from the Presence of.—Dr. Chapman gives the following case: I was called into consultation with Dr. Monges, to a boy who, with most of the symptoms of pthisis, particularly the copiousness of purulent expectoration, was so much reduced that the portions of the bones on which he rested, had protruded through the integuments in several places. Discovering that his abdomen was tumid, his tongue furred, his appetite capricious and depraved, and that he was subject occasionally to convulsions, I was led to suspect the existence of worms, and under such an impression, anthelmintics were administered. In less than one week, sixty-eight lumbricoides were evacuated, and from that moment he became convalescent and rapidly got well. *Part* xi., *p.* 55.

Ascarides—Of the Rectum.—An anonymous correspondent of " Amer. Jour. of Med. Sc." recommends to give an enema with five grains of Prussian blue, rubbed up in two ounces of rain water or mucilage, and let it be retained until the next regular stool. Repeat this daily, gradually increasing the qantity of the salt. *Part* xvi., *p.* 155.

Ascarides.—Give camphor in three or five-grain doses ; a convenient form is Sir James Murray's solution of camphor in his fluid magnesia. Or the same preparation may be given in the form of enema. *Part* xvii., *p.* 18.

Treatment of Worms in Children.—The symptoms said to indicate the presence of worms, are most of them, Dr. West remarks, of small value ; and nothing short of seeing the worms can be regarded as affording conclusive evidence of their existence. The general treatment is, to regulate the diet, and, give alteratives and ferruginous preparations, with occasionally a brisk cathartic. The special treatment for *ascarides* consists in giving a lime-water enema, with or without two drachms of muriated tincture of iron ; if they have occasioned much diarrhœa and tenesmus, the lime-water injection should be given daily for two or three days together, and small doses of castor oil mixture given every six or eight hours. For *tænia* give decoction of the bark of pomegranate root, in doses of ʒj. thrice a day, to a child seven years old, interrupting its administration twice in the week, in order to give a purge of calomel and scammony. *Part* xviii., *p.* 128.

Tape-worm treated by " Kousso."—The "kousso," or brayera anthelmintica (a plant of the natural order Rosaceæ), was introduced into notice by a pharmacien of Paris, and its properties as an anthelmintic were investigated by the Academy of Medicine so long ago as 1847. The report of the above-named body, as also of the Academy of Sciences, was extremely favorable.

The parts of the plants used are the flowers, which, being reduced to a fine powder, are macerated in lukewarm water for fifteen minutes. The infusion, with the powder suspended in it, is taken either in one, two, or three doses, quickly following each other. It is recommended that lemon juice should be taken freely before and after the kousso. The patient must be prepared by low diet for a day previously, and the medicine taken on an empty stomach before breakfast. The clear infusion has the color, and a somewhat similar taste, to very weak senna tea. It rarely causes any annoyance or uneasiness, except a slight nausea, and this but seldom. *Part* xxi., *p.* 153.

Lumbrici.—A combination of assafœtida with calomel, in the form of pills, says Dr. Cazin, has succeeded better than anything in expelling lumbrici. The dose of assafœtida is from four grains to half a drachm. The administration of three tablespoonfuls of cod oil, at intervals of an hour, has also been followed by the expulsion of lumbrici. *Part* xxi., *p.* 154.

Schmidt's Remedy for Tape-worm.—By the p   of Schmidt, the tape-worm is said to be expelled in from three to fivedays, without injury to the patient. A trial of it was made, under the authority of government, in the Berlin hospital, when the results were found to be so favorable, that the King of Prussia purchased the secret through a pension of several hundred dollars bestowed upon the originator. The plan substantiates the purely empirical fact, that vermifuge medicines, when exhibited separately, are less efficacious than when combined in complex formulæ. The patient commences by taking, in the morning, the following mixture : R. Pulv. rad. valer. min., ℨvj.; fol. senn., ℨij.; aq. ferv., ℥vj.; infunde et cola; adde sal. glauber. crystall., ℨiij.; syr. mannæ, ℥ij.; elaeosacch. tanaceti. ℨij., M.S. Two tablespoonfuls every two hours, drinking freely at intervals of sweetened coffee. With this he perseveres till seven in the evening. At noon he takes a thin gruel; and in the afternoon one or two herrings with the milt. At eight in the evening the patient has a herring salad, with minced raw ham, and oil, sweetened with sugar, plentifully added. Frequently portions of the tape-worm begin now to be discharged. At six in the ensuing morning, he commences the following pills, every hour : R. Assafœtidæ, extr. graminis, aa., ℨiij.; gambog., pulv. rhei, jalap. aa., ℨij.; pulv. pecac., digit. purp., sulph. antim. aurat. aa., Əss.; sub. muriat. hydr., Əij.; ol. tanacet., æther. anisi, aa., gt. xv. M. Divide into pills of two grains each, which are to be placed in a well-stoppered bottle ; of these, six pills are to be administered every hour with a teaspoonful of common sirup. Half an hour after the first dose, a tablespoonful of castor oil is also given. Sweetened coffee is again to be taken freely at intervals during the day. At two in the afternoon, the worm is usually wholly expelled, when the pills are to be discontinued. Should only separate portions be voided, however, the remedies are persisted with, and a second dose of castor oil becomes requisite. Meat soup is allowed at dinner, and in the evening. On the succeeding day, as an additional precaution, six pills are again exhibited at three different times—morning, noon, and evening. *Part* xxiii., *p.* 124.

Vermicularis (maw-worm.)—Dr. Merel uses injections of an infusion of red onion, mixed with half a grain of extract of aloes. *Part* xxvi., *p.* 90.

Tape-worm.—Prof. Osborne, of College of Physicians, Ireland, suggests tannic acid. This we might infer from analogy would be beneficial from its action on gelatine and albumen, both of which these parasites contain.

The seeds of the pumpkin contain a fixed oil ; Prof. Paterson, Philadelphia, recommends half an ounce of this given twice a day, followed by an ounce of castor oil. *Part* xxix., *p.* 120.

Tænifuge Medicines.—Prof. Strohl says : The fruits call *tatzé* and *zareh* are the produce of a shrub of the family of the myrsinaceæ, the " *myrsina Africana*."

This plant is found in Abyssinia, in moist, rocky places at the Cape of Good Hope, in the Azores, in Algeria, and other parts of Africa.

Tatzé is a powerful tænifuge, which has succeeded in all the six cases in which it was administered. This number is too small to draw any conclusion as regards the constancy of its action, but it is quite sufficient to assure us that it at least deserves to be placed among the resources of materia medica. Tatzé is less gentle in its action than saoria.

As to its mode of administration, it should be given in doses of about half an ounce, reduced to powder, and blended in a ptisan or aromatic infusion ; if after three hours it has not caused a motion from the bowels, or if in stools which have followed no traces of the worm are to be discovered, a dose of castor oil should be administered. *Part* xxx., *p.* 65.

Tape-worm.—Professor Bennett has found this to be the best remedy for tape-worm. Give ∋ij. of the ethereal extract of the male shield fern in the evening, and follow this in the morning by ʒj. of castor oil. If necessary, give another scruple of the extract the next evening, and another dose of castor oil the following morning These doses may be repeated according to circumstances. *Part* xxxi., *p.* 94.

Santonin as an Anthelmintic.—For round and thread-worms, Dr Perry gives to a child two years old, three grains of crystallized santonine, and about two hours after it a dose of calomel and jalap ; in the course of twelve or twenty-four hours the worms will be expelled. Santonine is a medicine which may be given with perfect safety, and its effects are certain and satisfactory *Part* xxxiv., *p.* 103.

Tape-worm.—The following mode of administration of male fern is recommended by Dr. Jenner, University College Hospital. You must first prepare the patient by clearing out the bowels and keeping on low diet. For an adult give two calomel and colocynth pills at night, and a dose of castor oil in the morning ; when the bowels have acted well give one drachm and a half of the oil of male fern on some aromatic water, and repeat in six hours if necessary. The dose of the oil must be the same for a child as an adult. No unpleasant results ever follow its use. *Part* xxxiv., *p.* 105.

Use of Kameela as an Anthelmintic.—*Kameela,* a native plant of India, is said to be much more efficacious than kousso, and is certainly much cheaper. It produces only the ordinary effect of a purging medicine and little or no griping. Dr. Gordon (surgeon to the 10th foot regiment) has never known it fail. A drachm may be given mixed with a little water, and repeated in about three hours—from one to five doses may be necessary. A spirituous tincture is more convenient, ʒiv. of the powder to Oj. of alcohol, and filtered. Only about ʒvj. will be obtained in this way. The dose necessary will be from ʒj. to ʒiij.—ʒij. being in most cases sufficient. *Part* xxxv., *p.* 263.

Nitrate of Silver in Ascarides.—Dr. Schultz states that he has employed enemata of this substance with great success for the removal of the *oxyuris vermicularis* which so frequently infest the anus in such large numbers. The clyster is formed of argent. nitrat. gr. x. ad xv. to aq. dest. ʒiv. Two, or at most three, of these suffice to effect a complete cure. The first one does not usually remain up long, and worms, some living and others dead, are returned with it. The next clyster remains from six to twenty-four hours, and the great mass of the dead worms are discharged with it. *Part* xxxviii., *p.* 91.

Tœnia.—Dr. Peacock, of St. Thomas' Hospital, considers kameela more efficient than kousso, but prefers the oil of male fern to either. The resinous principle of the oil is apt to be deposited from the ethereal solution, when the supernatant fluid is of course inefficacious. *Part* xxxviii., *p.* 334.

WOUNDS.

Hints on the Treatment of Wounds after Operations.—The following brief passages are extracted from a letter which M. Phillips, of Liege, a l-dressed to M. Baudens, the chief surgeon of the French army in Africa.

After an amputation in a joint, the flaps should be brought and kept together by a few stitches, in order to promote union by the first intention; but as adhesion rarely, or perhaps never, takes place between the surface of a cartilage and the contiguous flesh, we should not only remove so much of it (the cartilage) before closing the wound, but also place a small portion of lint upon it, so as to encourage suppuration at this point, while the rest is retained in exact contact. The annals of surgery afford scarcely one instance of complete and perfect union, without suppuration of a wound, after a disarticulating amputation. We are of opinion that whenever an amputation is performed at a joint, an issue or opening should always be left opposite to the cartilage, while the rest of the wound is retained together by sutures.

Even after ordinary amputation, where a bone has been sawn across, some surgeons have recommended that the same practice be pursued; but without positively admitting the propriety of so general a rule, it is worthy of remark that when the two ends of a bone are sawn off in cases of ununited fractures, not only is there a better chance of a union taking place, but this union is always much firmer and more solid, when suppuration has been established at the point of junction, than when immediate adhesion of the wound has occurred. Such was the opinion of M. Delpech; a high authority certainly on all subjects of practical surgery.

The success of M. Percy, after the battle of Neubourg, deserves to be alluded to, in consequence of certain circumstances. There was such a want of many of the most necessary articles, as lint, ointment, and bandages, in the French camp, that all the patients were dressed indiscriminately with merely cold water. It is probably to this very circumstance that the great success of the surgeons, in the results of their operations, was attributable on that occasion. For some years past, the same practice has been adopted by Mr. Liston at the London University Hospital, and M. Phillips has of late universally followed it with very marked benefit, after almost all his operations. In all severe injuries of, as well as after operations of the eye, M. P. always subjects the part to the action of the cold water for several days. Also after the extirpation of tumors, when the lips of the wound have been brought and kept together by several stitches, compresses wetted frequently with cold water, are laid invariably upon the part. M. Phillips mentions that in such cases he generally unties the ligature at the lower angle of the wound on the day after the operation, for the purpose of giving exit to any bloody or other kind of discharge, and after removing this, he again secures it. On the third or fourth day he removes one ligature, and another on each day successively; continuing the use of the cold application all the time. M. P. trusts to torsion of the arteries to arrest the hemorrhage, after many such operations. There is very little doubt that this simple expedient, if really sufficient as a hemostatic means, must contribute very materially to the speedy union of wounds, as each ligature on a blood-vessel must necessarily give rise to a point of suppuration and to a minute sinus or fistula extending from the tied vessel to the surface of the wound. ● *Part* i., *p.* 88.

Wounds after Amputation—Primary and Secondary Union of.—Baron Larrey was a surgeon eminently practical. In his work on the surgical cases of the campaigns of 1815, he takes the opportunity of noticing the mode of performing amputation in London, and whilst he admires the coolness and dexterity of the surgeons, he condemns their mode of dressing the stumps. This condemnation, however, is only applicable to those surgeons whose operations he witnessed, and not to many others who do not make a practice, as he supposes, of forcibly approximating the divided surfaces for the purpose of promoting union by the first intention. Larrey denies that the surgeon abridges the labor of nature by this process. He states that as the tissues or organs of the limb are divided more or less perpendicularly to the axis of the bone, there must necessarily remain at the bottom of the wound a cavity when the superficial parts are forcibly approximated. This will be especially the case when we remember the *conical* way in which the muscles are generally divided so as to produce a good flap to protect the extremity of the bone. In this cavity there will continue to accumulate the fluids that for some time are poured out of the contiguous surfaces, which will necessarily cause distention, and perhaps separation of the flaps or absorption of pus. The presence of pus in the veins is no proof of these vessels being inflamed; they may only be conveying this secretion from the wounded surfaces. In all amputations for chrome diseases of the extremities, he strongly recommends, as indeed is now adopted by many surgeons in this country, that the divided surfaces be not immediately united and kept together.

" When the tissues of an injured part are in a state of inflammation, they are not at all in an apt condition to unite; and the only way, in which they can become degorged, is by the process of suppuration being established. When the operation is performed for any chronic disease of the extremity, as for caries of the bones, white-swelling of the joints, or cancerous or other malignant degeneration of the soft parts, I consider it to be quite indispensable, if we hope to prevent local engorgement and purulent infection, that the divided surfaces be not immediately united and kept together; so that the effused fluids may not be retained or forced back upon the system, but may ooze out from the wound as they are formed."

He recommends nearly the same practice in those cases where amputation is adopted in consequence of recent injuries; and confirms his opinion by relating the want of success which followed many of the amputations at the siege of Antwerp, in consequence of attempting to heal the parts by the first intention, and the greater success of his own practice. In the former cases, the limbs were frequently not healed before the fiftieth or fifty-fifth day, whereas this was accomplished three weeks earlier by adopting his own method.

Most of our leading surgeons now adopt this practice to a greater or less extent—Liston, for example, says, " Surfaces are not disposed to unite for many hours after the division and separation have occurred. So long as oozing continues, there is no good end to be achieved by their close apposition. It is only when reaction has occurred, when vascular excitement around the solution of continuity has taken place, when the whole circulation has been roused, and when plastic matter begins to be secreted and thrown out, that the process can be expected to commence. The edges of a large wound, as that resulting from amputation of the extremities, may be approximated in part so soon as bleeding from the principal vessels and larger branches has been arrested. But the close apposition, and the application of all the retentive means, had better be delayed for six or eight hours at least. In the interval, extreme sensibility of the injured parts' may be abated, the oozing moderated, and the chance of secondary hemorrhage much diminished, by covering the parts with lint dipped in cold water, and frequently renewed; or a piece of lint may be placed on the wound, and a constant irrigation of the exposed surface kept for some time by threads passing from a vessel containing cold water. This plan is very useful when the whole surface of a wound is exposed. In cases where there is a deep cavity, where coagulated blood may collect, as at the bottom of the wound after amputation of the thigh, where the flaps, as they always should be, are very long, it is much better to change the lint frequently."

Mr. Fergusson, on the other hand, is an advocate for dressing the stump early. On this subject he says, "Whether an amputation is done by flap or circular incision, it is almost the invariable practice among British surgeons of the present day to promote union by the first intention; and for this purpose, as soon as the bleeding has been arrested by the application of ligatures and otherwise, the surfaces of the wound are brought into apposition, and retained thus by means of stitches, straps, and bandages. It is the custom of some to allow several hours to pass ere the edges or surfaces are finally adjusted; and this is done with the intention of making sure that all bleeding has actually ceased, and also under the conviction that union is not retarded by keeping the surfaces so long from each other. If the edges of such a wound are brought together immediately after the operation, and probably whilst the patient is faint from the shock, there is a chance of some vessel beginning to bleed after he has got warm in bed; and on this account it may be necessary to undo all the dressings. In general, however, if proper care be taken to apply a sufficient number of ligatures at the time of the operation, there will be no further trouble; and I do not hesitate to recommend that, as a common rule, the wound of an amputation should be dressed whilst the patient is on the operating table. I have tried both ways, and have always remarked the additional distress which any interference with the wound, four, six or eight hours afterward, has occasioned."

Larrey is a great enemy to the frequent dressing of all recent wounds, whether these be simple or complicated with fracture of bones. In the case of gun-shot wounds, the frequent renewal of the dressings is, we need scarcely say, often quite impracticable; it is therefore a matter of serious importance to know the best mode of proceeding under such circumstances. The authority of so experienced a writer will very properly command no ordinary attention. The main object of his instructions seems to be, to place the wound in such a position that nature is interfered with as little as possible in the reparation of the injury that has been inflicted. With this view he seeks to maintain the part in perfect quietude, guarding it from exposure to the outward air, and maintaining a proper temperature around it; and effecting these ends, without confining the patient to bed, or even to the house. He found by experience that in cold seasons wounds were, on the whole, more tardy of healing—especially if they were frequently exposed to the air—than in warm ones. He had too often occasion to verify the truth of this remark in the dreadful campaigns of Russia, Saxony, and France; especially when contrasted with the memorable one of Egypt. It was during these wars that the admirable effects of his "appareil inamovible" were most conspicuous. We were retreating, he says, all the while, and yet unwilling to leave our wounded behind. Accordingly, most of our patients, after they had their wounds dressed according to my plan, were immediately dispatched forward, and some of them even reached their homes in France before the original dressings of their wounds were removed. We give but one instance. A soldier, after having his arm amputated, at the shoulder joint, after the terrible battle of Moskowa, was advised to proceed direct on to his native place in Provence, and do nothing to the wound except keep it clean by sponging away any discharge from the outward dressings, and cover the limb with a good sheep's skin, to guard it from the cold and damp air. When he reached home, and the dressings were removed, the wound was found to be nearly cicatrized. This is one of many scores of similar cases, where the primary dressings were not removed for two, three, or even four weeks after they had been put on.

The following are the instructions given by Larrey how to arrange and apply his "appareil." If the fracture of the limb be complicated with a wound, we should first simplify it, as much as possible, by freely incising (débrider) its edges, extracting all foreign substances or pieces of broken bone, and arresting the hemorrhage. When all has been done, we should approximate the edges and keep them in apposition by means of a piece of linen (linge fenetré) on which some balsamic substance, such as the Styrax ointment, balsam of Mecca, etc., has been spread. Pledgets of lint, carded cotton or tow, are then to be placed over the dressing, and the anfractuosities that correspond to the wound; also, some square compresses dipped in a glutinous, strengthening fluid, that is prepared by beating up the white of two or three eggs with camphorated wine or vinegar, or, in lieu of these, with salt water. These compresses should be carefully applied over the whole of the injured part, while an assistant is engaged in maintaining the fractured bone or bones in exact apposition by appropriate extension and counter-extension. These compresses perform the service of immediate splints, without their inconvenience. They are kept in their place and are moreover strengthened by an eighteen-tailed bandage, which, when properly applied, maintains everything firmly together. The foot and ankle joint should previously be enveloped in long compresses, that have been wetted in the same fluid. A pad of tow, of a pyramidal shape, is to be placed under the tendo Achillis, to make all level and even, so that the pressure of the apparatus may be uniform throughout. The surgeon is then to take two cylindrical rolls of new rye straw, and, wrapping them up in the opposite edges of a towel or small sheet, which is to be stretched out under the leg, he applies them on each side, having previously interposed two or three flat cushions filled with oat chaff, to prevent the pressure of the straw rolls on the skin. These are secured in their place by a good many broad tapes or ribbons, which should be tied over the outer roll of straw, and in such a manner that they do not press directly upon the crest of the tibia. The advantage of the straw rolls is that they are so elastic, that, although they give way at first, to the swelling of the limb, they continue to remain in close contact with it as the swelling subsides, and no void ever exists between it and the apparatus—an objection to the paste-board splints, and other substitutes which have been suggested of late years As a substitute for the footboard, I use a piece of folded sheet placed like a stirrup under the sole, some tow being previously interposed to fill up the concavity; the two ends are brought up, crossed over the instep, and then secured to the straw rolls with strong pins.

The loose end of the sheet, stretched under the leg, which extends below the inferior ends of the straw-rolls, is to be folded under the foot and over the ends of the rolls, and then firmly secured by a few stitches or pins.

With such a simple, yet so efficient an apparatus, the reader will readily understand how a patient is able to walk about with the aid of crutches, the foot being merely suspended by a ribbon passed over the neck. The same apparatus is equally well suited for fractures of the body, or of the neck of the femur. We have only to lengthen the external straw-roll as far up as the pelvis, and secure it firmly by a belt passed round the body. The limb, in such cases, should be kept in the horizontal position, until the callus has become consolidated.

The camphorated albumino-vinous wash, which we have recommended, has the great advantage of increasing the tonic action of injured parts, and of preserving their natural heat, without obstructing the meshes of the linen or cotton cloth that is used in making the apparatus. The thinner portion of the discharge oozes out, and may be removed with a sponge, whenever it is necessary. *Part* xi., *p.* 120.

Punctured Wound and Ligature of the Posterior Tibial Artery.—Take the wound as a centre, and cut down upon the vessel, and tie it both above and below the seat of injury. (Arnott). If it be a case of secondary hemorrhage, and there is a good deal of coagulum in the parts surrounding the vessel, it will be advisable to tie the femoral artery. When there is a wound in the calf of the leg, with sufficient bleeding to warrant a belief that the posterior tibial artery is wounded, separate the soleus from its attachment to the tibia, cutting through the deep fascia, and secure the vessel. (Mr. B. B. Cooper.) *Part* xiii., *p.* 216.

Wounds of the Eyelids.—Diefenbach insists strongly on the advantages of his fine insect needles in producing union by the first intention. A sufficient number must be applied to effect exact apposition. If the edges do not correspond, they must be made to do so by the use of fine scissors. If a large piece of skin be lost and the edges cannot be united, subsequent ectropium is avoided by making an incision a quarter of an inch from the edge of the wound, which allows the edges then to be united. Opening of the lids during the healing process to be prevented by a strap of plaster, carried over them both. About the third or fourth day the needles are to be carefully removed, and the adherent wound supported by strips of plaster, to prevent reopening. If the needles are properly applied, no scar remains. *Part* xiii., *p.* 313.

Ergotine as a Styptic in Wounds of Arteries.—M. Bonjean has strongly advised the use of ergotine (ergot of rye) to arrest hemorrhage from wounded arteries. It is stated that in a recent experiment, he divided the right carotid artery of a horse by a transverse incision, which comprised one-third of the circumference of the vessel. The hemorrhage was speedily arrested by the application of ergotine. *Part* xiv., *p.* 192.

Severe Wounds of the Throat inflicted, for the purpose of Self-Destruction.—Dr. A. M. McWhinnie arranges them thus:

1st. Those in which the skin, superficial muscles, and vessels, are divided, and which are the most frequent in occurrence; 2nd, Those in which an opening is made either into the fauces, pharynx, larynx, trachea, or œsophagus, and which are next in point of frequency; and, 3d, Those in which blood-vessels of large calibre, or other parts, have been injured, so as to cause a sudden or speedy cessation of life, and which are comparatively rare in occurrence.

Treatment.—If the superficial parts are simply divided, and there is no mischief done to the air-passages, etc., a suture or two, aided by the approximation of the chin to the sternum, will generally suffice. Where the wound has opened the pharynx, larynx, or trachea, our first object must be to inquire as to the extent of the hemorrhage which may have taken place, and to spare no pains, even at the risk of enlarging the wound, to secure by ligature every divided vessel. Mr. John Bell says, that "they are often retracted among the cellular tissue, and that we are saved all trouble and care, except that of making our outward suture for uniting the external wound." These observations, coming from so eminent a surgeon, must carry with them considerable authority; but I cannot subscribe to so dangerous a proceeding. With regard to sutures, they should be employed only in superficial wounds; or, if allowable in deep ones, they must be confined to those cases in which the air-passages have escaped. In extensive wounds, where the cartilages of the larynx have been injured or separated from each other, sutures are irritating and hurtful. They cannot promote what never takes place in these parts, viz., union by the first intention; and by closing the outward wound, they will act in the most deleterious manner by confining the discharge, which should have as free an outlet as possible.

The wound is to be left freely open, and narrowly watched, in the event of any recurrence of the bleeding, when reaction has been established. The patient should be in a well-ventilated room, the head gently raised with pillows, and everything is to be avoided which may produce any bodily irritation or mental excitement. An elastic tube is to be introduced through the nostril, and, if the patient does not greatly object, should be allowed to remain in the œsophagus. Although it may at first produce some inconvenience, the patient will generally become accustomed to its presence. When the tube is passed, it should be quickly carried along the floor of the right nostril, and the finger of the left hand introduced, either through the mouth or wound, to guide its extremity into the pharynx. This is very important; for I have frequently seen the surgeon well-nigh foiled in his repeated attempts to introduce the instrument, in consequence of its hitching against, or passing into the aperture of, the glottis, which it will be liable to do, if not properly directed by the finger of the operator. The distress has been so great that every resistance has been offered to its employment. Much of the comfort to be derived from our treatment depends upon its use. All attempts at deglutition, and even speaking, are to be avoided, that these extremely movable parts may be kept as tranquil as possible. Every loose portion of cartilage or other tissue should be carefully removed, on account of the irritation and inconvenience produced. I have seen it necessary to take away the epiglottis, when nearly separated from its connections.

The lightest and simplest dressings will be found best adapted to these cases; water-dressing, with fine linen or muslin—occasionally a light poultice placed over the latter. The wound should be constantly cleansed; and if very extensive, and in the neighborhood of the glottis, the introduction and frequent renewal of soft portions of sponge will be found very useful in absorbing the purulent discharge which might otherwise flow into the larynx. The only nourishment allowed for some time should be fluids. The individual who has thus attempted suicide should be carefully watched; for the melancholy and deplorable condition in which he is placed urges him to resort to every possible means to accomplish his end; and the strictest restraint, during the treatment, is sometimes absolutely necessary, to prevent the infliction of further injury. Great advantage is derived from the administration of opium and other narcotics, introduced by the œsophagus tube, or by means of enemata.

With regard to other internal remedies, these will be few and simple; in the absence of cerebral and general febrile excitement, which, if present, must be combated by suitable treatment; and the great depression, both mental and physical, often supervening upon the cessation of the inflammatory symptoms, will demand the judicious employment of stimuli. Local and general bleeding, antimony, and mercurials, must be had recourse to, in the event of inflammation affecting the lining membrane of the air-passages and lungs.

[The plan suggested by Mr. Liston is now generally adopted, of introducing a tube through the glottis, when there is an œdematous state of the mucous membrane; and in those cases when dyspnœa has supervened after some time, in consequence of excrescences or granulations encroaching upon the air-tubes, Sir Charles Bell's plan of performing tracheotomy must be practised.]

In general, we may augur favorably of superficial wounds of the throat. When deep, their danger diminishes in proportion as they are remote from the aperture of the glottis. Thus, wounds entering the mouth above the os hyoides, or dividing the larynx below the glottis—i. e., through the lower part of the thyroid cartilage, or between it and the cricoid, will (as also wounds of the trachea, generally) do well; but, for reasons above mentioned, we should pronounce very unfavorably of a case where the incision has extended through the thyro-hyoid membrane, through the centre or upper part of the thyroid cartilage, or in any other direction toward the rima-glottidis, by which that part is exposed or injured.

Still, however, a great deal of comfort may be derived from proper treatment, and the chances of a favorable termination may thereby be much augmented. These wounds, from the great surface exposed, are extremely tedious in healing—a process which must take place almost wholly by granulations; and it has been shown that the patient must not be considered safe for a considerable time after the healing of the external wound.   *Part* xiv., *p.* 194.

Wound of Branches of the Palmar Arch of Arteries —-Gallic acid has proved a most useful addition to our use of astringents. Both as an external and internal remedy in hemorrhages its character stands high, and justly so; it is now generallly alleged to be the active principle in Ruspini's celebrated styptic, which Dr. Thompson is of opinion consists of gallic acid, sulphate of zinc, opium, alcohol, and rose-water; the gallic acid evidently being the active ingredient. Some time since, says Dr. Hughes, I saw the power of Ruspini's styptic put to the test in a case of a gentleman who had some of the branches of the palmar arch of arteries opened by the bursting of a bottle of soda water; profuse hemorrhage having ensued, and attempts to secure the bleeding vessels having been tried in vain, graduated pressure was applied, but to such an extent, and for such a length of time, that sloughing of the palm of the hand ensued, with inflammation extending up the forearm, and considerable fever, together with repeated periodical hemorrhages, by which the patient was considerably reduced; at this stage I saw the case in consultation, when it was agreed to give a trial to this powerful styptic, and a single application of it was followed by an immediate arrest of the hemorrhage, and recovery.   *Part* xv., *p.* 143.

Prevention of Infection from Dissecting Wounds.—Dr. Hargrave directs to wash the wound (on the fingers or thumb) for a few minutes in cold water; then suck it, and immediately tie a ligature on the cardiac side of the wound, so tightly as to induce numbness, and keep it on for at least twelve hours. The physiology of such treatment is explained by the ligature causing a permanent stasis in the fluids of the parts injured on its distal side, and producing a well-marked plethora in them; the greater the amount of it the greater will be the impediment to absorption, admitted by all. The constriction caused by the ligature will also oppose a barrier to the return of the venous and lymphatic fluids into the system, consequently to their being circulated through it, so that the poison is prevented entering into the constitution and destroying it, which will then be eliminated locally from the parts where it was first applied.
Part xvi., *p.* 299.

Treatment of Dissection Wounds.—Mr. B. Cooper advises not to apply caustic, unless infection has been received from a diseased subject. For an ordinary dissection wound, wash the part well, wrap up in a poultice, and keep the arm in a sling; take an aperient of calomel, James's powder, and rhubarb, followed by a saline, and go into the country for a week.

As precautionary measures, Dr. T. Cattell would apply sticking plaster to old abrasions, and anoint the whole surface of the hands, or wear india-rubber gloves. If wounded, immediately apply oil of turpentine, nitrate of silver, strong solution of alum, nitric acid with camphor, chloride of antimony, chloride of zinc, creasote, or concentrated solution of chloride of soda or lime.   *Part* xvi., *p.* 300.

Wounds of the Chest.—[Mr. Guthrie recommends the treatment of wounds of the chest in the following manner:]

1. All incised or penetrating wounds of the chest should be closed as quickly as possible, by a continuous suture through the skin only, and a compress supported by adhesive plasters, the patient being afterward placed on the wounded side.

2. If blood flows freely from a small opening, the wound should be enlarged, so as to show whether it does or does not flow from within the cavity. If it evidently proceed from a vessel external to the cavity, that vessel must be secured by torsion or by ligature.

3. If blood flow from within the chest, in a manner likely to endanger life, the wound should be instantly closed; but as the loss of a reasonable quantity of blood in such cases, say from two to three pounds, will be

beneficial rather than otherwise, this closure may be delayed until syncope takes place, or until a further loss of blood appears unadvisable.

4. If the wound in the chest have ceased to bleed, although a quantity of blood is manifestly effused into the cavity of the pleura, the wound may be left open, although covered, for a few hours, if the effused or extravasated blood should seem likely to be evacuated from it, when aided by position ; but as soon as this evacuation appears to have been effected, or cannot be accomplished, the wound should be closed. It must be borne in mind that the extravasation which does take place is usually less than is generally supposed—a point which auscultation and percussion will hereafter in all probability disclose.

5. If auscultation and percussion should indicate that the cavity of the pleura is full of blood, and the oppression of breathing and the distress are so great as to place the life of the patient in immediate danger, the wound, although recent, should be reopened.

6. As soon as the presence of even a serous fluid in the chest is ascertained to be in sufficient quantity to compress the lung against the spine, and time has been allowed for the closure of the vessel from which blood originally flowed, a counter-opening should be made in the place of election for its evacuation by the trocar and canula, which may be afterward enlarged, unless the reopening of the wound should be thought preferable, which will not be the case unless it should be low in the chest.

Part xvii., *p.* 149.

Solutions for Protecting the Skin against Contagion.—Mr. Acton has made various experiments with solutions of gun cotton, gutta percha, and caoutchouc, with a view of testing their property of protecting the surface from the influence, by contact, of contagious poisons, and the following are the conclusions at which he arrived : 1. That a solution of gun cotton, when dry, corrugates the skin too much to be available for the purposes required. 2. That gutta percha alone is devoid of elasticity and sufficient adhesive quality—that the solution of caoutchouc wants body and is too sticky, but that—3. The compound solution of caoutchouc and gutta percha possesses the requisite qualities to fulfill the purpose required. It is prepared by adding a drachm of gutta percha to an ounce of benzole, (the volatile principle of coal naphtha,) and ten grains of india-rubber to the same quantity of benzole, each being dissolved at a gentle heat, and then mixed in equal proportions. The author has employed this compound in painting the surface surrounding· a chancre, with the solution, and found that the acrid secretion had no effect upon it when dried, and warm or cold water may be applied with impunity. He considers that it may be employed advantageously in many and various ways, as in protecting the hands during post-mortem examinations, in preserving the cheek from excoriation in gonorrhœal ophthalmia, and in covering the parts contiguous to a sore where water-dressing is the application, etc. *Part* xix., *p.* 208.

Gunshot—Practice of "Debridement."—The question, as it now stands in Paris, says Dr. C. Shrimpton, may be rendered thus : Should large incisions be made to divide the aponeurotic membranes as a preventive means immedately on the receipt of a gunshot wound, or not ?

Larrey, the illustrious representative of French military surgery, and his son, the Baron, have, it is true, greatly recommended *débridement*, but this practice is not continued at the present day.

The potent antiphlogistic remedies, constant cold application, by means of ice or irrigations of cold water, so generally employed, have now completely superseded it.

In most cases, submitted to a proper treatment, the strangulation does not take place, and these large incisions may be avoided; but when the tumefaction does take place beneath the resisting membrane, it is time enough to open the aponeurosis and liberate the compressed tissues.

Part xix., *p.* 307.

Treatment of the Sting of a Bee.—The immediate application of honey is good; the use of indigo is better; and tobacco juice is thus recommended: " Apply the juice of tobacco as you find it in the mouth end of a smoked cigar, or in the reservoir of a German pipe. It not only immediately relieves the pain, but prevents swelling." The substance recommended is not, it must be remarked, the juice, but the empyreumatic oil which, according to Dr. Morris, is a much more energetic poison than the juice. *Part* xx., *p.* 283.

Wounds—Union of.—M. Vidal has contrived a number of minute forceps of different shapes, whereby the lips of the wounds, especially after the operation for phimosis, being gently kept in apposition by their self-applying pressure, the use of sutures is rendered unnecessary, the pressure exerted not being so great as to perforate the skin. The period for their application does not exceed twenty-four hours. *Part* xxii., *p.* 259.

Poisoned Wounds.—Dr. Maclagan, having removed the poison as much as possible by suction, encouraging the part to bleed, or excision of the whole tract of the wound, applies caustic to the surface freely. Venereal chancre may be regarded as a poisonous wound, and according to Ricord and others, if it is cauterized during the first three or four days, constitutional symptoms never follow, as the surface secreting the poison is destroyed, and the virus is thus prevented getting into the system.

Part xxii., *p.* 345.

Protection of Granulating Surfaces.—[Professor Miller protects raw granulating surfaces " from the influence of the atmosphere, by imitating the incrustation of nature." This he does by using " a thick semifluid aqueous solution of gum tragacanth." This is]

Laid gently and uniformly on the raw surface, so as completely to protect it; and if at any portion the envelope threaten to become imperfect, the attendant is directed to effect an immediate repair. The application is productive of no irritation; and, being translucent, permits a complete surveillance of the part. Atmospheric influence is completely excluded; and the raw surface would seem to be placed in circumstances somewhat analogous to its normal state, as if still invested by the integument. Should inflammation ensue, no harm has been done; on the contrary, action is likely to prove less intense than it otherwise would have been; the gum is loosened and washed away by the purulent secretion; and water-dressing may then be used, as in ordinary circumstances.

Part xxiii., *p.* 288.

New Forceps for Extraction of Bullets, etc.—These consist in the blades being separate, so that one blade at a time can be introduced into a sinus or cavity, and when the object is secured the handles can be locked like the midwifery forceps. *Part* xxxi., *p.* 312.

Glycerine as a Dressing for Wounds.—M. Demarquay considers glycerine a capital application to wounds of almost any description, and especially if sloughy. It is very clean, soft and comfortable to the patient, and it promotes cicatrization. The manner of applying it is by simply dipping a piece of lint into it, and placing it over the whole of the wound.

Part xxxiii., *p.* 238.

As formulæ frequently occur in this work, in which mention is made of French weights and measures, a table is here given of the value of those denominations which most frequently occur in pharmacy.

FRENCH MEASURES.

Millilitre	= 16.3 min. Brit. Apoth. Meas.	
Centilitre	= 2.705 fl. drs.	Do.
Decilitre	= 3.381 fl. oz.	Do.
Litre	= 1.7608 Imp. Pint.	

FRENCH WEIGHTS.

Milligramme	= .0154 grs.	English Troy.
Centigramme	= .1543 grs.	Do.
Decigramme	= 1.5434 grs.	Do.
Gramme	= 15.4340 grs.	Do.

Dr. W. S. Wells:

Dear Sir: I send you the following compilation, written several years ago for my own use. As it may be serviceable to students, it is at your option to publish. Yours, respectfully,

Samuel R. Percy, M.D., New York City.

A TABLE OF THE MUSCLES,

Showing the Origin, Insertion, and Action of the Muscles of one Longitudinal Median Section of the Human Body, not including the three Muscles of Hearing, the five of the Larynx, the Diaphragm, or Septum Medium, the six Inter-Spinal, eleven Inter-Transversal of the Neck, the five of the Loins, and the Cremaster.

Muscles of Facial Expression.

EPICRANIO-FRONTAL REGION, 3.

Name.	Origin.	Insertion.	Use.
1. Occipito-frontalis.	From the outer 2-3 of the superior curved line of the occipital bone, and from the mastoid portion of the temporal.	Into the orbicularis palpebrarum muscle and nasal tuberosity of the frontal bone.	To raise the eyebrows, thereby throwing the integuments of the forehead into transverse wrinkles.
2. Corrugator Supercilii.	From the inner extremity of the superciliary ridge.	Into the inner and inferior fleshy part of the occipito-frontalis, where it joins with the orbicularis palpebrarum.	To draw the eyebrow of that side toward the other, and make it project over the inner canthus of the eye. When both act they pull down the skin of the forehead and make it wrinkle, particularly between the eyebrows.
3. Pyramidalis Nasi.	Is a pyramidal slip of muscular fibres sent downward upon the nose by the occipito-frontalis.	Into the tendinous expansion of the compressores nasi.	Assists the occipito-frontalis in its action, draws down the inner angle of the eyebrow, and by its insertion fixes the aponeurosis of the compressores nasi.

AURICULAR REGION, 3.

Name.	Origin.	Insertion.	Use.
4. Retrahens Aurem (Auricularis posticus.)	By 2, 3, or 4 muscular slips from the mastoid process immediately above the insertion of the sterno-cleido mastoid muscle.	Into the back part of the ear, which is opposite to the septum that divides the scapha and concha.	To draw the ear back and stretch the concha.
5. Attollens Aurem.	From the tendon of the occipito-frontalis where it covers the aponeurosis of the temporal muscle.	Into the upper part of the concha.	To draw the ear upward, and make the parts into which it is inserted, tense.
6. Attrahens Aurem (Auricularis anticus.)	Thin and membranous near the posterior part of the zygoma at the edge of the aponeurosis of the occipito-frontalis.	Into a small eminence on the back of the helix, covering in the anterior and posterior temporal arteries.	To draw this eminence a little forward and upward.

PALPEBRAL REGION, 2.

	Origin	Insertion	Action
7. Orbicularis Palpebrarum (Palpebralis Anticus.)	From the internal angular process of the frontal bone, from the nasal process of the superior maxillary, and from a short tendon (tendo oculi), which extends from the nasal process of the superior maxillary bone to the inner extremities of the tarsal cartilages of the eyelids.	Into the lower border of the tendo oculi and nasal process of the superior maxillary bone.	To shut the eye by drawing both lids close together, the fibres contracting from the outer angle toward the inner, press the eyeball, squeeze the lachrymal gland, and convey the tears toward the puncta lachrymalia.
8. Levator Palpebræ Superioris.	From the under surface of the lesser wing of the sphenoid, immediately above the optic foramen, and from the fibrous sheath of the optic nerve.	Into the upper border of the superior tarsal cartilage.	To open the eye by drawing the eyelids upward, which it does completely by being fixed to the tarsus, pulling it below the eyebrow, and within the orbit.

CUBITO-OCULAR REGION, 6.

	Origin	Insertion	Action
9. Rectus superior Oculi (Attollens.)	From the margin of the optic foramen, and from the fibrous sheath of the optic nerve.	Into the upper surface of the globe of the eye.	The four recti, acting singly, pull the eyeball in the four directions of upward, downward, inward, and outward. Acting by pairs, they carry the eyeball in the diagonal of these directions—viz., upward and inward, upward and outward, downward and inward, downward and o... and... ding altogether they directly retract the globe within t.. orbit.
10. Rectus inferior Oculi (depressor.)	From the inferior margin of the optic foramen, by a tendon, which is common to it, and the internal and external rectus (ligament of Zinn), and from the fibrous sheath of the optic nerve.	Into the inferior surface of the globe of the eye.	
11. Rectus internus Oculi (Adductor.)	From the common tendon, and from the fibrous sheath of the optic nerve.	Into the inner surface of the globe of the eye.	
12. Rectus externus Oculi (Abductor.)	By two distinct heads, one from the common tendon, and the other with the origin of the superior rectus from the margin of the optic foramen; the nasal, third, and sixth, nerves passing between its heads.	Into the outer surface of the globe of the eye.	
13. Obliquus superior Oculi (trochlearis.)	From the margin of the optic foramen, and from the fibrous sheath of the optic nerve; it passes forward to the pulley beneath the internal angular process of the frontal bone; its tendon is then reflected beneath the superior rectus, to the outer and posterior part of the globe of the eye. The tendon is surrounded by a synovial membrane while passing through the cartilaginous pulley.	Into the tunica sclerotica, about half-way between the insertion of the attollens oculi and the optic nerve.	The superior oblique, acting alone, rolls the globe inward and forward, and carries the pupil outward and downward to the lower and outer angle of the orbit. The inferior oblique, acting alone, rolls the globe outward and backward, and carries the pupil outward and upward to the outer and upper angle of the eye. Both muscles acting together, draw the eyeball forward, and give the pupil that slight degree of eversion which enables it to admit the largest field of vision.
14. Obliquus inferior Oculi.	From the inner margin of the superior maxillary bone, immediately external to the lachrymal groove, and passes beneath the rectus inferior.	Into the outer and posterior part of the sclerotica at about two lines from the optic nerve.	

SUPRA MAXILLO NASAL REGION, 3.

Name.	Origin.	Insertion.	Use.
15. Compressor Nasi.	By its apex from the canine fossa of the superior maxillary bone, and spreads out upon the side of the nose.	Slightly into the interior extremity of the os nasi, and nasal process of the superior maxillary bone, which it meets with some of the fibres descending from the occipito-frontalis.	To compress the ala toward the septum nasi, particularly when we want to smell acutely, but if the fibres of the frontal muscle, which adhere to it, act, the upper part of this thin muscle assists to pull the ala outward. It also corrugates the skin of the nose, and assists in expressing certain passions.
16. Levator labii superioris alæque nasi.	By two distinct origins; the first from the external part of the orbital process of the superior maxillary bone, which forms the lower part of the orbit, immediately above the foramen infra orbitarium; the second portion arises from the nasal process of the superior maxillary bone, when it joins the os frontis at the inner canthus, descending along the edge of the groove for the lachrymal sac.	The first and shortest portion into the upper lip and orbicularis labiorum; the second and longest into the upper lip and outer part of ala nasi.	To raise the upper lip toward the orbit, and a little outward; the second portion serves to draw the skin of the nose upward and outward, by which the nostril is dilated.

SUPRA MAXILLO LABIAL, 4.

Name.	Origin.	Insertion.	Use.
17. Depressor labii inferioris alæque nasi (Myrtiformis).	Is seen by drawing upward the upper lip, and raising the mucous membrane; it is a small oval slip of muscle, situated on each side of the frænum, arising from the incisive fossa, and passing upward.	Into the upper lip and ala of the nose.	To draw the upper lip and ala nasi downward and backward.
18. Levator labii superioris proprius.	From the lower border of the external part of the orbital process of the superior maxillary bone.	Into the side of the upper lip. It covers in the infra orbital nerve and artery.	To raise the upper lip.
19. Levator anguli oris.	From the canine fossa of the superior maxillary bone, and passes outward.	Into the angle of the mouth, intermingling its fibres with those of the orbicularis, zygomaticl, and depressa anguli oris.	To draw the corner of the mouth upward.
20. Zygomaticus major.	From the os malæ near the zygomatic suture.	Into the angle of the mouth, continuous with the other muscles attached to this part.	To draw the corner of the mouth and under lip toward the origin of the muscle, and make the cheek prominent, as in laughing.
21. Zygomaticus minor.	From the upper prominent part of the os malæ above the origin of the former muscle.	Into the upper lip, near the corner of the mouth, along with the levator anguli oris.	To draw the corner of the mouth obliquely outward and upward toward the external canthus of the eye.

INTER MAXILLO LABIAL, 2.

	Origin	Insertion	Action
22. Buccinator (the Trumpeter's Muscle.)	From the lower jaw, as far back as the last dens molaris and part of the root of the upper jaw, between the last dens molaris and pterygoid process of the sphenoid bone and between both sides, to the constrictor pharyngis superior, with which it joins.	Into the angle of the mouth within the orbicularis oris. It is pierced opposite the second molar tooth of the upper jaw for the passage of Stenoni's duct.	To draw the angle of the mouth backward and outward, and to contract its cavity by pressing the cheek inward, by which the food is thrust between the teeth.
23. Orbicularis oris.	Is formed by the muscles that descending, one of the inferior ... the corner of the mouth, run along the lips to join one of the opposite side. It is a sphincter muscle. The upper segment is ... (labialis) to the columns of the nose.	one the lips, the fibres of the superior descending ... each other about the ... of the opposite side. ... by means of a small	To shut the mouth by contracting and drawing both lips together, and to counteract all the muscles that assist in forming it.

INFRA MAXILLO LABIAL, 3.

	Origin	Insertion	Action
24. Depressor anguli oris (triangularis oris.)	By a broad base from the external oblique ridge of the lower jaw.	Into the angle of the mouth, joining with the zygomaticus major and levator anguli oris.	To pull down the corner of the mouth.
25. Depressor labii inferioris (Quadratus menti vel genæ.	From the depression by the side of the symphysis of the lower jaw.	Into the orbicularis oris and integument of the lower lip.	To pull the under lip and the skin of the side of the chin downward and a little outward.
26. Levator labii inferioris,	From the incisive fossa of the lower jaw, a number of separate, slender, fleshy fibres.	Into the integuments of the chin.	To pull the parts into which it is inserted upward.

THORACO LABIAL.

	Origin	Insertion	Action
27. Platysma Myoïdes vel (Musculus Cutaneus.)	From the cellular substance that covers the upper parts of the deltoid and pectoral muscles; in their ascent they all unite to form a thin muscle which runs obliquely upward along the side of the neck, adhering to the skin.	Into the side of the chin, oblique line of the lower jaw, the angle of the mouth, and into the cellular tissues of the face.	To assist the depressor anguli oris in drawing the skin of the cheek downward. The entire muscle is analogous to the cutaneous muscles of brutes, the panniculus carnosus.

The Masticatory Muscles.

	Origin	Insertion	Action
28. Masseter.	Is composed of two planes of fibres, superficial and deep. The superficial layer arises by a strong aponeurosis from the tuberosity of the superior maxillary bone, and the lower border of the malar bone and zygoma, and passes backward. The deep layer arises from the posterior part of the zygoma, and passes forward.	Into the ramus and angle of the inferior maxillary. Into the upper half of the ramus.	To pull the lower to the upper jaw, and by means of its oblique decussation a little forward and backward. This muscle is crossed by a duct of the parotid gland, by the transverse facial artery, and by several branches of the facial nerve.

TEMPORA INFRA MAXILLARY, 2.

Name.	Origin.	Insertion.	Use.
29. Temporalis.	By tendinous fibres from the whole length of the temporal ridge, and by muscular fibres from the temporal fascia, and from the entire surface of the temporal fossa. Its fibres converge to a strong and narrow tendon.	Into the apex of the coronoid process, and for some way down upon its inner surface.	To pull the lower jaw upward and press it against the upper, at the same time drawing it a little backward. This muscle is covered in by a very dense fascia (temporal fascia.)

PTERYGO INFRA MAXILLARY, 2.

Name.	Origin.	Insertion.	Use.
30. Pterygoideus externus (minor.)	From the pterygoid ridge on the greater ala of the sphenoid, and from the external pterygoid plate, and tuberosity of the palate bone.	Into the neck of the lower jaw, and inter-articular fibro-cartilage.	To pull the lower jaw forward and to the opposite side, and to pull the ligament from the joint, that it may not be pinched during these motions. When both external pterygoid muscles act the fore teeth of the under jaw are pushed forward beyond those of the upper jaw.
31. Pterygoideus internus (major.)	From the inner and upper part of the internal plate of the pterygoid process, filling all the space between the two plates, and from the pterygoid process of the os palati between these plates.	Into the ramus and angle of the lower jaw internally.	To draw the jaw upward and obliquely toward the opposite side.

Muscles of Deglutition.

PTERYGO STAPHYLIN, 6.

Name.	Origin.	Insertion.	Use.
82. Levator palati (mollis.)	From the extremity of the pars petrosa of the temporal bone, where it is perforated by the eustachian tube, and also from the membranous part of the same tube.	Into the whole length of the velum pendulum palati, as far as the root of the uvula.	To draw the velum upward and backward, so as to shut the passage from the fauces into the mouth and nose.
83. Circumflexus, or tensor palati.	From the spinous process of the sphenoid bone behind the foramen ovale; from the eustachian tube not far from its osseous part, and then runs down the pterygoideus internus, passes over the hook of the internal plate of the pterygoid process, by a round tendon, which soon spreads into a broad membrane.	Into the velum pendulum palati, and the semi lunar edge of the os palati, and extends as far as the suture, which joins the two bones.	To stretch the velum, to draw it downward, and to a side toward the hook.
84. Azygos uvulae (levator uvulae.)	Is a pair of small muscles placed side by side in the middle line of the soft palate. They arise from the spine of the palate bone.	Into the apex of the uvula.	Raises the uvula upward and forward, and shortens it.
85. Palato pharyngeus.	From the middle of the velum pendulum	Into the muscular structure	Draws the uvula and velum downward and backward, and st

	Origin	Insertion	Use
86. Constrictor isthmi faucium (palato-glossus.)	palati, at the root of the uvula posteriorly, and from the tendinous expansion of the circumflexus palati.	of the pharynx and posterior border of the thyroid cartilage.	the same time pulls the thyroid cartilage and pharynx upward, and shortens it; with the constrictor superior and tongue it assists in shutting the passage into the nostrils; and, in swallowing, it thrusts the food from the fauces into the pharynx.
	From the side of the tongue near its root; runs upward within the anterior arch before the amygdala.	Into the middle of the velum pendulum palati at the root of the uvula anteriorly.	Draws the velum toward the root of the tongue, which it raises at the same time, and with its fellow contracts the passage between the two arches, by which it shuts the opening into the fauces.

PHARYNGEAL, 4.

	Origin	Insertion	Use
87. Constrictor pharyngis inferior.	From the side of the thyroid cartilage, near the attachment of the thyroideus and thyreo-hyoideus muscles; and from the cricoid cartilage near the crico-thyroides.	Into the white line in the middle of the pharynx.	To compress that part of the pharynx which it covers, and to raise it with the larynx a little upward.
88. Constrictor pharyngis medius.	From the appendix of the os hyoides; from the cornua of that bone, and from the ligament which connects it to the thyroid cartilage.	Into the middle of the cuneiform process of the os occipitis, and joined to its fellow at a white line in the middle back part of the pharynx.	To compress that part of the pharynx which it covers, and to draw it and the os hyoides upward.
89. Constrictor pharyngis superior.	Above the cuneiform process of the os occipitis, near the holes where the ninth pair of nerves pass out, lower down, from the pterygoid process of the sphenoidal bone; from the upper and under jaw near the roots of the last dentes molares; and between the jaws it is continued with the buccenator muscle and with some fibres from the root of the tongue and from the palate.	Into the middle of the pharynx, where it is overlapped inferiorly by the constrictor medius.	To compress the upper part of the pharynx, ward and upward.
40. Stylo-pharyngeus.	From the root of the styloid process.	Into the side of the pharynx and back part of the thyroid cartilage.	To dilate and raise the pharynx and thyroid cartilage upward.

GLOSSAL, 4.

	Origin	Insertion	Use
41. Lingualis.	From the root of the tongue laterally runs forward between the hyo-glossus and genio-glossus.	Into the tip of the tongue along with part of the stylo-glossus.	To contract the substance of the tongue and bring it backward, and to elevate the point of the tongue.
42. Genio-hyo-glossus.	From a rough protuberance in the inside of the middle of the lower jaw. Its fibres run like a fan, forward, upward, and backward.	Into the whole length of the tongue, from its base to the apex, and into the base of the os hyoides, near its cornua.	According to the direction of its fibres to draw the tip of the tongue backward into the mouth, the middle downward, and to render its dorsum concave, to draw its root and os hyoides forward, and to thrust the tongue out of the mouth.
43. Hyo-glossus.	From the base, cornua, and appendix of the os hyoides.	Into the side of the tongue between the stylo-glossus and lingualis.	To pull the tongue inward and downward.

Name.	Origin.	Insertion.	Use.
44. Stylo-glossus.	From the styloid process and stylo-maxillary ligament.	Into the root of the tongue, runs along its side, and is insensibly lost near its apex.	To draw the tongue laterally and backward.

SUPRA HYOIDAL, 4.

Name.	Origin.	Insertion.	Use.
45. Stylo-hyoideus.	By a round tendon, from the middle and inferior part of the styloid process it is pierced by the tendon of the digastricus muscle.	Into the os hyoides at the junction of the base and cornua.	To pull the os hyoides to one side and a little upward.
46. Digastricus.	From the digastric fossa immediately behind the mastoid process of the temporal bone; it is fleshy at each extremity, and tendinous in the middle.	Into a depression on the inner side of the lower jaw, close to the symphysis. The middle tendon is held in connection with the body of the os hyoides, by an aponeurotic loop through which it plays as through a pulley; the loop being lubricated by a synovial membrane	To open the mouth by pulling the lower jaw downward and backward, and when the jaws are shut to raise the os hyoides, and consequently the pharynx upward, as in deglutition.
47. Mylo-hyoideus.	From the molar ridge on the lower jaw, and proceeds obliquely inward; it is a broad triangular plane of muscular fibres, forming with its fellow of the opposite side the inferior wall or floor of the mouth.	Into the raphé of the two muscles, and into the base of the os hyoides.	To pull the os hyoides upward, forward, and to a side.
48. Genio-hyoideus.	From a small tubercle upon the inner side of the symphysis of the lower jaw.	Into the body of the os hyoides.	To pull the os hyoides toward the chin.

Muscles of the Neck.

HYOIDO-THYROIDAL, OR ANTERIOR SUPERFICIAL CERVICAL, 4.

Name.	Origin.	Insertion.	Use.
49. Thyro-hyoideus.	From the oblique line on the thyroid cartilage. It is a continuation upward of the sterno-thyroid.	Into the lower border of the body, and great cornua of the os hyoides.	To pull the os hyoides downward, or the thyroid cartilage upward.
50. Sterno-thyroideus.	From the posterior surface of the upper bone of the sternum, and from the cartilage of the first rib.	Into the oblique line on the great ala of the thyroid cartilage.	To draw the larynx downward.
51. Sterno-hyoideus.	From the cartilaginous extremity of the first rib, the upper and inner part of the sternum, and from the clavicle where it joins with the sternum.	Into the base of the os hyoides.	To pull the os hyoides downward.

	Origin	Insertion	Action
52. Omo-hyoideus.	From the upper border of the scapula, and from the transverse ligament of the supra scapular notch.	Into the base of the os hyoides between its cornua and the insertion of the sterno-hyoideus.	To pull the os hyoides obliquely downward.

ANTE-TRACHELIAN, OR DEEP ANTERIOR CERVICAL, 3.

	Origin	Insertion	Action
53. Rectus anticus major.	From the anterior tubercles of the transverse processes of the third, fourth, fifth, and sixth cervical vertebrae.	Into the basilar process of the occipital bone.	To bend the head forward.
54. Rectus anticus minor.	From the anterior border of the lateral mass of the atlas.	Into the basilar process.	To bend the head forward.
55. Longus colli.	The upper portion arises from the anterior tubercle of the atlas. The lower portion from the bodies of the second and third, and transverse processes of the fourth and fifth vertebrae.	Into the transverse processes of the third, fourth, and fifth cervical vertebrae, into the bodies of the three lower cervical and three upper dorsal vertebrae.	To bend the neck gradually forward and to one side.

LATERO-TRACHELIAN, OR LATERAL CERVICAL, 4.

	Origin	Insertion	Action
56. Rectus capitis lateralis.	From the transverse process of the atlas.	Into the os occipitis opposite the foramen stylo-mastoid curve of the temporal bone.	To bend the head a little to one side.
57. Scalenus anticus.	From the anterior tubercles of the transverse processes of the third, fourth, fifth, and sixth cervical vertebrae.	Into the tubercle upon the first rib. The inner border of the first rib. The phrenic nerve and subclavian vein lie on this side, and the subclavian artery behind it.	The scaleni muscles taking their fixed point from below are flexors of the vertebral column, and from above elevators of the ribs, and therefore inspiratory muscles.
58. Scalenus posticus.	From the posterior tubercles of all the cervical vertebrae, excepting the first.	By two fleshy stripe into the first and send ribs. Hence the scalenus medius and posticus of some anatomists.	
59. Sterno-cleido-mastoideus.	Arises by two distinct origins: the anterior from the top of the sternum, near its junction with the clavicle; the posterior from the upper and anterior part of the clavicle; both unite a little above the anterior articulation of the clavicle, to form one muscle which runs obliquely upward and outward.	By a thick strong tendon into the mastoid process, which it surrounds; and gradually turning thinner is inserted as far back as the lambdoid suture.	To draw the head to one side, and bend it forward. This is the great anterior muscle of connection between the thorax and the head. The anterior border of this muscle is the guide for the incisions in ligature of the carotid artery. It is pierced at its upper third by the spinal accessory nerve.

POST-TRACHELIAN, OR DEEP POSTERIOR CERVICAL, 4.

Names.	Origin.	Insertion.	Use.
60. Rectus posticus major (capitis.)	From the spinous process of the axis.	Into the inferior curved line of the os occipitis near the rectus capite lateralis, and the insertion of the obliquus capitis super.	To pull the head backward, and assist a little in its rotation.
61. Rectus posticus minor (capitis.)	From the spinous tubercle of the atlas.	Into a rough surface of the occipital bone, beneath the inferior curved line.	To assist the rectus major.
62. Obliquus superior (capitis)	From the extremity of the transverse process of the atlas.	Into the os occipitis near the rectus posticus major.	To draw the head backward.
63. Obliquus inferior.	From the spinous process of the axis.	Into the extremity of the transverse process of the atlas.	To give a rotary motion to the head.

POST-TRACHELIAN, OR MEDIAN POSTERIOR CERVICAL, 3.

Names.	Origin.	Insertion.	Use.
64. Splenius.	Is single at its origin, but divides soon after into two portions, which have different insertions. From the spinous processes of ten vertebræ, the four lower cervical and six upper dorsal, and divides, as it ascends the neck into the S. capitis and S. colli.	The splenius capitis into the rough surface of the occipital between the two curved lines, and into the said portion of the pal. The S. colli into the upper tubercles of the transverse processes of the four upper dorsal vertebræ.	To bring the head and upper vertebræ of the neck backward laterally, and when both act to pull the head directly backward.
65. Trachelo Mastoideus.	From the transverse processes of the four upper dorsal and four lower cervical vertebræ.	Into the mastoid process.	To assist the complexus, but it pulls the head more to one side.
6. Complexus.	From the transverse processes of the four upper dorsal and four lower cervical vertebræ. It is a large muscle, and with the splenius forms the great bulk of the back of the neck.	Into the rough surface on the occipital bone between the two curved lines, and near to the occipital spine.	To draw the head backward and to one side. A portion of the complexus is named bivender cervicis, from consisting of a central tendon, with two fleshy bellies.

Muscles of the Thorax.

ANTE-COSTAL OR ANTERIOR THORACIC, 3.

Names.	Origin.	Insertion.	Use.
67. Pectoralis major.	From the sternal 2-3 of the clavicle; from the breadth of sternum its whole length; and from the cartilages of all the true ribs, except the first.	By a broad tendon into the anterior bicipital ridge of the humerus.	To move the arm forward and obliquely upward, toward the sternum. That portion of the muscle which arises from the clavicle, is separated from that connected with the sternum, by a distinct cellular interspace; hence we speak of the clavicular portion and sternal portion of the pectoralis major.

68. Pectoralis minor.	From the upper edge of the third, fourth, and fifth ribs, near where they join with their cartilages.	Into the inner and upper surface of the coracoid process of the scapula.	To bring the scapula forward and downward, and to raise the ribs upward.
69. Subclavius.	By a round tendon from the cartilage of the first rib.	Into the under surface of the clavicle.	Draws the clavicle downward and forward, and thereby assists in steadying the shoulder. This muscle is concealed by the costo coracoid membrane, an extension of the deep cervical fascia, by which it is inserted. These three muscles are agents in forced respiration, but are unable to act until the shoulders are fixed.

LATERI COSTAL, 1.

70. Serratus magnus.	By fleshy serrations from the nine upper ribs, excepting the first, and extends backward upon the side of the chest.	Into the whole length of the base of the scapula.	Is the great external inspiratory muscle, raising the ribs when the shoulders are fixed, and thereby increasing the cavity of the chest. Acting upon the scapula it draws the shoulder forward, as we see to be the case in diseased lungs, where the chest has become almost fixed, from apprehensions of the expanding action of the respiratory muscles.

POST COSTAL, OR POSTERIOR THORACIC, 2.

71. Serratus posticus superior.	From the spinous processes of the two last cervical and two upper dorsal vertebræ.	By four serrations into the second, third, fourth, and fifth ribs.	To elevate the ribs and dilate the thorax.
72. Serratus posticus inferior.	From the spinous processes of the two last dorsal and two upper lumbar vertebræ.	By four serrations into the four lower ribs.	To depress the ribs into which it is inserted.

DEEP COSTAL, OR INTERNAL THORACIC, 23.

73. Inter-costales externi, 11 in number on each side.	From the inferior acute edge of each superior rib, and run obliquely forward, the whole length from the spine to near the joining of the ribs with their cartilages; from which to the sternum there is only a thin membrane covering the internal inter-costals.	Into the upper obtuse edge of each inferior rib, as far back as the spine, into which the posterior portion is fixed.	To raise the ribs when they act from above, and depress them when they take their fixed point from below. They are, therefore, both inspiratory and respiratory muscles.
74. Inter-costales interni, 11 on each side.	In the same manner as the external; but they begin at the sternum and run obliquely backward as far as the angle of the rib; from that to the spine they are wanting.	In the same manner as the external.	
75. Triangularis sterni.	By a thin aponeurosis from the side of the sternum, cuneiform cartilage, and sternal extremities of the costal cartilages.	Into the cartilages of the third, fourth, fifth, and sixth ribs, and often into the second.	To depress these cartilages and the extremities of the ribs, and consequently to assist in contracting the cavity of the thorax.

Scapular Muscles.

SUPRA AND INFRA SCAPULAR, 3.

Name.	Origin.	Insertion.	Use.
76. Trapezius, or (Cucularis.)	From the superior curved line of the occipital bone; from the ligamentum nuchæ, supra spinous ligament, and spinous processes of the last cervical and all the dorsal vertebræ. The fibres converge from these various points.	Into the scapular third of the clavicle, the acromion process, and the whole length of the upper border of the spine of the scapula.	Moves the scapula according to the three different directions of its fibres.
77. Rhomboideus, or inferior major.	From the spinous processes of the four, five, or six upper dorsal vertebræ, and from the supra spinous ligament.	Into the posterior border of the scapula, as far as its inferior angle below the spine.	To draw the scapula obliquely upward, and directly inward, or rotator of the scapula.
Or superior minor.	From the spinous processes of the two last cervical vertebræ and ligamentum nuchæ.	Into the edge of the triangular surface, on the posterior border of the scapula above the spine.	
78. Levator anguli scapulæ.	By distinct slips from the posterior tubercles of the transverse processes of the four upper cervical vertebræ, which soon unite.	Into the upper angle and the posterior border of the scapula as far as the triangular smooth surface at the root of its spine.	To pull the scapula upward and a little forward, and rotate.

SUPERFICIAL SCAPULAR, 4.

79. Supra spinatus.	From all that part of the base of the scapula that is above the spine; also from the spine and superior costa; passes under the acromion, and adheres to the capsular ligament of the os humeri.	Into that part of the large protuberance on the head of the os humeri, that is next the groove for lodging the tendon of the long head of the biceps.	To raise the arm upward, and at the same time to pull the capsular ligament from between the bones, that it may not be pinched.
80. Infra spinatus.	From all that part of the base of the scapula that is between its spine and inferior angle.	Into the middle depression upon the great tuberosity of the humerus.	To roll the humerus outward; to assist in raising and supporting it when raised, and to pull the ligament from between the bones.
81. Teres minor.	From all the round edge of the inferior border of the scapula.	Into the back part of the large protuberance on the head of the os humeri, a little behind and below the termination of the infra spinatus.	To roll the humerus outward, and draw it backward, and prevent the ligament being pinched.
82. Teres major.	From the lower third of the inferior border of the scapula, encroaching a little upon its dorsal aspect.	In common with the tendon of the latissimus dorsi into the posterior bicipital ridge.	To roll the humerus inward, and draw it backward and down ward.

DEEP SCAPULAR, 1.

83. Sub-scapularis.

From the whole of the under surface of the scapula, excepting the superior angle. The tendon of this muscle forms a part of the capsule of the joint, and communicates with the synovial membrane of the articulation.

Into the lesser tuberosity of the humerus.

To roll the humerus inward, and to draw it to the side of the body, and to prevent the capsular ligament being pinched.

Muscles of the Arm.

SUPRA HUMERAL, 1.

84. Deltoid.

Fleshy, from all the posterior part of the clavicle that the pectoralis major does not possess; tendinous and fleshy from the acromion, and lower margin of almost the whole spine of the scapula opposite to the insertion of the trapezius. The fibres from this broad origin converge to the middle of the outer side of the humerus.

Into a rough protuberance in the outer side of the os humeri, near its middle, where the fibres of this muscle intermix with some parts of the brachialis externus.

The Deltoid is the elevator of the arm in a direct line, and by means of its extensive origin can carry the arm forward or backward, so as to range with the hand a considerable segment of a large circle.

BT EL, OR ER EL, 1.

85. Triceps extensor cubiti.

Extensor of the forearm.

EL, OR ERIOR EL, 3.

86. Biceps flexor cubiti.

Flexor and supinator of the forearm.

Name.	Origin.	Insertion.	Use.
87. Coraco-brachialis,	From the forepart of the coracoid process of the scapula, adhering in its descent to the short head of the biceps.	About the middle of the internal part of the os humeri, near the origin of third head of the triceps, whence it sends down a thin tendinous expansion to the internal condyle of the os humeri.	Draws the humerus inward and assists in flexing it upon the scapula.
88. Brachialis anticus (Internus),	Fleshy, from the middle of the os humeri, at each side of the insertion of the deltoid, covering all the inferior and forepart of this bone, runs over the joint, and adheres firmly to the ligament.	By a strong tendon into the coronoid process of the ulna.	Flexor of the forearm. It is a powerful protection to the elbow joint.

Muscles of the Fore-Arm.

SUPERFICIAL ANTE-BRACHIAL, 10.

Name.	Origin.	Insertion.	Use.
89. Supinator Longus.	From the external condyloid ridge of the humerus, nearly as high as the insertion of the deltoid.	Into the base of the styloid process of the radius.	To roll the radius outward, and consequently the palm of the hand upward.
90. Extensor carpi radialis longior.	From the external condyloid ridge below the preceding. Its tendon passes through a groove in the radius immediately behind the styloid process.	Into the base of the metacarpal bone of the index finger.	To extend and bring the hand backward.
91. Extensor digitorum communis.	From the external condyle. Before it passes under the ligamentum carpi annulare externum it divides into four tendons. Opposite the first phalanx each tendon spreads out so as to form a broad aponeurosis, which covers the whole of the posterior aspect of the finger. At the first joint the aponeurosis divides into the three slips. The middle slip is inserted into the base of the second phalanx, and the two lateral portions are continued outward on each side of the joint, to be inserted into the last. Little oblique tendinous slips connect the tendons of this muscle as they cross the back of the hand.	Into the second and third phalanges of all the fingers.	Restores the fingers into the straight position, after being flexed by the two flexors—sublimis and profundis.
92. Extensor minimi digiti (auricularis),	Is an offset from the extensor communis. It assists in forming the tendinous expansion on the back of the little finger.	Into the two last phalanges.	It is to this muscle that the little finger owes its power of separate extension; and from being called into action when the point of the finger is introduced into the meatus of the ear for the purpose of removing unpleasant sensations; the muscle was called by old writers "Auricularis."
93. Extensor carpi ulnaris.	From the external condyle of the os humerus, and from the upper 2-3 of the border of the ulna. Its tendon passes through the posterior groove in the lower extremity of the ulna.	Into the base of the metacarpal bone of the little finger.	Assists in extending the hand.

94. Anconeus.	From the posterior part of the external condyle of the os humeri.	Into the olecranon and triangular surface on the upper extremity of the ulna.	Assists in extending the forearm.
95. Flexor carpi ulnaris.	By two heads—one from the inner condyle, and the other from the olecranon and upper, 2-3 of the inner border of the ulna. The ulnar nerve passes between its two heads.	Into the pisiform bone and base of the metacarpal bone of the little finger.	Flexor of the wrist.
96. Palmaris brevis.	From the palmar fascia, and passes transversely inward.	Into the integuments on the inner border of the hand.	To assist in contracting the palm of the hand.
97. Palmaris longus.	From the internal condyle of the os humeri, and from the sheath of fascia which surrounds it.	Into the palmar fascia.	Tensor of the palmar fascia.
98. Pronator radii teres.	By two heads—one from the inner condyle of the humerus and fascia of the forearm, the other from the coronoid process of the ulna. The median nerve passes between them.	Tendinous into the middle third of the oblique ridge of the radius.	Rotates the radius upon the ulna and the hand inward.

MIDDLE ANTE-BRACHIAL, 2.

99. Extensor carpi radialis brevior.	From the external condyle of the humerus. Its tendon is lodged in the same groove of the radius, with the extensor carpi radialis longior.	Into the base of the metacarpal bone of the middle finger.	To assist in extending the hand.
100. Flexor sublimis digitorum (perforatus).	From the inner condyle, coronoid process of the ulna, and oblique line of the radius. The median nerve and ulnar artery pass between its origins.	Divides into four tendons, which are inserted into the base of the second phalanges of the finger, splitting at their termination to give passage to the tendons of the deep flexors (thence perforatus.)	Flexors of the second phalanges.

RADIO-CUBITAL, OR DEEP ANTE-BRACHIAL, 8.

101. Flexor longus pollicis.	From the upper 2-3 of the radius, and part of the interosseous membrane. Its tendon passes beneath the annular ligament.	Into the base of the last phalanx of the thumb.	Flexor of the last phalanx of the thumb.
102. Extensor ossis metacarpi pollicis.	From the middle and posterior part of the ulna, immediately below the insertion of the anconeus, from the posterior part of the middle of the radius, and from the interosseous membrane.	Into the base of the meta-carpal bone of the thumb. Its tendon passes through the groove immediately in front of the styloid process of the radius	Extends the meta-carpal bones of the thumb.
103. Extensor primi internodii pollicis.	From the interosseous membrane and radius, and passes through the same groove as the former.	Into the base of the first phalanx of the thumb.	Extensor of the first phalanx of the thumb.

Name.	Origin.	Insertion.	Use.
104. Extensor secundi internodii pollicis.	From the ulna and interosseous membrane. Its tendon passes through a distinct canal in the annular ligament.	Into the base of the last phalanx of the thumb.	Extensor of the second phalanx of the thumb.
105. Extensor indicis.	From the ulna as high as the ex. ossis metac. pollicis, and from the interosseous membrane. Its tendon passes through a distinct groove in the radius.	Into the aponeuroses formed by the common extensor tendon of the index finger.	Extensor of the second phalanx of index finger.
106. Flexor profundus digitorum (perforans.)	From the upper 2-3 of the ulna, and part of the interosseous membrane, and terminates in four tendons, which pass beneath the annular ligament, and between the two slips of the tendons of the flexor sublimis (hence perforans.)	Into the base of the last phalanges.	Common flexor of the third phalanges of the fingers.
107. Supinator brevis.	From the external condyle and external lateral ligament, and winds round the upper part of the radius.	Into the head, neck, and tubercle of the radius.	Rotator of the fore-arm outward.
108. Pronator quadratus.	From the lower and inner part of the ulna.	Into the lower one-fourth of the oblique line of the radius.	Rotator of the fore-arm inward.

Muscles of the Hand.

METACARPO CARPAL, OR SUPERFICIAL PALMAR, 7.

Name.	Origin.	Insertion.	Use.
109. Abductor pollicis.	From the scaphoid bone and annular ligament.	Into the base of the first phalanx.	Bends the thumb toward the radius.
110. Flexor ossis metacarpi (opponens pollicis.)	From the trapezium and annular ligament.	Into the whole length of the metacarpal bone.	Rotates the thumb toward the palm.
111. Flexor brevis pollicis.	Consists of two portions, between which lies the tendon of the flexor longus pollicis. The external portion arises from the trapezium and annular ligament; the internal portion from the trapezoides and os magnum.	They are both inserted into the base of the first phalanx of the thumb, having a sesamoid bone in each of their tendons, to protect the joint.	Flexor of the first phalanx of the thumb.
112. Adductor pollicis.	Fleshy from almost the whole length of the metacarpal bone, that sustains the middle finger.	Into the inner part of the root of the 1st phalanx of the thumb.	To pull the thumb toward the fingers.
113. Abductor minimi digiti.	From the pisiform bone, and from that part of the ligamentum carpe annulare next to it.	Into the base of the first phalanx of the little finger.	Bends the little finger toward the ulna.
114. Flexor brevis minimi digiti.	From the unciform bone and annular ligament.	Into the inner and anterior part of first phalanx of the little finger.	Flexor of the first phalanx of little finger.

115. Flexor ossis metacarpi (adductor opponens.)	From the unciform bone and annular ligament.	Into the whole length of the metacarpal bone of little finger.	Rotates the little finger toward the palm.

METACARPO PHALANGEAN, OR DEEP PALMAR, 12.

116. Lumbricales (four in number.)	From the radial side of tendons of the deep flexor (four in number.)	Into the aponeurotic extension of the extensor tendons on the radial side of the fingers.	Coöperative with the flexors of the fingers.
117. Interossei palmares.		Into the base of the first phalanx and aponeurotic expansion of the extensor tendon of the same finger, the middle finger being excluded.	
Interossei pollicis.			Adducts the thumb, or inclines it toward the ulna.
8. Interossei indicis.			Adducts the fore finger and bends it toward the ulna.
19. Interossei annularis.	From the base of the metacarpal bone of one finger.		Adducts or bends the ring finger toward the radius.
20. Interossei auricularis.			Adducts or bends the little finger toward the radius.
21. Interossei dorsales.	Are bipeniform muscles, and arise by two heads from the adjoining sides of the base of the metacarpal bones.	Into the base of the first phalanges and aponeuroids of the extensor tendons. The first is inserted into the index finger; the second and third into the middle finger, compensating its exclusion from the palmar group; the fourth into the ring finger.	Adducts or bends the index finger toward the radius.
4.			Adducts or bends the middle finger toward the radius.
23.			Adducts or bends the middle finger toward the ulna.
24.			Abducts or bends the ring finger toward the ulna.

The radial artery passes into the palm of the hand between the two heads of the first dorsal interosseous muscle and the perforating branches of the deep palmar arch between the heads of the other dorsal interossei.

Muscles of the Abdomen.

TORSO PELVIC, OR ANTERIOR ABDOMINAL, 5.

125. Obliquus externus abdominis, descendens,	By eight fleshy digitations from the eight inferior ribs.	Into the outer lip of the crest of the ilium for one-half its length, the anterior superior spinous process of the ilium, spine of the pubis, pectineal line, front of the pubis and linea alba.	The external oblique muscle acting singly, would draw the thorax toward the pelvis, and twist the body to the opposite side. Both muscles acting together would flex the thorax directly on the pelvis. It is a muscle of expiration. Its name is derived from the obliquity of its direction, and the descending course of its fibres.
126. Obliquus internus abdominis, ascendens,	From the outer half of Poupart's ligament; from the middle of the crest of the ilium for two-thirds of its length, and by a thin aponeurosis from the spinous process of the lumbar	Into the pectineal line, crest of the pubis, linea alba and lower borders of the five inferior ribs.	Assists the former, but bends the trunk in the reverse direction. This is the middle flat muscle of the abdomen. It is a muscle of expiration.

Name.	Origin.	Insertion.	Uses.
184. Obliquus internus abdominis, ascendens (Continued.)	vertebræ. ... ligament ... of the ... with the ... of the ... In the spermatic cord.	... oblique ... is passage ... the ... this is the ... travel the ... ne of is	
187. Transversalis.	From the outer third of Poupart's ligament from the internal lip of the crest of the ilium, its anterior two-thirds; from the spinous and transverse processes of the lumbar vertebræ, and from the inner surfaces of the five inferior ribs, indigitating with the diaphragm. Its lower fibres curve downward.	With the ... is of the ... do the p... ... on the a... ... in. ri... it is ... et of the ... ... is in ... ... to the ... of ... is ... of the ... the p... ... n of ... th the ... r ... the final obli ue, lll.	To support and compress the abdominal viscera, and it is so particularly well adapted for that purpose that it might be called proper constrictor of the abdomen. This is the internal flat muscle of the abdomen. It is a muscle of expiration.
188. Rectus abdominis.	By two heads from the ligament of the cartilage, which joins the two ossa pubis to each other; runs upward the whole length of, and parallel to, the linea alba, growing broader and thinner as it ascends. It is transversed by several tendinous zig-zag lines called lineæ transversæ. One of these is usually situated at the umbilicus, two above that point, and sometimes one below.	Into the cartilages of the fifth, sixth, and seventh ribs and often intermixes with some fibres of the pectoral muscle.	Depresses the thorax and compresses the viscera muscle of expiration.
189. Pyramidalis abdominis.	From the crest of the pubis in front of the rectus.	Into the linea alba about midway between the umbilicus and the pubis.	Compresses, lowers, and extends the linea alba muscle of expiration.

SUPERFICIAL LUMBAR, 3.

Name.	Origin.	Insertion.	Uses.
190. Latissimus dorsi.	From the spinous processes of the six inferior dorsal vertebræ, all the sacral and lumbar, from the posterior third of the crest of the ilium, and from the three lower ribs by muscular slips which indigitate with the external oblique muscle of the abdomen. The inferior	With the teres major into the posterior bicipital ridge of the humerus.	Post-motor, adductor, and depressor of the arm, which it rotates inward.

	Origin	Insertion	Action
181. Sacro-lumbalis.	fibres ascend obliquely, and the superior run transversely over the inferior angle of the scapula toward the axilla, where they are collected, twisted, and folded. By a common origin from the posterior third of the crest of the ilium, from the posterior surface of the sacrum, and from the lumbar vertebræ. Opposite the last rib a line of separation begins to be marked between the two muscles.	By separate tendons into the angles of the six lower ribs.	Straightens the trunk and bends the thorax backward toward the pelvis.
182. Longissimus dorsi.	On turning the sacro-lumbalis a little outward a number of tendinous slips will be seen taking their origin from the ribs, and terminating in a muscular fasciculus, by which the sacro-lumbalis is prolonged to the upper part of the thorax.	Into all the ribs between their tubercles and angles.	Extends or straightens the trunk, or bends it backward and to one side.
Musculus accessorius (ad sacro lumbalem.)	This is the musculus accessorius ad sacro-lumbalem; it arises from the angles of the six lower ribs.	By separate tendons into the angles of the six upper ribs.	
Cervicalis ascendens.	Appears to be a continuation of the sacro-lumbalis upward into the neck. From the angles of the four upper ribs.	Into the transverse processes of the four lower cervical vertebræ.	

DEEP LUMBAR, 3.

	Origin	Insertion	Action
488. Psoas magnus.	From the intervertebra... læ, part of the bodies and sides of the transverse processes, and form a series of tendinous ...has, thrown across the constricted portion of the last dorsal and four upper lumbar vertebræ. These arches are added to protect the lumbar arteries and sympathetic filaments of a nerve from pressure in their passage each side. The tendon of the psoas agus ...ities with that of the ilius and the conjoined tendon.	Into the posterior part of the trochanter minor.	Flexes the thigh on the pelvis, and rotates it inward.
2. Psoas parvus.	From the tendinous arches and intervertebral substance of the last dorsal and first lumbar vertebræ, and terminates in a long, slender tendon.	Into the pectineal line of the pubis. The tendon is continuous by its outer border with the iliac fascia.	Bends down the loins forward on the pelvis.
3. Quadratus lumborum.	From the last rib, and from the transverse processes of the four upper lumbar vertebræ.	Into the crest of the ilium.	Depresses the last false rib, and bends the thorax to one side.

COCCYGEAL, OR ANAL, 3.

Name.	Origin.	Insertion.	Use.
136. Sphincter ani.	Is a thin elliptical plane of muscles closely adherent to the integument, and surrounding the opening of the anus. It arises posteriorly in the superficial fascia around the coccyx, and by a fibrous raphé from the apex of the bone. Internally it is a muscular ring embracing the extremity of the intestine, and formed by an aggregation of the circular muscular fibres of the rectum.	Anteriorly into the tendinous centre of the perineum, and into the raphé of the integument nearly as far forward as the commencement of the scrotum.	Constrictor of the anus.
137. Levator ani.	From the inner surface of the pubis; from the spine of the ischium, and between those points from the angle of division between the obturator and the pelvic fascia. Its fibres descend.	Into the extremity of the cox, into a fibrous raphé in front of that obe, into the lwer part of the rum and side of the oxter and prostate gland. In the female this muscle is inserted into the coxt and fibous raphé extremity of the tum and vagina.	Raises the anus. It is the antagonist of the diaphragm and the rest of the ... ry muscles, and serves to support the rum and vagina duri g th le expulsive efforts. It acts in unison with the diaphragm, and aises and falls like that muscle in bile respiration. Yielding to the propulsive tion of the us, it enables the tet of the puls to bear a greater for than a resisting rce, ard on the remission of such ...es it restores the perineum to its original rm.
138. Coccygeus.	From the spine of the ischium. It is in immediate contact with the lesser sacro-ischiatic ligament.	Into the side of the coxt and uer part of the sacrum.	The coccygic muscles restore the coccyx to its natural position after it has been pressed backward during defecation or during parturition.

GENITAL OF THE MALE, 3.

Name.	Origin.	Insertion.	Use.
139. Erector penis.	From the ramus and tuberosity of the ischium, and curves round the root of the penis.	The upper surface of the corpus cavernosum where it is continuous with a strong fascia which covers the dorsum of the organ, the fascia penis.	To compress the crura penis, by which the blood is pushed from it into the forepart of the corpora cavernosa. And the penis is by that means more completely distended.
140. Accelerator urinæ.	From a tendinous point in the centre of the perineum, and from the raphé. From these origins the fibres diverge like the plumes of a pen.	The posterior fibres are inserted into the ramus of the pubis and ischium; the middle to encircle the corpus spongiosum, and meet upon its upper side, and be inserted partly into its fibrous structure, and partly into the fascia of the penis.	Accelerator of the urine and semen.
141. Transversus perinæ.	From the tough, fatty membrane that covers the tuberosity of the os ischium.	Into the central tendinous part of the perineum.	Constrictor of the urethra.

GENITAL OF THE FEMALE. 2.

142. Erector clitoridis.	From the crus of the os ischium internally; and in its ascent covers the crus of the clitoris as far up as the os pubis.	Into the upper part of the crus and body of the clitoris.	Erector of the clitoris.
143. Constrictor vaginæ.	From the sphincter ani, and from the posterior side of the vagina, near the perineum; from thence it runs up the side of the vagina, near its external orifice, opposite to the nymphæ, and covers the corpus cavernosum vaginæ.	Into the crus and body, or union of the crura clitoridis.	Constrictor of the vagina.

Muscles of the Pelvis.

POSTERIOR ILIAC, OR GLUTEAL, 3.

144. Gluteus maximus.	From the posterior fifth of the external crest of the ilium; from the border of the sacrum and coccyx; and from the great sacro-ischiatic ligament. It passes obliquely outward and downward. This muscle forms the convexity of the nates.	Into the rough line leading from the trochanter major to the linea aspera, and is continuous by means of its tendon with the fascia lata covering the outer side of the thigh. A large bursa is situated between the broad tendon of the muscle and the femur.	Extensor or post-motor of the thigh, which it rotates outward.
145. Gluteus medius.	From the outer lip of the crest of the ilium, for four-fifths of its length from the surface of the bone between the border, and the superior curved line on the dorsum ilii, and from a deep and dense fascia.	Its fibres converge to the upper part of the trochanter major, into which its tendon is inserted.	Abductor, and slightly a rotator of the thigh outward.
146. Gluteus minimus.	Is a radiated muscle, arising from the surface of the dorsum ilii between the superior and inferior curved lines, and over the acetabulum.	Its fibres converge to the anterior border of the trochanter major, into which it is inserted, by means of a rounded tendon.	Assists the former.

ANTERIOR ILIAC, 1.

147. Iliacus internus.	Is a flat, radiated muscle; it arises from the inner concave surface of the ilium, and after joining with the tendon of the psoas magnus.	Into the posterior part of the trochanter minor.	Flexes the thigh on the pelvis.

PELVI-TROCHANTERIAL, 5.

Name.	Origin.	Insertion.	Use.
148. Obturator internus.	From the inner surface of the anterior wall of the pelvis, being attached to the margin of the and the obturator foramen, and to the other membrane. It passes out of the pelvis through the lesser sciatic foramen. The lesser sciatic notch over which this muscle plays as through a pulley, is faced with cartilage, and provided with a synovial bursa to facilitate its motion. The tendon of the obturator is supported on each side by the two gamelli muscles (so their names), which are inserted into the sides of the tendon, and appear to be auxiliaries or superadded portions of the obturator internus.	By a flattened tendon into the trochanteric fossa of the femur.	Rotator of the thigh outward.
149. Obturator externus.	From the obturate membrane, and from the lower surface of bone immediately surrounding it—viz., from the body and ramus of the os pubis and ischium; its tendon passes behind the neck of the femur.	With the external rotator muscles into the trochanteric fossa of the femur.	Idem.
150. Pyriformis.	From the anterior surface of the second, third, and fourth bones of the sacrum, by little slips that are interposed between the anterior sacral foramina. It passes out of the pelvis through the great sacro-ischiatic foramen.	By a rounded tendon into the trochanteric fossa.	Idem and abducting.
151. Gemellus superior.	From the spine of the ischium.	Into the upper border of the tendon of the obturator internus, and into the anterior trochanteric fossa.	Idem.
152. Quadratus femoris.	From the external border of the tuberosity of the ischium, anterior to the biceps semitendinosus and semi-membranosus.	Into a rough line on the posterior border of the trochanter major, which is thence named linea quadrati.	Idem.

Muscles of the Thigh.

FEMORO-ROTULAR, OR ANTERIOR FEMORAL, 2.

Name.	Origin.	Insertion.	Use.
153. Rectus femoris.	By two round tendons, one from the anterior inferior spinous process of the ilium, the other	By a broad and strong tendon, into the upper border of	Extensor of the leg and flexor of the thigh.

154. Triceps extensor femoris—viz.:	from the upper lip of the acetabulum. It is cuneiform in its shape, and bipenniform in the disposition of its fibres.	the patella. It is more correct to consider the patella as a sesamoid bone, developed within the tendon of the rectus; the ligamentum patellæ is the continuation of the tendon to its insertion into the spine of the tibia.	
Vastus externus.	From the outer border of the patella, narrow below and broad above.	Into the femur and outer side of the linea aspera, as high as the base of the trochanter major.
Vastus internus.	From the inner border of the patella, narrow above and broad below.	Into the femur and inner side of the linea aspera, as high as the anterior inter-trochanteric line.
Cruræus.	From the upper border of the patella.	Into the front aspect of the femur, as high as the anterior inter-trochanteric line.

Extensor of the leg.

FEMORO-ISCHIATIC, OR POSTERIOR FEMORAL, 2.

155. Semi-tendinosus.	In common with the long head of the biceps; from the tuberosity of the ischium, and sending down a long roundish tendon.	Into the inner tuberosity of the tibia.
156. Semi-membranosus.	Tendinous in common with the biceps and semi-tendinosus from the tuberosity of the os ischium, sends down a broad flat tendon, which ends in a fleshy belly, and in its descent runs at first on the forepart of the biceps, and, lower, between it and the semi-tendinosus.	Into the posterior part of the inner tuberosity of the tibia; at its insertion the tendon splits into three portions, one of which is inserted into a groove on the inner side of the head of the tibia, ... inth the ... inal ligament. The ... ned is ... ions with the aponeurotic expansion, that ... inds down the popliteus muscle—the popliteal ... ix, and the third ... nts upward and ... ward to the ... x ... imi ... de of the ... fer, ... ing the posterior ... ... gnt of the knee-joint (ligamentum ... poin. 1801 wir).

Post-motors and rotators of the thigh inward, and flexors of the thigh.

Name.	Origin.	Insertion.	Use.
157. Biceps flexor cruris.	By two distinct heads—one by a common tendon with the semi-tendinosus; the other, muscular and much shorter, from the lower two-thirds of the external border of the linea aspersia. This muscle forms the outer hamstring.	By a strong tendon into the head of the fibula, fascia and outer tuberosity of the tibia.	Post-motor of the thigh, flexor and rotator of the leg outward.

FEMERO-PUBAL, OR INTERNAL FEMORAL, 6.

Name.	Origin.	Insertion.	Use.
158. Sartorius (tailor's muscle)	Is a long ribbon-like muscle, arising from the notch, immediately beneath the anterior superior spinous process of the ilium; it crosses obliquely the upper third of the thigh, descends behind the inner condyle of the femur.	By an aponeurotic expansion into the inner tuberosity of the tibia. The inner border of the sartorius is the guide to the operation for tying the femoral artery in the middle of its course.	Flexor of the leg and thigh on the pelvis, rotates the thigh, and powerfully adducts the leg.
159. Pectineus.	From the pectineal line (pecten a crest) of the os pubis.	Into the line leading from the anterior inter-trochanteric line to the linea aspersia.	Adductor flexor and rotator inward of the thigh.
160. Gracilis.	By a broad but very thin tendon, from the edge of the ramus of the pubis and ischium. It is situated along the inner border of the thigh.	By a rounded tendon into the inner tuberosity of the tibia beneath the expansion of the sartorius.	Flexes and adducts the leg.
161. Adductor longus.	By a round tendon from the angle of the os pubis, assuming a flattened shape. It is the most superficial of the three adductors.	Into the middle third of the linea aspersia.	Adductor of the thigh.
162. Adductor brevis.	Placed between the pectineus and adductor longus, is fleshy and thicker than add. longus. Arises from the body and ramus of the os pubis.	Into the upper third of the linea aspersia. It is pierced by the middle perforating artery, and supports the anterior branch of the obturator nerve and artery.	Idem.
163. Adductor magnus.	Is a broad and extensive muscle, forming a septum of division between the muscles situated on the anterior, and those on the posterior aspect of the thigh. It arises by fleshy fibres from the ramus and side of the tuberosity of the ischium, and radiating in its passage outward.	Into the whole length of the linea aspersia and iher condyle of the femur. It is pierced by five openings; the three superior for the three perforating aries; the fourth for the termination of the profunda; the fifth is the large oval opening in the muscle, that gives passage to the femoral ...	Idem.

EXTERNAL FEMORAL, 1.

164. Tensor vaginæ femoris.	Is a short, flat muscle, situated on the outer side of the hip. It arises from the crest of the ilium, near to its anterior superior spinous process.	Between two layers of the fascia lata, at about one-fourth down the thigh.	Abductor and tensor of the aponeurosis called fascia lata.

Muscles of the Leg.

SUPERFICIAL TIBIO-PERONEAL OR TIBIAL, 4.

165. Tibialis anticus (flexor tarsi tibialis.)	From the upper two-thirds of the tibia, from the interosseous membrane, and from the deep fascia; its tendon passes through a distinct sheath in the annular ligament.	Into the inner side of the internal cuneiform bone and base of the metatarsal bone of the great toe.	Flexes and bends the foot inward.
166. Extensor longus communis digitorum.	From the head of the tibia; from the upper three-fourths of the fibula; from the interosseous membrane; and from the deep fascia. Below it divides into four tendons, which pass beneath the annular ligament. The mode of insertion of the extensor tendons both in the hand and in the foot, is remarkable; each tendon spreads into a broad aponeurosis over the first phalanx; this aponeurosis divides into three slips, the middle one is inserted into the base of the second phalanx, and the two lateral slips are continued onward, to be inserted into the base of the third.	Into the second and third phalanges of the four lesser toes.	Common extensor of the toes and flexor of the foot.
167. Peroneus longus (extensor tarsi fibularis longior).	From the upper third of the outer side of the fibula, and terminates in a long tendon, which passes behind the external malleolus, and obliquely across the sole of the foot, through the groove in the cuboid bone.	Into the base of the metatarsal bone of the great toe. The upper part of its origin is pierced by the peroneal nerve; its tendon is thickened where it glides behind the external malleolus, and a sesamoid bone is frequently developed in that part which plays upon the cuboid bone.	Extends the foot and elevates its outer edge.
168. Gastrocnemius.	By two heads from the two condyles of the femur, the inner head being the longest.	By means of the tendo Achillis into the lower part of the tuberosity of the os calcis, a synovial bursa being placed between that tendon and the upper part of the tuberosity.	Extensor of the foot and flexor of the leg.

MIDDLE TIBIO-PERONEAL, OR TIBIAL, 3.

169. Popliteus.	By a rounded tendon from a deep groove on the outer side of the external condyle of femur, beneath the external lateral ligament, spreads obliquely over the head of the tibia.	Into a ridge at the upper and internal edge of the tibia a little below its head.	Flexes the leg and rotates it inward.

Name.	Origin.	Insertion.	Use.
170. Soleus.	From the head and upper third of the fibula; from the oblique line and middle third of the tibia. It is a broad muscle, upon which the plantaris rests. Between the fibular and tibial regions of this muscle is a tendinous arch, beneath which the popliteal vessels and nerve pass into the leg.	Its fibres converge to the tendo Achillis, by which it is inserted into the tuberosity of the os calcis.	Extensor of the foot.
171. Plantaris.	Is a very small muscle, situate at its upper third, between the gastrocnemius and soleus; arises from the outer condyle of the femur, above the gastrocnemius.	By its long and delicately slender tendon into the inner side of the tuberosity of the os calcis, by the side of the tendo Achillis.	Extensor of foot and flexor of the leg.

DEEP TIBIO-PERONEAL, OR TIBIAL, 6.

Name.	Origin.	Insertion.	Use.
172. Extensor proprius pollicis pedis.	Lies between the tibialis anticus and extensor longus digitorum. Arises from the lower two-thirds fibula and interosseous membrane.	Its tendon passes through a distinct sheath in the annular ligament, and is inserted into the base of the last phalanx of the great toe.	Extends the great toe and flexes the foot.
173. Peroneus brevis.	Lies beneath the peroneus longus; arises from the upper 2-3 of the fibula.	Terminates in a tendon, passes behind the external malleolus, and passes through a groove in the os calcis, and is inserted into the base of the metatarsal bone of the little toe.	Extends the foot and raises its outer edge.
174. Peroneus tertius (flexor tarsi fibularis).	From the lower fourth of the fibula. Although apparently but a mere division of the extensor longus digitorum, this muscle may be looked upon as analogous to the flexor carpi ulnaris of the forearm. Sometimes it is altogether wanting.	Into the base of the metatarsal bone of the little toe.	Flexor of the foot, which it inclines outward.
175. Tibialis posticus (extensor tarsi tibialis).	Lies upon the interosseus membrane between the two bones of the leg. It arises by two heads from the adjacent sides of the tibia and fibula, their whole length, and from the interosseus membrane. Its tendon passes inward, beneath the tendon of the flexor longus digitorum, and runs in the same sheath, lying internally to it into the sole of the foot.	Into the tuberosity of the scaphoid bone and internal cuneiform bone.	Extensor of the tarsus upon the leg, and an antagonist to the tibialis anticus. It combines with the tibialis anticus in adduction of the foot.
176. Flexor longus pollicis (pedis).	From the posterior half of the fibula. Some way below its head, passes under the	Into the base of the last phalanx of the great toe.	Flexor of the great toe.

177. Flexor longus digitorum (pedis perforans).	From the surface of the tibia immediately below the popliteal line. Its tendon passes through a sheath common to it, and the tibialis posticus behind the inner malleolus into the sole of the foot, where it divides into four tendons.	Into the base of the last phalanx of the four lesser toes, perforating the tendons of the flexor brevis digitorum.	Common flexor of the toes and extensor of the foot.

Muscles of the Foot.

DORSAL, 1.

178. Extensor brevis digitorum.	From the outer side of the os calcis, crosses the foot obliquely, and terminates in four tendons.	The innermost of which is inserted into the base of the first phalanx of the great toe, and the other three into the sides of the long extensor tendons of the second, third, and fourth toes.	Common extensor of the toes.

SUPERFICIAL PLANTAR, 5.

179. Adductor pollicis.	From the cuboid bone; from the sheath of the tendon of the peroneus longus, and from the base of the third and fourth metatarsal bones.	Into the base of the first phalanx of the great toe.	Adductor and flexor of the great toe.
180. Flexor brevis pollicis.	By a pointed tendinous process from the os calcis, the side of the cuboid, and from the external and middle cuneiform bones.	By two heads into the base of the first phalanx of the great toe. Two sesamoid bones are developed in the tendons of insertion of these two heads, and the tendon of the flexor longus pollicis lies in the groove between them.	Flexor of the great toe.
181. Flexor brevis digitorum perforatus.	From the under surface of the os calcis, and plantar fascia.	By four tendons into the base of the second phalanx of the four lesser toes. Each tendon divides previously to its insertion, to give passage to the tendon of the long flexor (hence perforatus).	Common flexor of the toes.
182. Flexor brevis minimi digiti pedis.	From the base of the metatarsal bone of the little toe, and from the sheath of the tendon of the peroneus longus.	Into the base of the first phalanx of the little toe.	Flexor of the little toe.

Name.	Origin.	Insertion.	Use.
183. Abductor minimi digiti pedis.	From the outer side of the os calcis, and from the base of the metatarsal bone of the little toe. It lies along the outer border of the sole of the foot.	Into the base of the first phalanx of the little toe.	Abductor of the little toe.

DEEP PLANTAR, 14.

Name.	Origin.	Insertion.	Use.
184. Musculus accessorius (second portion of flexor long. com. digitorum—Massa carnea Jacobii Sylvii.)	By two slips from either side of the under surface of the os calcis, the inner slip being fleshy, the outer tendinous.	Into the outer side of the tendon of the flexor longus digitorum.	Rectifies the oblique action of the long flexor communis of the toes.
185. Four Lumbricales.	Are four small muscles arising from the tibial side of the tendons of the flexor longus digitorum.	Into the expansion of the extensor tendons, and into the base of the first phalanx of the four lesser toes.	Bend the phalanges upon the metatarsus.
186. Transversus pedis.	By fleshy slips from the heads of the metatarsal bone of the four lesser toes.	Tendinous into the base of the first phalanx of the great toe.	Abducts the great toe.
187. Interossei plantares.			
188. Idem.	From the base of the metatarsal bones of the toes.	Into the inner side of the extensor tendon and base of the first phalanx of the same toes.	Adds the great toe.
189. Idem.			Adds the third toe.
190. Idem.			Adds the fourth toe.
			Adds the fifth toe.
191. Interossei dorsales.	By two heads from the adjacent sides of the metatarsal bones.	Into the base of the first phalanx, and into the digital expansion of the tendons of the long extensor. The first is led into the inner side of the second, and is the outer side of the third toe, and is therefore abductors.	Adductor of the second toe. Adds the great toe. Adds the third toe. Adds the fourth toe.
192. Idem.			
" Idem.			
" Idem.			

A TABLE OF INCOMPATIBLES.

BY SAMUEL R. PERCY, M.D., NEW YORK.

Most of the articles here presented must be understood to be in solution. The formulæ given of them are as they are obtained in the dry state, and uncombined with water of crystallization. Many of the vegetable preparations prevent incompatibles with their infusions which are not incompatible with the alkaloids contained in their infusions, and it may be doubted if such re-agents injure their medicinal activity. The writer would respectfully suggest that there is as much, perhaps more, necessity for studying therapeutic incompatibles as chemical ones.

1. **Absinthium,** with acetate of lead, tartar emetic, nitrate of silver, sulphates of iron and zinc.

2. **Aoacia**—$C^{12} H^{10} O^{10}$—with alcohol, sulphuric ether and its compound spirits, strong acids, ammonia, subacetate of lead, tinct. mur. iron, nitrate of mercury.

3. **Acidum Aceticum**—$C^4 H^3 O^3$—with alkalies, alkaline and earthy carbonates, metallic oxides, etc.

4. **Acidum Arseniosum**—As O^3—with lime water, astringent vegetable infusions and decoctions, hydrated peroxide of iron, magnesia.

5. **Acidum Benzoicum**—$C^{14} H^5 O^3$ + Aq—with the mineral acids.

6. **Acidum Citricum**—$C^4 H^2 O^4$—with mineral acids, nitrate and acetate of mercury, acetate of lead, alkalies, alkaline carbonates and sulphurets, metallic oxides.

7. **Acidum Gallicum**—$C^7 H^3 O^5$—with the sulphate of copper, lime water, carbonates of iron and potash, acetate of lead, nitrate of silver, solutions of opium, Goulard's extract, iodide of iron, tartar emetic, and albumen.

8. **Acidum Hydriodicum**—HI—with atmospheric air, nitrate of silver, sulphate of copper and iron, nitric acid, chlorine, sulphuric acid.

9. **Acidum Hydrocyanicum**—HCy—with nitrate of silver, chlorine, mineral acids, metallic oxides.

10. **Acidum Hydrochloricum**—HCl—with alkalies, alkaline earths and their carbonates, with most metallic oxides and salts, especially those of silver, sulphuret of potassium, salifiable bases.

11. **Acidum Hydrosulphuricum**—HS—with nitrate of silver, acetate of lead, arsenious acid, sulphate of copper, metallic solutions, alkalies, etc.

12. **Acidum Lacticum**—HO, $C^6 H^5 O^5$—with mineral acids, alkalies.

13. **Acidum Nitricum**—NO^5—with alkalies, alkaline earths and their carbonates, essential oils, metallic oxides, salifiable bases.

14. **Acidum Oxalicum**—$C^2 O^3$, HO + Aq—with alkalies, alkaline earths and their carbonates, metallic oxides, lime-water, nitrate of silver, chloride of barium, sulphuric acid.

15. **Acidum Phosphoricum**—PO^5—with alkalies, alkaline earths and their carbonates, chloride of barium, sulphate of lime and magnesia, nitrate of silver, acetate of lead.

16. **Acidum Succinicum**—$C^4 H^2 O^3$—with sesquichloride of iron, oils, acetate of lead, chloride of barium, nitrates of silver and mercury, mucilage.

17. **Acidum Sulphuricum**—SO^3—with alkalies, alkaline earths and their carbonates, sul phurets, oxalic acid, phosphates, borates, hydrochlorates, nitrates, acetates, iodine, metallic iodides, baryta strontia, lead.

18. **Acidum Sulphurousum**—SO^2—with atmospheric air by which it is converted into sulphuric acid, hydrosulphuric acid. All the sulphites evolve sulphurous acid when treated with sulphuric or hydrochloric acid. Chlorine converts most sulphites to sulphates, chloride of barium precipitates neutral sulphites, but not free sulphurous acid.

19. **Acidum Tannicum**—$C^{18} H^8 O^{12}$—with albumen, gelatine, the persalts of iron, alka lies, alkaline earths and their carbonates, acetate of lead, tartar emetic, solutions of the vegetable alkaloids. (See Galla.)

20. **Acidum Tartaricum**—$C^4 H^2 O^5 + HO$—with alkalies, alkaline earths and their car bonates, salts of potassa, chloride of calcium.

21. **Aconitia**—$NC^{60} H^{47} O^{14}$—Precipitated from its solutions by potassa, soda and ammonia, but is redissolved by an excess of ammonia ; by the carbonates of these alkalies, which do not redissolve the precipitate ; by the vegetable astringents, magnesia and its carbonate, salts of iron, copper, zinc, silver lead.

The same will apply to the tinctures and extracts of aconite.

Tests of Purity.—It is fusible at a gentle heat; and is entirely dissipated, leaving no residue, at a high temperature. It is sparingly soluble in water, requiring for its solution 150 parts of cold and 50 parts of boiling water. Is perfectly soluble in the dilute mineral acids, from which solution it should be precipitated without loss of weight by ammonia, cautiously added. Is soluble in ether and alcohol.

22. **Æther Sulphuricus**—$C^4 H^5 O$.—Ether, as it evaporates, should leave but little foreign odor. When shaken with an equal volume of water, it should lose twenty-two per cent. of its volume. " In a test tube half filled and grasped in the hand for a short time, it should commence to boil very slowly on the addition of small fragments of broken glass." It should not redden litmus paper.

23. **Ætheris Spiritus Nitrici.**—Sulphate of protoxide of iron produces a deep olive color ; tincture of guaiacum, a blue changing to a green. It should boil if held in water at a temperature of 160°F., upon the addition of small fragments of broken glass.

24. **Albumen**—$C^{400} H^{310} N^{50} O^{120} S^2 P$—Nitric and hydrochloric acids, alcohol, corrosive sublimate, chloroform, creasote, heat, persulphate of iron, tannin, alum, nitrate silver.

25. **Alcohol**—$C^4 H^6 O^2$—with mucilages, nitrate of lime, chloride of barium.

26. **Aloe**, with galls, oak bark, and astringent vegetable infusions, chlorine, alum proto- chloride of tin, nitrates of silver and mercury, tartar emetic, acetate lead.

27. **Alumen**—$Al^2 O^3, 3SO^3 + KO, SO^3$—with alkalies and their carbonates, lime and lime- water, magnesia and its carbonate, tartarate of potassa, acetate of lead, astringent vegetable infusions, salts of mercury, ammonia.

28. **Ammonia**—NH^3—with acids, mineral salts, alum, the alkaloids, etc.

29. **Ammoniæ Acetas**—$NH^3, C^4 H^3 O^3$—(Ammonia Acetatis Liquor) with strong acids, alkalies, alkaline earths, nitrate of silver, corrosive sublimate, lime water, alum, sulphates of iron, copper, zinc and magnesia.

30. **Ammoniæ Bicarbonas**—$NH^3, 2CO^2$—with acids, fixed alkalies, lime-water, etc.

31. **Ammoniæ Carbonas**—NH^3, CO^2—with acids, fixed alkalies and their carbonates, lime-water, magnesia, chloride of calcium, alum, bitartrate and bisulphate of potassa, solutions of iron (except the tartrate of iron and potassa), corrosive sub- limate, acetate of lead, sulphate of zinc.

Test of Purity.—When heated on a piece of glass, it should evaporate without residue.

32. Ammoniæ Hydrochloras—NH^3, HCl—with nitric and sulphuric acids, acetate of lead, nitrate of silver, soda, potassa, lime and their carbonates.

33. Ammoniæ Hydrosulphuretum—NH^3 $2HS$—with acids, metallic salts.

34. Amygdalin—   —with the alkalies, alkaline earths and their carbonates, when mixed with emulsin or emulsion of sweet almonds, it forms hydrocyanic acid and volatile oil of bitter almonds; this is caused by a fermentation that takes place between them, that may be prevented by adding alcohol or acetic acid.

   Tests of Purity.—It should form a perfectly transparent solution with water; insoluble in ether; should leave no residue on incineration.

35. Amylum—C^{12} H^{10} O^{10}—Iodine, acids, lime water, baryta water, subacetate of lead, tannin, bromine.

36. Angustura, with sulphates of iron and copper, tartar emetic, acetate of lead, corrosive sublimate, nitrate of silver, potassa, ammonia, tannin.

37. Anthemis, with gelatine, gallic acid, salts of iron, nitrate silver, corrosive sublimate.

38. Antimonii Oxidum—SbO^3—Sulphureted hydrogen, tartaric acid, zinc, etc.

39. Antimonii et Potassæ Tartras—SbO^3, $KO2C^4$ H^2 O^5—with acids, alkalies, and their carbonates, most of the earths and metals, chloride of calcium, acetate of lead, astringent vegetable infusions and decoctions, soap, sulphureted hydrogen, impure water.

   Tests of Purity.—One hundred grains dissolved in water should yield forty-nine grains of ter-sulphuret of antimony to a solution of hydrosulphuric acid. A dilute solution should not be precipitated by chloride of barium, nitrate of silver, nor rendered blue by ferrocyanuret of potassium.

40. Antimonii Sulphuretum—SbS^3—with nitric and nitro-hydrochloric acids, tartaric acids.

41. Argenti Cyanuretum—$AgCy$—with hydrochloric acid, hydrosulphuric acid, etc.

42. Argenti Nitras—AgO, NO^5—with organic matter, impure water, the soluble chlorides; sulphuric, hydrosulphuric, hydrochloric, tartaric acids and their salts; the alkalies and their carbonates; lime water; astringent vegetable infusions.

   Tests of Purity.—If copper is present, its solution becomes blue on being supersaturated with ammonia. A solution of chloride of sodium, added in excess to one of nitrate of silver, throws down a white, curdy precipitate, and nothing besides; this precipitate should be entirely soluble in ammonia. To detect nitre, a very common adulteration, a solution of the suspected salt should be precipitated by hydrochloric acid, and sulphureted hydrogen; the filtered solution, if the salt be pure, will entirely evaporate by heat; if it contains nitre it will be left. "When a small piece of caustic is crushed to powder and spread evenly over a piece of paper, and the paper and powder then rolled up together, twisted, and burned as a match, it should leave a tasteless residue."

43. Argenti Oxidum—AgO—with hydrosulphuric and nitric acids, heat, etc.

44. Arnica, with sulphates of iron and zinc, acetate of lead, nitrate of silver.

45. Assafœtida, with the mineral acids, lime, hydrosulphuric acid, nitrate silver.

46. Atropa Belladonna, with alkalies, alkaline earths and their carbonates; vegetable astringents; lime water.

47. Atropia—NC^{34} H^{23} $O^6 = \overset{+}{At}$—with alkalies, alkaline earths and their carbonates, lime water, tannin, the salts of iron, zinc, lead and copper.

   Tests of Purity.—It is entirely soluble in absolute alcohol and ether; 100 parts of chloroform dissolves 51 parts of atropia. It is perfectly soluble in the dilute mineral acids, and is precipitated from its solution without loss of weight by ammonia, which should not be added in excess, as it redissolves the precipitate.

48. **Barii Chloridum**—BaCl—with the sulphates, oxalates, tartrates, borates, carbonates and alkaline phosphates, nitrate of silver, acetate of mercury, acetate of lead.

49. **Barytæ Carbonas**—BaO, CO^2—with sulphuric acid and sulphates, sesqui-oxide of iron, alumina.

50. **Belladonna**—(See Atropa Belladonna.)

51. **Benzole**—$C^{12} H^6$—Is mentioned here more for its great solvent powers; its incompatibles have not been sufficiently tested. It dissolves sulphur, phosphorus, iodine, mastic, camphor, wax, fatty and essential oils, caoutchouc, gutta percha. It dissolves quinia, but not cinchonia. Its boiling point is 176°F.

52. **Bismuthi Subnitras**—$BiO^{31} NO^5$—with hydrosulphuric acid. carbonate and chromate of potassa, vegetable astringents.

53. **Brominium**—Br—with chlorine, water, atmospheric air, nitrate of silver, starch.

54. **Brucia**—$C^{46} H^{26} N^2 O^8 = Br$—with potassa and carbonate of soda.

    Tests of Purity.—Ammonia produces a white precipitate in solution of salts of brucia which appears at first like a number of minute drops of oil, but changes subsequently—with absorption of water—to small needles. The precipitate redissolves, immediately after separation, very readily in an excess of the precipitant, but after a very short time—or, in dilute solutions after a longer time —the brucia combined with crystallization water, crystallizes from the ammoniacal fluid in small, concentrically grouped needles which addition of ammonia fails to redissolve.

    Bicarbonate of soda produces in neutral solutions of salts of brucia a precipitate of brucia, which separates into concentrically aggregated needles of silky lustre and are insoluble in an excess of the precipitant, but dissolve in free carbonic acid. Concentrated nitric acid dissolves brucia, and its salts to intensely red fluids, which subsequently acquire a yellowish-red tint and become completely yellow upon application of heat. Upon addition of protochloride of tin or sulphide of ammonium to this yellow fluid, it changes to a most intense violet. Chlorine water imparts to solutions of its salts a fine bright red tint, to which if ammonia is added, it changes to yellow brown.

55. **Cadmii Sulphas**—CdO, SO^3—with potassa ammonia and their carbonates, hydrosulphuric acid, lime water, the carbonates and sulphurets.

56. **Calcis Carbonas**—CaO, CO^2—with acids, acidulous salts, alum, vegetable astringents, soaps.

57. **Calcii Chloridum**—CaCl—with the soluble sulphates, the carbonates of potassa, soda, magnesia.

58. **Calcis Liquor**, with atmospheric air, mineral and vegetable acids, alkaline carbonates, and sulphates, soap, vegetable astringents, alum, acidulous and metallic salts, spirituous preparations.

59. **Calcis Phosphas**—$8CaO, 3PO^5$—with oxalate of lime, acetate of lead, nitrate of silver, carbonate of soda, potassa, ammonia.

60. **Calx Chlorinata**—CaO, Cl—with the acids, sulphate of iron, nitrate of silver, iodides.

61. **Camphora**—$C^{10} H^8 O$—with strong sulphuric and nitric acids, assafoetida, galbanum sagapenum, animé, tolu.

62. **Cantharis**, with strong acids, caustic alkalies.

63. **Capsicum**, with sulphate of iron, acetate of lead, nitrate of silver, corrosive sublimate, sulphates and sulphurets of the metals.

64. **Castoreum**, with strong acids, caustic alkalies, tannin.

65. **Catechu**, with gelatine, albumen, gluten, starch, the salts of the sesqui-oxides of iron, the salts of lead, copper, silver, mercury, tin.

66. **Cinchona**, with alkalies, sulphates of iron and zinc, sulphurets, lime, magnesia, nitrate of silver, tartar emetic.

67. **Cinchonia**—C^{40} H^{24} N^2 $O^2=\overline{Ci}$—with the alkalies, alkaline earths and their carbonates.

> *Tests of Purity.*—Cinchonia and its salts are insoluble in ether and benzole. Potassa, ammonia and their neutral carbonates produce in solution of cinchonia a white, loose precipitate, which does not redissolve in an excess of the precipitants. If chlorine water is added to a solution of the salts of cinchonia, it does not change the color, but if ammonia is added, a yellowish white precipitate is formed. 100 parts of chloroform dissolve but 4.31 of cinchonia. Cinchotina, with which it is sometimes admixed, is soluble in ether. (See Quinia.)

68. **Chloroformum**—C^2 HCl^3—with albumen. It would be improper to mix chloroform with any of the vegetable preparations whose alkaloid is soluble in chloroform, in any quantity more than sufficient for one dose, as the chloroform would dissolve the whole of the alkaloid.

> *Tests of purity.*—If equal parts of colorless, concentrated sulphuric acid and chloroform are shaken together in a glass-stoppered vial, there should be no color imparted to either liquid, nor any sensible heat developed at the time of mixing. If chloroform is dropped into water, it should not assume a milky appearance, but should be in transparent globules under the water. It should evaporate from the hand or bibulous paper without foreign odor.

69. **Cimicifuga,** with the sesqui salts of iron, with alkalies.

70. **Cocculus,** with alkalies and alkaline earths.

71. **Coccus,** with the salts of zinc, bismuth and nickel, which produce a lilac precipitate; with the salts of iron a dark purple; with the salts of tin a brilliant scarlet; with alumina the lakes.

72. **Colchicum,** with acetate of lead, nitrates of silver and mercury, tannin. Acids are said to render its preparations more drastic, and alkalies to render them milder in their operation, but as acids dissolve and alkalies precipitate its alkaloid, it will be seen that alkalies cannot be added but in extemporaneous mixtures.

73. **Colocynthis,** with sulphate of iron, acetate of lead, nitrate silver, tannin, alkalies.

74. **Conia**—NC^{16} $H^{15}=\overset{+}{Co}$—with tannin, albumen, salts of aluminum, copper, lead, zinc, manganese, iron, nitrate silver, alkalies.

75. **Creasotum**—C^{13} H^8 O^2—with nitric and sulphuric acids, nitrate and acetate of silver, albumen.

76. **Cupri Subacetas**—$2CuO$, C^4 H^3 O^3—with sulphuric acid, water which changes it to a neutral acetate and trisacetate, nitrate of silver, lime water.

77. **Cupri Sulphas**—CuO, SO^3—with potassa, soda and the alkaline carbonates; by ammonia, which, if added in excess, redissolves the precipitate; borax, acetates of lead and iron, nitrate silver, corrosive sublimate, tartrate of potassa, chloride of calcium, tannin, arsenites, hydrosulphuric acid, metallic iron.

78. **Cuprum Ammoniatum**—NH^3, SO^3+NH^3, $CuO+HO$—with potassa, soda, lime water, arsenious acid, acids; water and air on long exposure; tannin.

79. **Curcuma**—alkalies change its color to reddish-brown, as do also the concentrated mineral acids, pure boracic acid and numerous metallic salts, so that it cannot alone be relied upon as a test for alkalies. Its alcoholic solution produces colored precipitates with nitrate of silver, acetate of lead and other salts.

80. **Datura Stramonium,** with the salts of iron, lead, mercury, and silver, alkalies, alkaline earths and their carbonates, tannin.

81. **Daturia**—NC^{34} H^{23} O^6—with alkalies, tannin.

82. **Delphinia,** with alkalies, alkaline earths and their carbonates, tannin.

83. **Digitalis,** with sulphate of iron, acetate of lead, nitrate of silver, vegetable infusions or tinctures containing kinic, tannic or gallic acids.

84. **Digitalin,** with tannic and gallic acids, alkalies and their carbonates.

85. **Elaterium,** with alkalies and their carbonates, tannic and gallic acids.

86. **Elaterin,** with strong mineral acids, alkalies and their carbonates, tannin.

87. **Emetia,** with gallic and tannic acids, acetate of lead, corrosive sublimate, alkalies.

88. **Ergota,** with acetate of lead, nitrate of silver, astringent vegetable infusions and tinctures.

89. **Ferri Ammonio Citras,** with potassa, lime water, mineral acid, tannin.

90. **Ferri Chloridi Tinctura,** with alkalies, alkaline earths and their carbonates, astringent vegetable infusions and tinctures, mucilage of gum arabic, Fowler's solution.

91. **Ferri Citras—**$Fe^2 O^3, C^{12} H^5 O^{11}$—with mineral acids. alkalies, lime water, tannin.

92. **Ferri ferro-cyanuretum—**$Fe^7 Cy^9$—with nitric and hydrochloric acids, oxide of mercury with chromate of lead, it forms a beautiful green.

93. **Ferri Iodidi—**FeI—alkalies and their carbonates, and all other substances by which the sulphate of iron is decomposed.

94. **Ferri Liquor Perchloridi,** with atmospheric air, alkalies and their carbonates, metallic salts, vegetable astringents, nitrate silver, etc.

95. **Ferri Liquor Persulphatis** (Mousel's solution), albumen, fibrin, gluten, etc.

96. **Ferri Oxidum Hydratum—**$Fe^2 O^3 + 2HO$—used principally as an antidote to arsenic. is incompatible with the same substances as the other sesqui-oxides.

97 **Ferri Phosphas—**$FeO, PO^5 + Fe^2 O^5, PO^5$—same as sulphate of iron.

98. **Ferri Pulvis—**Fe—(iron reduced by hydrogen) atmospheric air, water, acids and acidulous salts, solutions of vegetable astringents, vegetable extracts.

99. **Ferri Pyrophosphas.—**This is a double salt, composed of about 49 per cent. of anhydrous pyrophosphate of iron, 35 per cent. of citrate of ammonia, and 16 per cent. of water. Robiquet states that it is not incompatible with the vegetable tonics and astringents, but this is not the case; but the changes do not take place quickly, therefore there is no objection to their mixture for extemporaneous administration.

100. **Ferri Subcarbonas** (Ferri Sesqui-oxidum)—$Fe^2 O^3$—with acids and acidulous salts.

101. **Ferri Sulphas—**FeO, SO^3—with alkalies, alkaline earths and their carbonates, lime-water, nitric acid, borax, iodide of potassium, acetate of lead, vegetable astringents, soap, muriate of barytes, nitrate of potassa, tartrate of soda and potassa, nitrate of silver, phosphate of soda.

102. **Ferri Sulphuretum—**$5FeS + Fe^2 S^3$—with acids which unite with the iron, with acidulous salts and vegetable astringents, etc. (See Potassii Sulphuretum.)

103. **Ferri Syrupus Superphosphatis,** is a double salt in solution like the last, the phosphoric acid being in excess. It is decomposed by the same substances that decompose most of the salts of iron.

104. **Ferri Valerianas,** with boiling water, mineral acids, alkalies and their carbonates, vegetable astringents, salts of copper and zinc, etc.

105. **Ferrum Ammoniatum,** with atmospheric air, alkalies and their carbonates, lime-water, acids and acidulous salts, astringent vegetable infusions and tinctures.

106. **Galla—**Sulphuric and hydrochloric acids, acetate of lead, sulphates of iron and copper, nitrates of silver and mercury, lime water, carbonates of ammonia and potassa, tartar emetic, corrosive sublimate, infusions of colombo, opium, peruvian bark and most other vegetables containing alkaloid principles, gelatin, albumen, gluten, alkalies and their carbonates. (See Acid. Tannicum.)

107. **Guaiaci Tinctura,** with mineral acids, spirits nitric ether, water.

108. **Hematoxylon,** with sulphuric, nitric, hydrochloric, and acetic acids, alum, sulphates of iron and copper, acetate lead, tartar emetic, gelatine, etc.

109. **Helleborus Niger,** with alkalies, alkaline earths and their carbonates, tannin.

110. **Hydrargyrum**—Hg—with the mineral acids, iodine, bromine.

111. **Hydrargyrum Ammoniatum**—HgCl, NH^2—with mineral acids, alkalies, protochloride of tin, boiling wa ter.

112. **Hydrargyrum cum Creta**, with acids, iodine, bromine, acidulous salts, alum, etc.

113. **Hydrargyri Chloridum Corrosivum**—$HgCl^2$—with many of the metals, alkalies and their carbonates, nitrate of silver, soap, lime water, tartar emetic, acetate of lead, sulphurets of potassium and sodium, sulphur, hydrosulphates, iodide of potassium, protochloride of tin, volatile oils, several vegetable infusions and decoctions, and animal and vegetable substances containing albumen, gelatine, or gluten, piperin.

> In some books this is called a chloride, in others a bichloride. It is better and safer, therefore, always to designate it by the epithet *Corrosivum.*

> *Tests of Purity.*—It should sublime, when heated, without residue. It should be readily and entirely soluble in ether, and in water.

114. **Hydrargyri Chloridum Mite**—HgCl—with alkalies, alkaline earths and their carbonates, hydrosulphates, hydrocyanic acid, bitter almonds, lime water, iodide of potassium, iodine, soap, citric acid, salts of iron, lead and copper, nitrate of silver.

> *Tests of Purity.*—It is completely sublimed by heat. Solutions of the fixed alkalies strike with it a black color free from a reddish tinge. Calomel washed with boiling distilled water, and the water tested with ammonia, will give no precipitate, if free from corrosive sublimate. If any is present there will be a white precipitate. Distilled water, with which calomel has been washed, should yield no precipitate to nitrate of silver, sulphureted hydrogen or iodide of potassium.

115. **Hydrargyri Cyanuretum**—$HgCy^2$—with the mineral acids, nitrate of silver, hydrosulphates, iodide of potassium, etc.

116. **Hydrargyri Iodidum**—HgI—with mineral acids, chloride of sodium, etc. It should completely sublime by heat. If it contains biniodide it may be separated by washing with alcohol.

117. **Hydrargyri Iodidum Rubrum** (Biniodidum)—HgI^2—with mineral acids, nitrate of silver, alkalies, acetate of lead, tartar emetic, sulphurets, etc.

> *Tests of Purity.*—It should completely sublime by heat. It is perfectly soluble in alcohol, and in solutions of iodide of potassium and chloride of sodium.

118. **Hydrargyri Oxidum Nigrum**—HgO—with mineral acids, acetic acid, iodine, etc.

119. **Hydrargyri Oxidum Rubrum**—HgO^2—with the mineral acids, ferrocyanurets.

120. **Hydrargyri Sulphas**—HgO^2 $2SO^3$—with the alkalies and their carbonates, chloride of sodium, lime water, etc.

121. **Hydrargyri Sulphas Flavus**—$3HgO^2$, $2SO^3$—with the alkalies, iodine, etc.

122. **Hyoscyamus**, with alkalies and their carbonates, nitrate of silver, sulphate of iron, tannin.

123. **Hyoscyamia**, with alkalies and their carbonates, tannin.

124. **Ichthyocolla Gelatine**—C^{96} H^{82} N^{15} O^{30}—Alcohol, tannin, and creasote, corrosive sublimate.

125. **Iodinum**—I—with starch and vegetable preparations containing it, magnesia.

126. **Ipecacuanha**, with acetate of lead, vegetable astringents, nitric acid, corrosive sublimate, alkalies.

127. **Jalapa**, with mineral acids, tannin, lime water.

128. **Jalapin**, with mineral acids.

129. **Kino**, with lime water, sesquichloride of iron, gelatine.

130. **Lactucarium**, with acetate lead, tannin, nitrate silver, corrosive sublimate, alkalies, lime water, oxalates

131. **Lobelia,** with alkalies, alkaline earths, and their carbonates, tannin, nitrate of silver, corrosive sublimate.

132. **Lobelina,** with tannin, alkalies, and their carbonates; it is decomposed by boiling water.

133. **Lupulin,** with the mineral acids, water.

134. **Magnesia**—MgO—with acids and acidulous salts, metallic salts.

135. **Magnesia Carbonas**—$3(MgOCO^2+HO)+NgO$, HO—with acids and acidulous salts, hydrochlorate of ammonia, nitrate of silver, corrosive sublimate, cream of tartar, acetate of lead, phosphate of soda.

136. **Magnesia Sulphas**—MgO, SO^3—with potassa, baryta, soda, and their carbonates, lime, strontia, baryta, and their soluble salts, ammonia partially forming with the remaining salt a double sulphate; carbonate of ammonia and bicarbonates of potassa and soda, do not decompose it when cold, but do upon boiling; phosphate of soda.

137. **Mangesii Binoxidum**—MnO^2—with acids.

138. **Maranta.** (See Amylum.)

139. **Mel,** with nitric acid.

140. **Mistura Ammoniaci,** with acids, ether, spirits of nitric ether, corrosive sublimate, nitrate silver, acetates potassa and lead

141. **Mistura Amygdalæ,** with alcohol, tinctures, oxymel and sirup of squills, spirits of nitric ether, hard water, cream of tartar, corrosive sublimate.

142. **Mistura Creta,** with cream of tartar acids and acidulous salts, etc

143. **Morphia**—$C^{34} H^{19} NO^6 \overset{+}{=} Mo$—precipitated from its solutions by potassa, soda, and ammonia, and redissolved by an excess of these alkalies; the carbonates of these alkalies precipitate but do not redissolve the morphia by vegetable astringents containing tannin, which precipitate is soluble in acetic acid; magnesia, the salts of iron, copper, zinc, silver, and lead, alum. (See also narcotina.)

   Tests of Purity.—It is almost insoluble in ether and chloroform, one hundred parts of chloroform dissolving but .57 of morphia, whereas one hundred parts of chloroform dissolve 31.17 of narcotina. It should be perfectly soluble in dilute nitric, hydrochloric, sulphuric, and acetic acids, and precipitated by potassa and ammonia, which precipitate should dissolve in an excess of these alkalies. Should leave no residue on incineration. A given weight of morphia, dissolved in dilute sulphuric acid, should be precipitated from its solution by potassa cautiously added, without loss of weight. It is but sparingly soluble in benzole.

144. **Moschus,** with corrosive sublimate, nitrate of silver, sulphates of iron and copper, mineral acid, infusion of cinchona, tannin.

145. **Mucilago.** (See Acacia, Tragacantha.)

146. **Narcein**—$NC^{28} H^{20} O^{12}$—with alkalies and their carbonates, tannin.

   Like morphia, it is insoluble in ether; it does not, like morphia, become blue by the action of the salts of iron, nor red by that of nitric acid. Mineral acids slightly diluted render it blue.

147. **Narcotina**—$C^{46} H^{26} NO^{14} \overset{+}{=} Na$—with alkalies, alkaline carbonates, and bicarbonates and the precipitate is insoluble in an excess of the precipitants; tannin. It is soluble in cold acetic acid, but is separated if the solution is heated.

   It may be distinguished from morphia by its solubility in chloroform and ether; by its insolubility in alkaline solutions when added in excess; by not forming a blue color with the salts of iron, and by not affecting vegetable colors.

   If the solution of a salt of narcotina is mixed with chlorine water, it acquires a yellowish green color, to which, if ammonia is added, it becomes yellowish red.

148. **Nickel**—(protoxide) NiO—with sulphide of ammonium, hydrosulphuric acid, potassa, soda, cyanide of potassium.

149. **Nicotia**—$N^2 C^{20} H_4^{14}$—with alkalies and their carbonates, tannin. It is soluble in alcohol, ether, water, oil of turpentine.

150. **Olea Destillata**, with alkalies, mineral acid, sulphur, heat and light, corrosive sublimate, nitrate of silver.

151. **Olea Expressa**, with alkalies and alkaline earths, chlorine, mineral acids, acidulous salts, corrosive sublimate, lime water.

152. **Opium**, with alkalies, alkaline earths and carbonates; nitrate of silver, salts of copper, iron, zinc, and lead, tannic and gallic acids. (See Chloroform.)

153. **Phosphorus**—P—atmospheric aid, heat, nitric and nitro-hydrochloric acids, alkaline solutions.

154. **Piper**, alkalies and their carbonates, corrosive sublimate.

155. **Piperin**—$N^2 C^{70} H^{37} O^{10}$—with corrosive sublimate, the alkalies and their carbonates. It is soluble in alcohol and ether, and is precipitated from these solutions by water, or the infusion of any substance in water. It is not precipitated by tannin in solutions of alcohol, or ether, or chloroform. It is very soluble in chloroform. With hydrochloric acid diluted with two parts of water, its solutions strike a brilliant yellow-green color, but do not precipitate the piperin. With nitric and sulphuric acids treated in the same manner, the color produced is a bright yellow. It is incompatible with soap, and therefore with the liniments containing it.

156. **Plumbi Acetas**—PbO, $C^4 H^3 O^3$—with sulphuric hydrochloric, citric and tartaric, lime-water, cream of tartar, alum, borax, metallic sulphates and sulphurets, soap, milk, infusion of opium, hard water, vegetable astringents, with iodide of potassium, it forms a yellow precipitate, with sulphureted hydrogen, a black precipitate; with carbonated alkalies, a white one; with chromate of potassa, a beautiful lemon-yellow; albumen.

157. **Plumbi Carbonas**—$2(PbO, CO^2) + PbO$, HO—with sulphureted hydrogen, the acids.

158. **Plumbi Iodidum**—PbI—with solution of potassa, sulphuric acid.

159. **Plumbi Liquor Subacetatis**—2PbO, $C^4 H^3 O^3$—with hard water, alkalies, alkaline earths, and their carbonates, sulphuric and hydrochloric acids, sulphates, sulphurets, hydrochlorates, the soluble iodides and chlorides, lime water, infusion of opium, vegetable astringents, soaps and liniments containing it, tartrates, chromate of potassa, solutions of acacia, albumen, gelatine.

160. **Podophillin**, as at present prepared, is a compound of two resinous principles, one soluble in ether and alcohol, the other in alcohol only. It is precipitated from its solution by hydrochloric acid; sulphuric acid darkens it; nitric acid produces a color much resembling tincture of iodine. Like jalapin, it is rendered milder in its operation by trituration, and by combination with an alkaline carbonate.

161. **Potassa**—KO—with acids and most acidulous salts, carbonic acid, ammonia and its salts.

162. **Potassæ Acetas**—KO, $C^4 H^3 O^3$—with mineral acids, sulphates of magnesia and soda, tartaric acid, nitrate of silver, corrosive sublimate, ammonia and its salts, lime water.

163. **Potassæ Arsenitis Liquor**, with acids, lime water, nitrate of silver, chloride of calcium, sulphate magnesia, alum, the salts of copper, tincture of chloride of iron, sulphureted hydrogen, vegetable astringents, piperin, infusions of vegetables containing alkaloids.

164 **Potassæ Bicarbonas**—KO, $2CO^2$—with acids, and acidulous salts, lime water, tincture of chloride of iron, nitrate of silver.

165. **Potassæ Bichromas**—KO, $2CrO^3$—with nitric, sulphuric, hydrosulphuric, tartaric and oxalic acids, nitrate of silver, acetate of lead, chloride of barium, sulphites.

166. **Potassæ Bisulphas**—KO 2SO³—with many of the metals and most oxides, with alkalies, alkaline earths, and their carbonates, lime water, etc.

167. **Potassæ Bitartras**—KO, 2C⁴ H² O⁵—with salifiable bases which form soluble tartrates, as soda, antimony, iron, etc., it gives rise to double salts. It is rendered very soluble by addition of boracic acid or borax. It is decomposed by strong acids, lime water, sulphate of magnesia, ammonia. carbonates of soda, potassa and magnesia, acetate of lead, nitrate of silver.

168. **Potassæ Carbonas**—KO, CO²—with acids and acidulous salts, sulphates of magnesia, copper, iron and zinc, lime and lime water, acetate and hydrochlorate, and carbonate of ammonia, chloride of calcium, iodine, tartar emetic, nitrate of silver, calomel, corrosive sublimate, tincture of chloride of iron, acetate of lead, alkaloids.

169. **Potass Citras**—3KO, C¹² H⁵ O¹¹—with sulphuric and other acids, the salts of lead, lime and silver.

170. **Potassæ Chloras**—KO, ClO⁵—with sulphuric and muriatic acids, sulphur, phosphorus, nitrate of silver.

171. **Potassæ Liquor**, with carbonic acid, acids and acidulous salts, and all metallic and earthy preparations held in solution by an acid, calomel, corrosive sublimate, ammoniacal salts, iodides of iron, zinc, mercury, silver; with all vegetable infusions containing an alkaloid principle. The neutral and acid solutions of potassa are precipitated of a yellow color by bichloride of platinum and of a white color by tartaric acid.

172. **Potassæ Nitras**—KO, NO⁵—with sulphuric acid sulphate of magnesia, and metallic sulphates, alum, tartaric acid

173. **Potassæ Sulphas**—KO, SO³—with nitric hydrochloric and tartaric acids, nitrate of silver, acetate of lead, corrosive sublimate, chloride of calcium and barium, sulphate of magnesia, chlorinated lime, chloride of platinum, nitrate of strontia.

174. **Potassæ Tartras**—KOC⁴ H² O⁵—with strong acids and many acidulous salts, chloride of barium and calcium, acetate of lead, lime water, nitrate of silver.

175. **Potassii Bromidum**—KBr—with acids, chlorine, nitrate of silver, starch.

176. **Potassii Cyanuretum**—KCy—with most of the salts with metallic oxides.

177. **Potassii Ferrocyanuretum**—2KCy, FeCy=2K, Cfy—with soluble salts of metallic oxides, chlorides, the salts of sesqui-oxide of iron, with which it strikes a deep blue color, a brown color with the salts of copper, and a white one with those of zinc.

178. **Potassii Iodidum**—KI—with nitrate of silver, acetate of lead, tartaric acid, metallic salts, corrosive sublimate, acids and acidulous salts except cream of tartar, chlorine.

179. **Potassii Sulphuretum**—K, S³—with acids, which unite with the potassium and set free the sulphur, precipitate part of it, and expel the other part in the form of sulphureted hydrogen gas; with metallic solutions, which unite with the sulphur and form sulphurets; with water, whose oxygen unites with the potassium of the bisulphuret forming potassa, and whose hydrogen unites with the sulphur, forming sulphureted hydrogen; when exposed to the air, oxygen combines with the ₛᵘₗₚₕᵘᵣ, forming sulphuric acid, and with the potassium of the bisulphuret, forming potassa, and these two new combinations unite and form sulphate of potassa.

180. **Populin**, with alkalies and their carbonates.

181. **Quassia**, with nitrate of silver, tannin; but as it contains no tannin, it is not incompatible with the salts of iron, copper, zinc, lead, corrosive sublimate, iodine, chlorine, gelatine.

182. **Quercus Tinctoria.** (See Acidum Tannicum.)

183. **Quinia**—C⁴⁰ H²⁴ N² O⁴ = Q̇—with tartaric acid, tartrate of potassa, lime water, tannin; with alkalies, their carbonates, alkaline earths, the precipitate redissolves to a very slight extent in potassa, but more freely in ammonia, the alkaline carbonates

do not redissolve it. Soluble salts of baryta and lead precipitate it from its solutions, and the precipitate from baryta is insoluble in the acids; concentrated nitric acid dissolves quinia to a colorless fluid, becoming yellowish upon the application of heat. The addition of chlorine water to a solution of a salt of quinia imparts no color, but if ammonia is added, the fluid acquires an emerald green color. If to the chlorine solution, ferrocyanide of potassium in solution is added, a dark red color is produced, which ultimately passes into green. This does not take place with cinchonia If a solution of quinia is precipitated with ammonia, ether added, and the mixture shaken, the quinia redissolves in the ether, and the clear fluid presents two distinct layers Such may also be done with benzole. This is not the case with cinchonia. Chloroform dissolves, to each 100 parts, 57.47 of quinia, whereas, of cinchonia, 100 parts dissolve but 4.31. (See Cinchonia.)

184. **Quinoidine,** or amorphous quinia, bears the same relation to quinia that uncrystallizable sugar does to crystallizable. It would probably be more used if it were not so much adulterated. It should be entirely soluble in alcohol and in dilute sulphuric acid, and its precipitate from these solutions, by ammonia, should weigh as much as the original substance.

185. **Rheum,** with the sesquioxide of iron and its salts, nitric acid, lime water, infusion of cinchonia, solution of quinia, acetate of lead, nitrates of silver and mercury, Goulard's extract, corrosive sublimate, tartar emetic.

186. **Sabadilla.** (See Veratria)

187. **Salicine**—$C^{26} H^{15} O^{14}$—is soluble in alcohol and water, and insoluble in ether. No reagent precipitates salicine as such. If salicine is treated with concentrated sulphuric acid, it agglutinates into a resinous lump, and acquires an intensely blood-red color without dissolving in the acid; the color of the acid is at first unaltered. If an aqueous solution of salicine is mixed with hydrochloric acid or dilute sulphuric acid, and the mixture boiled for a short time, the fluid suddenly becomes turbid, and deposits a finely granular crystalline precipitate (saliretine). It is not precipitated from its solutions by the alkalies. As silicine is frequently added to quinia as an adulteration, it may be readily distinguished by these tests.

188. **Salvia,** with the sesquisalts of iron, and vegetable infusions containing alkaloids.

189. **Sanguinaria,** with alkalies.

190. **Sapo**—and liniments containing it—with acids, earths, earthy and metallic salts.

191. **Scillæ,** with alkaline carbonates, nitrate of silver, acetate of lead, lime water.

192. **Senna,** with strong acids, tannin, solution of subacetate of lead.

193. **Soda**—NaO—with acids and most acidulous salts, carbonic acid, etc., etc.

194. **Sodæ Acetas**—NaO, $C^4 H^3 O^3$—with mineral acids, carbonate of lime, phosphate of sesqui-oxide of iron.

195. **Sodæ Bicarbonas**—NaO, $2CO^2$—with the same as the carbonate, excepting sulphate of magnesia in the cold.

196. **Sodæ Boras**—NaO, $2BO^3$—with acids, salts of ammonia, and many metallic oxides, carbonate of soda and potassa.

197. **Sodæ Carbonas**—NaO, CO^2—with acids, acidulous salts, lime water, earthy and metallic salts, hydrochlorate of ammonia, borax, vegetable acids, tartar emetic, sulphates, sulphureted hydrogen, calomel, corrosive sublimate, salts of iron, alkaloids, sulphate of magnesia.

198. **Sodæ Liquor,** with carbonic acid, acids and acidulous salts, and all metallic and earthy preparations held in solution by an acid; calomel, corrosive sublimate, ammoniacal salts, iodides of iron, zinc, mercury, silver; with all vegetable infusions containing an alkaloid principle.

199. **Sodæ Liquor Chlorinatæ,** with acids, lime water, carbonic acid, alum, nitrate of silver, iodides, calomel, sulphate of iron.

200. **Sodæ Phosphas**—2NaO, PO^5—with all the soluble salts of lime, and magnesia; mineral acids, nitrate of silver, alum, neutral metallic salts.

201. **Sodæ et Potassæ Tartras**—KO, $C^4 H^2 O^5$+NaO, $C^4 H^2 O^6$—with acids and acidulous salts except cream of tartar, soluble salts of lime and baryta, acetate and subacetate of lead, nitrate of silver.

202. **Sodæ Sulphas**—NaO, SO^3—with carbonates and acetates of potassa, chloride of calcium, nitrate of silver, acetate and subacetate of lead, lime water, ammonia, but not its subcarbonate, salts of barytes, chlorinated lime and soda.

203. **Sodii Chloridum**—NaCl—with nitrate of silver, nitric and sulphuric acids, carbonate of potassa, protoxide of mercury, sulphates of soda and potassa, salts of iron.

204. **Stramonium** (See Datura.)

205. **Stanni Protochloridum**—SnCl—chloride of mercury, hydrosulphuric acid, nitrate of silver, potassa, ammonia, and their carbonates, terchloride of gold, coccus cacti.

206. **Strychnia**—$C^{44} H^{24} N^2 O^4$=Sr—Potassa and carbonate of soda produce in solution of the salts of strychnia, precipitates of strychnia, which are insoluble in an excess of the precipitants. Ammonia produces the same precipitate which redissolves in an excess of ammonia, and after a time crystallizes in needles. Strong chlorine water produces a white precipitate which dissolves in ammonia to a colorless fluid.

Concentrated nitric acid dissolves strychnia to a colorless fluid, which becomes yellow by heat.

On putting a drop of concentrated sulphuric acid on a watch-glass, and adding to it a little strychnia or salt of strychnia, solution ensues without any particular reaction; but if a drop of solution of chromate of potassa is now added, it instantly acquires a deep blue color, which speedily changes to red. If the strychnia is rubbed together with binoxide of lead and concentrated sulphuric acid containing one per cent. of nitric acid, the mass acquires first a blue, then a violet color, which changes to red, and finally to yellowish green.

It is incompatible with tannic, but not with gallic acid, nor with sesqui-oxide of iron. One hundred parts of chloroform dissolve 20.16 of strychnia. It is but sparingly soluble in benzole.

207. **Sulphur**—S—with nitric and nitrohydrochloric acids, boiling solution of soda.

208. **Sulphuris Iodidum**—IS^2—with heat, boiling water, the acids, chlorine.

209. **Tobacum**, with oxides of mercury and antimony, nitrate of silver, sulphurets, chlorine, mineral acids.

210. **Toxicodendron**, with the sesquisalts of iron, alkalies, and alkaline carbonates, acetate of lead, sulphate, and valerianate of zinc.

211. **Tragacantha**, with sulphate of copper, iron, acetate of lead, alcohol, iodine.

212. **Uva Ursa**, with subacetate of lead, carbonate of potassa, gelatine.

213. **Valeriana**, with salts of iron and zinc, nitrate of silver.

214. **Veratrum Album**, with alkalies their carbonate, tannin.

215. **Veratrum Viride**, with alkalies their carbonates, tannin.

216. **Veratria**—$C^{34} H^{72} NO^6$=Ve—with alkalies, their carbonates, tannin, corrosive sublimate, chloride of gold, tincture of iodine. Veratria is insoluble in water, sparingly so in ether, freely in alcohol; 100 parts of chloroform dissolve 58.47 of veratria. It is soluble in the dilute acids. The alkalies and their carbonates and bicarbonates precipitate veratria from its solutions and the precipitate is not dissolved by an excess of the precipitants except ammonia in the cold, heat again causing a precipitate. Sulphuric acid produces with veratria a ruby or crimson-red color, nitric acid a yellow color, tincture of iodine a brownish red, soluble on boiling into clear red liquid, to which if ammonia was added while warm, it gave a yellow precipitate gradually changing to white. Solution of chloride of gold caused a yellow precipitate, insoluble in an excess of the precipitant until boiled, when it formed a greenish liquid, in which caustic potassa gave a purplish black precipitate.

Mr. Richardson has given a very elaborate treatise on veratria in the "American Journal of Pharmacy," 3d series, vol. v., No. 3, p. 209, in which he has proved the similarity of the veratria obtained from veratrum viride and V. alba, so far as they are amenable to chemical tests The writer has repeated these tests upon veratria from V. viride, made by himself, and veratria from V. album made by Merck, with the same results arrived at by Mr. Richardson, but although apparently identical in their chemical characteristics, they are not, according to the writer's observations, identical in their medicinal or therapeutic characteristics.

217. **Zinci Acetas**—ZnO, $C^4 H^3 O^3$—with the mineral acids and acidulous salts, carbonates of ammonia, potassa, and soda, lime water, vegetable astringents, ferrocyanuret of potassium, hydrosulphuric acid.

218. **Zinci Chloridum**—$ZnCl$—with nitrate of silver, carbonates of soda, potassa, and ammonia, ferrocyanuret of potassium; ammonia and potassa throw down a white precipitate which is dissolved in an excess of the precipitants.

219. **Zinci Oxidum**—ZnO—with ammonia, potassa, soda, acids, acidulous salts.

220. **Zinci Sulphas**—ZnO, SO^3—with alkalies and their carbonates, ferrocyanuret of potassium, hydrosulphate of ammonia, nitrate of silver, acetate of lead, lime water, chloride of barium, hydrosulphates, mucilages, milk, vegetable astringents.

221. **Zinci Valerianas**, with acids and acidulous salts, alkalies and their carbonates, metallic salts, vegetable astringents.

LATIN VOCABULARY.

Abdomen, is—The belly (abdominales).
Abduco, xi—To draw from (abductor).
Abluo, lui—To wash away (abluents)
Abnormis, e—Abnormal, out of the usual rule or order.
Abomasum, i—The fourth stomach of the Ruminantia.
Abortio, nis—Premature expulsion of the fetus.
Abrado, si—To rub off, abrasion.
Absedo—To separate (abscess)
Absente febre (abs. febr)—While the fever is absent.
Absorbeo—to suck up (absorbents).
Absorptio, onis—The function of the absorbents.
Abstineo, ui—To refrain from food, abstinence.
Ac (ac si, as if) (simul ac, as soon as)—And.
Acceleratio, onis—Increased rapidity of the pulse, respiration, etc.
Accelerator, oris—A muscle which contracts to accelerate the passage of the urine.
Accessio, onts—The approach of the pyrexial period in fevers.
Acclimatio, enis—Naturalization to a foreign climate.
Accurate—Accurately
Accurate misceantur—Mix them thoroughly.
Accurate pensi—Weigh them accurately.
Aciditas, or acidum (acer, sour)—Sourness, acescence.
Acini (pl. acinus, a grape stone)—The minute parts of the lobules of the liver, connected together by vessels.
Acme—The height of a disease
Acrimonia, æ—Sharpness of flavor.
Acutus, a, um—Disease or pain of a sharp character.
Acupungo, pupungi—To insert needles into the skin or flesh.
Ad—To, at, until
Ad libitum (ad lib.)—At pleasure.
Adde—Add.
Addantur—Let them be added.
Addendus—Being added
Addendo—By being added.
Adduco, xi—To draw to (adductor).
Adeps, ipis—Fat, animal oil.
Adhæreo, hæsi—To adhere, adhesion.
Adiposis—Hypertrophy of the adipose substance
Adjuvo, juvi—To assist or promote the operation of another (adjuvants).
Adjuvantia—Medicines which assist to relieve diseases.
Admoveatur (admov.)—Let it be applied.
Admoveantur—Let them be applied.
Adnascor—To grow to (adnata).
Adolescentia, æ—Youth, from the age of puberty to 25.
Adstante febre (ads. febr)—While the fever is present.
Adultus, a, um—Adult age from 25 to 50.
Adultero, avi—To adulterate, to corrupt.
Æger—A male patient.
Ægra—A female patient.
Ætas, atis—Age, term of life.
Afferens, tis—Afferent vessels that convey lymph to the lymphatic glands.
Affinitas, tis—Relationship, attraction, affinity.
Agglutino, avi—To form an adhesive union, agglutinate.
Aggressus—An attack
Aggressus febris—An attack of fever.
Agito—To shake.
Ala, æ—A wing (alæ nasi, etc.)
Albumen, inis—Albumen.
Albus—White (albino).
Alga, æ—Seaweed.
Alienatio, onis—Estrangement, mental derangement.
Aliformis, is—Wing-like.
Alimentum, i—Substances which nourish the body.
Aliquot—Some.
Aliquoties—Sometimes
Alter, a, um—The other (alteratives).
Alternæ—By turns, alternately.
Alternis horis—Every other hour.
Alternis diebus—Every other day.
Altrix, icis—A nurse.
Alumnus, i—He that is brought up a pupil.
Aluta—Soft leather.

900

Alvearium, i (a beehive)—The meatus auditorius externus
Alveolus, i (channels)—The alveolar processes or sockets of the teeth.
Alvus, i—The bowels, the belly (hence looseness, flux).
Alvo adstricta—The bowels being costive.
Alvo relax—The bowels being loose or relaxed.
Amentia, æ—Senseless, imbecility of intellect.
Amplus, a, um—Large
Ampullula, æ (a little bottle)—The extremity of each villus of the mucous coat of the intestines
Amputatio, onis—The removal of a limb or other part of the body by means of the knife.
Amuletum, i—A supposed charm against infection or disease.
Amylum, i—Starch
Anatomia, æ—A surgical dissection of the body.
Ancon, onis—The elbow.
Angina, æ—An inflammation of the throat.
Angina pectoris—Spasm of the chest.
Angor, oris—A strangling, a choking.
Anhelitus, us—Difficulty of breathing, dyspnœa.
Anima, æ—The vital principle, the soul.
Animal, is—A living creature.
Animalculus—Animalcule.
Annulus—A ring, a circle, a rounded margin.
Ante—Before.
Anteversio uteri—A morbid inclination of the fundus uteri forward.
Antidotum, i—A counter poison, antidote.
Anus, i—The fundament
Antrum Maxillare—A cavity above the molar teeth of the upper jaw.
Aperiens, cutis—Opening, mildly purgative.
Apex, icis—The extremity of a part.
Apotheca, æ—A place in which anything is laid up.
Apparatus, us—That with which preparation is made.
Apendix, icis—An appendage.
Appetitus, us—A longing or desire after anything.
Applicans, antis—Applying.
Applicantur—Let there be applied.
Aqua—Water
Aqua communis—Common well water.
Aqua bullientis (aq bul)—Boiling water.
Aqua ferventis—Hot water.
Aqua fluvialis—River water.
Aqua fontis—Spring water.
Aqua marina—Sea water.
Aquula, æ—A fatty tumor under the skin of the eyelid.
Arbor, oris—A tree (arborescent).
Arctatio, onis (narrow)—Constipation of the intestines, also preternatural straitness of the vagina
Arcus senilis (bow of old age)—An opacity round the margin of the cornea occurring in advanced age.
Ardor, oris—A heat, sense of heat, burning.
Ardor urinæ—A sense of scalding on passing the urine.
Area, æ—An open space.
Area differens, area serpens, area pellucida, area vasculosa
Areola, æ—The pink or brown circle which surrounds the nipple
Aridus, a, um—Dry, arid, without moisture.
Ars, artis—A knowledge acquired by learning.
Arteria, æ—An artery
Arthriticus, a. um—Afflicted with the gout.
Articularis, e—Relating to the joints.
As, assis—A pound weight.
Assimilatio, onis—Conversion of food into nutriment.
Astringo, inxi—To bend or draw together (astringent).
Athleticus, a, um—Athletic, strong.
Atomus, i—Any small invisible body, an atom.
Atque—And, also.
Atqui—But, however
Ater, tra, trum—Black, fatal, mortal.
Ater panis—Black bread.
Atra febris—A malignant fever.

Atrum venenum—Rank poison.
Attente—Carefully.
Attenuo, avi—To make thin, attenuate
Attollens, cutis—A muscle which draws any part upward.
Attondeo—To shave.
Attonsum caput—The head being shaved.
Attraho, xi—To draw toward oneself (attraction).
Atrahens auris—The muscle which draws the ear forward and upward.
Attritus—Rubbing, chafing.
Audio, ivi—To hear.
Auris, i (pl. es, ibus)—The ear.
Auriscalpium, i—An ear pick.
Aurium tinnitus—A ringing noise in the ears.
Auscultatio, onis—Listening by the application of the ear in the examination of disease.
Aut—Or.
Autem—But, notwithstanding.
Aviditas, atis—Eagerly, greedily.

Bacca—A berry.
Balneum arenæ—A sand bath.
Balneum maris—A sea bath.
Balneum vaporis—A vapor bath.
Balneum califeri jube—Order the bath to be made hot.
Balsamum—A balsam.
Barba, æ—The beard.
Basis, is—That on which anything rests.
Bene—Well.
Bene mane—Very early.
Bene multi—A great many, plenty.
Bibe—Drink.
Bibat (bibo)—Let him drink.
Bess, or bessis—Two thirds of a pound weight.
Biceps, ipitis—That has two heads.
Biduum—Two days.
(Omni biduo vel triduo)—Every two or three days.
Biduo continente—During two days.
Bifidus, a, um—Bifid, divided into two parts.
Bifer, a, um—That bears twice a year.
Biformis—Double formed.
Bifurcus—Bifurcated having two points.
Bilinguis—Double-tongued, treacherous.
Biliosus—Full of bile
Bimembris—Having double members.
Binominis—Having two names.
Binoctium—The space of two nights.
Bipartio—In two parts
Bipatens—Open on both sides.
Bipennis, e—Having two wings.
Bipes, edis—Two footed, biped.
Bis—Twice.
Bis in die—Twice daily.
Bis terve—Twice or thrice.
Bis quinque—Ten
Bis tanto—As much more.
Bolus—A bolus, a large pill.
Bonus, a, um—Good
Brevi—Soon after, shortly.
(Ad brevi)—A little while.
Bulliat—Let it boil
Blandimentum—Means of charming or soothing.
Blandus, a, um—Caressing, coaxing.
Blatero, ycis—A talk foolishly.
Bombyx, ycis—A silkworm.
Braca—A covering for the legs and thighs.
Brachialis—Of, or belonging to the arm.
Brachium—The arm from the wrist to the elbow.
Bubo—A swelling of the glands of the groin.
Bucca—A cheek.
Buccea—A mouthful.
Bucco—Chub-cheeked (hence a fool).
Bufo—A toad.
Bulla, æ—Blebs, vesicles raised by a watery fluid.
Butyrum—Butter.

Cachinno, are—To laugh immoderately.
Caco, avi—To go to stool.
Cadaver, eris—A corpse, a dead body.
Caduca—The deciduous membrane.
Cæco, avi—To blind (cæcum).
Cæche—Single, unmarried.
Cæruleus—Blue.
Cæteris paribus—Other things being equal.
Calcarius, a, um (calx)—Of, or belonging to lime.
Calculus, i—Stone in the bladder or kidney.
Calefacio—To make warm.
Calide—Hotly, warmly.
Calidus—Hot, scalding
Calix, icis—A drinking vessel, a cup.
Calix vitreus—A glass drinking vessel
Callide—Skillfully, cleverly
Callosus—Callous, having a hard thick skin.
Callus, i—Hard skin, want of feeling.
Calor, oris—Warmth, heat vehemence.
Calva, æ ; calvaria, æ—The skull.
Calveo, ere—To be bald.

Calvities, ei—Baldness.
Calyx, ycis—The bud or calyx of a flower.
Campa, æ, e, es—Canker worm, caterpillar.
Canalis, is—Canal, a conduit.
Cancello, avi—To make lattice-wise, cross-barred.
Cancer, cri—A crab.
Candefacio—To make red hot.
Caedela, æ—A taper, a candle.
Candesco, ere—To become of a glowing heat.
Canesco, ere—To become grey or white.
Canis, is—A dog.
Canities, ei—Grey hair.
Cannabis, is—Hemp.
Canula—A small tube.
Canus—Hoary, old.
Capillamentum, i—False hair, a peruke.
Capillus, i—The hair of the head (capillary).
Capito, onis—That hath a large head.
Capripes—Goat footed,
Capsula—A cover, a small chest.
Capto, avi—To snatch at, to catch.
Capularis, e (capulus)—Of, or belonging to a coffin.
Caput, itis—A head.
Capiat—Let him take.
Cap. coch magna—Take a tablespoonful.
Capiendus—To be taken.
Capiendus omni mane ac vespere—To be taken every morning and evening.
Carbo, onis—A coal.
Carbunculus—A carbuncle, anthrax.
Career—A prison, a gaol.
Carcinoma—A cancer.
Carcinosus, i—Cancerous.
Cardiacus—Belonging to the stomach.
Caries—Decay, rottenness.
Cariosus—Corrupt, rotten.
Carnifex, icis—A tormenter, a gaoler.
Carnivorus, a, um—Feeding on flesh.
Carnosus—Fleshy, muscular.
Carno, carnis—Flesh.
Carpus—The wrist.
Cartilago—Cartilage.
Caruncula—A small piece of flesh.
Caseus, i—Cheese.
Castitas, atis—Chastity, honesty.
Castro, avi—To castrate, geld.
Casus, us—A falling, an accident.
Catharticus, a—Cleansing, purgative.
Catharticum medicamentum—A purging medicine.
Cauda, æ—A tail.
Causarius, a, um—Sick, indisposed.
Causticus—Burning, caustic, biting.
Caute, ius, issime—Cautiously, carefully.
Cavea, æ—A cavity.
Caverna, æ—A hollow place.
Celeriter—Swiftly, quickly.
Centimanus—Having a hundred hands.
Centum—A hundred.
Cera—Wax.
Ceratum, i—Acerate made with wax.
Cerebellum—The little brain.
Cerebrum—The chief portion of the brain.
Ceroma—An ointment composed of wax.
Gerte—Certainly, surely.
Cervical—Of the neck.
Cervix—The neck.
Cerevisia, æ—Ale, beer.
Cestus—A band, a tie, a girdle.
Ceterus (et cetera)—The other
Ceu—As, like as, as if.
Chalceus—Brazen, of brass.
Chaos—Infinite empty space.
Charta—Paper.
Charta cerulea—Blue paper.
Chartula—A small paper, or letter.
Chart. in No. x. divide—Divide into ten papers, or powders.
Chiragra—The gout in the hand.
Chirurgia, æ—Surgery, chirurgery.
Chirurgicus, a, um—Of surgery.
Chirurgus, i—A surgeon.
Cholericus, a, um—Afflicted with a bilious complaint.
Cholera, æ—Bile, a bilious complaint.
Chorda, æ—A tendon, a gut, intestine, catgut.
Cibarius, a, um—Belonging to food.
Cibo—To feed.
Cibus, i—Anything which is eaten, food.
Cicada—A tree cricket.
Cicatricosus, a, um—Full of scars.
Cicatrix, icis—The scar of a wound.
Cilium, i—The eyelash.
Cimex, icis—A bug.
Cincinnus—Curled hair, a lock, a curl.
Cinctus—A girdle, a belt.
Cinefactus—Reduced to ashes.
Cingo—To bind, to dress.
Cinis—Ashes, lye.

Circa (circiter)—Around, about, near.
Circulatio, onis—The flow of blood through the heart, etc.
Circulatrix—A female mountebank, quackish.
Circumcido, idi—To circumcise.
Circumcisio, onis—Circumcision.
Circumligo, avi—To bind around, to encompass.
Circumplico, exi—To fold around.
Circumtondeo—To shave all round
Cirratus (cirrus)—Having curled or crisped hair.
Cis—On this side, within.
Citatim (cito)—Hastily, quickly.
Citissime—As quickly as possible.
Clam, or clanculum—Secretly, privately.
Claudico—To be lame, halt, limp.
Clando—To limp.
Clausus, a, um—Covered.
Clauso vase—In a covered vessel.
Clavicula, æ—The clavicle or collar bone.
Clementer—Mildly, gently.
Clinicus—A physician who visits patients who are confined to their beds.
Cloaca—A common sewer.
Clyster, eris—A clyster.
Coagulum, i—Curdled.
Coalesco, lui—To grow together
Coccyx—A cuckoo, the lower end of the spine.
Coetus—Boiled
Cochlearium—A spoon.
Cœcum—The cul de sac, cœcum
Cœliacus, a, um—Belonging to the stomach.
Cœna, æ—Dinner, the principal meal.
Cœnaturio, ire—To have an appetite for eating.
Cœnito—To take a meal frequently
Cœno—To eat at table, to take a meal,
Cœnula—A lunch, a lesser meal.
Cognatio, onis—Alliance by birth, relation by blood.
Cola—Strain, filter.
Colatus—Strained.
Cola trans chartam—Strain through paper.
Colato liquori—To the strained liquor.
Colentur—Let them be strained.
Collacrimo, avi—To weep together, to bewail.
Collaris—Belonging to the neck
Colliquefacio, feci—To make fluid, to melt.
Colloco, avi—To place, or put.
Collum—The neck
Colluo, ui—To wash, to wet.
Collyrium—A wash for the eyes.
Colo, avi—To sift, to strain.
Colon—The colon, the large intestine.
Color, oris—Color, complexion.
Colostrum—The first milk in the breasts after the birth of young
Colum—A strainer, colander.
Coma—The hair of the head.
Comans, tis—Having hair.
Combibor—To be drank together.
Comburor—To be burned
Comedo—To eat, eat away, eat up.
Commaculo, avi—Tc pollute.
Commendo, avi—To intrust to one's charge.
Commissura, æ—A commissure, a joint.
Commorior—To die at the same time.
Compar, aris—Equal
Compositus—Compound, put together.
Comprimens—Binding, pressing together.
Concaco—To bedaub, to pollute with ordure
Conceptio, onis—Conceiving, becoming pregnant.
Concerpo—To tear to pieces, to rend
Concha—A shell, a sea shell.
Conditorium, i—A coffin.
Condylus, i—A knuckle.
Congelo, avi—To freeze, to congeal.
Congius—A gallon.
Conjunctiva—The mucus membrane of the eye.
Conjugium, i—A union, marriage.
Connubialis, e—Relating to marriage.
Consanguineus, a, um—Related to blood.
Conscreor, ari—To spit, to hawk.
Consorbinus, a, um—Born of two sisters, cousins.
Conspergo, si—To sprinkle, bestrew.
Consipatio, onis—Costiveness of the bowels.
Consultum—Deliberation.
Consumptio, onis—Wasting away, phthisis.
Contactus—A touching contagion.
Contagio (contingo)—Contagion.
Contamino—To pollute, contaminate.
Contemero—To violate, dishonor.
Contero, trivi—To grind, crush, pound.
Continuantur remedia—Let the medicines be continued.
Contra—Over, against, opposite
Contra—Otherwise, on the other hand.
Contundo, tndi—To beat, to bruise.
Contusus—Bruised.
Contundo a bruise, a contusion.
Convalescentia—A regaining of health.
Convomo—To cover with vomiting.

Convoluto—To roll round.
Convulsus—Convulsed.
Copulatio, onis—Joining together.
Coquo—To cook.
Coque—Boil, cook.
Cor, dis—The heart.
Coram—Before, in the presence of.
Cordolium—Sorrow at heart.
Corium—Leather, the hide.
Corneus—Horny (cornea).
Cornipes—Horny feet, hoofed.
Cornu—A horn.
Cornu cervi ustum—Burnt hartshorn.
Corona, æ—A garland (coronal).
Corporeus, a, um—Corporeal, having a body
Corpulentus—Corpulent, fleshy.
Corpus—Body, anything not spiritual.
Corpusculum—A little body.
Corrodo—To corrode
Cortex, icis—The end, bark, peel.
Corvus—A raven, a surgical instrument.
Cosmeta, æ—A female slave, an adorner.
Costa, æ—A rib.
Coxa, æ, coxendrix—The hip bone.
Coxendrix luxa—Dislocation of the hip.
Cras—To-morrow.
Cras mane—To-morrow morning.
Cras mane sumendus—To be taken to-morrow morning.
Cras nocte—To-morrow night.
Crastinus—Of to-morrow.
    (In usum crastinum—For to-morrow's use.)
    (In crastinum differre—To put off till to-morrow.)
Crassamentum, i—The dregs, thickening.
Crepitus, us—A creaking.
Greta—Chalk.
Cribro, avi—To sift.
Cribrum—A sieve (cribriformis).
Crinalis—Of, or belong to the hair.
Crinis—Hair which is combed, a tress.
Crisis—Judgment, a state.
Croceus—Like saffron.
Crudesco—To grow raw, of wounds when they open.
Cruditas—Indigestion.
Cruor—Blood which runs out of a wound.
Cruralis—Of, or belonging to the shin or leg.
Crus—The leg from the knee to the ankle.
Crusta, æ—A hard rind, a scab.
Crypta, æ—A passage, a vault.
Crystallum, i—A crystal.
Cubicularis, i—Of a bedchamber.
Cubitalis—Belonging to the elbow.
Cubito, are (cubo)—To lie down.
Cujus—Of which.
Culus, i—The fundament.
Cum—With, when, although.
Cum minime—With the least.
Cum plurimum—Most frequently.
Cuneus—A wedge.
Cupreus—Of copper.
Curate—Carefully.
Curator—One who takes the management of a thing.
Curo—To take care of, heal, cure.
Cuticula, æ (cutis, is)—The skin.
Cyathus—A cup, a drinking vessel.
Cyathus vinarius—A wineglass.

Da, detur, dentur—Give, let it be given.
De—In respect of, about.
Deambulo—To walk abroad.
Deartuo—To rend limb from limb.
Deauro—To gild.
Debilitas, atis—Lameness, weakness.
Debilito—To lame, to maim.
Decem—Ten.
Deaurentur pilulæ—Let the pills be gilt.
De die in diem—From day to day.
Debitus—Due, proper.
    (Ad debitam spissitudinem—To the proper consistence.)
Decies—Ten times.
Deciduus—Deciduous, that falls off.
Decimo—To take out a tenth part, decimate.
Decoctus, us—A decoction.
Decoctor—One who decocts anything.
Decoquo, xi—To boil down.
Decumbo—To lie down to sleep.
    (Hora decubitus—At bed time.)
Defæco—To clean from dregs.
Deformis, e—Misshapen, deformed.
Deformo, avi—To disfigure, to deform.
Deglutio—To swallow.
Deglutietur—Let it be swallowed.
Dejectio, onis—A casting down, dejection.
    (Post duas dejectiones alvi—After two alvine evacuations.)
    (Donec alvus bis dejeciat—Until the bowels have been moved twice.)

Delinquo, liqui—To omit.
Deliquesco, cui—To melt down (deliquescent).
Deliquo, are—To strain, to render fluid.
Delirium, i—Madness, low of reason.
Delumbo, avi—To lame in the hip, or loins, to enervate.
Deluo—To wash, to cleanse.
Dementia—Madness, folly.
Demo, psi—To diminish, withdraw
Demum—At last, at length
Denaso—To deprive of a nose.
Denique—Finally, lastly.
Dens, tis—A tooth
Dentio, ire—To cut teeth.
Dentiscalpium—A toothpick.
Dentitio—The teething of children, dentition.
Dentifricium, ii—A dentifrice.
Denuo—Again, anew
Depilo, avi—To pull off hair.
Depilatus—Made bald
Depouo, sui—To lay aside.
Depuratus—Purified.
Desideratum—That which is desired.
Desperatus, a, um—Given over, past hope.
Despuo—To spit out.
Desquamo—To scale off, to desquamate.
Desterio—To cease snoring.
Destillo—To distill
Desudo—To sweat, so exude.
Detego—To lay open, to uncover.
Dexter—The right.
  (Manus dextra—The right hand.)
  (Auri dextro—The right ear.)
Diæta—Diet, food.
Diæteticus—Pertaining to food, or regimen.
Dico, avi—To say, to tell
Dictus, a, um—Spoken of, said.
Dies—A day
Die—In a day.
  (Bis dies—Twice a day.)
  (Tertius diebus—Every third day.)
  (De die—In the day time.)
Digestus, a, um—That has a good digestion.
Digitus—A finger
Digitalis—Of or belonging to a finger.
Digitulus—A little finger.
Dilutus—Thin, diluted.
Dilutium—An infusion or dilution.
Dimidius—The half
Diploma—A public document.
Directio, onis—Direction, order.
Directione propria—With the proper direction.
Discipulus—A scholar, a pupil per per
Dispenso—To weigh out, to dispense.
Dissectus (disseco)—Cut asunder, dissected.
Dissolutio—Separation, dissolution.
Dissolvo—To dissolve, to loosen.
Distincte—Distinctly.
Diu, diurnus—By day.
  (Tere diu—Rub for a long time).
Diuturnus—Lasting, durable.
Diuturna trituratione—By long continued trituration.
Divido, isi—To part, divide, separate.
Do, dedi, datum, dare—To give.
Doctor, oris—A teacher, instructor.
Doctrina, æ—Teaching, instruction.
Doctus, a, um—Learned, skillful.
Documentum—Anything by which one can learn, etc.
Dogma—An opinion or tenet of a philosopher.
Dolor, oris (dolens)—Pain.
Domus—Home, a dwelling place.
  (Domus et placens uxorcula.)
Donec (donicum)—Until.
Dormio, ivi—To sleep.
Dormitor, oris—A sleeper.
Dorsum, i—The back.
Drachma—A drachm.
Dropax, acis—An ointment that takes off the hair.
Ductus, us—A duct.
Dulcis, e—Sweet.
Dum—Whilst, during.
Duo, æ, o—Two.
Duodecem—Twelve.
Duodenum—A portion of the intestine,
Duplex—Double, twofold (duplicature).
Duplicatio, onis—A doubling.
Durante dolor—While the pain continues.
Duris, a, um—Hard
Dura mater—The outer membrane of the brain.

E, or ex—Out of, or from.
Ebullio—To bubble up (ebullition).
Edax, acis—Gluttonous, voracious.
Edento, avi—To deprive of teeth.
Edo, edi—To eat, to consume.
Edulis—Eatable.
Edulcorator (dulcis)—A wash bottle, for separating by washing.
Effeminatus—Womanish, delicate.

Effervesco, vi—To ferment, to effervesce.
Effetus—That has brought forth young.
Effligo, xi—To strike dead, to kill.
Effloresco—To blossom, to effloresce
Effundo, udi—To pour out.
Effluvium—Exhalation, vapor.
Egilidus—Coolish, lukewarm.
Ejaculator—To cast out (ejaculatores muscles).
Ejusmodi—Of that kind, like.
Elanguesco—To faint, to grow languid.
Elavo—To wash out, to bathe away.
Electe—With choice.
Elementum—Element, first principle.
Elephantus—An elephant (elephantiasis).
Elinguis—Speechless, dumb.
Elinguo, are—To deprive of the tongue.
Eliquo, are—To make liquid.
Emitto to send out, to send forth.
Emetica, æ—An emetic.
Emollio, avi—To soften.
Emorior—To die, to pass away.
Empirice, es—An art of healing founded on mere practice.
Empiricus, i—A physician instructed only by practice, a quack, an empiric.
Emplastrum—A plaster for a wound.
Emulsio—An emulsion
Eneco, cui—To kill, to torture.
Enema—A clyster.
Enervis, e—Weak enervated, feeble.
Enim—For, therefore.
Enimvero—Surely, of a truth.
Enitus, us—The act of bringing forth young.
Enterocele, es—A kind of rupture or hernia
Enterocelicus, a, um—Afflicted with rupture.
Enucleo, avi—To take out the kernel, enucleate.
Enudo, avi—To make bare.
Eo, avi—To go.
Eo, (adv.)—Thither, for that reason.
Eodem—To the same purpose.
Epiphora, æ—A stoppage of humors in the body.
Epitaphium, i—An epitaph.
Epulæ, arum—Upright.
Ergo—Therefore, because.
Erodo—To eat away.
Eratim—An error
Erubesco, bui—To redden, to blush.
Eructo, are—To belch or vomit forth (eructation).
Erudite, adv—Learnedly (tactus eruditus).
Eruptio, onis—A breaking out, an eruption.
Esculentus, a, um—Eatable.
Esse (est, sunt)—To be.
Esito, avi—To eat.
Estur—gormandizer.
Estrix—A female eater, a gormandizer.
Esurio, iro—To hunger, to be hungry.
Esuritor, oris—A hungry person.
Et—And.
Ethicus, a, um—Belonging to moral or manners.
Etiam—Also, although
Etiam atque etiam—Again and again.
Etsi—Although, yet, but
Eu! (euge, evax)—Well done, well, bravo.
Eunuchus, i—Eunuch.
Evaporatio, onis—Evaporation.
Evanesco—To vanish, to disappear.
Evigilo—To wake, be wakeful.
Eviro, avi—To castrate.
Evomo, ui—To vomit forth.
Exania—A falling down of the anus.
Exanimus, e—Without breath.
Exanthemata—An eruptive disease.
Excandescentia, iæ—Heat of passion, violent anger
Excelsus, a, um—High, lofty, elevated.
Excido, idi—To hue or cut out of, excise.
Excito—To stimulate (excitants).
Excrementum,—That which passes from the body.
Exempli gratia, (e. g.)—As for example.
Excorio—To take off the skin (excoriation).
Exedo—To eat out of, destroy.
Exhalatio, onis—An exhalation, an evaporation.
Exhalo, avi—To breath out, exhale, evaporate.
Exhibeo, ui—To exhibit, to give, to impart.
Exhumo—To disinter.
Exigue—Briefly, shortly.
Exoculo, avi—To deprive of eyes.
Exosis, ossis—Without bone.
Exosso, avi—To deprive of bone.
Exostosis, osis—A morbid enlargement of bone.
Exacerbo—To exasperate, (exacerbation).
Excresco—To grow from (excrescence).
Exfœtatio—Extra uterine fetation.
Exfoliatio—Separation of dead bone from the living.
Expectatio—To wait for (expectant).
Expectoratio—Expectoration.
Expedite—Easily, promptly, quickly.
Experientia, æ—Proof, trial, experience.
Experimentum—Experiment, trial.

Experto, ivi—To attain anything, to aim at.
Expiratio—Expiration, to breathe out.
Exploratio, onis—An examination, investigation.
Exsectio, onis—A cutting off or out.
Exsicco—To dry up, make dry.
Exspisso—To make thick, to exspissate.
Extendo—To stretch out, to extend.
Extensor—A muscle which extends.
Externus—External, outward.
Exturpo—To pluck up by the roots, extirpate.
Extractum—An extract.
Extravasatio—The passage of fluids out of their proper vessels.
Exudatio—Transpiration.
Exuviæ—The slough, the cast off covering of certain animals.

Fac—Make.
Facio, feci—To make, to do.
Facies—The face.
Facies hippocratica—A peculiar appearance of the face before death
Facies rubra—The old name for gutta rosacea, or acne.
Factitious, a, um—Artificial
Facultas—From facere, to make (faculty).
Pæcula, a—The dregs, the lees.
Fæx, cis (fæces pl)—Sediment, dregs, excrement.
Falciforma—Like a sythe.
Falx—A scythe, a sickle.
Falx cerebri, falx cerebelli—Processes of the dura mater.
Fama, æ—Fame, public opinion.
Fames, is—Hunger.
Far—Corn.
Farina—Meal, flour.
Farcimen—Farcy.
Fascia, æ—A long, narrow band.
Fascia lata—The aponeurosis of the thigh.
Fascia superficialis—A membrane extending over the abdomen
Fascialis—The tensor vaginæ femoris.
Fasciculus, i—A small bundle.
Fastidium. i—Nausea, or distaste for food.
Fatuus—Insipid, tasteless.
Faux, cis (fauces pl)—The throat, the gullet.
Favus, i—Honeycomb, a non-acuminated pustule.
Febris, is—A fever, pyrexia.
Febriculosus, a, um—Sick of a fever.
Febricula—A slight degree of fever.
Febrifugum—A febrifuge.
Febrifugum magnum—A name given to cold water as a drink in ardent fever.
Febris accessus—The accession of a fever.
Febris decessus—The decline of a fever.
Febre durante—While the fever continues.
Fecunde—Fruitfully.
Fecundo—To make fruitful, fertilize.
Fecundatio—Impregnation.
Fel, fellis—Gall, bile.
Fel, bovis—Ox gall.
Felis is—A cat (feline).
Felliflua passio—Ancient name for cholera (gall flux)
Femella—A little woman, a girl.
Femina, æ—A female.
Feminalis—Belonging to a woman.
Femineus—Womanlike
Femur, femoris—The thigh.
Fenestra—A window (fenestra ovalis, etc.)
Feralis, e—Of, or belonging to the dead, fatal.
Fere—Almost, nearly.
Fermento, avi—To cause, to ferment
Fermentum, i—That which causes anything to ferment, leaven.
Fermentatus panis—Leavened bread.
Ferrum, i—Iron.
Ferrugineus, a, um—Of, or pertaining to iron, the color of iron.
Fertilizatio—The function of the pollen of plants, etc.
Ferula, æ—An umbelliferous herb with a soft pith in which fire was easily harbored.
Fervefacio, eci—To cause to boil.
Fervefactus—Made hot.
Fervens, cutis—Hot, glowing.
Ferveo—To be hot, or heated, to burn.
Fervesco—To begin to boil, to grow hot.
Fessulus, a, um—Somewhat fatigued.
Fessus—Weary, tired
Fetura, æ—A treading, a bearing.
Fetus (fœtus)—Offspring, young.
Fibra—A fibre, a filament (fibrin, fibril).
Fibræ—The entrails (old).
Fibula, æ—A clasp or buckle, the lesser bone of the leg from its being opposite to where the knee buckle was attached.
Ficatio, or ficus—A fig-like tubercle about the anus.
Ficus—A fig.
Filia, æ—A daughter.
Filius, i—A son.

Filum, i—A thread.
Filamentus—A small thread, a filament.
Filaria—A thread-like parasitic worm.
Filix, icis—A fern
Filiformum—Thread-like.
Filtrum—A strainer.
Fimbra—A fringe, the fringe-like extremity of the Fallopian tube
Fimbriatus—Having the margin bordered with filiform processes
Fimus—Excrement of animals.
Finis—An end, limit
Fio fieri—To make, to become.
Fissura—A fissure, a groove.
Fistula—An ulcer, a fistula, a pipe.
Fistula, in ano—Fistula in the rectum.
Fistula lacrymalis—Fistula of the lacrymal sac.
Flabelliformis—Fan shaped, like the rays of a fan.
Flaccidus—Languid, without force.
Flagelliformis—Whip-like, long, taper.
Flamma, æ—A flame.
Flammatus—Inflamed.
Flatus—A blast, wind in the intestines.
Flavus—Yellow.
Flebilis—Tearful, mournful.
Flecto, xi—To bend
Flexio, onis—Bending (flexor).
Floccitatio—Picking of the bedclothes, forerunner of death.
Flocculus—Vel lobus nervi pneumogastrici.
Floreo (flores)—To flower, to blossom.
Fluctis—A flowing (flux).
Fluctuatio—Fluctuation, perceptible, motion on pressure.
Fluidus—Fluid, not solid.
Fœteo—To stink, to smell badly.
Fohum—A leaf, a herb.
Folicula—A minute secreting cavity.
Fomentum—A fomentation, an application.
Fomes, fomites pl —Substances imbued with contagion.
Fons, tis—A fountain.
Fontanella—Spaces left in the head of an infant.
Fonticulus—A little fountain, an issue.
Foramen (foro)—An opening, aperture.
Forceps, icis—A pair of tongs, pincers.
Formica—An ant, a creeping itching.
Formico—To raise in pimples, to creep.
Formidibalis—Terrible, formidable.
Formula—A prescription, a given form.
Fornix—An arch, a triangular lamina in the brain.
Fortis, e—Strong.
Fossa—A depression, a sinus
Fractus (frango)—Brittle, broken, (fracture).
Fragmentum—A piece broken off.
Frater, tris—A brother.
Frenum—A bridle (frenum lingue).
Frenum labiorum—The fourchette.
Fremitus—Vibration (in auscultation, etc)
Frigidus—Cold
Frigeo, xi—To freeze.
Frons, frontis—The forehead.
Fructus—Fruit
Frumentum—Corn or grain for making bread.
Fuligo—Soot or smoke (antimony guv)
Fuligo ligni—Soot of wood (fuliginous).
Pulmer—Lightning that strikes.
Fumigatio (fumo)—To smoke, to perfume.
Functio (fungor, to do)—To discharge an office, function
Fundus—The bottom of any viscera.
Fundamen—A foundation.
Funebris—Of, or belonging to a funeral.
Fungious (fungus)—A mushroom, a fungus.
Fungiformis—Like a fungus.
Funiculus—The spermatic cord.
Funis (umbelicus)—The umbilical cord.
Funus, eris—A dead body, a corpse.
Furfur—Bran, a desquamation of the cuticle.
Furor—Madness, vehement desire.
Furor uterinus—Old name for nymphomania.
Fusus—Melted, poured out, (fusibility).
Fusiformis—Spindleshaped,
Futurus—That shall or will be.
In futurum—Hereafter.

Galla—Galls.
Gelu (gelatus)—Frost (gelatine).
Gemellus—Double, twins, the name of two muscles.
Gemma—Precious stones, the leaf bud.
Gena—The cheek.
Genero, avi—To produce (generation).
Genesis—Generation, creation, birth,
Genu—The knee.
Genus—A race.
Germen—A bud (germinate).
Gestatio—A carrying, the state of pregnancy.
Glacies—Hardness, icy.
Glans, dis—An acorn, a gland.
Glandula—A small gland.

Glaucoma, atis—An optical illusion.
Globo, avi—To make round.
Globus, i—A globe, a ball, a pellet.
Globulus, i—A globule.
Globus hystericus—A sensation of hysteria.
Gluten, inis, glutinum, i—Glue, gluten.
Gradatim—Step by step, by degrees.
Gratus, a, um—Pleasing, agreeable.
Granum—A grain, a small portion.
Granula—A little grain.
Gravido, avi—To load, to impregnate.
Gravitas—Heaviness
Gula—The gullet, the esophagus.
Gulosus—Gluttonous
Gurgulio—The windpipe (hence gargle).
Gustatus—A tasting (gustatory).
Gutta—A drop
Guttifera—Drop bearing.
Guttatim—By drops.
Guttatus, a, um—Spotted, speckled.
Guttur—The throat.
Gymnas, adis—Exercise.
Gyrus, i—A circle, the spiral cavity of the internal ear, the convolutions of the brain.

Habendus—To be had or held.
Habeo, in—To have, to hold.
Hac—Here, thither.
Hæsitatio—Stammering, hesitation.
Halitus—An aqueous vapor, exhalation.
Hallucinatio—Erroneous imagination.
Halo—A circle surrounding a light, areola.
Hamulus—A little hook.
Hamulus cochleæ—A portion of the inner ear.
Haustus (haurio, to draw)—A draught.
Hemitritæus—A semitertian ague.
Hepar—The liver.
Hepatarius—Relating to the liver
Hepaticus—Diseased in the liver.
Herba, æ—Herbage, an herb.
Hereditas—Inheritance.
Heri—Yesterday.
Hesperus—The evening.
Hiatus—An opening, an aperture.
Hibrida, æ—Of ambiguous origin.
Hic, hæc, hoc—This, such.
Hiems, emis—Winter.
Hieto—To gape, to yawn.
Hilum—The base of a seed at its attachment.
Hilus lienis—A fissure in the spleen.
Hinc—Hence, from this place.
Hinc et hinc—On this part or that.
Hira, æ—A gut
Hircus—A he-goat, a goatish smell, the rank smell of the armpits.
Hirudo—A leech.
Hirsutus—Shaggy, superfluous growth of hair.
Hodie—To-day
Homicidium—Manslaughter, homicide.
Homo, inis—A human being, a man.
Hora—An hour.
Hora somni—At the hour of sleep.
Hora decubitus—At bed-time, or time of lying down.
Horis intermediis—At intermediate hours.
(In horas—Every hour.)
Hordeum—Barley.
Hornus—Of this year.
Horridus, a, um—Dreadful, terrible.
Humanitas, atis—Humanity, human nature.
Humanus, a um—Human.
Humerus, i—The upper bone of the arm.
Humidus, a, um—Moist, wet, damp.
Humo—To bury, to inter.
Humoris, oris—A moisture, a humor.
Humus, i—The earth, the ground.
Hyalus—Glass.
Hydraulicus, a, um—Relating to the scientific motion of the water.
Hydrocele, es—A watery rupture, a hydrocele.
Hydropsis, is—The dropsy.
Hydrargyrum, i—Mercury, quicksilver.
Hymen, inis—A membrane.
Hystericus, a, um—Hysterical.

Ibi—There, in that place.
Ibidem—In the same place.
Ictericus, a, um—Jaundiced,
Icterus—Jaundice, a small yellow bird, the sight of which was said to cure the jaundice.
Ictus solis (ictus, a blow)—Sun stroke, coup de soleil.
Idea, æ—An image, from (hence idea, notion).
Idiota—A senseless person.
Idolum, i—An image that is present to our eyes or mind, a spectre, a ghost.
Ignea—Fiery, burning.
Ignis fatuus—A luminous appearance.
Ignis sacer—(Old) St. Anthony's fire, erysipelas.
Ile, is—A small gut, the ilium.

Iliacum, os—Os coxarum, old name for os innomination.
Ille, a, ud—He, she, that
Illusio, onis—Deception as to the sight, imagination, etc.
Illutatio, onis—Mud bathing
Imago—Image, shadow, image of the mind,
Imbibo—To drink, imbibe.
Imbecills, e—Weak, infirm of mind.
Imberbis, e—Without a beard, beardless.
Imbibo—To drink, to suck in
Imbrex—A roof tile, (imbricated).
Immanis, e—Wild, savage, cruel, inhuman.
Immaturus—Untimely, unripe
Immergo—To dip, to plunge, immerse.
Immortalis, e—Immortal, divine.
Impar—Unequal, uneven
Impatientia, æ—Impatience, unability to suffer or endure.
Impenetrabilis, e—Impenetrable
Imperfectus—Incomplete, unfinished.
Impetigo (impeto to infest)—A pustular disease.
Implantatio, onis—Ingrafting.
Impluvium, i—A shower bath
Impono—To place, set, or apply upon.
Impotens—Powerless, weak, impotent.
Impransus—That has not taken any food, fasting.
Imponderabilis—Without weight.
Impregnatio—Impregnation, conception.
Imprimo—Principally, in the first place.
Impubes, eris—Beardless.
Impudicus—Shameless, unchaste.
Impure, (adv.)—Filthily, impurely.
In—In.
In die—In a day.
Indies—Every day, daily.
Inanimis—Without breath, lifeless.
Inanis—Void, empty, (inanition)
Inauris, is—An ear ring
Incandesco—To grow white, (incandescence).
Incauto—To enshant, to bewitch.
Incarcero—To imprison, to incarcerate.
Incarnatio (in carnis, flesh)—Granulation.
Inceptio—To begin
Inceste—Unchastely, impurely.
Incisio, onis—An incision
Incisorus, es ff—The front or cutting teeth.
Incontiens—Not holding together, incontinent.
Incoquo—To boil together.
Incubatio—Incubation.
Incuratus—Unhealed.
Incubus—Nightmare, oppressive sensation.
Incus, udis—An anvil, a small bone of the internal ear.
Inde—Hence, from that place.
Index (indico, to front out)—The forefinger.
Indicatio—A pointing out, indication
Indigena—A native of the country, indigenous.
Indigestio (indigero, to distribute)—Dyspepsia, indigestion.
Indolens—Indolent, slow in action.
Inductus—Persuaded, induction.
Induratio (induro)—Induration, hardening.
Inebrio, avi—To make drunk.
Inedia, æ—Abstinence from food,
Inertia—Inactivity.
Ineruditus—Unlearned, awkward, unskilled.
Infans—An infant, that cannot speak
Infanticido (infans cædo, to kill)—Infanticide.
Inficio, eci—To stain, to poison (infection).
Infirmitas—Weakness, infirmity (infirmary).
Infiltratio—Diffusion of fluid into the cellular tissue.
Inflammatio (to burn)—Inflammation.
Inflatio—A blowing up, inflation.
Infloresco—To flourish, inflorescence.
Infra—Beneath, below, under.
Infundibulum—A little funnel-shaped process.
Infusus—Pouring into, infusion.
Ingestus—A pouring in, ingesta.
Inguen, inis—The groin
Inhalo—To breath on (inhalation).
Inhumanus—Inhuman, not human.
Inhumo—To inter.
Inibi—Therein.
Injectus—A throwing in, an injection.
Injuria, æ—Hurt, injury, harm, damage.
Innominatus—Nameless.
Innuptis, a, um—Unmarried.
(Nuptiæ innuptiæ—An unfortunate marriage.)
Inoculatio—An insertion of virus.
Inopia—Poverty, need, destitution.
Inquietus, a, um—Restlessness, unquiet.
Inosculatio (osculum, a little mouth)—Union of vessels, anastomosis
Insaluber, bris—Unwholesome, not conducive to health.
Insanabilis, e—That cannot be cured or healed.
Insania, æ—Madness, phrenzy.
Insecta—An insect.
Inserto, avi—To put in, to insert.
Insiccatus—Undried.
Insidiosus, a, um—Dangerous.

Insolo, avi—To dry in the sun.
Insolubilis, e—That cannot be dissolved.
Insomnia, æ—Want of sleep, sleeplessness.
Insomnium, i—A dream.
Inspiro—To breathe upon, inhale (inspiration).
Inspergo—To sprinkle upon.
Inspico, exi—To inspect, examine.
Inspisso—To render thick, inspissate.
Instrumentum, i—Instrument, tool
Insufflatio—To blow into, insufflation.
Insulatio—Insulation
Integumentum, i—A covering, integument, cuticle.
Intelligens—Intelligent, sensible
Intemperans, tis—That cannot moderate himself.
Intente—With earnestness.
Inter—Between or among.
Interdie—By day, in the daytime.
Interim—In the meantime.
Intestinus, a, um—Internal, intestine.
Intume—Most intimately
Intra—Within, on the inside.
Intolero—That cannot be borne.
Intumesco—To swell, intumesence.
Intus susceptio (intus, within, suscipio, to receive)—The descent of a higher portion of intestine into a lower one
Invaginatio (in vagina, a sheath)—Synonymous with intus-susception.
Inverminatio—An affection in which worms or larvæ inhabit the stomach or intestines
Inverto—To turn, turn up or about.
Involucrum—The designation of membranes that cover any part.
Ipse—Self.
Ira—Anger, wrath, rage.
Irritabilis, e—Easily excited, irritable.
Irrito—To incite, to irritate, excite.
Irrigo—To irrigate, to apply cold water or lotion to an affected part.
Ita—Thus, even so.
Item—Also, likewise.
Iterum—Again, the second time.

Jactatio, vel jactitatio (jacto)—Restlessness, change of position
Jam—Now, at this time, at present.
Janitor, oris—A porter, a doorkeeper.
Jecur, oris—The liver
Jecusculum, i—A small liver.
Jejunum, i—The upper two-fifths of the small intestines, so called from this part being usually found empty.
Jejunus, a, um—Fasting, hungry, empty.
Jentaculum—A breakfast.
Jento, avi—To break one's fast.
Juba, æ—The mane, the flowing hair of an animal.
Jugulum, i—The throat.
Junctim—Unitedly, jointly.
Jus, juris—Broth, soup
Jusculum—Diminutive of jus.
Jureus—Consisting of broth, full of broth.
Jus ovilli—Mutton broth
Jusculum, coactum—Jelly.
Juxta—Near to, by.

Labium, i—A lip.
Labellum—Lip-like, used in botany.
Labor, oris—Work, toil, child-birth.
Lac, tis—Milk.
Lac vaccinum—Cow's milk.
Lac recens—New milk
Lacu depulsus—Weaned.
Lacero—To tear, (laceration).
Lacertus, i—The arm, (hence lacertus, a blow).
Lacryma, æ—A tear.
Lacrymo—To shed tears
Lactillo, are—To give milk, to suckle.
Lactuca, æ—A lettuce
Lacuna, æ—A lake, follicles in the mucous membrane of the urethra.
Lallo, are—To sing to sleep, to sing lulla, or lullaby.
Lamina, æ—A thin plate or leaf.
Lana—Flannel, wool.
Lana philosophica—White oxide of zinc.
Languor, oris—Faintness, feebleness, weariness.
Lancetta (lanca a shear)—A lancet.
Lapis, idis—A stone.
Larva, æ—A visor, a mask.
Lascivus—Wanton, lustful.
Lassitudo, inis—Faintness, weakness, fatigue.
Latus, eris—A side, a flank (lateral).
Lavo, avi—To wash, to bathe.
Laxo, avi—To loosen (laxatives).
Lectus, i—A bed.
Lectulus, i—A sofa, a lounge.
Lecto teneri—To be sick in bed.
Legumen, inis—Pulse.
Lenio ivi—To alleviate, to soften, to mitigate, (lenitives).

Lens, tis—A bean, a lentil (lenticular).
Lentigo—Freckles, yellow spots on the skin.
Lentus—Glutinous, clammy, (lentor of the blood).
Lesio—Hurt, injury, morbid change.
Lethe, es—Forgetfulness.
Leto—To kill
Letum, vel lethum—Death
Letum ibi, consciscere—To kill oneself
Levator—A lifter up.
Levigo—To polish, to smooth (levigation).
Liber, a, um—Free.
Liber, bri—A book
Libet, lent—It pleases, is agreeable.
Libet adlibitum—As you please)
Libitina—Any kind of furniture for funerals.
Libra, æ—A pound.
Libramen—A balance, counterpoise.
Lien, enis—The milt or spleen
Ligamentum—A band, a ligament.
Ligo, avi—To bind, to tie, (ligature).
Lignum—Wood
Limax (limus, slime)—A snail (cochlea terrestris).
Linamentum (linum, linen)—Lint, a tent for a wound.
Lineamentum, i—Features, lineaments, a line.
Linimentum (lino, to besmear)—A liniment, embrocation
Linum, i—Flax, lint.
Lippio—To have blear eyes.
Lippitudo, inis—An affection of the eyes.
Ligueo, qui—To be liquid or fluid.
Jaquefacio—To melt, to liquefy.
Liquor, oris—A liquid, fluid.
Lividus—Of a bluish color
Livor, oris—Black and blue, a mark produced by a blow.
Lix, licis—Lye, (lixivium).
Lobus (lobulus)—A lobe, a lobule.
Locales—Local diseases.
Locomotio—Moving from one place to another.
Lomentum, i—That which is used for washing, an emolent used for softening the skin.
Longus—Long.
Lotio—A lotion, a wash.
Lubrico, avi—To make smooth, to lubricate.
Lues, is—A contagious disease, a pestilence.
Lues Venerea—The plague of Venus, syphilis.
Lumbus, i—A loin
Lumbricalis—Muscles of the hand and foot.
Lumbricus—The earth worm
Luna—The moon (lunatic)
Lunula (a little moon)—The white semilunar mark at the base of the nails
Lupia—A wen, a tumor.
Lupus (a wolf)—A tubercular affection, noli me tangere.
Luseus—Blind in one eye
Lusciosus—Purblind, dimsighted (luscitas).
Luxus, us—A dislocation, luxation.
Lympha—Water (lymphatics).

Macero, avi—To make soft, to steep, to macerate.
Macies, ei—Leanness, thinness.
Macula, æ—A spot.
Magis—More.
Magnus, a, um—Large, great.
Magnesia—An earth, oxide of magnesium.
Mala, æ—A cheek bone, jaw.
Male—Badly, ill
Malignus—Of a bad kind, malignant.
Malleolus, i—A small hammer, the ankle bone.
Malleus—One of the small bones of the ear.
Malus, a, um—Bad, evil
Maliformis—Badly formed, malformed.
Malus, i, vel malum, i—An apple.
Mamma, æ—The breast.
Mammalia—Vertebrata with mammary glands.
Mamilla—Synonymous with papilla.
Mancus—Maimed, defective in limbs.
Mane—In the morning.
Mane primo—The first thing in the morning.
Maneo—To remain.
Manes, ium—The spirits of the dead.
Mania, æ—Madness, insanity, rage.
Manipulus, i—A handful.
Manubrium, i—A handle, the upper bone of the sternum.
Manus, us—A hand.
Mare, is—The sea.
Margo, inis—An edge, border.
Maritus, a, um—Of, or belonging to marriage.
Masculus, a, um—Male, masculine.
Massa—A lump, a mass.
Mastico—To chew, to masticate.
Matella, æ—A chamber pot, a night stool.
Masturbatio—Masturbation.
Mater—A mother
Materia medica—That branch of medical science which relates to medicines
Matrimonium, i—Marriage, matrimony.

Maturo—To ripen (maturation).
Maxilla—The cheek bone.
Maximus, a, um—The greatest, largest.
Meatus us—A passage.
Medicabilis, e—That can be healed or cured.
Medicamen, ints—Any remedy applied to diseases or wounds
Medicamentum, i—That heals diseases.
Medicinus, a, um—Of, or belonging to physic.
Medico—To heal, to cure.
Medicus—A physician
Medulla, æ—The marrow of bones, the pith of plants.
Mel, mellis—Honey
Melancholia, æ—Black bile, melancholy.
Membrana, æ—The skin or membrane that covers the separate members of the body.
Membratim—By members, limb by limb.
Membrum—A limb, a member of the body.
Mens—The mind.
Mensis, is—A month
Menstruus, a, um—That happens every month (menstruation)
Mensura, æ—A measure.
Mentum—The chin.
Mephitis, is—A noxious and pestilential vapor.
Meridies—Mid day, noon.
Metallicus—Of, or belonging to metals.
Metamorphosis, is—Transformation, change.
Miliaria—Miliary fever, vesiculæ
Milium—A millet seed, a small white tumor.
Mille—A thousand
Minimum—The least.
Misceo—To mix, to mingle.
Missus (mitto)—Sent.
Mistura, æ—A mixture.
Mitella, æ—A bandage around the head.
Mitigatio, onis—A mitigation, alleviation.
Mitto, misi—To send
Mitra—A mitre, a covering of the head (mitral).
Moderate—With moderation, temperately.
Modus, i—Way or manner, measure.
Modo præscripto—In the manner directed.
Molaris (mola, a millstone)—A double or grinding tooth.
Molestus—Troublesome.
Mollis, is—Soft.
Molluscum—A wen, a movable tumor (ord. tubercula).
Mons—A mountain.
Mons veneris—The eminence over the os pubis in women.
Monstrum, i—A monster, contrary to the usual course of nature
Mora, æ—A delay, tarrying.
Morbus, i—A disease.
Mordeo—To bite with the teeth.
Mordex—A tooth.
Moribundus—Dying, ready to die.
Morior—To die
Mors, tis—Death
Mortalis, e—Mortal, subject to death.
Morticinus—That has died through disease.
Morpheus—The God of sleep (morphia).
Morificatio (mors bo)—Morification.
Motio, onis—A moving, a modon.
Moveo, movi—To move, to set in motion, to stir.
Mucosus, a, um—Slimy, mucous.
Mucus, i—Mucus, the discharge from the nose.
Muliebris, e (mulier)—Womanly.
Mulier, eris—A woman.
Muluformis, e—Having many forms or shapes.
Multiplex, leis—That has many folds.
Multus, a, um—Many, numerous.
Musca, æ—A fly.
Muscæ volitantes—An appearance of motes or small bodies floating before the eyes.
Musculus, i—A muscle of the body
Muto, avi—To move, to change
Mutus, a, um—Dumb, silent, mute.

Nævus, i—A mark or mole on the body.
Nam—For.
Nanus—A dwarf.
Nares, ium, vel nasus, i—The nose.
Naris, is—A nostril.
Narthecium, i—A chest for unguents and medicines, a gallipot.
Nata, æ—A daughter.
Natalis, e—Of, or belonging to one's birth.
Natis, is—A buttock.
Natura, æ—Nature, birth, the universe.
Natus—A son.
Nausea, æ—Desire to vomit, nausea.
Nauseo, avi—To feel sick, to be ready to vomit, to loathe, to be disgusted with.
Naviculare, os—A boat-shaped bone of the carpus and tarsus.
Nebula, æ—A mist, vapor, cloud, haziness.
Nec—Neither, nor.
Nervus, i—A nerve.

Nex, necis—Death by violence.
Nicto, avi—To wink with the eyes (nictitation).
Niger, gra—Black
Nisi—If not, unless.
Nix, nivis—Snow.
Noceo, ni—To injure, to harm, to hurt.
Nocturnus, a, um—By night, nocturnal.
Noctambulatio, onis—Night-walking.
Nodo, avi—To knot
Nodus, i—A swelling of the bone, a node.
Nodula—A small bone.
Nodus cerebri—The pons varolii or tuber annulure of the brain.
Nolo—To be unwilling.
Noli me tangere—Touch me not, Lupus (tubercula).
Nomen, inis—A name, appellation.
Norma, æ—Rule, prescript (normal, abnormal).
Nostrum—Our own, a quack medicine.
Nothus, a, um—Spurious, counterfeit, not genuine.
Novo, avi—To make anything new, to renew.
Nox, noctus—Night.
Nocte (or de nocte)—By night.
(De multa nocte—Late at night.)
Noxius, a, um—Noxious, hurtful, harmful.
Nubes, is—A cloud.
Nebula, æ—A small cloud.
Nubilis, e—Marriageable.
Nubo, psi (to veil, to cover)—To marry, as the bride puts on a veil
Nupta, æ—A bride, a wife.
Nucleus, i—The kernel, the solid centre.
Nudus, a, um—Bare, naked.
Nullus, a um—None, nothing.
Numero, avi—To number, to reckon, to count.
Nunc—Now.
Nunquam—Never.
Nuptiæ, arum—Marriage, wedding.
Nurus, us—A daughter-in-law.
Nuto, avi—To nod
Nutrimentum, i—Nourishment, support.
Nutrio, avi—To give nourishment.
Nympha, æ—A veiled bride, the chrysalis of an insect.
Nymphæ—Labia minora
Nymphomania—Lascivious madness in females.

Obesus, a, um—Fat, corpulent (obesity).
Obliquus—Oblique, crooked, slanting.
Obluero, avi—To efface, to deface, to close.
Oblivio—Forgetfulness, failure of memory.
Obsoletus—Old, no longer new.
Obstetrix, leis—A midwife.
Obsto, iti—To stand before or against.
Obstructio—A stopping up, obstruction.
Obturo, avi—To stop up, (obturator).
Occiput, itis (ob. caput)—The back part of the head, occiput.
Occlusus, a, um—Shut, closed.
Occulto—To hide, to conceal.
Oceanus, i—The ocean.
Ocellus, i—A little eye.
Octies—Eight times.
Octo—Eight.
Oculatus, a, um—Furnished with, or having eyes.
Oculus, i—An eye (oculist).
Odor, oris—Scent, smell.
Odorifer, a, um—That brings an odor or scent.
Oestrus, i—The gad fly.
Officina, æ—A workshop (officinal).
Olea, æ—An olive.
Oleum, i—The expressed oil of olives, an oil.
Olfactorius, a, um (olfacio—That serves or belongs to smelling.
Olla, æ—A pot, a jar.
Ollaris, e—Preserved in jars.
Omasum, i—The third stomach of Ruminantia.
Omentum, i—The membrane which incloses the bowels.
Omitto, isi—To lay aside, to leave off, omit.
Omnis, e—All.
Onyx, ychis—A finger nail.
Onychia—An abscess near the finger nail.
Opacus—Shaded, opaque.
Operosus, a, um—Full of pains or endeavor.
Ophthalmicus, a, um—Of, or relating to the eyes.
Opposio, sui—To set or place against, oppose.
Optio, onis—Free will, choice.
Orbiculus, i—A small circle.
Orbis, is—Anything of a circular shape.
Orbita, æ—The cavity in which the eye is fixed.
Organum, i—A part which has a determinate office in the animal economy.
Origo, inis—An origin, beginning.
Orificium, i—An orifice, a mouth or entrance.
Os, oris—The mouth.
Os, ossis—A bone.
Osseus, a, um—Of, or pertaining to bone.
Ossificatio, onis—Becoming bone, formation of bone.
Ostium—The door of a chamber (osteum abdominale).
Ovis, is—A sheep.

Ovarium (ovum)—An organ containing the ova.
Ovulum, i—A little egg (ovula).
Ovum, i—An egg.

Pabulum, i—Food, nourishment, support.
Fœdor—Nastiness, by want of proper attention.
Palam—Openly, publicly
Palatum, i—The palate.
Pallidus, a, um—Pale, wan, pallid.
Palma, æ—The palm of the hand.
Palpebra, æ—An eyelid.
Palpatio, onis (palpo)—Manual examination, palpation.
Palpitatio, onis (palpito)—An action of the heart.
Panacea, æ—A herb said to cure all diseases.
Pants—Bread.
Pannus—(A rag, a cloth) a disease of the eye.
Papilla, æ—The nipple of the breast, a small eminence.
Papula. æ—A pimple, a papule.
Par, paris—Equal, even.
Parasitus, i—A parasite, a sponger.
Parate—Preparedly, carefully.
Parco, pepersi—To spare.
Parce—Sparingly, moderately.
Pareus, tis—A parent.
Paries, parietis—Partition wall, parietal.
Paro, avi—To prepare, to make.
Pats—Part, piece.
Parturio, ivi—To bring forth, to be in travail.
Parturifaciens, tis—A medicine which causes uterine pains.
Parvus—Small, little.
Pastillus, i—A perfumed or sweet ball.
Patella, æ—The knee pan.
Patens, tis—Open, passable.
Pater, tris—A father.
Patiens, tis—Patient, enduring.
Patulus, a, um—Open, standing open.
Pecco, avi—To do a thing wrongly, to be in fault (peccant).
Pecten, tinis—A comb (pectineus, pectenate).
Pectus, oris—The breast (pectoralia).
Pediculus—A louse.
Pediculosus, a, um—Full of lice, lousy.
Pediculatio, onis—An affection of the skin, phtheiriasis.
Pediluvium, i (pes lavo)—A foot bath.
Pedunculus—Splay footed, peduncle.
Pellicula, æ (pellis)—A thin skin, pellicle.
Pellis, is—A hide, or skin.
Pellucidus, a, um—Transparent, pellucid.
Pendeo, pependi—To hang down, to suspend.
Pendo, pependi—To hang down (pendent).
Pendulus, a, um—Hanging, hanging down.
Peniculum, i—(A painter's pencil) a tent, a pledget.
Penis, is—The male organ of generation, membrum virile
Penite—Inwardly, internally.
Penna, æ—A feather, a wing.
Pennatus, a, um—Winged, feathered.
Pennipes, edis—Feather-footed.
Penso, avi—To weigh, to weigh out.
Penus, us—Provision, store of food.
Per—Through, by.
Percolo, avi—To filter or strain through, to percolate.
Percutio, ussi—To strike through, percussion.
Perditus, a, um—Lost, hopeless.
Perennis, e—That lasts for a year or more, perennial.
Perfectus, a, um—Perfect, complete.
Perforo, avi—To bore through, to pierce through, to perforate.
Perfrico, cui—To rub over.
Periodus, i—A period.
Peritia, æ—Skill, practical knowledge.
Peritus, a um—Well versed or skilled, able, expert.
Permeo, avi—To pass through (permeate).
Perua, æ—The hip together with the leg.
Pernio, onis—A chilblain.
Permitto, issi—To permit, to allow.
Perscribo, psi—To write down, to write out at length.
Perscriptio, onis—Any written composition.
Persona, æ—A mask, a person, an individual.
Perspiro—To breath through (perspiration).
Pertineo, nui—To extend, to reach.
Perturbo, avi—To disturb (perturbation).
Pertussus—A cough, hooping cough.
Pervado, si—To pass through.
Pervigil, is—Very watchful, always wakeful.
Pervius, a, um—That may be passed through,
Pes, pedis—A foot.
Pestiferus, a, um—Causing or bringing pestilence.
Pestilens, tis—Pestilential, unwholesome.
Pestis, is—A plague, pestilence, infestion.
Petra, is—A rock, a stone.
Phalanga, æ—A phalanx, bones of the fingers and toes.
Phantasia, æ—A thought, an idea, phantasm, hallucination.
Phantasma, atis—An apparition, spectre.
Pharmaceutta, æ—(An enchantress) the compounding of drugs.

Pharmacopola, æ—A seller or dealer in medicines.
Phiala, æ—A drinking vessel, a small glass.
Philosophus, a, um—Philosophical, erudite.
Philtrum, i—A charm, a love potion.
Phlegmon, onis—A tense, painful swelling.
Phosphorus, i—A bringer of light.
Phrenesis, is—Phrenzy, madness.
Phthisis—A consumption.
Physica, æ—The science or study of nature.
Physice—Physically.
Physicus, a, um—An inquirer into nature.
Physiognomon, onis—One who judges of the character of men by their features.
Physiologia, æ—The science of natural philosophy.
Pica, æ—Depraved appetite, craving for improper substances.
Pico, avi—To bedaub with pitch.
Pigmentum, i (pungo)—A paint, a color, a pigment.
Pila, æ—A mortar.
Pilum, i—A pestle or pounder for a mortar.
Pilula, æ—A pill.
Pilus, i—A hair, a short hair.
Pingo, nxi—To paint.
Pinguis, e—Fat.
Pinna, æ—A feather.
Pinus, us—The fir tree.
Piper, eris—Pepper.
Pirum, i—A pear tree.
Picis, is—A fish.
Pisinnus, i—A little boy.
Pisinna, æ—A little girl.
Pisum, i—A pea.
Pisiformis—Pea like.
Pituita, æ—Phlegm, viscid mucus.
Pix, picis—Pitch.
Placenta, æ (a cake)—The afterbirth.
Placenta prævia—Presentation of the placenta
Placidus, a, um—Soft, gentle, mild.
Planta, æ—A vegetable, a plant.
Planta pedis—The sole of the foot.
Plantaris, e—Of, or belonging to the sole of the foot.
Planus, a, um—Smooth, plain, even.
Plenus, a, um—Full, loaded.
Plecto, xi—To plait, to braid, to weave.
Plexus—A net-work of blood vessels.
Plico, avi—To fold, to knit together.
Plica, æ—A fold, a duplicature, a plait.
Plica polonica—A disease of the hair.
(Sæpe sub pica latet seu fœtus seu plica.)
Ploro, avi—To cry, to weep, to bewail.
Pluma, æ—Down, soft feathers.
Plumbago, inis—Lead ore.
Plumbum, i—Lead.
Pluo, pluvi—To rain.
Pluries—Often, frequently, several times
Pluviometer—A rain gauge, pluvio.
Pneumaticus, a, um—Of, or belonging to the air.
Poculum, i—A little cup, a poisonous draught.
Podagra, æ—Gout in the feet.
Podex, icis—The fundament.
Polenta, æ—A prepared barley.
Pollen, inis—Very fine meal or flour, powdery matter.
Pollex, icis—The thumb.
Polluo, ni—To pollute, contaminate.
Polypus—A polypus, a swelling or excrescence.
Pomum, i—Fruit, an apple.
Pondus, eris—A weight.
Pono, posui—To set, lay, place.
Pons—A bridge.
Poples, itis—The leg behind the knee.
Populus, i—The people.
Populus, i—A poplar tree.
Porcus, i—A hog, swine.
Porrigo, inis (porrum, garlic)—A pustular disease of the skin.
Porta, æ—A gate, an entrance (portal).
Portio, onis—A part, a portion.
Porto, avi—To carry, to bear.
Possum, potui—To be able, to have the power.
Post—After, or since.
Post mortem—After death.
Postea—Afterward.
Posteritas, atis—Future times, future generations.
Potatio, onis—A drinking.
Potens, tis—Able, having power
Poto, potavi—To drink.
Potus, us—A draught, a potion.
Præ—Before.
Præcipito, avi—To throw or cast down, precipitate.
Præcise—Concisely, briefly.
Præcordia, orum—The diaphragm.
Prædico, xi—To say beforehand, predicate.
Prægnans, tis—With child, pregnant.
Præmaturus, a, um—Very early, untimely, premature.
Præparo, avi—To make ready beforehand, to prepare.
Præputium, i (puto, to cut off)—The prepuce, foreskin.
Præscribo, psi—To proscribe, order, appoint beforehand.

Præscriptio, onis—Order, rule, prescription.
Pranleo, di—(To eat before breakfast) to eat, to dine.
Piavus, a, um—Depraved, deformed.
Prehenso, avi—To take hold of, to seize.
Pressura, æ—Pressure, expressed.
Prima—The first.
Primæ viæ—The first passages, the stomach and intestines, as distinguished from the lacteals or secundæ viæ.
Primipara, æ—One who is delivered of her first child.
Priapus—Permanent rigidity of the penis, priapism.
Pro re nata—According to the nature of the case.
Probo, avi—To try, examine, inspect
Proboscis, idis—The snout of an animal proboscis.
Procedo, essi—To spring forth, proceed (processus).
Procreator, oris—One who brings forth, procreator.
Procreasco, ere—To grow forth, to spring up
Procurator, oris—One who superintends anything.
Produco, xi—To bring forth, to produce.
Professor, oris—A public teacher.
Proflatus, us—A snoring.
Progenero, are—To generate, beget, bring forth.
Progenitor, oris—The founder or progenitor of a family
Prognosticum, i—A sign or token of anything future (prognosis).
Progressus, ns—A going before, advancement.
Prohibeo, ui—To restrain, hinder, prohibit.
Prolapsus, a, um—A falling, a slipping down of a part.
Procidentia (cado, to fall)—Synonymous with prolapsus.
Proluvies, ei—Filth cast forth.
Promineus, tis—That which projects, a prominence.
Promiscuus, a, um—Mixed, in common.
Prompte—Without delay, quickly.
Vi onitas, atis—Pronation, a bending down.
'ronus, a, um—Bent, inclined.
'ropagatio, onis—A propagating, enlarging.
Propinquitas, atis—Relationship, nearness
Proscribo, psi—To make a thing publicly known by writing.
Proseda, æ—A common prostitute.
Prostibilis, e (pro, sto)—That publicly exposes itself for hire.
Protrudo—To thrust or put forward.
Prosector, oris—One who prepares subjects for anatomical lectures
Proximo, are—To approximate.
Prurigo, ins—An itching, severe itching (pruritus).
Psellismus—Misenunciation, stammering
Psilothrum, i—An ointment by means of which the hair falls off
Ptisanarium, i—A decoction of barley or rice, ptisan.
Pubeo, ui—To be pubescent.
Pubertas, ati—The age of puberty.
Pubes, is—Puberty, the pubis.
Pubis, os—The pubic bone.
Pudendum—The external parts of generation in the female.
Pudeo, ui—To be ashamed.
Puella, æ—A young woman, a girl.
Puellus, i—A little boy.
Puer, eri—A child, a boy.
Puerpera, æ—A woman recently delivered.
Puerperium, i—Child-birth, child-bed.
Pugnus, i—A fist.
Pulcher, chra—Beautiful.
Pulmo, onis—The lungs.
Pulmoneus, a, um—Of, or belonging to the lungs.
Pulpa, æ—The flesh with fat or bone
Puls, tis—A gruel or pottage made of pulse.
Pulsatio, onis—A beating, throbbing, pulsation.
Pulsus cordis—The impulse of the heart.
Pultatio, onis (puls.)—Substances having the consistence of porridge.
Pulvis, eris—Dust, powder.
Punctum, i—A small mole, a puncture.
Pungo, pupungi—To prick, to penetrate, to enter.
Pupula, æ—The pupil of the eye.
Purgatus, us—Cleansed, a purging.
Purgo, avi—To purge (purgatives).
Puriformis, is—Resembling pus.
Purpura, æ—An eruption of the skin.
Purus, a, um—Pure, clean.
Purifico, avi—To cleanse, to purify.
Pus, puris—Matter.
Pustula—A pimple containing matter, a pustule.
Puteo, ui—To stink, to rot.
Putresco—To rot, to putrefy.
Putrefactio, onis—Decomposition, putrefaction.
Putridus, a, um—Fetid, stinking.
Pyga, æ—The buttocks.
Pyramis, idis—A pyramid.
Pytessa, are—To spit out.
Pyriformis—Pear shaped.

Qui—How, in what manner.
Quadrans, tis—The fourth part, quarter (quadrant).
Quadratus, a, um—Square, four-cornered, the name of several muscles.

Quadrigeminus, (four double)—A term applied to four tubercules in the brain, nates, testes
Quadrupes, edis—Four-footed, quadruped.
Quam—How, as, as much as.
Quam, viæ—As much as you like
Quantitas, atis—Extent, quantity, number.
Quantus, a, um—How great, how much, as much as.
Quantum sufficit, Q. S.—As much as is sufficient.
Quies, etis—Rest, quiet, calm
Quiesco, evi—To be a rest, quiet.
Quarante—Forty (quarantine 40 days).
Quotidianus, a, um—Daily, every day, quotidian.

Rabies, ei—Maddess, phrenzy.
Rabide—Ravingly, madly.
Racemus, i—A bunch of grapes (raceme).
Radicula—A small root, radicle.
Radius, i—A rod, the small bone of the arm.
Radex, icis—A root
Radiatio, onis—Radiation.
Ramentum, i—Filings, shavings, scrapings,
Ramix, icis—The vessels of the lungs.
Ramus, i—A branch.
Rana, æ—A frog.
Ranula, æ—(A little frog, frog-tongue, a tumor under the tongue
Rancidus—Rancid, stinking.
Rapidus, a, um—Rapid, quick, swift.
Rare—Thinly.
Raptus, (rapio to seize)—Raptus nervosum, or cramp, raptus supinus, or opisthotonos.
Rarefacio—The act of making a substance less dense.
Ratio, onis—A reason, a principle, a maxim
Raucus, a, um—Hoarse, husky of voice, raucitas.
Ravio, ire—To speak oneself hoarse
Reago—To act again or upon (re-action, re-agent).
Recalvus, a, um—Bald-headed
Recedo, essi—To go back, recede.
Recens, tis—Fresh, recent, new.
Receptaculum, i—A receptacle.
Receptaculum chyli—The receptacle of the chyle.
Recipio, epi—To take, to secure, take back.
Recipe—Take
Reclino, avi—To lean or support onself upon, recline.
Recte—Rightly, directly.
Rectificatio, onis—Redistillation, rectification.
Rectum, i—The straight gut, the last portion of intestine.
Rectus, a, um—Straight, the name of several muscles
Recumbo, ui—To lie back, recline.
Recuperatio, onis—A recovering, obtaining again.
Recuro, avi—To heal or cure
Recurro cucurri—To run back, recurrent.
Reduco, xi—To take or draw back (reduction).
Reduvia—A whitlow, agnail.
Reflecto, xi—To bend back (reflection).
Refrigero—To make cool, refrigerate (refrigerants).
Regimen, inis—A rule of diet, etc., prescribed for a patient.
Regio, onis—Region, artificial divisions of the body.
Regurgitatio, onis—Regurgitation.
Relapsus—Relapse, recurrence.
Relaxo, avi—To loosen, to relax.
Remedium, i—Remedy, means of healing or cure.
Remissio, onis—A cessation of febrile symptoms.
Remitto—To remit (remittent, a class of fevers).
Remora, æ—A stoppage or obstacle.
Remotus, a, um—Remote, distant.
Ren, renis—A kidney, usually plural renes, kidneys.
Reniformis, is—Kidney shaped.
Repello, puli—To drive back (repellent)
Reproduco—Generation, continuation of the species.
Reptilia, æ—A reptile.
Requiesco, evi—To rest, repose, recreate.
Res—A matter or thing.
Resanesco, nui—To grow sound, or heal again.
Reseco, cui—To cut out, to cut off (resection).
Resina, æ—A resin.
Resolvo, solvi—To loosen again, to dissipate (resolvents).
Resono, avi—To reecho, resound (resonance)
Respiratio, onis—The act of fetching breath in and expiration.
Resuscitato, onis—The act of recovering life, or reviving
Restiformis—Cord-like, two cord-like process of the brain.
Retd, is—A net, a vascular net-work, or plexus of vesses.
Retentio, onis—A keeping back, retention.
Reticulum, i—A little network, the second stomach of the ruminantia.
Retiformis—Net-like.
Retina—A net-like expansion of the optic nerve, the retina.
Retraho, xi—To draw back (retractor, retrahens).
Retro—Behind, backwards.
Retrocedo, ere—To go back, to retrocede.

Retroversio, onis—A turning backwards
Retroversio uteri—A morbid inclination of the uterus backward.
Reverbero, avi—To beat back again.
Revulsus—A pulling away, revulsion.
Rhonchus, i—A snorting, a snoring, râle.
Rictus, i—The mouth wide open.
Rideo, si—To laugh.
Rigidus, a, um—Suff, inflexible, rigid.
Rigor, oris—Stiffness rigor.
Rigor mortus—The stiffness of death.
Rima, æ—A fissure, a cleft (rima, glottidis).
Risus—Laughter.
Risus sardonicus—A species of convulsive laughter.
Roboro, avi—To strengthen (roborans).
Robustus, a, um—Hardy, strong.
Rodo, si—To gnaw (rodentia).
Rosa, æ—A rose.
Rosalia, æ—Old term for scarlatina.
Roseola (roseus, rosy)—Rose colored efflorescence.
Rostrum i—The bill or beak of birds.
Rota, æ—A wheel, a circuit.
Roto, avi—To turn around (rotator, rotation, rotifera).
Rubefacio, eci—To make red, rubefacient.
Rubeola, æ (ruber, red)—Measles.
Rubigo—Rust.
Ructus, us—A belch, an act of belching.
Ruga, æ—A fold, a wrinkle.
Rugosus, a, um—Full of wrinkles (rugose, rugosity).
Ruminatio, onis—A chewing again, ruminating (ruminantia,
Ruptus, a, um—Broken, a rupture

Saccharum, i—Sugar.
Saccus, i—A sack or bag, a natural or morbid cavity.
Sacculus, i.—A little bag, minute vesicular bags.
Sacrum, i—The base of the vertebral column.
Sæpe—Often, frequently.
Sagitta, æ—An arrow (sagittalis, sagittae).
Sal, salis—Salt.
Salinus, a, um—Of, or belonging to salt, saline.
Saliva, æ—Spittle.
Salivatio, onis—Salivation, augmentation of the secretion of the saliva.
Saltus, us—A spring, a bound, a leap.
Salubritas, atis—Healthfulness, salubrity.
Salveo, ere—To be well, or in good health.
Salvatella, æ—A vein of the foot, the opening of which was said to preserve health, and cure melancholy.
Sanatio, onis—A curing, healing.
Sanate—Inviolably.
Sanguen, inis—Blood.
Sanguis, inis—Blood
Sanguificatio, onis—The process by which chyle is converted into blood.
Sanies ei—A thin, serous, fœtid matter.
Sanitas. atis—Soundness of body,
Sano, avi—To heal, to cure.
Sanus, a, um—Sound in body, in good health.
Sapo, onis—Soap
Sartor, oris—A tailor, a muscle of the leg
Sat, satis—Sufficient enough.
Satietas, atis—Fullness, satiety, disgust.
Saturo, avi—To satisfy (saturation).
Saucio, avi—To wound, to hurt mortally.
Scabies, ei—Scab, itch.
Scabo, bi—To scratch, to rub (scab).
Scala, æ—A ladder, a flight of stairs (scalæ of the cochlea).
Scalpellum, i—A scalpel.
Scalpo, psi—To rub, to scrape.
Scambus, a, um—Crooked-legged, bow-legged.
Scapula, æ—The shoulder-blade.
Scarabeus, i—A beetle.
Scarificio, avi—To lance, to scarify.
Sciens, tis—Knowing, skillful.
Scientia, æ—Knowledge, science.
Scintilla, æ—A small spark.
Scoria, æ—The dross or refuse of metals, excrement.
Scrobis, is, vel scrobs, is—A depression.
Scrobiculus cordis—The pit of the stomach.
Scrofa, æ—A sore (scrofula).
Scrotum, i—A leather bag, the envelope of the testes.
Scrupulus, i—A scruple, 20 grains.
Scutiformis—Shield-shaped
Sebum, vel sevum, i—Suet, tallow.
Secerno, crevi—To separate, remove (secernents).
Secretio, onis—A separating, parting, secretion.
Secta, æ—a party, set, faction.
Sectio, onis—A cutting off, section.
Seculum, i—A race, a generation.
Secundarius, a, um—The second in order (secundines).
Sedsmen, inis (sedo allay)—The means of allaying or composing, sedative
Sedimen, inis (sedo, to settle)—That which settles at the bottom of a liquid.
Seduco, xi—To lead aside, mislead, seduce.
Secundum—According to.

Segmentum, i—A cut, incision, segment.
Selectio, onis—A selecting, choosing
Sella, æ—A seat.
Sella Turcica—Part of the sphenoid bone
Semen, inis (seminum, i)—Seed, fecundating fluid.
Semi—Half.
Senesco, uui—To grow old.
Senex, senis—Old, aged (senilis)
Sentio, sensi—To perceive by the senses (sensation, sensibility, sensorium).
Separatus, a, um—Separated, divided.
Sepes, is—A hedge (septum)
Sepulcrum, i—A grave, a sepulchre.
Sequor, quutus—To follow or move after.
Sequela æ—A morbid affection which follows another.
Sequestrum, i—The portion of bone which is detached in necrosis.
Sericeus, a, um—Silky, covered with fine, long hairs, giving a silky appearance.
Serpens, tis—A serpent.
Serpigo, iginis (serpo)—Ringworm, tetter
Serratus, a, um—Serrated like a saw (serratus magnus posticus)
Serum, i—The watery part, serum
Serum lacris, serum sanguinis, serum chyli.
Sesqui—Half as much more
Sesqui-hora—One hour and a half.
Seta, æ—A bristle (seton)
Siccus, a, um—Dry. without moisture.
Sideratio, onis—An old name given to erysipelas of the face or scalp, from an idea of its being produced by the influence of the planets
Silentium, i—Silence, quietness.
Silex, icis—A flint.
Silus, a, um—Snub-nosed, nose turned up.
Silva, æ—A forest
Similes, e—Like, similar.
Simplex, leis—Simple, not mixed.
Sin—But if, if however.
Sine—Without.
Sinciput, itis—The fore part of the head.
Singulus, a, um—Single, one alone.
Singultus, us—A sobbing, hiccough
Sinister, tra—Left, to the left hand or side
Sinus, us—A hollow, a gulf, a cavity within the substance of bone. etc.
Sipho, onis—A siphon.
Situs, us—The situation
Sol, solis—The sun
Solamen, inis—Comfort, solace, consolation.
Solea, æ—The sole of the foot
Solidus, a, um—Solid, dense.
Solus, i—Alone, only
Solutio, onis—A loosening, dissolving, solution
Solvo, vi—To loosen, dissolve, solvent.
Somnus, i—Sleep.
Somniferus, a, um—That causes sleep.
Somnambulo—To walk in the sleep
Sono, ui—To sound, to make a noise.
Sophisticatio, onis—Adulteration
Sopor, oris—Profound sleep (soporific).
Sorbeo, ui—To suck in, absorb.
Sordes, is—Dirt, filth, viscid matter.
Spado, onis—A eunuch, a gelding.
Spargo, si—To strew, to sprinkle, to moisten.
Spatha, æ—A spatula.
Specto, avi—To look at anything
Spectrum, i—A form or image, whether real or imaginary.
Specularis, e—Like a mirror (speculum).
Sphæra, æ—Any round body.
Spica, æ—A point, an ear of corn, the name of a bandage.
Spina, æ—A thorn, the back bone.
Spira, æ—A spire, fold (spiral vessels.
Spiritus, us—Spirit
Spisso, avi—To make thick, to thicken.
Splen, enis—The spleen.
Spongia, æ—A sponge
Spumo, avi—To foam.
Spumo, avi—To foam.
Spuo, ui—To spit up or out.
Spuo, are—To spit.
Sputum, i—Spittle, expectoration.
Squamo, æ—The scale of a fish, scale-like substance.
Stagno, avi—To stagnate.
Stamen, inis—The male organ of flowering plants.
Statura, æ—Stature. size of body.
Stella, æ—A star (stellated)
Stercoreus, a, um—Of the nature of excrement, dung.
Sterilis, e—Unfruitful, barren.
Sternum, i—The breast bone.
Sterto, ui—To snore.
Sternutatio, onis—Sneezing (sternutatories).
Stigma, tis—A mark, a small red speck
Stigma—In plants, the upper extremity of the pistil.
Stillicidium, i—A liquid which falls by drops, strangury, a discharge of the urine guttatim.

Stimulo, avi—To goad, to increase the vital activity of an organ (stimulant).

Sto, steti—To stand.

Stoicus, a, um—Belonging to the Stoics or their philosophy.

Stomachus, a, um—Having a weak stomach

Stomachus, i—The stomach (stomachic).

Strabo, onis—Squint-eyed, one that has a cast in the eye (strabismus).

Stramen, inis—Straw, litter.

Stramentum, i—That which is spread, or strewed under.

Strangulo, avi—To strangle, to stifle.

Strangulatio, onis—The close constriction of a part.

Stranguria, æ—Strangury.

Stratum, i—A thing thrown upon another.

Strictura, æ—A contracted state of some part of a tube or duet

Stridor, oris—A grating, creaking.

Stridor dentium—A grinding or gnashing of the teeth, brygmus.

Stridulus, is—A hissing, goating, creaking

Strigilis, is—A scraper, or flesh brush used by the Romans in bathing.

Struma, æ—Scrofula, king's evil.

Studeo, ui—To apply the mind to a thing, to study.

Stupefacio, onis—To produce stupor or insensibility.

Stupor dentium—An affection called teeth on edge.

Stuprum, Disgrace, rape.

Suadeo, si—To persuade, to give advice.

Suavis, e—Pleasant, agreeable to the senses.

Sub—Under.

Subduo, didi—To put or lay under, subdue.

Subsultus—Twitching, sudden and irregular twitching of the tendons.

Succedaneus, a, um—A medicine substituted in place of another.

Succussus, us—A shaking, a mode of exploring the chest by shaking the patient's body and observing the sounds produced

Succus, i—Juice.

Sudo, avi—To sweat, perspire (sudorifics).

Suffio, ivi—To fumigate.

Suffitus—Fumes of burning substances used for inhalation.

Suffoco, avi—To suffocate, arrest of the respiratory function

Suffundo, fudi—To pour under, suffusion, (suffusio nigra)

Sugellatio, onis—Discoloration of the skin by a blow, ecchymosis.

Sulcus, i—A groove, furrow, depression.

Sulfur, sulphur, uris—Sulphur.

Sumo, ere—To take (by the mouth).

Super—Above, over, beyond.

Supercilium—The eyebrow.

Superficies, ei—A surface

Supino, avi—To bend backward, to lie on the back (supination, supinator).

Suppositus, a, um—Put in the place of, substitute, (suppository).

Supprimo, essi—To check, to stop, cessation of secretion.

Suppuro, avi—To suppurate, gather matter or pus.

Sura, æ—The calf of the leg.

Surditas, atis—Deafness, hardness of hearing.

Suspentio, di—To hang up (suspension, suspensory).

Suspiro, avi—To exhale, to draw a deep breath.

Susurrus, i—An acute, continuous hissing sound, a whisper.

Sutura (suo, to sew)—A seam, a suture.

Synthesis, is—The formation of any body from its elements.

Sirupus—A sirup.

Tabella, æ—A tablet.

Tabeo, ui—To waste away.

Tabes, is—A gradual wasting away by disease. Tabes mesenterica, tabes dorsales, tabes saturnia.

Tabula vitrea—A term applied to the dense internal plate of the skull

Tænia, æ—A tape-worm.

Tænia, æ—A ligature, a long narrow riband, (tenia hippocampi, etc)

Talipes, dis—Clubfoot, walking on the ankles.

Talus, i—The ankle bone.

Talpa, æ—A mole, a tumor under the skin.

Tango tetegi, tactum—To touch (tactus eruditus).

Tarsus—The instep ; also the thin cartilage situated at the edge of the eyelids.

Tegumentum, i (tego, to cover)—A covering of the body, as the cuticle.

Tela, æ—A web, a term applied to web-like tissues.

Tellus, uris—The earth

Temperatura, æ—Temperature, state of the atmosphere or a body, as to heat.

Tempus, oris—Time.

Tempora, æ—The temples (temporalis).

Temulentus, a, um—Drunk, intoxicated.

Tendo, tetendi—To stretch, extend (tensor)

Tenaculum, i—A hook to take hold of bleeding vessels.

Tenesmus, i—Painful and constant urgency to alvine discharges

Tenuo, avi—To make thin or weak, lessen.

Tepidus, a, um—Lukewarm, tepid

Teres, etis—Long and round (teres major and minor).

Terminatio, onis—A fixing of limits, an ending.

Tero, trivi—To rub, to make smooth.

Terra, æ—Earth

Testa, æ—A shell.

Testis, is—A testicle, testis virilitatis.

Tetro—Foully, shockingly.

Thalamus, i—A bedroom , that part of the brain from which the optic nerve arises

Theca, æ—A sheath, a case, an envelope.

Thorax, acis—The breast, the chest

Tibia, æ—The shin bone

Tibialis, e—The name of two muscles, anticus and posticus.

Tinea, æ—A gnawing worm, a disease of the scalp.

Tinnitus, us—A ringing.

Tinnitus aurium—Ringing in the ears

Titubatio, onis—General restlessness with a perpetual desire of changing the position fidgets

Toleratio, onis—A bearing, suffering, enduring.

Tonsilla, æ—A tonsil.

Tormen, inis—A griping pain in the intestines, tormina.

Torpor, oris—Numbness, torpor.

Torreo, torrui—To burn, to consume, inflame.

Tortus, a, um—Crooked, twisted.

Torticollis—Wry neck

Toxicum, i—Poison in which arrows were dipped, poison.

Trabecula, æ trabs, a beam—The small medullary fibres of the brain, which constitute the commissures.

Tractus, us—A line, a region, a space tractus opticus, etc.

Tranquillitas, atis—Calmness, tranquillity, rest.

Trans—Beyond, on the further side of

Transformatio, onis—Change from one shape to another.

Transversus, a, um—Lying across, transverse (transversalis.

Tremor, oris—A trembling, tremulous motion (tremor tendinum)

Triceps ipius—Three headed (several muscles)

Tricuspis, idis—Three points, three triangular folds between the right auricle and ventricle of the heart.

Tritura, æ—A rubbing or pounding, trituration.

Trochus, i—A lozenge, a round tablet

Truncus, i—The trunk of the body.

Tuba, æ—A tube, trumpet (tuba eustachiana).

Tuber, eris—A protuberance, excrescence

Tuberculum, i—A tubercle, a peculiar morbid product.

Tubulus, i—A little tube or pipe. (tubuli lactiferi).

Tumefacio, eci—To cause to swell, tumefaction.

Tumeo, ui—To swell, tumor.

Turbo, inis—That turns round in a circle, turbinated.

Turgidus, a, um—Swollen, inflated, turgid.

Tus, vel tus, uris—Frankincense.

Tussis, is—A cough.

Tuto—With safety.

Tympanum, i—The drum of the ear.

Uber cris—A teat, a nipple.

Ubi—Where.

Ulcis, eris—An ulcer, sore.

Ulna, æ—The elbow, the large bone of the fore-arm.

Umbilicus, i—The navel.

Uncia, æ—An ounce.

Unctus, a, um—Anointed, greasy.

Uncus, i—A hook

Unciformis—Formed like a hook, a bone of the carpus.

Unguentum, is—An ointment

Unguis, i—A nail of the finger or toe.

Unio, onis—Joining together, the growing together of opposite surfaces.

Urina, æ—Urine

Urtica, æ—A nettle, an itch.

Urticaria—Nettle rash.

Ustus, a, um—Burnt, scorched.

Uterus, i—The womb

Uva, æ—A berry, a grape

Uvula, æ—The pendulous body that hangs down from the middle of the soft palate.

Vaccinatio, onis—The act of inserting vaccine matter.

Vacuus, a, um—Empty, vacuum

Vagina, æ—A sheath, the membranous canal that extends from the os externum to the cervix uteri.

Valens, tis—In good health, strong.

Valetudinarius, a, um—Sickly, ill, infirm of health.

Valgus, a, um—Bent outward, bowed.

Valva, æ—The folding door, a valve.

Valvula, æ—A little valve

Vapor, oris—Steam, vapor, exhalation.

Varix, icis—A swollen or dilated vein in the leg.

Varus—A spot, a pimple eruption.

Vas, vasis—A vessel (vas deferens, vasa brevia etc.)

Vectis, is—An iron bar.

Vehiculum, i—Any vehicle.
Velum, i—A veil, a curtain.
Vena, æ—A vein.
Venesectio, onis—Blood-letting.
Ventriculus, i, (ventus)—The stomach (ventricles of the heart).
Vermis, is—A worm.
Vermiculus, i—A little worm.
Vermiformis—Worm-like.
Vermifugo—To expel worms, vermifuge.
Verminatio, onis—Breeding of worms, infestment by parasitic animalcules.
Verrucosus, a, um—Full of warts.
Veripellis, e—That changes its hide or skin.
Vertebra, æ—A bone of the spine.
Vertebrata, æ—Animals that have a vertebral column.
Verugo, ints—giddiness, dizziness.
Veru, u—A spit.
Veru montanum—A little eminence of the urethra, caput gallinaginis
Vesania, æ—Madness without coma or pyrexia.
Vesica, æ—A bladder, the urinary bladder (vesicate).
Vesicula, æ—A little bladder.
Vespera, æ—Evening.
Vestibulum, i—A threshold.
Veternus, a, um—Old, lethargic, sluggish.
Via, æ—A way, a passage.
Viæ lacrymales—The tear passages.
Vibro, avi—To move quickly, to vibrate.
Vibrissa, æ—The hair of the nostrils.
Vicarius, a, um—A substitute, vicarious.
Victus, us—(vivo)—Nourishment, provision.
Video, vidi—To see (vidian),
Vigilans, tis—Watchful, careful.
Vigor, oris (vigeo, to live)—Life, vigor, activity.
Villosus, a, um—Covered with long, soft, shaggy hair.
Villus, i—The shaggy hair of beasts, villi or villosities of the mucous membranes, resembling downy tissue.
Vinum, i—Wine.
Vir, i—A man, male person.
Virgo, inis—A virgin.
Viridis, e—Green.
Virilis—Of, or belonging to man.
Virus, i—Venom, poison, virus.

Vis, is—Force, power.
Vis a tergo, Vis medicatrix naturæ, Vis vitæ, etc.
Viscus, eris, viscera—Any organ which has an appropriate use.
Visio, ônis—A seeing, sight, vision.
Vita, æ—Life.
Vitalis, e—Of, or pertaining to life, vital.
Vitellus ovi—The yolk of an egg
Vitio, avi—To corrupt, spoil, vitiate.
Vitrum, i—Glass.
Vivo, vixi—To live, be alive.
Viviparie—Animals which bring forth their young alive and perfect, as distinguished from oviparous animals.
Vivisectio, onis—Dissection of living animals for the purpose of study.
Vocalis, e—That is heard vocal.
Vola, æ—The hollow of the hand or foot.
Volo, avi—To fly.
Volo, volui—To will, be willing.
Volsella, æ—Small pincers, tweezers.
Volvo, vi—To roll, to turn.
Volvulus—Intussusceptio
Vomer, eris—The middle bone of the nose.
Vomica, æ—An abcess of the lungs.
Vomicus, a, um—Purulent, nasty, noxious.
Vomito, are—To vomit, to spit up.
Voracitas, atis—Voracity, ravenousness.
Vorax, acis—That swallows greedily, consuming.
Vox, vocis—The voice.
Vulnero, avi—To wound (vulnerary)
Vulpis morbus—Alopecia, baldness, decay and fall of the hair.
Vulsus, a, um—Smooth, bald, without hair.
Vultus, us—The looks, the countenance.
Vulva, æ—The elliptic opening inclosed by the lahiæ majoræ of the pudendum.
Vulva cerebri—A small aperture of the brain.

Zona pellucida—A thick membrane constituting the external investment of the ovum
Zonula ciliaris—A thin vascular layer connecting the anterior margin of the retina with the circumference of the lens.
Zotheca, æ—A small private chamber for study.

PHARMACEUTICAL ABBREVIATIONS,

AND EXPLANATION OF TERMS USED IN PRESCRIPTIONS.

A, aa, ana, of each—Either by weight or measure.
Abdom , Abdomen—The belly.
Abs. feb., Absente febre—Fever being absent.
Ad du. vic., Ad duas vices—For two times.
Ad sec. vic , Ad secundum vices—To the second time.
Ad gr. acid., Ad gratam aciditatem—To an agreeable acidity.
Ad def. animi, Ad defectionem animi—To fainting.
Ad del. an , Ad deliquium animi—To fainting.
Ad lib., Ad libitum—At pleasure.
Add , Adde vel addentur—Add, or let them be added.
Adden , Addendus—To be added.
Adjac., Adjacens—Near, adjacent.
Admov., Admove, admoveatur, admoveantur—Apply, let it be applied, let them be applied.
Ads feb., Adstante febre—While the fever is present.
Alter. hor., Alternis horis—Every other hour.
Alvo adstr , Alvo adstrictâ—When the bowels are confined.
Aq. astr., Aqua astricta—Frozen water.
Aq. bull., Aqua bulliens—Boiling water.
Aq. com., Aqua communis—Common water.
Aq. dest , Aq destillata—Distilled water.
Aq. fluv , Aqua fluviatilis—River water.
Aq. mar., Aqua marina—Sea water.
Aq. niv., Aqua nivalis—Snow water.
Aq. pluv., Aqua pluvialis—Rain water.
Aq. ferv , Aqua fervens—Hot water.
Aq. font., Aqua fontana—Spring water.

Bis ind , Bis indies—Twice a day.
Bib., bibe—Drink.
Bbds , Barbadensis—Barbadoes (as aloe bbds.)
Baln. mar , Balneum maræ (or maris)—A salt water bath.
Baln. ar , Balneum arenæ—A sand bath
Baln. tep., Balneum tepidum—A tepid bath.

Baln. vap , Balneum vaporis—A vapor bath.
Bol , Bolus—A bolus
Bul , Bulliat—Let it boil.
But., Butyrum—Butter.

Cap , Capiat—Let him take.
Cærul., Cæruleus—Blue.
Calom , Calomelas—Calomel.
Cath., Catharticus—Cathartic
Cuc cru , Cucurbitula cruenta—Cupping glass.
Cochleat , Cochlearim—By spoonful
Coch ampl , Cochleare amplum—A tablespoonful, half fluid ounce.
Coch. mag , Cochleare magnum—A tablespoonful.
Coch. med , Cochleare medium ⎱ A medium sized or des-
Coch mod., Cochleare modicum ⎰ sert spoonful, 2 fld dr.
Coch. parv , Cochleare parvum—A teaspoonful, 1 fluid drachm.
Col , Cola, colatus—Strain, strained.
Colet , Coletur or colatur—Let it be strained.
Colaturæ—To the strained liquor
Colent , Colentur—Let them be strained.
Color., Coloretur—Let it be colored.
Comp., Compositus—Compounded.
Cong , Congius—A gallon.
Cons , Conserva—A conserve (also conservo, keep)
Cont. rem. vel med , Continuentur remedia vel medicamenta—Let the remedies or medicines be continued.
Cop , Copiosus—Plenteous.
Coq , Coque, boil, coquantur—Let them be boiled.
Coq ad med consumpt , Coquatur ad medietatis consumptionem—Let it be boiled to the consumption of one half.
Coq. s. a , Coque secundum artem—Boil according to art
Coq in s a , Coque in sufficiente quantitate aquæ—Boil in sufficient quantity of water.
Cort., Cortex—Bark.

Crast., Crastinus—For to-morrow.
C. n., Cras. nocte—To-morrow night.
C. m., Cras. mane—To-morrow morning.
C. v., Cras. vespere—To-morrow evening.
Cuj , Cujus—Of any.
Cujusl., Cujuslibet—Of any.
Cyath. the, Cyatho theæ—In a cup of tea.
Cyath. vin., Cyathus vinarius—A wineglass (about two fluid ounces.)

Deaur. pil., Deaurentur pilulæ—Let the pills be gilt.
Deb. spiss., Debita spissitudo—A proper consistence.
Dec , Decanta—Pour off.
Decub. hor., Decubitūs horā—At bed-time.
De d. in d , De die in diem—From day to day.
Deglut., Degluuatur—Let it be swallowed.
Dej. alv.—Dejectiones alvi—Stools.
Det., Detur—Let it be given.
Dieb. alt., Diebus alternis—Every other day.
Dieb. tert., Diebus tertiis—Every third day.
Dep , Depuratus—Purified.
Dex. lat., Dextra lateralis—The right side.
Dig., Digeratur—Let it be digested.
Dil., Dilutus—Diluted.
Diluc., Diluculo—A break of day.
Dim., Dimidius—One half.
Det. in dupl , Detur in duplo—Let it be given in twice the quantity.
Div. in p. e. (or æ), Divide in partes equales—Divide into equal parts.
Dir. pro., Directioue propria—With proper directions.
Donec alv. bis dej , Donec alvus bis dejecerit—Until the bowels have been twice opened.
Donee alv. sol. fuer., Donec alvus soluta fuerit—Until the bowels have been loosened.
Donec dol. neph. exulav , Donec dolor nephriticus exulaverit—Until the nephritic pain has been removed.
Dos., Dosis—A dose.
Dis., Distillata—Distilled.
Diuturn., Diuturnus—Long continued.
Div., Divide—Divide.
Dr., Drachma—A dram.

E. g., Exempli gratia—For example.
Eburn., Eburneus—Made of ivory.
Ed., Edulcora—Edulcorate.
Efferv., Effervescentia—Effervescence.
Ejusd., Ejusdem—The same.
Elect., Electuarium—An electuary.
Emp., Emplastrum—A plaster.
Enem., Enema—A clyster.
Exhib., Exhibeatur—Let it be administered.
Ext. sup. alut., Extende super alutam—Spread upon soft feather.
Extr., Extractum—An extract.

F., Fac, fiat, fiant—Make, let it be made, let them be made.
F. pil., Fiant pilulæ—Let pills be made.
Fasc., Fasciculus—A bundle.
Feb. dur., Febre durante—During the fever.
Fem. intern., Femoribus internis—To the inside of the thighs.
Ft. venæs., Fiat venæsectio—Let venesection be performed.
F. h., Fiat haustus—Let a draught be made.
Fict., Fictilis—Earthen
Fil., Filtrum—A filtre.
Fist. arm., Fistula armata—A clyster pipe or bladder fitted for use.
Fl., Fluidus—Fluid.
F. l. a., Fiat lege artis—Let it be made according to the rules of art.
F. m., Fiat mistura—Let a mixture be made.
F. s. a., Fiat secundum artem—Let it be made according to art.
Flor., Flores—Flowers.
Fol., Folium—A leaf.
Fontic . Fonticulus—An issue.
Fot., Fotus—A fomentation. .
Fruct., Fructus—Fruit.
Frust., Frustillatim—In small pieces.

Gel. quav., Geltina quavis—In any jelly.
Gr. Granum, grana—A grain, grains.
Gtt., Gutta, æ—A drop.
Gtt. quibusd., Guttis quibusdam—With some drops.
Guttat., Guttatim—By drops.
Garg., Gargarisma—A gargle.
Gum., Gummi—Gum.

Har. pil sum. tit , Harum pilularum sumantur tres—Of these pill let three be taken.
Hor. decub.. Hora decubitūs—At bed-time.
Haust. purg , Haustus purgans—A purging draught.
H. s , Hora somni—At the hour of going to sleep
Hor. un spa., Horæ unius spatio—At the expiration of an hour.

VOL. II.—58

Hor. interm., Horis intermediis—In the intermediate hours.
Hb., Herba—The plant.
Hebdom., Hebdomina—A week.
Hestern. Hesternus—Of yesterday.
Hirud., Hirudo—A leech.

Inc., Incide—Cut.
Ind., Indies—Daily.
In pulm., In pulmento—In gruel.
Inf., Infunde, infusum—Infuse, infusion.
Inj. enem., Injiciatur enema—Let an enema be given.
Inj. Injecto—Injection.

Jul., Julepus—A julep.

Lat. dol., Lateri dolenti—To the affected side.
Lb., Libra—A pound weight.
Lim., Limones—Lemons.
Liq., Liquor—Liquor, liquid.
Lot., Lotio—Lotion.

M., Misce—Mix.
Mac., Macera—Macerate.
Man., Maniplus—A handful.
Mane pr., Mane primo—Early in the morning.
Mass., Massa—A mass.
Mass. pil., Massa pilularum—A pill mass.
Mist., Mistura—A mixture.
Mic. pan , Mica panis—Crumb of bread.
Mitt., Mitte send, mittantur—Let them be sent.
Mod. præsc., Modo præscripto—In the manner directed.
Mor. dic., More dicto—In the way ordered.
Mor. sol., More solito—In the usual way.
Medioc , Mediocris—Middle sized.
Min., Minimum—A drop 60th part of a dram measure.
Muc., Mucilago—Mucilage.

Narth., Narthecium—A gallipot.
Ne tr. s. num., Ne tradas sine nummo—Do not deliver it without the money.
Noct., Nocte—By night.
No., Numero—A number.

O., Octarius—A pint.
Ol., Oleum—Oil.
Omn. hor. Omni hora—Every hour.
Omn. bid., Omni biduo—Every two days.
Omn. bih., Omni bihorio—Every two hours.
Omn. quadr. hor., Omni quadrante horæ—Every quarter of an hour.
Omn. man., Omni Mane—Every morning.
Omn. noct , Omni nocte.—Every night.
Ov., Ovum—An egg.
Ox.—Oxymel.
Oz.—The ounce avoirdupois.

P. æ., Partes æquales—Equal parts
P. d , Per deliquium—By deliquescence
Past., Pastillus—A pastil.
Pond., Pondere—By weight.
P. D., Pharmacopœia Dublinensis.
P. E., Pharmacopœia Edinensis.
P. L., Pharmacopœia Londinensis.
P. U. S., Pharmacopœia of the United States.
Part. vic., Partibus vicibus—In divided doses
Per. op. emet—Peractà operatione emetici—The operation of the emetic being over.
Pocul., Poculum—A cup.
Pocill., Pocillum—A small cup.
Paracent. abd., Paracentesis abdominis—Tapping.
Part. aff., Partem affectam—The part affected.
Part. dol., Partem dolentem—The part in pain.
Per salt , Per saltum—By leaps.
Pil., Pilula—A pill.
Plen. riv., Pleno rivo—In a full stream.
Post sing. sed, liq., Post singulas sedes liquidas—After every loose stool.
Ppt., Præparata—Prepared.
Pot., Potio—A potion.
P. r. n., Pro re nata—Occasionally.
P. rat. ætat., Pro ratione ætatis—According to the age.
P. pot. com., Pro potu communi—For a common drink.
Prox. luc., Proximà luce—The day before.
Pug., Pugillus—A pinch.
Pulp., Pulpa—The pulp.
Pulv., Pulvis—A powder.

Q. l., Quantum libet } As much as you please.
Q. p., Quantum placet }
Q. s., Quantum sufficiat—As much as much as may suffice.
Quor., Quorum—Of which.
Q v., Quantum vis—As much as you will.
Quadrihr , Quadrihorio—Every four hours.
Quamp , Quamprimum—Immediately.

Rad., Radix—Root.

Ras., Rasuræ—Shavings.
Rect , Rectificatus—Rectified.
  e . in pulv., Reductus in pulverem—Reduced to pow-
R der.
Redig. in pulv., Redigatur in pulverum—Let it be re-
  duced to powder.
Reg umbil., Regio umbilici—The umbilical region.
Rept., Repetatur, repetantur—Let it or them be re-
  peated.
Reg. hep., Regio hepatis—Region of the liver.

S a., Secundum artem—According to art.
Scat., Scatula—A box.
S. n., Secundum naturam—According to nature.
Sacch., Saccharum—Sugar.
Scap., Scapula—The shoulder blade.
Scrob. cord., Scrobiculus cordis—The pit of the stomach.
Sed., Sedes—A stool.
Sem., Semen—A seed.
Semidr., Semidrachma—A half a drachm.
Semih., Semihora—Half an hour.
Sesunc., Sesuncia—An ounce and a half.
Sesquih., Sesquihora—An hour and a half.
Sept., Septimana—A week.
Serv., Serva—Keep or preserve.
Sn n. val., Si non valeat—If it does not answer.
Si op. sit., Si opus sit—If it be necessary.
Si vir. perm., Si vires permittant—If the strength
  allows it.
Sign. n. pro., Signetur nomine proprio—Write the pro-
  per name upon it.
Signat., Signatura—A label.
Sing., Singulorum—Of each.
S. s. s., Stratum super stratum—Layer upon layer.
Sol., Solutio—Solution.
Solv., Solve—Dissolve.
Spt., Spiritus—Spirit.
Sq., Squama—A scale.
Ss., Semi—Half.
St., Stet, stent—Let it stand, let them stand.
Sub. fin. coct., Sub finem coctionis—When the boiling is
  nearly finished.
Subtep., Subtepidus—Lukewarm.
Succ., Succus—The juice.
Sum., Sumo, sumendus, take—To be taken.
Sum. tal., Sumat talem—Let the patient take one such as
  this.

Summ., Summitates—The tops or summits.
S. V., Spiritus vini—Spirits of wine.
S. V. R , Spiritus vini rectificatus—Rectified spirits of
  wine.
S. V. T., Spiritus vini tenuis—Proof spirits.
Syr., Syrupus—Syrup.

Tabel., Tabella—A lozenge.
Temp. dext., Tempori dextro—To the right temple.
Temp. sinis , Tempori sinistro—To the left temple.
Tr. tinct , Tinctura—A tincture.
Trit., Tritura—Triturate.
Troch., Trochiscus—A lozenge or troch.

Ult. præsc., Ultimo præscriptus—The last prescribed.
Umb., Umbilicus—The navel.
Ung., Unguentum—Ointment.
Utend., Utendus—To be used.

Vent., Ventriculus—The stomach.
V. O. S., Vitello ovi solutus—Dissolved in the yolk of an
  egg.
Vom. urg., Vomitione urgente—The vomiting being
  troublesome.
V. s., Venæsectio—Bleeding.

Zz., Zingiber—Ginger.

SYMBOLS USED IN PRESCRIPTIONS.

℞., Recipe—Take.
Gr., Granum—A grain.
Ɔ , Scrupulus—A scruple.
Ʒ , Drachma—A drachm.
℥ , Uncia—An ounce troy.
℔ , Libra—A pound.
♏., Minimum—A minim.
FƷ , Fluidrachma—A fluidrachm.
F℥ ., Fluiduncia—A fluidounce.
O., Octarius—A pint.
C., Congius—A gallon.

INDEX TO VOL. I.

INDEX TO VOL. II.

ADDENDA.